DENTISTRY FOR THE CHILD AND ADOLESCENT

DENTISTRY FOR THE CHILD AND ADOLESCENT

RALPH E. McDONALD, D.D.S., M.S.

Professor of Pedodontics and Dean,
Indiana University School of Dentistry,
Indianapolis, Indiana

DAVID R. AVERY, D.D.S., M.S.D.

Professor and Chairman of Pedodontics,
Indiana University School of Dentistry, and
Director of the Postdoctoral Pedodontic Program,
Indiana University School of Dentistry and
James Whitcomb Riley Hospital for Children,
Indianapolis, Indiana

FOURTH EDITION

with **1232** illustrations

The C. V. Mosby Company

ST. LOUIS · TORONTO · LONDON   1983

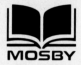

MOSBY

A TRADITION OF PUBLISHING EXCELLENCE

Editor: Darlene Warfel
Assistant editor: Melba Steube
Manuscript editor: Patricia Tannian
Book design: Kay M. Kramer
Production: Sue Soehngen, Barbara Merritt, Carol O'Leary

FOURTH EDITION

The C.V. Mosby Company
11830 Westline Industrial Drive, St. Louis, Missouri 63141

Library of Congress Cataloging in Publication Data

McDonald, Ralph E.
  Dentistry for the child and adolescent.

  Bibliography: p.
  Includes index.
  1. Pedodontics. I. Avery, David R. II. Title.
[DNLM: 1. Pedodontics. WU M135d]
RK55.C5M35 1983   617.6'45   82-14195
ISBN 0-8016-3277-3

TS/VH/VH 9 8 7 6 5 4 3 2 1 03/A/304

Contributors

DAVID R. AVERY, D.D.S., M.S.D.

Professor and Chairman of Pedodontics, Indiana University School of Dentistry, and Director of the Postdoctoral Pedodontic Program, Indiana University School of Dentistry and James Whitcomb Riley Hospital for Children, Indianapolis, Indiana

DAVID BIXLER, D.D.S., Ph.D.

Professor of Basic Science and Medical Genetics and Chairman of Oral Facial Genetics, Indiana University School of Dentistry and Indiana University School of Medicine, Indianapolis, Indiana

†DONALD M. CUNNINGHAM, D.D.S., M.S.D.

Former Professor and Co-Chairman, Fixed and Removable Partial Prosthodontics, Indiana University School of Dentistry, Indianapolis, Indiana

W. BAILEY DAVIS, D.D.S.

Professor of Pedodontics, Indiana University School of Dentistry, Indianapolis, Indiana

ROLAND W. DYKEMA, D.D.S., M.S.D.

Professor and Chairman, Fixed and Removable Partial Prosthodontics, Indiana University School of Dentistry, Indianapolis, Indiana

LaFORREST D. GARNER, D.D.S., M.S.D.

Professor and Chairman of Orthodontics, Indiana University School of Dentistry, Indianapolis, Indiana

---

†Deceased.

CHARLES W. GISH, D.D.S., M.S.D.

Co-Chairman of the Department of Community Dentistry and Professor of Community Dentistry and Pedodontics, Indiana University School of Dentistry, Indianapolis, Indiana

CHARLES J. GOODACRE, D.D.S., M.S.D.

Associate Professor of Fixed and Removable Partial Prosthodontics and Director, Undergraduate Fixed and Removable Partial Prosthodontics, Indiana University School of Dentistry, Indianapolis, Indiana

DAVID K. HENNON, D.D.S., M.S.D.

Professor of Pedodontics, Indiana University School of Dentistry, Indianapolis, Indiana

CHARLES E. HUTTON, D.D.S.

Professor and Chairman of Oral and Maxillofacial Surgery and Director of the Oral and Maxillofacial Surgery Internship-Residency Program, Indiana University School of Dentistry, Indianapolis, Indiana

JAMES E. JONES, D.M.D., M.S.

Assistant Professor of Pedodontics, Indiana University School of Dentistry, Indianapolis, Indiana; Adjunct Instructor, University of Louisville School of Dentistry, Louisville, Kentucky

MYRON J. KASLE, D.D.S., M.S.D.

Professor and Chairman, Department of Radiology, Indiana University School of Dentistry, Indianapolis, Indiana

THEODORE R. LYNCH, D.D.S.

Assistant Professor of Pedodontics, Indiana University School of Dentistry, and Dental Coordinator, Oral Facial Clinic, James Whitcomb Riley Hospital for Children, Indianapolis, Indiana

JAMES F. MATLOCK, D.D.S., M.S.D.

Associate Professor, Department of Radiology,
Indiana University School of Dentistry, Indianapolis,
Indiana

RALPH E. McDONALD, D.D.S., M.S.

Professor of Pedodontics and Dean, Indiana University
School of Dentistry, Indianapolis, Indiana

†WILLIAM W. MEROW, D.D.S.

Professor and Chairman of Orthodontics, West
Virginia University School of Dentistry, Morgantown,
West Virginia

RALPH W. PHILLIPS, M.S., D.Sc.

Research Professor of Dental Materials and Associate
Dean for Research, Indiana University School of
Dentistry, Indianapolis, Indiana

JAMES R. ROCHE, D.D.S.

Associate Dean for Faculty Development and
Professor of Pedodontics, Indiana University School of
Dentistry, Indianapolis, Indiana

WILLIAM G. SHAFER, D.D.S., M.S.

Distinguished Professor and Chairman of Oral
Pathology, Indiana University School of Dentistry,
Indianapolis, Indiana

PAUL E. STARKEY, D.D.S.

Professor and Former Chairman, Department of
Pedodontics, Indiana University School of Dentistry,
Indianapolis, Indiana

JAMES A. WEDDELL, D.D.S., M.S.D.

Assistant Professor of Pedodontics, Indiana University
School of Dentistry, and Acting Director, Riley Dental
Clinic, James Whitcomb Riley Hospital for Children,
Indianapolis, Indiana

BERND WEINBERG, Ph.D.

Adjunct Associate Professor of Otolaryngology,
Indiana University School of Medicine, Indianapolis,
Indiana; Professor and Head, Department of
Audiology and Speech Sciences, Purdue University,
Lafayette, Indiana

---

†Deceased.

Preface

This fourth edition of *Dentistry for the Child and Adolescent* represents a substantial revision of nearly all chapters of the text. A large portion of the revised material was developed in response to the many constructive suggestions received from our colleagues after publication of the third edition. We are grateful to our peers who invested their energy to review the book objectively and respond to the publisher's request for suggestions on improvement.

The basic structure and format of the text are similar to those of previous editions. The book provides current diagnostic and treatment recommendations based on research and clinical experience. The information is relevant to the practice of pedodontics. The book is designed to help undergraduate dental students and postdoctoral pedodontic students provide efficient and superior comprehensive oral health care for infants, children, and teenagers. It also gives the experienced dentist reference information on new developments and techniques.

As mentioned previously, the content of the fourth edition has changed considerably compared with the third edition. Chapter 1, "Examination of the Mouth and Other Relevant Structures," has been rewritten almost entirely. The topic of child abuse and neglect in Chapter 1 is new to this book. In view of the alarming statistics documenting the severity of this problem and dentists' potential for identifying possible child abuse or neglect, we believe the subject justifies our lengthy discussion. Three new chapters, 10, 11, and 23, have been developed for this edition. Chapter 9 of this edition is limited to local anesthesia, whereas this chapter also included sedation, analgesia, and general an-

esthesia in the previous edition. New Chapter 10 addresses sedation and analgesia, and new Chapter 11 discusses dentistry in the hospital setting and the use of general anesthesia. Chapter 23, "Dental Problems of the Handicapped Child," has been completely rewritten although it retains the same title as in the previous edition.

Several new treatment recommendations in the management of traumatic injuries of the teeth have been included. Current information related to the new emphasis on radiation hygiene in the dental office is included with appropriate illustrations. The new restorative procedures using laminate veneers are given expanded coverage.

Considerable emphasis is given throughout the book to preventive procedures recognized as effective in reducing the crippling effects of dental neglect that are often traced to childhood. In regard to dental caries control, we have included the currently recommended techniques for topical fluoride application. A revised discussion of the use of systemic fluorides is also included. The use of fluorides in dentistry is summarized with a new detailed outline.

The 20 authors who have joined us in the preparation of the revision of this book express a coordinated philosophy in the approach to the most modern concepts of dentistry for the child and the adolescent.

A textbook can be planned and written only with the supportive interest, encouragement, and tangible contributions of many people. Therefore it is a privilege to acknowledge the assistance of others in the preparation of this text. Typing and valuable editorial suggestions were provided by Marilyn Gruenhagen, Barbara Hagstrom, Elizabeth

Hatcher, JoAnn Heasley, and Lee McConnaughey. The photographic prints and many original photographs were provided by Richard Scott, Director of Dental Illustrations, and his staff, Alana Fears and Michael Halloran. The artwork was supplied by Dr. Rolando DeCastro, Director of Art. The faculties of the Department of Pedodontics and other departments have contributed substantially to this work. Many pedodontic postdoctoral students and pedodontic auxiliary staff have also assisted in numerous ways. Our heartfelt thanks is extended to all who played a role in helping us bring this project to a successful conclusion.

Ralph E. McDonald
David R. Avery

Contents

ix

DENTISTRY FOR THE
CHILD AND ADOLESCENT

1 Examination of the mouth and other relevant structures

RALPH E. McDONALD
DAVID R. AVERY

Dentists have traditionally been taught to perform a complete oral examination of the patient and to develop a treatment plan from the examination findings. Then the dentist makes a case presentation to the patient or parents outlining the recommended course of treatment. The dentist would be well advised to think of these procedures as the development and presentation of a prevention plan that outlines an ongoing comprehensive oral health care program for the patient. The plan should include recommendations designed to correct existing oral problems (or prevent their progression) and to prevent anticipated future problems. It is essential to obtain all relevant patient and family information, to secure parental consent, and to perform a complete examination before embarking on this comprehensive oral health care program for the child patient.

Each child patient should be given an opportunity to receive complete dental care. The dentist should not attempt to decide what the child, parents, or third-party agent will accept or can afford. If parents reject a portion or all of the recommendations, the dentist has at least fulfilled the obligation of educating the child and the parents about the importance of the recommended procedures. Parents of even moderate income will usually find the means to have oral health care completed if the dentist explains to them that the child's future oral health and even general health are related to the correction of oral defects.

Initial parental contact with the dental office

The parent usually makes the first contact with the dental office via the telephone. This initial conversation between the parent and the office receptionist is very important. It provides the first opportunity to attend to the parent's concerns by pleasantly and concisely responding to questions and by offering an office appointment. The receptionist must have a warm, friendly voice and the ability to communicate clearly. The receptionist's responses should assure the parent that the well-being of the child is the chief concern.

The information recorded by the receptionist during this conversation constitutes the initial dental record for the patient. Filling out a patient information form (Fig. 1-1) is a convenient method of collecting the necessary initial information. At the child's first office visit additional information may be obtained and the form is placed in the patient's permanent dental record. Additional discussion of the initial communication with parents is presented in Chapter 30.

The diagnostic method

According to Keller and Manson-Hing, before making a diagnosis the dentist must collect and evaluate the facts associated with the problem. Some pathognomonic signs may lead to an almost immediate diagnosis. For example, obvious gingival swelling and drainage may be associated with a single, badly carious, painful primary molar. Al-

1

Date _____ Patient no. _____

Patient _____ Birthdate_____ Race _____ Sex _____
      Last   First   Nickname   Mo. Day Yr.

Address _____
      Street   City   State   Zip

Telephone: Home_____ Business _____

Purpose of call:_____ Referred by whom:_____

Does child have any special medical, physical, or developmental problem?_____

_____Physician's name:_____

Last dental visit:_____ Dentist's name:_____

Appointment date & time:_____ Call taken by:_____

Father _____ Occupation _____

Mother _____ Occupation _____

Names and ages of other children _____, _____ , _____

Method of payment:

    ◻ DENTAL HEALTH CARE INSURANCE Insurance Company_____

    ◻ MEDICAID: Recipient _____
                      Patient's name as on card _____
                      Effective date _____ County _____
                      Medicaid number _____

    ◻ PERSONAL PAYMENT:
                      Guarantor (person responsible)_____
                      Relationship _____ Phone _____
                      Social Security number _____
                      Address _____
                          Street   City   State   Zip

                      Guarantor's employer_____
                      Address _____
                        Street   City   State   Zip   Phone

Date taken	NUMBER OF EXPOSURES						Total radio-graphs taken	Operator
	Periapical				BW	Other (Describe)		
	Max.		Mand.		R	L		
	R	L	R	L				

Fig. 1-1. Form that may be used to record information during the initial parental contact with the dental office. Only essential information is recorded during this first conversation, and the remainder of the form may be completed during the first office visit. (Courtesy Indiana University Pedodontic Faculty Committee, Dr. F.E. McCormick, Chairman.)

though the collection and evaluation of these associated facts are performed rapidly, they provide a diagnosis only for a single problem area and are not comprehensive. On the other hand, a comprehensive diagnosis of all the patient's problems or potential problems may sometimes need to be postponed until more urgent conditions are resolved. For example, a patient with acute necrotizing ulcerative gingivitis or a newly fractured crown needs immediate treatment, but the treatment would likely be only palliative and further diagnostic and treatment procedures would be required later.

The importance of thoroughly collecting and evaluating the facts concerning a patient's condition cannot be overemphasized. Moskow and Barr have described the following examination methods that aid the dentist in the process of collecting and evaluating the facts:

- History taking
- Inspection
- Palpation
- Exploration
- Radiographs
- Percussion
- Transillumination
- Vitality tests
- Study casts
- Laboratory tests
- Photography

In certain unusual cases all of these diagnostic aids may be necessary to arrive at a comprehensive diagnosis. Certainly no diagnosis could be comprehensive or complete unless the diagnostician had evaluated the facts obtained by history taking, inspection, palpation, exploration, and often radiographs.

Preliminary medical and dental history

It is important for the dentist to be familiar with the medical and dental history of the child patient. Familial history may also be relevant to the patient's oral condition and may provide important diagnostic information in some hereditary disorders. Before the dentist's examination of the child,

the dental assistant can obtain sufficient information to provide the dentist with a knowledge of the child's general health and to alert the dentist to the need for obtaining additional information from the parent or the child's physician. The form illustrated in Fig. 1-2 can be completed by the parent. However, it is more effective for the dental assistant to ask the questions informally and then to present the findings to the dentist and offer personal observations and a summary of the case. The questions included on the form will also provide information about any previous dental treatment.

Information regarding the child's social and psychologic development is important. Accurate information reflecting a child's learning, behavioral, or communication problems is sometimes difficult to obtain initially, especially if the parents are aware of their child's developmental disorder but reluctant to discuss it. Behavior problems in the dental office are often related to the child's inability to communicate with the dentist and to follow instructions, and this inability may be due to a low mental capacity. Parents often fail to volunteer the information that the child has a low IQ or is mentally retarded. An indication of mental retardation can usually be determined by the assistant while asking questions about the child's learning process.

A notation should be made if a young child has been hospitalized previously for general anesthetic and surgical procedures. Shaw has reported that hospitalization and a general anesthetic procedure can be a traumatic psychologic experience for a preschool child and may sensitize the youngster to procedures that will be encountered later in a dental office. If the dentist is aware of previous hospitalization and the child's fear of strangers in white, the necessary time and procedures can be planned to help the child overcome the fear and accept dental treatment.

Occasionally when the parents report significant disorders, it is best for the dentist to conduct the medical and dental history interview. When the parents meet with the dentist privately, they are more likely to discuss the child's problems openly

Text continued on p. 8.

MEDICAL-DENTAL HISTORY

Date_____

Child's Name_____
                              LAST   FIRST   NICKNAME

Place of Birth _____ Birth Date_____ Sex_____

Child's Physician/Pediatrician _____

Address_____ Telephone_____

Date of last medical examination _____

MEDICAL HISTORY

GROWTH AND DEVELOPMENT Any learning, behavioral or communication problems?	No ☐	Yes ☐
CENTRAL NERVOUS SYSTEM Any history of cerebral palsy, seizures, convulsions, fainting or loss of consciousness?	No ☐	Yes ☐
Any history of injury to the head?	No ☐	Yes ☐
Any sensory disorders? (Seeing, Hearing)	No ☐	Yes ☐
CARDIO-VASCULAR SYSTEM Any history of congenital heart disease or heart damage from rheumatic fever?	No ☐	Yes ☐
Any history of anemia, bleeding or other blood disorders?	No ☐	Yes ☐
RESPIRATORY SYSTEM Any history of pneumonia, asthma, shortness of breath or difficulty in breathing?	No ☐	Yes ☐
GASTRO-INTESTINAL SYSTEM Any history of stomach, intestinal or liver problems?	No ☐	Yes ☐
Any history of hepatitis or jaundice?	No ☐	Yes ☐
GENITO URINARY SYSTEM Any history of urinary tract infections, bladder or kidney problems?	No ☐	Yes ☐
ENDOCRINE SYSTEM Any history of diabetes?	No ☐	Yes ☐
Any history of thyroid disorder or other endocrine disorders?	No ☐	Yes ☐
SKIN Any history of skin problems?	No ☐	Yes ☐
EXTREMITIES Any limitations of use of arms or legs?	No ☐	Yes ☐
ALLERGIES Is your child allergic to any medications?	No ☐	Yes ☐

MEDICATIONS OR TREATMENTS
Is your child currently taking any medication?   No ☐   Yes ☐
If yes, Medication(s)   Dosage   Times Per Day

_____   _____   _____
_____   _____   _____

Has your child ever received radiation therapy (X-ray treatments?)   No ☐   Yes ☐

HOSPITALIZATIONS
Has your child been hospitalized?   No ☐   Yes ☐
Hospital 1) _____ 2) _____ 3) _____
Date   _____   _____   _____
Reason   _____   _____   _____

IMMUNIZATIONS Is your child presently protected by immunization against Diptheria, Whooping Cough, Tetanus	No ☐	Yes ☐
Polio	No ☐	Yes ☐
Measles and German Measles (Rubella)	No ☐	Yes ☐

Fig. 1-2. Form used in completing the preliminary medical and dental history. (Courtesy Indiana University Pedodontic Faculty Committee, Dr. F.E. McCormick, Chairman.)

DENTAL HISTORY

Does your child have a toothache or other immediate dental problem?	No ☐	Yes ☐
Has your child ever had a toothache?	No ☐	Yes ☐
Has your child had any injury to the mouth, teeth or jaws (fall, blow, etc.)?	No ☐	Yes ☐
Is this your child's first dental visit?	No ☐	Yes ☐

If no: Date_____Dentist _____

Reason _____

Has your child ever had an unfavorable dental experience?	No ☐	Yes ☐

Related comments:

DENTAL DISEASE PREVENTION

How often does your child brush?_____times per_____

Does your child use dental floss?	No ☐	Yes ☐

Does someone:

Assist your child with brushing and cleaning the teeth?	No ☐	Yes ☐
Inspect for thoroughness following the procedure?	No ☐	Yes ☐
Does your child use a fluoride toothpaste?	No ☐	Yes ☐
Has your child ever had a fluoride treatment?	No ☐	Yes ☐
Has your child ever taken a fluoride supplement or vitamins with fluoride?	No ☐	Yes ☐

Drinking water source:

City water supply ☐   Name of City_____

Private Well or other than city ☐ Has a fluoride analysis been done?	No ☐	Yes ☐

Date of analysis_____Fluoride content_____

_____
SIGNATURE (Parent or Guardian)

COMMENTS

MEDICAL CONSULTATION RECOMMENDED? No ☐   Yes ☐   Date Requested_____

PURPOSE FOR CONSULTATION:

ANNUAL REVIEW OF MEDICAL-DENTAL HISTORY

If history remains essentially unchanged, sign below.

Date_____Parent_____   Date_____Parent_____

Date_____Parent_____   Date_____Parent_____

Fig. 1-2, cont'd. For legend see opposite page.

ORAL EXAMINATION RECORD

Patient_____ Chart_____ Date_____
LAST   FIRST   NICKNAME

MEDICAL HISTORY SUMMARY

Last History Completed_____
Current medical status and medication:

DENTAL HISTORY SUMMARY

Date of: Last exam_____ Last radiographs F.M._____ B W_____ Other_____

Appliances: _____ Last Cemented_____

Describe any present problem:

Past treatment summarized:

EXTRA ORAL FINDINGS

Head
Neck
Face
Lips
Hands

INTRA ORAL FINDINGS

Palate and oropharynx
Tongue and floor of mouth
Buccal mucosa
Frena
Gingivae
Periodontium

PLAQUE SCORE

Today's score [   ]   Last score [   ]

OCCLUSION REVIEW

FACIAL PROFILE:_____

MOLAR RELATIONSHIP:

PERMANENT	R	L	PRIMARY	R	L
Unerupted	☐	☐	(Terminal Plane)		
End to end	☐	☐	Straight	☐	☐
Class	___	___	Mes. Step	☐	☐
			Dist. Step	☐	☐
			Primate Space	☐	☐

CANINE RELATIONSHIP: R L
    Class _____

INCISOR RELATIONSHIP:
    Overjet ____ mm.
    Overbite ____ %
    Openbite ____ mm.

MIDLINE: Normal ☐ Deviates ☐
    Maxilla R ☐ L ☐ mm.____
    Mandible R ☐ L ☐ mm.____
    Mandibular Shift No ☐ Yes ☐
        R ☐ L ☐ Ant. ☐ mm ____

ARCH LENGTH: (general impression)
    Maxilla: Mandible:
    Adequate   ☐   Adequate   ☐
    Inadequate ☐   Inadequate ☐

ANALYSIS RECOMMENDED: No ☐ Yes ☐

RELATED FINDINGS: (Describe abnormalities)

Eruption sequence

Crossbite

Oral habits

Supernumerary teeth

Congenitally missing teeth

Ectopic eruption

Other anomalies

Fig. 1-3. Chart that may be used to record the oral findings and the treatment proposed for the child patient. (Courtesy Indiana University Pedodontic Faculty Committee, Dr. F.E. McCormick, Chairman.)

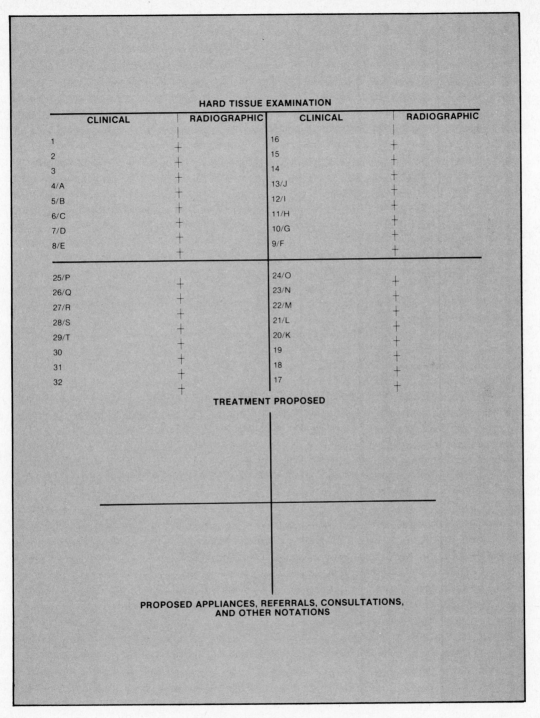

Fig. 1-3, cont'd. For legend see opposite page.

and there is less chance for misunderstandings regarding the nature of the disorders. In addition, the dentist's personal involvement at this early time strengthens the confidence of the parents of the "special" child. When there is indication of an acute or chronic systemic disease or anomaly, the dentist should consult the child's physician to learn the status of the condition, the long-range prognosis, and the current drug therapy.

Current illnesses or histories of significant allergic reactions, blood or lymphatic dyscrasias, cardiovascular problems, chronic kidney diseases, endocrine disorders, oncologic diseases, or severe respiratory distress signal the need for special attention during the history interview. In addition to consulting the child's physician, the dentist may decide to record additional data concerning the child's current physical condition that are not routinely recorded for healthy children. This information may include the patient's blood pressure, body temperature, heart sounds, height and weight, pulse, and respiration. Before treatment is initiated, certain laboratory tests may be indicated and special precautions may be necessary. A decision to provide treatment in a hospital and possibly under general anesthesia may be appropriate.

The dentist and the staff must also be alert to identify potentially communicable infectious conditions that threaten the health of the patient and others as well. It is advisable to postpone nonemergency dental care for a patient exhibiting signs or symptoms of acute infectious disease until the patient has recovered. A patient with a history of hepatitis requires determination of the patient's current status. The office staff should take special precautions when treating any patient with a history of hepatitis, even if the patient is fully recovered, unless it can be confirmed that the patient is not in a "carrier status." Except in a true dental emergency, dental treatment should be postponed for any patient with known active hepatitis (regardless of type) or with signs or symptoms of hepatitis. Further discussions of managing dental patients with special medical, physical, or behavior problems are presented in Chapters 10, 11, and 23.

The pertinent facts of the medical history can be transferred to the oral examination record (Fig. 1-3) for easy reference by the dentist. A brief summary of important medical information serves as a convenient reminder to the dentist and the staff, since they refer to this chart at each treatment visit.

The patient's dental history should also be summarized on the examination chart. This should include a record of previous care in the dentist's office and the facts related by the patient and the parent regarding previous care in another office. Information concerning the patient's current oral hygiene habits and the previous and current fluoride exposure will help the dentist develop an effective dental disease prevention program for the patient. If the family drinks well water, a sample may be sent to the state health department for determination of the fluoride content.

Clinical examination

Most facts needed for a comprehensive oral diagnosis in the young patient are obtained via a thorough clinical and radiographic examination. In addition to examining the structures in the oral cavity, the dentist may in some cases wish to note the patient's size, stature, gait, or involuntary movements. The first clue to malnutrition may come from observing a patient's abnormal size or stature. Similarly, the severity of a child's illness, whether oral or systemic, may be recognized by observing the weak, unsteady gait of lethargy and malaise as the patient walks into the office. All relevant information should be noted on the oral examination record (Fig. 1-3), which becomes a permanent part of the patient's chart.

Examination of the child patient, whether the first examination or a regular recall examination, should be all inclusive. Attention to the patient's hair, head, face, neck, and hands should be among the first observations made by the dentist after the patient is seated in the chair. The dentist can gather useful information while getting acquainted with a new patient.

The patient's hands may reveal information pertinent to the comprehensive diagnosis. The dentist may first detect an elevated temperature by holding the patient's hand. Cold, clammy hands or bitten fingernails may be the first indication of abnormal anxiety in the child. A callused or unusually clean digit suggests a persistent sucking habit. Clubbing of the fingers or a bluish color in the nail beds suggests congenital heart disease that may require special precautions during dental treatment.

Inspection and palpation of the patient's head and neck are also indicated. Unusual characteristics of the hair or skin should be noted. The dentist may observe head lice (Fig. 1-4), ringworm (Fig. 1-5), or impetigo (Fig. 1-6) during the examination. Proper referral is indicated immediately, since these conditions are contagious. After the child's physician has supervised the treatment to control the condition, the patient's dental appointment may be rescheduled. If a contagious condition is identified but the child also has a dental emergency, the dentist and the staff must take appropriate precautions to prevent spread of the disease to others while the emergency is alleviated. Further treatment should be postponed until the contagious condition is controlled.

Variations in size, shape, symmetry, or function of the head and neck structures should be recorded. Abnormalities of these structures may indicate various syndromes or conditions associated with oral abnormalities.

Temporomandibular joint (TMJ) function should be evaluated by palpating the head of each mandibular condyle and observing the patient while the mouth is closed (teeth clenched), at rest, and in various open positions (Fig. 1-7, *A* and *B*). Movements of the condyles or jaw that are not smooth flowing or that deviate from the expected norm should be noted. Similarly, any crepitus that may be heard or identified by palpation, or any other abnormal sounds, should be noted. Such deviations from normal TMJ function may require further evaluation and treatment. Follow-up is indicated when these deviations can be linked to symptoms identified by the patient. The extraoral examination continues with palpation of the patient's

neck and submandibular area (Fig. 1-7, *C* and *D*). Again, deviations from normal such as unusual tenderness or enlargement should be noted and follow-up tests or referrals made as indicated.

If the child is old enough to talk, speech should be evaluated. The positions of the tongue, lips, and paraoral musculature during speech, while swallowing, and at rest may provide useful diagnostic information.

The intraoral examination of a child patient should be comprehensive. There is a temptation to look first for obvious carious lesions. Certainly controlling carious lesions is important because they can progress rapidly in children and pulpal involvement can occur within a few months after their onset. However, the dentist should first evaluate the condition of the oral soft tissues and the status of the developing occlusion. If the soft tissues and the occlusion are not observed early in the examination, the dentist may become so engrossed in charting carious lesions and in planning for their restoration that other important anomalies in the mouth are overlooked. Any unusual breath odors and abnormal quantity or consistency of saliva should also be noted.

The buccal tissues, lips, floor of the mouth, palate, and gingivae should be carefully inspected and palpated (Fig. 1-8). A detailed periodontal evaluation is occasionally indicated even in young children. The tongue and oropharynx should be closely inspected. Enlarged tonsils accompanied by purulent exudate may be the initial sign of a streptococcal infection leading to rheumatic fever. When streptococcal throat infection is suspected, immediate referral to the child's physician is indicated. In some cases it may be helpful to the physician and convenient for the dentist to obtain a throat culture while the child is still in the dental office, thus contributing to an earlier definitive diagnosis of the infection. The diagnosis and treatment of soft tissue problems are discussed throughout this book, especially in Chapters 4 and 14.

After thoroughly examining the oral soft tissues, the dentist should inspect the occlusion and note any dental or skeletal irregularities. The dentition

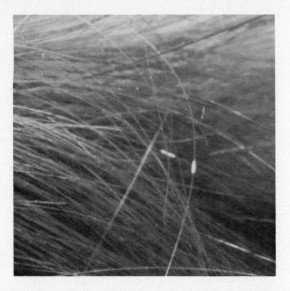

Fig. 1-4. Evidence of head lice infestation. Usually the insects are not seen, but their eggs or "nits" cling to hair filaments until they hatch. (Courtesy Dr. Hala Henderson.)

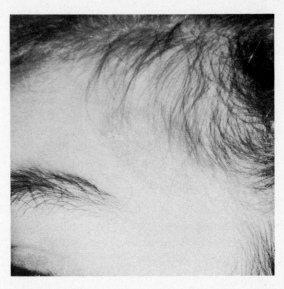

Fig. 1-5. Lesion on forehead above left eyebrow is due to ringworm infection. Several fungal species may cause the lesions on various areas of the body. The dentist may identify lesions on the head, face, or neck of a patient during a routine clinical examination. (Courtesy Dr. Hala Henderson.)

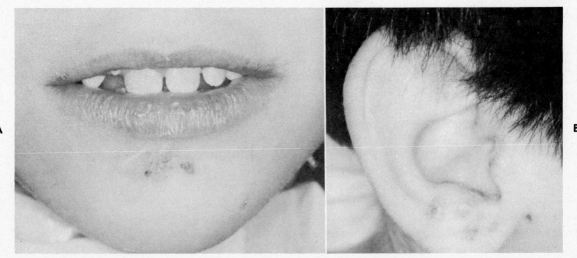

A

B

Fig. 1-6. Characteristic lesions of impetigo, **A,** on the lower face and, **B,** on the right ear. These lesions occur on various skin surfaces, but the dentist is most likely to encounter them on upper body areas. The infections are of bacterial (usually streptococcal) origin and usually require antibiotic therapy for control. The child often spreads the infection by scratching the lesions. (Courtesy Dr. Hala Henderson.)

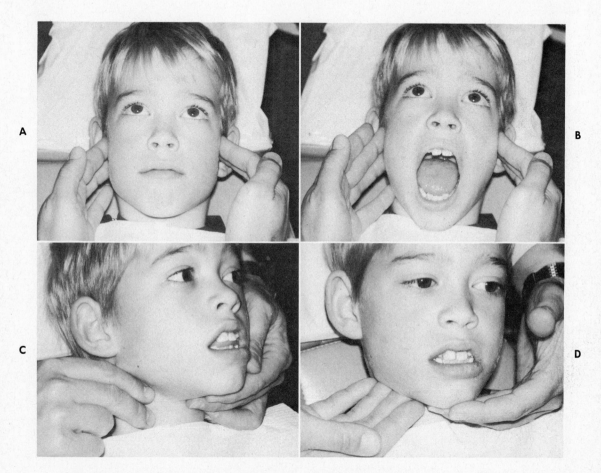

Fig. 1-7. A and **B,** Observation and palpation of TMJ function. **C** and **D,** Palpation of the neck and submandibular areas.

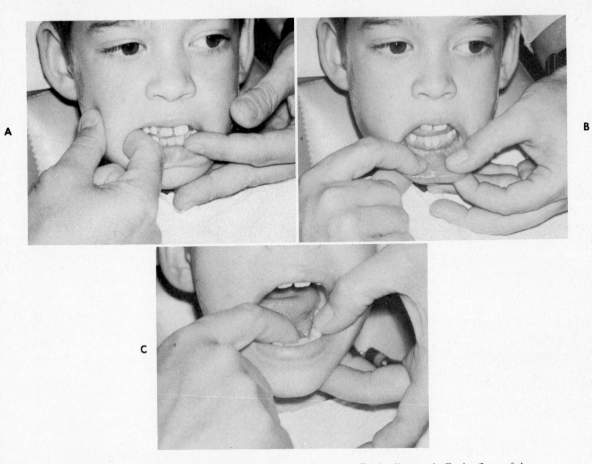

Fig. 1-8. Inspection and palpation of, **A,** the buccal tissues, **B,** the lips, and, **C,** the floor of the mouth.

and resulting occlusion may undergo considerable change during childhood and early adolescence. This dynamic developmental process occurs in all three planes of space, and with periodic evaluation the dentist can intercept and favorably influence undesirable changes. Monitoring of the patient's facial profile and symmetry; molar, canine, and anterior segment relationships; dental midlines; and arch length to tooth mass comparisons should be routinely included in the clinical examination. More detailed evaluation and analysis are indicated when significant discrepancies are found during critical stages of growth and development. Sometimes diagnostic cast and cephalometric analyses

are indicated relatively early in the mixed dentition stage. Detailed discussions of analyses of developing occlusions and interceptive treatment recommendations are presented in Chapters 18 to 21 and 24.

Finally, the teeth should be inspected carefully for evidence of carious lesions and hereditary or acquired anomalies. The teeth should also be counted and identified individually to ensure recognition of supernumerary or missing teeth. Identification of carious lesions is important in patients of all ages but is especially critical in young patients because the lesions tend to progress rapidly in children if not controlled. Eliminating the carious activity and restoring the teeth as needed prevent pain and the spread of infection and also contribute to the stability of the developing occlusion.

If the dentist prefers to perform the clinical examination of a new child patient before the radiographic and prophylaxis procedures, it may be necessary to correlate radiographic findings or other initially questionable findings with a second brief oral examination. This is especially true when the new patient has poor oral hygiene. Detailed inspection and exploration of the teeth and soft tissues cannot be adequately performed until the mouth is free of extraneous debris.

During the clinical examination for carious lesions each tooth should be dried individually and inspected under a good light. A definite routine for the examination should be established. For example, the dentist may always start in the upper right quadrant, work around the maxillary arch, move down to the lower left quadrant, and end the examination in the lower right quadrant. Sharp explorers providing different angles are necessary to detect proximal lesions, morphologic defects, and precarious areas in the enamel. If the sharpest exploring point sticks in a defect, it should be considered a carious or precarious lesion. Morphologic defects and incomplete coalescence of enamel at the base of pits and fissures in molar teeth can often be detected readily by visual examination after the teeth have been cleaned and dried. The decision of whether to restore a defect depends on the patient's history of dental caries, the parents' or patient's acceptance of a comprehensive preventive dentistry program (including dietary and oral hygiene control), and the patient's dependability in returning for recall appointments.

In patients with severe dental caries, caries activity tests and diet analysis may contribute to the diagnostic process by helping to define specific etiologic factors. These procedures probably have an even greater value in helping the patient or parents understand the carious disease process and in motivating them to make the behavioral changes needed to control the disease. The information provided the patient or parents should include instruction in plaque control and the appropriate recommendations for fluoride exposure. Dental caries susceptibility, the caries disease process, caries activity tests, diet analysis, and caries control are discussed in Chapters 4 and 7. Plaque control procedures and instructions are presented in detail in Chapter 15.

The dentist's comprehensive diagnosis depends on the completion of a number of procedures but requires a thorough, systematic, and critical clinical examination that includes at least inspection, palpation, and exploration. Any deviation from the expected or desired size, shape, color, and consistency of soft or hard tissues should be described in detail. The severity of associated problems and their causes must be clearly identified to the parents or the patient before success of a comprehensive oral health care program can be expected. The radiographic examination is an important supplement to these diagnostic procedures.

Uniform dental recording

Many different tooth charting systems are currently in use, including the universal system illustrated in the hard tissue examination section of Fig. 1-3. This system of marking teeth uses the numbers 1 to 32, beginning with the upper right third molar (No. 1) and progressing around the arch to the upper left third molar (No. 16), down to the lower left third molar (No. 17), and around the arch to the lower right third molar (No. 32). The primary teeth are identified in the universal system by the first 20 letters of the alphabet, A through T.

The Federation Dentaire International Special Committee on Uniform Dental Recording has specified the following basic requirements for a tooth charting system:

1. Simple to understand and teach
2. Easy to pronounce in conversation and dictation
3. Readily communicable in print and by wire
4. Easy to translate into computer input
5. Easily adaptable to standard charts used in general practice

The committee found that only one system, the two-digit system, seems to comply with these requirements. According to this system, the first digit indicates the quadrant and the second digit the type of tooth within the quadrant. Quadrants are allotted the digits 1 to 4 for the permanent teeth and 5 to 8 for the deciduous teeth in a clockwise sequence, starting at the upper right side; teeth within the same quadrant are allotted the digits 1 to 8 (deciduous teeth 1 to 5) from the midline backward. The digits should be pronounced separately; thus the permanent canines are teeth one-three, two-three, three-three, and four-three.

Permanent teeth

Upper right	Upper left
18 17 16 15 14 13 12 11	21 22 23 24 25 26 27 28
48 47 46 45 44 43 42 41	31 32 33 34 35 36 37 38
Lower right	Lower left

Deciduous teeth

Upper right	Upper left
55 54 53 52 51	61 62 63 64 65
85 84 83 82 81	71 72 73 74 75
Upper right	Lower left

The new system is gaining popularity in teaching institutions around the world, in the U.S. armed forces, and in private practice.

In the "Treatment proposed" section of the oral examination record (Fig. 1-3), the individual teeth that require restorative procedures, endodontic therapy, or extraction are listed. A check mark can be placed beside each listed tooth and procedure as the treatment is completed. Additional notations concerning treatment procedures completed and the date are recorded on supplemental treatment record pages.

Radiographic examination

When indicated, radiographic examination for children must be completed before the comprehensive oral health care plan can be developed, and subsequent radiographs at regular intervals are necessary to detect incipient carious lesions and other developing anomalies.

A complete mouth radiographic survey should be completed for each dental patient by 5 years of age. In some cases the clinical examination findings may justify an earlier radiographic survey. Isolated occlusal, periapical, or bite-wing films are often indicated in very young children (even in-

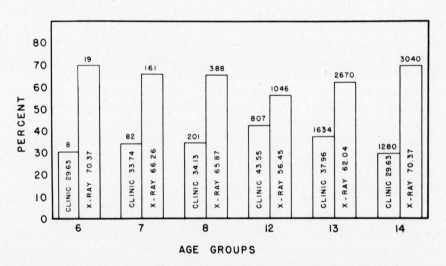

Fig. 1-9. Comparison of the number of carious lesions found on proximal surfaces of permanent teeth by direct observation and by radiographic examination in prefluoride year 1946. The figure at the top of each bar refers to the total number of lesions observed in each category. (From Blayney, J.R., and Hill, I.N.: J.A.D.A. **74:**233-302, 1967.)

fants) because of trauma, toothache, suspected developmental disturbances, or proximal caries.

The carious lesion always appears smaller on the radiograph than it actually is. Likewise, microscopic observation of ground sections of teeth reveals that progress of the lesion through the enamel and dentin is more extensive than is evident on the radiograph.

Blayney and Hill compared the number of proximal surface lesions found by direct examination with those too small to be observed clinically and visualized only on radiographs. In children of all ages the number of permanent tooth proximal surface lesions found only by radiographic examination surpassed those found only by direct observation (Figs. 1-9 and 1-10). In the group of children who had lifetime exposure to optimal fluoride levels the percentage of lesions observed by the use of radiographs increased, whereas those seen by direct observation decreased. Blayney and Hill emphasized the importance of recognizing hidden incipient lesions in the practice of preventive dentistry. The proximal lesion on a primary molar, even though it appears to be limited to the enamel, will almost always develop rapidly and within the normal recall period may progress to the extent that it endangers the pulp. If the child patient can be motivated to adopt a routine of good oral hygiene supported by competent supervision, many of the initial lesions will be arrested.

Radiographic techniques for the child patient are described in detail in Chapter 6.

Early examination

Roche has stated that historically, dental care for children has been designed primarily to prevent oral pain and infection, the occurrence and progress of dental caries, the premature loss of primary teeth, the loss of arch length, and the association between fear and dental care. Throughout pedodontic treatment the dentist is responsible for guiding the child and parent, resolving oral disor-

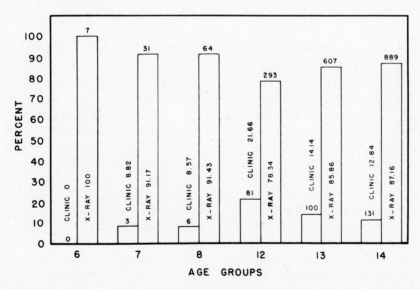

Fig. 1-10. Comparison of the number of carious lesions found on proximal surfaces of permanent teeth by direct observation and by radiographic examination after lifetime exposure to fluoridated water. The figure at the top of each bar refers to the total number of lesions found in each category. (From Blayney, J.R., and Hill, I.N.: J.A.D.A. **74:**233-302, 1967.)

ders before they can affect health and dental alignment, and preventing oral disease. The goals of pedodontic care therefore are primarily preventive.

Weddell and Klein studied oral disease in 441 children between 6 and 36 months of age who were born and reared in an area with a fluoridated water supply. They found no dental caries in children 6 to 11 months of age, but 4.2% of the children 12 to 17 months of age were found to have at least one carious lesion. Dental caries was identified in 19.8% of the children in the 24- to 29-month age group and in 36.4% of the 30- to 36-month age group. Of the 299 white children examined, gingivitis was present in 13.2% of those 6 to 17 months old, 33.9% of those 18 to 23 months old, and 38.5% of those 24 to 36 months old. Weddell and Klein observed that dental caries prevalence and the severity of gingivitis in children 6 to 36 months of age are independent of sex and socioeconomic status. They also found an increased prevalence of gingivitis in young children with dental caries compared to those without dental caries. They concluded that parent education by the dentist and preventive treatment are indicated very early in a child's life.

Some dentists like to counsel expectant parents before their child is born. Many prospective parents are interested in knowing what should be done to encourage optimum oral health from the very beginning of life. Parents of teething youngsters are also very interested in fostering favorable oral health and development in their children. Many family practitioners find it rewarding to offer infant dental care services. Others recommend early care but refer the very young children of their patients to pedodontists.

Dentists who treat children are encouraged to counsel prospective parents and parents of infants about their child's oral health and development. It is appropriate for a dentist to perform an oral examination for an infant of any age, even a newborn baby, and an examination is recommended anytime the parent or physician calls with questions concerning the appearance of an infant's oral tissues.

Even when there are no known problems, the child's first dental visit and oral examination should take place by at least 1 year of age (ideally about 9 months of age). This early dental visit enables the dentist and parents to discuss ways to nurture excellent oral health before any serious problems have had an opportunity to develop. An adequate oral examination for an infant is generally quite simple and very brief, but it may be the important first step toward a lifetime of excellent oral health.

Some dentists may prefer to ''preside'' during the entire first session with the infant and parents. Others may wish to delegate some of the educational aspects of the session to auxiliary members of the office staff and then conduct the examination and answer any unresolved questions. In either case it is sometimes necessary to have an assistant available to help hold the child's attention so that the parents can concentrate on the important information being provided.

It is not always necessary to conduct the infant oral examination in the dental operatory, but it should take place where there is adequate light for a visual examination. The dentist may find it convenient to conduct the examination in the private consultation room during the initial meeting with the child and the parents. The examination procedures may include only direct observation and digital palpation. However, if primary molars have erupted or if hand instruments may be needed, the examination should be performed at the dental chair to facilitate instrument transfers between the dental assistant and the dentist.

The parents should be informed before the examination that it will be necessary to gently restrain the child and that it is normal for the child to cry during the procedure. The infant is held on the lap of a parent, usually the mother. This direct involvement of the parent provides emotional support to the child and allows the parent to help restrain the child. Both parents may participate or at least be present during the examination.

The dentist should make a brief attempt to get acquainted with the child and to project warmth

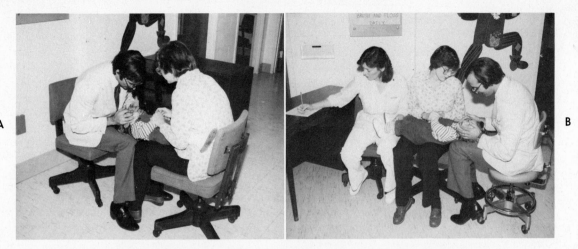

Fig. 1-11. A, One method of positioning a child for an oral examination in a small private consultation area. The dental assistant is nearby to record findings. **B,** If space allows three people to sit in a row, this method may be used to make it easier for the dental assistant to hear the findings dictated by the dentist. The dental assistant also helps restrain the child's legs.

and caring. However, many infants and toddlers are not particularly interested in developing new friendships with strangers, and the dentist should not be discouraged if the child shuns the friendly approach. Even if the child chooses to resist (which is common and normal), only negligible extra effort is necessary to perform the examination procedure. The dentist should not be flustered by the crying and resistant behavior and should proceed unhurriedly but efficiently with the examination. The dentist's voice should remain unstrained and pleasant during the examination. The dentist's behavior should reassure the child and alleviate the parent's anxiety concerning this first dental procedure.

One method of performing the examination in a private consultation area is illustrated in Fig. 1-11, *A*. The dentist and the parent are seated face to face with their knees touching. Their upper legs form the "examination table" for the child. The child's legs straddle the parent's body, allowing the parent to restrain the child's legs and hands. An assistant is present to record the dentist's examination findings as they are dictated and to help restrain the

child if needed. If adequate space is available in the consultation area, the approach illustrated in Fig. 1-11, *B*, may prove useful. The dental assistant is seated at a desk or writing stand near the child's feet. The dental assistant and the parent are facing the same direction side by side and at a right angle to the direction the dentist is facing. The dental assistant is in a good position to hear and record the dentist's findings as they are dictated, even if the child is crying loudly. These positions (Fig. 1-11) are also convenient for demonstrating oral hygiene procedures to the parents (see also p. 392).

When primary molars have erupted, the dentist will need an explorer and possibly a mouth mirror to complete the oral examination. If the parents express concern about the appearance of certain oral tissues, the dentist will probably prefer to conduct the examination at the dental chair where hand instruments can be transferred efficiently and safely and where light can be easily adjusted. The positions of the dentist, parent, child, and dental assistant during the examination at the dental chair are illustrated in Fig. 1-12. The dental assistant is seated higher to permit good visibility and to better

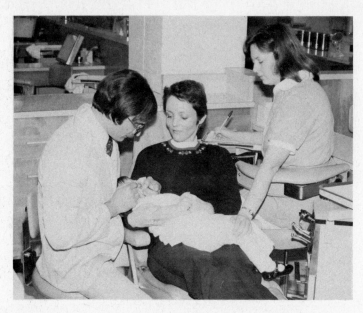

Fig. 1-12. Oral examination of a very young child in the dental operatory.

anticipate the dentist's needs. The assistant is also in a good position to hear and record the dentist's findings. The parent and the dental assistant restrain the child's arms and legs. The child's head is positioned in the bend of the parent's arm. The dentist establishes a chairside position so that not only the dentist's hands but also the lower arms and chest may be available for support of the child's head if necessary (see also pp. 778 and 779).

The initial oral examination may often be performed by careful direct observation and digital palpation. The dentist may need only good lighting for visibility and gauze for drying or debriding tissues. Sometimes a tongue blade and a soft-bristled toothbrush are also useful. At other times, as previously mentioned, the dentist will want the complete operatory available. In either case the examination should begin with a systematic and gentle digital exploration of the soft tissues without any instruments. The child may find this gentle palpation soothing, especially when alveolar ridges in teething areas are massaged. The digital examination may help relax the child and encourage less

resistance. If hand instruments are needed, the dentist must be sure to have a stable finger rest before inserting an instrument into the child's mouth.

A finger guard made of a double thickness of soft mouthguard material may facilitate the examination procedure (Fig. 1-13). This acts as a bite block to enable the child to rest the jaw in a mouth-open position, and it protects the dentist's fingers from the sharp cutting edges of young primary teeth. The finger guard may also be useful in examining or operating on patients who have poor motor control, such as spastic or mentally retarded patients. The finger guard may be fabricated with a vacuum adaptation technique similar to the one described for mouth guards on p. 734. A stone model of the dentist's second or third finger is made from an alginate impression using a small drinking cup as the impression tray. Martinez advocated impression tray material for the second layer of the finger guard. However, we prefer the softer polyvinyl mouthguard material.

Although there is little or no effective communication between the dentist and the infant or toddler,

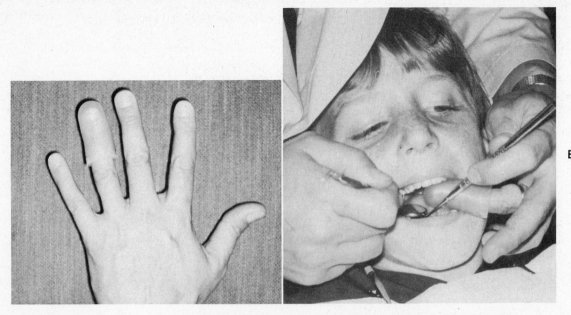

Fig. 1-13. A, Finger guard used to facilitate certain dental procedures and to protect the dentist's fingers from inadvertent biting by the patient. **B,** Actual use of the finger guard, which may be used on either hand.

the child realizes at the conclusion of the examination that nothing "bad" happened. The child also realizes that the procedure was permitted by the parents who remained and actually helped with the examination. The child will not hold a lasting grudge against anyone, and the experience will not have a detrimental effect on future behavior as a dental patient. On the contrary, our experiences suggest that such early examinations followed by regular recall examinations often contribute to the youngsters becoming excellent dental patients without fear at very young ages. These children's chances for enjoying excellent oral health throughout life are also enhanced.

Child abuse and neglect

Child abuse and neglect is a significant worldwide societal problem that threatens the physical or mental well-being of many defenseless children. Child abuse has been known since the beginning of recorded history; some forms of abuse have even been accepted in certain societies. Ironically, it was the Society for the Prevention of Cruelty to Animals that first defended the rights of abused children in the United States in 1871. Kempe and associates introduced the "battered child syndrome" to the medical literature in 1962, and the drive to protect children from abuse has continued to gain momentum since that time. Ellerstein reported that 1% to 3% of the children in the United States are abused or neglected. He also stated that child maltreatment causes more physical and psychologic morbidity than most pediatric illnesses and that more children die from child abuse each year than from leukemia. The dentist whose practice includes children should be aware of the signs and symptoms of abuse and neglect because the dentist may be in a key position to make the initial identification of such problems.

Nationwide legislation at state levels has established Child Protection Service Agencies through county welfare departments to ensure an immediate and appropriate response by professionals to reports of suspected cases of child abuse or neglect. In addition, the 1974 Child Abuse Prevention and Treatment Act mandated the creation of the National Center on Child Abuse and Neglect. This center is responsible for researching the causes, treatment, and prevention of child abuse and maintaining statistics on the incidence of abuse.

Child abuse. Child abuse may be defined as nonaccidental trauma to a child, inflicted by a caretaker, for which there is no reasonable explanation. Child abuse may be divided into physical abuse, sexual abuse, intentional drugging or poisoning, and emotional abuse. These categories overlap; all forms of abuse have emotional components, and sexual abuse and intentional drugging or poisoning are also categories of physical abuse.

Physical abuse is the category that dentists are most likely to encounter, since 65% or more of the injuries occur to the head, face, and neck. If child abuse is suspected, the only body areas considered inappropriate for a dentist to examine are the genitalia and buttocks. Examination of body areas normally covered by clothing should be witnessed by at least one other staff member.

The list of possible signs of physical abuse is almost inexhaustible, but the following are some of the more common types:

- Bite marks
- Broken bones, especially jaw, nasal, or other facial fractures but also fractures of the digits, limbs, or ribs
- Broken, discolored, displaced, loosened, or missing teeth
- Bruises, especially if multiple and in places not usually seen in common accidents
- Bumps on the head or swellings of other body parts
- Burns (for example, from cigarettes, hot liquids, hot metal, or ropes)
- Choke marks on the neck (may be bruises)
- Cuts, especially if multiple and in unusual places
- Hematomas (for example, on the earlobes from pinching)
- Lacerations of the face or lips

- Patchy baldness (for example, from burns or hair pulling)
- Retinal hemorrhages (for example, from violent shaking)
- Scars or welts (for example, from beatings with straps, switches, or whips)
- Sores or abrasions at the lip commissures (for example, from a mouth gag)
- Tongue injuries (for example, from a blow forcibly occluding the teeth)
- Torn oral frena

The dentist should always obtain the history of an injury. If the injury is of a suspicious nature, the dentist may find the history to be equally suspicious. During an interview with the child, parents, or other caretakers about the cause of the injury, the dentist may find their explanations to be implausible or may notice discrepancies between two individual accounts of the injury. Children are not likely to get a "black eye" or an oral injury from falling out of bed, and bilateral "black eyes" are unusual in any type of accident that could not be easily confirmed. Multiple cigarette burns cannot be accidental. Logic and common sense are important in correlating the findings with the history of the injury.

Sexual abuse is probably the most underdiagnosed form of child abuse, and it is feared that sexual abuse is often not reported by other family members. Sexual abuse of children most often affects girls, but young boys have also been subjected to this trauma. The list of offenses is long and includes any form of sexual activity with children from exhibitionism and fondling to child pornography, forced prostitution, incest, rape, and sodomy. The dentist is not likely to suspect sexual abuse unless oral venereal disease is identified. A male dentist may suspect sexual abuse if a girl patient exhibits an atypical reluctance to cooperate for a simple oral examination and is especially concerned about being touched. Bite marks constitute physical abuse but are often associated with sexual abuse.

Intentional drugging or poisoning occurs when a caretaker administers prescription drugs to a child for whom they were not intended, deliberately gives a child an overdose of any drug, shares illegal drugs with a child, or knowingly administers toxic agents to a child. Unless the victim exhibits overt signs or symptoms of drug overdose or poisoning while in the dental office, the dentist would probably not suspect this form of abuse.

Emotional abuse is the most difficult form of child abuse to prove, but it may be quite damaging psychologically. Examples include:

• Continual belittling, rejection, or scapegoating
• Lack of love, support, or guidance
• Severe and inappropriate punishment (nonphysical) or psychologic terrorism (for example, locking a child in a dark closet or threatening mutilation)
• Severe and frequent verbal abuse or berating

The dentist may identify severe psychopathology resulting from emotional abuse, but the diagnosis must be confirmed by a psychiatrist. If the parents or caretakers persist in refusing to cooperate with treatment for the child, emotional abuse may be established.

Child neglect. Child neglect may be defined as the caretaker's failure to provide the basic emotional, physical, and psychologic needs of a child. Child neglect may be caused by a caretaker's ignorance, but it probably results more often from immaturity, irresponsibility, or negligence. Neglect is considered a somewhat less serious offense than abuse because there is no overt or willful attempt to harm the child. However, there is a fine line between abuse and neglect, and some forms of abuse can be proved only as neglect.

Underfeeding or negligence in feeding is the most common cause for failure to thrive in infants. This problem may be accidental in the case of a parent who did not learn to mix the baby formula properly, but it is believed to result more often from negligence or as a direct attack (conscious or unconscious) on the child produced from an unwanted pregnancy. Water deprivation leading to serious dehydration is a related form of neglect. Deliberate underfeeding or water deprivation constitutes child abuse.

Inadequate attention to a child's safety, physical well-being, and education is also neglect. Child abandonment is the most severe offense in this category. Gross lack of supervision of the child (especially if 2 years old or younger), providing totally inadequate hygiene, clothing, or shelter, and failing to send the child to school at the proper time are other examples.

Failure to obtain needed dental care and certain needed medical care is a form of child neglect that is easily identified by the dentist. Neglect should always be reported when parents or guardians refuse to accept lifesaving treatment for their child or if the caretakers seem to be apathetic or unconcerned about treatment known to improve the child's health and quality of life. Inability to pay for health care is a problem that must be resolved by the caretakers and the health care provider, but it should not prevent essential care for the child. The caretakers should exhibit a sincere interest in the child's welfare.

The dentist's responsibilities in suspected cases of abuse and neglect. As health care professionals, dentists should be especially sensitive to the need for protecting children from abuse or neglect. They must, of course, treat dentally related injuries. It is also important for dentists, and all other citizens, to know that they are legally mandated to report suspected child abuse or neglect. Reporting is initiated simply with a telephone call to the appropriate Child Protection Service Agency. Local agencies operate 24-hour "hotlines" listed in the telephone directory under "Child Protection Service" or a similar title. The telephone call initiates an immediate response by appropriately trained professionals, but the dentist should follow the call with a brief written report. Dentists are mandated to report on the basis of "reasonable suspicion," and they are not responsible for any further investigation. Cases of abuse and neglect are usually resolved without litigation, but the reporting dentist will not necessarily be called to testify even if the case does go to court.

Any person who in good faith reports child abuse or neglect is immune from civil or criminal liability that might otherwise result from such action. The privileged quality of communication between the caretakers or the patient and the practitioner is not grounds for excluding evidence in a judicial proceeding resulting from a report or for failing to make a report as required by law. Strict confidentiality of records is maintained. Reports and any other information obtained in reference to a report are confidential and available only to persons authorized by the Juvenile Code. Some state statutes stipulate that a mandated reporter who fails to make a report when abuse or neglect is suspected may be liable for proximate damages caused by the failure to report. In 1972 a suit was filed against a group of pediatricians who had failed to report a documented case of child abuse. The suit was settled out of court against the pediatricians for $600,000.

As mentioned previously, the dentist's only legal obligation may be to report suspected child abuse or neglect. The reporter is guaranteed anonymity. However, several experts believe that it is professionally appropriate and possibly therapeutic to discuss the suspicion with the caretakers. The dentist should not accuse a specific individual. (In fact, the dentist probably would not have sufficient information to accuse anyone.) However, the dentist could state that ''someone'' is suspected of injuring the child. Abusers are often cooperative after learning that nonaccidental injury is suspected, even though they do not usually offer incriminating information before the child's examination. It would seem that most abusers do want help.

The dentist must maintain a calm and nonthreatening attitude during the discussion. The dentist should not exhibit anger but rather concern for the child's welfare and a desire to help. If the caretaker becomes hostile, the dentist should emphasize that the suspicion of abuse is based on the signs and symptoms observed (which often do not correlate with the history) and that possible abuse must be reported as mandated by law. Then the dentist must follow through immediately with a telephone report. Some professionals advise telephoning the report on the basis of the facts observed before discussing it with the caretakers, to ensure that an unexpectedly pleasant conversation with the care-

takers does not sway the earlier decision to make a report. Such a decision rests with the individual practitioner.

In some cases the dentist may wish to have a pediatrician or family physician corroborate the findings. If the physician is nearby (next door or in the same building), the consultation can take place immediately without the prior knowledge of the caretakers. If referral is necessary, it is probably not advisable to discuss any suspicion of abuse with the caretakers. Rather the dentist should identify concern for the child's welfare and the medical implications of the injury that require follow-up by the physician. The dentist may explain that arrangements have been made for the child to be seen as soon as the caretakers can bring the child to the physician's office or hospital. The dentist should maintain contact with the physician's office, and the Child Protection Service Agency should be notified if the patient has not arrived by the anticipated time. Occasionally it may be appropriate to admit a child to the hospital to afford immediate protection.

Early intervention in child abuse and neglect helps everyone. It provides the best opportunity to obtain the necessary treatment and supportive services in time to preserve and strengthen the family unit. Without intervention the problem grows and may culminate in morbid results. For these reasons, calling attention to a possible case of child abuse or neglect is justified on the basis of well-founded suspicion alone.

Drug abuse

The prevalence of child abuse and neglect begins to diminish as children grow older, but the problem of voluntary drug abuse by the youngsters themselves begins to intensify. The dentist who treats preteenage and teenage patients should be aware of drug abuse in these age groups. In addition, the dentist should have a basic knowledge of the signs and symptoms of drug abuse to help identify drug-abusing patients and should be prepared to take appropriate precautionary measures when drug abusers are treated in the dental office.

Rosenbaum states that it may be difficult for the

dentist to identify a drug abuser unless the patient offers the information voluntarily. He offers the following clues to identification of such a patient:

- A tendency to look off into space
- Moodiness
- Carelessness in appearance, especially if well dressed on previous appointments
- Drowsiness
- Frivolous laughter, espcially when things are not funny
- Apparent intoxication without the odor of alcohol of the patient's breath
- A "hopped-up" appearance (bright, shiny eyes)
- Changes in pupillary dilation that are inconsistent with changes in light intensity
- Possession of pills, capsules, or injection equipment
- Hallucinations or convulsions (a signal for immediate medical attention)

Rosenbaum further points out that a drug abuser should not receive dental treatment while under the influence of the drug(s). Addicts tend to seek only emergency dental care, and they may try to obtain drug prescriptions from the dentist. Drug addicts who inject drugs into their bodies are potential hepatitis carriers. Appropriate precautionary measures should be taken during and after the treatment of such a patient. Drug addicts also seem to have a higher susceptibility to subacute bacterial endocarditis, which is attributed to the response of the heart valves to the agents used to dilute the drugs. Prophylactic antibiotic therapy is indicated for these patients before dental treatment.

Emergency dental treatment

All too often a patient's initial dental appointment is prompted by an emergency situation. The diagnostic procedures necessary for an emergency dental appointment have already been outlined in this chapter. However, the emergency appointment tends to focus on and resolve a single problem or a single set of related problems rather than provide a comprehensive oral diagnosis and management of the patient. Once the emergency problem is under control, the dentist should offer comprehensive services to the patient or parents.

The remainder of this book presents information for dentists and dental students to augment their diagnostic and management skills in providing oral health care services to children and adolescents during both emergency and preplanned dental visits.

REFERENCES

Avery, D.R.: Integrated dental treatment in children: diagnosis, Quintessence Int. **2:**59-62, 1980.

Berson, R.B.: Head lice infestation and pedodontic practice, J. Dent. Child. **48:**201-204, 1981.

Blayney, J.R., and Hill, I.N.: Fluorine and dental caries, J.A.D.A. **74:**233-302, 1967.

Bureau of Economic and Behavioral Research for the Council on Dental Practice: The dentist's responsibility in recognizing and reporting child abuse: a report, Chicago, 1980, American Dental Association.

Croll, T.P., Menna, V.J., and Evans, C.A.: Primary identification of an abused child in a dental office: a case report, Pediatr. Dent. **3:**339-342, 1981.

Ellerstein, N.S.: Child abuse and neglect, New York, 1981, John Wiley & Sons, Inc.

Keller, S.E., and Manson-Hing, L.R.: Diagnosis and treatment planning for the child patient. In Finn, S.B.: Clinical pedodontics, ed. 4, Philadelphia, 1973, W.B. Saunders Co.

Kempe, C.H., and others: The battered child syndrome, J.A.M.A. **181:**17-24, 1962.

Kittle, P.E., Richardson, D.S., and Parker, J.W.: Two child abuse/child neglect examinations for the dentist, J. Dent. Child. **48:**175-180, 1981.

Little, J.W., and Falace, D.A.: Dental management of the medically compromised patient, St. Louis, 1980, The C.V. Mosby Co.

Malecz, R.E.: Child abuse: its relationship to pedodontics; a survey, J. Dent. Child. **46:**193-194, 1979.

Martinez, C.R.: Custom finger guard-mouth prop as an alternative to conventional mouth props, J.A.D.A. **95:**804-806, 1977.

Moskow, B.S., and Barr, C.E.: Examination of the patient. In Goldman, H.M., and others, editors: Current therapy in dentistry, vol. 4, St. Louis, 1970, The C.V. Mosby Co.

Nelson, W.E., and others: Nelson's textbook of pediatrics, ed. 11, Philadelphia, 1979, W.B. Saunders Co.

Nowak, A.J.: The infant patient: initial appointment management. In McDonald, R.E., and others, editors: Current therapy in dentistry, vol. 7, St. Louis, 1980, The C.V. Mosby Co.

Robinson, H.B.G.: Diagnosis of oral lesions, Dent. Surv. **37:**1443-1446, 1587-1590, 1961.

Roche, J.R.: Preventive pedodontics. In Bernier, J.L., and Muhler, J.C., editors: Improving dental practice through preventive measures, ed. 2, St. Louis, 1970, The C.V. Mosby Co.

Rosenbaum, C.H.: Dental precautions in treating drug addicts: a hidden problem among teens and preteens, Pediatr. Dent. **2:**94-96, 1980.

Shafer, W.G., Hine, M.K., and Levy, B.M.: Textbook of oral pathology, ed. 3, Philadelphia, 1982, W.B. Saunders Co.

Shaw, O.: Dental anxiety in children, Br. Dent. J. **139:**134-139, 1975.

Smith, D.W.: Introduction to clinical pediatrics, ed. 2, Philadelphia, 1977, W.B. Saunders Co.

Snawder, K.D.: Handbook of clinical pedodontics, St. Louis, 1980, The C.V. Mosby Co.

ten Bensel, R.W. and King, K.J.: Neglect and abuse of children: historical aspects, identification and management, J. Dent. Child. **42:**348-358, 1975.

Updegrave, W.J.: The role of panoramic radiography in diagnosis, Oral Surg. **22:**49-57, 1966.

Weddell, J.A., and Klein, A.I.: Socioeconomic correlation or oral disease in six- to thirty-six month children, Pediatr. Dent. **3:**306-310, 1981.

2 Psychologic approach to behavior guidance

RALPH E. McDONALD
DAVID R. AVERY

It is generally agreed that the proper guidance of a child's behavior in the dental office is prerequisite for complete dental care. Until only recently little research had been undertaken to provide answers to even common problems associated with such guidance. Weinstein and associates have demonstrated that dentists often react to a child's fear-related behavior with responses that are counterproductive. Coercion, coaxing, and negative remarks by the dentist were shown to increase negative behavior, while guiding the child toward desirable behavior by patting the child and asking questions about feelings greatly increase the probability of reducing fear-related behavior. They point out that, in general, dentists who treat children should, in addition to demonstrating a sincere personal interest in the child, become more adept in providing direction and reinforcement.

Many dentists agree with Chambers' statement that the fragmented nature of dental behavioral research can be traced directly to a preoccupation with techniques instead of goals or standards. Virtually all research in the field is technique oriented—typically, a comparison of one particular behavioral technique with a control group to prove that the technique is effective in some statistically significant fashion. Chambers also believes there is no shortage of proven effective techniques for managing children in the dental office. What is lacking, however, is profession-wide standards for child behavior. Perhaps the wide variety of tech-

niques used in private practice today is based on this lack of definition concerning appropriate child dental behavior.

In recent years the profession has witnessed an increase in practical behavior modification research. Although freudian psychosexual interpretations are still important, there has been a trend away from this approach. Several new techniques have been developed from the social sciences, some of which are behavior modification, desensitization, hypnosis, modeling, and performance contracting. Most of these methods have proved to be at least partially successful in modifying some behavior of the child patient, and several of them are discussed in this chapter. Chambers also notes that the literature contains accounts of individual successes with tell-show-do, hand-over-mouth exercise, token reinforcement, voice control, and restraint. These methods are also discussed here.

Pinkham emphasizes that the dentist who treats children should develop proficiency in observing and analyzing child behavior. The development of these skills is enhanced by experience, the ability to assess nonverbal aspects of communication, a knowledge of children's fears and anxieties about the dental situation, and a knowledge of the social, cultural, and personal aspects of child behavior. The dentist who can integrate the information gained from observed child behavior with the personal, social, and historical information acquired from the parents may more accurately predict a child's behavior and then select the best method of managing that behavior during the clinical experience.

In spite of an often limited knowledge of child psychology, dentists in general get along well with children and are able to treat them with the same degree of efficiency as adult patients. The real problem child in the dental office is the exception. However, the dentist would find it much easier to accept each child knowing that a behavior problem or anxiety state could be readily diagnosed and solved. Such acceptance will occur only as a result of continued study and research in the field of child psychology as it relates to dental practice.

Few parents realize the difficult position of the dentist introduced to a child who is afraid, anxious, or actually resistant to the initial examination and dental procedures. Only rarely does the dentist understand the psychologic development of the young child or know anything about the preparation provided by the child's parents for the first visit or whether there has been a previous unfortunate experience. Almost without exception, however, the parents expect the dentist to be the complete master of all situations and to provide a health service for their child regardless of the child's reaction.

This chapter outlines considerations that are generally agreed to be important in guiding the young child through the dental experience. It seems imperative that both the student and the practitioner acquaint themselves with problems of behavior guidance, as well as of diagnosis and treatment procedures, in order that they may do their part in meeting this dental health challenge. Individuals with a particular interest in behavior guidance are referred to textbooks by Wright and by Ripa and Barenie.

Role of the dentist

Although the dentist's primary function is to provide the necessary preventive dental care and treatment, competence should not be limited to technical efficiency alone. By cultivating a sensitive and understanding approach, the dentist can do a great deal to help the patient cope with the experience. Furthermore, dental treatment is an event that the child must attempt to accept. Children who have learned to cope with their role as dental patients exhibit some flexibility of behavior and an interest in what is going on around them. They show a capacity to trust and to respond to the dentist and demonstrate confidence in their ability to meet the demands of the situation.

The dentist who limits dental services to children or the general practitioner who treats many children is often asked, "Why do you have such an interest in this phase of dental practice?" Many assume it is because the dentist has a genuine liking for children. Most authorities agree that liking children is extremely important in managing them successfully in the dental office, and this love of children should be evident at all times. More important, however, should be the desire to provide a good health service because of an appreciation of its importance to the child. This phase of dental practice probably presents a greater challenge than some others. Its rewards are that the dentist can see the long-term benefits of early and adequate care: reducing the national accumulation of dental needs to a manageable size for the future, particularly when the treatment program encompasses preventive dentistry in its broadest aspect.

There are times when anyone working with children will feel insecure in the management of a particular child. This insecurity is more likely to occur when a person is faced with an unfamiliar problem. That is why the dentist who treats children must continually study dentistry and become familiar with the wide variety of situations and anomalies that must be diagnosed and managed. Perhaps insecurity must be accepted as a part of the practice of modern dentistry. Dentists must realize, however, that there are weaknesses in their own profession and that they do not have the answers to all the problems related to child management.

It is important for dentists to understand child behavior because it will help them understand their own behavior and reactions to problems in the dental office, as well as realize that control of the child or guidance during the dental situation often deviates from a fixed pattern. It is difficult or even impossible for one dentist to tell another how to proceed with a given behavior problem. The reactions of a child will differ from time to time, and so will the approach of the dentist. Thus if behavior control deteriorates occasionally, it is not necessarily a reflection on the dentist's adequacy. There may not have been sufficient time to determine the cause of abnormal behavior. An instance of failure may merely mean that the dentist should reconsider the problem or use a different approach.

It is extremely important that the dentist learn to mask emotional reactions to situations. Even the young child can quickly sense indecision or anxiety. As the dentist's apprehension grows, it will be reflected in the child. The dentist should never show anger, regardless of provocation. In fact, it will be helpful to mask any type of emotional involvement and to create a controlled, understanding atmosphere.

Psychologic growth

The dentist who successfully guides children through a dental experience realizes that a normal child undergoes intellectual as well as physical growth. The dentist further realizes that the child is constantly acquiring, shedding, or modifying habits. This change is perhaps one reason that the child's reaction in the dental office may differ from one appointment to the next. Every child has a rhythm and a style of growth. No two children, even in the same family, develop in exactly the same pattern. Furthermore, everyone who works with children must realize that the child's psychologic age may not always correspond to chronologic age. While chronologic age is relatively unimportant to the dentist, the psychologic and physiologic age of the child must be considered in the diagnosis of behavior problems as well as treatment planning.

The learning process

According to Yarrow, data suggest that simple learning mechanisms operate even before birth.

There is no question that simple associative learning occurs from the moment of birth. Through learning, the infant becomes sensitized to specific experiences and becomes conditioned to environmental events.

Children's behavior is a function of learning and is often classified by identifying the types of behavior that represent the "norm" for certain age groups. Such a classification at least provides a basis for discussing various behaviors. However, the dentist should not be overly influenced by the child's chronologic age in trying to predict or deal with behavior. When behavior is classified in categories by chronologic age, it must be remembered that it is also "normal" to encounter some 4-year-old children who behave like 2-year-olds in the dental environment. Conversely, the dentist will meet some 2- or 3-year-old children who are advanced in psychosocial development and may behave in the dental chair at a higher age level than the "norm." A categorical discussion of normal child behavior by chronologic age is relevant only if one remembers the wide range of variation that is possible. The dentist's management of undesirable behavior in the operatory should focus on the behavior itself rather than on the child's age.

Infancy and toddler ages. A great deal of learning occurs during the first 2 years of life. However, the toddler or infant has little or no ability to comprehend the need for a dental examination or dental treatment, nor is the dentist able to communicate effectively with the child. Occasionally the dentist may encounter a 15-month-old child who will cooperate even for restorative procedures, but such an occurrence represents the exception rather than the rule. Even without cooperation, oral examinations and certain treatment procedures may be accomplished on very young children efficiently and without sedation.

Two years of age. At 2 years of age children differ greatly in their ability to communicate, primarily because there is considerable difference in the development of vocabulary at that age. According to Gesell and Ilg, the 2-year-old's vocabulary may vary from 12 to 1000 words. If the child has a limited vocabulary, it will make communication difficult. For this reason work can be successfully completed for some 2-year-old children, while with others there will be limited cooperation. The 2-year-old child is often referred to as being in the "precooperative stage." Usually the child has not learned to play with other children and seems to prefer solitary play. The child is too young to be reached by words alone and must handle and touch objects to fully understand their meaning. At this age the child must be allowed to handle the mirror, to smell the toothpaste, or to feel the rubber cup. By so doing, the child will have a better idea of what the dentist is attempting to do, especially since the 2-year-old child is often intrigued by water and washing. Since the child at this early age is shy of new people and places and finds separation from parents difficult, almost without exception the child should be accompanied by a parent to the treatment room.

Three years of age. The dentist can usually communicate and reason with the 3-year-old child during the dental experience. The 3-year-old has a great desire to talk and will often enjoy telling stories to the dentist and the assistants. At this stage the dental personnel can begin to use the positive approach with the child although it is a good idea to point out the positive rather than the negative factors with children at any age. This is particularly true with the young child, who is more likely to do the very things that have been specifically pointed out as undesirable.

Hymes has reported that children 3 years of age and under, in times of stress or when they are hurt, fatigued, or frightened, will automatically turn to the mother or her substitute for comfort, support, and assurance. They have difficulty taking someone else's word for anything, and they feel more secure if the parent is allowed to remain with them until they become fully acquainted with the personnel and the procedures.

Four years of age. The 4-year-old child will usually listen with interest to explanations and normally will be responsive to verbal directions. Children at this age tend to have lively minds and may

be great talkers, although they often exaggerate in their conversation. In some situations the 4-year-old may become defiant and may resort to name-calling. In general, however, the 4-year-old child who has had a happy home life with a normal amount of training and discipline will be a cooperative dental patient.

Five years of age. The 5-year-old child is ready to accept group activities and community experience. At this age personal and social relationships are better defined, and the child usually has no fear of leaving one of the parents for the dental appointment. If 5-year-old children have been properly prepared by their parents, they will have no fear of new experiences, such as those related to going to kindergarten or to the physician's or dentist's office. The children in this age group are usually proud of their possessions and their clothes and are responsive to comments about their personal appearance. Comments about clothing can often be effectively used in establishing communication with a new patient.

Six years of age. At 6 years of age most children move away from the close ties of the family. It is still, however, a time of important transition that may cause considerable anxiety. Gesell and Ilg refer to the 6-year-old as a changed child. The tensional manifestations rise to a peak at this age, and they may include outbursts of screaming, violent temper tantrums, and striking at the parents. At this age there is often a marked increase in fear responses. Many children have a fear of dogs, the elements, or even other human beings. Some children at this age are afraid of injury to their bodies. Thus a slight scratch or the sight of blood may produce a response out of all proportion to the cause. With the proper indoctrination to the dental experience, however, the 6-year-old can be expected to respond in a satisfactory manner.

Introducing the child to dentistry

The indoctrination to dentistry consists primarily of teaching the child to meet a new situation and to follow the instructions of the dental personnel. The process is usually accomplished easily if the dentist allows the child to survey the dental office and the environment casually but at the same time attempts to impress the child with the necessity and the importance of the occasion. The dentist and office personnel should remember that the child, particularly the first-time patient, is totally unaware that a painful tooth or a periapical infection poses a health threat. Instead, the child may look on the dentist and staff as the real threat. If the dental personnel keep this fact in mind, it will help them understand the reaction of the normal child in the dental office.

The first objective in the successful management of young children is to establish communication and to make them believe that the dentist and the assistants are their friends and are interested in helping them. The dentist and staff can do this by making children aware of the importance of the dental appointment and the various procedures.

The learning process should be recognized as irregular, with ascents, plateaus, and perhaps even periods of regression. This irregular process is, of course, related to environmental changes and psychologic states. Irregularities in the learning process may be observed by parents in the home. Periods when children learn quickly or accomplish a great many tasks may be followed by a period when they actually accomplish little or perhaps even seem to regress. The same is true of their play habits, their table manners, their speech, and certainly their relationships with the dentist and the office staff.

A number of situations can influence the learning process. However, one that the dentist should be fully aware of is a state of prolonged physical illness. Long-term confinement in the home or in the hospital can definitely influence the learning pattern. The period of interrupted activity and socialization creates an abnormal pattern. A child confined to a children's hospital ward for a long period often has a more positive attitude and is perhaps more receptive owing to the active social environment there than a child who has been either at home or in a private room in a hospital for a long period of time.

Larson observed that the preschool experiences of physically handicapped children were below normal in nearly every area, even in areas where adequacy did not depend on physical ability. In no case did the difference favor the handicapped group. In spite of this fact, most children with a history of prolonged physical illness are fairly cooperative. However, they exhibit varying degrees of rejection depending on the anxiety state created at home or in the hospital by overprotective or anxious parents. A detailed discussion of dentistry for the handicapped is included in Chapter 23.

The dentist may occasionally note a negative reaction in the young patient. Benjamin calls this the "period of resistance" and refers to it as a normal period in the growing up or learning process of the child. The child may react against any procedure because of inability to communicate with the dentist or the office personnel. It is important that the dentist be aware that this is a normal part of the learning process and not a reaction the dentist or staff stimulated. With this in mind the dentist should work rapidly, gently, and yet firmly, perhaps not expecting complete cooperation.

Frankl and associates, in their categorizing of behavior, refer to the child's negative response. Frankl's rating scale of four categories is commonly used to record the behavior of children in the dental office. By the use of this scale, it is possible to maintain a record of a child's reaction to specific dental procedures.

Categories of behavior

Rating 1: Definitely negative. Refuses treatment, cries forcefully, is fearful, or portrays any other overt evidence of extreme negativism.

Rating 2: Negative. Is reluctant to accept treatment, is uncooperative, portrays some evidence of negative attitude but not pronounced, that is, sullen or withdrawn.

Rating 3: Positive. Accepts treatment; at times is cautious, is willing to comply with the dentist, at times with reservation but follows the dentist's directions cooperatively.

Rating 4: Definitely positive. Has good rapport with the dentist, interested in the dental procedures, laughs and enjoys the situation.

Reactions to the dental experience

There are at least four negative reactions to the dental experience: fear, anxiety, resistance, and timidity. The dentist who routinely treats young children, however, will quickly realize that the child does not always demonstrate one clear-cut reaction. Instead, there may be a combination of several reactions to the dental experience. This combination of reactions makes the problem more complex, particularly since the dentist must diagnose the reaction quickly and without the advantage of complete knowledge of the child's previous experience with members of the health profession.

Fear. Fear is one of the most frequently experienced childhood emotions. Its effect on the physical and mental well-being of the child can be extremely harmful. Morgan and associates refer to surveys indicating that fear of dentistry, which often results in avoidance of dental care, is present in 5% to 6% of the population. Prevalence of fear may be as high as 16% among school-age children. Research suggests that the acquisition and perpetuation of negative attitudes toward dentistry are a cyclic process that has its genesis in childhood. Numerous factors have been identified as contributing to the development of such attitudes in children. Shoben and Borland demonstrated many years ago that parents can and do convey their negative attitudes to their children.

Watson and Lowery also believe that fear, for the most part, is "home grown," just like love and temper outbursts. They further believe that by the age of 3 years the child's emotional life has been established and the parents' behavior has already determined whether the child will be a happy, wholesome, and good-natured person or a whining and complaining person, one whose every move in life is controlled by fear. The young child, however, seems to have certain native fears, such as those associated with insecurity or the threat of insecurity.

Gesell and Ilg state that babies will cry if they hear a door slam, if there is an abrupt movement, or if they experience a sudden loss of support.

Older children experience a second type of fear, an acquired fear developed through the imitation of those who are afraid. The individual they imitate may be afraid of thunderstorms, of a visit to the dentist, or of a wide variety of experiences. A third type of fear expressed by a child is the result of an unpleasant experience—with an animal, a playmate, or perhaps a previous dentist or physician.

We should not assume, therefore, that all children have a fear of the dental office. Those who do show this reaction may be imitating someone else or they may have acquired the fear as the result of an actual experience.

In the management of the fearful child in the dental office, the dentist should first attempt to determine the degree of fear and the factors that may be responsible for it. Some children come to the dentist ready to respond with tension and fear, primarily because of the way dentistry has been presented to them in the home or by other relatives, friends, or peers. In isolated cases the fear of a dentist may be the result of a traumatic dental or medical experience that may sensitize a child and, by association, cause generalized fear from an isolated incident.

Numerous approaches to the problem of removing fear have been recommended to the dental profession. They involve delaying the appointment, attempting to reason with the child, ridiculing or reprimanding, or allowing the child to observe another dental procedure. None of these approaches has been entirely successful in solving the problem. Most children who come to the dental office need some type of immediate treatment or preventive care; therefore it is impractical to delay treatment for fearful children in hope that they will eventually outgrow their fear of dentistry and become more cooperative. Since fear is controlled by the autonomic nervous system, it is impossible to reason with the truly frightened child. Ridicule or comparison with a normal child who went through the dental experience in an uneventful manner may only complicate the emotional life of a frightened child and will usually not lead to a satisfactory degree of cooperation. Most dentists have also found that it is highly impractical to allow fearful children to watch someone else receive dental treatment. Rarely are they less fearful or more cooperative when their turn comes to face the situation. Therefore the most logical approach seems to be a reconditioning of the fearful child.

If the child is truly fearful, the slow approach to the problem will pay great dividends. Half the battle will be won if the dentist engages the child in conversation and attempts to learn the cause of the fear. Often the child will express the fear of a certain procedure or will tell of hearing something frightening about the dental experience. In this case the dentist can overcome this apprehension through demonstration and explanation.

During the first appointment the dentist should perform simple procedures, carefully explaining each one as well as the use of all the instruments, gradually building up to normal routine procedures that are necessary for the health service. Although voice control is usually sufficient in overcoming the child's fears, it may occasionally be necessary to use some form of restraint, particularly in a dental emergency, to override the child's fears. The parents, however, should be informed and give their consent to having the child restrained for dental procedures. Forcing the fearful child to accept an oral examination or other dental procedure often proves to the child that the procedure is nothing to be feared. Children with fears acquired from peers or others must experience the dental procedure to learn that it is different from their expectations.

Anxiety. Anxiety or insecurity is probably closely related to the fearful state. Edelston believes that some children develop the necessary assurance slowly and remain insecure and anxious long after they should have outgrown such feelings. Anxious children are essentially fearful of new experiences, and the anxious child's reaction may be violently aggressive, such as a display of temper tantrums in the dental office. Benjamin believes that a child's temper tantrum is usually a "behind the scene" spite reaction and is always associated with an anxiety state or state of insecurity. If a child who has temper tantrums at home is

rewarded, the tantrums may become a habit. When this child behaves similarly in the dental office, the dentist must determine whether the reaction is one of acute fear or a tantrum. Of course, if the child is truly fearful, the dentist may be sympathetic and may work slowly. If the child is definitely demonstrating a temper tantrum, however, the dentist must demonstrate authority and mastery of the situation.

Several studies have indicated a direct relationship between maternal anxiety and levels of anxiety in the child dental patient. Klorman and associates have suggested that the relationship between maternal anxiety and the child's anxiety may be limited to the initial treatment appointment when the child still lacks direct personal experience with dental treatment. Their studies show that the mother's anxiety does not seem to correlate with the experienced pedodontic patient's uncooperativeness during treatment.

Resistance. Resistance is one manifestation of anxiety or insecurity in which the child actually rebels against the environment. The child may display temper tantrums or head beating or may develop vomiting habits to avoid conforming. Regression may be another manifestation. Such a child may continue to wet the bed or follow infantile play habits or may make no attempt to talk plainly. Withdrawal may be another manifestation of resistant anxiety, in which case the child refuses to participate in play and will not talk to strangers or even to acquaintances. The dentist has difficulty communicating with this type of patient; the child is easily hurt and cries on almost any occasion.

Although it is not the dentist's responsibility to treat these psychologic states, it will be helpful to recognize them and realize that the child's reaction in the dental office is prompted by previous experience, home training, and environment.

Wright and Alpern have studied variables influencing children's cooperative behavior at the first dental visit. They found that the chances for negative behavior increase if the child believes a dental problem exists. They reasoned that a child who is aware of a dental problem might approach the appointment with a higher level of apprehension than a child who is unaware of one. The apprehension may have been transmitted to the child by the mother, particularly if she first recognized the problem as one requiring dental treatment.

Timidity. Timidity is another reaction that is occasionally observed, particularly in the case of the first-time patient. This reaction may be related to the child's limited social experience. The child who is timid needs to go through a warming-up period. This is one instance when it may be helpful to allow the child to be accompanied to the treatment room by a well-adjusted child patient. The timid child needs to gain self-confidence and confidence in the dentist. On the other hand, timidity may reflect tension resulting from the parents expecting too much from the child or even overprotecting the child.

The first-time dental patient

It is recognized that thoughtful preparation of the child patient and the parents before the first visit will result in a better behavior pattern in the dental office. The preparation may begin at the time of the receptionist's telephone contact with the parent. The receptionist will explain that unless an emergency exists, the dentist will want to make an appointment at a time that will permit a complete examination and introduce the child to dentistry in an unhurried manner.

The dentist may prefer that the parents avoid any form of home preparation of the child for the first visit, believing that acquainting the child with dentistry and the dental office is best achieved by the dentist and the office staff. Some dentists prefer to send a form letter to the parents, outlining the office policy and indicating what is to be accomplished at the time of the first visit. Parents appreciate receiving pamphlets to use in explaining how the dentist plans to help their child enjoy good dental health. Wright and Alpern found that a preappointment letter was effective in lowering the mother's anxiety and helpful in preparing her children for their first dental visits. The letter described what the dentist planned to accomplish for each

child during the first visit. It assured the mother that the dentist's staff looked forward to serving her children and discussing with her the essential factors related to good dental health.

Machen and Johnson observed significantly less negative behavior in a group of 3- to 5-year-old children who were exposed to either "desensitization" or "model learning therapy" before undergoing restorative dental treatment than in children given more customary initial dental experiences. In desensitization therapy anxiety-producing stimuli were presented gradually. Least anxiety-producing stimuli (prophylaxis, contra-angle, and polishing paste) were presented first, whereas high-anxiety evokers (anesthetic and handpiece) were presented as the child was able to tolerate them.

The model learning therapy consisted of viewing an 11-minute videotape of a child exhibiting positive behavior during dental treatment. The use of a filmed peer model displaying positive coping behavior during a dental visit has been described by Melamed and associates as successful in reducing disruptive behavior in children who are experiencing their first dental treatment. This method of preparation for the dental procedure can be implemented easily in the office by a dental auxiliary.

Time of the appointment. The time of day at which the child, especially the young child, is seen, may influence behavior. Generally, early morning hours should be reserved for young children. Parents will almost always cooperate if the dentist explains that young children are better able to accept dental treatment early in the day before they are tired. The dentist, too, is more alert and is best able to handle the unpredictable reactions of the child early in the day. Further, the dentist is more likely to be on schedule. Waiting in the reception room often gives the child a chance to develop an uncooperative frame of mind or become frightened by an unusual sound or observation. There are, of course, exceptions to early morning appointments for children, such as the child who is known to be uncooperative or handicapped in some manner that makes it difficult to conform to the usual office routine. For this type of child the last appointment in the morning should be considered or some time when the office will be clear of children and other patients who might be influenced by a disturbance.

Length of the appointment. Appointments for the young child or the child who is apprehensive or fearful should be relatively short until the child becomes fully indoctrinated into the procedures and gains confidence.

Lenchner carried out a study in a private office to determine if the scheduling of longer-than-customary appointments placed an undue burden on young patients. A long appointment was considered 45 minutes or more. Lenchner's evaluation showed no significant difference in the child's behavior during long (as opposed to short) appointments. However, there did seem to be a trend toward deterioration of behavior during long appointments. Lenchner concluded that in the treatment of the child patient undue consideration need not be given to the length of any particular appointment; instead, length of appointments may be based on procedures involved in the dental treatment, the individual practitioner and staff, personal idiosyncrasies of the child patient, and external factors such as school excuses, weather, transportation, baby-sitters, fees, and availability of time. When the mothers were questioned, the majority preferred long appointments for themselves and for their children. Reasons included the physical and psychologic well-being of the child, convenience for parent and child, and concern about acquiring excuses from school for frequent dental visits.

Dental treatment during school hours. Excusing children for dental appointments does not seem to be a problem if a plan has been agreed on by the local dental society and the board of school commissioners. Moen reported the results of a questionnaire sent to school superintendents in 3529 cities of more than 2000 population. Approximately 92% of the superintendents indicated that they excused children for dental appointments, 4% did not excuse children, and another 4% excused them only in the case of an emergency or a toothache. A

series of conferences with the school superintendent, the superintendent's representatives, and members of the board of school commissioners resulted in the adoption of an excuse form (Fig. 2-1) and policy and procedures for dental appointments during school time in Indianapolis. The plan has worked successfully for more than 30 years, and teachers have been enthusiastic about the form because they know in advance the days that the child will be absent from school.

Greeting the child and gaining control and cooperation. When the dentist can expect a normal reaction from the first-time dental patient to the invitation to enter the office, the assistant should greet the child and the parent. The dentist should stay in the background rather than make a hasty appearance. The assistant should address the child by the name he or she is accustomed to, usually the first name or a nickname. If the appointment is for the first examination, the assistant may invite the child and the parents to come into the treatment room or a consultation room. Many dentists prefer to see the communicative child, even for the initial examination, without the presence of the parents. However, it is recommended that the dentist meet the child and the parents in a consultation room before the actual examination procedure because the parents can often provide information that will be meaningful during the examination.

The dentist should review the medical and dental history (previously filled out) with the parents and briefly reiterate what will be done during the examination. Unless the child has a significant medical problem or developmental disorder, this portion of the meeting should be very brief because the office staff would have already discussed these matters with the parents. Next the dentist should ask the mother or father if there is anything either one is particularly concerned about in regard to the child's mouth or teeth. (A parent may have identified a chief concern to other office personnel, so the dentist may already have a clue.) Since most parents will have made some previous observation or will have a question that seems important to them, they should be given time to talk and also to

DENTAL TREATMENT DURING SCHOOL HOURS

_____ had an appointment at this

office on the _____ of _____ at _____
                Day   Month   Hour

o'clock. His treatment plan calls for the following future appointments:

Day	Month	Hour
Day	Month	Hour
Day	Month	Hour
Day	Month	Hour

If there is any reason why this schedule should be changed, will you please get in touch with me?

_____
                                         D.D.S.

Telephone no. _____

(This form has been approved by the Indianapolis District Dental Society and the Indianapolis Board of School Commissioners.)

POLICY AND PROCEDURES FOR
DENTAL APPOINTMENTS DURING SCHOOL HOURS

1. In general, it is legitimate to excuse children from school to keep dental appointments for two reasons: (1) when properly conducted, the dental appointment is a matter of dental education as well as dental repair, and (2) the child who needs dental care can be excused from school under the illness clause just as if he had a cold or a fever.

2. Suggestions for scheduling of dental appointments.

   A. Appointments for high school students should be alternated so that they do not come at the same hour, whereas appointments for elementary school students should be scheduled so that they do not come on the same day.

   B. A special effort should be made to use Christmas vacation, spring vacation, and summer vacation for extensive treatment of a continuous nature.

   C. Appointments should be scheduled so that not all appointments are made during school hours.

   D. Appointments should be held to not more than one per week unless emergencies occur.

   E. The school would be helped if the dentist would schedule a number of appointments in accordance with a treatment plan. This would indicate to the school that a pattern of treatment is involved.

   F. Dentists should see that the time is not used exclusively for repair or treatment. This is an ideal time to discuss dental health.

Fig. 2-1

present a brief history of any previous dental care. The dentist may be able to offer information related to the parent's question or concern, but it is also appropriate to suggest that further discussion be postponed until after the examination of the child. The dentist should, however, mentally note the parental concern, keep it in mind during the examination, and comment about it when the findings are summarized after the examination.

At the conclusion of this usually brief conversation, the dentist speaks directly to the child in a pleasant and clear manner. The dentist should say something like, ''Lisa, we are going to look at your teeth now in my other room where I have a brighter light that helps me see better. After we are finished, we will call your parents in so we can all talk together again about your mouth and your teeth.'' At this point the dentist stands and without delay or hesitation, but in a pleasant and calm manner, takes the child by the hand and leads him or her to the treatment room while reassuring the parents that they will be invited there in a few minutes. (Reassuring the parents is really more reassurance for the child because the parents, and possibly the child, have already been informed that the dentist would probably examine the child without the presence of the parents.) A dental assistant should be available to politely direct the parents back to the reception room. If the child is cooperative but reluctant or fearful, continued reassurance and positive reinforcement will help during the walk to the treatment room; maintaining a conversation centered on the child is appropriate. If the child vigorously resists or becomes defiant, the dentist must remain calm and pleasant but take firm and immediate control of the situation, reassuring the parents as the child is taken to the treatment room.

If the dentist prefers to have the parents with the child during the initial examination, both the brief conversation with them just described and the examination can take place in the treatment room. In this case the dental assistant greets the child and parents and escorts them directly to the treatment room to meet the dentist. There should be enough chairs or stools surrounding the dental chair to allow the dentist and the parents to be seated while they talk. Usually the child sits on a parent's lap. After the initial review and discussion the child may be transferred to the dental chair by a parent, with assistance by the dentist if needed. If the child is uncooperative, the dentist can explain that the parents may remain in the room only if the child is a ''good helper'' during the examination. The receptionist should have previously told the parents that they might be asked to leave the treatment room.

We do not advise separating the very young child (2 years or younger and sometimes older) from the parents, at least during the first appointment. In this situation the parents and the child should be escorted into the room where the dentist will conduct the initial examination. If the appointment is for a nonemergency first examination of an infant or toddler, the dentist may find it more desirable to meet in a private office or consultation room, provided there is adequate light. If it is known that the parents have a specific concern about the child's mouth, if the child is 14 months or older, or if the appointment is an emergency visit, it is advisable to conduct the first visit consultation and examination in the treatment room at the dental chair. If the child is 2 years of age or younger, a parent should sit in the dental chair holding the child (see ''Early examination'' in Chapter 1).

During subsequent treatment appointments the parents should remain in the reception room. Exceptions to this policy may be appropriate in the case of the handicapped or severely ill child and possibly (but not routinely) the very young child. When parents do accompany the child to the operatory for treatment, they should understand that it is important for the dentist to be in control of the situation. Therefore the parents should remain passive, offering support to the child only by their presence, unless requested by the dentist to take a more active role. The dentist's attention should be directed toward the child and the child's toward the dentist. It is most important for the parents to understand that their presence and behavior should not distract either the dentist or the child.

Generally, for subsequent treatment appointments the assistant greets the child pleasantly (at eye level) in the reception room by saying something like, "Scotty, Dr. Doe is ready to see you now. He will explain what we need to do today. When we are finished, we will call Mother in to talk and to show her what we did." By making such a statement, the assistant once again notifies the parents and the child that the child is the center of attention now and that the adults should remain in the reception room until later. At the same time the assistant extends a hand and begins leading the child toward the treatment area. If the child is mildly reluctant, the assistant may need to gently but firmly grasp the child's shoulders to offer more positive encouragement while guiding the child toward the treatment area and, at the same time, providing positive reinforcement through conversation.

If the child refuses to accompany the assistant into the operatory, the dentist may appear on the scene and, using a firm but pleasant approach, take the child into the room. The dentist has been in the background and perhaps has been able to diagnose the behavior problem and can manage it accordingly. Perhaps the dentist has been able to learn whether the child is really frightened or is unwilling or unable to cooperate. It can often be determined whether this is a child who lacks discipline at home and has not previously had to cooperate.

Rand and associates suggest some rules for obtaining obedience that are often helpful in managing children in the dental office. The first rule is to gain the child's attention. For example, the screaming or crying child must first hear the dentist's commands. A second rule is to phrase the command in a language the child can understand. Since a 4-year-old child will not know the meaning of "saliva ejector" or the names of most other instruments, the dentist must talk in a language that the child can interpret and understand. Berson, Brostoff, and Martinoff have identified over 200 names and phrases used in dental practices to facilitate communication about dental procedures for child patients.

It is important to pronounce words slowly and clearly. The child is then better able to follow the commands. It is also important to give only a few commands at one time. At the age of 5 years, a child can carry out three simple commands at one time but only with concentrated attention. The dentist and other personnel should be reasonable in their requests. They cannot expect cooperation if the child is uncomfortable or in pain.

The use of threats or bribes is a poor means of gaining obedience. A statement such as, "When you leave, I will give you a book or a present or a toy" is preferable to, "If you are good, I will give you a book or toy when you leave." Then the child will not interpret the gift as a bribe.

If the child is truly frightened, an attempt to overcome the fear by the use of the approach previously presented should be made. However, many of the reactions of children are not clear cut, and the child who merely does not want to cooperate may also be somewhat fearful or apprehensive. Apprehension can be alleviated by taking time to explain the dental instruments in words that the child can understand. Only a few instruments should be visible at one time. In fact, when examining first-time patients, we merely ask the children to open their mouths and, with our fingers, we retract the lips and make the initial inspection of the teeth. After that, a mouth mirror or perhaps an explorer can be introduced. The need and use of each instrument, however, should be explained and demonstrated. This tell-show-do approach is very effective in introducing most communicative children to initial dental procedures.

If a child does not want to cooperate for the oral examination or a simple procedure such as the dental prophylaxis, a degree of restraint to gain control of the situation and also to make the child realize that the procedure is not associated with pain or discomfort is justified. Perhaps a consultation with the parents at this time is desirable to inform them that the child is unwilling to cooperate, to impress them with the need for the examination or treatment, and to gain their permission to proceed in a kind yet firm manner.

When all the psychologic approaches to managing the child and gaining cooperation have failed, the dentist may choose to use a restraint measure that involves placing the hand over the child's mouth to extinguish an unacceptable response to the dental treatment. This technique has been referred to by several names, such as "aversion," reported by Kramer; "restraint discipline," mentioned by Wright and Feasby; "HOME: hand-over-mouth exercise," described by Levitas; and more recently, "flooding," proposed by Davis and Rombom. Craig has reported on the controversy related to this technique; however, it is generally agreed that it can be a successful means of controlling the child's crying.

Levitas describes the technique as placing the hand over the child's mouth to muffle the noise. The dentist's face is positioned close to the child so the dentist can talk directly into the child's ear. The dentist makes such comments as, "If you want me to take my hand away, you must stop screaming and listen to me. I only want to talk to you and look at your teeth." After a few seconds, the procedure is repeated, and then the dentist adds, "Are you ready for me to remove my hand?" Almost invariably there is a nodding of the head. With a final word of caution to be quiet, the hand is removed, and the dentist proceeds with the treatment.

Davis and Rombom sent questionnaires to administrators of all postdoctoral pedodontic training programs in the United States to survey the teaching of certain behavior management techniques. The responses confirmed widespread acceptance of both restraint and hand-over-mouth (HOM) techniques. HOM was identified as a "flooding" technique that prevents the "avoidance response" of the child. Since it has been suggested that HOM may create dental phobia, the authors point out that the technique should not be used in a punitive or vicious manner or without appropriate verbalization. They suggest that the chances are greater for creating a dental phobia if the child is allowed to consistently avoid the dental experience.

In a later publication, Rombom points out that most children treated in the dental office are cooperative and relaxed. However, occasionally the dentist will encounter a child patient who has the ability to cooperate but refuses to do so. The behavior of such children may be disruptive and defiant and include temper tantrums, kicking, screaming, and flailing about. It is for these few children that extraordinary behavior management techniques such as HOM may be indicated.

Indoctrination to dentistry. If the parents accompanied the child to the treatment room at the time of the first appointment for the purpose of providing information to the dentist, it is advisable to describe briefly the conditions noted in the child's mouth. The dentist should emphasize, however, that the presentation of the dental findings and the treatment plan will be made at a subsequent visit after the necessary records have been completed. The dentist may then prefer to excuse the parents while proceeding with the initial part of the examination and treatment routine.

Some dentists make the mistake of trying to do too much for the first-time patient. If a child does not have a toothache, the first appointment should be limited to simple procedures. A toothache, of course, will have to be treated, but that is one of the few exceptions. Performing an initial dental prophylaxis and inspection allows the child to gain confidence both in accepting dental procedures and in the dentist. These procedures also give the dentist an opportunity to begin planning an orderly sequence of treatment for the child on subsequent visits. If the examination and prophylaxis go smoothly, as they will in most cases, the dentist may want to take dental radiographs at the first visit. The type of survey selected will, of course, depend on the age of the child and the condition of the dentition.

After all initial procedures are completed, the dentist should invite the parents back into the operatory and briefly discuss the findings. The dentist should discuss any significant problem areas specifically, make a general statement about the severity of the case, and suggest the time that will be necessary to restore the mouth to a healthy condition. Then the dentist may inform the parents that before the child's next visit the radiographs will be carefully restudied and a comprehensive dental health care plan will be developed for recommendation to them when they return for the next appointment. The dentist again thanks the child for being "a good helper" as the parents and child leave the treatment room.

If the dentist follows a procedure similar to that which has been outlined, a number of objectives will be accomplished. First, the child has been introduced to dentistry. There has been an opportunity to observe the child's reaction in the dental office, which is important in determining the time that will be required to complete the treatment and in establishing a fee for the service. Radiographs have been taken, if needed, that will enable the dentist to complete a treatment plan before the next visit. Most important of all, a true health service has been performed for which the dentist should request a fee comparable to any other service requiring a similar amount of time.

The following statements summarize the areas considered in child behavior guidance:

1. Successful management of the child depends on kindness, firmness, a sense of humor, and the dentist's ability to overlook initial demonstrations of uncooperativeness.
2. The dentist should approach the situation in a positive, friendly manner but should convey the idea that the work is essential to the well-being of the child.
3. Some psychologists have stated that the members of the health team should avoid a conflict or a fight with the child. If the child resists dental treatment, however, the "fight" is on, and the dentist must win. In other words, something must be accomplished at the time of the dental appointment.
4. If the child demonstrates a bad habit, it should be rejected or overcome at the start.
5. The dentist should encourage all good habits with praise and should look for the appropriate time to compliment the child.
6. An attempt should be made to transfer the confidence, security, and enthusiasm of the dentist and other office staff to the child patient. Constant conversation from the dentist or assistant will aid in the realization of this endeavor.
7. If the child does not want to concede that there is important work to be done, the dentist should maintain a positive approach, first using voice control. If this is unsuccessful, some form of restraint should be used to let the child know there will be a consistent endeavor to provide a health service. A child who is lacking in discipline at home many times will respect the dentist who supplies it.

In 1980 the American Association of Pedodontic Diplomates surveyed more than 1000 members of the American Academy of Pedodontics to determine attitudes in practices of child and behavior management. The responses to the questionnaire provide additional information that will be helpful to the dentist in the management of children. Behavior can be managed by personal interaction alone, according to 93% of the respondents, although 56% indicated that behavior management is one of the most trying aspects of pedodontics. Parents are always allowed in the operatory by 7% of the pedodontists, while 87% allow it only in selected cases, usually with children under 3 years of age or with handicapped or ill children.

Ninety-one percent use the hand-over-mouth airway open technique in selected cases, usually with children above the age of 2, and generally to gain the child's attention or cooperation. The hand-over-mouth airway closed technique is used selectively by 54%, generally for children 3 years and older and usually to control temper tantrums, hysteria, aggression, and resistance. In the opinion of 48% of the respondents, restricting the airway is not potentially harmful psychologically. Eighty-seven percent of the pedodontists occasionally use physical restraint other than hand over mouth—for example, a Papoose Board* or a Pedi-Wrap.†

---

* Olympic Medical Corp., Seattle, Wash. 98108.
† Clark Associates, Charlton City, Mass. 01508.

In selected cases, nitrous oxide analgesia is used by 73%, premedication by 85%, and general anesthesia by 77%. The average respondent uses general anesthesia for 6 to 20 patients a year.

Hypnodontics

Hennon points out that most dentists use soothing words to allay patients' fears and apprehensions about dental procedures. As previously mentioned, the use of properly selected words with a positive, confident approach will often produce the desired patient response. In some instances, however, the clinician may desire another method to enhance patients' responses. Hypnosis offers this possibility. The use of hypnosis in dentistry is sometimes referred to as "hypnodontics."

Hennon also comments that hypnodontics can become an extension of an already established chairside manner. The technique has no significant disadvantages if the practitioner regards it as an alternative to behavior management and not as the ultimate solution to all management problems. Hennon states that inducing a hypnotic trance is simple, but learning to use the trance state properly is difficult until sufficient clinical training is attained. For this reason, those who use hypnosis agree that a practitioner should obtain training from a recognized professional group such as the American Society of Clinical Hypnosis, the Society for Clinical and Experimental Hypnosis, or one of their affiliates.

Generally, hypnodontics may be applicable for child patients with whom communication is possible. Communicative children and teenagers are good hypnotic subjects because they are familiar with pretend games and readily influenced by suggestions from adults. Hennon offers the following list of uses of hypnosis in pedodontics:

1. To reduce or eliminate nervousness and apprehension
2. To eliminate defense mechanisms patients use to postpone actual dental work
3. To control functional or psychosomatic gagging
4. To prevent thumbsucking
5. To prevent bruxism
6. To facilitate obtaining impressions and occlusal records
7. To control hemorrhage and salivation
8. To provide acclimation to surgery and postoperative adjustment and to introduce intraoral appliances
9. To reinforce home care and oral hygiene procedures
10. To induce anesthesia
11. To effect distortion
12. To promote postoperative healing
13. To reduce operator fatigue
14. To induce posthypnotic suggestions
    a. Reinduction
    b. Removal of discomfort
    c. Time limit to anesthesia
    d. Pleasant memories
    e. Reminder for recall or return appointment

Neiburger conducted a study in which 150 children 3 to 12 years of age were evaluated during 302 prophylaxis appointments in a private dental office to determine the effects of suggestion on their reactions to and behavior during a dental prophylaxis. The dentist made comments to the patients, such as, "When I brush your teeth it will tickle and make you laugh even more. You don't have to laugh too much, but many children do." It was found that such suggestions generally influence children toward a more positive reaction and better behavior during the prophylaxis than when no suggestions are made. The children in the 5-, 6-, 7-, 11-, and 12-year age groups were most readily influenced by the suggestions. Neiburger believes that this study demonstrates the significance and benefits of light hypnosis in actual treatment.

Few if any dentists who treat children would deny the value of carefully chosen suggestive phrases to positively influence the dental behavior of children.

REFERENCES

Association of Pedodontic Diplomates: Survey of attitudes and practices in behavior management, Pediatr. Dent. **3**:246-250, 1981.

Bailey, P.M., Talbot, A., and Taylor, P.P.: A comparison of maternal anxiety levels with anxiety levels manifested in the child dental patient, J. Dent. Child. **40**:277-284, 1973.

Benjamin, E.: The period of resistance in early childhood, J. Pediatr. **18**:659-669, 1941.

Berson, R.B., Brostoff, D., and Martinoff, J.T.: A survey of dental office terminology in pediatric dental practice, Pediatr. Dent. **2**:110-116, 1980.

Braham, R.L.: Control of behavior and anxiety in the child patient. In McDonald, R.E., and others, editors: Current therapy in dentistry, vol. 7, St. Louis, 1980, The C.V. Mosby Co.

Chambers, D.W.: Behavior management techniques for pediatric dentists: an embarrassment of riches, J. Dent. Child. **44**:30-34, 1977.

Christopher, A., and Hawthorne, E.: Management of the preschool dental patient, J. Dent. Child. **48**:42-45, 1981.

Craig, W.: Hand over mouth technique, J. Dent. Child. **38**:387-389, 1971.

Davis, M.J., and Rombom, H.M.: Survey of the utilization of and rationale for hand-over-mouth (HOM) and restraint in postdoctoral pedodontic education, Pediatr. Dent. **1**:87-90, 1979.

Edelston, H.: The anxious child, Br. Dent. J. **108**:345-349, 1960.

Frankl, S.N., Shiere, F.W., and Fogels, H.R.: Should the parent remain with the child in the dental operatory? J. Dent. Child. **29**:150-163, 1962.

Gesell, A., and Ilg, F.L.: The child from five to ten, New York, 1946, Harper & Row, Publishers.

Gesell, A., and Ilg, F.L.: Child development: an introduction to the study of human growth, New York, 1949, Harper & Row, Publishers.

Hennon, D.K.: Hypnosis in pedodontics. In Wright, G.Z., editor: Solving behavior management problems in dentistry for children, St. Louis, 1983, The C.V. Mosby Co.

Hymes, J.L.: Early childhood, Children **7**:111, 1960.

Johnson, R., and Baldwin, D.C.: Maternal anxiety and child behavior, J. Dent. Child. **36**:87-92, 1969.

Johnson, R., and Machen, J.B.: Behavior modification techniques and maternal anxiety, J. Dent. Child. **40**:272-276, 1973.

Klorman, R., and others: Predicting the child's uncooperativeness in dental treatment from maternal trait, state, and dental anxiety, J. Dent. Child. **45**:62-67, 1978.

Kramer, W.C.: Aversion: a method for modifying child behavior, American Academy of Pedodontics, Annual Meeting, Los Angeles, 1973.

Larson, L.: Preschool experiences of physically handicapped children, Except. Child. **24**:310-312, 1958.

Lenchner, V.: Effect of appointment length on behavior of the pedodontic patient and his attitude toward dentistry, J. Dent. Child. **33**:61-73, 1966.

Levitas, T.C.: HOME: hand over mouth exercise, J. Dent. Child. **41**:178-182, 1974.

Machen, J.B., and Johnson, R.: Desensitization, model learning, and the dental behavior of children, J. Dent. Res. **53**:83-87, 1974.

Melamed, B.G., and others: Use of filmed modeling to reduce uncooperative behavior of children during dental treatment, J. Dent. Res. **54**:797-801, 1975.

Moen, B.D.: Bureau of economic research and statistics: survey of public school dental programs, J.A.D.A. **51**:594-599, 1955.

Morgan, P.H., Jr., and others: Children's perceptions of the dental experience, J. Dent. Child. **47**:243-245, 1980.

Neiburger, E.J.: Child response to suggestion, J. Dent. Child. **45**:395-402, 1978.

Olsen, N.H.: Behavior control of the child patient, J.A.D.A. **68**:873-877, 1964.

Pinkham, J.R.: Observation and interpretation of the child dental patient's behavior, Pediatr. Dent. **1**:21-26, 1979.

Rand, W., Sweeney, M.E., and Vincent, E.L.: Growth and development of the young child, ed. 4, Philadelphia, 1946, W.B. Saunders Co.

Ripa, L.W., and Barenie, J.T.: Management of dental behavior in children, Littleton, Mass., 1979, PSG Publishing Co.

Rombom, H.M.: Behavioral techniques in pedodontics: the hand-over-mouth technique, J. Dent. Child. **48**:208-210, 1981.

Shoben, E.J., and Borland, L.R.: Empirical study of the etiology of dental fears, J. Clin. Psychol. **10**:171, 1954.

Watson, E.H., and Lowery, G.H.: Growth and development of children, ed. 2, Chicago, 1954, Year Book Medical Publishers, Inc.

Weinstein, P., and others: The effect of dentists' behaviors on fear-related behaviors in children, J.A.D.A. **104**:32-38, 1982.

Weinstein, P., and others: Dentists' responses to fear- and nonfear-related behaviors in children, J.A.D.A. **104**:38-40, 1982.

Wright, G.Z.: Behavior management in dentistry for children, Philadelphia, 1975, W.B. Saunders Co.

Wright, G.Z., and Alpern, G.D.: Variables influencing children's cooperative behavior at the first dental visit, J. Dent. Child. **38**:124-128, 1971.

Wright, G.Z., and Feasby, W.H.: Control of anxiety, videotape, London, Ont., 1972, University of Western Ontario.

Wright, G.Z., Alpern, G.D., and Leake, J.L.: The modifiability of maternal anxiety as it relates to children's cooperative dental behavior, J. Dent. Child. **40**:265-271, 1973.

Yarrow, L.J.: The infancy period, Children **8**:110-111, 1960.

SUGGESTED ADDITIONAL READINGS

Dobson, J.: The strong-willed child, Wheaton, Ill., 1978, Tyndale House Publishers.

Erikson, E.H.: Childhood and society, ed. 2, New York, 1963, W.W. Norton & Co., Inc.

3 Development and morphology of the primary teeth

RALPH E. McDONALD
DAVID R. AVERY

The purpose of this chapter is to present a brief review of the development of the teeth. An accurate chronology of primary tooth calcification is of clinical significance to the dentist. There is often a need to explain to parents the time sequence of calcification in utero and during infancy. The common observation of tetracycline pigmentation, developmental enamel defects, and generalized hereditary anomalies can be explained if there is a knowledge of the calcification schedule. A brief consideration of the morphology of the primary teeth is also appropriate before a consideration of restorative procedures for children.

A much more complete review is available in the reference texts on oral histology, dental anatomy, and developmental anatomy listed at the end of the chapter.

Life cycle of the tooth

Initiation (bud stage). Evidence of development of the human tooth can be observed as early as the sixth week of embryonic life. Cells in the basal layer of the oral epithelium undergo proliferation at a more rapid rate than do the adjacent cells. The result is an epithelial thickening in the region of the future dental arch that extends along the entire free margin of the jaws. This event is referred to as the "primordium of the ectodermal portion of the teeth" and what results is called the "dental lamina." At the same time, 10 round or ovoid swellings occur in each jaw in the position to be occupied by the primary teeth.

Certain cells of the basal layer begin to proliferate at a more rapid rate than do the adjacent cells (Fig. 3-1, *A*). These proliferating cells contain the entire growth potential of the teeth. The permanent molars, like the primary teeth, rise from the dental lamina. The permanent incisors, canines, and premolars develop from the buds of their primary predecessors. The congenital absence of a tooth is the result of a lack of initiation or an arrest in the proliferation of cells. The presence of supernumerary teeth is a result of a continued budding of the enamel organ.

Proliferation (cap stage). Proliferation of the cells continues during the cap stage. As a result of unequal growth in the different parts of the bud, a cap is formed (Fig. 3-1, *B*). A shallow invagination appears on the deep surface of the bud. The peripheral cells of the cap later form the outer and inner enamel epithelium.

As with a deficiency in initiation, a deficiency in proliferation will result in failure of the tooth germ to develop and in less than the normal number of teeth. Excessive proliferation of cells may result in epithelial rests. These rests may remain inactive or become activated as a result of an irritation or stimulus. If the cells become partially differentiated or detached from the enamel organ in their partially differentiated state, they assume the secretory functions common to all epithelial cells and a cyst develops. If the cells become more fully differentiated or detached from the enamel organ, they produce enamel and dentin, resulting in an odon-

41

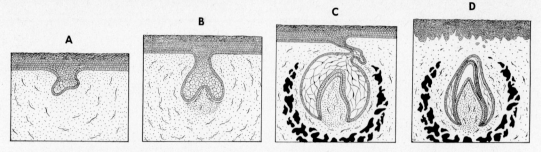

Fig. 3-1. Life cycle of the tooth. **A,** Initiation (bud stage). **B,** Proliferation (cap stage). **C,** Histodifferentiation and morphodifferentiation (bell stage). **D,** Apposition and calcification. (Modified from Schour, I., and Massler, M.: J.A.D.A. **27:**1785, 1940.)

toma (see Fig. 4-5) or a supernumerary tooth. The degree of differentiation of the cells determines whether a cyst, an odontoma, or a supernumerary tooth develops (see Figs. 21-1 and 21-3).

Histodifferentiation and morphodifferentiation (bell stage). The epithelium continues to invaginate and deepen until the enamel organ takes on the shape of a bell (Fig. 3-1, *C*). It is during this stage that there is a differentiation of the cells of the dental papilla into odontoblasts and of the cells of the inner enamel epithelium into ameloblasts.

Histodifferentiation marks the end of the proliferative stage as the cells lose their capacity to multiply. This stage is the forerunner of appositional activity. Disturbances in the differentiation of the formative cells of the tooth germ result in abnormal structure of the dentin or enamel. One clinical example of ameloblasts failing to differentiate properly is amelogenesis imperfecta (see Fig. 4-35). The failure of the odontoblasts to differentiate properly, with the resultant abnormal dentin structure, will result in the clinical entity dentinogenesis imperfecta (see Fig. 4-32).

In the morphodifferentiation stage the formative cells are arranged to outline the form and size of the tooth. This process occurs before matrix deposition. The morphologic pattern of the tooth becomes established when the inner enamel epithelium is arranged so that the boundary between it and the odontoblasts outlines the future dentinoenamel junction. Disturbances and aberrations in morphodifferentiation will result in abnormal forms

and sizes of teeth. Some of the resulting conditions are peg teeth, other types of microdontia, and macrodontia.

Apposition

Appositional growth is the result of a layerlike deposition of a nonvital extracellular secretion in the form of a tissue matrix. This matrix is deposited by the formative cells, ameloblasts and odontoblasts, which line up along the future dentinoenamel and dentinocemental junction at the stage of morphodifferentiation. These cells deposit the enamel and dentin matrix according to a definite pattern and at a definite rate. The formative cells begin their work at specific sites referred to as ''growth centers'' as soon as the blueprint, the dentinoenamel junction, is completed (Fig. 3-1, *D*).

Any systemic disturbance or local trauma that injures the ameloblasts during enamel formation can cause an interruption or an arrest in matrix apposition, resulting in enamel hypoplasia (see Fig. 4-27). Hypoplasia of the dentin is less common than enamel hypoplasia and occurs only after severe systemic disturbances.

Calcification

Calcification (mineralization) takes place following matrix deposition and involves the precipitation of inorganic calcium salts within the deposited matrix. The process begins with the precipitation of a small nidus about which further precipitation occurs. The original nidus increases in size by the addition of concentric laminations. There is an eventual approximation and fusion of these individual calcospherites into a homogeneously mineralized layer of tissue matrix. If the calcification process is disturbed, there is a lack of fusion of the calcospherites. These deficiencies are not readily identified in the enamel, but in the dentin they are evident microscopically and are referred to as interglobular dentin.

Early development and calcification of the anterior primary teeth

Kraus and Jordan have found that the first macroscopic indication of morphologic development occurs at approximately 11 weeks in utero. The maxillary and mandibular central incisor crowns appear identical at this early stage as tiny, hemispheric, moundlike structures.

The lateral incisors begin to develop morphologic characteristics between 13 and 14 weeks. There is evidence of the developing canines between 14 and 16 weeks. Calcification of the central incisor begins at approximately 14 weeks in utero, the upper central incisor slightly preceding the lower central. The initial calcification of the lateral incisor occurs at 16 weeks and the canine at 17 weeks.

It is interesting to note that the developmental dates listed precede by 3 to 4 weeks the dates that appear in the chronology of the human dentition, as developed by Logan and Kronfeld. This observation has been confirmed by Lunt and Law.

Early development and calcification of the posterior primary teeth and the first permanent molar

The maxillary first primary molar appears macroscopically at 12½ weeks in utero. Kraus and Jordan have observed that as early as 15½ weeks the apex of the mesiobuccal cusp may undergo calcification. At approximately 34 weeks the entire occlusal surface is covered by calcified tissue. At birth, calcification includes roughly three fourths of the occlusal gingival height of the crown.

The maxillary second primary molar also appears macroscopically at about 12½ weeks in utero. There is evidence of calcification of the mesiobuccal cusp as early as 19 weeks. At birth, calcification extends occlusogingivally to include approximately one fourth of the height of the crown.

The mandibular first primary molar first becomes evident macroscopically at about 12 weeks in utero. Calcification may be observed as early as 15½ weeks at the apex of the mesiobuccal cusp. At birth a completely calcified cap covers the occlusal surface.

The mandibular second primary molar also becomes evident macroscopically at 12½ weeks in utero. According to Kraus and Jordan, calcification may begin at 18 weeks. At the time of birth the five centers have coalesced and only a small area of uncalcified tissue remains in the middle of the occlusal surface. There are sharp conical cusps, angular ridges, and a smooth occlusal surface, all of which indicate that calcification of these areas is incomplete at birth. Thus there is a calcification sequence of central incisor, first molar, lateral incisor, canine, and second molar.

The work of Kraus and Jordan would indicate that the adjacent second primary and the first permanent molars undergo identical patterns of morphodifferentiation but at different times and that the initial development of the first permanent molar occurs slightly later. The excellent research of these two workers has also shown that the first permanent molars are uncalcified before 28 weeks of age; at any time thereafter calcification may begin. Some degree of calcification is always present at birth.

Morphology of individual primary teeth

Maxillary central incisor. The mesiodistal diameter of the crown of the maxillary central incisor is greater than the cervicoincisal length. Developmental lines are usually not evident in the crown; thus the labial surface is smooth. The incisal edge is nearly straight even before abrasion becomes evident. There are well-developed marginal ridges on the lingual surface and a distinctly developed cingulum (Figs. 3-2 and 3-3). The root of the incisor is cone shaped with tapered sides.

Maxillary lateral incisor. The outline of the maxillary lateral incisor is similar to that of the central, but the crown is smaller in all dimensions. The length of the crown from the cervical to the incisal edge is greater than the mesiodistal width. The root outline is similar to that of the central incisor but is longer in proportion to the crown.

Maxillary canine. The crown of the maxillary canine is more constricted at the cervical region than are the incisors, and the incisal and distal surfaces are more convex. There is a well-developed sharp cusp rather than a relatively straight incisal edge. The canine has a long, slender, tapering root that is more than twice the length of the crown. The root is usually inclined distally, apical to the middle third.

Mandibular central incisor. The mandibular central incisor is smaller than the maxillary central, but its labiolingual measurement is usually only 1 mm less. The labial aspect presents a flat surface

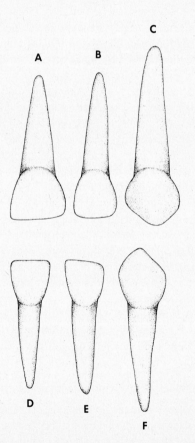

Fig. 3-2. Primary left anterior teeth, labial aspect. **A,** Maxillary central incisor. **B,** Maxillary lateral incisor. **C,** Maxillary canine. **D,** Mandibular central incisor. **E,** Mandibular lateral incisor. **F,** Mandibular canine. (From Wheeler, R.C.: Dental anatomy, physiology and occlusion, ed. 5, Philadelphia, 1974, W.B. Saunders Co.)

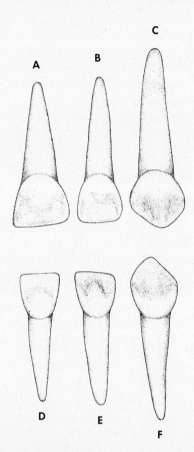

Fig. 3-3. Primary right anterior teeth, lingual aspect. **A,** Maxillary central incisor. **B,** Maxillary lateral incisor. **C,** Maxillary canine. **D,** Mandibular central incisor. **E,** Mandibular lateral incisor. **F,** Mandibular canine. (From Wheeler, R.C.: Dental anatomy, physiology and occlusion, ed. 5, Philadelphia, 1974, W.B. Saunders Co.)

without developmental grooves. The lingual surface presents marginal ridges and a cingulum. The middle third and the incisal third on the lingual surface may have a flattened surface level with the marginal ridges, or there may be a slight concavity. The incisal edge is straight, and it bisects the crown labiolingually. The root is approximately twice the length of the crown.

Mandibular lateral incisor. The outline of the mandibular lateral incisor is similar to that of the central incisor but is somewhat larger in all dimensions except labiolingually. The lingual surface may have greater concavity between the marginal ridges. The incisal edge slopes toward the distal aspect of the tooth.

Mandibular canine. The form of the mandibular canine is similar to the maxillary canine, with a few exceptions. The crown is slightly shorter, and the root may be as much as 2 mm shorter than the maxillary tooth. The mandibular canine is not as large labiolingually as its maxillary opponent.

Maxillary first molar. The greatest dimension

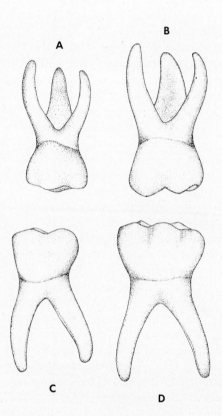

Fig. 3-4. Primary left molars, buccal aspect. **A,** Maxillary first molar. **B,** Maxillary second molar. **C,** Mandibular first molar. **D,** Mandibular second molar. (From Wheeler, R.C.: Dental anatomy, physiology and occlusion, ed. 5, Philadelphia, 1974, W.B. Saunders Co.)

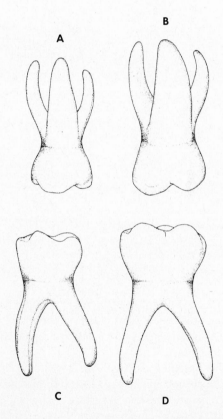

Fig. 3-5. Primary right molars, lingual aspect. **A,** Maxillary first molar. **B,** Maxillary second molar. **C,** Mandibular first molar. **D,** Mandibular second molar. (From Wheeler, R.C.: Dental anatomy, physiology and occlusion, ed. 5, Philadelphia, 1974, W.B. Saunders Co.)

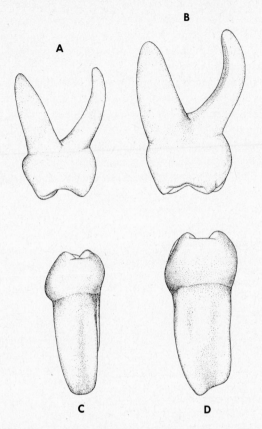

Fig. 3-6. Primary right molars, mesial aspect. **A,** Maxillary first molar. **B,** Maxillary second molar. **C,** Mandibular first molar. **D,** Mandibular second molar. (From Wheeler, R.C.: Dental anatomy, physiology and occlusion, ed. 5, Philadelphia, 1974, W.B. Saunders Co.)

of the crown of the maxillary first molar is at the mesiodistal contact areas, and from these areas the crown converges toward the cervical region (Figs. 3-4 to 3-6).

The mesiolingual cusp is the largest and sharpest. The distolingual cusp is poorly defined, small, and rounded. The buccal surface is smooth, with little evidence of developmental grooves. The three roots are long, slender, and widely spread.

Maxillary second molar. There is considerable resemblance between the maxillary primary second molar and the maxillary first permanent molar. There are two well-defined buccal cusps, with a developmental groove between them. The crown of the second molar is considerably larger than that of the first molar.

The bifurcation between the buccal roots is close to the cervical region. The roots are longer and heavier than those of the first primary molar, the lingual root being large and thick compared with the other roots (Figs. 3-4 and 3-5).

The lingual surface has three cusps: a mesiolingual cusp that is large and well developed, a distolingual cusp, and a third and smaller supplemental cusp (cusp of Carabelli). A well-defined groove separates the mesiolingual cusp from the distolingual cusp. On the occlusal surface a prominent oblique ridge connects the mesiolingual cusp with the distobuccal cusp (Fig. 3-7).

Mandibular first molar. Unlike the other primary teeth, the first primary molar does not resemble any of the permanent teeth. The mesial outline of the tooth, when viewed from the buccal aspect, is almost straight from the contact area to the cervical region. The distal area of the tooth is shorter than the mesial area.

The two distinct buccal cusps have no evidence of a distinct developmental groove between them; the mesial cusp is the larger of the two.

There is a marked lingual convergence of the crown on the mesial aspect, with a rhomboid outline present on the distal aspect. The mesiolingual cusp is long and sharp at the tip; a developmental groove separates this cusp from the distolingual cusp, which is rounded and well developed. The mesial marginal ridge is well developed, to the extent that it appears as another small cusp lingually. When the tooth is viewed from the mesial aspect, there is an extreme curvature buccally at the cervical third. The crown length is greater in the mesiobuccal area than in the mesiolingual; thus the cervical line slants upward from the buccal to the lingual surface.

The longer slender roots spread considerably at the apical third, extending beyond the outline of the crown. The mesial root, when viewed from the mesial aspect, does not resemble any other primary root. The buccal and lingual outlines of the root

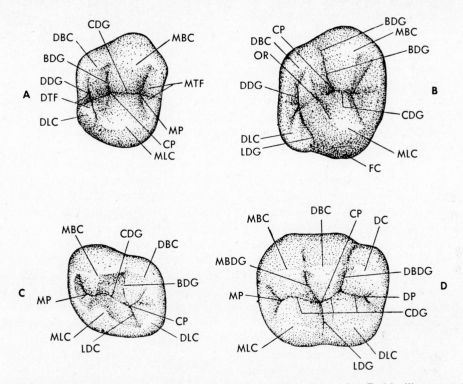

Fig. 3-7. Primary right molars, occlusal aspect. **A,** Maxillary first molar. **B,** Maxillary second molar. **C,** Mandibular first molar. **D,** Mandibular second molar. *MBC,* Mesiobuccal cusp; *MTF,* mesial triangular fossa; *MP,* mesial pit; *CP,* central pit; *MLC,* mesiolingual cusp; *DLC,* distolingual cusp; *DTF,* distal triangular fossa; *DDG,* distal developmental groove; *BDG,* buccal developmental groove; *DBC,* distobuccal cusp; *CDG,* central developmental groove; *FC,* fifth cusp; *LDG,* lingual developmental groove; *OR,* oblique ridge; *DC,* distal cusp; *DBDG,* distobuccal developmental groove; *DP,* distal pit; *MBDG,* mesiobuccal developmental groove. (From Wheeler, R.C.: Dental anatomy, physiology and occlusion, ed. 5, Philadelphia, 1974, W.B. Saunders Co.)

drop straight down from the crown, being essentially parallel for over half their length. The end of the root is flat and almost square.

Mandibular second molar. The mandibular second molar resembles the mandibular first permanent molar, except that the primary tooth is smaller in all its dimensions. The buccal surface is divided into three cusps that are separated by a mesiobuccal and distobuccal developmental groove. The cusps are almost equal in size. Two cusps of almost equal size are evident on the lingual surface and are divided by a short lingual groove.

The primary second molar, when viewed from the occlusal surface, appears rectangular with a slight distal convergence of the crown. The mesial marginal ridge is developed to a greater extent than the distal marginal ridge.

One difference between the crown of the primary molar and that of the first permanent molar is in the distobuccal cusp; the distal cusp of the permanent molar is smaller than the other two buccal cusps.

The roots of the primary second molar are long and slender, with a characteristic flare mesiodistally at the middle and apical thirds.

Morphologic differences between primary and permanent teeth

Wheeler has listed the following differences in form between the primary and permanent teeth:

1. The crowns of the primary teeth are wider mesiodistally in comparison with their crown length than are the permanent teeth.
2. The roots of primary anterior teeth are narrow and long in comparison with crown width and length.
3. The roots of the primary molars are relatively longer and more slender than the roots of the permanent teeth. There is also a greater extension of the primary roots mesiodistally. This "flaring" allows more room between the roots for the development of the premolar tooth crowns.
4. The cervical ridge of enamel at the cervical third of the anterior crowns is much more prominent labially and lingually in the primary than in the permanent teeth.
5. The crowns and roots of primary molars are more slender mesiodistally at the cervical third than those of the permanent molars.
6. The cervical ridge on the buccal aspect of the primary molars is much more definite, particularly on the maxillary and mandibular first molars, than on the permanent molars.
7. The buccal and lingual surfaces of the primary molars are flatter above the cervical curvatures than those of the permanent molars, thus making the occlusal surface narrower as compared with permanent teeth.
8. The primary teeth are usually lighter in color than the permanent teeth.

Size and morphology of the primary tooth pulp chamber

Considerable individual variation exists in the size of the pulp chamber and pulp canal of the primary teeth. Immediately after the eruption of the teeth the pulp chambers are large, and in general they follow the outline of the crown. The pulp chamber will decrease in size with an increase in age and under the influence of function and of abrasion of the occlusal and incisal surfaces of the teeth.

Rather than attempt to describe in detail each pulp chamber outline, it is suggested that the dentist examine critically the bite-wing radiographs of the child before undertaking operative procedures. Just as there are individual differences in the calcification time of teeth and also in eruption time, so are there individual differences in the morphology of the crowns and the size of the pulp chamber. It should be remembered, however, that the radiograph will not demonstrate completely the extent of pulp horn into the cuspal area. If the principles of cavity preparation for primary teeth described in Chapter 12 are followed, the mechanical exposure of the pulp will not be a problem.

REFERENCES

Bhaskar, S.N.: Orban's oral histology and embryology, ed. 9, St. Louis, 1979, The C.V. Mosby Co.

Brauer, J.C., and others: Dentistry for children, ed. 5, New York, 1964, McGraw-Hill Book Co.

Kraus, B.S., and Jordan, R.E.: The human dentition before birth, Philadelphia, 1965, Lea & Febiger.

Logan, W.H.G., and Kronfeld, R.: Development of the human jaws and surrounding structures from birth to the age of fifteen years, J.A.D.A. **20:**379-427, 1933.

Lunt, R.C., and Law, D.B.: A review of the chronology of calcification of deciduous teeth, J.A.D.A. **89:**599-606, 1974.

Schour, I., and Massler, M.: Studies in tooth development: the growth pattern of human teeth, J.A.D.A. **27:**1778-1793, 1940.

Wheeler, R.C.: Dental anatomy, physiology and occlusion, ed. 5, Philadelphia, 1974, W.B. Saunders Co.

4 Acquired and developmental disturbances of the teeth and associated oral structures

RALPH E. McDONALD
DAVID R. AVERY

Common disturbances in children

It has long been recognized that the most common physical defect found in school-age children is dental caries, a fact substantiated in Schiffer and Hunt's National Health Survey in 1963. Since that time, dental care services have become more readily available to children, and caries prevention programs have become more effective. Therefore there has been a steady decline from year to year in the incidence and prevalence of dental caries among U.S. children (see Chapter 7). However, dental caries remains one of the most prevalent diseases of children in our society. Periodontal disturbances are also quite common. Although severe forms of periodontal disease are rare in children, all experience at least mild gingivitis on occasion. Both caries and periodontal diseases are, for the most part, acquired and preventable disturbances of the teeth and jaws. Other chapters of this book are devoted to a more in-depth discussion of the cause, prevention, and management of dental caries (Chapters 7, 8, and 12) and periodontal disturbances (Chapters 14 and 15). Traumatic injuries to the teeth and supporting tissues represent another large category of acquired disturbances (see Chapter 17).

Greene reported that 60% of American children have orthodontic conditions that justify corrective treatment, and for 20% of them the condition is serious enough to be categorized as deforming or crippling. Approximately 1 in every 700 children is born with a cleft lip or palate. These conditions are primarily developmental disturbances and are discussed in greater detail in Chapters 18 to 21 and 24.

Alveolar abscess

During the examination procedure the dentist may observe evidence of an acute or chronic alveolar abscess. An alveolar abscess associated with the pulpless permanent tooth is usually a specific lesion localized by a fibrous capsule produced by fibroblasts that differentiate from the periodontal membrane. The primary tooth abscess is usually evident as a more diffuse infection, and the surrounding tissue is less able to wall off the process.

The most common microorganism associated with a periapical infection, as verified by Turner, Moore, and Shaw, is *Streptococcus viridans*. It is susceptible to all antibiotics commonly recommended in dental practice, except the tetracyclines. The virulence of the microorganisms and the ability of the tissues to react to the infection probably determine whether the infection will be acute or chronic.

In the early stages the acute alveolar abscess can be diagnosed on the basis of radiographic evidence

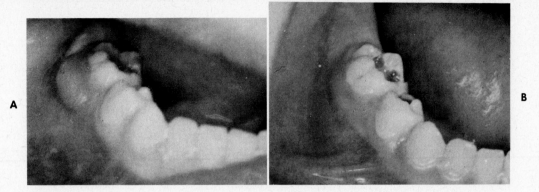

Fig. 4-1. A, Acute alveolar abscess associated with a pulpless second primary molar. **B,** Removal of the roof of the pulp chamber to allow drainage resulted in immediate relief of pain. After the swelling has been reduced, it can be decided whether the tooth is to be treated or extracted.

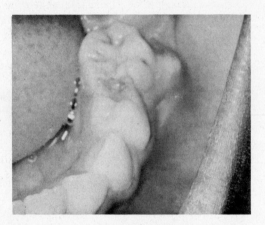

Fig. 4-2. Chronic alveolar abscess associated with a pulpless second primary molar that is also a candidate for incision and drainage, in addition to removal of the roof of the pulp chamber to initiate root canal therapy if the tooth is to be saved.

of a thickened periodontal membrane. The tooth will be sensitive to percussion and movement, and the patient may have a slight fever. The acute symptoms of an alveolar abscess can be relieved by establishing drainage and using an antibiotic that is effective against *S. viridans* (Fig. 4-1). A large opening should be made into the pulp chamber to permit drainage to continue until the acute symptoms have subsided. In 24 to 48 hours it can be determined if the tooth can be treated endodontically or if extraction is necessary. Should pain occur during the cutting of tooth structure to estab-

lish drainage, the discomfort can be lessened if the tooth is stabilized either by holding it or by a splint of impression compound.

Warm saline mouthrinses often aid in localizing the infection and maintaining adequate drainage before endodontic treatment or extraction.

Chronic alveolar abscess, characterized by less soreness, is often a better defined radiographic lesion. The patient will likely have some lymphadenopathy as well. Draining fistulas are also frequently associated with chronic alveolar abscesses. Usually antibiotic therapy is unnecessary unless

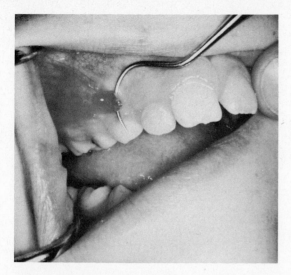

Fig. 4-3. A pedunculated granulomatous lesion overlying the canine but associated with a chronic draining alveolar abscess of the maxillary right first primary molar.

there is an overriding systemic problem (for example, susceptibility to subacute bacterial endocarditis). Again, drainage and sterilization of the infected local area are necessary through root canal therapy for the involved tooth or through extraction. If the lesion has only recently passed the acute stage, there may be a pointing soft tissue abscess. In this situation incision and drainage of the soft tissue may be indicated in addition to opening the tooth, especially if the tooth is to be treated endodontically (Fig. 4-2). If the lesion is in an advanced chronic stage, drainage may already be established as a natural reaction (Fig. 4-3).

Cellulitis

Cellulitis is a diffuse type of infection of the soft tissues caused by a pulpless primary or permanent tooth. It often causes considerable swelling of the face or neck, and the tissue appears discolored.

Cellulitis is a very serious infection. It can be life threatening, and it is a potential complication of all acute dental infections. It is usually a result of severe untreated caries in patients who do not receive regular dental care or who may have had dental care only for treatment of dental emergencies. It is not unusual for the parents to take the child suffering from cellulitis to the hospital emergency room although they may not always appreciate the seriousness and urgency of the situation. The child will appear acutely ill and may have an alarmingly high temperature with malaise and lethargy.

If a maxillary tooth is the problem, the swelling and redness may involve the eye (Fig. 4-4). If cellulitis is treated too late, serious complications, such as involvement of the central nervous system or a cavernous sinus thrombosis, could result. If cellulitis results from an infected mandibular tooth, the diffuse swelling and infection will spread in the floor of the mouth along facial planes, nerves, and vessels. If the infection involves the submandibular, sublingual, and submental spaces, it is called Ludwig angina. In this condition the tongue and floor of the mouth become elevated to the extent that the patient's airway is obstructed and swallowing is impossible.

The establishment of drainage, if possible, by opening into the pulp chamber of the offending tooth will be helpful in reducing the acute symptoms of cellulitis. However, the child may have difficulty opening the mouth to permit the procedure. Incision of soft tissue to establish drainage is not indicated in the early stages of cellulitis because of the diffuse, nonlocalized nature of the infection.

The offending organisms in cellulitis from dental infections are usually streptococci capable of producing hyaluronidase (''spreading factor'') and fibrinolysins. These agents break down the intercellular cementing substance (hyaluronic acid) and fibrin, permitting the rapid spread of the infection. Some hyaluronidase-producing staphylococci may also give rise to cellulitis. Penicillin or other broad-spectrum antibiotics (if there is penicillin allergy)

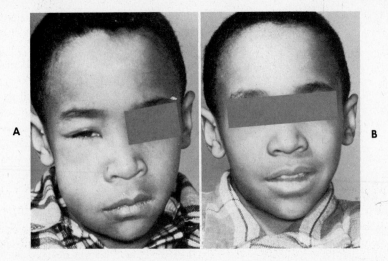

Fig. 4-4. A, Patient appears to be acutely ill because of an infected permanent molar and resultant cellulitis. **B,** Use of broad-spectrum antibiotics reduced the acute symptoms of the disease and prevented extraoral drainage.

should be prescribed early to reduce the possibility of the infection localizing and draining on the outer surface of the face (Fig. 4-4, *B*). It should be emphasized to the parents or patient that antibiotics will not heal the condition completely and that follow-up treatment of the tooth is essential.

If the infection is already severe when the parent or patient seeks treatment, a blood culture or a culture of exudate is indicated to identify the infecting organisms. Thus if the infection does not respond to the initial antibiotic therapy, a second, more appropriate antibiotic may be selected after the causative organisms have been identified.

The child with cellulitis should be hospitalized if the clinical signs or symptoms warrant very close monitoring or if there is any question about the parents or patient following through with the prescribed treatment. Hospitalization is recommended especially in the case of Ludwig angina, since maintaining a patent airway may be dependent on professional personnel. In these severe cases the parenteral administration of antibiotics is also recommended, at least initially.

Developmental anomalies of the teeth

Odontoma. The abnormal proliferation of cells of the enamel organ may result in an odontogenic tumor, commonly referred to as an "odontoma." An odontoma may form as a result of continued budding of the primary or permanent tooth germ or as a result of an abnormal proliferation of the cells of the tooth germ, in which case an odontoma replaces the normal tooth (Figs. 4-5 and 4-6). The anomaly is discussed in detail in Chapter 28. An odontoma should be surgically removed before it can interfere with eruption of teeth in the area.

Fusion of teeth. Fusion represents the union of two independently developing primary or permanent teeth. The condition is almost always limited to the anterior teeth and, like gemination (see the following discussion), may follow a familial tendency.

The radiograph may show that the fusion is limited to the crowns and roots. Fused teeth will have separate pulp chambers and separate pulp canals (Fig. 4-7). Dental caries often develops in the line of fusion of the crowns, necessitating the place-

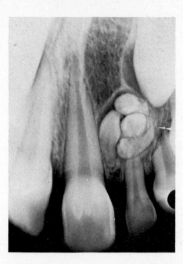

Fig. 4-5. Compound composite odontoma. The anomalous structure consists of small structures resembling teeth.

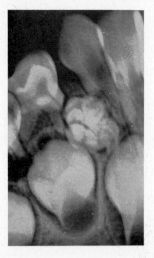

Fig. 4-6. Complex composite odontoma.

ment of a restoration. A frequent finding in fusion of primary teeth is the congenital absence of one of the corresponding permanent teeth.

Delaney and Goldblatt recently reported an interesting case to illustrate the multidisciplinary approach that may be indicated in the clinical management of certain problems associated with fused teeth. The disciplines of pedodontics, endodontics, surgery, restorative dentistry, and orthodontics were all represented in the initial management of the case, and a post and core and a crown restoration were anticipated for the future. Yet excellent results were obtained in only 6 months with an organized approach to a complex problem that involved the fusion of a supernumerary tooth to a maxillary central incisor, severe crowding, and a palatally displaced lateral incisor. One root of the fused teeth was treated endodontically. The fused teeth were then hemisectioned, and the endodontically treated tooth was restored while the separated tooth was sacrificed. Orthodontic repositioning of the palatally displaced lateral incisor and alignment of the anterior segment concluded the management

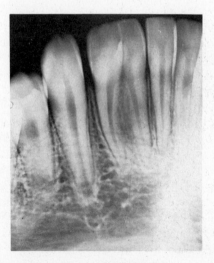

Fig. 4-7. Fusion of a permanent central and lateral incisor.

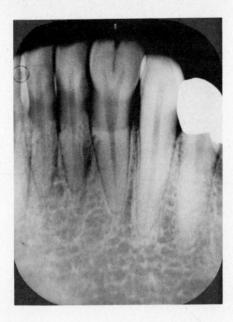

Fig. 4-8. Gemination of a mandibular lateral incisor. The crown has a groove on the labial surface and is wider than normal.

of the problem. A case of bilateral fusion of primary incisors has also recently been reported by Eidelman.

Gemination. A geminated tooth represents an attempted division of a single tooth germ by invagination occurring during the proliferation stage of the growth cycle of the tooth. The geminated tooth appears clinically as a bifid crown on a single root (Fig. 4-8). The crown is usually wider than normal, with a shallow groove extending from the incisal edge to the cervical region. The anomaly, which may follow a hereditary pattern, is seen in both primary and permanent teeth, although it probably occurs more frequently in primary teeth.

The treatment of a permanent anterior geminated tooth may involve reduction of the mesiodistal width of the tooth to allow normal development of the occlusion. Periodic disking of the tooth, when the crown is not excessively large, can be recommended, as can eventual preparation of the tooth for restoration if dentin is exposed. Secondary dentin formation and pulpal recession will follow judicial periodic reduction of crown size. Devitalization of the tooth and root canal therapy followed by the construction of a post crown may be necessary when the geminated tooth is large and malformed.

Dens in dente. The diagnosis of a dens in dente (tooth within a tooth) can be verified by a radiograph. The developmental anomaly has been described as a lingual invagination of the enamel. This condition can occur in primary and permanent teeth; however, it is most often seen in the permanent maxillary lateral incisors. The condition should be suspected whenever deep lingual pits are observed in maxillary permanent lateral incisors.

The cause of the condition is not well established. Those factors most often considered are related to increased localized external pressure, focal growth retardation, and focal growth stimulation.

Anterior teeth with dens are usually of normal shape and size. In other areas of the mouth, however, the tooth can have an anomalous appearance. A dens in dente is characterized by an invagination lined with enamel and the presence of a foramen cecum with the probability of a communication between the cavity of the invagination and the pulp chamber (Fig. 4-9).

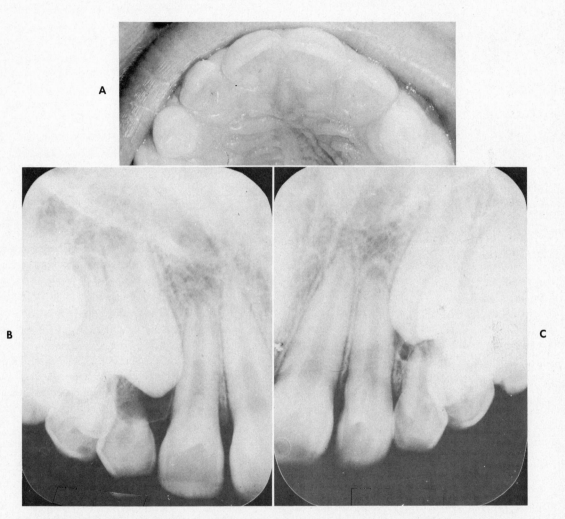

Fig. 4-9. A, Small, "nonsticky" pits on the lingual surfaces of the maxillary lateral incisors were the only clues to the dens in dente condition of the teeth revealed radiographically in **B** and **C.**

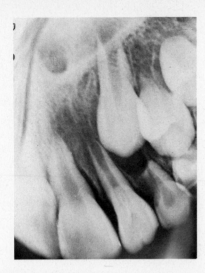

Fig. 4-10. Dens in dente in a maxillary lateral incisor. A communication between the invagination and the pulp chamber apparently caused necrosis of the pulp.

Thomas has reported the finding of 146 instances of dens in dente in 1886 radiographic surveys, or a prevalence of 7.7%, which is a higher percentage than previously described. Of these surveys 278 were of dental students, and in that group the number of individuals with dens in dente was much higher (17.2%).

Prophylactic restorations of the opening to the invagination and pulp are the recommended treatment to prevent pulpal involvement. If the condition is detected before complete eruption of the tooth, the removal of gingival tissue to facilitate cavity preparation and restoration is indicated.

Endodontic procedures on teeth that have pulpal degeneration are dependent on pulp chamber morphology (Fig. 4-10).

Early exfoliation of teeth

Variations in the time of eruption of the primary teeth and in the time of exfoliation are frequently observed in the child patient. A variation of as much as 18 months in the exfoliation time of primary teeth may be considered normal. However, this pattern must be consistent with other aspects of the dental development. The early exfoliation of teeth merits special attention because it can be related to pathologic conditions of local and systemic origin.

The early exfoliation of primary teeth resulting from periodontosis has been observed occasionally in young children (Chapter 14). The widespread loss of supporting alveolar bone with loosening, migration, and spontaneous loss of teeth or the necessity for premature extraction is characteristic of periodontosis in children.

Familial fibrous dysplasia (cherubism). Fibrous dysplasia of the jaws is a rare disease that may occur in childhood. Although the cause has not been clearly established, the disease may follow a familial pattern and may represent a local disturbance in the embryonic development of tissues.

A symmetric or asymmetric enlargement of the jaws may be noted at an early age. Numerous sharp, well-defined multilocular areas of bone destruction and thinning of the cortical plate are evident in the radiograph (Fig. 4-11). Teeth in the involved area are frequently exfoliated prematurely as a result of the loss of support or root resorption or, in permanent teeth, as a result of an interference in the development of roots. Spontaneous loss of the teeth may occur, or the child may pick the teeth out of the soft tissue.

McDonald and Shafer reported a case in which the mandible and maxillae of a 5-year-old girl were symmetrically enlarged. Radiographs showed multilocular cystic involvement of both mandible and maxillae. A complete skeletal survey failed to reveal similar lesions in other bones. Microscopic examination of a segment of soft tissue, as well as of a small segment of bone, showed a large number of multinucleated giant cells scattered diffusely throughout a cellular stroma. The giant cells were large and irregular in shape and contained 30 to 40 nuclei. During a 10-year observation period the bony lesions had not progressed appreciably.

The patient illustrated in Fig. 4-11 was followed into adult life and her mouth was restored in a very satisfactory manner. A comparison of the full-face photographs in Fig. 4-11 (*A* and *I*) illustrate that as the face increases in height, the "cherub" appearance caused by the bilateral bulging of the bone of

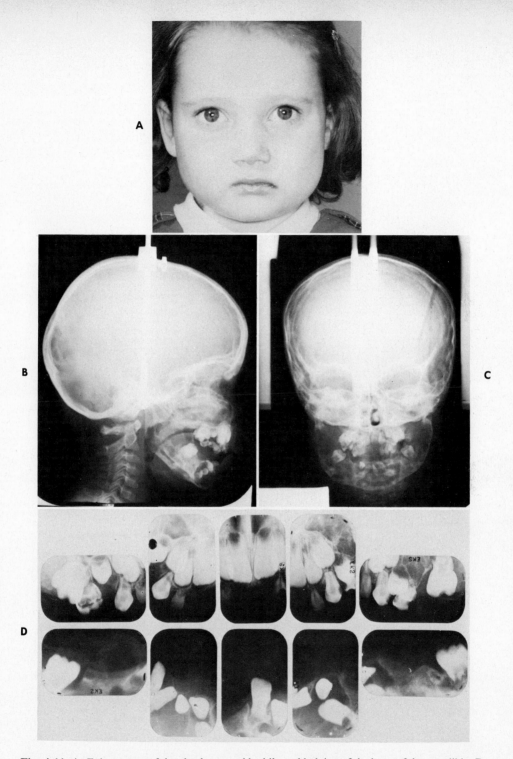

Fig. 4-11. A, Enlargement of the cheeks caused by bilateral bulging of the bone of the mandible. **B** and **C,** Lateral and anteroposterior cephalometric radiographs. Note the displacement of the mandibular anterior teeth in a large area of bone destruction, the locular cystic involvement of the mandible and maxillae, and the number of missing teeth. **D,** Full-mouth radiographs demonstrating large areas of bone destruction and several missing teeth.

Continued.

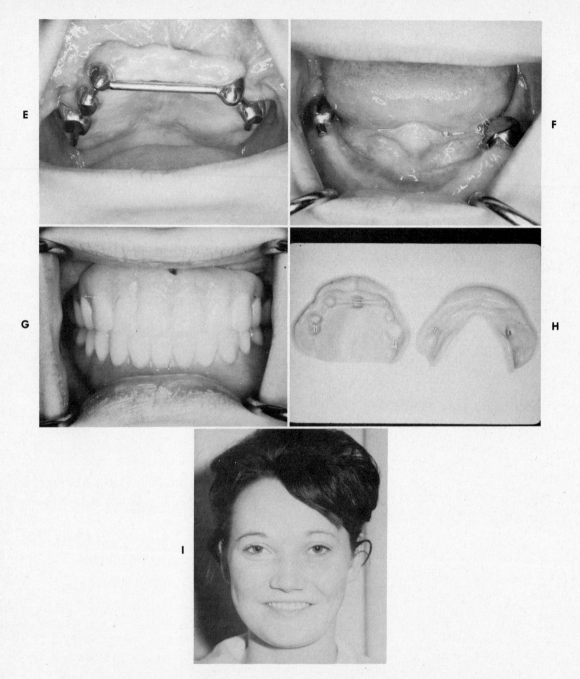

Fig. 4-11, cont'd. E to H, At age 18 the permanent teeth that had good support were prepared for Baker attachments, and complete dentures were constructed. (Courtesy Dr. Donald Cunningham.) **I,** The restored mouth and improved appearance of the young adult.

the mandible is less apparent. Seven permanent teeth in the upper and lower arches were retained and prepared for Baker attachments. Complete dentures were constructed to restore function and an improved appearance.

Although the treatment of choice for a true giant cell tumor is curettage, that type of treatment is not practical in familial fibrous dysplasia because the lesions are widespread.

Peters has reported a study of 20 cases of cherubism from one family that confirmed an autosomal dominant pattern of inheritance and penetrance of 80%. In this study males were affected twice as often as females. The author also emphasized that a conservative approach is indicated in managing the giant cell lesions, since they tend to resolve with maturity.

Acrodynia. The exposure of young children to minute amounts of mercury is responsible for a condition referred to as ''acrodynia'' or ''pink disease.'' Ointments, diaper rinses, and medication are the usual sources of the mercury.

The clinical features of the disease include fever, anorexia, desquamation of the soles and palms, sweating, tachycardia, gastrointestinal disturbance, and hypotonia. The oral findings include inflammation and ulceration of the mucous membrane, excessive salivation, loss of alveolar bone, and premature exfoliation of teeth.

Hypophosphatasia. The clinical dental finding diagnostic of hypophosphatasia in children is premature exfoliation of the anterior primary teeth. The loss of teeth in the young child may be spontaneous or may result from a slight traumatic injury. There will be an absence of severe gingival inflammation. The loss of alveolar bone may be limited to the anterior region. Baer, Brown, and Hammer have reported a low alkaline phosphatase level (7 King-Armstrong units; normal is 13 to 17 units) in a 2½-year-old child. The child's mother had a serum alkaline phosphatase score below the lower limit of normal. The histologic evidence of hypocementosis of the affected teeth is characteristic. The disease has been reported to be an inborn error of metabolism inherited via an autosomal recessive gene. However, Poland and associates report that at least two and perhaps three different inheritance patterns have been described for families with hypophosphatasia. Diagnostic tests should include the determination of serum alkaline phosphatase levels for parents and siblings.

Pseudohypophosphatasia. Pseudohypophosphatasia, which seems to be hereditary, resembles hypophosphatasia and results in premature loss of the primary teeth. However, the serum alkaline phosphatase level is normal. Patients afflicted with pseudohypophosphatasia exhibit osteopathy of the long bones and skull.

Nonlipid reticuloendothelioses. The nonlipid reticuloendothelioses, also known as the histiocytosis X group of diseases, represent a group of metabolic diseases of the reticuloendothelial system. Their cause is unknown. The three diseases comprising this group are Letterer-Siwe disease, Hand-Schüller-Christian disease, and eosinophilic granuloma of bone. Most authorities regard these as a single disease entity, with the three forms of the disease representing only a variable clinical expression. Cranin and Rockman have reported three cases of histiocytosis X in which the prodromal symptoms of the disease occurred in the oral cavity. Tooth mobility was present in all three cases. In the case of an infant 10 months old, precocious tooth eruption, ectopic tooth position and mobility, abnormal gingival bleeding, and soft spongy gingival folds were noted during the oral examination. The mother reported that tooth eruption and gingival bleeding began at 4 weeks of age and were the first signs of an unusual condition. The child was found to have Letterer-Siwe disease.

Letterer-Siwe disease is an acute fulminating form of the disease that chiefly affects infants and young children. These patients typically develop lesions of the spleen, liver, lymph nodes, skin, and skeleton manifested by hepatosplenomegaly, lymphadenopathy, skin nodules, and destructive lesions of bone, including the jaw. Fever and malaise are commonly present. The lesions themselves consist basically of the accumulation and proliferation of huge numbers of histiocytes, often intermingled with focal collections of eosinophils. The intracellular accumulation of the lipid cholesterol within the histiocytes is usually not as prominent as it is in the other two forms of histiocytosis X.

The lesions of the jaw are characterized by a diffuse destruction of bone, usually resulting in loosening and premature exfoliation of teeth. The clinical and radiographic appearance of the jaw lesions is not characteristic, however, since many other diseases may produce a similar destruction of bone and loss of teeth. Ulceration of oral tissue and pain are also common findings.

Letterer-Siwe disease has a poor prognosis because of its fulminating course. Most individuals with the disease die within a relatively short time.

Hand-Schüller-Christian disease is another variation of the same basic disease that occurs in somewhat older children and young adolescents, has a more subacute course, and presents a more favorable prognosis.

Clinically, visceral involvement similar to that in Letterer-Siwe disease may occur but is not usually as diffuse and widespread. A somewhat more common finding is skeletal involvement, although the extent of such involvement will vary markedly. Skull involvement is a particularly common finding, often resulting in dyspituitarism and ensuing diabetes insipidus. Retro-orbital involvement producing exophthalmos is also common.

The jaw is involved as in Letterer-Siwe disease, with severe destruction of bone, loosening of teeth, and premature loss of teeth. Extensive oral ulceration with pain, fetid breath, and excessive salivation is also common. On dental radiographs the teeth often appear to be situated completely within soft tissue.

The microscopic appearance of the soft tissue and bone lesions is one of sheets of histiocytes, with or without lipid material intracellularly, often intermingled with focal collections of eosinophils. When the histiocytes contain abundant cholesterol, they present a characteristic vacuolated or foamy appearance and are often referred to as "foam cells."

The prognosis of Hand-Schüller-Christian disease is somewhat better than that of Letterer-Siwe disease, although many individuals with the former die. The prognosis appears to depend chiefly on the extent of the disease with respect to organ and skeletal involvement. X-radiation and corticosteroid therapy are both of definite value in treatment.

Eosinophilic granuloma of bone is the third form of histiocytosis X disease. It occurs chiefly in young adults, runs a chronic course, and is limited in extent, often involving only one bone. Because of this limitation, the disease has an excellent prognosis.

Any bone in the skeleton may be involved, and lesions of the jaw are common. These lesions are often asymptomatic and are discovered during routine radiographic examination. Some lesions produce mild swelling and occasional pain. Loss of superficial alveolar bone, often mimicking periodontosis or localized periodontitis, is a common early manifestation of the disease.

These solitary lesions are treated by surgical excision, and the prognosis is excellent. When such a solitary lesion is discovered and diagnosed, however, a skeletal radiographic survey should be carried out to make certain that additional lesions are not present in other bones.

Anomalous dental development. Defective root development, as observed in cases of dentinal dysplasia and in shell teeth, can cause early exfoliation of primary and permanent teeth. Other anomalous conditions are occasionally observed in which the teeth exfoliate early (Fig. 4-12). Bruce reported a case that represents the strictly dental anomaly involving both the primary and permanent teeth. Early maturation, early eruption, early exfoliation, and microdontia were noted. The condition was unrelated to systemic disease or abnormality. The microscopic appearance of the enamel was normal, but the dentin and cementum appeared to deviate from the usual pattern. Bruce theorized that the absence of cementum from the root surface may have accounted for the rapid eruption and also for the early exfoliation of the teeth. Since the thin layer of cementum covering the roots provided the

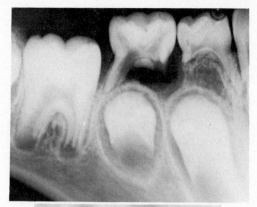

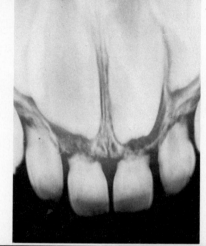

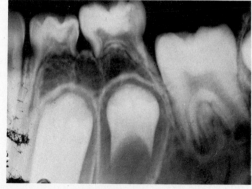

Fig. 4-12. Dental radiographs of a 5-year-old boy. The atypical premature resorption of the roots of the primary teeth was followed by early exfoliation. (Courtesy Dr. Roger L. Parrott.)

terminal fibrils of the periodontal membrane with little area for secure anchorage, adequate function and retention of the tooth were not possible.

Cyclic neutropenia. Cyclic neutropenia, an unusual form of agranulocytosis, is characterized by a periodic or cyclic diminution in polymorphonuclear neutrophilic leukocytes and is accompanied by mild clinical manifestations. This condition spontaneously regresses, only to recur subsequently in a rhythmic pattern. The cause of this disease is unknown. Although the role of hormonal factors has been suggested, there is no sound evidence to indicate that this is the case. Similarly, a hereditary feature has been suggested but has not been proved.

The condition occurs at any age. Numerous cases have been reported in children. The patients manifest a fever, malaise, sore throat, stomatitis, and regional lymphadenopathy, as well as headache, cutaneous infection, and conjunctivitis. A bacterial infection is not a serious feature, presumably because the neutrophil count is low for such a short time.

Children exhibit a severe gingivitis with ulceration. With a return of the neutrophil count to normal, the gingiva assumes a nearly normal clinical appearance. In children with repeated insults of the infection there is a considerable loss of supporting bone around the teeth. This has sometimes been termed "prepubertal periodontitis."

Other disorders. Premature exfoliation of teeth has been linked to other systemic disorders including acatalasia, hyperpituitarism, juvenile diabetes, leukemia, and progeria.

Enamel hypoplasia

Amelogenesis occurs in two stages. In the first stage the enamel matrix forms, and in the second stage the matrix undergoes calcification. Local or systemic factors that interfere with the normal matrix formation cause enamel surface defects and irregularities referred to as "enamel hypoplasia." Factors that interfere with calcification and maturation of the enamel produce a condition referred to as "enamel hypocalcification."

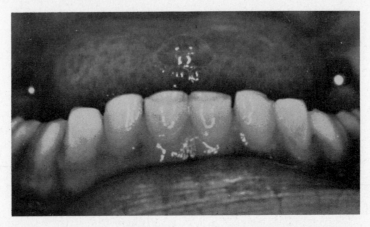

Fig. 4-13. Prenatal enamel hypoplasia. The medical history revealed that the patient suffered from cerebral palsy as the result of a premature birth (gestation, 6 months; birth weight, 2 pounds, 5 ounces). (Courtesy Dr. Stanley C. Herman.)

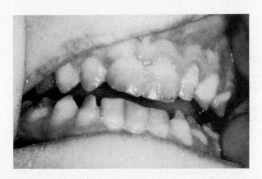

Fig. 4-14. Neonatal enamel hypoplasia. Only the most cervical parts of the intrinsically stained areas are hypoplastic. The child experienced severe nutritional deficiency during the first month of extrauterine life. (Courtesy Dr. Stanley C. Herman.)

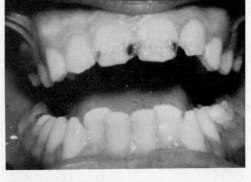

Fig. 4-15. Enamel hypoplasia that occurred during infancy. A wide band of pitted enamel is evident on the maxillary and mandibular permanent incisors and first permanent molars. The child was severely affected with pneumonia at 6 months of age. (Courtesy Dr. Stanley C. Herman.)

Enamel hypoplasia may be mild and may result in a pitting of the enamel surface or in the development of a horizontal line across the enamel of the crown. If ameloblastic activity has been disrupted for a long period of time, gross areas of irregular or imperfect enamel formation occur.

Postnatal hypoplasia of the primary teeth is probably as common as hypoplasia of the permanent teeth, although the former usually does not occur in as severe a form. However, hypoplasia of the primary enamel that forms before birth is rare (Fig. 4-13). Kronfeld and Schour state that neonatal hypoplasia represents a disturbance in formation rather than in the calcification of enamel and dentin that originated during the neonatal period. In its mildest form, a prenatal disturbance is reflected as an accentuated neonatal ring in the primary tooth. In the severe type of neonatal disturbance, enamel

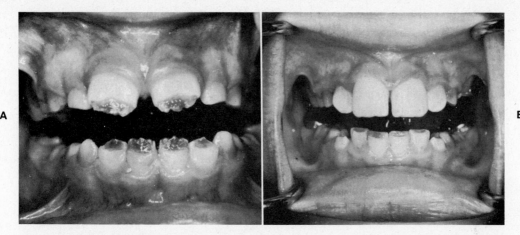

Fig. 4-16. A, Enamel hypoplasia that developed as the result of a nutritional deficiency during infancy. The first permanent molars, maxillary central incisors, and mandibular incisors show hypoplastic enamel and dentin. **B,** At age 10½ years, acrylic jacket crowns were constructed for the maxillary incisors. The acid etch resin technique described in Chapter 17 has been accepted as an excellent procedure for improving the appearance of hypoplastic teeth. The defect on the incisal edge of the lower incisors was reduced to improve the appearance.

formation is sometimes arrested at birth or during the neonatal period (Fig. 4-14). Postnatal amelogenesis is confined to the portion of the crown located cervically from the enamel area present at birth (Fig. 4-15).

Stein reported that 50% of children born prematurely (at about the seventh month of pregnancy) had enamel hypoplasia in the primary teeth. The position of the defect on the teeth corresponded in time of development with the time of their birth.

Hypoplasia resulting from nutritional deficiencies. Many clinical investigations have been undertaken to determine the relationship between hypoplastic defects of enamel and systemic disabilities. Relatively little importance has been placed on exanthematous fevers, but deficiency states—particularly those related to deficiencies in vitamins A, C, and D, calcium, and phosphorus—can often be related to the occurrence of enamel hypoplasia.

Sarnat and Schour observed that in a group of 60 children who had adequate medical histories, two thirds of the hypoplastic disturbances occurred during infancy (birth to the end of the first year) (Fig.

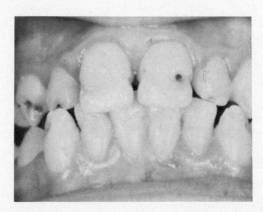

Fig. 4-17. Enamel hypoplasia occurred during early childhood. Enamel formation on the incisal third of the lower incisors and the maxillary central incisors is normal.

4-16). Approximately one third of enamel hypoplasia was found in the portion of teeth formed during early childhood (13 to 34 months) (Fig. 4-17). Less than 2% of enamel defects found originated in late childhood (35 to 80 months).

Sheldon, Bibby, and Bales sought to determine whether defects in enamel were related to the occurrence of systemic ailments. They examined ground sections of 95 teeth from 34 patients with detailed medical histories. In more than 70% of the individuals a positive correlation between the time of formation of a band of defective enamel and the existence of some systemic disability was established. However, defects occurred in the enamel of 23% of patients who had no history of systemic conditions that might have produced enamel defects. No enamel changes occurred in 6% of patients who had histories of disabilities that had produced enamel changes in other patients. Deficiencies of vitamins A, C, and D, calcium, and phosphorus were the most common causes of defective enamel formation.

Purvis and associates, in a study of 112 infants with neonatal tetany in Edinburgh, observed that 63 (56%) later showed severe enamel hypoplasia of the deciduous teeth. Histologic examinations revealed a prolonged disturbance of enamel formation in the 3 months before birth. An inverse relationship was demonstrated between the mean daily hours of bright sunshine in each calendar month and the incidence of neonatal tetany 3 months later. This observation suggested that enamel hypoplasia and neonatal tetany can be manifestations of a vitamin D deficiency during pregnancy and are most likely the result of secondary hyperparathyroidism in the mother. There was also a significantly higher mean maternal age and a preponderance of lower social class mothers in the tetany group. Another study in Edinburgh indicated that only 1% of pregnant mothers took vitamin D supplements.

Apparently in some children a mild deficiency state or systemic condition without clinical symptoms can interfere with ameloblastic activity and can produce a permanent defect in the developing enamel.

Hypoplasia related to brain injury and neurologic defects. Herman and McDonald studied 120 cerebral palsied children between the ages of 2½ and 10½ years (for whom complete medical records were available) to determine the incidence of dental hypoplasia. The researchers compared them with 117 normal children in the same age group and observed enamel hypoplasia in 36% of the cerebral palsied group and in 6% of the normal group. A definite relationship between the time of the possible factors that could have caused brain damage and the apparent time of the enamel defect (based on its location in the enamel on the crown of the tooth) was established (Fig. 4-13) in 70% of the affected teeth of children with cerebral palsy. Evidence of enamel hypoplasia is an aid to the clinician and the research worker in determining when brain injury occurred in patients in whom the etiology is not clearly defined.

Cohen and Diner observed that enamel defects occurred with greatest frequency in children with low IQ scores and a high incidence of neurologic defects. They found that chronologically distributed enamel defects were a valuable aid in neurologic diagnosis, since they occur commonly in brain-damaged children. In addition, the defects indicate the time of insult to the developing fetus or infant even when the history is reportedly negative.

Hypoplasia associated with nephrotic syndrome. Oliver and Owings observed enamel hypoplasia in permanent teeth in a high percentage of children with nephrotic syndrome and found a correlation between the time of severe renal disease and the estimated time at which the defective enamel formation occurred.

Hypoplasia associated with allergies. Rattner and Myers discovered a correlation between enamel defects of the primary dentition and the presence of severe allergic reactions. Enamel defects were present 26 of 45 children with congenital allergies. The enamel lesions were localized in the occlusal third of the primary canines and first molars.

Hypoplasia associated with chronic pediatric lead poisoning. In Chicago about 3500 cases of lead poisoning (plumbism) are reported annually, and in some industrial areas lead salts may account for up to 79% of all childhood deaths caused by accidental poisoning. Many mild cases of pediatric lead poisoning undoubtedly go undetected.

Lawson and Stout observed that in areas of

Charleston, South Carolina, containing very old frame buildings, the incidence of pitting hypoplasia was approximately 100% greater than published standards or the findings in their control group of children. They suggest that dentists treating children with unexplained pitting hypoplasia should consider previous exposure to lead poisoning as a part of their health evaluation, particularly if the child is from a family in a low economic stratum.

Pearl and Roland have pointed out that the fetus of a lead-poisoned mother can be affected because lead readily crosses the placenta during pregnancy. They observed significant delays in development and eruption of the primary teeth of the child of a lead-poisoned mother. They also listed pica (ingesting unusual objects to satisfy an abnormal craving) as the common cause of plumbism in children 1 to 6 years old, as well as in their mothers. One mother admitted eating plaster from her apartment walls during several months of pregnancy.

Hypoplasia caused by local infection and trauma. Enamel hypoplasia resulting from a deficiency state or a systemic condition will be evident on all the teeth that were undergoing matrix formation and calcification at the time. The hypoplasia will follow a definite pattern. Individual permanent teeth will often have hypoplastic or hypocalcified areas on the crown resulting from infection or trauma (Figs. 4-18 and 4-19).

Turner first described the localized type of hypoplasia. He noted defects in the enamel of two premolars and traced the defects to apical infection of the nearest primary molar. Enamel hypoplasia resulting from local infection is referred to as "Turner tooth."

Bauer concluded from a study of autopsy material that the periapical inflammatory processes of primary teeth extend toward the buds of the pertinent permanent teeth and affect them during their prefunctional stage of eruption. The infection fails to stimulate the development of a fibrous wall that would localize the lesion. Instead, the infection spreads diffusely through the bone around the buds of the successors, thereby affecting the important

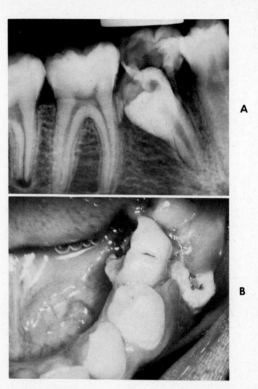

Fig. 4-18. A, Infected mandibular second primary molar has caused hypoplasia of the second premolar and delayed eruption of the tooth. **B,** Hypoplasia is evident in the occlusal third of the second premolar.

protective layer of the young enamel, the united enamel epithelium.

Bauer found that in some cases the united enamel epithelium was destroyed and the enamel was exposed to inflammatory edema and to granulation tissue. The granulation tissue later eroded the enamel and deposited a well-calcified, metaplastic, cementum-like substance on the surface of the deep excavation.

A traumatic injury to an anterior primary tooth that causes its displacement apically can interfere with matrix formation or calcification of the underlying permanent tooth. The trauma or subsequent periapical infection frequently produces defects on the labial surface of the permanent incisor (Fig. 4-20). The retention of infected primary teeth,

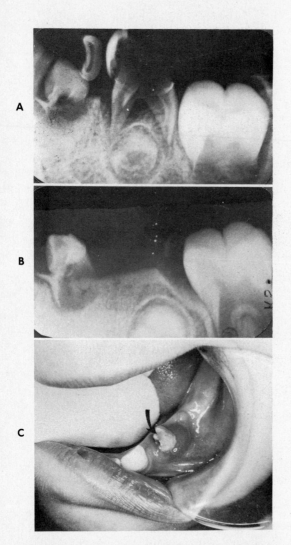

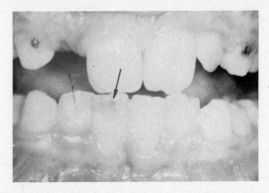

Fig. 4-20. Hypoplastic defect on the labial surface of a mandibular permanent central incisor *(arrow)*. There was a history of trauma to the primary tooth.

Fig. 4-19. A, Only a root fragment remains as evidence of a pulpless first primary molar. The infection has affected the development of the first premolar. **B,** The second primary molar has been exfoliated prematurely. The first premolar is malformed as a result of the infection in the area. **C,** The malformed calcified mass *(arrow)* is surrounded by inflamed tissue.

even though they are asymptomatic, is unjustifiable. The development of hypoplastic defects on the permanent tooth, its deflection from the normal path of eruption because of the pressure of the inflammatory exudate, or even death of the developing tooth may result.

Hypoplasia-associated repaired cleft lip and palate. Mink studied the incidence of enamel hypoplasia of the maxillary anterior teeth in 98 repaired bilateral and unilateral complete cleft lip and palate patients ranging in age from 1½ to 18 years. In the repaired unilateral and bilateral complete cleft lip and palate group with maxillary anterior primary teeth, 66% had one or more primary teeth affected with enamel hypoplasia. In the repaired unilateral and bilateral complete cleft lip and palate group with erupted maxillary anterior permanent teeth, 92% had one or more permanent teeth affected with enamel hypoplasia (Fig. 4-21). Mink concluded that the permanent teeth are in earlier stages of development at the time of the surgical procedure and are more subject to damage when severely disturbed.

Hypoplasia caused by x-radiation. Children who receive excessive x-radiation in the treatment of a malignancy have developed rampant caries in the irradiated area. The cause is generally believed

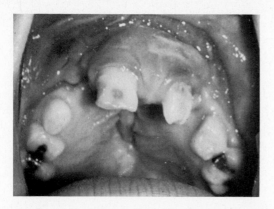

Fig. 4-21. Enamel hypoplasia of the permanent central incisors caused by the surgical repair of the cleft lip and palate. (Courtesy Dr. John Mink.)

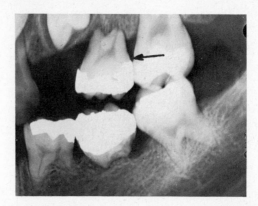

Fig. 4-22. X-radiation caused hypoplastic defect on the crown of the first permanent molar *(arrow)* and stunting of root development.

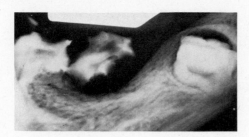

Fig. 4-23. Absence of developing premolars and the malformed second permanent molar were caused by excessive x-radiation.

to be changes in the salivary glands and is discussed in Chapter 7.

Ameloblasts are generally resistant to x-radiation. However, a line of hypoplastic enamel that corresponds to the time of the stage of development during therapy may be seen (Fig. 4-22). A more severe effect on the development of the dentin will occur, and root formation will be stunted. Occasionally development of the permanent teeth will be arrested (Fig. 4-23).

Hypoplasia resulting from rubella embryopathy. Musselman examined 50 children (average age 2½ years) with congenital anomalies attributed to in utero infection with rubella. Enamel hypoplasia was found in 90% of the affected children, as compared with only 13% of unaffected children in a control group. Tapered teeth also occurred in 78% of the children with a history of rubella (Figs.

4-24 and 4-25). Nine of the children in the study group had notched teeth, but this defect was not present in any of the control group children.

Treatment of hypoplastic teeth. The contention that hypoplastic teeth are more susceptible to dental caries than are normal teeth has little evidence to support it. Carious lesions do develop, however, in the enamel defects and in areas of the clinical crown where dentin is exposed. Small carious and precarious areas can be restored with amalgam, silicate cement, or resin. The restoration is usually confined to the area of involvement (Figs. 4-26 and 4-27).

The occlusal third of the first permanent molar frequently shows gross evidence of hypoplasia, and treatment is necessary before the tooth erupts sufficiently to permit restoration with a gold inlay or gold crown. The chrome steel crown will suffice

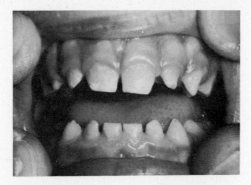

Fig. 4-24. Enamel hypoplasia in a 2½-year-old child. The child's mother had rubella in the sixth week of pregnancy. (Courtesy Dr. Robert Musselman.)

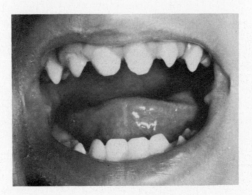

Fig. 4-25. Mother of this child had rubella in the eighth week of pregnancy. The primary teeth were tapered and presented a rough hypoplastic surface. The child had a patent ductus arteriosus, pulmonary stenosis, and mental retardation. There was also a history of difficult feeding and dehydration at age 2 months. (Courtesy Dr. Robert Musselman.)

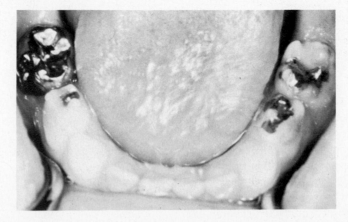

Fig. 4-26. Amalgam has been used to restore hypoplastic defects that have become carious on primary molars. A chrome steel crown was used to restore a tooth that was more severely affected.

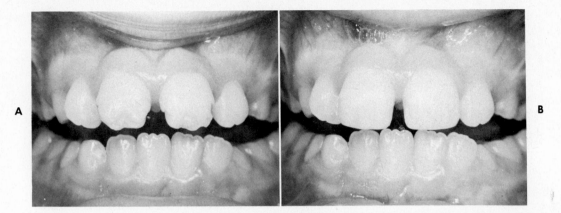

Fig. 4-27. A, Hypoplasia of the incisal third of the maxillary permanent central incisors. The lower incisors were unaffected, suggesting that there had been trauma to the maxillary primary incisors and resulting interference of matrix formation and calcification of the permanent incisors. **B,** The hypoplastic teeth have been restored with the acid etch resin technique.

as a restoration until a more adequate restoration can be made. Restorative procedures, referred to as the "acid etch resin techniques," have been shown to be effective in restoring anterior permanent teeth with hypoplastic defects in the incisal half of the crown. The techniques are described later in this chapter and also in Chapter 17. Acid etch resin techniques with the newer composite resins may also be used to provide interim restorations for many hypoplastic permanent molars to produce well-contoured restorations and to prevent gingival insult from steel crowns. Since the coronal pulp usually recedes more rapidly in hypoplastic teeth, preparation for a jacket crown or a cast crown if necessary is usually possible at an early age.

Hypoplastic primary and permanent teeth with large areas of defective enamel and exposed dentin may be sensitive as soon as they erupt. Satisfactory restoration is often impossible at this time. The topical application of 8% stannous fluoride has been found to decrease the sensitivity of the tooth. The application should be repeated as often as necessary to reduce sensitivity to thermal change and acid foods.

Hypoplasia caused by fluoride (dental fluorosis). Drinking water that contains in excess of 1 part per million (*ppm*) fluoride can affect the ameloblasts during the tooth formation stage and can cause the clinical entity referred to as "mottled enamel."

The appearance of enamel, which is affected in its formation by excessive fluoride in the water, varies considerably. Although the more severe cases of dental fluorosis are associated with a high level of fluoride consumption, there is apparently a great deal of individual variation. The enamel may have a white, opaque, or pitted appearance. The maxillary anterior teeth frequently have brown pigmentation.

Bhussry demonstrated in ground sections that the pigmentation is essentially limited to the outer third of the enamel. In these regions the structures of the rod sheath and the incremental lines were obscured by pigmentation. Bhussry also observed that the nitrogen content of the enamel was higher than normal. Ockerse and Wasserstein presented evidence that manganese is present in moderately and severely mottled enamel but not in normal enamel. It is not known whether only manganese compounds cause the mottling or whether stains from food and saliva are also causative factors. Attempts to remove brown stain from mottled teeth

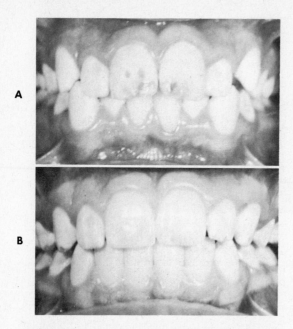

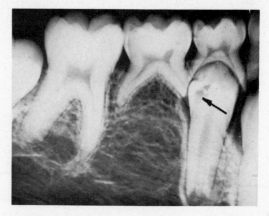

Fig. 4-29. Preeruptive "caries" on the crown of an unerupted first premolar *(arrow)*.

Fig. 4-28. A, Mottled enamel. The drinking water contained 9 ppm fluoride. Since the brown pigmentation was objectionable, the teeth were bleached. **B,** Much of the pigment has been removed by the bleaching process.

by bleaching have been somewhat successful, although the pigmentation tends to return gradually. Laminate veneer restorations have also been used successfully to mask the pigmentation. The bleaching and laminate veneer techniques are described in this chapter in the discussion of tetracycline discoloration of teeth. Several bleaching treatments will be necessary in order to bring about the desired result (Fig. 4-28).

Preeruptive "caries"

Occasionally defects on the crowns of developing permanent teeth are evident radiographically, even though no infection of the primary tooth or surrounding area is apparent (Fig. 4-29). Muhler refers to this condition as preeruptive "caries." Such a lesion does resemble caries when it is observed clinically, and the destructive nature of the lesion progresses if it is not restored. As soon as

the lesion is reasonably accessible, the tooth should be uncovered by removal of the overlying primary tooth or by surgical exposure. The carious-like dentin is then excavated and the tooth is restored with amalgam or a durable temporary restorative material. In some cases the lesion may be so extensive that indirect pulp therapy is justified (Fig. 4-30). Mueller and associates have reported "caries-like" resorption bilaterally in mandibular permanent second molars of a 12-year-old patient. Both lesions were successfully treated in a fashion similar to the treatment illustrated in Fig. 4-30.

Dentinogenesis imperfecta (hereditary opalescent dentin)

Dentinogenesis imperfecta is inherited as a simple autosomal dominant trait. Bixler, Conneally, and Christen observed this pattern in a six-generation family in which 34 members were studied. There was a 100% penetrance and consistent gene expression within a sibship. In a survey of 96,000 Michigan children, Witkop (1961) reported a prevalence of 1 in 8000 with the trait. The anomaly may be seen in conjunction with osteogenesis imperfecta (Fig. 4-31). A decade later, Witkop suggested that there are two distinct diseases. He recommends the term "hereditary opalescent dentin" for the disease that occurs as an isolated trait

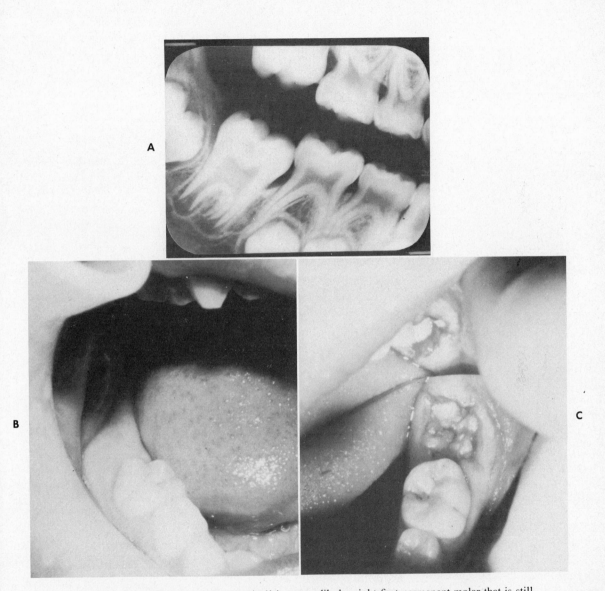

Fig. 4-30. A and **B,** Preeruptive "caries" in a mandibular right first permanent molar that is still unerupted. **C,** Mirror view of the lesion on the occlusal surface of the unerupted tooth.

Continued.

Fig. 4-30, cont'd. D, Mirror view of excavated cavity after gross "caries" removal. **E,** Mirror view of temporary restoration 1 week postoperatively (dark spot on mesial marginal ridge area is an artifact). **F,** Nine months postoperatively patient had continued normal root development and eruption of the tooth. The temporary restoration remained 3 months before the tooth was reentered and restored with amalgam. (Courtesy Drs. George E. Krull and James R. Roche.)

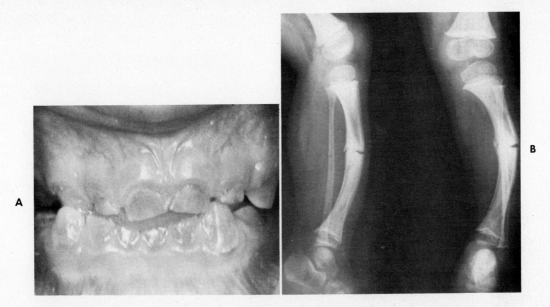

Fig. 4-31. A, Five-year-old girl with dentinogenesis imperfecta and osteogenesis imperfecta. The child had sustained numerous fractures of the long bones. **B,** A fracture of the tibia is evident in the radiograph.

and the term "dentinogenesis imperfecta" for that which occurs in conjunction with osteogenesis imperfecta. Shields, Bixler, and El-Kafrawy recognized the difference and proposed a new classification: the dentin defect that occurs in association with osteogenesis imperfecta is termed "type I dentinogenesis imperfecta" and that which occurs as an isolated trait is termed "type II dentinogenesis imperfecta."

The clinical picture of dentinogenesis imperfecta is one in which the primary and permanent teeth are a characteristic reddish brown to gray opalescent color. Soon after the primary dentition is complete, enamel often breaks away from the incisal edge of the anterior teeth and the occlusal surface of the posterior teeth. The exposed soft dentin abrades rapidly, occasionally to the extent that the smooth polished dentin surface is continuous with the gingival tissue (Fig. 4-32).

Radiographs show slender roots and bulbous crowns. The pulp chamber is small or entirely absent, and the pulp canals are small and ribbonlike (Fig. 4-33). These conditions emphasize the primary mesodermal defect. Periapical rarefaction in the primary dentition is occasionally observed. However, no satisfactory explanation has been offered, since the condition apparently is not related to pulp exposures and pulpal necrosis. Multiple root fractures are often seen, particularly in older patients.

The permanent teeth often seem to be of better quality and have less destruction. Occasionally they appear essentially normal clinically (Fig. 4-34). A histologic examination shows enamel and dentin of normal structure, and the dentinoenamel junction is not unlike that found in normal teeth. However, some have related the fracturing of the enamel to a lack of scalloping at the dentinoenamel junction. The dentinal tubules are greatly reduced in number, and they appear to be irregular and branching.

Hursey and associates described the mantle layer

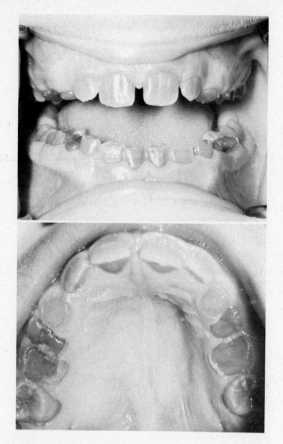

Fig. 4-32. Dentinogenesis imperfecta. The primary teeth are severely abraded. Enamel is breaking away from the incisal edge of the lower permanent central incisors.

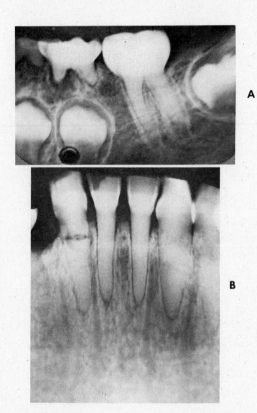

Fig. 4-33. A, Slender roots with ribbonlike pulp canals and bulbous crowns are characteristic of dentinogenesis imperfecta. The primary molars show periapical rarefaction. **B,** Root fractures are common in older patients.

of dentin as resembling that seen in normal teeth. The remainder of the dentin shows prominent incremental lines. The cells, cell remnants, and tubules are located for the most part in the path of these lines. As a result of the histologic study of these teeth, the authors concluded that the primary odontoblasts form normal-appearing dentin for only a limited time. Then they probably degenerate and become incorporated in a matrix in various stages of preservation. The presence of these cell remnants and tubules in the matrix causes a weakening of the tooth at this point. The mesenchymal cells of pulp differentiate from odontoblast-like

cells, which have a limited capacity to form a fully organized dental matrix. These cells then degenerate after a short period and are incorporated in the matrix of the dentin. This process is repeated until obliteration of the pulp chamber results.

The treatment of dentinogenesis imperfecta in both the primary and permanent dentitions is difficult. The placement of chrome steel crowns on the primary posterior teeth may be considered a means of preventing gross abrasion of the tooth structure. Chapter 26 describes the full restoration of the permanent dentition affected by the hereditary anomaly. Full cast crowns are placed on the molars. The

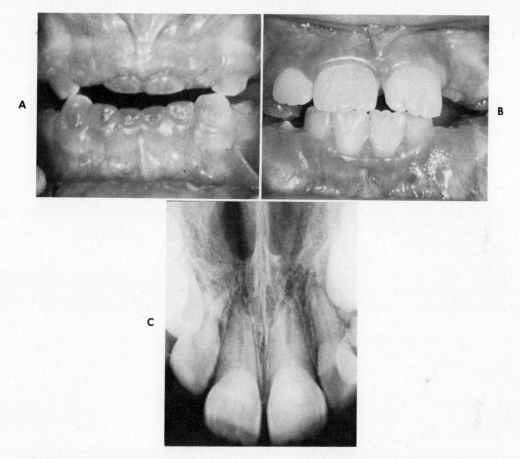

Fig. 4-34. A, Four-year-old child with dentinogenesis imperfecta. **B,** The permanent teeth, in contrast to the primary teeth, are normal in color. **C,** The radiograph shows the typical picture of dentinogenesis imperfecta.

premolar teeth and those anterior to them are covered with metal-ceramic restorations. This approach to restoring the teeth to functional and esthetic standards represents a major achievement in helping patients with this dental anomaly. Laminate veneer restorations on anterior teeth have also been successful in esthetic improvement for patients with dentinogenesis imperfecta when full coverage restorations were unnecessary.

Teeth that have periapical rarefaction and root fracture should be removed. Extraction of the affected teeth is difficult because of the brittleness of the dentin.

True carious lesions have been observed in affected teeth. However, the caries process seems to progress slowly and to be influenced by the abrasion of the tooth surface.

Amelogenesis imperfecta

Amelogenesis imperfecta that affects the enamel of both the primary and permanent dentition is generally accepted as a hereditary defect. The anomaly occurs in the general population in the range of 1 in 14,000 to 1 in 16,000 and has a wide range of clinical appearances. At least three different clinical variations of amelogenesis imperfecta are ob-

Table 4-1. Amelogenesis imperfecta and modes of inheritance

Amelogenesis imperfecta type	Mode of inheritance*
Hypocalcified	AD and AR
Hypomaturation	XLR, AR, and AD (?)
Hypoplastic	AD and XLD

*AD, autosomal dominant; AR, autosomal recessive; XLR, sex-linked recessive; XLD, sex-linked dominant.

served: the hypocalcified type, the hypomaturation type, and the hypoplastic type. Burzynski, Gougalez, and Snawder have suggested several modes of inheritance for amelogenesis imperfecta (Table 4-1). Chaudhry and associates (1959), however, have reported that a few children have been observed to demonstrate enamel dysplasia without hereditary background.

Congleton and Burkes reported three cases of amelogenesis imperfecta in which the patients also demonstrated taurodontism of the teeth. Others have identified the occurrence of amelogenesis imperfecta and taurodontism along with anomalies of the hair and bones (tricho-dento-osseous syndrome).

The defective tooth structure is limited to the enamel. On radiographic examination the pulpal outline appears to be normal, and the root morphology is not unlike that of normal teeth. The difference in the appearance and quality of the enamel is thought to be due to the state of enamel development at the time the defect occurs. In the hypoplastic type the enamel matrix appears to be imperfectly formed; although calcification subsequently occurs in the matrix and the enamel is hard, it is defective in amount and has a roughened, pitted surface (Fig. 4-35). In the hypocalcified type, matrix formation appears to be of normal thickness, but calcification is deficient and the enamel is soft (Fig. 4-36). In both of these more common types of the defect the enamel becomes stained because of the roughness of the surface and the increased permeability.

In still another variation of amelogenesis imperfecta there is a thin, smooth covering of brownish

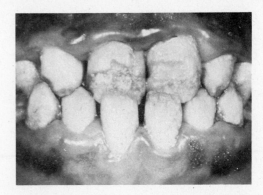

Fig. 4-35. Both the primary and permanent teeth are affected by the hereditary anomaly amelogenesis imperfecta. The enamel is pitted but hard.

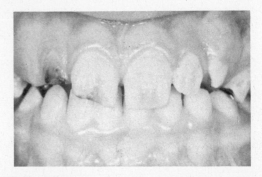

Fig. 4-36. Hypocalcification type of amelogenesis imperfecta. The primary teeth were similarly affected. The enamel surface is soft.

yellow enamel. In this type the enamel does not seem excessively susceptible to abrasion or caries (Figs. 4-37 and 4-38).

The treatment of amelogenesis imperfecta depends on the severity and the demands for esthetic improvement. Since the dentin structure is normal, the teeth can be prepared for porcelain jacket crowns. The coronal pulp seems to recede more rapidly than in normal teeth, possibly as the result of a thin, imperfectly formed enamel covering. Therefore, jacket crown preparations can often be made for relatively young patients. Laminate veneer restorations may offer a more conservative alternative for the management of the esthetic problem of the anterior teeth.

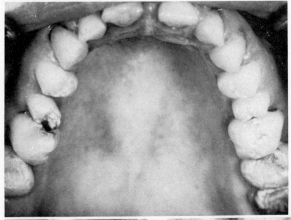

A

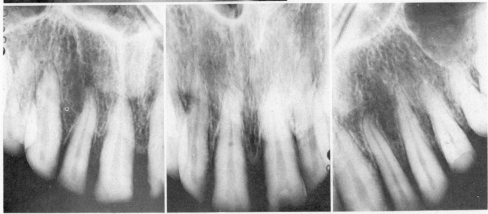

B

Fig. 4-37. A, Case diagnosed as amelogenesis imperfecta. The permanent teeth have a thin covering of pigmented enamel. **B,** The radiographs show essentially normal root morphology. The crowns have a thin covering of enamel.

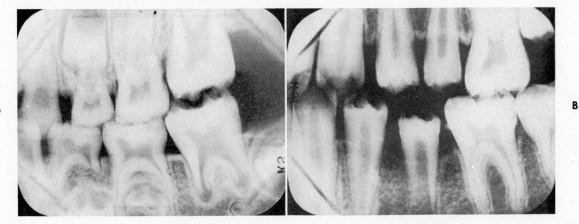

A

B

Fig. 4-38. A and **B,** Left bite-wing radiographs of a patient with amelogenesis imperfecta. Radiograph in **B** was made 6 years after radiograph in **A** and demonstrates the maintenance of a caries-free dentition in spite of the thin enamel.

Enamel and dentin aplasia

Observation of teeth that have some characteristics of both dentinogenesis imperfecta and amelogenesis imperfecta has been reported in the literature. Chaudhry and associates (1961) reported such an observation and referred to it as "odontogenesis imperfecta."

Schimmelpfennig and McDonald observed a similar dentition and referred to it as "enamel and dentin aplasia." The primary teeth were essentially devoid of enamel, and the smooth, severely abraded dentin was reddish brown. Radiographs showed normal alveolar bone around the roots of the teeth. Two teeth had pulp exposure and pulpal degeneration (Fig. 4-39). Radiolucent areas were present at the apices of the two primary teeth with exposed and degenerated pulps. The pulp chambers and canals in all the primary teeth were extremely large, with no evidence that the pulp chambers and canals were becoming obliterated. In ground sections of the primary teeth the dentinal tubules showed little evidence of a normal growth pattern. They were few and irregular, with a tendency toward branching (Fig. 4-40). The cementum appeared normal and was acellular. There was no evidence of secondary dentin formation. A few fragments of enamel adhering to the dentin appeared thinner than normal, and few normal morphologic characteristics were present. The dentinoenamel junction was atypical in that it lacked the characteristic scalloping.

The permanent teeth, when they erupted, were partially covered with a thin, gray, poorly coalesced coating of enamel. Brown dentin could be seen on the labial aspect of the central incisors and at the base of the fissures of the first permanent molars.

Gold overlays were constructed for the remaining primary teeth to prevent continued abrasion and pulp exposure. Chrome steel crowns were placed on the first permanent molars and the lower permanent incisors (Fig. 4-41).

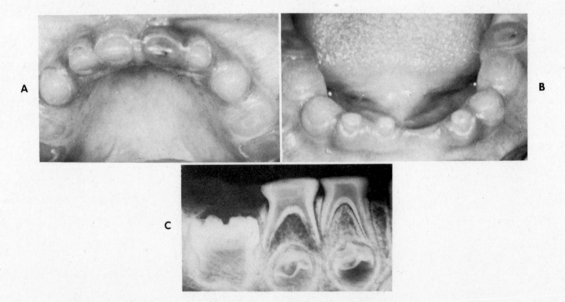

Fig. 4-39. A and **B,** Severely abraded teeth are almost entirely devoid of enamel. The outline of a large pulp chamber can be seen through a thin covering of dentin. The mandibular second primary molars have pulp exposure. **C,** Radiograph shows large pulp canals and large pulp chambers. Apical rarefaction is associated with pulp exposure of the second primary molar.

Shell teeth

Rushton reported an anomalous type of dental development in which the pulp chambers and canals were so enlarged that little more than a shell of enamel and dentin remained. This condition, which has some of the characteristics of dentinogenesis imperfecta, is referred to as "shell teeth" (Fig. 4-42). In this condition normal dentin formation is confined to a thin layer next to the enamel and cementum, followed by a layer of disorderly dentin containing few tubules. The roots of shell teeth are short, and the primary teeth may be exfoliated prematurely.

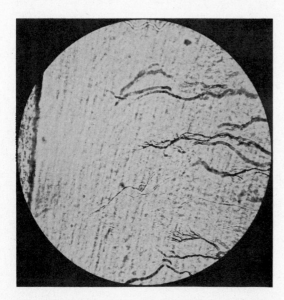

Fig. 4-40. Ground section of an extracted primary tooth. The dentinal tubules are sparse, irregular, and branching.

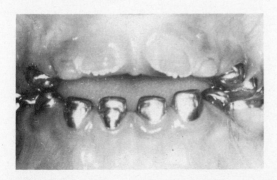

Fig. 4-41. Permanent incisors had an incomplete covering of enamel. Chrome steel crowns and gold overlays were constructed to protect the teeth from continual abrasion.

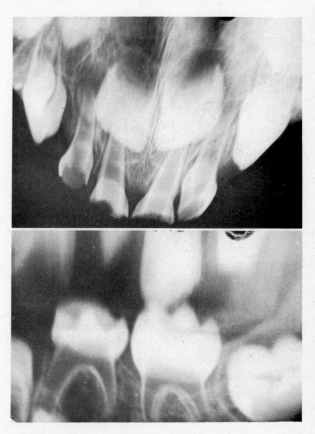

Fig. 4-42. Shell teeth. The large size of the pulp cavities indicates the nonexistence of secondary dentin.

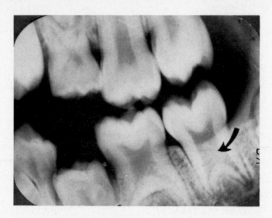

Fig. 4-43. Taurodontism. Note the elongated pulp chamber and short root canals *(arrow).*

Taurodontism

A survey of the literature on this anomaly by Lysell credits Keith with giving the name to the phenomenon known as "taurodontism." There is a tendency for the body of the tooth to enlarge at the expense of the roots. The pulp chamber is elongated and extends deeply into the region of the roots (Fig. 4-43). A similar condition is seen in the teeth of cud-chewing animals such as the ox (Latin, *taurus*).

Mena observed a mother and seven children, four of whom showed evidence of taurodontism in the permanent and/or primary teeth. His was probably the first report of taurodontism of the primary dentition as a definite family trait in black children.

The clinical significance of the condition becomes apparent if vital pulp therapy or root canal therapy is necessary.

Congenital absence of teeth

Anodontia. Anodontia, which implies complete failure of the teeth to develop, is a rare condition. It has been reported as one of the manifestations of a severe form of ectodermal dysplasia. The other manifestations are hypotrichosis, anhidrosis, and asteatosis. Secondary characteristics of ectodermal dysplasia include a deficiency in salivary flow,

protuberant lips, and a saddle nose appearance. The skin is often dry and scaly, and there is fissuring at the corners of the mouth.

Since the absence of teeth predisposes the child to a lack of growth of the alveolar process, the construction of dentures is complicated. However, as might be expected in an ectodermal dysplasia, skeletal structures are normal.

Serial headplate radiographs during childhood and adolescence have shown that the development of the jaw occurs in an essentially normal manner. A deficiency in sweat glands causes an increased body temperature, and children with ectodermal dysplasia are extremely uncomfortable during hot weather. Many of them must reside in cool climates. Children with ectodermal dysplasia have normal mentality and a normal life expectancy.

Oligodontia (partial anodontia). The congenital absence of primary teeth is relatively rare. When a number of the primary teeth fail to develop, other ectodermal deficiencies are usually evident. Children with a number of missing primary and permanent teeth may have some or all of the signs of ectodermal dysplasia.

Observations at Indiana University indicate that oligodontia with associated ectodermal dysplasia, like color blindness, may be inherited as a sex-linked recessive characteristic. The gene is transmitted from an affected man to all his daughters because it is in his X chromosome. These daughters will be normal, although heterozygous, because the gene for anodontia is recessive and is dominated by the corresponding normal gene in the homologous chromosome. However, half of the daughters' sons by a normal man will receive an affected chromosome from their mother and will have the defect. In contrast to a sex-linked inheritance, an autosomal recessive gene may be transmitted through several generations without the defect being evident. Consanguineous marriages in a family carrying the recessive gene may cause it to be dominant. For ectodermal dysplasia to occur in the female individual, it is generally believed that the affected person would have to inherit two affected chromosomes, one from each parent. Thus

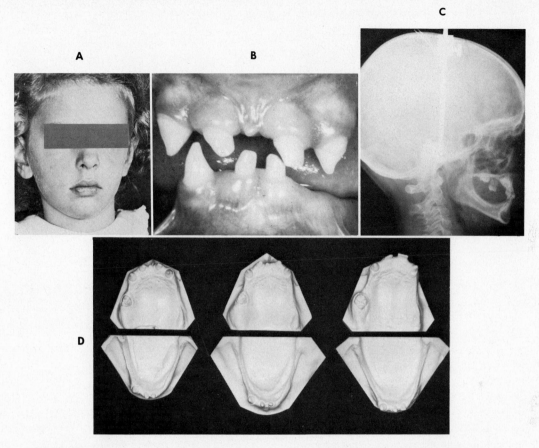

Fig. 4-44. A, Four-year-old girl with many features of ectodermal dysplasia. There was a history of consanguinity. **B,** The anterior teeth were small and conical in shape. The lack of development of the alveolar process is evident in the photograph. **C,** The facial pattern was good even though many primary and permanent teeth were missing. **D,** Partial dentures were constructed, modified, and remade as additional teeth erupted. The models show how growth has occurred in the mandible and maxilla.

inbreeding makes this condition much more likely (Fig. 4-44). Bartlett indicates that a number of females showing all the typical manifestations of ectodermal dysplasia have been reported.

The size of the primary teeth that are present may be normal or reduced. The anterior teeth are often conical, which is characteristic of oligodontia associated with an ectodermal dysplasia. The primary molars without permanent successors have an unexplained tendency to become ankylosed.

Children with a large number of missing primary teeth can have partial dentures constructed at an early age; 2-year-old and 3-year-old children have worn partial dentures successfully. Their ability to masticate food has increased, and their nutritional status has definitely improved. A partial denture may be adjusted or remade at intervals to allow for the eruption of permanent teeth. Thus there is no need for concern that the partial dentures will cause an unfavorable change in the growth pattern.

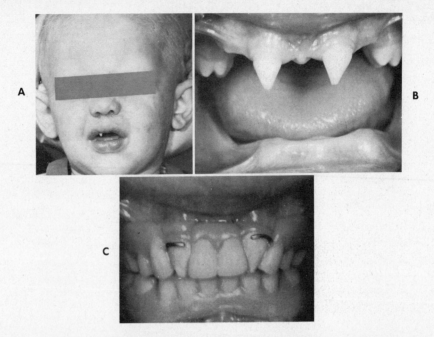

Fig. 4-45. A, Two-year-old boy with characteristics of ectodermal dysplasia. Many primary and permanent teeth are congenitally missing. The skin is dry, and the hair is sparse. **B,** The anterior primary teeth are typically conical. **C,** A full mandibular denture and a partial maxillary denture were constructed at 2½ years of age.

Growth of the arches will progress along a fairly normal pattern with or without the dentures in place. Denture construction at an early age is desirable, however, to reduce the psychologic problem that may cause the child to feel ''different'' and to ensure masticatory efficiency (Fig. 4-45).

If the permanent teeth erupt in good position and in favorable relationship to each other, partial dentures may serve until the child is old enough for fixed bridgework. Orthodontic treatment may be necessary before this procedure, as described in Chapter 26.

Swallow reported an 11-year-old boy who had a complete primary dentition but no permanent dentition. A comparable situation is shown in Fig. 4-46. Laird reported a similar case with a complete primary dentition, but the only permanent teeth were maxillary first permanent molars. It appears that there is no predetermined pattern for the miss-ing primary or permanent teeth. Congenital absence of one or more of the permanent teeth without evidence of ectodermal dysplasia is a common occurrence. When one tooth or only a few teeth are missing, the condition is known as ''hypodontia.''

A ''tooth and nail'' type of autosomal dominant ectodermal dysplasia is described in reports by Giansanti, Long, and Rankin. The ectodermal dysplasia demonstrated a familial pattern and was characterized by hypoplastic nails, hypodontia, and fine-textured hair.

Bennett and Ronk reported an unusual case of a 4-year-old boy with three missing primary teeth. The mother related that the two missing mandibular central incisors erupted a few days after birth (neonatal teeth) and were removed because of a lack of root formation. The maxillary left first primary molar was congenitally missing as well. A

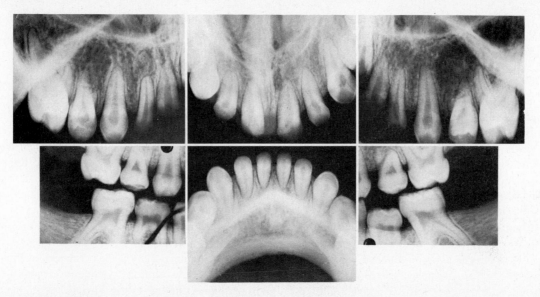

Fig. 4-46. Fourteen-year-old girl with a complete primary dentition but without evidence of permanent teeth.

panoramic radiograph of the patient also revealed the absence of multiple permanent tooth buds. The child did not exhibit any other signs or symptoms of ectodermal dysplasia, he appeared normal in every other way, and there was no known familial history of missing teeth.

Any one of the 32 permanent teeth may be missing. However, those most frequently missing in children are the mandibular second premolars, maxillary lateral incisors, and maxillary second premolars. This order of frequency has been confirmed in studies by Glenn and by Grahnen. The absence of teeth may be unilateral or bilateral. Glenn observed during an examination of 1702 children that 5% had a missing permanent tooth other than a third molar. Glenn's study suggests that there has been an increase in the prevalence of missing permanent teeth when compared with estimates 30 years ago. In 97% of the children the formation of the second premolar could be detected radiographically at 5½ years of age and that of the lateral incisor at 3½ years of age.

Acid etch resin techniques have improved the ability to provide esthetic interim restorations and greater function for patients with conical teeth with or without oligodontia or hypodontia. Goepferd and Carroll reported on the esthetic and prosthetic management of a patient with ectodermal dysplasia. There was anodontia in the mandible. The patient had two permanent molars, one primary molar (all microdonts), and four peg-shaped and widely spaced permanent incisors. Habilitative treatment with excellent results consisted of acid etch resin restorations and orthodontic repositioning of the incisors, a maxillary partial denture, and a mandibular complete denture. Goepferd and Carroll reported no complications from the appliances in over 2 years of use. The restoration of conical teeth has also been successfully achieved with laminate veneer restorations. The treatment of patients with congenitally missing premolars is discussed further in Chapters 20, 21, and 26.

When maxillary lateral incisors are missing, the occlusion and arches must be analyzed carefully to determine whether there is sufficient room within the arch to maintain space and to provide fixed bridgework. If space for a normal-sized lateral incisor replacement is insufficient, the orthodontist may choose to move the canine forward into the lateral position and reshape it to make it appear more like a permanent lateral incisor.

Pigmentation of teeth (intrinsic)

The primary teeth occasionally have unusual pigmentation. Certain conditions arising from the pulp can cause the whole tooth to appear discolored. Factors causing these conditions include blood-borne pigment, blood decomposition within the pulp, and drugs used in procedures such as root canal therapy. Color changes related to traumatic injury are discussed in Chapter 17.

Pigmentation in erythroblastosis fetalis. The condition of erythroblastosis is characterized by an excessive destruction of erythrocytes. The peripheral blood has many nucleated red cells, whereas anemia develops from excessive hemolysis.

Nelson and others believe that erythroblastosis fetalis is based on immunization of an Rh-negative mother by Rh-positive red cells of the fetus or perhaps by previous transfusion of Rh-positive blood cells. The mother produces an anti-Rh agglutinin. The passage of this soluble substance into the circulation of the infant causes the complete destruction of the fetal erythrocytes. Immunization of the mother occurs slowly. Usually one or more pregnancies with an Rh-positive fetus are necessary for the development of a sufficient amount of anti-Rh agglutinin to harm the fetus.

If an infant has had severe, persistent jaundice during the neonatal period, the primary teeth may have a characteristic blue-green color (Fig. 4-47), although in a few instances brown teeth have been observed. The color of the pigmented tooth is gradually reduced. The fading in color is particularly noticeable in the anterior teeth.

Via stated that there is no evidence for the existence of prenatal jaundice in children with Rh incompatibility. The staining of the dentin, which occurs after birth and is probably a matter of profusion of bilirubin and biliverdin into the dentin, is similar to the internal staining of the tooth after the rupture of vessels as a result of trauma.

Pigmentation in porphyria. A rare genetic disturbance of porphyria metabolism occurring in humans and animals is characterized by the excessive production of pigment in the body. The condition is often observed at birth, or it may develop during infancy.

Children with congenital porphyria have red-colored urine, are hypersensitive to light, and develop blisters on their hands and face. Their teeth are purplish brown as a result of the deposition of porphyrin in the developing structures. Dunsky, Freeman, and Gibson reported that a 17-month-old girl passed red urine several hours after birth. When her primary teeth erupted, they were purplish brown.

In congenital porphyria the permanent teeth also show evidence of intrinsic staining (Fig. 4-48).

Pigmentation in cystic fibrosis. A high percentage of children with cystic fibrosis have teeth that are dark in color, ranging from yellowish gray to dark brown. Zegarelli and associates have suggested that tooth discoloration in persons with cystic fibrosis is a result of the disease alone or therapeutic agents, especially tetracyclines, or a combination of the two factors. Patients afflicted with cystic fibrosis are usually subjected to large amounts of tetracyclines during childhood. Primosch reported on tetracycline tooth discolorations, enamel defects, and dental caries in 86 young patients with cystic fibrosis. The incidence of dental caries in these patients was compared to control subjects matched for sex, race, exposure to optimally fluoridated water, chronologic age, and dental age. The findings indicated a high prevalence of tooth discolorations and enamel defects but a significantly reduced caries experience in the patients with cystic fibrosis who had received the tetracycline drugs. Cohen and Parkins have reported success in the bleaching of tetracycline-stained teeth in children with cystic fibrosis in a preliminary study, using a technique similar to that described in this chapter.

Pigmentation in tetracycline therapy. In recent years dentists and physicians have observed

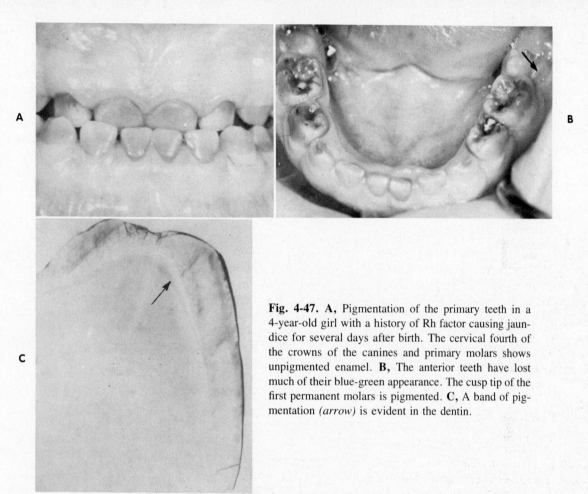

Fig. 4-47. A, Pigmentation of the primary teeth in a 4-year-old girl with a history of Rh factor causing jaundice for several days after birth. The cervical fourth of the crowns of the canines and primary molars shows unpigmented enamel. **B,** The anterior teeth have lost much of their blue-green appearance. The cusp tip of the first permanent molars is pigmented. **C,** A band of pigmentation *(arrow)* is evident in the dentin.

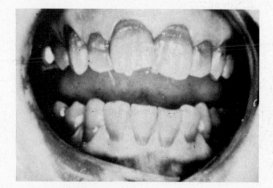

Fig. 4-48. In congenital porphyria the primary and permanent teeth have a purplish brown color. (From Finn, S.E., and others: Clinical pedodontics, ed. 3, Philadelphia, 1967, W.B. Saunders Co.)

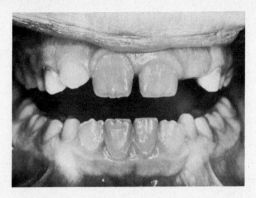

Fig. 4-49. Pigmentation in tetracycline therapy. The permanent incisors that have erupted demonstrate an objectionable yellowish brown color.

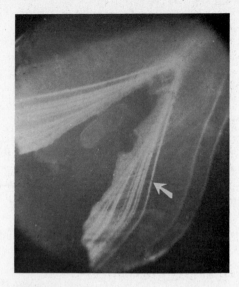

Fig. 4-50. Ground section of a primary tooth. Tetracycline has been deposited in the dentin *(arrow)* and to a lesser extent in the enamel.

that children who have received tetracycline during the period of calcification of the primary or permanent teeth show a degree of pigmentation of the clinical crowns of the teeth. The crowns of the teeth are discolored, ranging from yellow to brown and from gray to black (Fig. 4-49).

Mull has reported that the deposition of the drug in the teeth is thought to be the result of its chelating properties with the formation of a tetracycline–calcium orthophosphate complex. The exposure of the teeth to light results in slow oxidation, with a change in color of the pigment from yellow to brown. The larger the dose of drug relative to body weight, the deeper the pigmentation. The duration of exposure to the drug may be less important than the total dose relative to body weight. Hennon has reported that a survey of 1707 children, 5 to 11 years of age, revealed that 3.5% exhibited tetracycline pigmentation of the teeth.

The tetracycline will be deposited in the dentin and to a lesser extent in the enamel of teeth that are calcifying during the time the drug is administered. The location of the pigment in the tooth can be correlated with the stage of development of the tooth and time and duration of drug administration. The tetracyclines, yellow in color, fluoresce under ultraviolet light (Fig. 4-50). The compounds undergo oxidation on exposure to light. When tetracyclines in the dental structures darken from yellow to brown, the fluorescence diminishes because of the destruction of the fluorophore.

Since tetracyclines can be transferred through the placenta, the crowns of the primary teeth may also show marked discoloration if tetracyclines are administered during pregnancy. Moffitt and associates have observed that the critical period for tetracycline-related discoloration in the primary dentition is 4 months in utero to 3 months postpartum for maxillary and mandibular incisors and 5 months in utero to 9 months postpartum for maxillary and mandibular canines. The sensitive period for tetracycline-induced discoloration in the permanent maxillary and mandibular incisors and canines is 3 to 5 months postpartum to about the seventh year of the child's life. The maxillary lateral incisors are an exception because they begin to calcify at 10 to 12 months postpartum.

Several tetracycline analogues available to the practitioner can induce different degrees of discoloration in intact teeth. Tetracyclines can be grouped in two categories: those causing severe tooth discoloration (epianhydrotetracycline, demethylchlortetracycline, tetracycline hydrochloride, and tetracycline-L-methylene lysine) and those causing less tooth discoloration (chlortetracycline, methacycline, doxycycline, oxytetracycline, and anhydrotetracycline).

Teeth with tetracycline pigmentation occasionally show evidence of enamel hypoplasia. This is true for both the primary and the permanent teeth. It may be that the illness for which the drug is given rather than the tetracycline drug itself is responsible for the enamel hypoplasia, but this has not yet been proved.

Although pediatric tetracycline drops were withdrawn from the market in 1978, they continue to be used frequently in children, according to a 1979 report by the Food and Drug Administration. Other liquid forms of tetracyclines were allowed to remain on the market because they are needed for geriatric patients. However, the figures from the *National Disease and Therapeutic Index* (July 1978 to June 1979) show that 60% of the prescriptions for tetracycline liquid were written for children from birth to 9 years, while patients over age 65 account for only 6% of the drug's consumption. Similarly, 80% of the prescriptions for tetracycline congener liquid were written for children under the age of 9. The report also pointed out that tetracycline liquids and tetracycline congener liquids may cause depression of bone growth, permanent discoloration of the teeth, and enamel hypoplasia if administered to women during the last half of pregnancy or to children under 9 years of age. The report concluded that tetracyclines should not be used in this age group unless other drugs are not likely to be effective or are contraindicated. Ray, Federspiel, and Schaffner corroborate the reports of excessive use of tetracycline drugs in children, and they also recommend using alternative drugs whenever possible. Dentists should discreetly discourage their medical colleagues from prescribing tetracycline drugs to pregnant women and children 9 years of age or younger.

Clinical studies at Indiana University, using a technique described by Arens, Rich, and Healey, have been successful in improving the appearance of tetracycline-stained teeth. The armamentarium and technique for bleaching vital teeth are as follows. After a careful polishing of the clinical crowns of the affected anterior teeth, the gingival tissue in the upper arch is covered with a petrolatum jelly. A rubber dam is placed over the maxillary anterior teeth, and clamps are placed over the rubber dam on the first premolars. Each tooth is separately ligated to prevent leakage of the 35% hydrogen peroxide* onto the gingival tissues, which could result in a surface burn. The teeth are then scrubbed with cotton matting saturated with a mixture of equal parts chloroform and ethyl alcohol to dissolve any surface stain remaining on the teeth. The teeth should then be dried with warm air.

The bleaching solution is a mixture of 35% hydrogen peroxide (Superoxol) and ethyl ether (5 parts peroxide to 1 part ether). Because ethyl ether is volatile and peroxide decomposes rapidly at room temperature, the drugs should be refrigerated and mixed immediately before each bleaching procedure. An open flame as a heat source is to be avoided if ether is used.

The ether-peroxide preparation may be placed in a small glass container, and a mass of cotton approximately 6 cm long and 1.5 cm wide is placed in the container and saturated with bleaching fluid. The wet cotton may then be placed over the labial surfaces of the isolated teeth. The cotton should be kept moist but not to the extent that the liquid runs off. A Union Broach–Indiana University bleaching instrument† (Fig. 4-51) should be preset at about 120° F (49° C) with the gold-plated spoon attached to the handle. The spoon should be placed on the cotton and gently pressed against each tooth surface for several seconds at a time. If the patient experiences discomfort, the spoon should be removed. The procedure should be continued for

---

*It is essential that a fresh solution of hydrogen peroxide be used for each bleaching procedure. The solution, which has a 30-day shelf life, is available in 4-ounce bottles from the Union Broach Co., 36-40 Thirty-Seventh Street, Long Island City, N.Y. 11101.

†Union Broach Dental Specialties Catalogue, 1970.

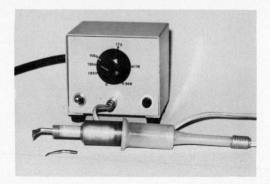

Fig. 4-51. Union Broach–Indiana University bleaching instrument.

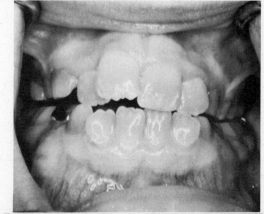

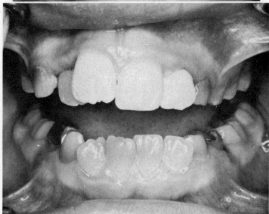

Fig. 4-52. A, Tetracycline-pigmented teeth. **B,** The maxillary incisors have been bleached; the lower mandibular incisors are untreated.

approximately 20 to 30 minutes with frequent reapplication of the solution and the intermittent application of heat. A comparison of the lingual tooth color will give an indication of the degree of bleaching. It is usually desirable to repeat the procedure on the lingual surface.

At the end of the bleaching procedure the patient's head is lowered over an emesis basin and the teeth and rubber dam are sprayed with warm water. With the rubber dam and ligates removed, the mouth can be cleansed of the lubricant. The patient may experience a transitory sensitivity of the teeth. Usually two or more treatments are necessary at weekly intervals to bring about desired results.

If the lower teeth are visible during conversation, it is desirable to carry out the same procedure in the mandibular arch (Fig. 4-52).

This bleaching procedure has been known to be most effective for the yellow-brown discolorations. Teeth affected with gray-black shades may become lighter after bleaching, but the color usually persists. However, bleaching the teeth reduces the pigment oxidation process as the teeth continue to be exposed to light, thereby minimizing their continued darkening with time.

Seale, McIntosh, and Taylor evaluated the effects of 35% hydrogen peroxide and heat, as used in the bleaching technique, on the pulps of dogs' teeth. The histologic examinations demonstrated the reversible nature of the pulpal irritation created

by the bleaching procedure. The heat alone was not detrimental to the pulp tissue. Hydrogen peroxide applied to enamel surfaces alone or in combination with heat caused some obliteration of odontoblasts, hemorrhage, resorption, and inflammatory infiltration in the pulp tissue. These pulpal changes demonstrated evidence of reversibility after 60 days. The pulpal reaction is undoubtedly responsible for the patient's sensitivity soon after the bleaching procedures.

If the discoloration is severe and bleaching does not adequately improve the condition, the dentist may consider masking the labial surfaces with laminate veneer restorations (Fig. 4-53). A common

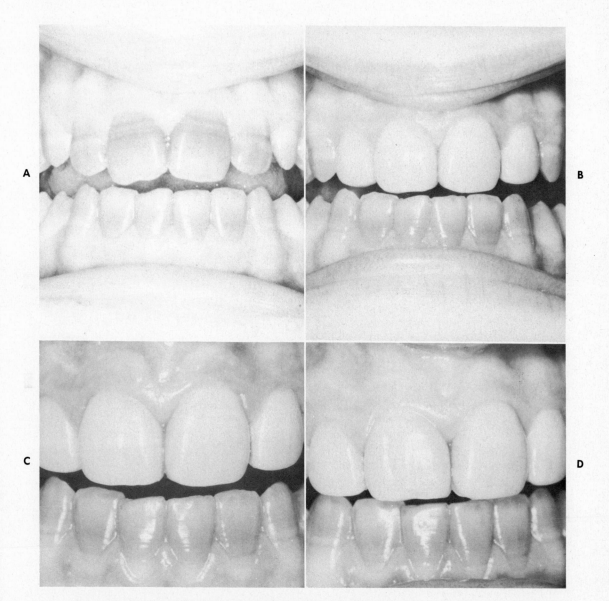

Fig. 4-53. A, The vital bleaching procedure did not significantly improve the gray tetracycline discoloration shown here. **B,** The four maxillary incisors were restored 6 months earlier with laminate veneer restorations. **C,** Close-up view of the restorations 6 months postoperatively. Oral hygiene instructions concerning plaque control at the gingival margins were reemphasized. **D,** The restorations 2 years postoperatively. The gingival health has been compromised somewhat (compared with preoperative health), but the gingival sulcus depths are still acceptable.

problem confronting dentists who treat children is the esthetic management of anterior teeth that are discolored, developmentally malformed, or fractured. Dentists recognize that esthetic impairments of the teeth often adversely affect the social and psychologic development of the growing child. The frustration associated with solving this problem has been significantly alleviated in recent years with the development of improved restorative resin systems and the acid etch technique. A recent advance is the use of thin, prefitted plastic facings (laminate veneers) that are bonded to the labial surfaces of affected anterior teeth.

Interest in laminate veneer restorations has grown steadily since their introduction by Faunce. These restorations for maxillary anterior teeth are now being recognized as conservative, esthetically satisfactory alternatives to the more traditional full-coverage restorations, especially in children and young adults. The successful use of laminate veneers on mandibular anterior teeth has also been reported, but occlusal interferences and increased stress on the mandibular restorations during function could limit their application in the lower arch.

The laminate veneer technique offers esthetic improvement because the restored teeth project the natural hue and appearance of normal healthy tooth structure. When properly finished, the laminate restorations are well tolerated by the gingival tissues even though their contour is slightly excessive. Immaculate oral hygiene is essential, but experience has shown the maintenance of gingival health around the restorations is certainly possible in cooperative patients.

The basic procedure, which has several variations, involves luting custom-fitted resin veneers onto etched enamel of labial surfaces of teeth. The luting materials must be tooth-colored restorative resin systems designed for use in enamel etching techniques and chemically compatible with the plastic veneers to achieve adequate bonding at both the tooth-resin and resin-resin interfaces. The materials may be autopolymerizing or light poly-

merizing, depending on the dentist's preference. If the teeth being treated are severely discolored, a resin opaquing agent may be cured to the etched surface to mask the dark areas before luting the veneer to the tooth. The laminate veneer procedure is not complicated, but it requires meticulous attention to detail for success.

The veneers are thin (less than 0.5 mm) and heat and pressure cured. Their highly polished acrylic facings provide better esthetic effect and surface durability than conventional direct restorative resin materials. They are custom fitted to the surfaces to which they will be luted. Fitting the veneers may be accomplished by laboratory fabrication on a stone model, by hollow grinding selected acrylic denture teeth or facings, or by custom grinding selected preformed labial veneers* that have been specifically designed for the laminate technique. This last approach offers a more time- and cost-efficient procedure and is available in a self-cure kit, an ultraviolet light–cure kit, and a visible light–cure kit. The visible light–cure system is recommended because it seems to offer more advantages.

Preformed laminate veneers of the appropriate size are selected for each tooth by first measuring the incisocervical and mesiodistal dimensions of the tooth and then referring to the veneer mold guide in the kit. Next, the selected veneers are adapted to fit the labial surfaces of the teeth by shaping their peripheral outline and grinding the inside of the veneers with a small white stone. Although the veneers may be adapted directly on the patient's teeth at chairside, an indirect adaptation on an accurate stone model of the teeth is recommended. The indirect method can be performed by a dental auxiliary. It also allows the opportunity to obtain closer adaptation of the veneers when needed by heat treating the thermoplastic veneers directly against the replicated labial surfaces on the stone model.

---

*Mastique Laminate Veneer System, L.D. Caulk Co., Milford, Del. 19963.

Ideally a veneer should completely cover the labial surface. It should fit just to the gingival margin without causing tissue blanching—flush with the incisal edge and just slightly beyond the proximal line angles of the tooth. In other words, it should cover all visible areas of the tooth from an anterior view.

The teeth to be veneered are thoroughly cleaned with a pumice slurry and rubber cup. The shade of composite luting material is selected, and the teeth are isolated. Rubber dam isolation is ideal, but often the rubber dam material will interfere with the proper adaptation of the veneer cervically, especially when the teeth have not fully erupted. Thorough cotton roll isolation or lip retractors* may be used instead of the rubber dam; however, special attention must be given to controlling crevicular fluid that may otherwise flow onto the labial surfaces.

Next, the close adaptation of the laminates to the labial tooth surfaces is confirmed by trial fit; usually no additional grinding is necessary. The inside surface of each laminate is then swabbed with laminate cleaner and painted with two thin coatings of laminate primer. Then they should be set aside to dry for 5 minutes.

While the laminates are drying, the labial enamel of each tooth is conditioned (etched) with the phosphoric acid tooth conditioner. The conditioner may be applied with a small brush or saturated cotton pellet. Pressure should be avoided during the application, and the surfaces should be kept moist during the 60-second conditioning process. The teeth are then thoroughly washed with an air-water spray and dried with clean, oil-free air. The enamel should have a dull, frosted appearance. It is important to keep the labial surfaces clean and dry from this point until the veneers are placed and cured.

A thin layer of sealant or opaquer is painted onto the etched and dry enamel surfaces and cured with the visible light instrument.* The opaquer material is needed to mask severely discolored areas. Additional layers of the opaquing agent may be added and cured over the first layer until the desired amount of masking is obtained. Clear plastic matrix strips may be used to separate the adjacent teeth and prevent bonding them together when the sealant or opaquer is cured. The strips are not necessary if the operator clears each proximal contact area with unwaxed dental floss before the material is cured.

Next, the inside surfaces of the fitted veneers (previously set aside to dry) are completely but sparingly coated with the selected shade of composite paste. Different shades may be blended and incisal toner may also be used to achieve the desired hues. The paste should be spread evenly and without entrapment of air. Each veneer is then individually and gently pressed onto its corresponding labial surface until it is properly positioned and comes to a positive stop against the tooth. During this procedure, the excess paste will be forced out at the veneer margins and removed with hand instruments. Again, the use of plastic matrix strips or unwaxed dental floss to clear proximal contacts will prevent tooth-to-tooth bonding. After the excess paste has been removed, the restoration is exposed to the visible light instrument to complete polymerization of the materials. This procedure is repeated for each laminate veneer restoration. Multiple restorations may be placed at one time after the operator has gained experience with the technique.

The margins of the restorations are finished to a smooth feather edge in the conventional manner. A No. 7901 finishing bur is recommended for the gingival, incisal, and embrasure areas (Fig. 4-54). The proximal contact areas are finished with interproximal strips. The margins are further refined with a rubber cup polisher, using a slurry of flour of pumice followed by a composite polishing

---

*Clear and Dry, L.D. Caulk Co., Milford, Del. 19963.

*Prisma-Lite, L.D. Caulk Co., Milford, Del. 19963.

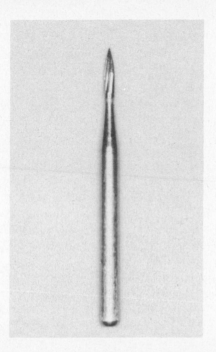

Fig. 4-54. The No. 7901 finishing bur is made of carbide steel, has 12 flutes, and fits the friction grip handpiece. Most of the marginal trimming of the laminate restoration may be done with this bur.

paste. Esthetically pleasing restorations are the result (Figs. 4-55 to 4-57).

Micrognathia

Micrognathia is usually considered a congenital anomaly; however, the condition may be acquired in later life. The mandible is most often affected (Fig. 4-58). The cause of congenital micrognathia is unknown. However, deficient nutrition of the mother and intrauterine injury resulting from pressure or trauma have been suggested.

Infants with mandibular micrognathia have difficulty in breathing and episodes of cyanosis and must be kept in a ventral position as much as possible. The anterior portion of the mandible is positioned so far back that the tongue has little if any support and can fall backward, causing an obstruction.

The treatment of congenital micrognathia is directed toward adequate function of the mandible. Since the infant should be made to reach for the nipple of the nursing bottle, the bottle should never be allowed to rest against the mandible. Davis and Dunn devised an extension for the nursing bottle

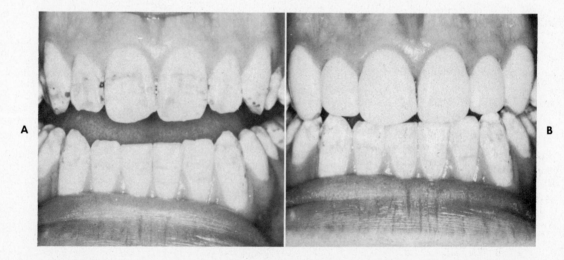

Fig. 4-55. A, Severe mottled enamel caused by dental fluorosis. **B,** Immediate postoperative result with laminate restorations. The mesial incisal angle of the maxillary right central incisor could have been restored to more normal contour as well. Minimal tissue damage occurred during finishing.

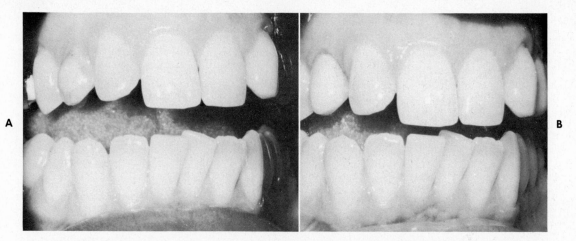

Fig. 4-56. A, This patient has congenitally missing maxillary lateral incisors, and the permanent canines erupted into the lateral incisor positions leaving unsightly retained primary canines. **B,** One restored primary canine immediately after restoration. The laminate should have extended farther into the mesial embrasure.

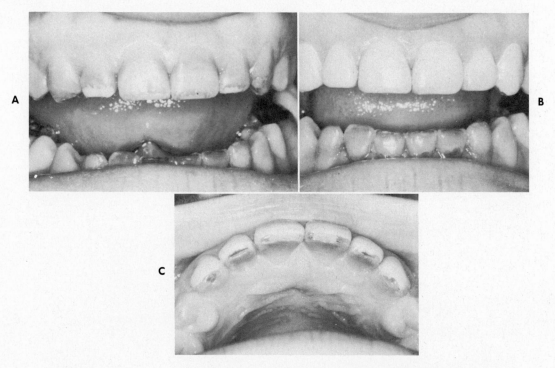

Fig. 4-57. A, Severe tetracycline discoloration with hypoplastic defects. The incisal areas of the four maxillary incisors had been previously restored with resin. **B,** Result with laminate restorations 6 months postoperatively. **C,** Incisal view of the restorations illustrates their excessive labial contour.

that rests against the maxilla and holds the bottle away from the mouth. Thus the infant must extend the mandible in order to feed.

Pruzansky and Richmond reported as a result of longitudinal growth studies that in most instances of congenital micrognathia the increment in mandibular growth as related to total facial growth is sufficient to overcome the extreme recessiveness of the chin at birth. Since mandibular growth continues until late adolescence, it is possible to hope for an esthetically pleasing profile in adulthood.

Acquired micrognathia may develop gradually and may not be evident until 4 to 6 years of age. This anomaly in growth is usually related to heredity. Ankylosis of the jaw caused by a birth injury or trauma in later life may result in an acquired type of micrognathia. Infection in the temporomandibular joint area can also cause arrested growth at the head of the condyle, and the acquired pattern of micrognathia develops. In cases of true ankylosis of the mandible, arthroplasty or ostearthrotomy should be recommended.

Anomalies of the tongue

Child patients rarely complain of symptomatic tongue lesions. However, the tongue should be inspected carefully during the examination procedure. A number of benign conditions may be evident that should be brought to the attention of the parents.

Burket described four main types of papillae on the dorsum of the tongue. Large circumvallate papillae, 8 to 12 in number, may be found on the posterior border of the dorsum. These papillae have a blood supply and are the site of a large number of taste buds. Mushroom-shaped fungiform papillae may be distributed over the entire dorsum of the tongue; however, they are present in a greater number at the tip and toward the lateral margins of the tongue. Inflammatory and atrophic changes occurring on the dorsum of the tongue may involve the vascularized fungiform papillae. The most numerous papillae of the tongue are the filiform, which are thin and hairlike and are evenly distributed over the dorsal surface. The filiform

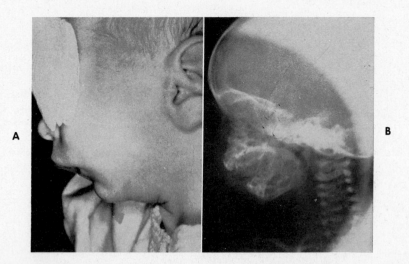

Fig. 4-58. A, Micrognathia in a girl 1 month old. The chin was noticeably recessive. **B,** The radiograph shows the extent of the development of the dentition at birth. At 1 year of age the micrognathia was less noticeable.

papillae are without a vascular core, and their continuous growth is slight. The foliate papillae represent a fourth type and are arranged in folds along the lateral margins of the tongue; the taste sensation is associated with these papillae.

Macroglossia. Macroglossia refers to a tongue that is larger than normal; this condition may be either congenital or acquired in type. Congenital macroglossia, which is due to an overdevelopment

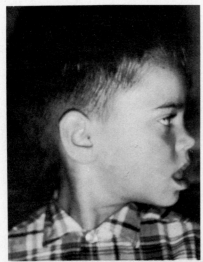

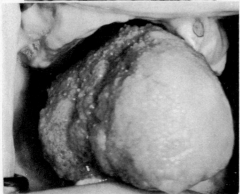

Fig. 4-59. Congenital macroglossia. The tongue can be observed to protrude from the mouth. There was a flaring of the lower anterior teeth. (Courtesy Dr. W.B. Davis.)

of the lingual musculature, becomes increasingly apparent as the child develops (Fig. 4-59).

An abnormally large tongue is characteristic of cretinism, in which case the tongue is fissured and may extend from the mouth. Macroglossia may also be evident to a lesser degree in Down syndrome. Occasionally an allergic reation will cause a transitory enlargement of the tongue (angioneurotic edema). Both the allergic reaction and the traumatic injury can cause such severe enlargement of the tongue that a tracheotomy is necessary to maintain an airway.

A disproportionately large tongue may cause both an abnormal growth pattern of the jaw and malocclusion. Flaring of the lower anterior teeth and an Angle Class III malocclusion are occasionally the result of macroglossia.

The treatment of macroglossia depends on its cause. Surgical removal of a wedge-shaped portion of the tongue is occasionally necessary.

Ankyloglossia (tongue-tie). A short lingual frenum extending from the tip of the tongue to the floor of the mouth and onto the lingual gingival tissue limits movements of the tongue and causes speech difficulties (Fig. 4-60). Stripping of the lingual tissues may occur if the tongue-tie is not corrected (Fig. 4-61). Surgical reduction of the abnormal lingual frenum is indicated if it interferes with the infant's nursing. In the older child a reduction of the frenum should be recommended only if local conditions warrant the treatment.

Ayers and Hilton reported a case of ankyloglossia in a 7-year-old boy who had been evaluated at his school for a speech problem. The patient had previously had routine dental examinations, but no treatment had been suggested by the dentist. Tongue mobility and speech patterns improved markedly after the frenum attachment was released surgically (lingual frenectomy). The patient and parents reported very little postoperative discomfort. This history and the results are similar to those of the 6-year-old girl with ankyloglossia illustrated in Fig. 4-62.

Fissured tongue. A fissured tongue is seen in a

small number of children and may be of no clinical significance, although it is sometimes associated with cretinism and Down syndrome. The fissures on the dorsum of the tongue usually have a symmetric pattern and may be longitudinal in direction or at right angles to the margin of the tongue. Robinson suggested that vitamin B complex deficiency may be associated with the fissuring. Treatment of the fissured tongue is generally unnecessary unless a mild inflammation develops at the base of the fissures from an accumulation of food debris. Brushing of the tongue and improved oral hygiene aid in reducing the inflammation and soreness.

Coated tongue. A white coating of the tongue is usually associated with local factors rather than with a disturbance of the gastrointestinal system, as was originally believed. The amount of coating on the tongue varies with the time of the day and is related to oral hygiene and the character of the diet. The coating consists of food debris, microorganisms, and keratinized epithelium found on and around the filiform papillae (Fig. 4-63).

Children who have a congenital or acquired deficiency in salivary flow will have a coated tongue, occasionally to the extent that a dry crust appears on the dorsum of the tongue. Systemic disease with associated fever and dehydration will also cause a coating that is usually white but may become stained with foods or drugs.

White strawberry tongue. An enlargement of the fungiform papillae extending above the level of the white desquamating filiform papillae gives an appearance of an unripe strawberry. The condition is seen in at least half the cases of scarlet fever in young children. During the course of scarlet fever and other acute febrile conditions the coating disappears, and the enlarged red papillae extend above a smooth denuded surface, giving the appearance of a red strawberry or raspberry. The tongue will return to normal after recovery from the systemic condition.

Black hairy tongue. The condition referred to as black hairy tongue is rarely seen in children but occurs in young adults and has been related to the oral and systemic intake of antibiotics (Fig. 4-64). The filiform papillae on the middle third of the

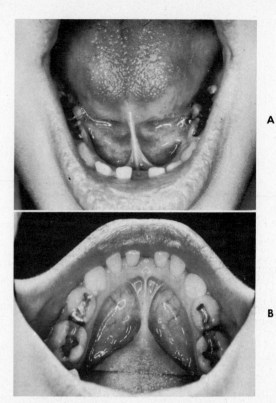

Fig. 4-60. A, Ankyloglossia (tongue-tie). A short, heavy lingual frenum extends from the top of the tongue to the floor of the mouth and onto the lingual tissue. **B,** A mirror view of the abnormal frenum.

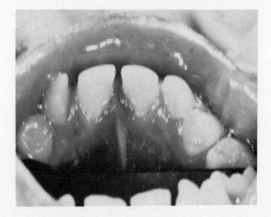

Fig. 4-61. Stripping of the lingual gingival tissue caused by the short lingual frenum extending into the area.

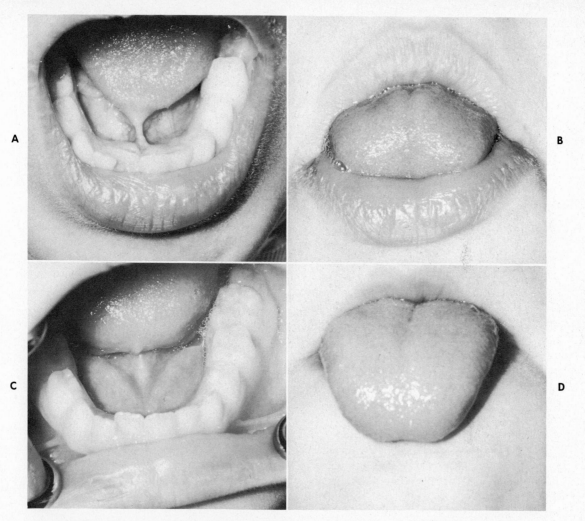

Fig. 4-62. A, Ankyloglossia in a 6-year-old girl. **B,** Patient had limited tongue mobility and speech problems. **C,** Two weeks after surgical release. **D,** Tongue mobility and speech improved spontaneously.

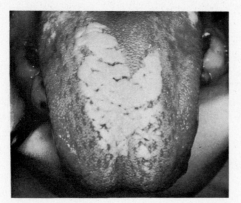

Fig. 4-63. White coating of the tongue is usually associated with local factors.

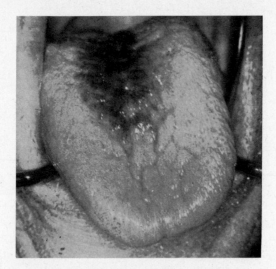

Fig. 4-64. Black hairy tongue. This condition usually has no clinical significance.

tongue become elongated into hairlike processes, sometimes as long as 1 inch. Certain antibiotics, including penicillin and tetracyclines, suppress the drug-sensitive microorganisms and allow the resistant bacilli, cocci, and fungi to multiply. Heavy keratin tips develop on the filiform papillae and are not shed in the acid environment of the protective covering that develops on the tongue as a result of a change in the oral flora. The condition is asymptomatic, is without real significance, and usually disappears without treatment.

Geographic tongue (benign migratory glossitis). A wandering-type lesion, which is essentially limited to children and is probably the most common tongue anomaly, is known as geographic tongue. Rahaminioff and Muhsam observed a 14% prevalence of migratory glossitis in 5000 children 2 years old and younger. Meskin, Redman, and Gorlin have observed the incidence of geographic tongue among college students to be 1.1%.

Although the cause of geographic tongue is unknown, Burket suggested that the condition is caused by a bacterial or fungoid infection. Banoczy, Szabo, and Csiba have indicated that gastrointestinal disturbances associated with anemia may

be related to tongue symptoms. In addition, a psychosomatic background should be considered as a possible etiologic factor. Histologically, the process appears to be superficial with desquamation of the keratin layers of papilla and inflammation of the corium.

Geographic tongue is often detected during routine dental examination of child patients, who often are unaware of the condition. Red, smooth areas devoid of filiform papillae appear on the dorsum of the tongue. The margins of the lesion are well developed and slightly raised. The involved areas enlarge and migrate by extension of the desquamation of the papillae at one margin of the lesion and regeneration at the other (Fig. 4-65). Every few days a change can be noted in the pattern of the lesions. The condition is self-limited, however, and no treatment is necessary.

Indentation of the tongue margin (crenation). During the examination of the child patient the dentist may notice a scalloping or crenation along the lingual periphery of the tongue. Careful examination will reveal the markings to be caused by the tongue lying against the lingual surfaces of the mandibular teeth. Although it is not usually possible to attach any significance to these crenations, they have been related to pressure habits, macroglossia, vitamin B complex deficiency, and systemic disease that causes a reduction of muscle tone.

Median rhomboid glossitis. Median rhomboid glossitis is a congenital abnormality of the tongue that appears clinically as an oval, rhomboid, or diamond-shaped reddish patch or plaque on the dorsal surface immediately anterior to the circumvallate papillae. A flat or slightly raised area, sometimes mamillated, it stands out distinctly from the rest of the tongue because it has no filiform papillae.

The term "glossitis" is misleading, since the lesion is not inflammatory. It is presumably caused by failure of the tuberculum impar to retract or withdraw before fusion of the lateral halves of the tongue, so that a structure devoid of papillae is interposed between them. It is most obvious clini-

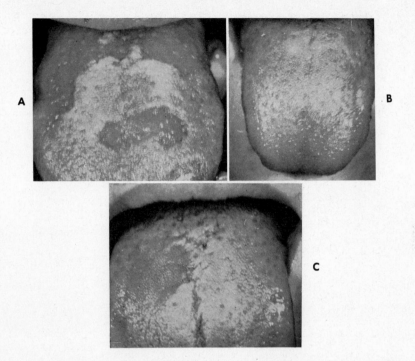

Fig. 4-65. A, Geographic tongue. The smooth areas are devoid of filiform papillae. **B,** The pattern observed at the initial visit is indistinguishable 4 weeks later. **C,** In 1 year a new pattern is developing on the dorsum of the tongue.

cally when the rest of the tongue appears coated or when the papillae are heavy and matted.

Traumatic injury to the tongue. A child may bite his or her tongue as a result of a traumatic injury or a fall. The dentist may inadvertently traumatize the tongue with a disk or bur during operative procedures. The copious flow of blood that usually follows such an injury is probably one reason for a low incidence of infection.

Deep laceration of the tongue requires suturing to minimize the scarring and to aid in the control of hemorrhage. In cases of severe traumatic injury the tongue should be examined carefully to detect any enlargement that might interfere with the maintenance of an open airway.

Abnormal labial frenum

A maxillary midline diastema is frequently seen in preschool children and in those in the mixed den-

tition stage. It is important to determine whether the diastema is normal for that particular time of development or is related to an abnormal maxillary labial frenum.

A midline diastema may be considered normal for many children during the time of eruption of the permanent maxillary central incisors. When the incisors first erupt, they may be separated by bone, and the crowns incline distally because of the crowding of the roots. With the eruption of the lateral incisors and the permanent canines, the midline diastema will be reduced, and in most cases normal contact between the central incisors will develop.

Insufficient tooth mass in the maxillary anterior region, the presence of peg lateral incisors, or the congenital absence of lateral incisors may cause a diastema. Other factors and anomalies, including a midline supernumerary tooth, an oral habit, macro-

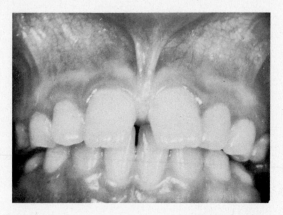

Fig. 4-66. Abnormal labial frenum. There is blanching of the free marginal tissue between the central incisors and also of the palatine papilla. A frenectomy is indicated.

glossia, and abnormally large mandibular anterior teeth, should be considered as possible causes (in addition to an abnormal labial frenum) of the midline diastema.

The labial frenum is composed of two layers of epithelium enclosing a loose vascular connective tissue. Muscle fibers, if present, are derived from the orbicularis oris muscle.

The origin of the maxillary frenum is at the midline on the inner surface of the lip. The origin is often wide, but the tissue of the frenum itself narrows in width and is inserted in the midline into the outer layer of periosteum and into the connective tissue of the internal maxillary suture and the alveolar process. The exact attachment site is variable. It can be several millimeters above the crest of the ridge or on the ridge, or the fibers may pass between the central incisors and attach to the palatine papilla.

Walls suggested that the frenum may be attached to the palatine papilla at birth, but that with the development of the alveolar ridge and teeth the position of the frenum changes. As growth progresses, the frenum may atrophy and may assume a higher position or maintain its attachment to the papilla. The assumption that an abnormal frenum can be diagnosed in the infant and that surgical

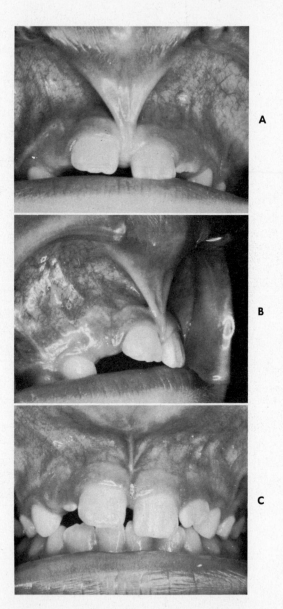

Fig. 4-67. A, Abnormal labial frenum in an 8-year-old child. The heavy, fan-shaped band of tissue interfered with speech and presented an undesirable appearance. **B,** An oblique view of the abnormal frenum. **C,** A much more desirable appearance is noted 6 months after the frenectomy.

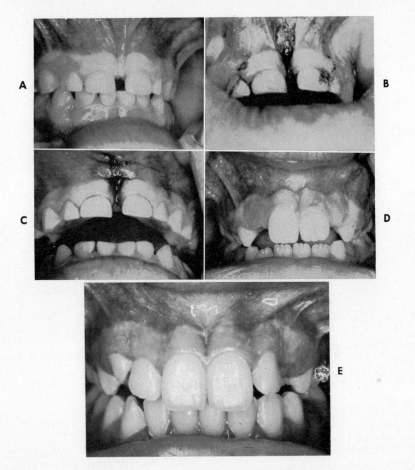

Fig. 4-68. A, Abnormal labial frenum observed in a preschool-age child is causing a diastema between the primary central incisors and is interfering with normal movement of the upper lip. **B,** A wedge-shaped section of tissue including the frenum has been removed. **C,** Two sutures have been placed to approximate the tissue margins. **D,** The permanent incisors have erupted. No reattachment of the frenum fibers has occurred. **E,** A desirable result of the frenectomy is evident 5 years after the surgical procedure.

reduction is necessary at this age cannot be substantiated. In the past, many dentists delayed considering an abnormal labial frenum as the cause of the diastema until all the maxillary permanent anterior teeth, including the canines, had erupted. This approach may be considered generally correct. However, other diagnostic points should be kept in mind.

A simple diagnostic test for an abnormal frenum can be carried out by observing the location of the alveolar attachment when intermittent pressure is exerted on the frenum. If a heavy band of tissue with a broad, fanlike base is attached to the palatine papilla and produces blanching of the papilla, it is safe to predict that the frenum will unfavorably influence the development of the anterior occlusion (Fig. 4-66).

The abnormal labial frenum, in addition to causing a midline diastema, can produce other undesirable clinical conditions. The heavy band of tissue and low attachment can interfere with toothbrushing by making it difficult to place the brush at the proper level in the vestibule to brush in the conventional manner. If fibers of the frenum attach into the free marginal tissue, stretching of the lip during mastication and speech may cause stripping of the tissue from the neck of the tooth. Such attachment may also cause the accumulation of food particles and eventual pocket formation. The abnormal frenum may restrict movements of the lip, may interfere with speech, and may produce an undesirable cosmetic result (Fig. 4-67).

Frenectomy. The decision regarding treatment of the labial frenum should be made only after a careful evaluation to determine whether the result will be undesirable if the condition is allowed to remain.

In the surgical technique a wedge-shaped section of tissue is removed, including the tissue between the central incisors and the tissue extending palatally to the nasal palatine papilla (Figs. 4-67 and 4-68). Lateral incisions are made on either side of the frenum to the depth of the underlying bone. The free marginal tissue on the mesial side of the central incisors should not be disturbed. The wedge of tissue can be picked up with tissue forceps and excised with tissue shears at an area close enough to the origin of the frenum to provide a desirable cosmetic effect. Sutures are placed inside the lip to approximate the free margin of the tissue. It is generally unnecessary to suture or pack the tissue between the incisors.

REFERENCES

American Dental Association: Accepted dental therapeutics, ed. 38, Chicago, 1979, The Association.

Arens, D.E., Rich, J.J., and Healey, H.J.: A practical method of bleaching tetracycline-stained teeth, Oral Surg. **34**:812-817, 1972.

Avery, D.R.: Improving esthetics with laminate veneers. In McDonald, R.E., and others, editors: Current therapy in dentistry, vol. 7, St. Louis, 1980, The C.V. Mosby Co.

Avery, D.R.: The use of preformed acrylic veneers for the aesthetic treatment of severely discolored anterior permanent teeth, Int. Dent. J. **30**(1):49-53, 1980.

Ayers, F.J., and Hilton, L.M.: Treatment of ankyloglossia: report of case, J. Dent. Child. **44**:237-239, 1977.

Baer, P.N., Brown, N.C., and Hammer, J.E., III: Hypophosphatasia: report of two cases with dental findings, Periodontics **2**:209-215, 1964.

Banoczy, J., Szabo, L., and Csiba, A.: Migratory glossitis: a clinical-histologic review of seventy cases, Oral Surg. **39**:113-121, 1975.

Bartlett, R.C., Eversole, L.R., and Adkins, R.S.: Autosomal recessive hypohidrotic ectodermal dysplasia: dental manifestations, Oral Surg. **33**:736-742, 1972.

Bauer, W.H.: Effect of periapical processes of deciduous teeth on the buds of permanent teeth, Am. J. Orthod. **32**:232-241, 1946.

Bennett, C.G., and Ronk, S.L.: Congenitally missing primary teeth: report of case, J. Dent. Child. **47**:346-348, 1980.

Bhussry, B.R.: Studies on mottled enamel, I.A.D.R. (abstract), March 21, 1957, p. 9.

Bixler, D., Conneally, P.M., and Christen, A.G.: Dentinogenesis imperfecta: genetic variations in a six-generation family, J. Dent. Res. **69**:1196-1199, 1969.

Briggs, P.C.: Submandibular duct stenosis as a complication of Ludwig's angina, Oral Surg. **47**:14-15, 1979.

Bruce, K.W.: Dental anomaly: early exfoliation of deciduous and permanent teeth, J.A.D.A. **48**:414-421, 1954.

Burket, L.W.: Oral medicine: diagnosis and treatment, ed. 4, Philadelphia, 1961, J.B. Lippincott Co.

Burzynski, N.J., Gougalez, W.E., Jr., and Snawder, K.D.: Autosomal dominant smooth hypoplastic amelogenesis imperfecta, Oral Surg. **36**:818-823, 1973.

Chaudhry, A.P., and others: Hereditary enamel dysplasia, J. Pediatr. **54**:776-785, 1959.

Chaudhry, A.P., and others: Odontogenesis imperfecta: report of a case, Oral Surg. **14**:1099-1103, 1961.

Cohen, H.J., and Diner, H.: The significance of developmental dental enamel defects in neurological diagnosis, Pediatrics **46**:737-747, 1970.

Cohen, S., and Parkins, F.M.: Bleaching tetracycline-stained teeth, Oral Surg. **29**:465-471, 1970.

Congleton, J., and Burkes, E.J.: Amelogenesis imperfecta with taurodontism, Oral Surg. **48**:540-544, 1979.

Cranin, A.N., and Rockman, R.: Oral symptoms in histiocytosis X, J.A.D.A. **103**:412-416, 1981.

Davis, A.D., and Dunn, R.: Micrognathia: suggested treatment for correction in early infancy, Am. J. Dis. Child. **45**:799-806, 1933.

Delaney, G.M., and Goldblatt, L.I.: Fused teeth: a multidisciplinary approach to treatment, J.A.D.A. **103**:732-734, 1981.

Dunsky, I., Freeman, S., and Gibson, S.: Porphyria and porphyrinuria: report of a case; review of porphyrin metabolism with a study of congenital porphyria, Am. J. Dis. Child. **74**:305-320, 1947.

Eidelman, E.: Fusion of maxillary primary central and lateral incisors bilaterally, Pediatr. Dent. **3:**346-347, 1981.

Faunce, F.R., and Faunce, A.R.: The use of laminate veneers for restoration of fractured or discolored teeth, Tex. Dent. J. **93**(8):6-7, 1975.

Faunce, F.R., and Myers, D.R.: Laminate veneer restoration of permanent incisors, J.A.D.A. **93:**790-792, 1976.

Giansanti, J.S., Long, S.M., and Rankin, J.L.: The "tooth and nail" type of autosomal dominant ectodermal dysplasia, Oral Surg. **37:**576-582, 1974.

Glenn, F.B.: A consecutive six-year study of the prevalence of congenitally missing teeth in private practice of two geographically separated areas, J. Dent. Child. **31:**269-270, 1964.

Goepferd, S.J., and Carroll, C.E.: Hypohidrotic ectodermal dysplasia: a unique approach to esthetic and prosthetic management, J.A.D.A. **102:**867-869, 1981.

Goyan, J.E., and others: Pediatric tetracycline use, FDA Drug Bull. **9:**29-30, 1979.

Grahnen, H.: Hypodontia in the permanent dentition, Dent. Abs. **3:**308-309, 1957.

Greene, J.C.: Dimensions of unmet dental needs in U.S., Dent. Abs. **16:**385, 1971.

Gulmen, S., Pullon, P.A., and O'Brien, L.W.: Tricho-dento-osseous syndrome, J. Endodont. **2:**117-120, 1976.

Hennon, D.K.: Dental aspects of tetracycline therapy: literature review and results of a prevalence survey, J. Ind. Dent. Assoc. **44:**482-492, 1965.

Herman, S.C., and McDonald, R.E.: Enamel hypoplasia in cerebral palsied children, J. Dent. Child. **30:**46-49, 1963.

Hursey, R.J., Jr., and others: Dentinogenesis imperfecta in a racial isolate with multiple hereditary defects, Oral Surg. **9:**641-658, 1956.

Jorgenson, R.J., and Warson, R.W.: Dental abnormalities in tricho-dento-osseous syndrome, Oral Surg. **36:**693-700, 1973.

Kronfeld, R., and Schour, I.: Neonatal dental hypoplasia, J.A.D.A. **26:**18-32, 1939.

Laird, G.S.: Congenital anodontia, J.A.D.A. **51:**722, 1955.

Lawson, B.F., and Stout, F.W.: The incidence of enamel hypoplasia associated with chronic lead poisoning, S.C. Dent. J. **29:**5-10, 1971.

Lysell, L.: Taurodontism: a case report and a survey of the literature, Odontol. Rev. **13**(2):158-174, 1962.

McDonald, R.E., and Shafer, W.G.: Disseminated juvenile fibrous dysplasia of the jaws, Am. J. Dis. Child. **89:**354-358, 1955.

McKusick, V.A.: Heritable disorders of connective tissue, ed. 4, St. Louis, 1972, The C.V. Mosby Co.

Mena, C.A.: Taurodontism, Oral Surg. **32:**812-823, 1971.

Meskin, L.H., Redman, R.S., and Gorlin, R.J.: Incidence of geographic tongue among 3,668 students at the University of Minnesota, J. Dent. Res. **42:**895, 1963.

Mink, J.R.: Relationship of enamel hypoplasia and trauma in repaired cleft lip and palate, thesis, Indianapolis, 1961, Indiana University School of Dentistry.

Mitchell, D.F., Standish, S.M., and Fast, T.B.: Oral diagnosis/oral medicine, ed. 3, Philadelphia, 1978, Lea & Febiger.

Moffitt, J.M., and others: Prediction of tetracycline-induced tooth discoloration, J.A.D.A. **88:**547-552, 1974.

Mueller, B.H., and others: "Caries-like" resorption of unerupted permanent teeth, J. Pedod. **4:**166-172, 1980.

Muhler, J.C.: Effect of apical inflammation of the primary teeth on dental caries in the permanent teeth, J. Dent. Child. **24:**209-210, 1957.

Mull, M.M.: The tetracyclines and the teeth, Dent. Abs. **12:**346-350, 1967.

Musselman, R.J.: Dental defects and rubella embryopathy: a clinical study of fifty children, thesis, Indianapolis, 1968, Indiana University School of Dentistry.

Nelson, W.E., and others: Nelson's textbook of pediatrics, ed. 11, Philadelphia, 1979, W.B. Saunders Co.

Ockerse, T., and Wasserstein, B.: Stain in mottled enamel, J.A.D.A. **50:**536-538, 1955.

Oliver, W.J., and Owings, C.L.: Hypoplastic enamel associated with the nephrotic syndrome, Pediatrics **32:**399-406, 1963.

Pearl, M., and Roland, N.M.: Delayed primary dentition in a case of congenital lead poisoning, J. Dent. Child. **47:**269-271, 1980.

Peters, W.J.N.: Cherubism: a study of twenty cases from one family, Oral Surg. **47:**307-311, 1979.

Poland, C., III, and others: Histochemical observations of hypophosphatasia, J. Dent. Res. **51:**333-338, 1972.

Primosch, R.E.: Tetracycline discoloration, enamel defects, and dental caries in patients with cystic fibrosis, Oral Surg. **50:**301-308, 1980.

Pruzansky, S., and Richmond, J.B.: Growth of mandible in infants with micrognathia: clinical implications, Am. J. Dis. Child. **88:**29-42, 1954.

Purvis, R.J., and others: Enamel hypoplasia of the teeth associated with neonatal tetany: a manifestation of maternal vitamin D deficiency, Lancet **2:**811-814, 1973.

Rahaminioff, P., and Muhsam, H.F.: Some observations on 1,245 cases of geographic tongue, Am. J. Dis. Child. **93:**519-525, 1957.

Rattner, L.J., and Myers, H.M.: Occurrence of enamel hypoplasia in children with congenital allergies, J. Dent. Res. **41:**646-649, 1962.

Ray, W.A., Federspiel, C.F., and Schaffner, W.: The malprescribing of liquid tetracycline preparations, Am. J. Public Health **67:**762-763, 1977.

Ray, W.A., Federspiel, C.F., and Schaffner, W.: Prescribing of tetracycline to children less than 8 years old, J.A.M.A. **237:**2069-2074, 1977.

Robinson, H.B.G.: Diagnosis of oral lesions, Dent. Surv. **37:**1443-1446, 1587-1590, 1961.

Rushton, M.A.: New form of dentinal dysplasia: shell teeth,

Oral Surg. **7:**543-549, 1954.

Sarnat, B.G., and Schour, I.: Enamel hypoplasia (chronologic enamel aplasia) in relation to systemic disease: a chronologic, morphologic, and etiologic classification, J.A.D.A. **28:**1989-2000, 1941; **29:**67-75, 1942.

Schiffer, C.G., and Hunt, E.P.: Illness among children, Pub. No. 405, Washington, D.C., 1963, U.S. National Health Survey, U.S. Children's Bureau.

Schimmelpfennig, C.B., and McDonald, R.E.: Enamel and dentin aplasia: report of a case, Oral Surg. **6:**1444-1449, 1953.

Seale, N.S., McIntosh, J.E., and Taylor, A.N.: Pulpal reaction to bleaching of teeth in dogs, J. Dent. Res. **60:**948-953, 1981.

Sheldon, M., Bibby, B.G., and Bales, M.S.: Relationship between microscopic enamel defects and infantile disabilities, J. Dent. Res. **24:**109-116, 1945.

Shields, S.D., Bixler, D., and El-Kafrawy, A.M.: A proposal classification for heritable human dentin defects with a description of a new entity, Arch. Oral Biol. **18:**543-554, 1973.

Stein, G.: Enamel damage of systemic origin in premature birth and diseases of early infancy, Am. J. Orthod. **33:**831-841, 1947.

Swallow, J.N.: Complete anodontia of the permanent dentition, Br. Dent. J. **107:**143-145, 1959.

Thomas, J.G.: A study of dens in dente, Oral Surg. **38:**653-655, 1974.

Turner, J.E., Moore, D.W., and Shaw, M.T.: Prevalence and antibiotic susceptibility of organisms isolated from acute soft-tissue abscesses secondary to dental caries, Oral Surg. **39:**848-859, 1975.

Turner, J.G.: Two cases of hypoplasia of enamel, Br. J. Dent. Sci. **55:**227-228, 1912.

Via, W.F.: Personal communication.

Walls, J.T.: Indications and contra-indications for removal of the labial frenum, J. Oreg. Dent. Assoc. **15:**7-8, 1946.

Witkop, C.J., Jr.: Genetics and dental health, New York, 1961, McGraw-Hill Book Co., pp. 227-234.

Witkop, C.J., Jr.: Manifestations of genetic diseases in the human pulp, Oral Surg. **32:**278-316, 1971.

Zegarelli, E.V., and others: Discoloration of teeth in a 24-year-old patient with cystic fibrosis of the pancreas not primarily associated with tetracycline therapy, Oral Surg. **24:**62-64, 1967.

5 Eruption of the teeth: local, systemic, and congenital factors that influence the process

RALPH E. McDONALD

DAVID R. AVERY

Development of the teeth

A variety of developmental defects that are evident after eruption of the primary and permanent teeth can be related to systemic and local factors that influence the matrix formation and the calcification process. Thus it is important that the dentist be able to explain to the parents time factors related to the early stages of tooth calcification both in utero and during infancy.

Lunt and Law made a careful review of the literature on the calcification of the primary teeth. They compared their findings with the values shown in Table 5-1 of Logan and Kronfeld's chronology of the human dentition, which has been an accepted standard for many years. They offered a revised table that establishes earlier ages than the previously accepted value for initial calcification and a corrected sequence for calcification (Table 5-2). A similar review was carried out for the ages at which the primary teeth erupt.

Lunt and Law concluded after reviewing the work of Kraus and Jordan and of Nomata that the old table used in previous editions of this book should be modified. The sequence of calcification of the primary teeth should be changed to central incisor, first molar, lateral incisor, canine, and second molar. They determined that the times of initial calcification of the primary teeth are 2 to 6 weeks earlier than those used in Table 5-1. They also concluded that the maxillary teeth are generally ahead of the mandibular teeth in development. Exceptions are the second molars, which generally are advanced in the mandible, and the lateral incisors and canines, which at times may be ahead in the mandible.

Lunt and Law believe that their suggested modifications in the times of initial calcification should be confirmed with additional research using fetal specimens with accurate clinical histories for determination of age. For this reason we continue to include the original chronology chart while adding the important newer data of Lunt and Law.

In the past, the ages at which the primary teeth erupt have appeared as fixed values in a typical order, with mandibular teeth erupting first (Table 5-1). Lunt and Law suggest that this schedule also be modified. They conclude that the lateral incisor, first molar, and canine tend to erupt earlier in the maxilla than in the mandible; the Logan and Kronfeld table suggests eruption in the mandible to be generally ahead of that in the maxilla. The ages at which primary teeth erupt are confirmed in the recent literature to be later by 2 months or more than suggested in the Logan and Kronfeld table.

It should be remembered that the time of eruption of both primary and permanent teeth varies

Table 5-1. Chronology of the human dentition

	Tooth	Hard tissue formation begins	Amount of enamel formed at birth	Enamel completed	Eruption	Root completed
Deciduous dentition						
Maxillary	Central incisor	4 mo in utero	Five sixths	1½ mo	7½ mo	1½ yr
	Lateral incisor	4½ mo in utero	Two thirds	2½ mo	9 mo	2 yr
	Cuspid	5 mo in utero	One third	9 mo	18 mo	3¼ yr
	First molar	5 mo in utero	Cusps united	6 mo	14 mo	2½ yr
	Second molar	6 mo in utero	Cusp tips still isolated	11 mo	24 mo	3 yr
Mandibular	Central incisor	4½ mo in utero	Three fifths	2½ mo	6 mo	1½ yr
	Lateral incisor	4½ mo in utero	Three fifths	3 mo	7 mo	1½ yr
	Cuspid	5 mo in utero	One third	9 mo	16 mo	3¼ yr
	First molar	5 mo in utero	Cusps united	5½ mo	12 mo	2¼ yr
	Second molar	6 mo in utero	Cusp tips still isolated	10 mo	20 mo	3 yr
Permanent dentition						
Maxillary	Central incisor	3 - 4 mo		4 - 5 yr	7- 8 yr	10 yr
	Lateral incisor	10 -12 mo		4 - 5 yr	8- 9 yr	11 yr
	Cuspid	4 - 5 mo		6 - 7 yr	11-12 yr	13-15 yr
	First bicuspid	1½- 1¾ yr		5 - 6 yr	10-11 yr	12-13 yr
	Second bicuspid	2 - 2¼ yr		6 - 7 yr	10-12 yr	12-14 yr
	First molar	At birth	Sometimes a trace	2½- 3 yr	6- 7 yr	9-10 yr
	Second molar	2½- 3 yr		7 - 8 yr	12-13 yr	14-16 yr
	Third molar	7 - 9 yr		12 -16 yr	17-21 yr	18-25 yr
Mandibular	Central incisor	3 - 4 mo		4 - 5 yr	6- 7 yr	9 yr
	Lateral incisor	3 - 4 mo		4 - 5 yr	7- 8 yr	10 yr
	Cuspid	4 - 5 mo		6 - 7 yr	9-10 yr	12-14 yr
	First bicuspid	1¾- 2 yr		5 - 6 yr	10-12 yr	12-13 yr
	Second bicuspid	2¼-2½ yr		6 - 7 yr	11-12 yr	13-14 yr
	First molar	At birth	Sometimes a trace	2½- 3 yr	6- 7 yr	9-10 yr
	Second molar	2½- 3 yr		7 - 8 yr	11-13 yr	14-15 yr
	Third molar	8 -10 yr		12 -16 yr	17-21 yr	18-25 yr

From Logan, W.H.G., and Kronfeld, R.: J.A.D.A. **20:**379, 1933; modified by McCall and Schour.

Table 5-2. Modification of the table "Chronology of the Human Dentition" (Logan and Kronfeld, modified by McCall and Schour), suggested by Lunt and Law, for the calcification and eruption of the primary dentition

Deciduous tooth		Hard tissue formation begins (fertilization age in utero in wk)	Amount of enamel formed at birth	Enamel completed (mo after birth)	Eruption (mean age in mo, ± 1 SD)	Root completed (yr)
Maxillary						
Central incisor	14	(13-16)	Five sixths	1½	10 (8-12)	1½
Lateral incisor	16	(14⅔-16½)	Two thirds	2½	11 (9-13)	2
Canine	17	(15-18)	One third	9	19 (16-22)	3¼
First molar	15½	(14½-17)	Cusps united; occlusal completely calcified plus a half to three fourths crown height	6	16 (13-19) boys (14-18) girls	2½
Second molar	19	(16-23½)	Cusps united; occlusal incompletely calcified; calcified tissue covers a fifth to a fourth crown height	11	29 (25-33)	3
Mandibular						
Central incisor	14	(13-16)	Three fifths	2½	8 (6-10)	1½
Lateral incisor	16	(14⅔-)	Three fifths	3	13 (10-16)	1½
Canine	17	(16-)	One third	9	20 (17-23)	3¼
First molar	15½	(14½-17)	Cusps united; occlusal completely calcified	5½	16 (14-18)	2¼
Second molar	18	(17-19½)	Cusps united; occlusal incompletely calcified	10	27 (23-31) boys (24-30) girls	3

From Lunt, R.C., and Law, D.B.: J.A.D.A. **89:**878, 1974.

greatly. Variations of 6 months on either side of the usual eruption date may be considered normal for a given child.

The results of most clinical studies indicate that the teeth of girls erupt slightly earlier than those of boys. Garn and associates, who investigated sex differences in the time of tooth calcification in 255 children, developed five stages of calcification and eruption. In general, they found that girls were more advanced in each stage, especially in the later stages. The average amount of tooth development for girls was 3% ahead of boys.

Normal eruption process

Although many theories have been advanced, the factors responsible for the eruption of the teeth are not fully understood. The developmental processes and factors that have been related to the eruption of teeth include elongation of the root, forces exerted by the vascular tissues around and beneath the root, growth of the alveolar bone, growth of dentin, pulpal constriction, growth and pull of the periodontal membrane, pressure from the muscular action, and resorption of the alveolar crest.

Sicher proposed that the axial movement of a continuously growing tooth is the expression of its longitudinal growth. The most important factor causing the tooth to move occlusally is the elongation of the pulp resulting from pulpal growth in a proliferation ring at its basal end. The proliferation zone is separated from the periapical tissue by an infolding of Hertwig's epithelial sheath referred to as the "epithelial diaphragm." The pulpal growth is normally considered to be simultaneous with and equal to the elongation of Hertwig's sheath.

At the basal end of the tooth is a "hammock" ligament that acts to direct the growth of the tooth. Sicher suggested that continuous changes in this ligament, stimulated by the expansion of the pulp, are an integral part of the process of eruption. These changes take place in the intermediate layer of the periodontal membrane, which consists of a plexus of precollagenous fibers.

Baume, Becks, and Evans reported evidence that tooth eruption is influenced by the pituitary growth hormone and the thyroid hormone. Although the theory that hormones play a major role in tooth eruption is supported by considerable evidence, probably normal physiologic eruption is the result of a combination of the factors that have been mentioned.

Shumaker and El Hadary observed in a radiographic study that each tooth starts to move toward occlusion at approximately the time of crown completion. The interval between crown completion and beginning of eruption until the tooth is in full occlusion is approximately 5 years for permanent teeth.

Gron observed in her study of 874 Boston children that tooth emergence appeared to be more closely associated with the stage of root formation than with the chronologic or skeletal age of the child. By the time of clinical emergence approximately three fourths of root formation had occurred. Teeth reach occlusion before the root development is complete.

Demirjian and Levesque have presented a large sample of 5437 radiographs from a homogeneous (French-Canadian) population. They used this sample to investigate the sexual differences in the development of mandibular teeth from the early stages of calcification to closure of the apex. The analysis of the developmental curves of individual teeth shows a common pattern, namely the similarity in timing between sexes for the early stages of development. For the first stages of crown formation, which they refer to as A, B, and C, there was no difference in the chronology of the dental calcification between boys and girls in the majority of teeth. For the fourth stage, D, which represents the completion of crown development, girls were more advanced than boys by an average of 0.35 year for four teeth. For the stages of root development the mean difference between sexes for all teeth was 0.54 year, the largest difference being with the canine (0.90 year). The data from Demirjian and Levesque show the importance of sexual dimorphism during the period of root development rather than during the period of crown development.

The eruption pattern of human primary molars, premolars, and permanent molars was studied by Darling and Levers in a cross section of patients between 2 and 22 years of age. Measurements were made on Orthopantomographic radiographs using the inferior dental canal as a fixed reference structure. They determined that eruption can be divided into five stages. Concentric follicular growth is followed by a phase of active eruption. When the first radiographic evidence of the forming root is detected, the occlusal surface of the tooth and the vertical center of the follicle begin to move toward the occlusal plane. Once occlusion is reached and equilibrium established, the occlusal plane remains the same distance from the inferior dental canal for periods that vary from 2 to 8 years, depending on the tooth observed. The adolescent growth spurt is accompanied by a second phase of active eruption. Because this stage can occur after root completion, it cannot be a result of root growth. A second equilibrium is established at about 18 years of age and maintained for the remainder of the period of observation.

Influence of premature loss of primary molars on eruption time of their successors. Posen, after a review of the records of children in the Burlington study who had undergone unilateral extraction of primary molars, made the following conclusions. Eruption of the premolar teeth will be delayed in children who lose primary molars at 4 or 5 years of age and before. If extraction of the primary molars occurs after the age of 5 years, there will be a decrease in the delay of premolar eruption. At 8, 9, and 10 years of age, premolar eruption resulting from premature loss of primary teeth is greatly accelerated.

Variations in the sequence of eruption. The mandibular first permanent molars are often the first permanent teeth to erupt. They are quickly followed by the mandibular central incisors. Lo and Moyers found little or no clinical significance in the eruption of the incisors before the molars.

After analyzing serial records of 16,000 children in Newburgh and Kingston, New York, Carlos and Gittelsohn concluded that the average eruption time of the lower central incisors was earlier than that of the first molars by about 1½ months in both boys and girls. Of considerable interest was the sex difference in the eruption sequence of permanent teeth. The mandibular canine erupted before the maxillary and mandibular first premolars in girls. In boys the eruption order was reversed—the maxillary and mandibular first premolars erupted before the mandibular canine.

Moyers stated that the most favorable sequence of eruption of permanent teeth in the mandible is first molar, central incisor, lateral incisor, canine, first premolar, second premolar, and second molar. The most favorable sequence for the eruption of the maxillary permanent teeth is first molar, central incisor, lateral incisor, first premolar, second premolar, canine, and second molar (Fig. 5-1).

It is desirable that the mandibular canine erupt before the first and second premolars. This sequence will aid in maintaining adequate arch length and in preventing lingual tipping of the incisors. Lingual tipping of the incisors not only will cause a loss of arch length but also will allow the development of an increased overbite. An abnormal lip musculature or an oral habit that causes a greater

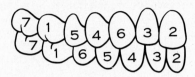

Fig. 5-1. Desirable eruption sequence for the permanent teeth.

force on the lower incisors than can be compensated by the tongue will allow a collapse of the anterior segment. For this reason a passive lingual arch appliance is often indicated when the primary canines have been lost prematurely or when the sequence of eruption is undesirable.

A deficiency in arch length can occur if the mandibular second permanent molar develops and erupts before the second premolar. The second permanent molar's erupting out of sequence will exert a strong force on the first permanent molar and will cause its mesial migration and encroachment on the space needed for the second premolar. The importance of maintaining the second primary molar until its replacement by the second premolar is discussed in Chapter 20.

In the maxillary arch the first premolar ideally should erupt before the second premolar, and they should be followed by the canine. The untimely loss of primary molars in the maxillary arch, allowing the first permanent molar to drift and tip mesially, will result in the permanent canine being blocked out of the arch, usually to the labial side. The position of the developing second permanent molar in the maxillary arch and its relationship to the first permanent molar should be given special attention. Its eruption before the premolars and canine can cause a loss of arch length, just as in the mandibular arch.

The eruption of the maxillary canine is often delayed because of an abnormal position or devious eruption path. This delayed eruption should be considered along with its possible effect on the alignment of the maxillary teeth. The significance of the sequence of the eruption of permanent teeth is considered further in Chapter 20.

Lingual eruption of mandibular permanent incisors

The eruption of mandibular permanent incisors lingual to retained primary incisors is often a source of concern for parents. The primary teeth may have undergone extensive root resorption and may be held only by soft tissues. In other instances the root may not have undergone normal resorption and the tooth remains solidly in place. Lingual eruption of one or more of the mandibular incisors has been estimated to occur from approximately 10% of the time (Berland and Seyler) to about 50% of the time (McDonald). Regardless of the actual frequency, it is common for mandibular permanent incisors to erupt lingually, and this pattern should be considered essentially normal. It is seen both in patients with an obvious arch length inadequacy (Fig. 5-2) and in those with a desirable amount of spacing of the primary incisors (Fig. 5-3). In either case the tongue and continued alveolar growth seem to play an important role in influencing the permanent incisor into a more normal position with time. Although there may be insufficient room in the arch for the newly erupted permanent tooth, its position will improve over several months. In some cases there is justification for removing the corresponding primary tooth. Extraction of other primary teeth in the area, however, is not recommended because it will only temporarily relieve the crowding and may even contribute to the development of a more severe arch length inadequacy.

Gellin has emphasized the anxiety created when the parents discover a double row of teeth. He suggested that if the condition is identified before the age of 7½ years, it is unnecessary to subject the child to the trauma of removing the primary teeth because the problem is almost always self-correcting within a few months. However, he warned that when lingually erupted permanent mandibular incisors are seen in an older child and the radiograph shows no root resorption of the primary teeth, self-correction has not been achieved and the corresponding primary teeth should be removed.

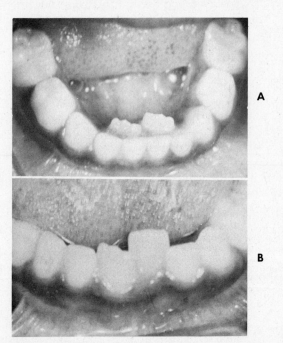

Fig. 5-2. A, The permanent central incisors are erupting lingual to the retained primary central incisors, which were extracted. **B,** The arch length is inadequate to accommodate the permanent incisors. However, they have moved forward into a more favorable position as a result of the force exerted on them by the tongue.

Gellin and Haley recently conducted a clinical study to determine if removal of the corresponding primary tooth is necessary when the lingual eruption pattern of the mandibular permanent incisor is identified. They monitored 57 lingually positioned mandibular permanent central or lateral incisors in 44 children. The children were selected for the study if they had one or more permanent mandibular incisors erupting immediately lingual to the corresponding primary incisor. Other criteria required for the study included the presence of both primary mandibular canines, the absence of any other anomalies of the mandibular primary or per-

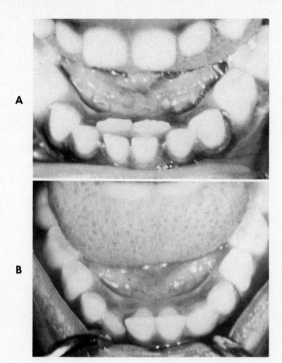

Fig. 5-3. A, The primary teeth are desirably spaced, with sufficient room for the permanent central incisors. However, the permanent teeth erupted lingually to the primary teeth. **B,** Extraction of the primary central incisors resulted in a desirable positioning of the permanent teeth. Given enough time this condition would have probably been self-correcting.

manent incisors, and the absence of severe crowding of the permanent mandibular incisors characterized by the lateral incisors erupting directly behind the central incisors. The mean age of the children at their first observation was 6 years, 4 months, and the ages ranged from 4 years, 10 months to 8 years, 8 months. There were 22 boys and 22 girls in the study. Of the permanent teeth studied, 47 were central incisors and 10 were lateral incisors.

In all cases labial migration occurred naturally and extraction of the corresponding primary incisor was unnecessary. Gellin and Haley reported that

spontaneous correction of lingually erupted mandibular permanent central incisors occurred by age 8 years, 2 months in 95% of the cases that met the criteria of their study. They also observed that spontaneous correction of lingually erupted lateral incisors occurred by at least 8 years, 4 months of age. Although the sample of the lateral incisors was too small to draw specific conclusions, correction occurred in all cases and central incisors migrated labially at an earlier age. Gellin and Haley recommended a conservative approach of waiting and periodic observation to spare the child a surgical procedure. They suggested that if labial migration of the permanent incisor had not occurred by 8.2 years for central incisors and 8.4 years for lateral incisors, overretention of the primary incisor should be suspected and removal of the primary tooth considered. However, they recommended removal only if the primary incisor remained firm and the root had failed to resorb.

We recognize that spontaneous correction of lingually erupted permanent incisors is likely to occur given enough time, particularly in cases where there is not severe crowding. A watchful waiting approach may be justified, especially when the patient is first seen in the dentist's office for this specific problem. Removal of a tooth during the first dental appointment of a child 6 to 8 years old probably compromises the dentist's ability to develop rapport with the child. However, the extraction procedure in such cases is quite simple, and we believe there may be many times when it is appropriate. The parents' feelings should not be ignored in the decision; even a 95% chance that correction will occur may not satisfy all parents. The dentist may find that some "experienced" dental patients prefer to have the primary tooth extracted and the problem laid to rest. Although monitoring the condition without extraction is acceptable under the conditions outlined by Gellin and Haley, we know of no significant contraindications to early removal of the offending primary incisor even in spaced dentitions, if specific conditions warrant its consideration.

Even when mandibular permanent incisors erupt uneventfully, they often appear rotated and staggered in position. The molding action of the tongue and the lips improves their relationship within a few months.

Difficult eruption

In most children the eruption of primary teeth is preceded by increased salivation, and the child will want to put the hand and fingers into the mouth. These observations may be the only indication that the teeth will soon erupt.

Some young children become restless and fretful during the time of eruption of the primary teeth. In the past, many conditions, including croup, diarrhea, fever, and even convulsions, were incorrectly attributed to eruption.

Illingworth made a thorough search of the world literature and failed to produce evidence that teething causes fever, convulsions, bronchitis, or diarrhea. His findings are supported by Tasanen's unique study of teething, in which 192 tooth eruptions were observed in 126 infants and in 107 controls with a total of 1538 examinations in Finland. The infants were in a nursery or were living at home but attended a child welfare center. All the babies were seen on the day of the eruption of the tooth, and records were kept of the temperature, incidence of infection, erythrocyte sedimentation rate (ESR), white blood cell count, behavior (including sleep), color of the mucosa, sensitivity of the tissue covering the erupting tooth, and pain resulting from pressure on the tooth. In addition, a questionnaire was sent to 200 mothers of 720 children asking their views on the symptoms of teething. Tasanen concluded that teething does not increase the incidence of infection, does not cause any rise in temperature, ESR, or white blood cell count, and does not cause diarrhea, cough, sleep disturbance, or rubbing of the ear or cheek, but that it does cause daytime restlessness, an increase in the amount of finger sucking or rubbing of the gum, an increase in drooling, and possibly some loss of appetite. In one third of the children there

was no change in the color of the mucosa in the area of the erupting tooth, in one third of the children the change was slight, and in the remainder of the children there was a marked change in the mucosa, often with small hemorrhages.

Since the eruption of teeth is a normal physiologic process, the association with fever and systemic disturbances is not justified. A fever or respiratory tract infection during this time should be considered coincidental to the eruption process rather than related to it.

Inflammation of the gingival tissues before complete emergence of the crown may cause a temporary painful condition that subsides within a few days. The surgical removal of the tissue covering the tooth to facilitate eruption is not indicated. If the child is having extreme difficulty, the application of a nonirritating topical anesthetic may bring temporary relief. The parent can apply the anesthetic to the affected tissue over the erupting tooth three or four times a day. Tanner and Kitchen have found that a salve compounded of equal parts of lidocaine ointment and Orabase is effective. The eruption process may be hastened by allowing the child to chew on a piece of toast or a clean teething object.

Eruption hematoma (eruption cyst). A bluish purple, elevated area of tissue, commonly called "eruption hematoma," occasionally develops a few weeks before the eruption of a primary or permanent tooth. The blood-filled "cyst" is most frequently seen in primary second molar or first permanent molar regions. This fact substantiates the belief that the condition develops as a result of trauma (Fig. 5-4). Usually within a few days the tooth breaks through the tissue, and the hematoma subsides. Since the condition is almost always self-limited, treatment of an eruption hematoma is rarely necessary. However, surgically uncovering the crown may occasionally be justified (see p. 764 and Fig. 29-18).

When the parents discover an eruption hematoma, they may fear that the child has a serious disease such as a malignant tumor. The dentist

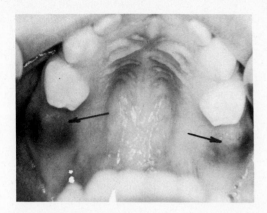

Fig. 5-4. Eruption hematomas *(arrows)* have developed before the eruption of the second primary molars.

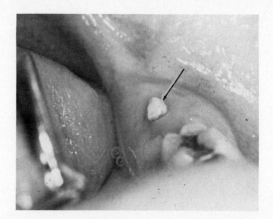

Fig. 5-5. Arrow points to an eruption sequestrum in a girl 5 years, 11 months of age. It appears clinically as a white spicule of nonviable bone overlying the central fossa of a mandibular first permanent molar, which is just beginning to erupt through the mucosa. (Courtesy Drs. Paul E. Starkey and William G. Shafer.)

must be understanding and sensitive to their anxiety while reassuring them that the lesion is not serious.

Eruption sequestrum. The eruption sequestrum is seen occasionally in children at the time of the eruption of the first permanent molar (Figs. 5-5 and 5-6). Starkey and Shafer have described the sequestrum as a tiny spicule of bone overlying the crown of an erupting permanent molar just before or immediately after the emergence of the tips of the cusps through the oral mucosa. Generally, the position of the fragment of nonviable bone is directly overlying the central occlusal fossa but contoured within the soft tissue. As the tooth continues to erupt and the cusps emerge, the fragment of bone sequestrates through the mucosa. The finding is of little clinical significance.

When an eruption sequestrum has "surfaced" through the mucosa, it should be removed to control the local irritation usually associated with it. The base of the sequestrum is often still well embedded in gingival tissue when it is discovered, and a topical anesthetic or infiltration of a few drops of a local anesthetic may be necessary to avoid discomfort during removal.

Ectopic eruption. Arch length inadequacy, tooth mass redundancy, or a variety of local factors

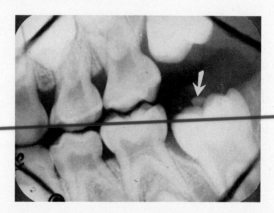

Fig. 5-6. Radiographic appearance of an eruption sequestrum *(arrow)* at age 6 years, 9 months. No treatment is indicated. (Courtesy Drs. Paul E. Starkey and William G. Shafer.)

may influence a tooth to erupt or "try" to erupt in an abnormal position. Occasionally this condition may be so severe that actual transposition of teeth takes place. Several problems associated with ectopic eruption of teeth and the management of these problems are presented in Chapter 21.

Natal and neonatal teeth

The incidence of natal teeth (teeth present at birth) and neonatal teeth (teeth that erupt during the first 30 days) is probably low. Massler and Savara reported that the incidence in two Chicago hospitals was one baby with a neonatal tooth in approximately 2000 births. About 85% of natal or neonatal teeth are lower primary incisors, and only a small percentage have been observed to be supernumerary teeth. An unusual occurrence of a natal mandibular primary canine and a maxillary second primary molar was reported in a 34-day-old Malay child. Both teeth were loosely attached and, as reported by the child's mother, had been present since birth.

Sponge and Feasby believe that the terms "natal teeth" and "neonatal teeth" constitute a relatively artificial distinction and should be further qualified to provide a more practical clinical significance. They have suggested that the terms "mature" and "immature" are more in keeping with the varying prognoses associated with such teeth.

The cause of the early eruption of primary teeth is often obscure, although early eruption seems to be familial. Many parents volunteer the information that their teeth erupted early. Bodenhoff and Gorlin found that 15% of the children with natal or neonatal teeth had parents, siblings, or other near relatives with a history of such teeth. Evidence of a relationship between early eruption and a systemic condition or a syndrome is not conclusive. This possibility should be considered, however, in the diagnosis and treatment of a natal or neonatal tooth.

A radiograph should be made to determine the amount of root development and the relationship of a prematurely erupted tooth to its adjacent teeth. One of the parents can hold the x-ray film in the infant's mouth during the exposure.

Most prematurely erupted teeth (immature type) are hypermobile because of the limited root development. Some teeth may be mobile to the extent that there is danger of displacement of the tooth and possible aspiration, in which case the removal of the tooth is indicated. In exceptionally rare cases in

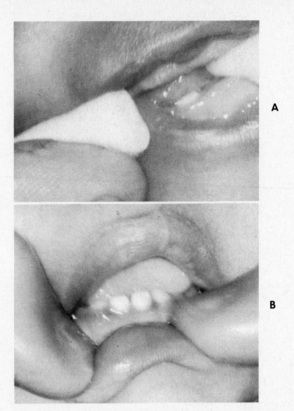

Fig. 5-7. A, Natal tooth in a 3-day-old infant. Since the tooth was not excessively mobile, there was no reason to recommend its removal. **B,** Within 2 months other teeth in the mandibular anterior region erupted.

which the sharp incisal edge of the tooth may cause laceration of the lingual surface of the tongue or may interfere with nursing, the tooth may have to be removed. The more desirable approach, however, is to leave the tooth in place and to explain to the parents the desirability of maintaining this tooth in the mouth because of its importance in the growth and uncomplicated eruption of the adjacent teeth. Within a relatively short time the prematurely erupted tooth will become stabilized, and the other teeth in the arch will erupt (Fig. 5-7).

Eruption of teeth during the neonatal period presents less of a problem. These teeth can usually be maintained even though root development is limited (Figs. 5-8 and 5-9).

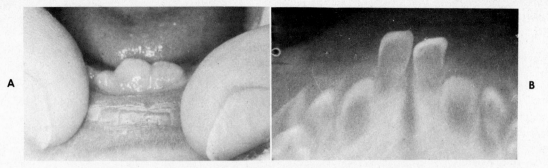

Fig. 5-8. A, Parents of a 3-week-old infant were concerned about the elevated mass of tissue on the lower ridge. **B,** Radiograph revealed two primary central incisors that would soon erupt.

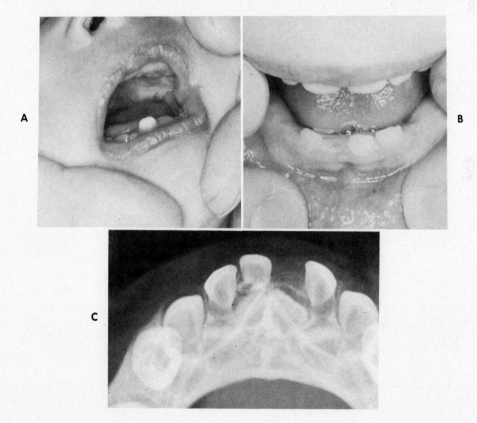

Fig. 5-9. A, Eruption of one of the primary central incisors occurred at 4 weeks of age. The tooth was mobile because of limited root formation, but it was not extracted. **B,** One of the prematurely erupted central incisors was subsequently lost as the result of a fall, but the other was retained. **C,** Dilacerated root formation on one of the neonatal teeth.

A retained natal or neonatal tooth may cause difficulty for a mother who wishes to breast-feed her infant. If breast-feeding is too painful for the mother initially, the use of a breast pump and storing the milk are recommended. However, the infant may be conditioned not to "bite" during suckling in a relatively short time if the mother persists with breast-feeding. It seems that the infant senses the mother's discomfort and learns to avoid causing it.

Epstein's pearls, Bohn's nodules, and inclusion cysts

Small white or grayish white lesions on the alveolar mucosa of the newborn may on rare occasions be incorrectly diagnosed as "natal teeth." The lesions are usually multiple but do not increase in size (Fig. 5-10). No treatment is indicated, since the lesions are spontaneously shed a few weeks after birth.

Fromm has reported that clinically visible cysts were found in 1028 of 1367 newborn infants. He noted and classified the following three types of inclusion cysts:

1. Epstein's pearls are formed along the midpalatine raphe. They are considered remnants of epithelial tissue trapped along the raphe as the fetus grew.

2. Bohn's nodules are formed along the buccal and lingual aspects of the dental ridges and on the palate away from the raphe. The nodules are considered remnants of mucous gland tissue and histologically different from Epstein's pearls.

3. Dental lamina cysts are found on the crest of the maxillary and mandibular dental ridges. The cysts apparently originated from remnants of the dental lamina.

Local and systemic factors that influence eruption

Ankylosed teeth. The problem of ankylosed primary molars deserves much attention by dentists. The term "submerged molar" as applied to this condition is unacceptable, even though the tooth may appear to be submerging into the mandible or maxillae. This misconception results from the fact that the ankylosed tooth is in a state of static retention, whereas in the adjacent areas eruption and alveolar growth continue. Henderson pointed out that ankylosis should be considered an interruption in the rhythm of eruption and further observed that a patient who has one or two ankylosed teeth is more likely to have other teeth become ankylosed.

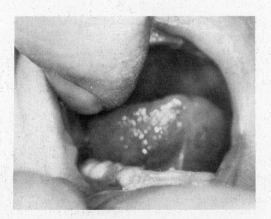

Fig. 5-10. Bohn's nodules. No treatment is indicated, since the lesions disappear within a few weeks after birth. (Courtesy Dr. Alfred Fromm.)

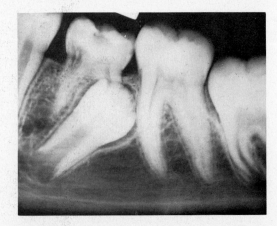

Fig. 5-11. The second primary molar is ankylosed and below the normal plane of occlusion. There is evidence of root resorption and deposition of bone into the resorbed areas.

The mandibular primary molars are the teeth most often observed to be ankylosed (Figs. 5-11 and 5-12). In unusual cases all the primary molars may become firmly attached to the alveolar bone before their normal exfoliation time. Such a case was recently reported by Alexander and associates, and a similar case is illustrated in this chapter (see Fig. 5-17). Ankylosis of the anterior primary teeth does not occur unless there has been a traumatic injury.

The cause of ankylosis in the primary molar areas is unknown, but at least three theories have been proposed. The observation of ankylosis in several members of the same family lends support to the theory that it follows a familial pattern. Via has reported that the condition has greater occurrence among siblings of children with the characteristics. The occurrence is noted to have a familial tendency and is probably a non-sex-linked trait. Krakowiak has observed the prevalence of ankylosis among black children to be much lower (0.93%) than among white children (4.10%).

Darling and Levers (1973) observed that in a group of children with 108 ankylosed teeth, 21 of the affected primary teeth had no permanent successors. Brown also reported a higher prevalence of developmentally absent premolar teeth in patients with ankylosis. It is often suggested that there is a relationship between congenital absence of permanent teeth and ankylosed primary teeth. Steigman, Koyoumdjisky-Kaye, and Matrai have discounted this relationship. On the basis of observation and a careful review of the literature, they reported that there appears to be no causal relationship between ankylosed precursors and congenital absence of their successors.

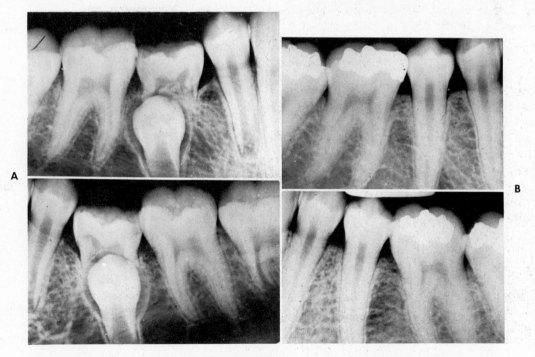

Fig. 5-12. A, Bilateral ankylosis of second primary molars. **B,** The ankylosed molars were eventually shed, and the second premolars erupted into good occlusion. Frequently the ankylosed teeth must be removed surgically.

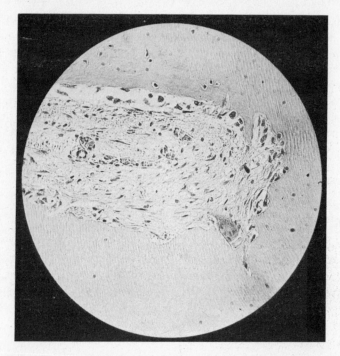

Fig. 5-13. A multinucleated giant cell is seen in the lower portion of the photomicrograph, whereas osteoid tissue has been laid down only a short distance away.

Normal resorption of the primary molar begins on the inner surface or the lingual surface of the roots. The resorption process is not continuous but is interrupted by periods of inactivity or rest. A reparative process follows periods of resorption. In the course of this reparative phase a solid union often develops between the bone and the primary tooth (Fig. 5-13). This intermittent resorption and repair may explain the varying degrees of firmness of the primary teeth before their exfoliation. Extensive bony ankylosis of the primary tooth may prevent normal exfoliation, as well as the eruption of the permanent successor.

Ankylosis of the primary molar to the alveolar bone does not usually occur until after resorption begins at the age of 4 years. If ankylosis occurs early, eruption of adjacent teeth may progress enough that the ankylosed tooth is far below the normal plane of occlusion and may even be partially covered with soft tissue (Fig. 5-14). An

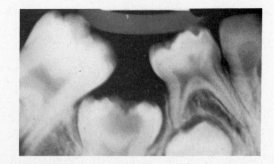

Fig. 5-14. Ankylosed second primary molar with a carious lesion in the occlusal surface. This tooth probably became ankylosed soon after root resorption began.

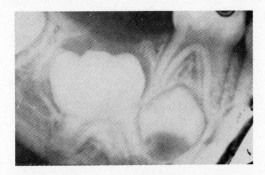

Fig. 5-15. An ankylosed, deeply embedded second primary molar. Surgical removal of this tooth is indicated.

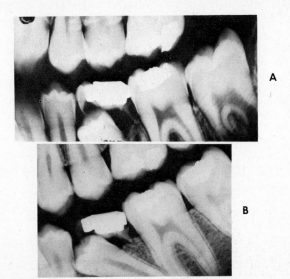

Fig. 5-16. A, A small spicule of root of the primary tooth is ankylosed to the alveolar bone. This was overlooked at the time of the routine examination. **B,** One year later the second primary molar is still retained, and the second premolar has moved into an unfavorable position.

epithelium-lined track will, however, extend from the oral cavity to the tooth. Ankylosis may occasionally occur even before the eruption and complete root formation of the primary tooth (Fig. 5-15). Ankylosis can also occur late in the resorption of the primary roots and even then can interfere with the eruption of the underlying permanent tooth (Fig. 5-16).

The histologic picture in ankylosis is one of hyperactivity. The osseous ankylosis lies between the dentin and bone and is closely associated with osteoclastic activity (Fig. 5-13). In one area of the root osteoclastic activity in old dentin is prevalent, whereas a short distance away osteoblasts are laying down new osteoid tissue that is hyperplastic and is not entirely unlike alveolar bone. Resorption occurs in an area of increased vascularity. Formation of dentin and calcification, as well as rebuilding of bone, are evident in histologic sections.

The diagnosis of an ankylosed tooth is not difficult to make. Because eruption has not occurred and the alveolar process has not developed in normal occlusion, the opposing molars in the area appear to be out of occlusion. The ankylosed tooth is not mobile, even in cases of advanced root resorption. Ankylosis can be partially confirmed by tapping the suspected tooth and an adjacent normal tooth with a blunt instrument and then comparing the sounds. The ankylosed tooth will have a solid sound, whereas the normal tooth will have a

cushioned sound because it has an intact periodontal membrane that absorbs some of the shock of the blow.

The radiograph is a valuable aid in making a diagnosis. A break in the continuity of the periodontal membrane indicating an area of ankylosis is usually evident radiographically.

In the management of an ankylosed tooth, early recognition and diagnosis are extremely important (Fig. 5-17). The eventual treatment usually involves surgical removal. However, unless the caries problem is unusual or loss of arch length is evident, the dentist may choose to keep the tooth under observation. A tooth that is definitely ankylosed may at some future time undergo root resorption and be normally exfoliated. When patient cooperation is good and recall periods are regular, a watchful waiting approach is best.

The recent observations of Messer and Cline indicate that failure to carry out timed extraction of severely infraoccluded molars results in reduced

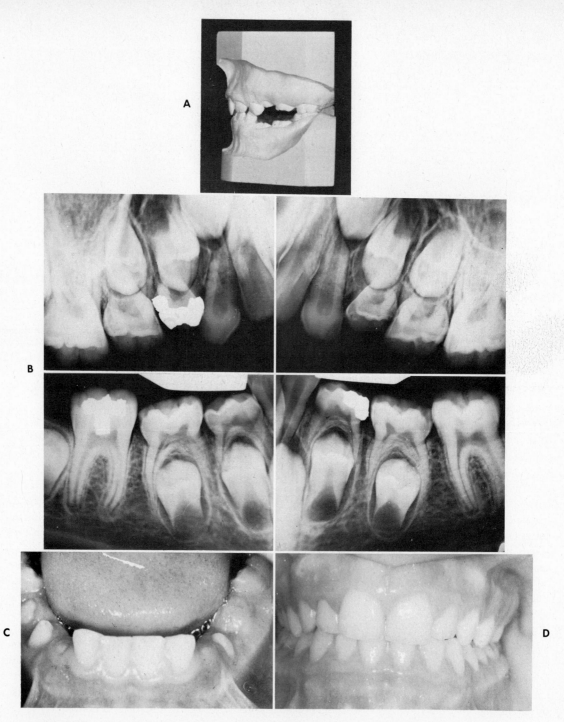

Fig. 5-17. A, All eight of the primary molars were ankylosed. Continuing eruption of the adjacent teeth has caused a loss of arch length. **B,** Radiographs aided in the diagnosis of the ankylosed primary molars. The recommended treatment was surgical removal of the ankylosed teeth. **C,** Space maintainers were constructed after removal of the ankylosed teeth and were worn until the permanent teeth erupted. **D,** Ideal occlusion was achieved as a result of early diagnosis and the removal of the ankylosed teeth at the proper time.

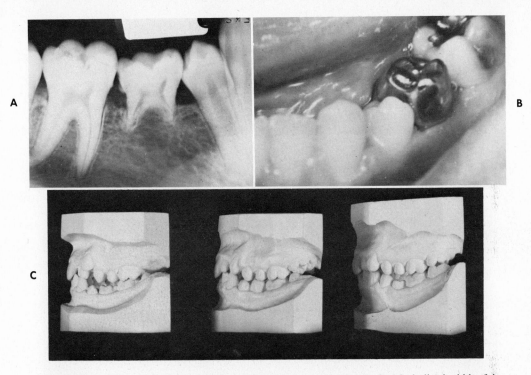

Fig. 5-18. A, Ankylosed primary molar without a permanent successor. **B,** Mesiodistal width of the primary molar was reduced to allow the premolar to erupt, and an overlay was constructed to establish occlusion with the opposing teeth. **C,** Models at the left show the original condition. Center models show the occlusion at the time the overlay was placed on the ankylosed tooth. Models at the right show the continued eruption of the adjacent teeth that occurred in the subsequent 18-month period.

alveolar bone support for the premolars. In children in whom the permanent successor of the ankylosed primary tooth is missing, attempts have been made to construct overlays for ankylosed molars to establish normal occlusion. This treatment is successful only if maximum eruption of permanent teeth in the arch has occurred. If adjacent teeth are still in a state of active eruption, they will soon bypass the ankylosed tooth (Fig. 5-18).

Ankylosed permanent teeth. The incomplete eruption of a permanent molar may be related to a small area of root ankylosis. The removal of soft tissue and bone covering the occlusal aspect of the crown should be attempted first, and the area should be packed with surgical cement to provide a pathway for the developing permanent tooth (Fig.

5-19). If the permanent tooth is exposed in the oral cavity and at a lower occlusal plane than the adjacent teeth, ankylosis is the probable cause. Biederman, and more recently Skolnick, have described a luxation technique as often effective in breaking the bony ankylosis. If the rocking technique is not immediately successful, it should be repeated in 6 months. A delay in treatment may result in a permanently ankylosed molar (Fig. 5-20).

Unerupted permanent teeth may become ankylosed by inostosis of enamel. According to Franklin, the process follows the irritation of the follicular or periodontal tissue resulting from chronic infection. The close association of an infected apex to an unerupted tooth may give rise to the process. In the unerupted tooth, enamel is protected by

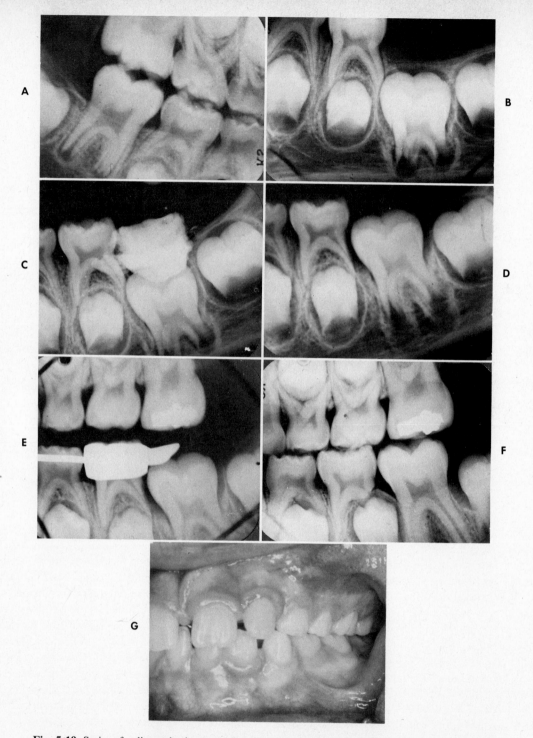

Fig. 5-19. Series of radiographs demonstrating the successful treatment of delayed eruption of a first permanent molar. **A,** The first permanent molar has erupted on the right side. **B,** The left first permanent molar remains embedded in bone and is probably ankylosed. **C,** Soft tissue and bone have been removed, and surgical cement has been placed over the unerupted tooth. **D,** Within 3 months the first permanent molar has moved occlusally. **E,** The lingual arch and distal extension hold the surgical cement in position and prevent continued eruption of the opposing molar. **F** and **G,** The first permanent molar has erupted, and the occlusion is good.

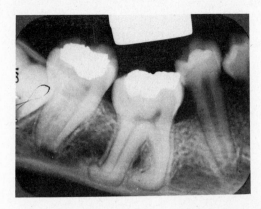

Fig. 5-20. Ankylosed first permanent molar. The tooth must be removed surgically.

enamel epithelium. The enamel epithelium may disintegrate as a result of infection (or trauma), the enamel may subsequently be resorbed, and bone or "coronal cementum" may be deposited in its place. The result is solid fixation of the tooth in its unerupted position (Fig. 5-21).

21-Trisomy syndrome (Down syndrome or mongolism). 21-Trisomy syndrome is one of the congenital anomalies in which delayed eruption of the teeth frequently occurs. The first primary teeth may not appear until 2 years of age, and the dentition may not be complete until 4 to 5 years of age. The eruption often follows an abnormal sequence, and some of the primary teeth may be retained until 14 to 15 years of age.

Although the cause remains obscure, the defect is apparently initiated between the sixth and eighth weeks of development, as evidenced by other abnormal conditions, including congenital heart defects and anomalies of the eye and external ear. Down syndrome is apparently related to some extent to maternal age. Benda reported the frequency of this syndrome to be approximately 1.5 per 1000 births of mothers in the 18- to 29-year age group. The frequency increases after the maternal age of 30 years, reaching 29 per 1000 in the 40-year and older age group, and a high of 91 per 1000 in the 44-year age group.

LeJeune provided additional insight into the etiology of Down syndrome when a careful analysis of the chromosomes of affected children demonstrated an extra autosomal chromosome, approximating the number 21 chromosome. Of all the theories of etiology of Down syndrome, trisomy of the twenty-first chromosome is the most consistent. (Trisomy is the presence in an otherwise diploid complement of an extra member of a particular chromosome pair.)

The diagnosis of a mongoloid child is not difficult to make because of the characteristic facial pattern (Fig. 5-22). The orbits are small, the eyes slope upward, and the bridge of the nose is more depressed than normal. In addition, Cohen reported that in a study of 194 mongoloid children 54% demonstrated anomalies in the formation of the external ear, characterized by outstanding "lap" ear with flat or absent helix. Mental retardation is a characteristic finding, although a few mongoloid children have an IQ greater than 50. Landau made a cephalometric comparison of children with Down syndrome and their normal siblings. Retardation in the growth of the maxillae and mandible was evident. Both the maxillae and mandible were positioned anteriorly under the cranial base. The upper facial height was found to be significantly smaller in the mongoloid children. The midface was also found to be small in the vertical and horizontal dimensions.

Many mongoloid children have chronic inflammation of the conjunctiva and a history of repeated respiratory tract infection. The use of antibiotics has reduced the incidence of chronic infection and has resulted in fewer deaths from infection.

Tannenbaum and also Baer and Benjamin have observed that the prevalence and severity of periodontal disease in mongoloid children are much higher than in the "normal" population. A high prevalence of acute necrotizing ulcerative gingivitis, affecting more than 30% of the individuals, was also observed. Brown and Cunningham have reported that as many as 90% of mongoloid individuals have periodontal disease, at least in the anterior region.

Dental caries susceptibility is usually low in

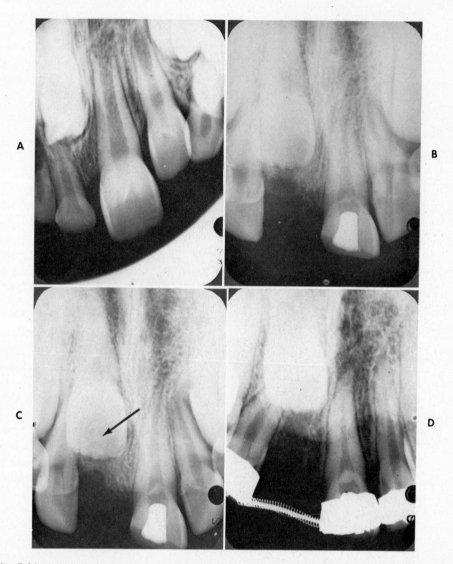

Fig. 5-21. Ankylosis by inostosis. **A,** A mesiodens has delayed the eruption of the maxillary left permanent central incisor. **B,** The primary incisors and the mesiodens were removed. During the surgical removal of the mesiodens, there was apparently damage to the enamel epithelium. **C,** There is evidence of resorption of the enamel of the unerupted incisor and ankylosis of the tooth. **D,** The right central incisor crown sustained a fracture and pulp exposure. A calcium hydroxide pulpotomy was successfully performed, resulting in continued root development.

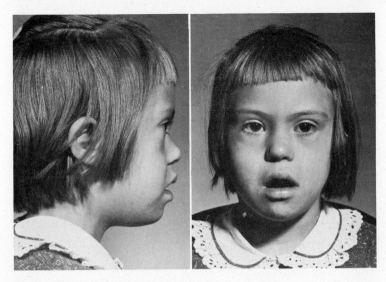

Fig. 5-22. Child with Down syndrome, age 8 years. (Courtesy Dr. Mace Landau.)

those with Down syndrome. This fact has been reported by Johnson, Young, and Gallios, who found a much lower dental caries incidence in both the primary and the permanent dentition. Brown and Cunningham in a study of mongoloid children found that 44% were caries free. Although some mongoloid children with a low mentality are unmanageable for dental procedures, most are pleasant, cheerful, affectionate, and well behaved. They can often be managed in the dental office in the same way as normal children The possibility of reduced resistance to infection should be considered in the dental management of the mongoloid child.

Cleidocranial dysostosis. A rare congenital syndrome that has dental significance is cleidocranial dysostosis. Transmission of the condition, which has also been referred to as osteodentin dysplasia, cleidocranial dysplasia, mutational dysostosis, and Marie-Sainton syndrome, is by either parent to a child of either sex, thus following a true mendelian dominant pattern. The syndrome can also occur sporadically with no apparent hereditary influence and with no predilection for race. The diagnosis is based on the finding of an absence of

clavicles, although there may be remnants of the clavicles, as evidenced by the presence of the sternal and acromial ends. The fontanels are large, and radiographs of the head show open sutures, even late in the child's life. The sinuses, particularly the frontal sinus, are usually small.

Jarvinen has indicated that the skeletal development of the face in this syndrome may be characterized by marked individual variation. Many previous reports refer to retrusion of the maxilla and pseudoprognathism. However, Jarvinen observed individuals with real maxillary prominence in addition to those with mandibular prognathism.

The development of the dentition is delayed. Complete primary dentition at 15 years of age resulting from delayed resorption of the deciduous teeth and delayed eruption of the permanent teeth is not uncommon (Fig. 5-23). One of the important distinguishing characteristics is the presence of supernumerary teeth. In some children there may be only a few supernumerary teeth in the anterior region of the mouth; others may have a large number of extra teeth throughout the mouth. Even with removal of the primary and supernumerary teeth, eruption of the permanent dentition is often de-

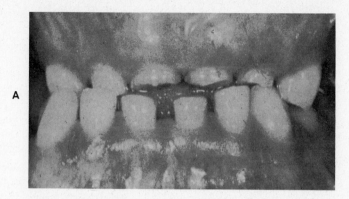

Fig. 5-23. Cleidocranial dysostosis. **A,** Primary dentition is still present at 15 years of age.

layed and irregular. Children who have only a few supernumerary teeth can be successfully treated by surgical removal of the extra teeth, complete uncovering of the crowns of the permanent teeth, and the construction of space-maintaining appliances to maintain the relationship of the teeth in the arch until the delayed teeth can erupt.

Hutton, Bixler, and Garner have reported the successful dental management of a patient with cleidocranial dysostosis over a 15-year period. The patient was first seen at 2 years of age. Treatment consisted of timed extractions of primary and supernumerary teeth and conservative uncovering of the permanent teeth. The surgical procedures were planned according to progressive radiographic evidence of the development of the permanent teeth. This management resulted in a nearly normal but slightly delayed eruption sequence. Orthodontic treatment was begun at 14 years of age, and by 16 years of age the patient displayed acceptable occlusion and normal vertical dimension, root development, and periodontal bone support.

Kelly and Nakamoto have reported that in older patients the only successful approach to improving occlusion and appearance is to remove all teeth and construct full dentures. Retaining a few teeth and then constructing overdentures for them has also been successful.

Delayed eruption has also been reported in other forms of osteopetroses.

Hypothyroidism. The assumption that all delayed eruption in the apparently normal, healthy child is related to a hypofunction of the thyroid gland is incorrect. However, hypothyroidism should be considered one of the possible causes of delayed eruption. Patients in whom the function of the thyroid gland is extremely deficient will have characteristic dental findings.

Congenital hypothyroidism (cretinism). Hypothyroidism occurring at birth and during the period of most rapid growth causes a condition known as cretinism. Congenital hypothyroidism is the result of an absence or underdevelopment of the thyroid gland. Cretinism, which if severe can often be diagnosed in the early weeks of life, is the result of insufficient thyroxine (Fig. 5-24). The cretin is a small and disproportionate person, often referred to as a dwarf because of abnormally short arms and legs. The head is disproportionately large, although the trunk shows less deviation from normal. Obesity is common. Some mental retardation is invariably associated with cretinism.

The dentition of the cretin is delayed in all stages, including eruption of the primary teeth, exfoliation of the primary teeth, and eruption of the permanent teeth. The teeth are normal in size but

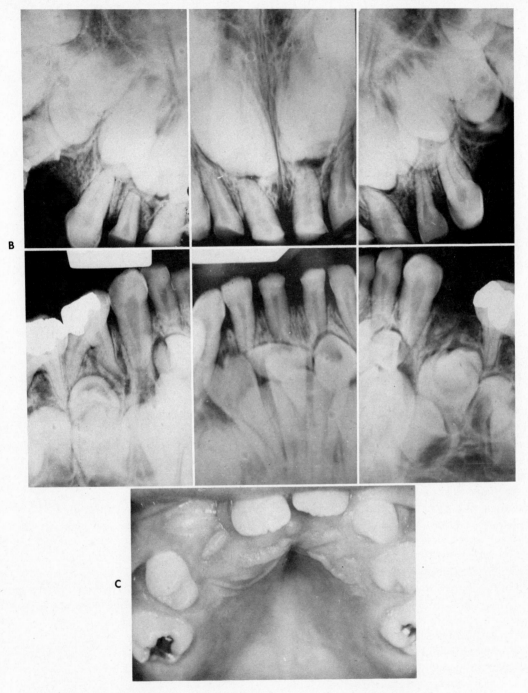

Fig. 5-23, cont'd. B, Delayed dentition and the presence of many supernumerary teeth. **C,** Removal of supernumerary teeth in the maxillary arch caused irregular and delayed eruption of some of the permanent teeth.

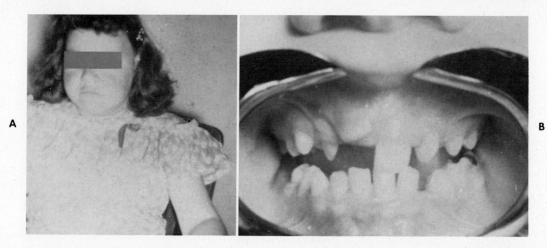

Fig. 5-24. A, A 24-year-old patient with congenital hypothyroidism. **B,** Dentition is markedly delayed. With the administration of thyroxine the eruption of the permanent teeth was accelerated. (Courtesy Dr. David F. Mitchell.)

are crowded in jaws that are smaller than normal. The tongue of the cretin is large and may protrude from the mouth. The abnormal size of the tongue and its position often cause an anterior open bite and flaring of the anterior teeth. The crowding of the teeth, malocclusion, and mouth breathing cause a chronic hyperplastic type of gingivitis.

Juvenile hypothyroidism (acquired hypothyroidism). Juvenile hypothyroidism results from a malfunction of the thyroid gland, usually between the ages of 6 and 12 years. Since the deficiency occurs after the period of rapid growth, there is not the unusual facial and body pattern that is characteristic of the cretin; however, obesity is evident to a lesser degree. In the untreated case of juvenile hypothyroidism, delayed exfoliation of the primary teeth and delayed eruption of the permanent teeth are characteristic. A child with a chronologic age of 14 years may have a dentition in a stage of development comparable with that of a child 9 or 10 years of age (Fig. 5-25).

Hypopituitarism. A marked deceleration of the growth of the bones and soft tissues of the body will result from a deficiency in the secretion of the growth hormone. The pituitary dwarf is the result of an early hypofunction of the pituitary gland. Since pituitary dysfunction does not usually occur before 4 years of age, a diagnosis cannot be made as early as in the case of congenital hypothyroidism.

The pituitary dwarf is a well-proportioned individual but resembles a child of considerably lower chronologic age (Fig. 5-26). Since the crowns of the permanent teeth are well along in their development by the time of the onset of the dysfunction, the dentition is essentially normal in size.

Delayed eruption of the dentition is characteristic. In severe cases the primary teeth do not undergo resorption but instead may be retained throughout the life of the individual. The underlying permanent teeth continue to develop but do not erupt. Extraction of the deciduous teeth is not indicated, since eruption of the permanent teeth cannot be assured. Some degree of mental retardation often occurs.

Achondroplastic dwarfism. The achondroplastic dwarf has few characteristic dental findings. Unlike cretinism, achondroplastic dwarfism is easily diagnosed at birth. Many achondroplastic children die during the first year of life.

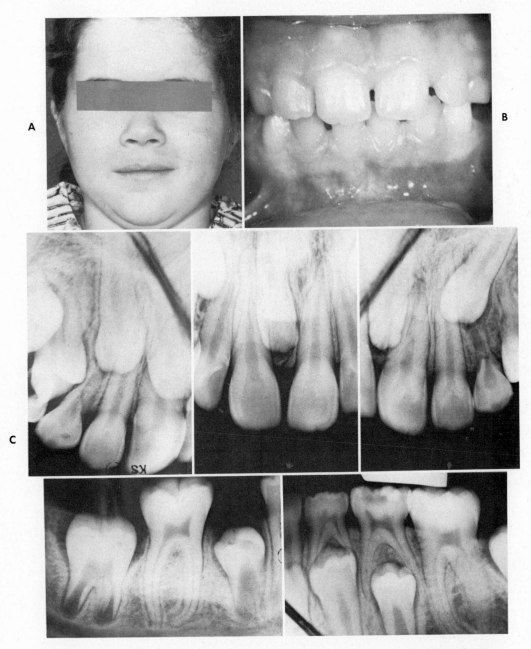

Fig. 5-25. A, A 14-year-old girl who was diagnosed as having juvenile hypothyroidism. **B,** The occlusion was essentially normal but was delayed in its development. **C,** Delayed development of the teeth in juvenile hypothroidism. The maxillary midline supernumerary tooth is a coincidental finding.

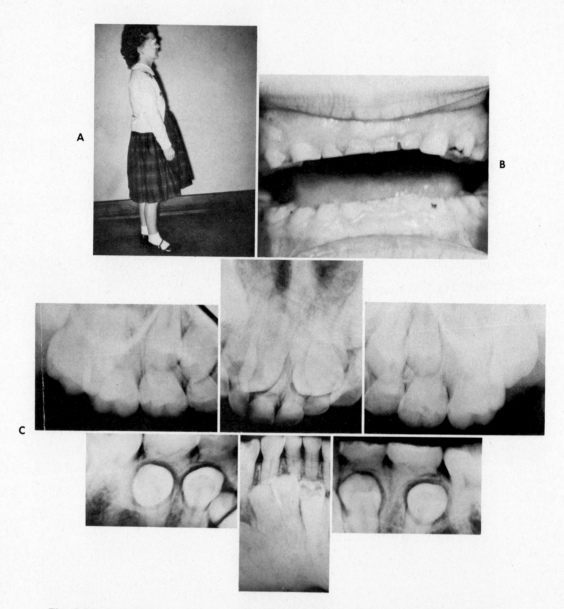

Fig. 5-26. A, A 28-year-old woman diagnosed as a hypopituitary dwarf. **B,** Complete primary dentition at 28 years of age. The first permanent molars have erupted. **C,** The roots of the primary teeth have not been resorbed to an appreciable degree, although some permanent teeth show complete development.

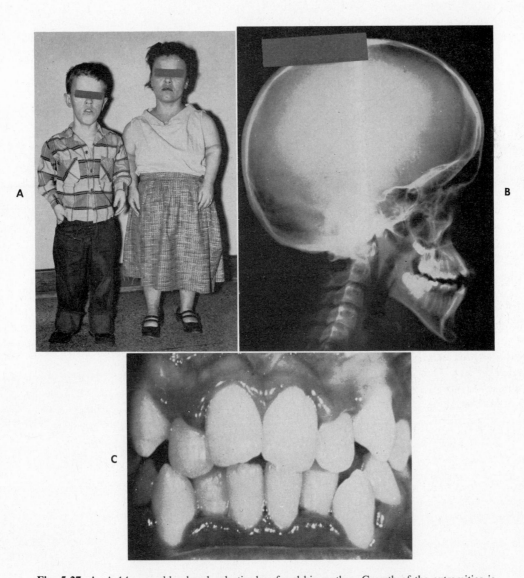

Fig. 5-27. A, A 14-year-old achondroplastic dwarf and his mother. Growth of the extremities is limited in both. **B,** The upper face is markedly underdeveloped. **C,** The arch length is inadequate, and the teeth are crowded. (**A** and **B** courtesy Dr. Ralph E. McDonald. **C** from Shafer, W., Hine, M.K., and Levy, B.M.: A textbook of oral pathology, Philadelphia, 1958, W.B. Saunders Co.)

Growth of the extremities is limited because of a lack of calcification in the cartilage of the long bones. The head is disproportionately large, although the trunk is normal in size. The fingers may be of almost equal length, and the hands are plump. The fontanels are open at birth. The upper face is underdeveloped, and the bridge of the nose is depressed.

The etiology of achondroplastic dwarfism is unknown, although some cases have a genetic background. The condition occurs as a dominant mendelian trait in these cases. There is some evidence that the condition is more likely to occur when the ages of the parents are greatly different. In contrast to Down syndrome, the increased age of the father may be related to the occurrence of the condition.

No adequate study of the oral condition of achondroplastic dwarfs has been made. Deficient growth in the cranial base is evident in many. The maxilla may be small, with resultant crowding of the teeth. A chronic gingivitis is usually present. However, this condition may well be related to the malocclusion and crowding of the teeth. In the patient in Fig. 5-27, the development of the dentition was slightly delayed.

Other causes. Delayed eruption of teeth has been linked to other disorders including fibromatosis gingivae (p. 361), chondroectodermal dysplasia (Ellis-van Creveld syndrome), Gardner syndrome, and rickets.

REFERENCES

Alexander, S.A., and others: Multiple ankylosed teeth, J. Pedod. **4:**354-359, 1980.

Baer, P.N., and Benjamin, S.D.: Periodontal disease in children and adolescents, Philadelphia, 1974, J.B. Lippincott Co., p. 199.

Baume, L.J., Becks, H., and Evans, H.M.: Hormonal control of tooth eruption. I. The effect of thyroidectomy on the upper rat incisor and the response to growth hormone, thyroxin, or the combination of both, J. Dent. Res. **33:**80-90, 1954.

Benda, C.E.: The child with mongolism, New York, 1960, Grune & Stratton, Inc.

Berland, T., and Seyler, A.E.: Your children's teeth, New York, 1968, Meredith Co., p. 87.

Biederman, W.: Etiology and treatment of tooth ankylosis, Am. J. Orthod. **48:**670-684, 1962.

Bodenhoff, J., and Gorlin, R.J.: Natal and neonatal teeth: folklore and fact, Pediatrics **32:**1087-1093, 1963.

Brown, I.D.: Some further observations on submerging deciduous molars, Br. J. Orthod. **8**(2):99-107, 1981.

Brown, R.H., and Cunningham, W.M.: Some manifestations of mongolism, Oral Surg. **14:**664-676, 1961.

Carlos, J.P., and Gittelsohn, A.M.: Longitudinal studies of the natural history of caries. I. Eruption patterns of the permanent teeth, J. Dent. Res. **44:**509-516, 1965.

Cohen, M.M.: Variability of facial and dental characteristics in trisomy G, South. Med. J. **64:**51-55, 1971.

Darling, A.I., and Levers, B.G.H.: Submerged human deciduous molars and ankylosis, Arch. Oral Biol. **18:**1021-1040, 1973.

Darling, A.I., and Levers, B.G.H.: The pattern of eruption of some human teeth, Arch. Oral Biol. **20:**89-96, 1975.

Demirjian, A., and Levesque, G.Y.: Sexual differences in dental development and prediction of emergence, J. Dent. Res. **59:**1110-1122, 1980.

Franklin, C.D.: Ankylosis of an unerupted third molar by inostosis of enamel, Br. Dent. J. **133:**346-347, 1972.

Fromm, A.: Epstein's pearls, Bohn's nodules and inclusion cysts of the oral cavity, J. Dent. Child. **34:**275-287, 1967.

Garn, S.M., and others: Sex difference in tooth calcification, J. Dent. Res. **37:**561-567, 1958.

Gellin, M.E.: Indications and contraindications for the removal of primary teeth, Dent. Clin. North Am. **13:**899-911, 1969.

Gellin, M.E., and Haley, J.V.: Managing cases of overretention of mandibular primary incisors where their permanent successors erupt lingually, J. Dent. Child. **49:**118-122, 1982.

Gron, A.M.P.: Prediction of tooth emergence, J. Dent. Res. **41:**573-585, 1962.

Henderson, H.Z.: Ankylosis of primary molars: a clinical, radiographic, and histologic study, J. Dent. Child. **46:**117-122, 1979.

Hutton, C.E., Bixler, D., and Garner, L.D.: Cleidocranial dysplasia—treatment of dental problems: report of case, J. Dent. Child. **48:**456-462, 1981.

Illingworth, R.S.: Teething, Dev. Med. Child. Neurol. **11:**376-377, 1969.

Jarvinen, S.: Cephalometric findings in three cases of cleidocranial dysostosis, Am. J. Orthod. **79**(2):184-191, 1981.

Johnson, N.P., Young, M.A., and Gallios, J.A.: Dental caries experience of mongoloid children, Dent. Abs. **6:**371, 1961.

Kelly, E., and Nakamoto, R.Y.: Cleidocranial dysostosis: a prosthodontic problem, J. Prosthet. Dent. **31:**518-526, 1974.

Krakowiak, F.J.: Ankylosed primary molars, J. Dent. Child. **45:**288-292, 1978.

Kraus, B.S., and Jordan, R.E.: The human dentition before birth, Philadelphia, 1965, Lea & Febiger.

Landau, M.J.: A cephalometric comparison of children with Down's syndrome and their normal siblings, thesis, Indianapolis, 1966, Indiana University School of Dentistry.

LeJeune, J.: Le mongolisme trisomie dégressive, Ann. Genet. **2:**1-38, 1960.

Lo, R.T., and Moyers, R.E.: Studies in the etiology and prevention of malocclusion. I. The sequence of eruption of the permanent dentition, Am. J. Orthod. **39:**460-467, 1953.

Lunt, R.C., and Law, D.B.: A review of the chronology of calcification of deciduous teeth, J.A.D.A. **89:**599-606, 1974.

Lunt, R.C., and Law, D.B.: A review of the chronology of eruption of deciduous teeth, J.A.D.A. **89:**872-879, 1974.

Massler, M., and Savara, B.S.: Natal and neonatal teeth, J. Pediatr. **36:**349-359, 1950.

McDonald, R.E.: Pedodontics, St. Louis, 1963, The C.V. Mosby Co., p. 124.

Messer, L.B., and Cline, J.T.: Ankylosed primary molars: results and treatment recommendations from an eight-year longitudinal study, Pediatr. Dent. **2:**37-47, 1980.

Mitchell, D.F., Standish, S.M., and Fast, T.B.: Oral diagnosis/oral medicine, ed. 3, Philadelphia, 1978, Lea & Febiger.

Moyers, R.E.: Handbook of orthodontics, Chicago, 1960, Year Book Medical Publishers, Inc.

Nelson, W.E., and others: Nelson's textbook of pediatrics, ed. 11, Philadelphia, 1979, W.B. Saunders Co.

Nomata, N.: Chronological study on the crown formation of the human deciduous dentition, Bull. Tokyo Med. Dent. Univ. **11:**55-76, 1964.

Posen, A.L.: The effect of premature loss of deciduous molars on premolar eruption, Angle Orthod. **35:**249-252, 1965.

Shumaker, D.B., and El Hadary, M.S.: Roentgenographic study of eruption, J.A.D.A. **61:**535-541, 1960.

Sicher, H.: Tooth eruption: the axial movement of continuously growing teeth, J. Dent. Res. **21:**201-210; **21:**395-402, 1942.

Skolnick, I.M.: Ankylosis of maxillary permanent first molar, J.A.D.A. **100:**558-560, 1980.

Sponge, J.D., and Feasby, W.H.: Erupted teeth in the newborn, Oral Surg. **22:**198-208, 1966.

Starkey, P.E., and Shafer, W.G.: Eruption sequestra in children, J. Dent. Child. **30:**84-86, 1963.

Steigman, S., Koyoumdjisky-Kaye, E., and Matrai, Y.: Submerged deciduous molars and congenital absence of premolars, J. Dent. Res. **52:**842, 1973.

Tannenbaum, K.A.: The oral aspects of mongolism, J. Public Health Dent. **35:**95-108, 1975.

Tanner, H.A., and Kitchen, R.N.: An effective treatment for pain in the eruption of primary and permanent teeth, J. Dent. Child. **31:**289-292, 1964.

Tasanen, A.: General and local effects of the eruption of deciduous teeth, Ann. Paedrit. Fenn. **14** (suppl. 29):1-40, 1968.

Tay, W.M.: Natal canine and molar in an infant, Oral Surg. **29:**598-602, 1970.

Via, W.F., Jr.: Submerged deciduous molars: familial tendencies, J.A.D.A. **69:**128-129, 1964.

6 Radiographic techniques

MYRON J. KASLE

JAMES F. MATLOCK

The most important diagnostic aid in dentistry was Professor Roentgen's discovery of the "x-ray" in 1895. This newly revealed form of energy could now be used to cast shadows or images on a photographic film. Those in dentistry can take pride that 6 weeks after Roentgen's astonishing announcement, a dentist attempted to record shadows of oral structures on a film. Although they were crude images at first, dental radiography had its beginning at that time.

This important diagnostic tool is essential if we are to treat children successfully. Prima facie evidence indicates that unless caries is discovered early, the primary teeth cannot be retained to their normal exfoliation time. The literature abounds with statistical data demonstrating how often carious lesions go undetected without radiographic examination. The early diagnosis of caries prevents the young patient from being exposed to dental pain or extraction and the emotional stress resulting from these experiences. In addition, eruptive or developmental problems can be discovered in the radiographs, and early treatment of these problems will reduce the need for prolonged orthodontic procedures. Some operative procedures require an accurate registration of the outline of pulpal tissue in its relation to the surrounding hard tissue, and only a radiograph will reveal this information.

Less common but not less important is the detection of metabolic disturbances by dental radiographic examination. In many instances the first detection of bone calcification in a child is the dental radiograph. Certainly any deviation from the normal trabecular pattern should be investigated. Signs of periodontal disease in the dental radiograph of a young patient may be indicative of a systemic physiologic aberration. Genetic defects also produce numerous dental anomalies, and it is not uncommon for the dental examination to uncover a congenital disease.

The anomalies that a good radiographic technique should disclose have been classified by Brown as follows:

1. *Anomalies of number.* Congenitally missing teeth, partial or total anodontia, and supernumerary teeth are examples of such pathologic deviations.
2. *Anomalies of shape.* This classification encompasses such conditions as peg teeth, Hutchinson incisors, mulberry molars, Turner hypoplasia, dilaceration, dens in dente, supernumerary roots, macrodontia or microdontia, and gemination.
3. *Anomalies of position.* The most common ectopic eruption occurs with the first permanent molars and usually involves a concurrent ectopic resorption of the second primary molar.
4. *Anomalies of texture.* The most common anomaly of texture is caries. Others are amelogenesis imperfecta and dentinogenesis imperfecta.

We gratefully acknowledge the assistance of Gail F. Williamson, R.D.H., in the preparation of this chapter.

In addition to these anomalies, radiographs reveal calculus, internal resorption, fractured roots or crowns, periapical involvement, dentigerous cysts, neoplasia, fractures of the alveolar process, periodontal disease, clefts, fissural cysts, taurodontia, and dentinal bridges.

The selection of a good technique for obtaining radiographs of a child depends on age, mouth size, and patient cooperation. The ideal technique should expose the patient to a minimum amount of radiation, require as few radiographs as possible without sacrificing diagnostic quality, consume as little time as possible, and obtain an adequate examination of the dentition and surrounding structures. The child patient's cooperation is as essential to a good radiographic examination as selecting the correct radiographic technique, since it will increase the probability of success and help reduce any additional radiation exposures resulting from patient movement. Since the emotionally disturbed and the mentally or physically incapacitated child require special handling, they are discussed later in the chapter.

The majority of normal children become the radiologist's helpful partners if they are treated warmly and cheerfully. It is important to greet them intimately and address them by first name or even by a nickname. A running conversation before the radiographic procedure helps to initiate the relationship even though it is usually a monologue. Topics that focus on children's interests, such as pets, clothing, school, sports, and birthday gifts, are usually good openers.

The dental x-ray equipment can be awesome, or it can generate curiosity, depending on the child. It is wise to allow the patient to run a hand over the x-ray head and become acquainted with the "camera." The patient might hold one of the films and be shown where it will be placed. If it is a film that requires occlusion for fixation, the patient should be shown how to bite on the film. Radiographing the easiest region first may ensure success in filming the more difficult areas. This is particularly important if the child has an exaggerated gag reflex or objects to the placement of films into the sensitive portion of the floor of the mouth. Topical anesthetic agents are beneficial in both situations.

The dentist should be patient with the child in obtaining radiographs. Repeated attempts at film placement may be necessary before the actual radiation exposure is made. In the case of the uncooperative child, firmness, voice control, and tender loving care are often effective.

Preschool radiographic survey

The preschool radiographic survey is designed to facilitate procurement of an adequate radiographic examination of children between the ages of 3 and 6 years. Intraorally, this survey includes maxillary and mandibular anterior occlusal films and maxillary right and left posterior occlusal films taken with No. 2 periapical film. For extraoral use, right and left 5 × 7 inch Ready Pack Kodak Lateral Jaw films are used.

The lateral jaw radiograph affords an excellent view of the developing mandibular and maxillary first permanent molars, as well as of the mandibular primary molars and their succeeding premolars. Because of the difficulty of positioning the young patient, the lateral jaw film does not always produce a usable view of the maxillary primary molars; therefore the posterior maxillary occlusal radiographs are incorporated into the survey. These films offer an acceptable view of the maxillary primary molars, the permanent premolars, and the primary and permanent canines. The anterior occlusal films furnish a view of the maxillary and mandibular anterior teeth.

The advantages of this technique are that (1) it eliminates most of the behavioral problems encountered in obtaining intraoral periapical films, (2) the intraoral films used in this survey are more stable because film stabilization is not dependent on digital pressure, (3) more complete coverage is obtained of the molar regions than is possible with intraoral periapical films, and (4) it provides a good introduction to the dental office. The disadvantages are that (1) the films are not adequate to determine the presence of proximal caries in primary molars and (2) these films should not be

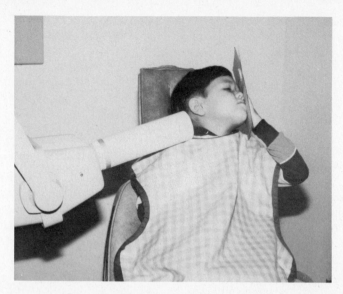

Fig. 6-1. Lateral jaw technique demonstrating the proper position of the patient's head and proper placement of the 5 × 7 inch film. The vertical angle is −17 degrees.

relied on for the diagnosis of early periapical lesions. Therefore if the primary molars are in proximal contact, making visual or explorer detection of caries impossible, right and left bite-wing radiographs should be included. If the dentist suspects the presence of a periapical pathologic lesion, a periapical film should be obtained of the area in question. Since intraoral periapical and bite-wing films are difficult for some children and may cause a behavior problem, these supplemental radiographs should be obtained after the survey films have been exposed.

Lateral jaw technique. A 5 × 7 inch Kodak nonscreen medical x-ray film is used for the lateral jaw technique (Fig. 6-1). The film is marked with a right or left lead identification letter placed on the film packet slightly anterior and superior to the central portion of the film. When the film is finally positioned, this letter should be located in the orbit area. A cardboard backing behind the film, secured with a rubber band, will support the film and reduce image distortion. The exposure timer is set at $^{24}/_{60}$ second with a 90-kV(p), 15-ma setting using a 12-inch open end cone.

To begin, the patient's head is positioned so that the occlusal plane is parallel to the floor and the sagittal plane is perpendicular to the floor. The long axis of the film, also perpendicular to the floor, rests on the patient's shoulder and against the face. The patient is instructed to rotate the head toward the film until the nose rests against it. Then the patient raises the chin and tilts the head approximately 15 degrees toward the film. The patient secures the film with the palm of the hand, fingers extended. The cone is positioned so that the central x-ray beam enters at a point ½ inch behind and below the angle of the mandible on the side opposite the film. The vertical angle is −17 degrees. The central x-ray beam is perpendicular to the horizontal plane of the film. For optimum processing results, lateral jaw films should be developed and fixed for twice the normal time of intraoral radiographs.

Anterior maxillary occlusal technique. For the

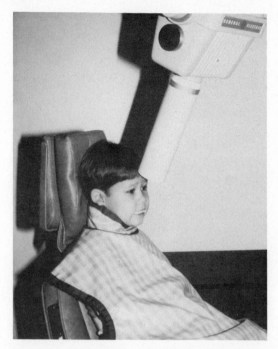

Fig. 6-2. Anterior maxillary occlusal technique demonstrating the proper position of the patient's head and proper placement of the No. 2 periapical film. The vertical angle is +60 degrees.

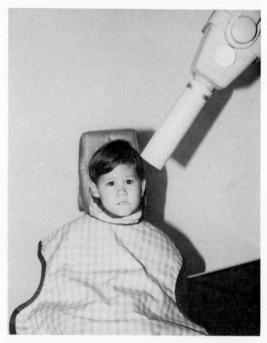

Fig. 6-3. Posterior maxillary occlusal technique demonstrating the proper position of patient's head and proper placement of the No. 2 periapical film. The central ray is directed to the apices of the primary molars. The vertical angle is +50 degrees.

anterior maxillary occlusal technique, the patient's occlusal plane should be parallel to the floor, and the sagittal plane should be perpendicular to the floor (Fig. 6-2). A No. 2 periapical film is placed in the patient's mouth so that the long axis of the film runs from left to right rather than anteroposteriorly and the midsagittal plane bisects the film. The patient is instructed to bite lightly to hold the film. The anterior edge of the film should extend approximately 2 mm in front of the incisal edge of the central incisors. The central ray is directed to the apices of the central incisors and ½ inch above the tip of the nose and through the midline. The vertical angle is +60 degrees. This film is exposed at the usual setting for maxillary incisor periapical films.

Posterior maxillary occlusal technique. In the posterior maxillary occlusal technique, the patient's occlusal plane should be parallel to the floor, and the sagittal plane should be perpendicular to the floor (Fig. 6-3). A No. 2 periapical film is placed in the patient's mouth so that the long axis of the film is parallel to the floor. The anterior edge of the film should extend just mesial to the canine. The outer buccal edge of the film should extend approximately 2 mm beyond the primary molar crowns. The patient is instructed to bite lightly to hold the film. The central ray is directed toward the apices of the primary molars as well as interproximally. The vertical angle is +50 degrees. The film is exposed at the usual setting for maxillary premolar periapical films.

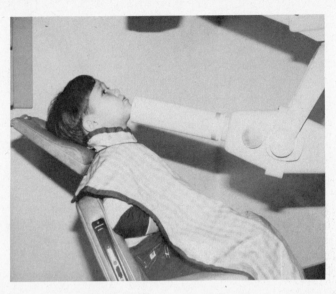

Fig. 6-4. Anterior mandibular occlusal technique demonstrating the proper position of patient's head and proper placement of the No. 2 periapical film. The occlusal plane is 45 degrees from the vertical. The vertical angle is −15 degrees.

Anterior mandibular occlusal technique. The film placement for the anterior mandibular occlusal technique is identical to that for the anterior maxillary occlusal technique, except that the film must be placed so that the tube side faces the x-ray source (Fig. 6-4). In addition, when the patient occludes on the film, the anterior edge of the film is 2 mm beyond the incisal edge of the lower incisors. The patient's head is positioned so that the occlusal plane is at a −45-degree angle. The cone is then aligned at a −15-degree vertical angle, and the central ray is directed through the symphysis.

Bite-wing radiograph technique. A No. 0 bite-wing film is usually the most suitable size for the pedodontic patient. Some children's mouths are large enough to receive a No. 2 bite-wing film. The film is placed horizontally, lingual to the mandibular primary molars, so that the tab rests on the occlusal surface. The dentist holds the tab with an index finger and directs the patient to slowly bite. As the patient is closing, the superior edge of the film should be guided lingual to the maxillary teeth. The central ray enters the middle of the tab at a +8-degree angle, perpendicular to the buccal plane of the teeth.

Exposure times and film processing. The following exposure times are based on a 12-inch focal film distance, using 90 kV(p) and 15 ma:

Lateral jaw	$^{24}/_{60}$ second
Posterior maxillary occlusal	$^{12}/_{60}$ second
Anterior maxillary occlusal	$^{12}/_{60}$ second
Anterior mandibular occlusal	$^{10}/_{60}$ second
Bite-wings	$^{10}/_{60}$ second

The developing time is 4½ minutes at 68° F (20° C) for the occlusal and bite-wing films. Since the lateral jaw film has a thicker emulsion, developing time and fixing time must be increased. Fig. 6-5 shows the completed radiographs comprising the preschool survey.

Intraoral periapical and bite-wing techniques

Maxillary permanent molar periapical radiographs. The child's head is positioned so that the midsagittal plane is vertical to the floor. The ala-tragus line is parallel to the floor (Fig. 6-6).

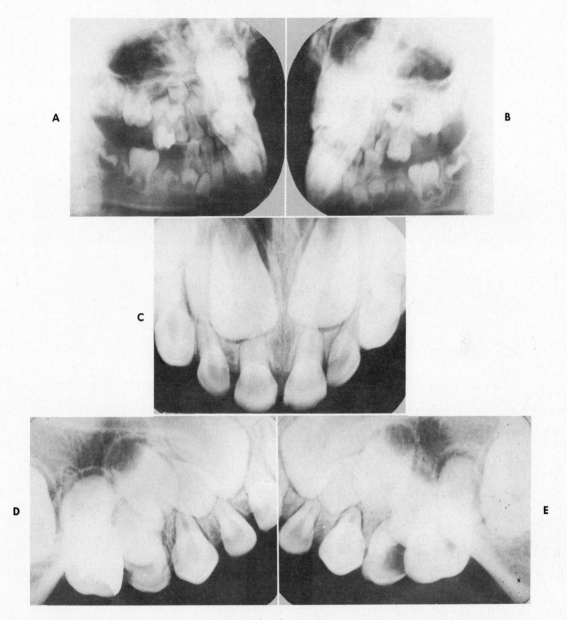

Fig. 6-5. Preschool survey with supplemental bite-wing films. **A** and **B**, Right and left lateral jaw films. **C**, Anterior maxillary occlusal film. **D** and **E**, Right and left posterior maxillary occlusal films.

Continued.

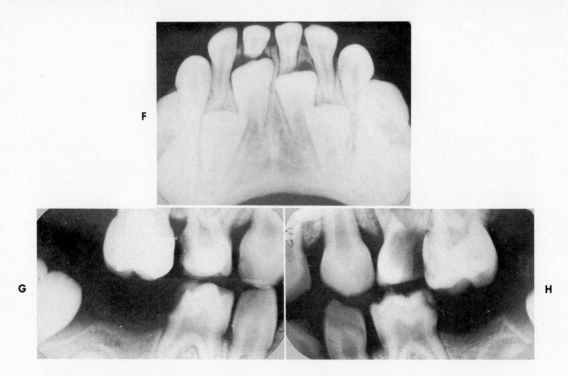

Fig. 6-5, cont'd. F, Anterior mandibular occlusal film. **G** and **H,** Right and left bite-wing films.

The unfolded film packet is positioned so that all of the maxillary tuberosity, the third molar, the second molar, and all or part of the first molar are recorded. The identification dot is placed toward the occlusal plane. The superior edge of the film packet is near or at the midline of the palate, and the tips of the palatal cusps are about ¼ inch from the occlusal edge. Light thumb pressure is applied against the film packet to maintain the desired film position. The left hand is used for the right side and the right hand for the left side. The fingers are extended and held back against the side of the patient's face. Since the film retention force must not cause the film packet to bend, the patient should be instructed to hold it lightly. The central ray enters below the outer canthus of the eye on the ala-tragus line (Fig. 6-6). The recommended starting vertical angle is +30 degrees (Fig. 6-6). The horizontal diameter of the end of the open end cone is parallel to the occlusal edge of the film packet or the mesiodistal tangent of the buccal surfaces of the molars (Fig. 6-7).

Maxillary premolar or primary molar periapical radiographs. The child's head is positioned so that the midsagittal plane is vertical. The ala-tragus line is parallel to the floor (Fig. 6-6). The film packet is folded and positioned so that the first molar, the first and second premolars or first and second primary molars, and the distal surface of the canine are recorded. The tips of the lingual cusps are ¼ inch from the occlusal edge of the film packet. The identification dot is placed toward the occlusal plane. The superior edge of the film packet usually lies near or at the midline of the palate, and the folded anterosuperior corner lies as far anteriorly as possible (Fig. 6-8).

Light thumb pressure is applied against the lower or upper third of the film packet to retain it

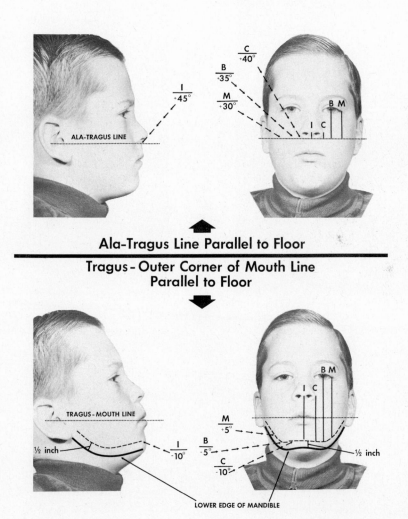

Fig. 6-6. Head position, vertical angles, and central ray entry points for the intraoral periapical techniques. *I,* Incisor technique; *C,* canine technique; *B,* premolar or primary molar technique; *M,* permanent molar technique.

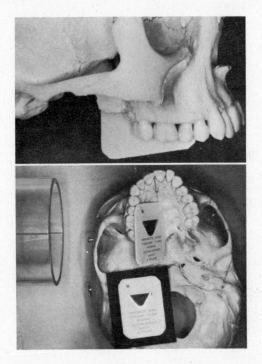

Fig. 6-7. Film placement and proper horizontal angulation for the maxillary permanent molar radiograph.

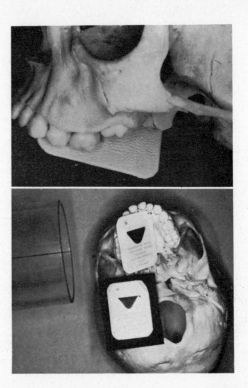

Fig. 6-8. Film placement and proper horizontal angulation for the maxillary premolar or primary molar periapical radiograph.

during exposure. Since the film retention force must not cause the film packet to bend, the patient should be instructed to hold it lightly. The left hand is used for the right side and the right hand for the left side. The fingers are extended and held back out of the x-ray beam against the side of the patient's face. The central ray enters at a point below the pupil of the eye on the ala-tragus line (Fig. 6-6). The vertical angle is +35 degrees. The horizontal diameter of the end of the open end cone is parallel to the occlusal edge of the film packet or the mesiodistal tangent of the buccal surfaces of the premolars or primary molars. The central ray is thus perpendicular to the mesiodistal axis of the film packet or the mesiodistal tangent of the buccal surfaces of the premolars or primary molars (Fig. 6-8).

Maxillary permanent or primary canine periapical radiographs. The child's head is positioned so that the midsagittal plane is vertical to the floor. The ala-tragus line is parallel to the floor (Fig. 6-6). The film packet is folded as illustrated in Fig. 6-9 and is positioned diagonally so that the posteroinferior corner is under the tip of the canine crown. The canine and lateral incisors are to be recorded in their entirety. The anteroinferior corner usually extends beyond the incisal edge of the central incisors. The anterosuperior corner usually lies palatal to the contralateral premolars or primary molars. The identification dot is toward the occlusal plane.

Light thumb pressure is applied against the film packet so that it remains unbent in the desired position. The left hand is used for the right side and the

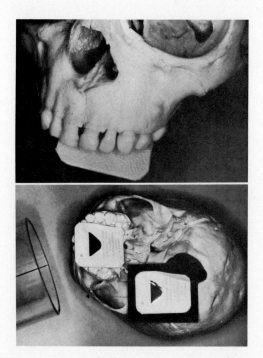

Fig. 6-9. Film placement and proper horizontal angulation for the maxillary permanent or primary canine periapical radiograph.

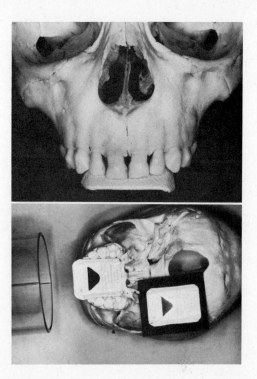

Fig. 6-10. Film placement and proper horizontal angulation for the maxillary permanent or primary central incisor periapical radiograph.

right hand for the left side. The fingers are extended and held back out of the x-ray beam against the side of the patient's face. The central ray enters through the ala (Fig. 6-6). The recommended starting vertical angle is +40 to 50 degrees (Fig. 6-6). The central ray should be parallel to the proximal surfaces of the canine and lateral incisor. The objective is to record some superimposition of the distal surface of the canine and the lingual cusp of the first premolar or the first primary molar without any superimposition of the mesial aspect of the canine and the distal aspect of the lateral incisor (Fig. 6-9).

Maxillary permanent or primary incisor periapical radiographs. The head is positioned so that the midsagittal plane is vertical. The ala-tragus line is parallel to the floor (Fig. 6-6). If the film packet

must be folded because of the narrowness of the arch, a ⅛-inch bend should be made throughout the entire length of the film on the sides that parallel the long axis of the film. The film packet is placed so that the central incisors are centered mesiodistally on the film. The incisal edge of the central incisors is ¼ inch from the incisal edge of the film packet. The identification dot is down toward the occlusal plane (Fig. 6-10).

Light thumb pressure is applied against the film packet so that it remains in the desired position and is not curved to conform to the shape of the arch. The right or left hand may be used, and the patient should be instructed to hold the film packet lightly. The fingers are extended and held back out of the x-ray beam against the side of the patient's face. The central ray is directed through the tip of the nose. The recommended starting vertical angle is +45 to 55 degrees. The horizontal diameter of the end of the open end cone is parallel to the mesiodistal axis (or the incisal edge) of the film packet (Fig. 6-10).

Mandibular permanent or primary incisor periapical radiographs. The head is positioned so that the midsagittal plane is vertical. The tragus corner of the mouth line is parallel to the floor (Fig. 6-6). The film packet is not usually folded. For small children, however, it may be necessary to fold the inferior corners and to use a short bite block. In addition, the No. 0 children's periapical film may have to be used for this exposure, as well as in all the mandibular techniques, if the child is small. In some instances digital fixation may be necessary. The bite block is centered on the incisal edge of the film packet. The inferior edge of the film packet is placed as far under the tongue as possible before the anterior end of the bite block is placed on the incisal edges of the incisors. The identification dot is located toward the occlusal plane (Fig. 6-11).

With the anterior end of the bite block resting on the mandibular incisors, the patient is instructed to close on the bite block with enough occlusal force to retain the bite block and film packet in the desired position. The central ray enters about ½ inch above the inferior border of the mandible at a point below the tip of the nose (Fig. 6-6). The recommended starting vertical angle is −10 degrees (Fig. 6-6). The horizontal diameter of the end of the open cone is parallel to the mesiodistal axis (or the incisal edge) of the film packet (Fig. 6-11).

Mandibular permanent or primary canine periapical radiographs. The child's head is positioned so that the midsagittal plan is vertical. The tragus corner of the mouth line is parallel to the floor (Fig. 6-6). The film packet is not folded. The bite block is usually attached slightly mesial to the center of the film packet. This position employs the flat incisal edges of the maxillary central and lateral incisors to hold the bite block, ensuring greater stability than if the incisal points of the maxillary and mandibular canines are used. The

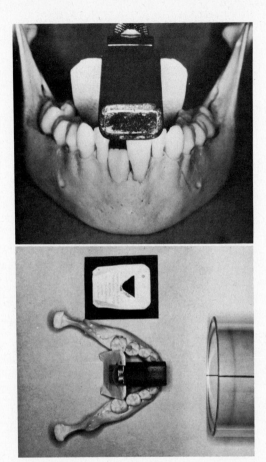

Fig. 6-11. Film placement and proper horizontal angulation for the mandibular permanent or primary incisor periapical radiograph.

inferior edge of the film packet is placed as far under the tongue as possible before the anterior end of the bite block is placed on the incisal aspect of the mandibular canine. The identification dot is toward the occlusal plane (Fig. 6-12).

With the anterior end of the bite block resting on the incisal aspect of the mandibular canine, the patient is instructed to close on the bite block with enough occlusal force to retain the bite block and film packet in the desired position. The central ray enters about ½ inch above the inferior border of the mandible at a point below the ala of the nose (Fig.

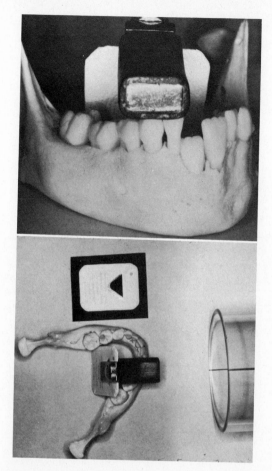

Fig. 6-12. Film placement and proper horizontal angulation for the mandibular permanent or primary canine periapical radiograph.

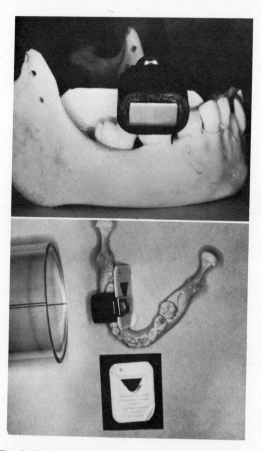

Fig. 6-13. Film placement and proper horizontal angulation for the mandibular premolar or primary molar periapical radiograph.

6-6). The recommended starting vertical angle is −10 degrees. The horizontal diameter of the end of the open end cone is parallel to the occlusal edge of the film packet (Fig. 6-12).

Mandibular premolar or primary molar periapical radiographs. The head is positioned so that the midsagittal plane is vertical. The tragus corner of the mouth line is parallel to the floor (Fig. 6-6). The lower anterior corner of the film packet is folded, and the film packet is positioned so the distal surface of the canine, first and second premolars or first and second primary molars, and the first

permanent molar are recorded. The bite block is attached to the anterior third of the film packet so that the bite block rests primarily on the mandibular premolars or primary molars. The folded lower anterior corner of the film packet is placed as far anteriorly as possible in the midline near or on the lingual frenum. The identification dot is toward the occlusal plane (Fig. 6-13).

With the bite block resting on the occlusal surface of the mandibular premolars or primary molars, the patient is instructed to close on the bite block with enough occlusal force to retain the bite block and film packet in the desired position. The central ray enters about ½ inch above the inferior border of the mandible at a point below the pupil of the eye (Fig. 6-6). The recommended starting vertical angle is −5 degrees (Fig. 6-6). The horizontal diameter of the end of the open end cone is parallel to the occlusal edge of the film packet (Fig. 6-13).

Mandibular permanent molar periapical radiographs. The child's head is positioned so that the midsagittal plane is vertical. The tragus corner of the mouth line is parallel to the floor (Fig. 6-6). The film packet is not folded and is positioned so that the retromolar area (or the anterior border of the ascending ramus), the third molar, and the sec-

ond molar are recorded in their entirety. The bite block is usually attached to the anterior third of the film packet so that it can be placed further posteriorly. When the curve of Spee is great or the third molar is malpositioned, the posterior aspect of the film packet is tilted slightly upward to record the retromolar area and the third molar more completely. For the right mandibular molar radiograph the identification dot is oriented apically to obtain an unobstructed view of the third molar crown. For the left mandibular molar radiograph the identification dot is oriented occlusally (Fig. 6-14).

With the bite block resting on the occlusal surface of the mandibular molars, the patient is instructed to close on the bite block with just enough occlusal force to retain it and the film packet in the desired position. The central ray enters about ½ inch above the inferior border of the mandible at a point below the outer canthus of the eye (Fig. 6-6). The vertical angle is +5 degrees (Fig. 6-6). The horizontal diameter of the end of the open end cone is parallel to the occlusal edge of the film packet or to the mesiodistobuccal tangent of the molars (Fig. 6-14).

Posterior bite-wing radiographs. The head is positioned so that the midsagittal plane is vertical—as for the periapical radiographs. The ala-

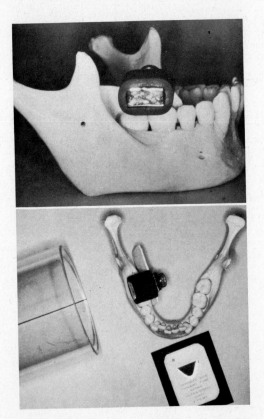

Fig. 6-14. Film placement and proper horizontal angulation for the mandibular permanent molar periapical radiograph.

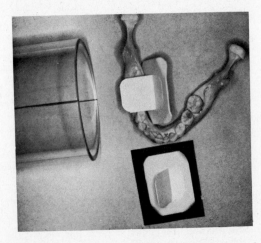

Fig. 6-15. Film placement and proper horizontal angulation for the posterior bite-wing radiograph.

tragus line is horizontal. The inferior edge of the bite-wing film packet is placed in the floor of the mouth between the tongue and the lingual aspect of the mandible, and the bite-tab is placed on the occlusal surfaces of the mandibular teeth (Fig. 6-15). The anterior edge of the film packet is located as far anteriorly as possible in the region of the canine so that the distal aspect of the tooth will be recorded. The lower anterior corner of the film packet is bent sharply toward the lingual to facili-

tate film placement and to decrease possible discomfort of the patient. In addition, the anterosuperior corner is bent to conform to the palate, and the anteroposterior corner is bent to prevent irritation of the gag reflex. The anteroinferior corner of the film packet usually lies near or at the attachment of the lingual frenum in the midline.

The dentist firmly holds the bite-tab against the occlusal surfaces of the patient's mandibular teeth with an index finger, and the patient is instructed to

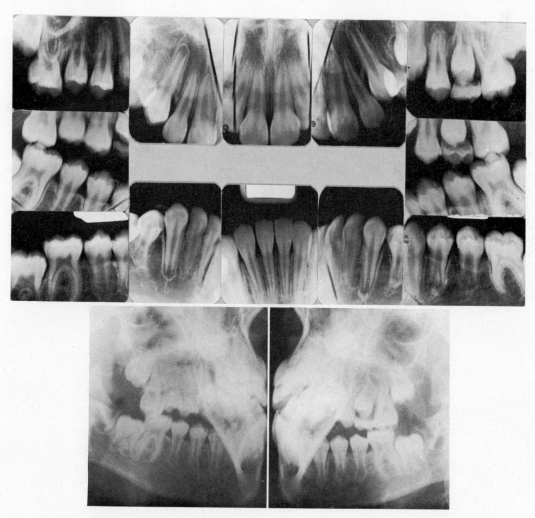

Fig. 6-16. Right and left lateral jaw radiographs supplementing the 12-film intraoral radiographic examination.

slowly close. The finger is rolled out of the way onto the buccal surfaces of the teeth as the patient closes in centric occlusion. The central ray enters through the occlusal plane at a point below the pupil of the eye. The vertical angle is +8 degrees. The horizontal diameter of the open end cone is parallel to the end of the bite-tab or to the mean tangent of the buccal surfaces of the posterior teeth being radiographed.

Twelve-film intraoral radiographic examination

The 12-film technique is used for obtaining radiographs of children between the ages of 6 and 12 years. It includes four primary molar periapical radiographs, four canine periapical radiographs, two incisor periapical radiographs, and two posterior bite-wing radiographs (Fig. 6-16). The No. 2 size periapical film should be used in this exami-

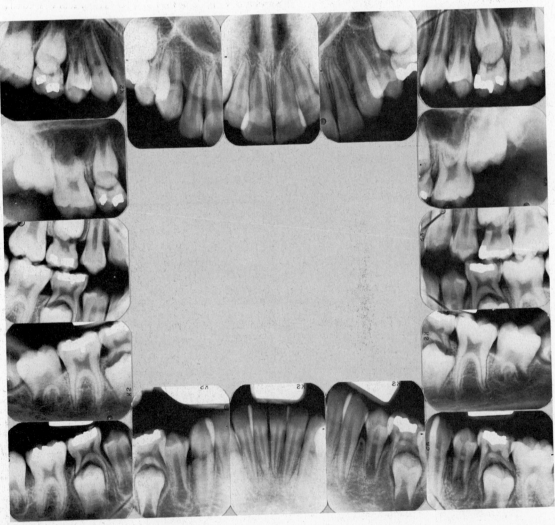

Fig. 6-17. Sixteen-film intraoral radiographic examination.

nation. If the child's mouth is small or if a behavior problem exists, however, the dentist may elect to use the No. 0 size periapical film in the mandible. Since it is desirable to obtain an adequate view of the second and third molars, it may be necessary to augment the 12-film examination with right and left lateral jaw films (Fig. 6-16). The techniques used in this examination are outlined on p. 136.

Sixteen-film intraoral radiographic examination

The 16-film examination is used to obtain radiographs of children 12 years of age and older. This survey includes 14 periapical films and two posterior bite-wing films. The periapical radiographs are four molar views, four premolar views, four canine views, and two incisor views (Fig. 6-17). The No. 2 adult-size films should be used in this examination. If the child's mouth is small or if the patient is uncooperative and adequate radiographs of the molar areas cannot be obtained, however, right and left lateral jaw radiographs may be used to supplement the intraoral films.

Paralleling technique

An alternative technique of taking intraoral radiographs for the older child patient employs the principles of the paralleling technique. Using film-holding devices with cone and angle guides such as the Rinn XCP holder (Fig. 6-18) helps reduce radiation exposure to the patient. However, because of the shallowness of the child's palate and floor of the mouth, film placement is somewhat compromised. Despite this, the resulting films are quite satisfactory.

Panoramic radiography

A fairly recent innovation in dental radiology has been the application of body section radiography. Numerous panoramic x-ray units are available today. Fig. 6-19 demonstrates the use of the Panelipse panoramic unit.* Body section radiography employs a mechanism in which the x-ray film and

---

*General Electric Dental Systems, Milwaukee, Wis. 53201.

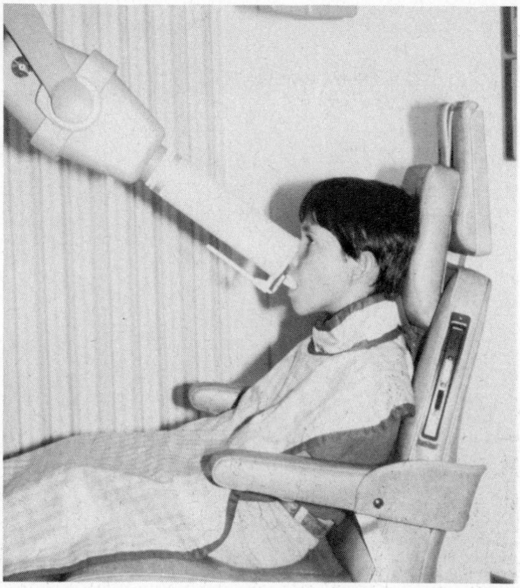

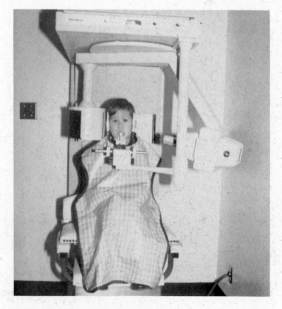

Fig. 6-18. Use of the Rinn XCP holder. This view depicts the proper alignment for the maxillary incisor periapical radiograph.

Fig. 6-19. Patient positioned in a General Electric Panelipse panoramic unit.

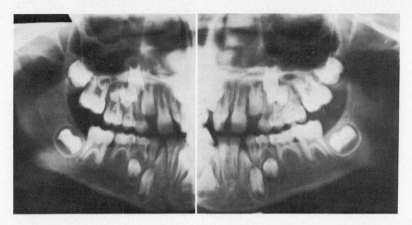

Fig. 6-20. Radiograph obtained with the S.S. White Panorex x-ray unit. Note the congenitally missing mandibular second premolars.

the source of x-rays are moving simultaneously in opposite directions at the same speed. The x-ray film and the x-ray tube revolve around a fixed point of rotation. This fixed point is stationary relative to the moving x-ray film and the narrow beam of x-rays. Therefore any structure being radiographed at the fixed point is distinctly recorded.

A panoramic radiographic unit can be used for examination of children. Since this examination can be obtained without placing anything in the mouth, it eliminates the problem of alarming the nervous or disturbed child who may refuse an intraoral film. Moreover, the young patient feels some exhilaration from "taking a ride" in the chair. The diversion of being momentarily entertained invites cooperation. However, the necessity for sustaining complete immobility for 15 to 22 seconds may not be possible with some young children.

Although panoramic radiography is considered a supplement to, rather than a substitute for, the intraoral periapical radiographic series, it does provide excellent coverage of the structures that are viewed during pedodontic diagnosis. A diagnostic film includes the teeth, the supporting structures, the maxillary region extending to the superior third of the orbit, and the entire mandible including the temporomandibular joint region. Pedodontists who

have used the panoramic radiographic technique routinely for a period of time have discovered condylar fractures, traumatic cysts, and anomalies that might have gone undetected with the routine periapical series of radiographs (Fig. 6-20).

Panoramic radiology can be valuable in examining handicapped patients. If the patient can sit in a chair and hold his or her head in position, this examination is usable. It may be necessary to administer relaxants or sedation to palsied or spastic patients, who are more difficult to control when they are emotionally charged by the dental visit.

There are some inherent drawbacks with the use of panoramic radiographs. A loss of image detail is probably the greatest limitation. Since these films are not suitable for diagnosing early carious lesions, adjunct bite-wing radiographs and selected periapical radiographs are required.

Localization techniques

One method of localizing embedded or unerupted teeth employs the buccal object rule, which states that the image of any buccally oriented object appears to move in the opposite direction from a moving x-ray source. Conversely, the image of any lingually oriented object appears to move in the same direction as a moving x-ray source (Fig. 6-21).

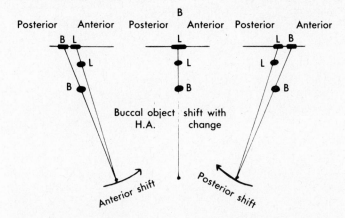

Fig. 6-21. The buccal object rule. *B,* Buccal; *L,* lingual; *H.A.,* horizontal angle.

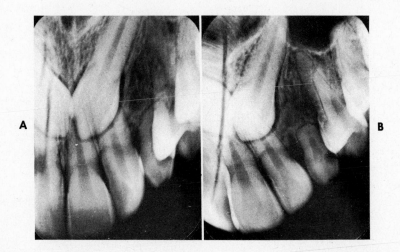

Fig. 6-22. A, Shadow of the maxillary permanent canine is superimposed over the central incisor root. **B,** When the horizontal angle of the x-ray tube is shifted posteriorly, the crown of the unerupted canine appears to move posteriorly. The canine is lingually placed.

Using this principle for localization, the radiologist makes two radiographs of the area of the unerupted tooth. The technique consists of positioning the patient's head so that the sagittal plane is perpendicular to the floor and the ala-tragus line is parallel to the floor. An intraoral periapical film is placed in the mouth and then exposed. A second film is placed in the mouth in the same position as the first film, with the patient's head position remaining the same. The second film is then exposed. The vertical angulation should be the same for each exposure. However, the horizontal angle is shifted either anteriorly or posteriorly, depending on the area being examined, for the second view.

Fig. 6-22, *A,* shows an unerupted maxillary permanent canine. The shadow of this tooth is superimposed over the central incisor root. When the

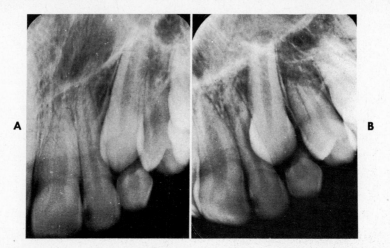

Fig. 6-23. A, Shadow of the maxillary permanent canine covers a small portion of the lateral incisor root on its distal aspect. **B,** When the horizontal angle of the x-ray tube is shifted posteriorly, the canine appears to move anteriorly. The canine lies buccal to the erupted teeth.

horizontal angle of the x-ray tube is shifted posteriorly (Fig. 6-22, *B*), the crown of the unerupted canine also seems to move posteriorly and the image of the canine crown is no longer superimposed over the central incisor root. If the buccal object rule is applied, it can be seen that the embedded canine is *lingually* oriented to the erupted teeth.

Fig. 6-23, *A,* shows an embedded maxillary permanent canine. The shadow of the crown of this tooth covers a small portion of the lateral incisor root on its distal aspect. When the horizontal angle is shifted posteriorly (Fig. 6-23, *B*), the unerupted crown appears to move anteriorly or in a direction opposite to the shift of the x-ray source. The unerupted canine is *buccally* oriented to the erupted teeth.

Another localization technique is the *cross section* occlusal radiograph. Depending on the size of the child's mouth, either the adult occlusal or a No. 2 periapical film may be used. To obtain a cross section occlusal radiograph of the maxilla, the patient's sagittal plane is perpendicular to the floor, and the ala-tragus line is parallel to the floor. The patient is asked to occlude lightly on the film. The

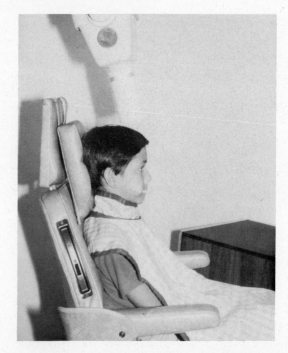

Fig. 6-24. Cross section maxillary occlusal technique demonstrating the proper position of the patient's head and the proper central ray entry point. The central ray is directed coincidentally with the long axes of the central incisor roots.

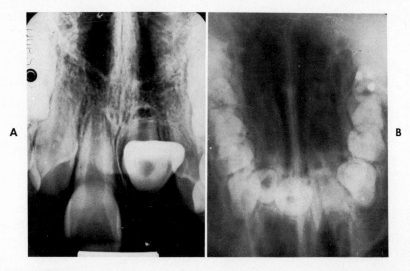

Fig. 6-25. A, Dilacerated maxillary central incisor. **B,** The crown of the dilacerated central incisor lies labially.

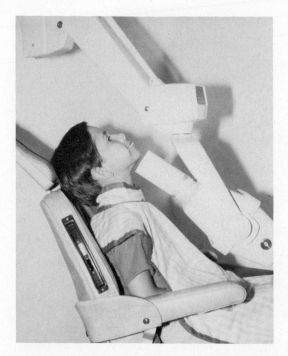

Fig. 6-26. Cross section mandibular occlusal technique demonstrating the proper position of patient's head and the proper vertical angulation of the x-ray head.

central ray is projected through the midsagittal plane and enters the skull 1 cm posterior to bregma. (Bregma is the point at which the sagittal suture meets the coronal suture.) The proper vertical angulation is determined by directing the central ray through the long axes of the maxillary central incisor roots (Fig. 6-24).

A maxillary central incisor periapical radiograph demonstrating a grossly dilacerated central incisor may be seen in Fig. 6-25, *A.* It is important to determine before a surgical procedure if the crown of such a tooth is in a labial or a lingual position. In this instance a cross section occlusal film reveals that the crown is positioned labially (Fig. 6-25, *B*).

The cross section occlusal film can be employed for localization of anomalies in the mandible. Either the adult occlusal or a No. 2 periapical film can be used. The patient's head is tilted backward sufficiently to direct the central ray through the long axes of the erupted teeth (Fig. 6-26). The patient's head must be tilted on its long axis to accommodate positioning of the x-ray tube. If determination of the buccal or lingual position of an impacted mandibular third molar is desired, the

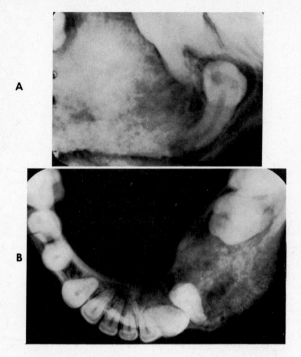

Fig. 6-27. A, Unerupted mandibular premolar displaced by an ossifying fibroma. **B,** The crown of the unerupted premolar is lingually oriented.

central ray should be projected through the long axis of the mandibular second molar. If it is necessary to localize an unerupted second premolar, the central ray should be directed through the long axis of the first premolar. Fig. 6-27, *A,* reveals an unerupted mandibular premolar that has been displaced by an ossifying fibroma. In Fig. 6-27, *B,* a cross section occlusal radiograph demonstrates that the crown of the premolar is lingually placed.

Radiation safety

In the 1950s the dental profession began a massive effort to reduce the hazards of ionizing radiation. This campaign has resulted in reducing radiation hazards to a minimum. In the 1950s most of the effort was directed toward educating dentists. They were instructed in such areas as why and how to collimate an x-ray beam, why and how to filter an x-ray beam, and why to use fast films.

The success of these programs is indicated by the following statistics: 80% of the dental units in the United States in 1964 met or exceeded the proper requirements of collimation and filtration. This represented a 50% increase in acceptable x-ray units from 1960. The reader should consult the reference materials for information concerning dosage and radiation measurements.

One characteristic of x-rays is their ability to cause changes that will result in biologic defects. The earliest detectable biologic change, which is completely reversible, is skin erythema. The skin erythema dose (SED) is 165 to 350 roentgens (r) in a single dose. The skin dose received in the preschool radiographic survey is approximately 3 r. The skin dose for the 12-film children's examination is 4 r, and the skin dose for the 16-film examination is approximately 5 r. The Panorex radiographic unit* produces a skin dose ranging from 6 to 203 millirad/millirem to the skin on the back of the patient's neck. All of these skin doses are well below the SED.

Much attention has been focused on gonadal doses of x-rays. The allowable gonadal dose is 10 r from conception to 30 years of age. It is interesting to note that the gonads receive 0.125 r per year from natural background radiation emanating from the earth's crust and outer space. This type of irradiation is unavoidable, and humans have always been exposed to it.

The male gonadal doses for the various techniques are as follows: preschool survey—0.0003 r; 12-film examination—0.0004 r; 16-film examination—0.0005 r. The Panorex produces a gonadal dose of 0.0001 r, which is smaller than that of the other techniques because the x-ray source is never directed toward the gonads. The male gonadal dose is approximately $1/10,000$ of the skin dose from dental radiographs. The female gonadal dose is slightly lower because the female gonads are located internally. With proper use of a protective lead apron, these low radiation doses to the gonads can be reduced even more.

---

*S.S. White Dental Products, Div. of Pennwalt Corp., Philadelphia, Pa. 19102.

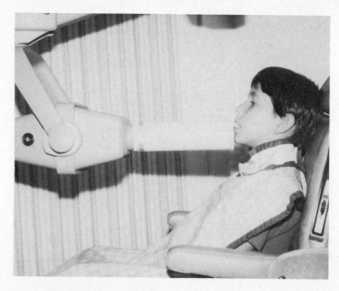

Fig. 6-28. Patient with lead apron and thyroid collar.

If a patient has a yearly full-mouth radiographic examination from ages 3 to 30, the gonadal dose from these radiographs would approximate the amount of background irradiation the individual would be exposed to in 1 month. This is a total of 27 full-mouth radiographs, which is more than would normally be recommended. In the routine practice of dentistry it is doubtful if a patient receives even a third of this number of radiographs from ages 3 to 30 years. However, dental x-ray films may be only a part of the total x-rays to which a patient is exposed during the reproductive years. For example, a posteroanterior view of the chest produces a gonadal dose of 0.0005 r, and a lateral head plate exposes the gonads to 0.0002 r.

The dental practitioner should be judicious in the use of the radiographic examination. The use of fast films, a properly collimated and filtered x-ray beam, correct exposure and processing times, and good radiographic technique will minimize retakes and reduce radiation exposure of the patient. For greater protection from radiation, all children should be covered with a lead apron and a lead thyroid collar during radiographic examination (Fig. 6-28).

Special radiographic technique for handicapped children

The physically handicapped child usually cannot hold a film in his or her mouth with the fingers or hold an extraoral film with a hand. Such a child may be an amputee, a paralytic, or an arthritic; may be disabled by congenital anomalies; or may be unconscious as the result of an accident. There are several radiographic techniques that may be used to obtain films of these patients—for example, intraoral radiographs with the parent or guardian holding the films in place. Film-holding devices, such as bite blocks or a hemostat extended through a rubber stopper, may also be employed to retain the film. In addition, the films can be retained with the patient's occlusion and are not dependent on digital fixation. The panoramic technique is also adaptable to the physically handicapped child, as is the preschool radiographic survey. However, the parent or guardian must hold the lateral jaw films in the preschool survey (Fig. 6-29).

Trismus must be considered a physically handicapping condition, since affected patients cannot open their mouths. For patients with trismus the only techniques available are extraoral radiographs.

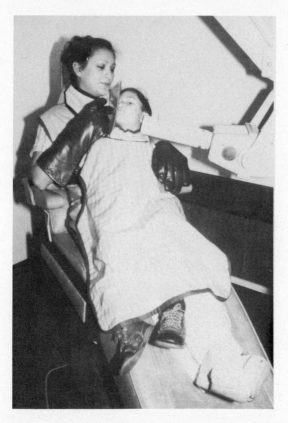

Fig. 6-29. Parent holding the lateral jaw film for the child during radiation exposure. Both the parent and the child are shielded from extraneous exposure.

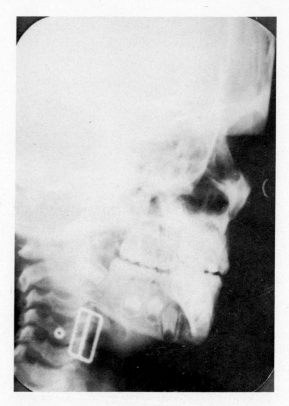

Fig. 6-30. Forty-five-degree oblique head plate. The patient's head is positioned in a cephalostat.

The dentist who wishes to obtain radiographs of mentally handicapped children or young children must be willing to accept films of less desirable quality. Many mentally handicapped children will not allow an intraoral film to be placed in their mouths. Therefore intraoral radiographs for these children are usually obtained with the parent holding the film in position while an assistant restrains the child. The assistant is frequently exposed to x-rays and therefore must wear a lead apron, thyroid collar, protective glasses, and lead gloves during the radiographic examination. A holding device that fixes the film in position while the patient occludes is more effective than trying to hold the film by digital placement. Some mentally handicapped patients will accept a film placed in the mucobuccal fold rather than in the floor of the mouth. When a film is placed in the mucobuccal fold, the dentist must use a lateral jaw technique in which the x-rays are projected below the lower border of the mandible of the side not being radiographed.

If in spite of all efforts the patient still refuses an intraoral film, extraoral views can usually be obtained. The child may still have to be restrained. It is wise to use a short exposure time; this can be accomplished by employing an x-ray unit with high kilovoltage and a cassette with an intensifying

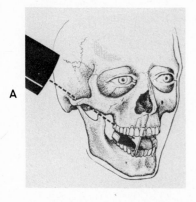

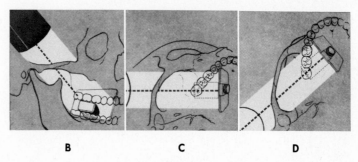

Fig. 6-31. A, Cone position. **B,** Relationship of zygomatic arch and cone. **C,** Inferior view showing relationship of film and third molar. **D,** Disto-oblique angle.

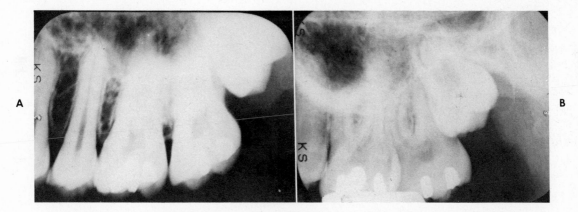

Fig. 6-32. A, Inadequate view of an unerupted maxillary third molar employing the conventional molar technique. **B,** Excellent view of an unerupted maxillary third molar employing the disto-oblique technique.

screen. The 45-degree oblique head plate shown in Fig. 6-30 requires an exposure time of 0.5 second using a 60-inch focal film distance, 15 ma, and 90 kV(p). This extremely short exposure time is useful in radiographing mentally retarded, cerebral palsied, or uncooperative patients.

Disto-oblique technique for unerupted maxillary third molars

The disto-oblique technique is excellent for radiographing unerupted maxillary third molars that cannot be viewed using the conventional maxillary

molar periapical procedure. The film is positioned with the posterosuperior corner of the film resting against the palate on the opposite side of the arch and the anterosuperior corner lying just above the maxillary premolars of the side being radiographed. A long wooden or metal bite block is used for film stabilization. The vertical angle is +35 degrees. The central ray, directed perpendicular to the long axis of the film, passes through the sigmoid notch. The exposure time should be 50% greater than the conventional molar exposure time (Figs. 6-31 and 6-32).

REFERENCES

Block, A.J., Goepp, R.A., and Mason, E.W.: Thyroid radiation dose during panoramic and cephalometric dental x-ray examinations, Angle Orthod. **47:**17-24, 1977.

Brown, W.E.: The utilization of radiology in a children's practice, N.J. State Dent. Soc. J. **23:**17-27, 1952.

General Electric Co.: Panelipse Panoramic X-Ray System user manual, Milwaukee, 1979.

Kasle, M.J.: Radiography: cross-fire localization technic, Dent. Surv. **45:**29-31, 1969.

Kasle, M.J.: Radiographic technique for difficult maxillary third molar views, J.A.D.A. **83:**1104-1105, 1971.

Kasle, M.J., and Langlais, R.P.: Basic principles of oral radiology, vol. 4, Exercises in dental radiology, Philadelphia, 1981, W.B. Saunders Co.

Langland, O.E., Langlais, R.P., and Morris, C.R.: Principles and practice of panoramic radiology, Philadelphia, 1982, W.B. Saunders Co.

Myers, D.R., and others: Radiation exposure during panoramic radiography in children, Oral Surg. **46:**588-593, 1978.

National Council on Radiation Protection and Measurements: Radiation protection in pediatric radiology, Report No. 68, Washington, D.C., 1981, The Council.

7 Dental caries in the child and adolescent

RALPH E. McDONALD
DAVID R. AVERY

Dental caries continues to be a major problem in dentistry and should receive significant attention in everyday practice, not only from the standpoint of restorative procedures but also in terms of preventive practices designed to reduce the problem. It is estimated that dental caries affects 98% of the U.S. population, creating a dental disease problem of massive proportions. By 17 years of age, 94% of all children have had caries in their permanent teeth. On the average, 17-year-olds have had about nine permanent teeth affected. Children from low-income families have about four times as many untreated decayed teeth as children from high-income families. Forty-seven percent of children under age 12 have never been to a dentist. About 31 million adults aged 18 to 74 years have lost all their upper or lower natural teeth. This figure includes about 19 million adults who have lost all of their teeth.*

The annual expenditure for dental care in 1970 was $4.8 billion. The *American Dental Association News* reported that Americans spent nearly $16 billion on dental services in 1980, which represents an increase of approximately 18% over the $13.5 billion spent in 1979. Much of this cost is due to the ravages of dental caries. In addition, the number of people covered by dental insurance increased by more than 50% between 1976 and 1979.

According to Infante and Owen, little informa-

tion is available regarding the prevalence and distribution of dental caries activity and levels of treatment in preschool children in the United States. Estimates of the number of carious teeth have ranged from 0.60 for the average 2-year-old to 4.75 for the average 5-year-old. For children of these same ages, levels of treatment have ranged from 3% to 39%. Infante and Owen's analysis of data from 1155 probability-selected preschool children representing 36 states and the District of Columbia indicated the following conclusions:

1. No significant difference in caries experience exists by geographic region, although children in the West had significantly higher levels of treatment.
2. Compared with children in the middle socioeconomic group, the lower status children of both urban and rural areas and within each geographic region had significantly greater caries incidence and significantly lower levels of treatment either by restoration or by extraction of teeth.
3. Compared with urban children, rural children had a significantly greater incidence of caries and a significantly lower level of treatment.
4. Compared with white children, black children had a significantly greater caries incidence and significantly less treatment.

Hennon, Stookey, and Muhler (1969) made a survey of 915 white children between 18 and 39 months of age, which showed that 8.3% of the 18- to 23-month-old children had dental caries. The

---

*Data from U.S. Department of Health and Human Services: Promoting health—preventing disease, Washington, D.C., 1981, U.S. Government Printing Office.

Table 7-1. Mean DMFS for U.S. children aged 5 to 17 from 1971-1973 National Center for Health Statistics Survey and the 1979-1980 National Institute of Dental Research Survey

Age	NCHS* (1971-1973)		NIDR (1979-1980)	
	Number in thousands†	Mean DMFS	Number in thousands†	Mean DMFS
5	1068	0.15	1055	0.11
6	2825	0.41	2750	0.20
7	3704	0.69	3525	0.58
8	3661	1.86	3453	1.25
9	4036	3.59	3420	1.90
10	4378	4.14	3515	2.60
11	4088	4.58	3479	3.00
12	4116	6.36	3601	4.18
13	4153	8.67	3822	5.41
14	4046	9.60	4063	6.53
15	4256	11.67	4171	8.07
16	4164	15.12	4195	9.58
17	3898	16.90	4267	11.04
All ages	48393	7.06	45315	4.77

Reprinted from The prevalence of dental caries in United States children, 1979-1980, The National Dental Caries Prevalence Survey, NIH Pub. No. 82-2245, Washington, D.C., Dec. 1981, with permission of the National Institutes of Health, U.S. Department of Health and Human Services.

*Decayed, missing and filled surfaces among children. National Health Survey, 1971-1973. Hanes 1 special dental tape, National Center for Health Statistics. June 1978. Unpublished.

†Sample weighted to represent total U.S. children.

number of children afflicted with dental caries by 36 to 39 months of age increased to 57.2%. The average decayed, exfoliated, or filled primary (def) teeth and def surface values for these older children were 4.65 and 6.16, respectively.

Research indicates that the prevalence of dental caries in some areas of the United States has dropped 40% to 50% in the past 30 years. This decrease is due, at least in part, to the fact that approximately 110 million people drink water to which fluoride has been added or that naturally contains fluoride at an adequate level. The three-decade-old program of water fluoridation has had a dramatic impact on caries formation. The federal Centers for Disease Control in Atlanta estimates that about 20% of all teenagers in communities with a fluoridated water supply are caries free.

According to the American Dental Association's survey in 1975, 50% of the U.S. population resides in communities with fluoridated water. These reports are the result of work completed by Scholle and Schrotenboer.

The National Caries Program of the National Institute of Dental Research, in cooperation with the National Center for Health Statistics, designed the National Dental Caries Prevalence Survey, which was conducted during the 1979-1980 school year. The continental United States was divided into seven geographic regions, and a large sample of schoolchildren (aged 5 to 17 years) from each region was given oral examinations. Over 5000 children from 25 to 33 communities in each region were examined. The findings are no doubt conservative, since the tactile-visual examinations were

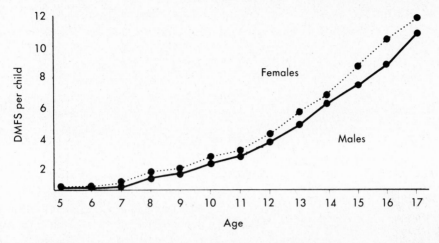

Fig. 7-1. Age- and sex-specific prevalence of dental caries in permanent teeth for the United States, 1979-1980. (Reprinted from The prevalence of dental caries in United States children, 1979-1980, The National Dental Caries Prevalence Survey, NIH Pub. No. 82-2245, Washington, D.C., Dec. 1981, with permission of the National Institutes of Health, U.S. Department of Health and Human Services.)

confined to the use of explorers, mouth mirrors, and transilluminated light (no radiographs were taken). Nevertheless, the findings are meaningful, especially when they are compared with a similar National Health Survey conducted from 1971 to 1973. These new data indicate a definite downward trend in the prevalence of decayed, missing, or filled permanent tooth surfaces (DMFS) among the nation's schoolchildren (Table 7-1).

The results of the survey translate to an estimated 4.77 DMFS per child among the nation's 45.3 million schoolchildren 5 to 17 years of age. The average number of decayed, missing, or filled permanent teeth (DMFT) per child was calculated to be 2.91. The average DMFS scores increase with age, ranging from 0.11 in 5-year-olds to 11.04 by age 17. Yet 36.6% of all children examined were scored (without bite-wing radiographs) as completely caries free in permanent teeth. Obviously the majority of caries-free permanent teeth are found in the younger children, and many older children have very high DMFS scores. The average score (4.77) compares favorably with the 1971-1973 survey when DMFS figures ranged from 0.15

to 16.90, with an overall average of 7.06. Thus the prevalence of caries in schoolchildren in the continental United States has decreased substantially in the last decade.

The 1979-1980 data also suggest that the level of restorative dental care for children is high. Only 7.1% of the permanent teeth were found to have been extracted because of caries and 16.8% were found to be decayed and unfilled, while 76.1% of the DMF scored surfaces had been restored by dental treatment.

Fig. 7-1 illustrates the progressive increase in DMFS with age for both boys and girls, and Fig. 7-2 shows the percent distribution of DMFT among children in the United States, according to the 1979-1980 survey. The greatest prevalence of caries in DMFS was found in the northeastern (5.56) and far western states (5.12), while children in the southwestern states showed the least prevalence of caries (3.41). These findings are consistent with previous national surveys.

Additional data revealed that in the primary dentition of children 5 to 9 years of age, there was an average of 5.31 decayed or filled surfaces (dfs) and

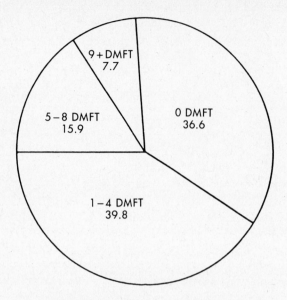

Fig. 7-2. Percent distribution of U.S. children according to DMFT status, 1979-1980. (Reprinted from The prevalence of dental caries in United States children, 1979-1980, The National Dental Caries Prevalence Survey, NIH Pub. No. 82-2245, Washington, D.C., Dec. 1981, with permission of the National Institutes of Health, U.S. Department of Health and Human Services.)

2.55 decayed or filled teeth (dft). The regional data suggest that these averages are reasonably representative of the estimated 16.7 million schoolchildren in the 5- to 9-year age group. Interestingly, however, the dfs average for these children in the southwestern states was 5.80 (second highest) while the dfs average was 4.73 for northeastern states and 5.01 for the far western states. (These regional data show an opposite trend when compared with the DMFS scores.) The children in the northwestern states had the highest dfs average, 6.12. However, these data do not account for the number of missing primary teeth lost as a result of caries.

As might be expected, children residing in urban areas, because of their access to fluoridated public water supplies, have a lower caries prevalence than children in rural areas.

In addition, unpublished data from dental health surveys made by the Dental Division of the Indiana State Board of Health show a 37% reduction in first permanent molar mortality in children participating in the 4-H Club summer program. This reduction has been attributed to an educational program emphasizing adequate diet and good oral hygiene as important factors in improving dental health. The reduction was also a result of both referral of those children with dental defects to their family dentist for corrective work and the excellent quality of dental care they received.

Gish reported that in Indianapolis in 1951, before fluoridation, the missing permanent tooth rate was 14.1 teeth per 100 children for the 6-, 7-, and 9-year-old groups. In 1964, after 12 years of fluoridation, the missing permanent tooth rate was 2.8 per 100 children, representing a significant reduction in tooth mortality.

A statewide survey conducted by the Dental Division of the Indiana State Board of Health in 1972 revealed that there had been a 55% reduction in the number of missing permanent teeth per 100 children as compared with the 1959 figures. Another 10-year-cycle survey is being conducted, and it is anticipated that the results will demonstrate a continued reduction in the prevalence of dental caries in Indiana. Despite this progressive decline, meeting the dental restorative needs of children remains a formidable task.

Currently accepted theories of the cause of dental caries

There are three general theories regarding the mechanism of dental caries. The proteolysis theory, with its identification of protein in human enamel, received attention from such proponents as Gottlieb and Frisbie. Even some who do not subscribe to the theory admit that proteolysis may play a role in the dental caries process.

The proteolytic-chelation theory has received considerable attention. This theory postulates that oral bacteria attack organic components of enamel and that the breakdown products have chelating ability and thus dissolve the tooth minerals.

The chemicoparasitic or acidogenic theory was

advanced by Miller in the latter part of the last century. This theory has been the most popular over the years and is probably the one most widely accepted today. Evidence in support of decalcification as the mechanism of caries attack is greater than evidence for the other two theories. It is generally agreed that dental caries is caused by acid resulting from the action of microorganisms on carbohydrates. It is characterized by a decalcification of the inorganic portion and is accompanied or followed by a disintegration of the organic substance of the tooth.

When Miller in 1890 pronounced his theory of caries, he assumed that there was no one microorganism directly associated with dental caries but that every acidogenic organism in the coating of the teeth contributed to the process of fermentation that resulted in the decalcification of the enamel surface.

Studies by Orland and by Fitzgerald, Jordan, and Achard demonstrated that dental caries will not occur in the absence of microorganisms. Animals maintained in a germ-free environment did not develop caries even when fed a high-carbohydrate diet. However, dental caries did develop in these animals when they were inoculated with microorganisms from caries-active animals and then fed cariogenic diets.

A number of microorganisms can produce enough acid to decalcify tooth structure, particularly aciduric streptococci, lactobacilli, diphtheroids, yeasts, staphylococci, and certain strains of sarcinae. Gnotobiotic studies have shown that the main agents of caries production are streptococci, including *S. mutans, S. sanguis,* and *S. salivarius.* In recent years *S. mutans* has been implicated as the major and most virulent of the caries-producing organisms.

The acids that initially decalcify the enamel have a pH of 5.2 or less and are formed in the plaque material, which has been described as an organic nitrogenous mass of microorganisms firmly attached to the tooth structure. The dental plaque is present on all teeth, whether susceptible or immune to dental caries. This film that exists primarily in the susceptible areas of the teeth has received a great deal of attention since the chemicoparasitic theory of dental caries was first proposed.

Considerable emphasis is currently being given to plaque and its relationship to oral disease. Methods of chemical plaque control are being investigated. Perhaps in the future it will be possible to make enamel resistant to bacterial colonization (plaque formation) and consequently reduce both caries and gingival disease.

The acids involved in the caries process are derived from carbohydrate substances after they have been acted on by microbial enzymes. The enzymes are produced by the microorganisms in the plaque material. If enough acid is formed and is held in contact with the tooth structure long enough, the enamel will be decalcified, and the carious lesion will be initiated. The process will continue until the acid is neutralized by the dissolved tooth minerals or saliva or both.

Dental caries depends on the presence of the plaque material containing the acidogenic microorganisms. The microorganisms readily provide the enzymes necessary to act on food material (carbohydrates) to produce an acid that, if sufficient in quantity and held in contact with the tooth structure long enough, will initiate the development of the carious lesion. The tooth itself, however, must be susceptible to the acid attack. Several factors influence the degree of vulnerability of the tooth.

Areas of caries susceptibility in the primary dentition

In the primary dentition the sequence of caries attack follows a specific pattern: mandibular molars, maxillary molars, and maxillary anterior teeth. Seldom are the mandibular anterior teeth or the buccal and lingual surfaces of the primary teeth involved, except in instances of rampant caries.

The first primary molars in both the mandibular and maxillary arches are much less susceptible to caries than the second primary molars, even though the first primary molars erupt earlier. Walsh and Smart observed that in 8-year-old patients, 50% of the second primary molars had occlusal caries, but

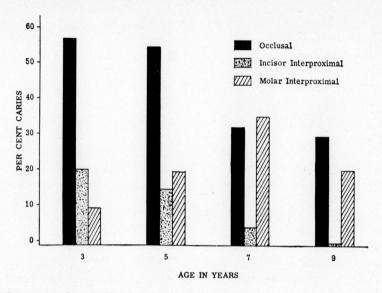

Fig. 7-3. Percentage of proximal and occlusal caries in primary teeth. (From data by Parfitt, G.J.: J. Dent. Child. **23:**31-39, 1956.)

only 20% of the first primary molars had occlusal involvement. This difference in caries susceptibility is no doubt related to differences in morphology of the occlusal surface. The second primary molar usually has deeper, less completely coalesced pits and fissures.

Interproximal caries in both the anterior and buccal segments of the primary dentition usually does not occur until proximal contact develops. Parfitt reported that, before the age of 7 years, a greater number of involved occlusal surfaces than proximal surfaces is seen (Fig. 7-3). However, proximal caries progresses more rapidly than occlusal caries and causes a higher percentage of pulp exposures. This fact makes periodic routine radiographs imperative after proximal contact is established between the primary molars.

The susceptibility of the distal surface of the first primary molar and the mesial surface of the second primary molar is essentially the same. However, clinical observation has established that caries on the mesial surface of the second primary molar is more extensive and more likely to cause pulpal involvement.

The previously mentioned survey by Hennon, Stookey, and Muhler of 915 children between 18 and 39 months of age showed that the mandibular and maxillary second molars and the maxillary central incisors are most often carious. A surface-by-surface comparison showed the following surfaces of the individually named teeth to be most often carious:

	Maxillary	**Mandibular**
Second molar	Occlusal and lingual	Occlusal and buccal
First molar	Occlusal	Occlusal and buccal
Canine	Buccal	Buccal
Lateral	Mesial	Mesial
Central	Mesial	Mesial

Radiographic findings indicate that 75% of all posterior interproximal carious lesions in this age group would not have been detected without the aid of radiographs. This study emphasized the need to develop effective techniques to prevent, diagnose, and treat dental caries in children from 18 to 39 months of age.

Areas of caries susceptibility in the mixed dentition

With the eruption of the first permanent molar, the dentist can expect to find frequent carious involvement of the occlusal pits and fissures and morphologic defects that must be restored to prevent the development of extensive carious lesions. Walsh and Smart found that at the age of 7 years, approximately 25% of the mandibular first permanent molars had caries on the occlusal surface, whereas at the same age approximately 12% of the maxillary first permanent molars were carious. By the age of 9 years, 50% of the mandibular first permanent molars and 35% of the maxillary first permanent molars were carious. At the age of 12 years, 70% of the mandibular molars and 52% of the maxillary first permanent molars were carious.

The observations of Blayney and Hill have given support to the belief that the mandibular first permanent molars decay first and have a higher caries occurrence rate than their maxillary counterparts. Conversely, they found that the caries-free rate is greater for the maxillary molars, with the exception of the 13-year-old group.

The distal surface of the second primary molar is a common site for caries after the eruption of the first permanent molar. If a lesion of even the incipient type develops on the distal surface of the second primary molar, the mesial surface of the first permanent molar will almost invariably be decalcified, even though it cannot be detected on the radiograph.

The maxillary permanent central and lateral incisors are not highly susceptible to caries attack, except in children who have rampant caries caused by high-carbohydrate diet, mouth breathing, or salivary deficiency. At the age of 8 years, approximately 1% of these teeth will be carious. However, by the age of 12 years, the carious involvement can be expected to increase to approximately 15%. Much of this increase is probably due to exposure of the lingual pits on lateral incisors as they complete eruption. Carious involvement of the lower incisors is minimal, except in cases of rampant car-

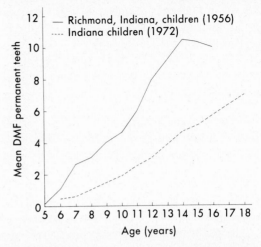

Fig. 7-4. Dental caries prevalence in permanent teeth in children 5 to 18 years of age. The 1972 survey revealed a marked reduction in DMFT rate when compared with a 1956 survey.

ies. In fact, involvement of these teeth is often considered an indication of essentially uncontrollable caries activity. At the end of the transitional dentition period (age 12), less than 20% of the mandibular incisors will have caries involvement.

Areas of caries susceptibility in the permanent dentition

A sharp rise in the caries attack rate continues with the eruption of the second permanent molars and the premolars. A survey of more than 11,000 Indiana children in grades 1 through 12 was conducted by Bell. Fig. 7-4 shows the increase in permanent tooth involvement between ages 6 and 18 years. A surprising finding was the fact that there was no significant difference in the total number of DMFT between high and low income groups. However, tooth mortality was four times as great in the lowest income group as it was in the highest income group.

An interesting observation can be made when these survey results are compared with the study reported by Waterman in 1956 involving 6000 Richmond, Indiana, children. The DMFT rate at age 10 in Waterman's study was 4.5, whereas in Bell's study the DMFT rate was only 2. In the 14-year-old group the DMFT rate was reduced from 10.5 to 4.7. These reductions reflect the benefits of 30 years of fluoridation and dental health education in Indiana communities.

The mandibular second permanent molars, like the first permanent molars, have a high occlusal surface attack rate (20%), whereas 10% of the maxillary second permanent molars have carious involvement within a year after they erupt. These teeth require careful attention to prevent rapid caries penetration of the underlying dentin and pulp exposure.

The maxillary lateral incisors frequently erupt with a defect in the lingual surface. The progression of caries can be rapid in this area and can involve the pulp before the child or the dentist is aware of the presence of the cavity. A prophylactic cavity preparation and a restoration or a sealant are indicated if the sharpest exploring point can be engaged in the lingual pit.

The cervical portions of the buccal grooves of the mandibular first and second permanent molars and the lingual grooves of the maxillary first and second permanent molars are also sites of morphologic defects and incomplete enamel formation. Early restoration of these areas or the placement of sealants is imperative if the sharp exploring point can be made to stick in the defect.

Secondary factors in dental caries

Clinical observation and laboratory investigation often support the theory that dental caries is influenced by a number of secondary factors.

Anatomic characteristics of the teeth. The teeth of many patients, particularly permanent teeth, seem predisposed to dental caries and may show evidence of the attack almost coincident with their eruption into the oral cavity. First permanent molars often have incompletely coalesced pits and fissures that allow the dental plaque material to be retained at the base of the defect in contact with exposed dentin. These defects or anatomic characteristics can readily be seen if the tooth is dried and the debris and plaque material are removed with a sharp explorer point. Lingual pits on the maxillary first permanent molars, buccal pits on the mandibular first permanent molars, and lingual pits on the maxillary incisors are vulnerable areas in which the process of dental caries can proceed in a rapid and uninterrupted manner.

Tooth morphology and enamel defects apparently follow a familial pattern. In a study of the dental arches of identical twins, Goldberg concluded that heredity influences dental caries indirectly by influencing tooth morphology, especially the pit-fissure formation. Therefore it might be said that morphology is one indirect relationship between susceptibility to dental caries and heredity.

Arrangement of the teeth in the arch. Crowded and irregular teeth are not readily cleansed during the natural masticatory process. It is likewise difficult for the patient to clean the mouth properly with a toothbrush if the teeth are crowded or overlapped. This condition therefore may contribute to the problem of dental caries.

Presence of dental appliances. Partial dentures, space maintainers, and orthodontic appliances often encourage the retention of food debris and plaque material and have been shown to result in an increase in the bacterial population. Few patients keep their mouths meticulously clean, and even those who make an attempt may be hampered by the presence of dental appliances that retain plaque material between brushings. Patients who have had moderate dental caries activity in the past might be expected to have increased caries activity after the placement of appliances in the mouth unless they practice unusually good oral hygiene.

Hereditary factors. Although parents of children with excessive or rampant caries have a tendency to blame the condition on hereditary factors or tendencies, there is little scientific evidence to support this contention. The fact that children often acquire their dietary habits and habits related to oral hygiene from their parents makes dental caries more an environmental than a hereditary disease.

After a study of 224 pairs of twins of the same sex between the ages of 5 and 17 years, Mansbridge concluded that environmental factors clearly have a greater influence on dental caries than genetic factors, but the genetic factors also contribute to the causation of dental caries.

Shaw and Murray compared the caries status and dietary habits of the families of 44 caries-resistant and 37 caries-susceptible English schoolchildren between the ages of 13 and 15. Questionnaires and clinical examinations were completed for 147 parents and 132 siblings living in their homes. The mean age of the parents in both groups was almost the same, but only 8% of the parents of the caries-resistant children were edentulous as compared with 37% of the parents of the caries-susceptible children. The mean DMFS for the dentulous parents of caries-resistant children was 43.6 compared with a mean DMFS of 64.2 for dentulous parents of the caries-susceptible children ($P = .001$). The corresponding mean DMFS scores for the siblings of each group were 7.6 and 21.3 ($P = .001$). The intake of refined sugars did not vary widely between groups. However, the parents and siblings in the caries-susceptible group did consume more snacks—1.7 snacks per day compared with 1.2 for the caries-resistant group ($P = .01$). The authors suggested that the effects of genetic and environmental factors on dental caries in humans cannot be readily separated for analysis. They concluded that caries-immune and caries-susceptible individuals are affected by some genetic and environmental factors that were not addressed by their study, even though a familial pattern of caries susceptibility was demonstrated.

Of unusual interest is the work of Hunt, Hoppert, and Rosen, who showed in laboratory rats that heredity is a factor in determining resistance or susceptibility to dental caries. By selective breeding, they produced two distinct strains of albino rats, one caries susceptible and the other caries resistant. The caries-resistant rats were studied for many generations and continued to be free of the disease even when fed a caries-producing diet.

Rampant dental caries

There is no complete agreement on the definition of "rampant caries" or on the clinical picture of this condition. It has been generally accepted, however, that the disease referred to as rampant caries is, in the terms of human history, relatively new. Rampant caries has been defined by Massler as a suddenly appearing, widespread, rapidly burrowing type of caries, resulting in early involvement of the pulp and affecting those teeth usually regarded as immune to ordinary decay.

There is no evidence that the mechanism of the decay process is different in rampant caries or that it occurs only in teeth that are malformed or inferior in composition. On the contrary, rampant caries can occur suddenly in teeth that were for many years relatively immune to decay. Some factor in the caries process seems to accelerate the process to the extent that it becomes uncontrollable, and it is then referred to as "rampant caries."

When a patient has what is considered an excessive amount of tooth decay, it must be determined whether that individual actually has a high susceptibility and truly rampant caries of sudden onset or whether the oral condition represents years of neglect and inadequate dental care.

Some believe that the term "rampant caries" should be applied to a caries rate of 10 or more new lesions per year. Davies thinks that the distinguishing characteristics of rampant caries are the involvement of the proximal surface of the lower anterior teeth and the development of cervical-type caries. Young teenagers seem to be particularly susceptible to rampant caries, although it has been observed in both children and adults of all ages (Figs. 7-5 to 7-7).

Some believe that rampant caries is due to primary and secondary nutritional inadequacies. However, it is more generally agreed that rampant caries is not a deficiency disease or one associated with malnutrition. Massler and Schour observed that in spite of severe malnutrition, dental caries incidence in children in postwar Italy was much lower than that in well-nourished children of simi-

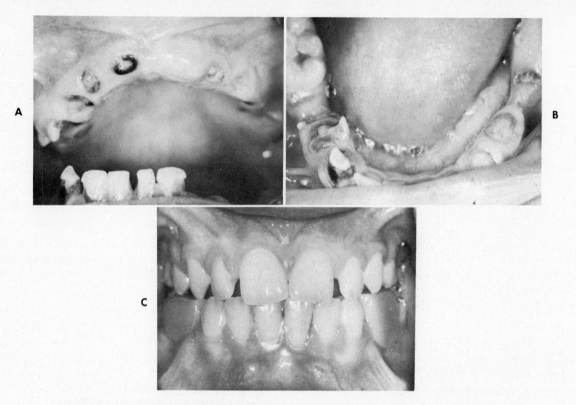

Fig. 7-5. A, Rampant dental caries and evidence of dental neglect in a preschool child. There has been gross destruction of the clinical crowns of the primary teeth. **B,** Recently erupted first permanent molar with an extensive carious lesion. The destruction process evident in the primary teeth at an early age would be expected to continue in the permanent teeth. **C,** Same patient at 10 years of age. A preventive and corrective program has maintained the permanent teeth.

lar ages living in the United States. The low intake of refined sugar, however, could possibly explain the low prevalence of dental caries in the Italian group. Jay stated that there is indisputable evidence that rampant caries is caused by too much sugar in the diet and that it can be brought under control by careful regulation of refined sugar intake. Additional evidence that rampant caries is not associated with malnutrition has been presented by Mann and associates. They observed that a group of individuals with symptoms of nutritional deficiency had, on the average, 30% less caries than those who were well nourished.

Keyes believes there are sufficient clinical and laboratory findings to indicate that sucrose, more than other carbohydrates, fosters certain types of caries-conducive processes. Under laboratory conditions sucrose is more likely to cause rampant multisurface cavitation than glucose, fructose, sorbitol, hydrogenated starch, and starch. The difference, Keyes suggests, is related to insoluble, gummy polysaccharides (high molecular weight dextrans) that are formed during the metabolism of sucrose by *S. mutans.*

There is considerable evidence that emotional disturbances may be the causative factor in some

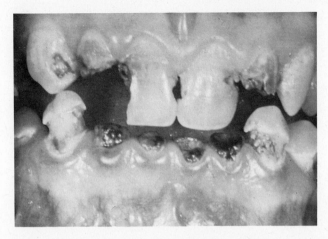

Fig. 7-6. Teenage patient with rampant caries. Occasionally a full-mouth extraction must be recommended if there is gross destruction with pulpal involvement. Partial dentures are of little value without a determination of the etiologic factors and without complete patient cooperation.

cases of rampant caries. Repressed emotions and fears, dissatisfaction with achievement, rebellion against a home situation, a feeling of inferiority, a traumatic school experience, and continuous general tension and anxiety have been observed in children and adults who have rampant dental caries. Since adolescence is often considered to be a time of difficult adjustment, the increased incidence of rampant caries in this age group lends support to the theory. An emotional disturbance may initiate an unusual craving for sweets or the habit of snacking, which in turn might influence the incidence of dental caries. On the other hand, a marked salivary deficiency is not an uncommon finding in tense, nervous, or disturbed persons. The role of saliva in rampant dental caries is discussed in the consideration of the natural protective mechanism.

Nursing caries

In recent years it has been recognized that prolonged bottle feeding, beyond the usual time when the child is weaned from the bottle and introduced to solid food, may result in early and rampant caries. The clinical appearance of the teeth in "bottle

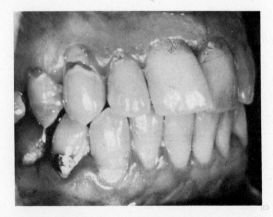

Fig. 7-7. Rampant caries in an adult patient. Extensive carious lesions have developed on smooth surfaces and on surfaces adjacent to well-placed restorations. (From McDonald, R.E.: Management of rampant dental caries in children, Practical Dental Monographs, Chicago, 1961, Year Book Medical Publishers, Inc.)

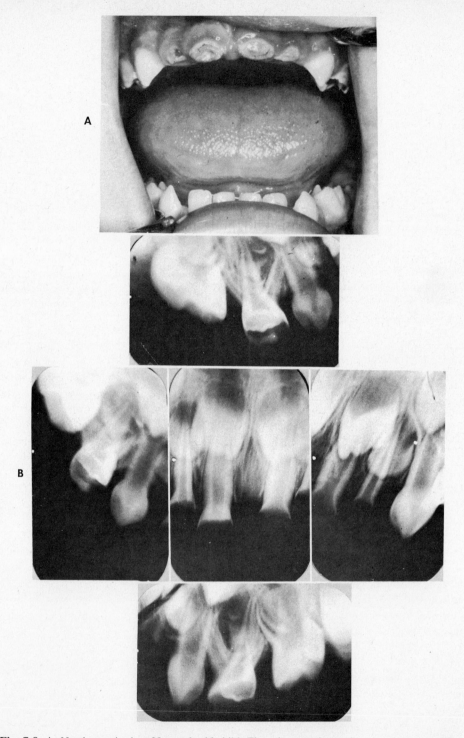

Fig. 7-8. A, Nursing caries in a 20-month-old child. There is extensive carious involvement of the maxillary primary incisors and first molars. **B,** Radiographs of the maxillary arch. Maxillary incisors are indicated for extraction. Note the deep caries in the first primary molars. The primary second molars have not erupted.

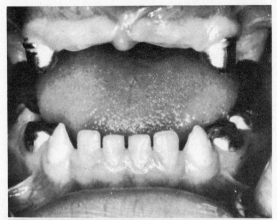

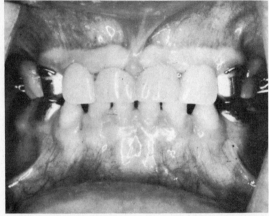

C

Fig. 7-8, cont'd. C, At 2½ years of age a partial denture was constructed for the maxillary arch.

caries'' in a child 2, 3, or 4 years of age is typical and follows a definite pattern. There is early carious involvement of the maxillary anterior teeth, the maxillary and mandibular first primary molars, and the mandibular canines. The mandibular incisors are usually unaffected (Fig. 7-8). A discussion with the parents reveals a common factor: the child has been put to bed at afternoon nap time or at night with a nursing bottle containing milk or a sugar-containing beverage. The child falls asleep, and the milk or sweetened liquid becomes pooled around the maxillary anterior teeth. The carbohydrate-containing liquid provides an excellent culture medium for acidogenic microorganisms. Salivary

flow is decreased during sleep, and clearance of the liquid from the oral cavity is slowed.

Gardner, Norwood, and Eisenson reported four case histories in which the same pattern of caries was observed, and in each child the condition was attributed to a specific breast-feeding habit. This observation is supporting evidence that the lactose content of human milk, as well as that of bovine milk, can be cariogenic if the milk is allowed to stagnate on the teeth. In each case the mother explained that human milk was the main source of nutrition. The investigators recommend that from birth the infant should be held while feeding. The child who falls asleep while nursing should be burped and then placed in bed. In addition, the parent should start brushing the child's teeth as soon as they erupt and discontinue nursing as soon as the child can drink from a cup—at approximately 12 to 15 months of age.

Kotlow also reported three such cases of severe caries associated with breast-feeding. Dilley, Dilley, and Machen observed a large number of children with prolonged nursing-habit caries and concluded that there was no association between the nursing habit and the family background with the exception of predominantly lower socioeconomic conditions. All subjects demonstrated prolonged breast-feeding or bottle feeding, with milk reported to be the liquid most often used in the bottle. Parents indicated that they did not know when weaning should occur and when oral hygiene should be instituted. Dilley and associates also observed the nearly symmetric caries pattern.

Bottle caries and the similar type of caries resulting from at-will breast-feeding can be prevented by early counseling of the parents. This is one reason for suggesting that children receive their first dental examination by at least 9 months of age, when nursing caries will not likely have developed. Parents should be cautioned about prolonged and frequent infant feeding habits.

Control of dental caries

Many practical measures for the control of dental caries are applicable to private practice. For the most part they are not new. Most practitioners have tried these control measures with varying degrees of success. It is impossible, however, to emphasize too strongly that no one measure for the control of dental caries will be entirely satisfactory. At the present time all possible preventive measures and approaches must be considered in the hope of successfully combating dental caries, which is often referred to as the most widespread human disease.

Pedodontists who see patients on a referral basis may hear a parent remark, ''My child has so many cavities that my dentist doesn't know where to start.'' Although it is true that the problem may at first seem overwhelming, a systematic, understanding approach can usually result in a gratifying response. An outline of procedure in the control of rampant caries follows. With this approach and with patient cooperation, the problem can usually be explained and brought under control. The successful management of a dental caries problem, however, depends on the parents' or patient's interest in maintaining the patient's teeth and their cooperativeness in a preventive program.

Control of all active carious lesions. The first step is the initial treatment of all carious lesions. The problem may then be approached in a systematic manner. Many practitioners have become discouraged when following a plan of restoring one tooth at a time to its normal contour, only to observe new carious lesions developing so rapidly that full restoration is never actually completed. A more logical approach is the gross excavation of each carious lesion, the technique for which is described in detail in Chapter 8. The gross caries removal (indirect pulp treatment) can usually be accomplished easily in one appointment. If there are a large number of extensive carious lesions, however, a second appointment may be necessary.

Gross excavation as an initial approach in the control of rampant dental caries has several advantages. The removal of the superficial caries and the filling of the cavity with zinc oxide–eugenol mate-

rial (IRM*) will at least temporarily arrest the caries process and prevent its rapid progression to the dental pulp (Fig. 7-9). This procedure gives the dentist time to take a history and complete tests to determine the cause of the rapid destructive process. It will also provide an opportunity to outline a preventive and restorative approach to the problem. Furthermore, this approach will increase the chances of success in the treatment of vital pulp exposures. The dressing of zinc oxide and eugenol not only arrests the caries process but also aids in the sterilization of the remaining carious material and perhaps reduces the inflammation of the pulp that has been invaded by the caries process and microorganisms. The elimination of the gross carious material, the temporary filling of the teeth, and the elimination of food traps also result in a reduction in the number of oral microorganisms, which in itself plays an important role in the caries control program. Elliott observed a 76% reduction in the number of oral lactobacilli in children 1 week after complete mouth rehabilitation.

Reduction in the intake of freely fermentable carbohydrates. Coincident with the removal of the gross caries and the attempt to slow the caries attack rate should be an attempt to determine the dietary habits of all patients who have a dental caries problem. Some excellent studies have been reported in recent years that show a relationship between diet and dental caries. As a result of these studies, considerable emphasis has been given to this phase of the caries control program. There is also increasing evidence that between-meal eating and the frequency of eating are related to dental caries incidence.

Gustafsson and associates conducted a well-controlled study of dental caries and observed that a group of patients whose diet was high in fat, low in carbohydrate, and practically free from sugar had low caries activity. When refined sugar was added to the diet in the form of a mealtime supple-

---

*Intermediate Restorative Material, L.D. Caulk Co., Milford, Del. 19963.

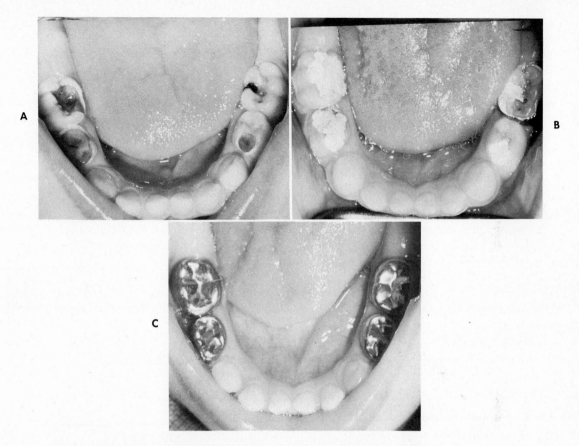

Fig. 7-9. A, Mandibular primary teeth with extensive carious lesions and without a history of painful pulpitis. **B,** Following gross caries removal the lesions were filled with zinc oxide–eugenol. It is sometimes necessary to support the dressing with a steel band. **C,** After a waiting period of 6 to 8 weeks the teeth are restored. (Courtesy Dr. James R. Roche.)

ment, there was still little or no caries activity. However, when caramels were given between meals, a statistically significant increase in the number of new carious lesions occurred. It was concluded from these studies that dental caries activity could be increased by the consumption of sugar if the sugar was in a form easily retained on the tooth surface. The more frequently this form of sugar was consumed between meals, the greater was the tendency for an increase in dental caries.

Mack studied a group of institutionalized chil-

dren whose diet was adequate and included sugar only at mealtime. The addition of more carbohydrate to the diet in the form of candy did not significantly increase dental caries activity, but the children did not eat candy between meals and were encouraged to brush their teeth after meals.

Potgieter and associates surveyed the dental status in relation to diet as determined from records of weekly food intake of 864 Connecticut schoolchildren. Those who consumed more fruits and vegetables and who had better basic diets had a lower incidence rate of DMFT. The frequency of between-meal snacks also showed a slight positive relationship to the dental caries activity.

In reviewing the dietary records of 200 children between the ages of 5 and 13 years, Zita, McDonald, and Andrews found that the mean weekly sugar equivalent was 164 teaspoons and the between-meal sugar equivalent was 55 teaspoons. Approximately one third of the free sugar or freely fermentable carbohydrate was consumed in the form of between-meal snacks. These authors found little relationship between the total sugar intake and the dental caries incidence. However, there was a high correlation between the sugar consumed between meals and dental caries.

Weiss and Trithart reported additional evidence of the relationship of between-meal eating habits and incidence of dental caries. In a group of preschool children it was found that most between-meal snacks were of high sugar content or were high in adhesiveness. The children who did not eat between meals had 3.3 def teeth, whereas those who ate four or more items between meals had a def rate of 9.8. The most popular types of between-meal items consumed, in descending order of popularity, were gum, candy, soft drinks, pastries, and ice cream.

In view of the results of these well-controlled studies, the first consideration in the clinical control of dental caries should be a determination of eating habits by having the patient keep a 7-day record of all food eaten at mealtime and between meals. The record should then be evaluated to determine the adequacy of the diet and the amount of freely fermentable carbohydrate. The number of servings of food in the four basic groups—dairy foods, meat, vegetables and fruit, and bread and cereals—should be determined and compared with the recommended number of servings outlined in

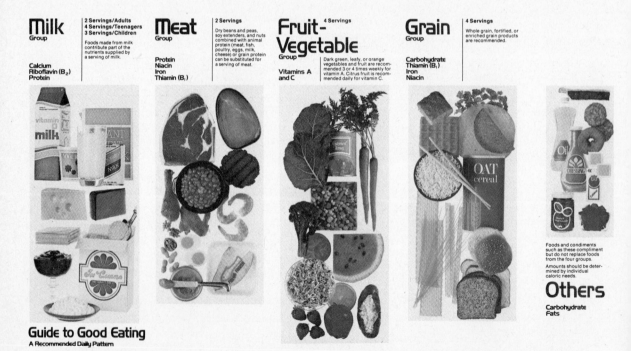

Fig. 7-10. "A Guide to Good Eating." (Reprinted by permission of the National Dairy Council, Rosemont, Ill.)

Fig. 7-10. The basic four analysis form (see boxed material below) has been found to be helpful in evaluating the adequacy of the diet.

Henderson has reported that a number of computer-facilitated dietary analysis systems are commercially available but that not all of them are based on the same type of data input. One computer-assisted dietary analysis of a 5-day food intake record is based on the recommended dietary allowances (RDA).* The patient's age and sex are taken into consideration, and the analysis provides information regarding the patient's average daily intake compared to recommended intake of calories; protein, fat, polyunsaturated fatty acids, and carbohydrates (in grams); calcium, phosphorus, iron, niacin, and ascorbic acid (in milligrams); thiamin and riboflavin (in micrograms); and vitamin A (in international units). A second evaluation of

---

*Analysis system available from Dr. George R. Young, University of Missouri–Kansas City School of Dentistry, 650 East 25th St., Kansas City, Mo. 64608.

the diet on this printout uses the basic four food groups as a standard. The vegetable-fruit group is divided into subgroup sources of vitamin A and vitamin C. The patient's total sugar intake in teaspoons of sugar and number of exposures is also provided. The exposures are further categorized according to the time of intake (either during or between meals) and the physical form (retentive or in solution). Properly used, these systems can be of diagnostic and therapeutic value in counseling individual patients and in helping to clarify the role of dietary factors other than sugar that may affect the dental caries status of an individual patient.

Luke, Ostergard, and Hunt have demonstrated that a computerized diet analysis is more consistent than those performed by individuals. They also point out that the computerized method offers the advantage of specific nutrient analysis but that all analyses should be used only as a general guide to improving the nutritional level and reducing the cariogenic potential of the patient's diet.

It has been observed from evaluating 500 consecutive records of children coming to the Indiana University Clinic that only a small percentage have adequate diets. The majority of children with inadequate diets have a gross deficiency of fruits and vegetables, and at least 50% receive inadequate amounts of dairy foods. Dunham, who determined the eating habits of schoolchildren in a high socioeconomic area, has reported that only 13% had diets that could be classified as good. In a study of 1269 children by Koss, 42% were found to eat unsatisfactory breakfasts, and 10% were found to be routinely omitting this meal. Harris determined the quality of breakfast eaten by 336 El Paso high school students whose ages ranged from 16 to 18 years. He found that only 12% of the girls and 14% of the boys ate breakfasts that adequately met their nutritional requirements. The addition of milk, citrus fruit, or both would have improved the nutritional quality of the breakfasts eaten by these students. Over 50% of the students said they were hungry soon after 10 AM.

Basic four analysis

Weekly requirement	Total servings consumed	Actual deficiency	Percent of total received
Milk group 28 servings (teenagers) 21 servings (children) 14 servings (adults)			
Meat group 14 servings			
Vegetable-fruit group 28 servings			
Bread-cereal (whole grain) 28 servings			

The physical state of carbohydrates and frequency of ingestion contribute to the initiation and extension of caries. Fermentable carbohydrate-containing foods taken in adherent solid form are considerably more cariogenic than those consumed in soluble form. Carbohydrate-containing foods that are rapidly cleared from the oral cavity have a low caries potential in comparison with those slowly cleared.

A list of fermentable carbohydrate-containing foods has been compiled for use in the Pedodontic Department of Indiana University School of Dentistry:

Foods containing sugar in solution
Soft drinks, soda pop, drink mixes such as Kool-Aid
Sweetened condensed milk
Sweetened sauces, such as chocolate and butterscotch
Chocolate milk, hot chocolate, cocoa
Milk shakes, malts
Popsicles

Foods containing solid or retentive sugars
Cakes, doughnuts, cookies, marshmallows, candy bars, brownies, chocolate
Pastries, puddings, muffins, sweet rolls, pies
Sugar-coated cereals, sugar-coated gum
Dried fruits such as raisins, dates, apricots
Fruits cooked in sugar
Ice cream, jams, jellies
Vegetables glazed with sugar such as candied sweet potatoes
Vegetables cooked with sugar or molasses such as Boston baked beans
Hard candy, Life Savers, lollipops, peanut brittle, jelly beans
Frosting, honey
Cough drops

This list does not include every type of food containing sugars in solution or retentive sugars. However, it does present an adequate guide for analyzing the fermentable carbohydrate exposures.

Katz has suggested the following substitute foods for those containing sugar:

Peanuts, walnuts, pecans, almonds, and other types of nuts*
Popcorn, corn chips,† potato chips,† whole wheat biscuits, unsweetened cereals
Cold cuts of meat (unsweetened)
Cubes of cheese*
Pizza, tacos, toast
Fresh fruits, salads
Vegetables such as carrot slices, celery sticks, cucumber slices
Baked potatoes, fried potatoes
Hamburgers, hot dogs
Unsweetened fruit juices, freshly squeezed fruit juices
Sugarless chewing gum
Sandwiches

Dreizen reports that direct measurement of acid production within the dental plaque shows that tooth demineralizing concentrations are reached within 4 minutes and maintained for 30 to 45 minutes after ingestion of a carbohydrate-containing meal. Since, in diet analysis, foods containing sugars in solution as well as retentive sugars are included, 20 minutes may be considered as the average time each exposure permits acid concentrations to be available in the bacterial plaque (Fig. 7-11).

The following can be used in an explanation of the dental caries process to a parent or child:

Fermentable carbohydrate + Oral bacteria
within plaque → Acid within plaque
Acid + Susceptible tooth → Tooth decay

DiOrio and Madsen point out that merely giving the patient or parent facts related to diet in the prevention of dental disease does not change established habits. Discussion enables the patient to define his or her own dental and diet problem and to discover solutions. Listening to the patient and

---

*According to Katz, research indicates that nuts and cheese tend to diminish the pH drop in plaque after the ingestion of acidic foods or those containing sugar.
†It is advisable to read the list of ingredients on packaged products. Some foods, particularly "chip" products, have highly cariogenic additives.

Fermentable carbohydrate exposures									
Form	*Day of week*								*Total number of exposures*
Sugar in solution	During meal								
	End of meal								
	Between meals								
Solid and retentive sugar-containing foods	During meal								
	End of meal								
	Between meals								

Grand total: _____

Total exposures $\times$ 20 min. = _____

Which specific food items are the offenders?

Suggested substitutes:

1._____

1._____

2._____

2._____

3._____

3._____

4._____

4._____

Fig. 7-11. Form for analysis of ingested fermentable carbohydrate.

allowing the youngster to contribute to the discussion help establish the rapport critical for patient cooperation.

Foods in the basic four groups should not be included in the fermentable carbohydrate calculation (with some exceptions) unless free sugar is added during the preparation. One exception is dry cereal, since it is considered a refined food. Cereals may be retained on the teeth for long periods of time; in addition, many of them are sugar coated, and some are high in sucrose content. Evidence is accumulating that sucrose concentration is important. Shannon analyzed 78 cereals for sucrose and glucose content (Table 7-2). The cereals are listed in order of increasing sucrose concentration. Although the cariogenicity of a food may be related to its consistency, the time of consumption, and the conditions under which it is eaten, sucrose con-

Table 7-2. Sucrose and glucose content of commercially available breakfast cereals

Commercial cereal product	Sucrose content (%)	Glucose content (%)	Commercial cereal product	Sucrose content (%)	Glucose content (%)
Shredded wheat (large biscuit)	1.0	0.2	All Bran	20.0	1.6
Shredded wheat (spoon size biscuit)	1.3	0.3	Granola (with almonds and filberts)	21.4	1.2
Cheerios	2.2	0.5	Fortified Oat Flakes	22.2	1.2
Puffed Rice	2.4	0.4	Heartland	23.1	3.2
Uncle Sam Cereal	2.4	1.2	Super Sugar Chex	24.5	0.8
Wheat Chex	2.6	0.9	Sugar Frosted Flakes	29.0	1.8
Grape Nut Flakes	3.3	0.6	Bran Buds	30.2	2.1
Puffed Wheat	3.5	0.7	Sugar Sparkled Corn Flakes	32.2	1.8
Alpen	3.8	4.7	Frosted Mini Wheats	33.6	0.4
Post Toasties	4.1	1.7	Sugar Pops	37.8	2.9
Product 19	4.1	1.7	Alpha Bits	40.3	0.6
Corn Total	4.4	1.4	Sir Grapefellow	40.7	3.1
Special K	4.4	6.4	Super Sugar Crisp	40.7	4.5
Wheaties	4.7	4.2	Cocoa Puffs	43.0	3.5
Corn Flakes (Kroger)	5.1	1.5	Cap'n Crunch	43.3	0.8
Peanut Butter	5.2	1.1	Crunch Berries	43.4	1.0
Grape Nuts	6.6	1.1	Kaboom	43.8	3.0
Corn Flakes (Food Club)	7.0	2.1	Frankenberry	44.0	2.6
Crispy Rice	7.3	1.5	Frosted Flakes	44.0	2.9
Corn Chex	7.5	0.9	Count Chocula	44.2	3.7
Corn Flakes (Kellogg)	7.8	6.4	Orange Quangaroos	44.7	0.6
Total	8.1	1.3	Quisp	44.9	0.6
Rice Chex	8.5	1.8	Boo Berry	45.7	2.8
Crisp Rice	8.8	2.1	Vanilly Crunch	45.8	0.7
Raisin Bran (Skinner)	9.6	9.3	Baron Von Redberry	45.8	1.5
Concentrate	9.9	2.4	Cocoa Krispies	45.9	0.8
Rice Krispies (Kellogg)	10.0	2.9	Trix	46.6	4.1
Raisin Bran (Kellogg)	10.6	14.1	Froot Loops	47.4	0.5
Heartland (with raisins)	13.5	5.6	Honeycomb	48.8	2.8
Buck Wheat	13.6	1.5	Pink Panther	49.2	1.3
Life	14.5	2.5	Cinnamon Crunch	50.3	3.2
Granola (with dates)	14.5	3.2	Lucky Charms	50.4	7.6
Granola (with raisins)	14.5	3.8	Cocoa Pebbles	53.5	0.6
Sugar Frosted Corn Flakes	15.6	1.8	Apple Jacks	55.0	0.5
40% Bran Flakes (Post)	15.8	3.0	Fruity Pebbles	55.1	1.1
Team	15.9	1.1	King Vitamin	58.5	3.1
Brown Sugar-Cinnamon Frosted Mini Wheats	16.0	0.3	Sugar Smacks	61.3	2.4
40% Bran Flakes (Kellogg)	16.2	2.1	Super Orange Crisp	68.0	2.8
Granola	16.6	0.6	MEAN	25.1	2.3
100% Bran	18.4	0.8	S.D.	19.16	2.21

From Shannon, I.L.: J. Dent. Child. **41:**348, 1974.

Table 7-3. Food retention and decalcification potentials of representative food

Food	Total carbohydrate (%)	Free sugar* (%)	Food retained (mg)	4-hr acid formation (ml 0.1 normal sodium hydroxide)	Decalcification potential
Cookie (fig)	70.0	27.6	678	1.2	814
Date	77.5	33.8	507	1.6	811
Chocolate	50.0	39.0	370	2.1	777
Ice cream	17.0	—	423	1.6	677
Cookie (shortbread)	59.5	24.8	370	1.3	481
Danish pastry†	53.8	40.0	181	1.6	434
Cracker (salted)	70.0	11.0	340	1.2	408
Caramel†	56.8	43.0	219	1.8	394
Chocolate pudding†	35.0	18.5	300	1.3	390
Cracker (oil sprayed)	71.0	12.1	310	1.2	372
Toffee	90.0	—	266	1.3	346
White bread	49.0	13.0	188	1.8	338
Potato (boiled)†	18.2	4.0	128	2.4	307
Cola drink	10.5	10.5	237	1.0	237
Apple	17.5	11.0	228	1.0	228
Orange soda	10.5	10.5	219	1.0	219
Orange juice (fresh)	8.5	—	177	1.2	212
Potato chip†	48.2	12.7	61	1.9	116
Carrot (fresh)†	9.5	—	73	1.2	88
Carrot (cooked)†	8.3	6.8	2	1.5	3

From Bibby, B.G.: J.A.D.A. **51**:298, 1955.
*Sugar recovered in water filtrate.
†Values from Bibby, B.G., Goldberg, H.J.V., and Chen, E.: J.A.D.A. **42**:491, 1951.

sumption should be considered during dietary counseling.

Shannon and McCartney affirmed that accurate and reproducible analytic methods are now available for measuring sugar in foods. They also pointed out that presweetened cereals, which are popular snacks, are potential dental hazards. They suggested, however, that this tendency of prolonged intraoral retention is neutralized when these products are eaten at mealtime with milk.

Dried fruits, including raisins, prunes, peaches, apricots, and dates, have a high sugar content; therefore their sugar equivalents should also be included in the diet analysis. These are foods commonly eaten by children between meals, and there is no reason to believe that they are any less cariogenic than refined foods. Although honey is con-

sidered a natural food, its sugar equivalent should be calculated in addition to syrups and other spreads for bread.

Bowen (1978) discussed the controversy regarding the relative cariogenicity of different carbohydrates, stating that sucrose is usually regarded as the most cariogenic of sugars, probably because it is the sugar most frequently ingested. Results of animal investigation appear to indicate little difference in the cariogenicity of sucrose, glucose, and fructose.

Caries-producing potential of foodstuffs. Bibby has carried out extensive research related to food retention in the oral cavity and the decalcification potential of commonly eaten foods (Table 7-3). His work has shown that the persistence of sugar in the mouth, the acid formed in the mouth, and the other theoretic caries-producing indexes of foods are not determined solely by the concentration of sugar in the foods. The nature of the materials with which the sugar is mixed (and their consistency) is an important factor. The rate of sugar clearance from the mouth, the teeth, or saliva and the duration of acid persistence in saliva or plaque material all indicate that the effects of sugar last for a shorter time when contained in liquid form than in a solid or semisolid form. Bibby also postulates that sugar taken in liquid form should less often initiate caries than sugar taken in a solid state or in combination with adhesive substances.

Of interest to the dental profession in the consideration of dental caries control is the per capita consumption of refined cane and beet sugar and corn sweeteners. Walter has reported that consumption of cane and beet sugars increased from 75.4 pounds per person in 1910 to a high of 102.8 pounds in 1972. There was a slight decrease to 94.7 pounds in 1976, the last year for which figures are available. Corn sweetener consumption increased from 6.5 pounds in 1910 to 29.9 pounds in 1976. Furthermore, candy sales in 1974 reached $2.8 billion with an annual consumption of 17.8 pounds per person.

Rather than insist that the patient follow a strict dietary routine severely restricted in carbohydrates, the dentist should suggest a basic diet. The purpose of limiting a diet to the basic four food groups is twofold. An adequate diet is essential to general health and is, of course, essential during the period of tooth formation to help ensure the development of normal tooth structure. In addition, however, it is a well-established fact that if children and adults closely follow the recommended basic diet and consume a diet containing adequate amounts of protein, fresh fruits, and vegetables, there will be a decreased appetite for snacks between meals. Although there is inconclusive evidence to indicate that the frequency of eating is related to an increase in dental caries experience, there seems to be general agreement that if the foods contain sugar in a form that is easily retained

on the teeth, there will be an increase in dental caries.

Low-calorie beverages. Many dentists recommend low-calorie beverages to their child patients as one means of reducing the refined carbohydrate intake. Hennon has stated that although the use of low-calorie beverages will not be detrimental to the average person, the unrestricted use of these beverages by growing children is potentially harmful. First, a calorie deficiency may result. During the growth period sufficient amounts of energy are required for optimum physical and metabolic activity. Second, the ingestion of such beverages provides little nutritive value in terms of supplying calories, vitamins, or bulk. Drinking these beverages between meals will depress the appetite and will prevent the ingestion of a well-balanced diet at regular mealtime. Although the facts are inconclusive at this time, indications are that artificially sweetened beverages may be damaging to the teeth because of their high content of carboxylic acid.

Reduction in the number of oral microorganisms. Over 30 years ago Fosdick reported a 50% reduction over a 2-year period in the caries attack rate in 523 students who were instructed to brush their teeth within 10 minutes after each meal. Berenie, Ripa, and Leske studied the relationship of frequency of toothbrushing, oral hygiene, gingival health, and caries in 384 children, 9 to 13 years of age, residing in a fluoride-deficient western New York community. Of the children studied, 37% brushed their teeth once a day, 37% brushed twice a day, and 13% brushed less than once a day. The remaining children in the group, approximately 13%, brushed their teeth three or more times each day. A trend toward decreased scores for DMFT and DMFS accompanied increased daily brushing. The increased frequency of daily toothbrushing had its most significant positive effect on the level of oral hygiene.

We have demonstrated that toothbrushing reduces the number of oral microorganisms, particularly if the teeth are brushed after each meal. Toothbrushing also removes gross amounts of food debris and plaque material. Clinical observation can substantiate the statement that removal of this material will often result in a reduction of smooth surface lesions commonly seen in children with rampant caries.

Beal and associates studied the caries incidence and gingival health of children who were 11 to 12 years old at the start of the study. The children's dental cleanliness was evaluated at yearly examinations for a 3-year period. The children whose dental cleanliness was consistently good had lower caries increments than those whose dental cleanliness was consistently bad. A.M. Horowitz and associates have demonstrated the benefits of a school-based plaque removal program in a 3-year study among children in grades 5 to 8. At the end of the study the adjusted mean DMFS scores were 13% lower in the supervised plaque removal group than in the control group. The difference between groups was accounted for entirely by a 26% difference in affected mesial and distal surfaces, a figure approaching statistical significance ($P = .07$). Similarly, Tsamtsouris, White, and Clark have demonstrated that supervised toothbrushing with instruction produces significantly and consistently lower plaque scores, even in preschool children, than were achieved through a control test of the same children when they were neither supervised nor instructed. The investigators concluded that constant reinforcement is necessary to maintain effective plaque control in preschool children.

Wright, Banting, and Feasby conducted a clinical study to evaluate the effect of frequent interdental flossing on the incidence of proximal dental caries. Schoolchildren from a fluoride-deficient area were studied after clinical and radiographic examinations. Based on the observations of this study, the authors concluded that frequent interdental flossing resulted in a significant reduction (50%) in the incidence of proximal caries in deciduous teeth during a 20-month period. The longer the period of interdental flossing, the greater the benefit; however, there was little residual effect after flossing was discontinued.

Encouragement of good oral hygiene. An interesting study has been conducted to determine what motivates children to practice good oral hygiene. For many years the profession has supported the concept that clean teeth are associated with a decreased incidence of dental decay. Dudding and Muhler estimated the level of oral hygiene of 374 schoolchildren between the ages of 6 and 14 years. Only 22% were classified as having good oral hygiene, and the remaining 78% were classified as having poor oral hygiene. Sixty-one percent of those children with good oral hygiene indicated that they learned this practice from their dentist, whereas 33% of the group with poor oral hygiene stated that they had received instructions from their dentist. This finding should stimulate those who routinely counsel children on good oral hygiene to continue this practice and to encourage their auxiliary personnel to emphasize the importance of good oral health.

Use of fluorides

Communal water fluoridation. Recent research studies and observations in private practice continue to support the contention that fluoridation of the communal water supply is the most effective method of reducing the dental caries problem in the general population. According to an American Dental Association survey in 1975, 50% of the U.S. population resides in communities with fluoridated water. Several states have adopted a mandatory fluoridation law, and other states are considering legislation that would require fluoridation of all municipal water supplies. On a worldwide basis, more than 150 million people in more than 30 countries are drinking optimally fluoridated water.

Cohen has cited observations in Philadelphia, the first city with a population over 1 million to fluoridate its water supply. The reduction in DMFT has averaged 75% at age 6 years, 54.5% at age 8 years, 42.6% at age 12 years, and 46.7% at age 14 years. A 50% reduction in the decay rate has been noted in the primary teeth.

Murray and Rugg-Gunn reviewed 94 studies,

conducted in 20 countries, to help clarify varying reports on the benefits to primary teeth of communal water fluoridation. A thorough review of the data clearly showed that water fluoridation provides protection to primary teeth against dental caries but to a somewhat lesser degree than permanent teeth. The caries reduction benefits to primary teeth ranged between 40% and 50%, while the range for permanent teeth was between 50% and 60%.

Documented evidence that water fluoridation is an effective public health measure continues to grow. Carmichael and associates and Rock, Gordon, and Bradnock have recently reported data in separate studies comparing the caries incidence of children living in two fluoridated communities with children living in two nonfluoridated communities in England. The role of fluoridation in reducing dental caries is obvious in both studies. The study by Carmichael and associates also demonstrates that children in lower social classes gain an even greater caries prevention benefit than children in higher social classes. This is because, as a group, the children in the lower social classes have a higher prevalence of proximal carious lesions, and proximal tooth surfaces derive the greatest benefit from fluoridation.

The protection afforded by fluoridation carries over into adult life. Arnold and associates, as well as Hayes, Littleton, and White, have found that the posteruptive benefits of drinking fluoridated water can result in caries reduction as great as 30%.

When fluoridation is discontinued in a community, there is a dramatic increase in the dental caries incidence. Way has reported that after a lapse of 2 years, children drinking fluoride-free water in Galesburg, Illinois, experienced as much as a 38% increase in tooth decay. Lemke, Doherty, and Arra have reported that in Antigo, Wisconsin, a city of 9600, tooth decay rose 92% among kindergarten children, 183% among second graders, and 100% among fourth graders when fluoridation was discontinued. The findings substantiate previous studies regarding the withdrawal of fluorides from the water supply.

In a summary of long observations, Blayney and Hill refer to the economic value of fluoridation. In Evanston, Illinois, families with children in the 6- to 8-year-old group experienced a reduction in dental costs of 35% to 40% as a result of fluoridation. Families with children 12 to 14 years of age had a reduction of at least 50% in dental costs.

Eichenbaum, Dunn, and Tinanoff reported interesting information related to the long-term impact of communal fluoridation on the private practice of pedodontics. A survey conducted from 1948 to 1950 showed that 86% of the child patients in a private pedodontic practice needed restorative treatment, and nearly half of these children required pulp therapy. The results of this survey encouraged the city health officials to implement dental health education and preventive programs that included communal water fluoridation. A survey of the same practice almost 30 years later (1977 to 1979) revealed a dramatic change in the restorative needs of the children. The majority of children needed no restorations, and the number of teeth with pulp involvement was negligible.

Smith has estimated that the average annual cost of fluoridating communal water supplies is approximately 25 cents per person. Gish has pointed out that the annual cost varies with the size of the community and may range from approximately $1.50 per person for very small communities to as low as 10 cents per person in larger metropolitan areas. Communal water fluoridation remains by far the most cost-effective caries prevention measure.

H.S. Horowitz and associates have reported findings that have relevance for the millions of Americans who are deprived of the benefits of community water fluoridation because they live in areas not served by central water supplies. The water supply of a rural school was fluoridated for 12 years at a level of 5 ppm, which is 4.5 times the optimum level for community fluoridation in the area. In the final survey, children who had attended the school continuously during the study had 39%

fewer DMFT than did their counterparts who had not attended the school continuously. Late-erupting teeth (canines, premolars, and second molars) demonstrated twice as much caries protection as early-erupting teeth (incisors and first molars). In both categories of teeth the greatest benefits were observed on proximal surfaces, with as much as 69% less caries for late-erupting teeth.

The research related to the effect of school water fluoridation on dental caries has continued, using even higher concentrations of fluoride. Heifetz, Horowitz, and Driscoll are conducting a long-term study in Seagrove, North Carolina, where school water is fluoridated at the level of 6.3 ppm, or approximately seven times the optimum recommended for community water fluoridation. Observations after 8 years show only a slight improvement in DMFS reduction compared to an earlier study using 5 ppm. However, the researchers point out that the full potential of school water fluoridation at seven times the optimum level cannot be adequately determined until children in all grades will have been exposed since entering the first grade (a 12-year study).

Fluoride-containing dentifrices. During the past decade the stannous fluoride–calcium pyrophosphate dentifrice* has been repeatedly documented to have cariostatic properties. Its effectiveness as a means of contributing to the control of dental caries was recognized and reported in *Accepted Dental Therapeutics* (1979) by the Council on Dental Therapeutics of the American Dental Association (ADA). The favorable effect of the home use of a stannous fluoride dentifrice in combination with the professional application of a 10% stannous fluoride solution has been recently reported by Powell, Barnard, and Craig. However, the stannous fluoride dentifrice is not readily available to the public. At this writing the following dentifrices have been approved by the ADA's Council on Dental Therapeutics: Improved Crest and Gleem

---

*Crest, Procter & Gamble, Cincinnati, Ohio 45202.

(both containing sodium fluoride) and Colgate, Maclean's Fluoride, Aqua-Fresh, and Aim (all of which contain sodium monofluorophosphate).

A recent clinical study of 3 years' duration was conducted by Beiswanger, Gish, and Mallat to determine the effect of a sodium fluoride–silica abrasive dentifrice on dental caries. The dentifrice, containing 0.243% sodium fluoride, was compared with stannous fluoride in a study group of 1824 schoolchildren aged 6 to 14 years in Indiana cities where water supplies were fluoride deficient (containing less than 0.35 ppm fluoride). After 3 years the group brushing with the sodium fluoride dentifrice had significantly lower DMFT and DMFS increments than the group brushing with the stannous fluoride dentifrice. Two independent examiners found that the reductions for DMFT were 14.8% and 10.5% and, for DMFS, 16.4% and 13.1%. These results are consistent with those reported by Zacherl. Data are not available regarding the effect of the sodium fluoride dentifrice on the arrest of incipient carious lesions.

Topical fluorides. This section provides a history of the use of topical fluorides and describes currently accepted procedures.

The topical application of fluorides for dental caries control became popular in the 1940s. The recommended procedure of four applications of a 2% sodium fluoride solution in large numbers of children resulted in a 40% reduction in dental caries.

In 1955 Howell and associates reported on the superiority of the topical application of stannous fluoride. They found that four applications of a 2% sodium fluoride solution resulted in a 36% reduction in dental caries, whereas four applications of a 4% stannous fluoride solution resulted in at least a 58% reduction. If the solution was applied continuously during a 4-minute period, the reduction was as great as 65%. Howell and associates also reported reversals in diagnosis. Stannous fluoride, in some patients at least, seemed to have the ability to arrest the caries activity in small smooth-surface lesions. At the time of the second examination, these lesions were no longer considered to be active.

In a study by McDonald and Muhler, stannous fluoride was evaluated on primary teeth in three groups of children receiving either four applications of 2% solution of sodium fluoride, four applications of 4% stannous fluoride, or no treatment. When the two treatment groups were compared with the control group, which received only a prophylaxis, the group treated with sodium fluoride had a 12% reduction in new carious surfaces after 1 year, whereas the group treated with stannous fluoride had a 37% reduction. The effect of the stannous fluoride treatment was statistically significant and that of the sodium fluoride treatment was not.

Gish, Howell, and Muhler reported encouraging results with one application of an 8% solution of stannous fluoride, which in well-controlled studies has been found to be at least 21% more effective, and often as much as 59% more effective, than four applications of a 2% sodium fluoride solution.

A stannous fluoride compound is available in powder form, in either bulk containers or pre-weighed capsules. Currently the recommended concentration is 8%. This concentration is obtained by dissolving 0.8 g of powder in 10 ml of distilled water. Stannous fluoride solutions are acidic, with a pH of about 2.4 to 2.8. Aqueous solutions of stannous fluoride are not stable but lead to the formation of stannous hydroxide and, subsequently, stannic oxide, which is visible as a white precipitate. As a result, solutions of this compound for topical application must be prepared immediately before use.

The one-application technique using stannous fluoride fits ideally into the private office routine, and it may be beneficial both before and immediately after the completion of all restorative work. Since the application is usually repeated at recall appointments, the patient receives at least two applications of the 8% solution each year. The technique, which allows the dentist to apply the fluoride to half of the mouth at one time, was developed by Gish, Howell, and Muhler. A thor-

ough prophylaxis should be performed before using the topical solution. Extreme care must be taken to clean and polish thoroughly each available tooth surface, using a therapeutic prophylaxis paste. A 2-inch No. 2 cotton roll is securely attached to the lingual prong of the cotton roll holder. The distal extension of the cotton roll should be flush with the lingual extension of the holder to prevent the tongue from pushing the distal part of the lingual cotton roll against the mandibular first permanent molar and absorbing the fluoride solution. The anterior extension may be folded back to absorb secretions from the sublingual duct. A 6-inch No. 2 cotton roll is used for the buccal extension. Approximately 1 inch of the cotton roll should extend forward to facilitate holding the lip away from the anterior teeth. The long cotton roll is then doubled back and held with the index finger as the holder is carried to the mouth. The patient's head should be in an upright position to prevent stretching the buccal cheek muscles. This position will also reduce the possibility of the fluoride solution flowing back into the posterior part of the mouth and throat. Fig. 7-12 shows the preparation of the cotton rolls and the application of the fluoride solution to the clean, dry teeth in half the mouth. The 8% stannous fluoride is applied with a cotton applicator, and the teeth are kept moist with the solution throughout the treatment period. This usually requires one reapplication.

Acidulated phosphate fluoride (APF) is available as either a solution or a gel, both of which are stable and ready to use. APF systems consist essentially of mixtures of sodium fluoride, hydrofluoric acid, and phosphoric acid with concentrations of 1.23% fluoride and 0.98% phosphoric acid, and a pH of 3 to 3.5. Flavoring, coloring, and sweetening agents are added, and thickening agents are used in APF gels. The systems are chemically stable for at least 2 years when stored in plastic containers, but there may be a decrease in the viscosity of the gels after several months of storage.

The rationale for the use of topical APF solution and gels, based originally on studies by Brudevold and DePaola, is that these agents result in a signif-

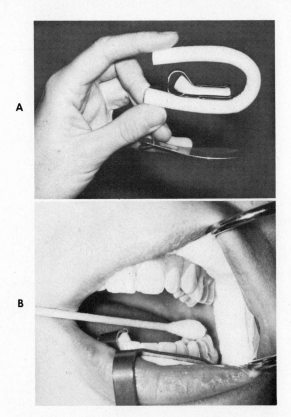

Fig. 7-12. A, A No. 2 cotton roll, 2 inches long, has been securely attached to the lingal prong of the cotton roll holder. A 6-inch No. 2 cotton roll has been attached to the buccal extension of the cotton roll holder. The cotton roll has been doubled back before placement in the mouth. **B,** Stannous fluoride is applied to the clean, dry teeth in half the mouth.

icant and beneficial increase in the fluoride content of the enamel surface. A number of reports indicate an inverse relationship between the fluoride content of the enamel and the prevalence of caries. Horowitz and Heifetz have reported the results of a study in which children given a semiannual application of a flavored APF solution developed 41% fewer DMFS than did the controls after 3 years.

A 4-minute treatment time, preceded by a thorough prophylaxis, is recommended for either solution or gel. Topical applications of APF gel or solu-

tion should be repeated at least every 6 months. With solution, care should be taken to see that it reaches the interproximal surfaces. The technique for the 4-minute application of APF solution is the same as that recommended for the topical stannous fluoride solution.

If gel is used with a tray technique, an ample ribbon of gel will force the substance into the proximal areas. Usually both trays are inserted at once to complete the topical fluoride treatment in one 4-minute application (Fig. 7-13). The patient sits in an upright position with the head tipped slightly forward to allow excess saliva and gel to flow toward the lips. Patients who follow instructions well may be provided with the high-velocity evacuator tip to help control the drooling themselves, or they may be given a plastic ''drool bag'' that enables them to tip the head forward even more and catch the drooled liquid in the bag, which is later discarded. The dentist or an office auxiliary should supervise the treatment and provide assistance as needed. If necessary the auxiliary may manipulate the evacuator tip or help hold the patient's head forward and the trays in place over the drool bag. Patients requiring assistance also often need positive reinforcement during the procedure.

Topical fluorides for the general anesthetic patient. Complete dentistry for very young children or handicapped individuals under general anesthesia has become an accepted procedure. The application of 8% or 10% stannous fluoride to the teeth of children under a general anesthetic, after the placement of restorations, has been widely practiced. An unfavorable oral tissue reaction to the stannous fluoride, evidenced as sloughing or ulceration, may occur unless the dentist alters the usual application technique. The occasional unfavorable reaction has been attributed to the dehydration of the oral tissues and the caustic properties of the fluoride solution. However, it is generally agreed that even with the occasional unfavorable reaction, the benefit of the procedure—the reduction of caries—far outweighs the disadvantages.

A thorough prophylaxis should precede the placement of the rubber dam for a quadrant of res-

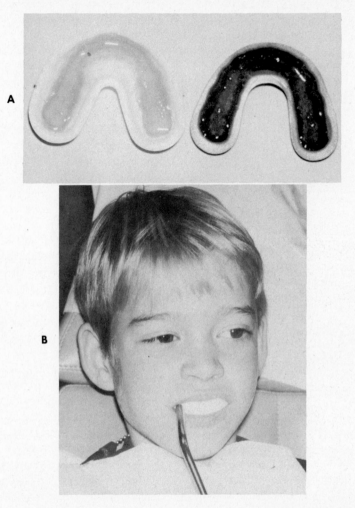

Fig. 7-13. A, Sufficient APF gel is placed in the upper and lower trays so that each tray is approximately one-third full. **B,** The teeth are dried and both trays are inserted in the patient's mouth to provide a complete mouth topical fluoride treatment in a single 4-minute application. The evacuator tip is positioned to remove the excess saliva and gel as the liquids flow toward the lips.

torations. Stannous fluoride should be applied after the restorative work has been completed for that quadrant but before removal of the rubber dam. If a rubber dam is not used for operative procedures, it is suggested that an oral evacuator be used at the time of the topical application to limit the amount of solution that flows over the tissue and to prevent possible saturation of the throat pack with solution.

Fluoride mouthrinses. There is increasing interest in the use of oral fluoride rinses as an additional dental caries control measure. Children under 4 years of age may not have full control over their swallowing reflexes; therefore caution should be exercised in recommending rinses for home use. However, some small children can expectorate rinses quite reliably under proper supervision. In nonfluoridated areas it may be desirable to have the child swallow the rinse after "swishing" it to gain the systemic fluoride effect as well. Some rinses (acidulated or aqueous solutions that do not contain alcohol) are prepared to provide the necessary supplemental systemic dose of fluoride if the child does not drink fluoridated water.

Radike and associates observed schoolchildren who rinsed their mouths once each school day for 2 school years with stannous fluoride mouthrinse containing 250 ppm fluoride (about 0.1% stannous fluoride). There was a significant reduction in dental caries at the end of the first and second school years. Two independent examiners showed caries reductions of 33% and 43% in DMFS scores. The anticaries benefit from the stannous fluoride mouthrinse was especially encouraging because the children already were receiving the optimum benefit of fluoridation.

APF mouthwashes in concentrations of either 100 or 200 ppm fluoride ion used twice daily have been shown by Finn and associates to be effective. They reported that during a 26-month period the APF rinses containing relatively small amounts of fluoride were effective in reducing dental caries.

Miller (1977) made a preliminary report on the National Caries Program sponsored by the National Institute of Dental Research. A nationwide school-based fluoride mouthrinse program that included 85,000 children in 17 states and Guam produced encouraging results. The schoolchildren rinsed their mouths for 60 seconds once weekly with 5 ml of a 0.2% neutral sodium fluoride solution. Children in the 7-, 11-, and 13-year-old groups experienced a reduction in dental decay. There was also evidence of caries decrease in the primary teeth.

Leske and others have reported recently on results of a fluoride rinsing program that was begun in 1975 in the Three Village Central School District of Long Island, New York. The program was one of 17 demonstration projects sponsored by the National Institute of Dental Research, which initially enrolled approximately 4500 elementary schoolchildren (kindergarten through the sixth grade), who rinsed once a week with a 0.2% neutral sodium fluoride solution under the supervision of homeroom teachers. The prevalence of caries in the children who participated in the rinse program was 20.4% DMFT and 24.4% DMFS less than that of children who had never rinsed. The reduction in proximal caries was 49.6%. The reductions in occlusal and buccolingual caries were 21.0% and 18.8%, respectively. The examination of exfoliated teeth also indicated that fluoride rinsing may produce a residual benefit.

Extensive field research in the use of fluoride mouthrinses has been conducted in recent years. Most studies incorporate the use of a 0.2% sodium fluoride rinse once weekly or a 0.05% sodium fluoride rinse once daily. In addition to the work previously summarized, these other studies show unquestionable caries prevention benefits of the regular use of self-administered fluoride rinses when properly supervised. These benefits accrue to primary and permanent teeth and seem to be helpful both in fluoridated areas and in areas with non-fluoridated water. Additional references of such studies are offered at the end of this chapter.

Dietary fluoride supplements. A review of the literature on the value of fluorides administered during pregnancy fails to disclose any valid evidence to support such use even in nonfluoridated areas. In 1966 the U.S. Food and Drug Administration (FDA) banned the manufacturers of fluoride supplements from marketing products bearing a claim that dental caries would be prevented in the offspring of women who used such products during pregnancy. The FDA took this action because of insufficient clinical evidence to substantiate such a claim. There was no question of safety. Although some medical and dental practitioners have continued to prescribe dietary fluoride supplements for pregnant women since the FDA's advertising ban, generally there is unanimity among research experts and public health officials that fluoride ingested by gravid women does not benefit the teeth of their offspring, at least not the permanent teeth.

Participants in a recent symposium concerning the use of prenatal fluorides agreed that transfer of fluoride does occur from the mother to the fetus through the placenta. Only in recent years has such a transfer been generally acknowledged. How much fluoride is transferred, however, from the blood of the mother to the blood of the fetus remains uncertain. Nevertheless, the members of the symposium generally agreed that some benefit of caries prevention accrues to the primary teeth when the fetus is subjected to fluoride. There is considerable doubt about the benefit to the permanent teeth. The symposium discussions seemed to lead to the conclusion that additional well-controlled research efforts are needed to more clearly define the possible benefits of prenatal fluoride administration.

A study by Katz and Muhler suggests that the effect of fluoride on primary teeth is mainly postnatal. To determine the effect of waterborne fluoride on dental caries in primary teeth, 890 children from 4 to 7 years of age were examined in one Indiana city having a communal water supply with only 0.05 ppm fluoride and in three cities having a concentration of 1 ppm fluoride. Children living in the cities with fluoridated water had between 35% and 65% fewer dental caries in their primary teeth than those living in the fluoride-deficient city. Comparisons of dental caries incidence in primary teeth of children living in the same city and exposed, either prenatally and postnatally or exclusively postnatally, showed no difference between the groups.

In recent years a number of studies have demonstrated the anticariogenic effectiveness of fluoride supplements. If children do not have the benefit of drinking water containing an optimum fluoride concentration, supplements should be prescribed.

Hennon, Stookey, and Muhler (1966) conducted a clinical study that included 815 children between 18 and 39 months of age residing in three fluoride-deficient Indiana communities. The children received chewable tablets containing vitamins, vitamins plus fluoride, or fluoride alone (1 mg as sodium fluoride) and were examined for dental caries initially and at 6-month intervals. The findings during the first 2 years of the 5-year study indicate a significant reduction, about 37%, in the incidence of dental caries after 6 months in the children ingesting either the fluoride or vitamin-fluoride supplements. This degree of protection increased to about 55% and 63%, respectively, after the children had used the supplement for 1 and 2 years. The important finding was the significant reduction in the incidence of dental caries after use of the tablets for only 6 months. This observation indicates a highly effective topical benefit of the chewable tablets, since most of the primary teeth had already erupted when the study began.

The administration of fluoride supplements should commence shortly after birth and should continue through the time of the eruption of the second permanent molars. The natural fluoride content of the water should first be determined. If the natural fluoride content is 0.7 ppm or more, supplements should not be administered.

Summary. The following outline* of the use of fluorides identifies the current recommended dosages for supplemental fluoride:

I. General considerations for a fluoride regimen in children
   A. It should be custom designed for each individual patient.
      1. Avoid adopting routine procedures for all patients. Take into account each individual's dental health status and dental needs.
      2. Use agents and procedures that have proved safe and effective.
      3. Select appropriate therapeutic agents and methods that appear in the latest edition of *Accepted Dental Therapeutics* (ADA).
      4. Exercise extreme caution in applying fluorides to children under 3 years of age because of the increased possibility that they may ingest excessive amounts of fluoride. Use high-volume evacuation and permit rinsing with water following the procedure.
   B. Fluoride effects are additive; no single treatment

---

*Courtesy of a joint faculty committee of the Pedodontic Department and Preventive Dentistry Department, Dr. A.G. Christen and Dr. F.E. McCormick, Co-Chairmen, Indiana University School of Dentistry.

or procedure provides maximum disease control.

1. Fluorides are beneficial when properly used.
   a. Consider multiple fluoride therapy for each patient.
   b. Dental office and home use of fluorides are recommended.
2. Since fluoride usage has the potential of producing dental fluorosis and systemic overdose, all forms of fluorides must be used with care under professional supervision.
   a. Be aware of the fluoride content of drinking water and other sources of fluoride *before* prescribing dietary fluoride supplements.
   b. Always consider the patient's age, and prescribe according to ADA guidelines.
3. Multiple fluoride therapy includes the following.
   a. Systemic fluorides (one source only)
      (1) Communal, home, or school water fluoridation, *or*
      (2) Pediatric fluoride supplements
   b. Topical fluorides in several forms
      (1) Prophylaxis paste in office
      (2) Office-applied topicals (gels or solutions)
      (3) Fluoride dentifrices
      (4) Self-applied fluorides (rinses, pastes, brush-ins)

II. Office fluoride regimen
   A. Prophylaxis. Always use fluoride-containing prophylaxis paste before applying topical fluoride solution or gel to make enamel surfaces readily accessible and more reactive to the fluoride agent.
      1. No prophylaxis paste has been proved clinically effective, and no products have been accepted by either the FDA or the ADA.
      2. Most effective at this time appear to be the following.
         a. Compatible lava pumice–8% stannous fluoride mixture
            (1) Place a small amount (1.5 g) of heat-treated, compatible, flavored flour of lava pumice in a dappen dish or container.
            (2) Prepare a fresh 8% SnF_2 solution,

and wet the pumice with the fluoride solution to obtain a suitable working consistency.
         b. Luride APF paste
         c. Preventodontic APF paste
      3. The function of prophylaxis paste is to clean, polish, and replenish fluoride lost from the enamel surface during a prophylactic procedure.
      4. Because of the taste factor, APF systems are usually preferable for use with children under 15 years of age.
      5. *Always* follow with a topical application in children.
   B. Clinical procedures for using prophylaxis paste
      1. Apply to the tooth surfaces with rotating rubber cup in logical, orderly sequence for at least 5 seconds on each surface.
      2. Use a prophylaxis brush for occlusal surfaces.
      3. Use unwaxed floss to draw the paste through interproximal contacts.
      4. Caution patients not to swallow the prophylaxis paste.
         a. Although limited ingestion of prophylaxis pastes is not dangerous, it may cause nausea in some patients.
         b. Have patient rinse and expectorate frequently, or provide continuous use of high-velocity evacuation.
   C. Topical fluoride applications—office applied
      1. Stannous fluoride—8% solution*
         a. Advantages
            (1) More effective than NaF
            (2) Equivalent in effectiveness to APF gel
            (3) Will arrest incipient lesions
         b. Disadvantages
            (1) Bad taste (especially pronounced if splashed on the tongue)
            (2) Pigmentation of arrested lesions

---

*To prepare this solution, use a premeasured scoop and graduated cylinder (0.8 g SnF_2 in 10 ml water provides 8% SnF_2) or a 16% flavored stock solution of SnF_2 in a jug with a pump. Dilute an equal amount of stock solution with distilled water to prepare an 8% solution. Ten milliliters of an 8% SnF_2 solution is sufficient to treat a single patient.

(3) Possible gingival blanching in individuals with severe gingivitis (blanching is reversible in 1 to 3 days)

(4) Stains silicate restorations (does not stain plastics or composites)

(5) Potentially harmful if swallowed in excessive quantities

c. Procedure for topical SnF_2 application

(1) The treatment should be immediately preceded by a thorough prophylaxis with a fluoride prophylaxis paste.

(2) Seat the patient upright and isolate both an upper and lower right or left quadrant from salivary contamination, using cotton roll isolation (half-mouth technique).

(3) Dry isolated teeth thoroughly with compressed air.

(4) Keep the tooth surfaces continuously soaked with fluoride solution for 4-minute application if active caries is present, 30 seconds to 1 minute application if caries inactive. Commence timing when the last tooth in the half-mouth area is wet with the SnF_2 solution. If necessary, carefully reapply solution during timing period.

(5) Repeat procedure on the opposite side of the mouth.

(6) Have the patient rinse thoroughly with water and expectorate immediately on completion of the topical treatment.*

2. APF (acidulated phosphate fluoride)—1.23% (fluoride ion) gel. If an APF gel is to be used, be sure to obtain a product bearing an ADA acceptance label.

a. Advantages

(1) More acceptable taste than SnF_2

(2) No staining or pigmentation; little blanching of gingival tissues

(3) More effective than NaF (equivalent to 8% SnF_2)

(4) Can be applied to both complete arches simultaneously

b. Disadvantages

(1) May damage porcelain restorations

(2) Potentially harmful if swallowed in large quantities

c. Procedure for topical APF application

(1) Use gels only in trays. Use careful technique to reduce swallowing.

(2) Technique for topical APF gel application

(a) Application should be immediately preceded by a thorough prophylaxis with a fluoride prophylaxis paste.

(b) Teeth must be dried and free of saliva.

(c) Pleace enough of the APF gel to fill one third of the trough area of the trays that properly fit over each dental arch. Avoid overloading tray to reduce oozing of the gel, which could lead to excessive ingestion.

(d) Place loaded tray over the arch, and squeeze the buccal and lingual surfaces; force gel between teeth.

(e) With light biting pressure, allow the tray to remain in the mouth for *4 minutes*.

(f) Provide the patient with a "drool bag" or saliva ejector to prevent the patient from swallowing excessive saliva.

(g) After the 4-minute treatment period, remove the tray(s) and use a high-volume evacuator to thoroughly remove the gel that remains on the teeth.

(h) Have the patient rinse thoroughly with water and expectorate on completion of the topical treatment.

3. Frequency of topical applications—SnF_2 or APF

---

*Previous guidelines have suggested that patients not eat or rinse for 30 minutes following a topical fluoride application. However, there now appears to be no scientific basis for such a recommendation.

a. Rampant caries: four to five applications for 4- to 6-week period, repeating single application every 3 months until caries is under control. The patient should brush teeth with a fluoride dentifrice immediately before receiving subsequent, follow-up fluoride treatments.

b. Moderate caries: single application at 2- to 3-month intervals

c. Minimal or no caries activity: single application every 6 months

III. Other topical fluoride measures

A. Fluoride dentifrices

1. Recommend the use of an ADA or FDA approved fluoride dentifrice as listed below.

a. Improved Crest (NaF)	Approved 1981
b. Aim (MFP)	Approved 1980
c. Colgate (MFP)	Approved 1980
d. Aqua-Fresh (MFP)	Approved 1978
e. Maclean's Fluoride (MFP)	Approved 1976
f. Gleem (NaF)	Documented (FDA) 1973

2. At least 25% caries reduction can be expected.

3. Increased benefit results from two to three brushings each day as compared to one brushing.

B. Fluoride mouthrinses

1. Public health situations (for example, school rinse programs) show 35% caries reduction with daily or weekly supervised rinses.

2. The following are recommended for home use for patients with rampant caries or poor oral hygiene.

a. Not to serve as a replacement for other fluoride applications performed in the office

b. Rinsing after thorough brushing, especially before retiring at night

c. Daily use of one of the following commercially available mouthrinses (as opposed to weekly)

Name of product	Percentage of fluoride	F-ions available
Fluoriguard	0.05% NaF	0.023%
Fluorinse	0.05% NaF	0.023%
Stan Care	0.10% SnF_2	0.024%

IV. Systemic fluoride measures

A. Communal fluoridation: addition of low concentrations of fluoride to public water supply

1. The optimum concentration varies with the mean annual area temperature (in Indiana, 1 ppm is considered optimum).

2. Water fluoridation is the single most effective public health procedure for caries prevention.

a. Overall caries reduction in children residing in fluoridated area during enamel-forming years: 50% to 60%

(1) Protection on anterior teeth (smooth surface caries): 80% to 100%

(2) Protection on premolars: 55% to 75%

(3) Protection on posterior teeth (lesser effect on pit and fissure caries): 30% to 50%

B. School water fluoridation

1. The optimum concentration is 4.5 times that of city water supplies because of lower water consumption at school.

2. Overall caries reduction of 40%

C. Pediatric fluoride supplements (fluoride or fluoride-vitamin preparations)

1. Offer 50% to 60% caries reduction

2. To be prescribed only if the water fluoride content is less than 0.7 ppm

3. Fluoride-vitamin preparation to be prescribed only if the child *really* needs vitamins

4. Dosage dependent on age and water fluoride content (Table 7-4)

5. Not indicated beyond the age of 13

Table 7-4. Fluoride supplement (in mg F/day)

Fluoride content of drinking water (ppm)	Birth to age 2 yr (mg)	Age 2 to 3 yr (mg)	Age 3 to 13 yr (mg)
Less than 0.3	0.25	0.50	1.00
0.3-0.7	—	0.25	0.50
0.7 and over	Fluoride supplements not indicated		

Modified from American Dental Association Council on Dental Therapeutics: Accepted dental therapeutics, ed. 38, Chicago, 1979, The Association.

6. Appropriate dosages to be carefully dispensed under supervision of conscientious parent
   a. It is considered safe to dispense up to 120 mg fluoride (264 mg of NaF), even if all of it is accidentally ingested at one time by the child.
   b. Alert parents to the need for keeping medications in secure place.

Fluoride is the most effective caries prevention agent available today. It is considered completely safe when properly used. However, the ingestion of high concentrations can lead to nausea, vomiting, dental fluorosis (mottling), or in extreme cases, even death, especially in children. Thus it is imperative that the dental profession have full awareness of the hazards accompanying the use of fluoride and yet be prepared to use it to maximum advantage through careful consideration of each patient's individual situation.

Restorative dentistry in the control program. Excellent operative dentistry is also valuable as a preventive measure in the dental caries control program. For patients who do not respond to nonrestorative caries control recommendations (for example, use of fluorides, diet, and plaque control), the restoration of even the smallest proximal lesion is indicated. Restoring such a lesion, often referred to as an "etching" or "initial decalcification," will protect the dental pulp against the often rapid progress of the lesion and will reduce the possibility of a lesion developing on the proximal surface of the adjacent tooth.

Something that must not be overlooked in the evaluation of operative intervention in the control of dental caries is the quality or thorough application of operative principles. Unfortunately, there is no standard by which an evaluation can be made, at least for statistical studies. However, by observation it can be noted that when sound operative dentistry is performed early in the course of the caries attack in a manner that controls or affects some of the etiologic factors, certain beneficial results occur—that is, the caries activity in the respective regions is stopped or altered.

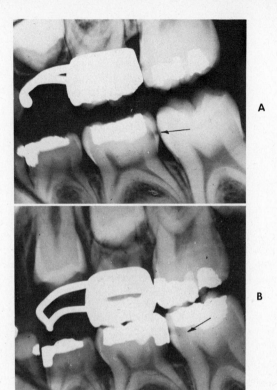

Fig. 7-14. A, Radiograph of an incipient carious lesion on the mesial surface of a first permanent molar. **B,** During a 6-month period, the carious lesion on the mesial surface of the first permanent molar has progressed to the degree that it endangers the pulp horn.

It can also be shown that the removal of the carious material and the restoration of the tooth will result in a reduction in the number of oral microorganisms. The restoration of the tooth to a comfortable masticating surface, making it possible for the patient to eat coarser, more detergent foods, will result in a cleaner mouth and will indirectly reduce the dental caries problem.

Application of cariostatic agents. Although it is now generally agreed that the once-practiced application of silver nitrate to deep carious lesions is ineffective in arresting the caries process and may result in serious pulpal irritation, some have observed its effectiveness in temporarily arresting initial carious lesions limited to the enamel.

Table 7-5. Effect of topical application of 8% stannous fluoride and silver nitrate in the arrest of small carious lesions

Treatment	Number of teeth	Percent in which carious lesion remained un-changed	
		12 mo	24 mo
Control	92	54	26
Stannous fluoride	88	93	43
Silver nitrate	72	75	43

We have completed a 2-year study designed to compare the effectiveness of an 8% stannous fluoride solution and ammoniacal silver nitrate in arresting caries. Patients were selected with at least bilateral involvement of the distal surface of the second primary molars and with radiographic evidence of superficial involvement of the enamel on the mesial surface of the first permanent molar (Fig. 7-14).

All operative procedures were completed with a rubber dam in place. Before the placement of a restoration in the primary molar, however, the etching on the mesial surface of the first permanent molar was observed. Eight percent stannous fluoride was applied to the etched area of a third of the teeth, a third of the teeth were treated with ammoniacal silver nitrate that was precipitated with eugenol, and the remaining third served as controls. Bite-wing radiographs were taken at 6-month intervals, and observations were made regarding the progress, if any, of the lesion on the first permanent molars. The results of the study can be seen in Table 7-5. Approximately half the untreated (control) lesions increased in size during the first year, and 74% were larger by the end of the second year; 93% of the lesions treated with stannous fluoride appeared identical in size at the end of the first year (Fig. 7-15). At the end of the second year, with no additional treatment in the interim, 43% remained unchanged. This finding seems to confirm the ob-

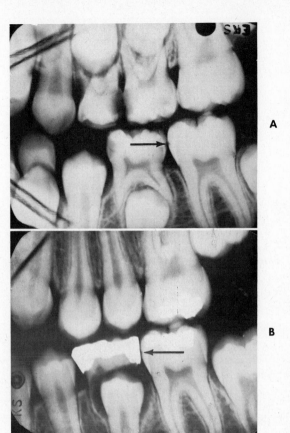

Fig. 7-15. A, A carious lesion that has penetrated the dentin can be seen in the lower second primary molar *(arrow)*. Before a restoration was placed in the primary molar, the initial lesion on the mesial surface of the first permanent molar was treated with 8% stannous fluoride. **B,** Two years after the application of stannous fluoride to the carious lesion on the mesial surface of the lower first permanent molar, the lesion remains unchanged *(arrow)*.

servation that stannous fluoride loses much of its protective power after 1 year. Therefore topical applications must be repeated at regular intervals.

An unexpected observation was the apparent cariostatic effect of silver nitrate. Although silver nitrate is not as effective as stannous fluoride, 75% of the treated lesions remained unchanged during

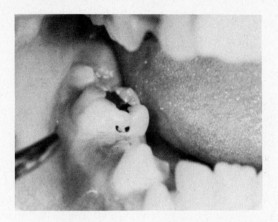

Fig. 7-16. Eight percent stannous flouride was applied to the mesial surface of the first permanent molar at the time of the restoration of a distal cavity in the second primary molar. Two years later, the lesion in the permanent molar remains pigmented and inactive.

the first year. At the end of the second year the protective effect of silver nitrate was identical to that of stannous fluoride—that is, 43% of the lesions appeared unchanged.

As a result of the findings in this study it seems advantageous to recommend the routine application of 8% stannous fluoride to a quadrant of isolated teeth before the placement of restorations. The caries-arresting effect of the application of stannous fluoride can be seen in Fig. 7-16.

Pit and fissure sealants. For many years attempts have been made to eliminate pit and fissure caries. In 1923 Hyatt recommended that all pits and fissures be opened with a bur and filled with amalgam. Attempts have been made to prevent pit and fissure caries by applying a variety of different chemical solutions, including silver nitrate and potassium ferrocyanide with zinc chloride, and by covering the depressions with various types of dental cement. To date, none of these methods has proved successful.

In recent years pit and fissure sealants have been used by many dentists. A variety of sealant types are available, all marketed by reputable dental manufacturing companies and all offering satisfactory results when used according to their instruc-tions. Thus the decision regarding which type to use is determined largely by individual preference. Sealants are available as clear, colorless materials, as clear, tinted materials, and as opaque, colored materials. They are also marketed in chemical self-cured or light-cured systems to further accommodate dentists' preferences. No one type of material or curing system is perfect. They all offer certain different advantages and are limited by different disadvantages. Their one common benefit, when they are properly used, is a reduction in the incidence of pit and fissure caries. However, the use of sealants in preventing occlusal caries may not be as cost effective for dentists in a private practice as it is in public health programs unless the sealants are applied by dental auxiliaries.

Handelman, Washburn, and Whopper have published a preliminary report on the effect of fissure sealants on bacteria in dental caries. The results of this study support the idea that treating naturally occurring debris or caries in the teeth with an occlusal sealant may retard and perhaps prevent the progress of decay. The investigators caution, however, that studies of the long-term sealant effect on bacteria present in the carious lesion are needed to provide information on the duration of the seal and a better understanding of the role of bacteria in dental caries.

It should be recognized that the clinical diagnosis of incipient carious lesions in posterior permanent teeth is complicated by the depth, narrowness, and complexity of the pits and fissures. Jeronimus, Till, and Sveen caution that such lesions may remain undetected and may inadvertently be sealed with a dental sealant. Their studies indicate that the sealing of incipient lesions extending to the deepest limit of the incipient classification (with the extension less than one fourth of the distance from the dentinoenamel junction to the pulp) did not reduce the viability of microorganisms in the carious dentin. This was true regardless of the sealant product used.

Numerous recent studies attest to the long-term retention and effectiveness of pit and fissure sealants as a caries prevention measure. Simonsen has

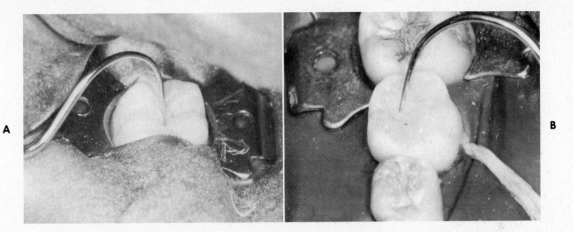

Fig. 7-17. A, Mandibular first permanent molar isolated to receive a sealant application. The tooth is judged to be noncarious, but the occlusal surface is caries susceptible as determined by the penetrance of a sharp explorer into the deep pit and fissure areas. **B,** After placement of an occlusal sealant, the explorer no longer penetrates the pits and fissures of this mandibular second primary molar but slides along the smooth resin surface. There are no "catches" or ledges along the margins. (**B** courtesy Dr. Hala Z. Henderson.)

demonstrated very favorable results of a colored pit and fissure sealant after a 3-year evaluation. Mertz-Fairhurst and associates have completed a 6-year clinical evaluation of a clear, chemical self-cure sealant material, and they observed 67% complete retention on the 161 teeth treated originally. They found the single application of sealant material to be 52% effective in caries prevention for the 6-year period. It is now recognized that reapplication of sealant material when it becomes lost or partially lost will increase the caries prevention effectiveness of the sealant procedure. Other studies demonstrating the benefits of pit and fissure sealants are listed in the references for this chapter. It becomes obvious from reviewing the literature that the newer sealants, when applied according to the manufacturer's instructions, should have a much longer life than sealants introduced in the late 1960s or early 1970s.

Ideally, the teeth to receive the sealant should be isolated with a rubber dam. The acid-conditioning agent is applied to the occlusal surface for a full 60 seconds. The area, after it is rinsed and dried, should appear frosty, indicating that the enamel prisms are roughened and have a microscopic honeycomb-like structure. Frequent oral and radiographic examinations should be made to determine the effectiveness of the sealant in controlling and preventing caries on the occlusal surfaces of the teeth (Fig. 7-17).

Caries vaccine. A vaccine to prevent the disease of dental caries has been an anticipated scientific breakthrough since at least the early 1940s. More recent research supports the belief that *S. mutans* is the principal etiologic organism of dental caries, and the development of a method of immunization specifically targeted at neutralizing *S. mutans* has been a major thrust of caries vaccine research. Bowen has reported that monkeys remained caries free for over 6 years after the animals received intraoral injections of killed *S. mutans,* even though the monkeys were fed highly cariogenic diets and had severe malocclusion that would predispose them to caries. Attention is also being directed toward the development of a caries vaccine that may be taken orally. However, Carlos has reported that research must be undertaken to identify the most potent antigens and the optimum route and frequency of vaccination and to establish safety of the procedure before full-scale clinical trials can begin. Although at least partial prevention of dental caries by vaccination in humans will probably become a reality, a readily available caries vaccine for humans is not imminent. Therefore this discussion focuses on the methods already available and proved to be effective and safe in pedodontic practice.

Natural protective mechanism of the mouth

It is generally accepted that the dental caries process is controlled to some extent by a natural protective mechanism inherent within the saliva. Many properties of saliva have been investigated to learn their possible role in the caries process. Considerable importance has been placed on the salivary pH, the acid-neutralizing power, and the calcium and phosphorus content. It has long been suggested that in addition to these properties the rate of flow and the viscosity of saliva may influence the development of caries. The normal salivary flow aids in the solution of food debris on which microorganisms thrive. In addition, the saliva manifests a variety of antibacterial and other anti-infectious properties. These have been ascribed to mucus, lysozyme, and other bacteriostatic inhibins and bacteriolytic and bactericidal substances. In the management of rampant caries these considerations have become increasingly important.

Saliva is secreted by three paired masses of cells—the submaxillary, the sublingual, and the parotid glands. There are also small glands that secrete mucoid fluid scattered over the buccal mucous membranes. Each of these has its own duct. The submaxillary gland secretes a mixed type of fluid—a thin, watery type and a thick, viscid juice rich in mucin. The sublingual alveoli are predominantly of the mucous type, although a few serous alveoli are present. The secretion may be thin and watery or viscid, depending on the nature of the secretory stimulus. However, it is usually of the mucous type. The parotid secretion is thin and watery and is low in organic content.

The salivary glands are under the control of the autonomic (involuntary) nervous system, receiving fibers from both its parasympathetic and sympathetic divisions. Stimulation of either the parasympathetic (chorda tympani) fibers or the sympathetic fibers to the submaxillary or sublingual gland causes a secretion of saliva. The secretion resulting from the parasympathetic stimulation is profuse and watery in consistency in most animals. Sympathetic stimulation, however, causes a scanty secretion of a thick, mucinous juice. Stimulation of the parasympathetic fibers to the parotid gland causes a profuse, watery secretion, but stimulation of the sympathetic fibers causes no secretion.

Salivary deficiency. One of the first reports of a severe salivary deficiency with its deleterious effect on the dentition was made by Hutchinson in 1888. Since that time many reports have emphasized the importance of a normal flow of saliva in preventing a breakdown of the dental apparatus. A reduction in the salivary flow may be of a temporary or a permanent nature. When the quantity is only moderately reduced, the oral structures may appear normal. A marked reduction or complete absence of saliva, however, will result in a septic mouth with rampant caries (Fig. 7-18). In addition to the rapid destruction of the teeth, there may be dryness and cracking of the lips, with fissuring at

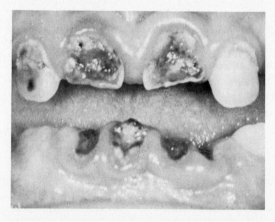

Fig. 7-18. Rampant dental caries in a boy 9 years of age. There was a septic dry mouth caused by the congenital absence of salivary glands.

the corners of the mouth, burning and soreness of the mucous membranes, crusting of the tongue and palate, and sometimes paresthesia of the tongue or mucous membrane. Often the first symptom of salivary deficiency is the rapid deterioration of the teeth, even to the extent that they cannot be repaired. This deterioration is doubly unfortunate because it may be difficult for a person with a salivary deficiency to wear dentures satisfactorily.

There are many reasons for a reduction in salivary flow. Acquired salivary dysfunction may be the result of a psychic or emotional disturbance and may be either temporary or permanent in nature. During the acute stages mumps may cause a temporary reduction in salivary flow. Both Furstenberg and Morris reported that specific diseases, such as syphilis, tuberculosis, and actinomycosis, as well as acute suppurative infection or infiltration, may inhibit the function of one or all of the salivary glands. Shafer reported histologic changes in the parotid gland of rats after x-radiation. In humans, irradiation for the treatment of hypertrichosis and malignancy has resulted in mouth dryness. An interruption in the central pathways of the secretory nerves has been suggested as a cause of salivary failure, but this is usually overshadowed by definite neurologic signs and symptoms. Similarly, the deficiency in vitamin B complex, especially nicotinic acid, has been reported by Burket as a cause of salivary gland dysfunction.

A study we made indicated that the minimum effective dose of many of the antihistaminic drugs can reduce salivary flow as much as 50%. Scopp and associates have found that dryness of the mouth may occur after the use of a tranquilizer drug such as chlorpromazine (Thorazine). It has likewise been observed that dry mouth and rampant caries may accompany a systemic condition such as myasthenia gravis. In this disease the acetylcholine that is necessary for the proper transmission of nerve impulses is destroyed, with the result that the salivary glands do not receive adequate stimulation.

Previous work has shown a great deal of individual variation in the amount of saliva produced by

stimulation of the glands. The range is from less than a measurable amount in patients with acquired or congenital dysfunction of the salivary glands to 65 ml during a 15-minute period of stimulation and collection. Patients with deficient salivary flow almost without exception showed excessive or rampant caries. In contrast, patients with greater than average salivary flow had relative freedom from dental caries.

Determination of salivary flow. The procedure for determining the stimulated salivary flow of anyone over 8 years of age is relatively simple. Because children under 8 years frequently have difficulty in following directions, an accurate indication of the salivary flow in the younger age group may be impossible to obtain.

Since a minimum amount of equipment is needed (Fig. 7-19), the procedure can be included in the series of dental caries activity tests. The

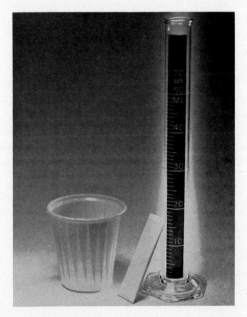

Fig. 7-19. Materials needed to determine the stimulated salivary flow include a piece of unflavored paraffin, a paper cup for collecting the saliva, a stopwatch, and a 50-ml graduated cylinder for measuring the volume of saliva.

patient is provided with a piece of unflavored paraffin (approximately 1 g) and is instructed to hold it in the mouth until it becomes soft. Then the patient is instructed to chew continuously for 15 minutes, spitting all of the secreted saliva into a paper cup. At the end of the chewing period, the saliva is poured into a graduated cylinder to determine the amount secreted. Although there is little daily or seasonal variation in the salivary flow of an individual, when comparative evaluations in salivary flow are to be made, the saliva should be collected at the same time each day—for example, at least 1½ hours after a meal.

Since salivary flow usually increases 0.78 ml each year up to the age of 35, the normal stimulated flow for individuals of different ages can be calculated with the following equation:

$$0.78 \times \text{Age} + 5.6* = \text{Stimulated flow/15 min}$$

It is not unusual to find a salivary deficiency ranging from slightly below normal to practically a dry mouth. If there is a deficiency of saliva or a dry mouth, the cause should be sought. Sometimes the cause is readily determinable; sometimes it is obscure. An emotional disturbance should not be overlooked as a cause in a patient of any age. Psychotherapy may be helpful in these cases. If the cause cannot readily be determined, perhaps it should be assumed that the sparse flow is related to inadequacies in the diet, particularly a vitamin deficiency or excessive sugar consumption to the exclusion of needed foods. Monthly quantitative analyses of the saliva should be made to determine whether dietary improvement is accompanied by an increased flow.

If the salivary glands have not undergone degenerative or metaplastic change and if the nerve pathways between the central nervous system and the salivary glands are still intact, salivary stimulants may be recommended. If dryness of the mouth is due to dehydration, increased fluid intake should be recommended. Cholinergic drugs such as pilocarpine and neostigmine bromide (Prostigmin)

---

*Estimated stimulated salivary flow of the infant.

may be beneficial, but their undesirable effects on other body systems generally contraindicate their use for promoting salivation. The use of gustatory stimulants (sugar-free candy) or masticatory stimulants (sugar-free gum) have been suggested as adjuncts to encourage salivation. Salivary substitutes have been suggested by Shannon, McCrary, and Starcke as helpful in preventing soft tissue problems associated with dry mouth. These saliva substitutes are also reported to enhance remineralization of tooth surfaces and may help prevent radiation-induced caries.

Viscosity of saliva. It has long been suggested that there is a relationship between the viscosity of saliva and the rate of dental decay. Both thick, ropy saliva and thin, watery saliva have been blamed for rampant dental caries. Previous work conducted at Indiana University has shown a statistically significant direct relationship between the viscosity of saliva and the number of DMFT. This relationship held true for all members of the observation group, regardless of age. Patients with thick, ropy saliva invariably had poor oral hygiene. The teeth were covered with stain or plaque, and the rate of dental caries ranged from greater than average to the rampant type.

There is no evidence that under normal conditions viscosity changes with age. This property of the saliva is governed not only by the particular set of glands stimulated but also by the type of nervous stimulation and the amount of mucin (glycoprotein) present.

Hewat observed a relationship between viscous saliva and excessive sugar consumption. We have also observed that children who consume excessive amounts of carbohydrates often have not only a sparse flow but also a viscous saliva. Even minimal doses of some antihistaminic drugs will result in a greatly increased viscosity of saliva in some individuals.

There are apparently only a limited number of ways to alter the viscosity of saliva. Reduction of refined sugar intake may be effective in some patients. A slight reduction of viscosity may be noted after pilocarpine therapy.

Dental caries activity tests

Lactobacillus count. The lactobacillus count was introduced by Hadley in 1933, and for years it was used routinely by many dentists as an aid in determining the current dental caries susceptibility and in predicting the future incidence of dental caries. Although the present use of lactobacillus count tests is probably limited primarily to research, the discussion is being retained in this edition because of its historical interest.

Jay stated that lactobacillus counts under 2000, as a rule, should be considered unimportant in determining caries activity. On the other hand, counts from 2000 to 10,000 are usually indicative of moderate caries activity, and counts over 10,000 generally are associated with high caries activity and an indication of a need for strict dietary treatment or restriction.

Rovelstad, Geller, and Cohen reported a direct relationship between the salivary lactobacillus count and dental caries as revealed by the number of DMFT and the number of carious teeth at the time of the test. The greater the lactobacillus count, the greater the amount of caries.

Green and Weisenstein, however, after making counts of lactobacilli and other oral microorganisms and comparing them with the previous caries attack, current dental conditions, and later caries attacks, concluded that although some associations were found, none was clear and consistent enough to permit accurate prognosis of the future caries experience in individuals. A study by Carter and Wells corroborated the finding of Green and Weisenstein that the extent of previous caries attacks is not related to any specific current conditions regarding the number of salivary lactobacilli. They also added support to the previous observation that in mouths in which the carious lesions have been restored there will be a general reduction in salivary lactobacilli. Shklair and associates also reported that the restoration of all carious lesions reduced lactobacillus counts sharply over a 7- to 8-week period, whereas in control patients no change in the lactobacillus counts occurred.

The practical value of the lactobacillus count and other caries activity tests depends on the use the dentist intends to make of them. Although their reliability in predicting the number of new carious lesions that will develop in a specified time has been questioned, the lactobacillus count and other activity tests may be useful tools in determining the patient's acceptance of recommended improved oral measures and dietary changes, particularly those involving the restriction of freely fermentable carbohydrate.

Lactobacillus count technique. The patient is given sterile bottles and pieces of paraffin and is instructed to collect saliva samples on two or three successive mornings before the teeth have been brushed and before any food or water has been taken. Continuous chewing of the unflavored paraffin for 5 minutes will stimulate a sufficient quantity of saliva.

The saliva is thoroughly shaken, and 1 ml is mixed with 4 ml of beef extract broth adjusted to pH 5. Then 0.1 ml of the diluted solution is transferred to plated tomato juice agar, to which 1:10,000 sodium azide has been added (pH adjusted to 5); the diluted solution is distributed evenly with a glass spreader. The plate is incubated at 98.6° F (37° C) for 72 hours, after which time the colonies are counted.

Snyder test. Snyder introduced the relatively simple colorimetric test for the estimation of relative numbers of lactobacilli in saliva. In actuality the test was designed to give a quantitative determination of the number of acid-producing microorganisms in the saliva. The test has been widely used as a diagnostic tool as well as a way to evaluate the patient's acceptance of dietary changes and preventive measures designed to reduce dental caries.

Alban test. In recent years the Alban test, a simplified substitute for the Snyder test, has been used. Because of its simplicity, its low cost, its diagnostic value when negative results are obtained, and most of all, its motivational value, the Alban test is recommended for all patients prone to caries. Practically all children fall into this group, especially those who are undergoing orthodontic

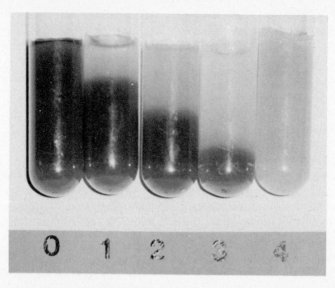

Fig. 7-20. Alban test scale. Instead of the degree of color change as in the classical Snyder test, the Alban test measures the depth to which the medium has turned yellow. From left to right the tubes of medium illustrate scores ranging from 0 to +4. (Courtesy Drs. Simon Katz, James L. McDonald, and George K. Stookey.)

treatment or who wear removable appliances in the mouth.

The main features of the Alban test are (1) use of a somewhat softer medium that permits the diffusion of saliva and acids without the necessity of melting the medium and (2) use of a simpler sampling procedure in which the patient expectorates directly into tubes that contain the medium.

To prepare the Alban test medium the following are required: Snyder test agar, a small scale to measure 60 g (2.12 ounces), a 2-liter Pyrex glass or stainless steel container to melt the medium, a funnel to dispense the medium into test tubes, and 100 × 16-mm test tubes with screw caps. Sixty grams of Snyder test agar is placed in 1 liter of water, and the suspension is brought to a boil over a low flame or a hot plate at medium heat (excessive heating should be avoided to prevent scorching the medium). When thoroughly melted, the agar is distributed, using about 5 ml per tube. The tubes should be autoclaved for 15 minutes, allowed to cool, and stored in a refrigerator. To avoid the need

for measuring the amount of medium when dispensing it into the tubes, it is convenient to mark the height of 5 ml of medium in one tube and use it as a reference for dispensing the medium into the remaining tubes. A small variation in the content of the tubes is unimportant.

To complete the test procedure, two tubes of Alban medium are taken from the refrigerator (since it is convenient to conduct the test in duplicate), and the patient is asked to expectorate a small amount of saliva directly into the tubes. The use of a sterilized glass funnel simplifies the collection. The volume of saliva should be sufficient to cover the surface of the test medium. According to Alban, the volume of saliva, the time of day at which the samples are taken, and the proximity of this time to the time of eating do not affect the results significantly. The tubes are labeled and incubated at 98.6° F (37° C) for up to 4 days. The tubes are observed daily for (1) change of color from bluish green (pH of around 5) to definite yellow (pH 4 or below) and (2) the depth in the medium to which the change has occurred. As recommended by Alban, the daily results collected for a 4-day period should be recorded on the patient's chart.

Alban suggests the following scale for scoring purposes (Fig. 7-20):

1. No color change (negative)   —
2. Beginning color change (from top to medium down)   +
3. One-half color change (from top down)   + +
4. Three-fourths color change (from top down)   + + +
5. Total color change to yellow   + + + +

The following method is used for the final recordings (after 72 or 96 hours' incubation):

1. Readings negative for the entire incubation period are labeled "negative."
2. All other readings are labeled "positive" whether +, + +, + + +, or + + + +.
3. Slower change or less color change (when compared with previous test) is labeled "improved."
4. Faster change or more pronounced color change when compared with previous test is labeled "worse."
5. When consecutive readings are nearly identical, they are labeled "no change."

Sources for the media used for the Snyder and Alban tests include Difco Laboratories* and Baltimore Biological Laboratories.† Those who wish to prepare the media themselves may use the following composition: Bacto peptone, 20 g; dextrose, 20 g; sodium chloride, 5 g; agar, 16 g; and bromcresol green, 0.02 g.

Disclosing agents in measuring tooth cleanliness. A number of commercially available disclosing agents in both chewable tablet form and solution can be used to discolor plaque and hard deposits on the clinical crowns of the teeth. The disclosing agent may be used immediately after the child brushes the teeth to demonstrate the effective-

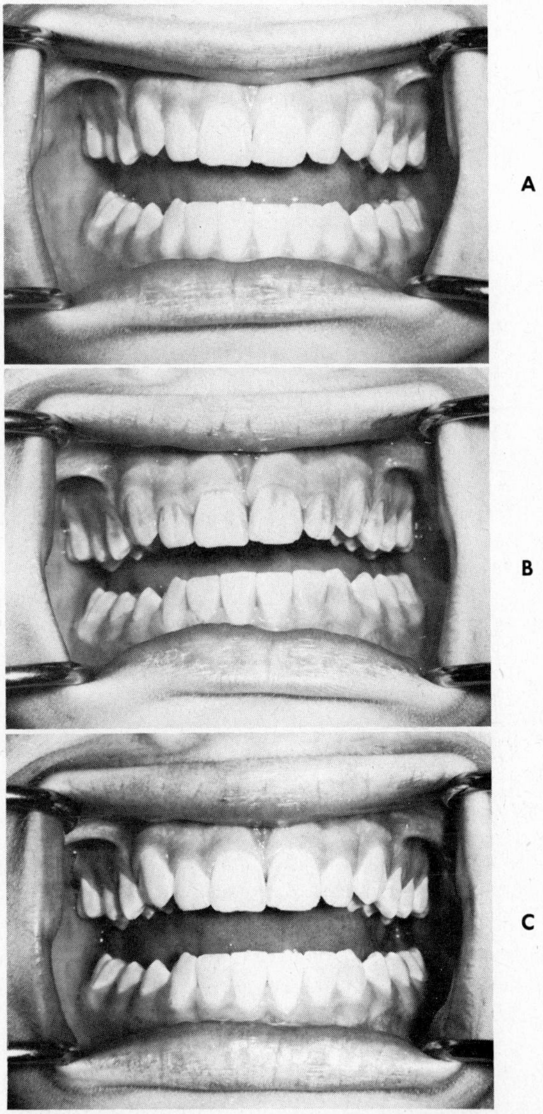

Fig. 7-21. A, Apparently clean mouth before the chewing of disclosing wafer. **B,** Plaque material is now evident as a result of staining with erythrosine dye. **C,** The patient has used a toothbrush and dentifrice to remove the stain.

*Difco Laboratories, Detroit, Mich. 48232.
†Baltimore Biological Laboratories, Baltimore, Md. 21030.

ness of the brushing procedure, or it may be used after chewing and swallowing a high-carbohydrate food to demonstrate the adhesive properties of the food (Fig. 7-21).

Some of the dyes used in the past for disclosing solutions have recently been removed from the market by the FDA. An acceptable and effective disclosing solution is one composed of 0.5% basic fuchsin to which can be added a sweetening agent and a flavor to improve the taste. The following prescription can be given to patients for home use:

Rx

Basic fuchsin	0.5 g
Ethyl alcohol, 95%	2.5 ml
Sodium saccharin	0.2 g
Flavoring agent to taste	
Water	100.0 ml

The basic fuchsin is dissolved in alcohol, and then the other ingredients are added.

Use: Apply to the teeth with a cotton applicator, or rinse the mouth with a small amount of this solution. Then rinse twice with clean water, and observe the teeth for plaque.

WARNING: This solution stains the clothes. Use with care.

The dentist's role in the caries control program

The success of a dental caries control program depends to a great extent on the interest and cooperation of the patient. Rampant caries should not be looked on as a hopeless problem. Diagnostic and preventive measures are available to control it. In the clinical management of rampant caries, the dentist's role consists of seeking the cause, correcting bad habits or deficiency states that may be contributing factors, restoring the teeth, and finally, making use of all available preventive and control measures.

During an informal discussion with the child and the parents, the dentist can often find a clue to the cause of excessive or rampant caries: evidence of nervousness, possible family conflict, the pattern of eating habits, the patient's appreciation of oral and general health, and the past experience with members of the dental profession. All of these factors may have a bearing on the cause of the problem and its successful management. Such informal discussions in a private office, where everyone is more relaxed, will invariably provide the dentist with more information than the usual procedure of chairside questioning.

Successful management of the dental caries problem demands a carefully completed history, the use of currently accepted diagnostic aids, the application of sound principles of operative dentistry, a comprehensive preventive program, and regular recall appointments for maintenance work and reemphasis of the preventive procedures.

REFERENCES

Alban, A.L.: Putting prevention into practice: laboratory test of value to the dentist and the patient for control of dental disease, Natl. Dent. Health Conf. **21**:440-450, 1970.

American Dental Association: Accepted dental therapeutics, Chicago, 1979, The Association, pp. 321-329.

American Dental Association Bureau of Economic Research and Statistics: Expenditures and prices for dental and other health care, 1935 to 1970, J.A.D.A. **83**:1334, 1971.

Arnold, F.A., and others: Effect of fluoridated public water supplies on dental caries prevalence: tenth year of the Grand Rapids–Muskegon study, Bull. Am. Assoc. Public Health Dent. **17**:32-38, 1957.

Beal, J.F., and others: The relationship between dental cleanliness, dental caries incidence and gingival health, Br. Dent. J. **146**:111-114, 1979.

Beiswanger, B.B., Gish, C.W., and Mallatt, M.E.: A three year study of the effect of a sodium fluoride–silica abrasive dentifrice on dental caries, Pharmacol. Ther. Dent. **6**:9-16, 1981.

Bell, C.D.: Survey of dental health of Indiana school children, 1970-1972 (unpublished report), Indiana Dental Health Task Force Project, Library, Indianapolis, Indiana University School of Dentistry.

Berenie, J., Ripa, L.W., and Leske, G.: The relationship of frequency of toothbrushing, oral hygiene, gingival health, and caries experience in school children, J. Public Health Dent. **33**:160-171, 1973.

Bibby, B.G.: Effect of sugar content of foodstuffs on their caries-producing potentials, J.A.D.A. **51**:293-306, 1955.

Bibby, B.G., Goldberg, H.J.V., and Chen, E.: Evaluation of caries-producing potentialities of various foodstuffs, J.A.D.A. **42**:491-509, 1951.

Blayney, J.R., and Hill, I.N.: Fluorine and dental caries, J.A.D.A. **74**:233-302, 1967.

Bowen, W.H.: Role of carbohydrates in dental caries. In Shaw,

J.H., and Roussos, G.G., editors: Proceedings of a meeting on sweeteners and dental caries, Feeding, Weight, Obesity Abs. (special suppl.) pp. 147-155, 1978.

Bowen, W.H.: Relevance of caries vaccine investigations in rodents, primates, and humans: critical assessment, Immunol. Abs. (special suppl.) pp. 11-20, 1976.

Brudevold, F., and DePaola, P.: Studies on topically applied acidulated phosphate fluoride at Forsyth Dental Center, Dent. Clin. North Am. **10:**299-308, 1966.

Burket, L.W.: Oral medicine, diagnosis, and treatment, Philadelphia, 1946, J.B. Lippincott Co.

Carlos, J.P.: The prevention of dental caries: ten years later, J.A.D.A. **104:**193-197, 1982.

Carmichael, C.L., and others: The effect of fluoridation upon the relationship between caries experience and social class in 5-year-old children in Newcastle and Northumberland, Br. Dent. J. **149:**163-167, 1980.

Carter, W.J., and Wells, J.E.: Changes in salivary lactobacilli counts following dental procedures in children, J. Dent. Child. **27:**65-67, 1960.

Cohen, A.: Fluoridation in Philadelphia, Dent. Abs. **11:**552, 1966.

Davies, G.N.: Management of rampant dental caries, Aust. Dent. J. **26:**57-69, 1954.

Dennison, J.B., and others: A clinical comparison of sealant and amalgam in the treatment of pits and fissures. I. Clinical performance after 18 months, Pediatr. Dent. **2:**167-175, 1980.

Dennison, J.B., and others: A clinical comparison of sealant and amalgam in the treatment of pits and fissures. II. Clinical application and maintenance during an 18-month period, Pediatr. Dent. **2:**176-183, 1980.

Dilley, G.J., Dilley, D.H., and Machen, J.B.: Prolonged nursing habit: a profile of parents and their families, J. Dent. Child. **47:**102-108, 1980.

DiOrio, L.P., and Madsen, K.O.: A personalized approach: discussing food in prevention of dental disease, Nutr. News **33:**1, 4, 1970.

Dreizen, S.: The role of diet in dental decay, Nutr. News **29:**1-2, 1966.

Driscoll, W.S., and others: Caries-preventive effects of daily and weekly fluoride mouthrinsing in an optimally fluoridated community: findings after eighteen months, Pediatr. Dent. **3:**316-320, 1981.

Dudding, N., and Muhler, J.C.: What motivates children to practice good oral hygiene? J. Periodont. **31:**141-142, 1960.

Dunham, M.: A good diet for every child, Month. Bull. Ind. State Board of Health **62:**12-15, 1960.

Eichenbaum, I.W., Dunn, N.A., and Tinanoff, N.: Impact of fluoridation in a private pedodontic practice: thirty years later, J. Dent. Child. **48:**211-214, 1981.

Elliott, R.P.: Full-mouth rehabilitation retards oral lactobacilli, J. Tenn. Dent. Assoc. **44:**13-19, 1964.

Finn, S.B., and others: The clinical cariostatic effectiveness of two concentrations of acidulated phosphate–fluoride mouthwash, J.A.D.A. **90:**398-402, 1975.

Fitzgerald, R.J., Jordan, H.V., and Archard, H.O.: Dental caries in gnotobiotic rats infected with a variety of *Lactobacillus acidophilus,* Arch. Oral Biol. **11:**473-476, 1966.

Fosdick, L.S.: Reduction of the incidence of dental caries. I. Immediate toothbrushing with a neutral dentifrice, J.A.D.A. **40:**133-143, 1950.

Frisbie, H.E.: Modern concept of the etiology of dental caries: proteolytic theories, Int. Dent. J. **1:**15-31, 1950.

Furstenberg, A.C.: The parotid gland: its common disorders, J.A.M.A. **117:**1594-1598, 1941.

Gardner, D.E., Norwood, J.R., and Eisenson, J.E.: At-will breast feeding and dental caries: four case reports, J. Dent. Child. **44:**186-191, 1977.

Gish, C.W.: Personal communication, 1951.

Gish, C.W.: The dollar and cents of prevention, J. Ind. Dent. Assoc. **58**(2)**:** 12-14, 1979.

Gish, C.W., Howell, C.L., and Muhler, J.C.: A new approach to the topical application of fluorides for the reduction of dental caries in children: a preliminary report, J. Dent. Res. **36:**784-786, 1957.

Goldberg, S.: The dental arches of identical twins, Dent. Cosmos **72:**869-881, 1930.

Gottlieb, B.: Dental caries, Philadelphia, 1947, Lea & Febiger.

Green, G.E., and Weisenstein, P.R.: Salivary and plaque lactobacilli in the prognosis of human dental caries, J. Dent. Res. **38:**951-960, 1959.

Gustafsson, B.E., and others: The Vipeholm dental caries studies: the effect of different levels of carbohydrate intake on caries activity in 436 individuals observed for five years (Sweden), Acta Odontol. Scand. **11:**232-364, 1954.

Hadley, F.P.: A quantitative method for estimating baccillus acidophilus in saliva, J. Dent. Res. **13:**415-428, 1933.

Handelman, S.L., Washburn, F., and Whopper, P.: Two-year report of sealant effect on bacteria in dental caries, J.A.D.A. **93:**967-970, 1976.

Harris, W.H.: A survey of breakfasts eaten by high school students, J. Sch. Health **40:**323-325, 1970.

Hayes, R.L., Littleton, N.W., and White, C.L.: Posteruptive effects of fluoridation on first permanent molars of children in Grand Rapids, Michigan, Dent. Abs. **2:**615, 1957.

Heifetz, S.B., Horowitz, H.S., and Driscoll, W.S.: Effect of school water fluoridation on dental caries: results in Seagrove, NC, after eight years, J.A.D.A. **97:**193-196, 1978.

Heifetz, S.B., Meyers, R., and Kingman, A.: A comparison of the anticaries effectiveness of daily and weekly rinsing with sodium fluoride solutions: findings after two years, Pediatr. Dent. **3:**17-20, 1981.

Henderson, H.Z.: The diet survey for your child patient. In McDonald, R.E., and others: Current therapy in dentistry, vol. 7, St. Louis, 1980, The C.V. Mosby Co.

Hennon, D.K.: Low-caloric beverages and dental health, J. Ind. Dent. Assoc. **44:**275, 1965.

Hennon, D.K., Stookey, G.K., and Muhler, J.C.: The clinical anticariogenic effectiveness of supplementary fluoride-vitamin preparation: results at the end of three years, J. Dent. Child. **33:**3-12, 1966.

Hennon, D.K., Stookey, G.K., and Muhler, J.C.: A survey of the prevalence and distribution of dental caries in preschool children, J.A.D.A. **79:**1405-1414, 1969.

Hennon, D.K., Stookey, G.K., and Muhler, J.C.: The clinical anticariogenic effectiveness of supplementary fluoride-vitamin preparations: results at the end of five and a half years, Pharmacol. Ther. Dent. **1**(1):1-6, 1970.

Hewat, R.E.T.: Dental caries: an investigation in search of determining factors in its manifestation, N.Z. Dent. J. **28:**45-59, 1932.

Horowitz, A.M., and Thomas, H.B., editors: Dental caries prevention in public health programs. Proceedings of a Conference, Oct. 27-28, 1980, NIH Publ. No. 81-2235. Sponsored by the National Caries Program, National Institute of Dental Research, Washington, D.C., August 1981.

Horowitz, A.M., and others: Effects of supervised daily plaque removal by children after 3 years, Community Dent. Oral Epidemiol. **8:**171-176, 1980.

Horowitz, H.S.: Pit and fissure sealants in private practice and public health programmes: analysis of cost-effectiveness, Int. Dent. J. **30:**117-126, 1980.

Horowitz, H.S., and Heifetz, S.B.: The current status of topical fluorides in preventive dentistry, J.A.D.A. **81:**166-177, 1970.

Horowitz, H.S., Heifetz, S.B., and Law, F.E.: Effect of school water fluoridation on dental caries: final results in Elk Lake, Pa. after 12 years, J.A.D.A. **84:**832-838, 1972.

Horowitz, H.S., and others: A program of self-administered fluorides in a rural school system, Community Dent. Oral Epidemiol. **8:**177-183, 1980.

Houpt, M., and Shey, Z.: Clinical effectiveness of an autopolymerized fissure sealant (Delton) after thirty-three months, Pediatr. Dent. **1:**165-168, 1979.

Howell, C.L., and others: Effect of topically applied stannous fluoride on dental caries experience in children, J.A.D.A. **50:**14-17, 1955.

Hunt, H.R., Hoppert, C.A., and Rosen, S.: The role of heredity in the causation of dental caries in rats. In Muhler, J.C., and Hine, M.K., editors: A symposium on preventive dentistry, St. Louis, 1956, The C.V. Mosby Co.

Hutchinson, J.: A case of dry mouth, Trans. Clin. Soc. London **21:**180-181, 1888.

Hyatt, T.P.: Prophylactic odontotomy: the cutting into the tooth for the prevention of disease, Dent. Cosmos **65:**234-241, 1923.

Infante, P.F., and Owen, G.M.: Dental caries and levels of treatment for school children by geographical region, socio-economic status, race, and size of community, J. Public Health Dent. **35:**19-27, 1975.

Jay, P.: The role of carbohydrate in the control of dental caries. In Muhler, J.C., and Hine, M.K., editors: A symposium on preventive dentistry, St. Louis, 1956, The C.V. Mosby Co.

Jeronimus, D.J., Till, M.J., and Sveen, O.B.: Reduced viability of microorganisms under dental sealants, J. Dent. Child. **42:**275-280, 1975.

Katz, S.: Clinical evaluation of the use of fluoridated water on the deciduous dentition, thesis, Indianapolis, 1966, Indiana University.

Katz, S.: A diet counseling program, J.A.D.A. **102:**840-845, 1981.

Katz, S., and Muhler, J.C.: Prenatal and postnatal fluoride and dental caries experience in deciduous teeth, J.A.D.A. **76:**305-311, 1968.

Keyes, P.H.: Present and future measures for dental caries control, J.A.D.A. **79:**1395-1404, 1969.

Koss, B.J.: Personal communication, 1960.

Kotlow, L.A.: Breast feeding: a cause of dental caries in children, J. Dent. Child. **44:**192-193, 1977.

Lemke, C.W., Doherty, J.M., and Arra, M.C.: Controlled fluoridation: the dental effects of discontinuation in Antigo, Wis., J.A.D.A. **80:**782-786, 1970.

Leske, G.S., and others: Post-treatment benefits from participating in a school-based fluoride mouthrinsing program, J. Public Health Dent. **41:**103-108, 1981.

Luke, L.S., Ostergard, N.J., and Hunt, I.F.: Analysis of nutrient intakes, J. Pedod. **3:**207-215, 1979.

Mack, P.B.: A study of institutional children with particular reference to the caloric value as well as other factors of the dietary, Monogr. Soc. Res. Child Dev. **13:**1, 1948.

Mann, A.W., and others: Comparison of dental caries activity in malnourished and well-nourished patients, J.A.D.A. **34:**244-252, 1947.

Mansbridge, J.N.: Heredity and dental caries, J. Dent. Res. **38:**337-347, 1959.

Massler, M.: Teen-age caries, J. Dent. Child. **12:**57-64, 1945.

Massler, M., and Schour, I.: Dental caries experience in postwar Italy, J. Dent. Child. **14:**6-11, 1947.

McDonald, R.E., and Muhler, J.C.: Superiority of topical application of stannous fluoride on primary teeth, J. Dent. Child. **24:**84-86, 1957.

Mertz-Fairhurst, E.J., and others: Six-year clinical evaluation of two pit and fissure sealants, J. Dent. Res. **60** (Spec. Issue A):313, Abs. No. 9, 1981.

Meurman, J.H., Helminen, S.K.J., and Luoma, H.: Caries reduction over 5 years from a single application of a fissure sealant, Scand. J. Dent. Res. **86:**153-156, 1978.

Miller, A.J.: National caries program, National Institutes of Health, American Academy of Pedodontics meeting, Miami Beach, Fla., 1977.

Miller, W.D.: Microorganisms of the human teeth, Philadelphia, 1890, S.S. White Dental Manufacturing Co.

Morris, S.A.: Salivary glands: pathological conditions affecting them, Calif. West. Med. **57:**190-192, 1942.

Murray, J.J., and Rugg-Gunn, A.J.: A review of the effectiveness of artificial water fluoridation throughout the world, ORCA XXVI Congress, Abs. No. 65, 1979.

National Institute of Dental Research: The prevalence of dental caries in United States children, 1979-1980, National Dental Caries Prevalence Survey, NIH Pub. No. 82-2245, Washington, D.C., December 1981, U.S. Department of Health and Human Services.

Nikiforuk, G., and Fraser, D.: Fluoride supplements for prophylaxis of dental caries, Am. J. Dis. Child. **107:**111-118, 1964; J. Can. Dent. Assoc. **30:**67-76, 1964.

1980 dental spending nears $16 billion, A.D.A. News **12:**1, 3, 1981.

Orland, F.J.: Bacteriology of dental caries: formal discussion, J. Dent. Res. **43:**1045-1047, 1964.

Parfitt, G.J.: Conditions influencing the incidence of occlusal and interstitial caries in children, J. Dent. Child. **23:**31-39, 1956.

Potgieter, M., and others: Food habits and dental status of some Connecticut children, J. Dent. Res. **35:**638-644, 1956.

Powell, K.R., Barnard, P.D., and Craig, G.G.: Effect of stannous fluoride treatments on the progression of initial lesions in approximal surfaces of permanent posterior teeth, J. Dent. Res. **60:**1648-1654, 1981.

Radike, A.W., and others: Clinical evaluation of stannous fluoride as an anticaries mouth rinse, J.A.D.A. **86:**404-408, 1973.

Report on dentist busyness in *Wall Street Journal*, A.D.A. News **11:**8, 10, 1980.

Richardson, A.S., and others: The effectiveness of a chemically polymerized sealant: four-year results, Pediatr. Dent. **2:**24-26, 1980.

Ripa, L.W., and Leske, G.: Effect on the primary dentition of mouthrinsing with a 0.2 percent neutral NaF solution: results from a demonstration program after four school years, Pediatr. Dent. **3:**311-315, 1981.

Rock, W.P., Gordon, P.H., and Bradnock, G.: Dental caries experience in Birmingham and Wolverhampton school children following the fluoridation of Birmingham water in 1964, Br. Dent. J. **150:**61-66, 1981.

Rovelstad, G.N., Geller, J.H., and Cohen, A.H.: Caries susceptibility tests, hyaluronidase activity of saliva and dental caries experience, J. Dent. Res. **37:**306-311, 1958.

Scholle, R.H.: Caries prevention—second thoughts, J.A.D.A. **102:**602, 1981.

Schrotenboer, G.H.: Fluoride benefits—after 36 years, J.A.D.A. **102:**473-474, 1981.

Scopp, I.W., and others: Dryness of the mouth with the use of tranquilizers: chlorpromazine, J.A.D.A. **71:**66-69, 1965.

Shafer, W.G.: The effect of single and fractional doses of selectively applied x-ray irradiation on the histologic structure of the major salivary glands of the rat, J. Dent. Res. **32:**796-806, 1953.

Shannon, I.L.: Sucrose and glucose in dry breakfast cereals, J. Dent. Child. **41:**347-350, 1974.

Shannon, I.L., and McCartney, J.C.: Presweetened dry breakfast cereals: potential for dental danger, J. Dent. Child. **48:**215-218, 1981.

Shannon, I.L., McCrary, B.R., and Starcke, E.N.: A saliva substitute for use by xerostomic patients undergoing radiotherapy of the head and neck, Oral Surg. **44:**656-666, 1977.

Shaw, L., and Murray, J.J.: A family history study of caries-resistance and caries-susceptibility, Br. Dent. J. **148:**231-234, 1980.

Shklair, I.L., and others: Preliminary report on the effect of complete mouth rehabilitation on oral lactobacilli counts, J.A.D.A. **53:**155-158, 1956.

Simonsen, R.J.: The clinical effectiveness of a colored pit and fissure sealant at 36 months, J.A.D.A. **102:**323-327, 1981.

Smith, C.E.: Personal communication, 1982.

Snyder, M.L.: A simple colorimetric method for the estimation of relative numbers of lactobacilli in the saliva, J. Dent. Res. **19:**349-355, 1940.

Statistical abstract of the United States, National Data Book and Guide to Sources, U.S. Department of Commerce, Bureau of the Census, Washington, D.C., 1975, U.S. Government Printing Office.

Symposium: Perspectives on the use of prenatal fluorides, J. Dent. Child. **48:**100-133, 1981.

Tsamtsouris, A., White, G.E., and Clark, E.R.: The effect of instruction and supervised toothbrushing on the reduction of dental plaque in kindergarten children, J. Dent. Child. **46:**204-209, 1979.

U.S. Department of Health and Human Services: Promoting health—preventing disease, Washington D.C., Fall 1980, U.S. Government Printing Office, p. 51.

Walsh, J.P., and Smart, R.S.: Relative susceptibility of tooth surfaces to dental caries and other comparative studies, N.Z. Dent. J. **44:**17-35, 1948.

Walter, B.J.: Sweetener economics: analysis and forecasts. In Shaw, J.H., and Roussos, G.G., editors: Sweeteners and dental caries, Feeding, Weight, Obesity Abs. (special suppl.), 1978.

Waterman, G.E.: Richmond-Woonsocket studies on dental care services for school children, J.A.D.A. **52:**676-684, 1956.

Way, R.M.: The effect on dental caries of a change from a naturally fluoridated to a fluoride-free communal water, J. Dent. Child. **31:**151-157, 1964.

Weiss, R.L., and Trithart, A.H.: Between-meal eating habits and dental caries experience in preschool children, Am. J. Public Health **50:**1097-1104, 1960.

Wright, G.Z., Banting, D.W., and Feasby, W.H.: The Dorchester dental flossing study: final report, Clin. Prev. Dent. **1**(3):23-26, 1979.

Young, G.R.: Personal communication, 1982.

Young, G.R., and others: Computer-assisted dietary analysis (unpublished report).

Zacherl, W.G.: A three year clinical caries evaluation of a sodium fluoride–silica abrasive dentifrice, Pharmacol. Ther. Dent. **6**:1-7, 1981.

Zita, A., McDonald, R.E., and Andrews, A.L.: Dietary habits and the dental caries experience in 200 children, J. Dent. Res. **38**:860-865, 1959.

8 Treatment of deep caries, vital pulp exposure, and pulpless teeth

RALPH E. McDONALD
DAVID R. AVERY

The treatment of the dental pulp exposed by the caries process, by accident during cavity preparation, or even as a result of traumatic injury and fracture of the tooth has long presented a challenge in treatment. As early as 1756 Pfaff reported placing a small piece of gold over a vital exposure in an attempt to promote healing.

From the time of the first report of pulp therapy, many claims of successful treatment have unfortunately been based on other than scientific evidence. In the early studies little attention was given to the importance of a preoperative diagnosis, adequate controls, and critical postoperative observation.

In recent years a number of studies involving observations of pulp healing in experimental animals and in humans have had an influence on the currently accepted methods of treating the exposed pulp. A few of these studies are cited in this chapter as reference is made to the various methods of pulp therapy.

Although it has been established that the pulp is capable of healing, there is need for continued research. Current methods of diagnosing the extent of pulpal injury are inadequate. Certainly there is still much to be learned regarding the control of infection in the vital pulp. More effective pulp-capping drugs and materials must be found that will result in a higher percentage of successful treatments.

Diagnostic aids in the selection of teeth for vital pulp therapy

History of pain. The history of either presence or absence of pain may not be as reliable in the differential diagnosis of the condition of the exposed primary pulp as it is in permanent teeth. Degeneration of primary pulps even to the point of abscess formation without the child recalling pain or discomfort is not uncommon. Nevertheless, the history of a toothache should be the first consideration in the selection of teeth for vital pulp therapy. A toothache coincident with or immediately after a meal may not mean extensive pulpal inflammation. The pain may be caused by an accumulation of food within the carious lesion, by pressure, or by a chemical irritation to the vital pulp protected by only a thin layer of intact dentin.

Mitchell and Tarplee found in a study of teeth with painful pulpitis that severity of pain and the extent of pulp involvement were not correlated. Subjective complaints of pain resulting from the intake of hot foods or drink were indicative of pulpitis, but they were not as reliable as careful tests made by the dentist. No real difference in response to heat or cold was detected. Testing showed most patients to be sensitive to both. Mitchell and Tarplee further observed that most teeth with pulp exposure were sensitive to percussion even though thickening of the apical periodontal membrane was not evident radiographically.

A severe toothache at night usually means extensive degeneration of the pulp and calls for other than a conservative type of pulp therapy. Likewise, a spontaneous toothache of more than momentary duration occurring at any time during the day or night usually means that involvement of the pulp has progressed too far for treatment with even a successful pulpotomy.

Clinical signs and symptoms. A gingival abscess or a draining fistula associated with a tooth with a deep carious lesion is an obvious clinical sign of an irreversibly diseased pulp. Such infections can be resolved only by successful endodontic therapy or extraction of the tooth.

Abnormal tooth mobility is another clinical sign that may be indicative of a severely diseased pulp. When such a tooth is evaluated for mobility, the manipulation may elicit localized pain in the area, but this is not always the case. If pain is absent or minimal during manipulation of the diseased, mobile tooth, the pulp is probably in a more advanced and chronic degenerative condition. Pathologic mobility must be distinguished from normal mobility in primary teeth near exfoliation.

Sensitivity to percussion or pressure is a clinical symptom suggesting at least some degree of pulpal disease, but the degenerative stage of the pulp is probably of the acute inflammatory type. Tooth mobility or sensitivity to percussion or pressure may be a clinical signal of other dental problems as well, such as a "high" restoration or advanced periodontal disease. However, when this clinical information is identified in a child and is associated with a tooth having a deep carious lesion, the problem is most likely to be from pulpal disease and possible inflammatory involvement of the periodontal ligament.

Radiographic interpretation. A recent x-ray film must be available to examine for evidence of periapical changes, such as thickening of the periodontal ligament or rarefaction of the supporting bone. These conditions rule out treatment other than an endodontic procedure or extraction of the tooth. Radiographic interpretation in children is more difficult than in adults. The permanent teeth

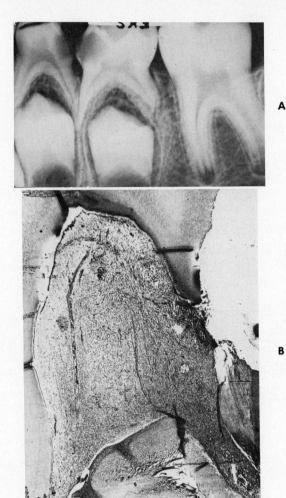

Fig. 8-1. A, First primary molar appears to have an intact dentinal barrier beneath the carious lesion. **B,** Histologic section shows a perforation of the barrier with necrotic material at the exposure site. There is advanced inflammation of the pulp tissue, which is likely to evoke a spontaneous pain response.

may have incompletely formed root ends, giving an impression of periapical radiolucency, and the roots of the primary teeth undergoing even normal physiologic resorption often present a misleading picture or one suggesting pathologic change.

The proximity of carious lesions to the pulp cannot always be determined accurately in the x-ray film. What often appears to be an intact barrier of secondary dentin protecting the pulp may actually be a perforated mass of irregularly calcified and carious material. The pulp beneath this material may have extensive inflammation (Fig. 8-1). Radiographic evidence of calcified masses within the pulp chamber is diagnostically important. Zander reported that if the irritation to the pulp is relatively mild and chronic, the pulp will respond with inflammation and will attempt to eliminate the irritation by blocking with irregular dentin those tubules through which the irritating factors are transmitted. If the irritation is intense and acute and if the carious lesion is developing rapidly, the defense mechanism may not have a chance to lay down the secondary dentin barrier, and the disease process may reach the pulp. In this instance the pulp will attempt to erect a barrier at some distance from the exposure site. These calcified masses are sometimes evident in the pulp horn or even in the region of the pulp canal entrance. A histologic examination of these teeth shows irregular, amorphous masses of calcified material that are not like pulp stones (Fig. 8-2). The masses bear no resemblance to dentin or to a dentinal barrier. In every instance they are associated with advanced degenerative changes of the coronal pulp and inflammation of the tissue in the canal.

Pulp testing. The value of the electric pulp test in determining the condition of the pulp of primary teeth is questionable, although it will give an indication of whether the pulp is vital. The test does not give reliable evidence of the degree of inflammation of the pulp. A complicating factor is the occasional positive response to the test in a tooth with a necrotic pulp if the content of the canals is liquid. The reliability of the pulp test for the young child can also be questioned because of the child's apprehension associated with the test itself.

A study by Reynolds failed to show a correlation between thermal response and response to the electric pulp tester except in nonvital (pulpless) teeth, in which all responses were negative, and in vital teeth with small pulp chambers, in which negative

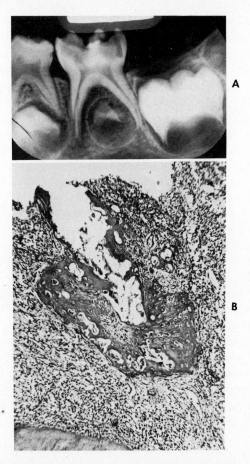

Fig. 8-2. A, Calcified mass in the pulp chamber beneath the exposure site is associated with extensive inflammation of the pulp in the coronal area and in the pulp canals. **B,** The amorphous mass is surrounded by pulp tissue with advanced inflammation.

thermal responses corresponded to high readings with the electric pulp tester. The size of the pulp chamber was the most important factor in determining the thermal response, with small pulp chambers making thermal stimulation of the pulp difficult.

Physical condition of the patient. Although the local observations are of extreme importance in the selection of cases for vital pulp therapy, the dentist must also consider the physical condition of the patient. Glickman and Shklar believe that successful pulp capping is dependent, in some measure at least, on the absence of systemic disturbances that might exert a deleterious effect on the pulp. In experimental animals suffering from systemic disturbances, they noted a degeneration of the odontoblasts and assumed that this would ultimately cause a disturbance in the formation of new dentin.

In the case of chronically ill children, extraction of the involved tooth, after proper premedication with antibiotics, rather than pulp therapy should be the treatment of choice. Children with conditions that render them susceptible to subacute bacterial endocarditis or those with nephritis, leukemia, solid tumors, idiopathic cyclic neutropenia, or any condition that causes cyclic or chronic depression of granulocyte and polymorphonuclear leukocyte counts should not be subjected to the possibility of an acute infection resulting from pulp therapy. Occasionally, a pulpectomy and root canal filling may be justified in a permanent tooth of a chronically ill child but only after careful consideration is given to the prognosis of the child's general condition, the prognosis of the endodontic therapy, and the relative importance of retaining the involved tooth.

Evaluation of treatment prognosis before pulp therapy

The diagnostic process of selecting teeth that are good candidates for vital pulp therapy has at least two dimensions. First, the dentist must decide that the tooth has a good chance of responding favorably to the pulp therapy procedure indicated. Second, the advisability of performing the pulp therapy and restoring the tooth must be weighed against extraction and space management. For example, nothing is gained by successful pulp therapy if the crown of the involved tooth is nonrestorable or if the periodontal structures are irreversibly diseased. By the same rationale, a dentist is likely to invest more time and effort to save a pulpally involved second primary molar in a 4-year-old

child with unerupted first permanent molars than to save a pulpally involved first primary molar in an 8-year-old child.

Other factors to consider include the following:

1. The level of patient and parent cooperation and motivation in receiving the treatment
2. The level of patient and parent desire and motivation in maintaining oral health and hygiene
3. The caries activity of the individual and the overall prognosis of oral rehabilitation
4. The stage of dental development of the patient
5. The degree of difficulty anticipated in adequately performing the pulp therapy (instrumentation) in the particular case
6. Space management considerations resulting from previous extractions, preexisting malocclusion, ankylosis, congenitally missing teeth, and space loss caused by the extensive carious destruction of teeth and subsequent drifting
7. Excessive extrusion of the pulpally involved tooth resulting from missing opposing teeth

These examples illustrate the almost infinite number of treatment considerations that could be important in an individual patient with pulpal pathosis.

Treatment of the deep carious lesion

Children and young adults who have not received early and adequate dental care and whose drinking water does not contain an optimum amount of fluoride often have a large number of deep carious lesions in the primary and permanent teeth. Many of the lesions appear radiographically to be dangerously close to the pulp or to actually involve the dental pulp. Approximately 75% of the teeth with deep caries have been found from clinical observations to have pulpal exposures. Work by Dimaggio and Hawes supports this observation. They also showed that well over 90% of the asymptomatic teeth with deep carious lesions could be successfully treated without pulp exposure using indirect pulp therapy techniques. This procedure will be described in the following pages.

Reeves and Stanley's research supports the common clinical observation that the dentist cannot initially predict with certainty the state of health of the pulp. When dealing with a deep cavity, however, the dentist can probably be assured that the caries has invaded the reparative dentin. Therefore the dentist should take every precaution to minimize the trauma of the operative procedure, for, in the presence of established pulpal pathosis resulting from caries, the addition of operative trauma can provide sufficient irritation to compound the pathosis. This can lead to the establishment of irreversible pulpal lesions. In view of the direct relationship between caries depth and pulpal pathosis, early excavation of what might appear to be superficial caries in the dentin is advocated as sound preventive treatment to minimize pulpal exposure.

If carious exposures discovered at the time of the initial caries excavation could be routinely treated with consistently good results, a major problem in dentistry would be solved. Unfortunately, the treatment of vital exposures, especially in primary teeth, has not been entirely successful. For this reason care must be taken to prevent pulp exposure during the removal of deep caries.

Indirect pulp therapy (gross caries removal or indirect pulp treatment). The procedure in which only the gross caries is removed from the lesion and the cavity is sealed for a time with a bactericidal agent is referred to as "indirect pulp therapy" (Fig. 8-3). Indirect pulp treatment is not a new procedure but has attracted renewed interest. Laboratory studies and favorable clinical evidence justify its routine use. Only teeth with deep caries that are free of symptoms of painful pulpitis should be selected for this procedure.

The clinical procedure involves the removal of the gross caries with large round burs or sharp spoon excavators, allowing sufficient caries to remain over the pulp horn to avoid exposure of the

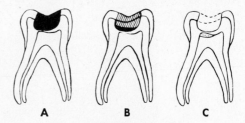

Fig. 8-3. Indirect pulp therapy. **A,** A primary or permanent tooth with deep caries. **B,** The gross caries has been removed and the cavity sealed with a treatment of zinc oxide–eugenol. **C,** Six to 8 weeks later the zinc oxide–eugenol has been removed and the remaining caries excavated. A sound dentin barrier protects the pulp. The tooth may now be restored. (Courtesy Dr. Paul E. Starkey.)

pulp. Because the procedure usually results in some discomfort to the child, it is advisable to use a local anesthetic. The placement of a rubber dam is a further advantage.

The walls of the cavity are planed back with a fissure bur. Carious enamel and dentin at the margins of the cavity will interfere with the establishment of an adequate seal during the period of repair. The remaining thin layer of caries in the base of the cavity is dried and covered with a bactericidal dressing of calcium hydroxide. Some dentists prefer to place a dressing of zinc oxide–eugenol over the remaining caries, and this material is as effective as calcium hydroxide. However, if the dentist suspects that the excavated lesion could have an undetected, microscopic pulp exposure, a calcium hydroxide dressing is indicated and is therefore recommended routinely. The dressing should be covered with a stiff mix of zinc oxide–eugenol.

The contour of the treatment restoration is adjusted to receive no stress in mastication. The procedure should be repeated for all teeth with deep accessible carious lesions (Fig. 8-4). The use of a reinforced zinc oxide–eugenol composition as an intermediate restorative material (IRM*) to cover

---

*L.D. Caulk Co., Milford, Del. 19963.

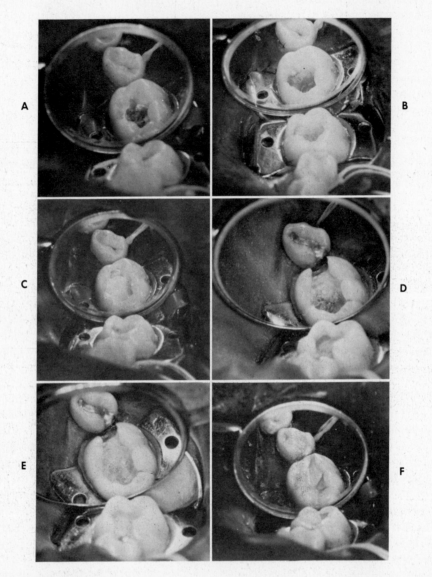

Fig. 8-4. A, Second primary molar with deep occlusal caries. Because the tooth was free of symptoms of painful pulpitis, indirect pulp therapy was completed. **B,** The gross caries has been removed. A small amount of soft carious dentin remains at the base of the cavity. **C,** Calcium hydroxide has been placed over the remaining caries. The cavity may be filled with a stiff mix of zinc oxide–eugenol or some other intermediate restorative material. **D,** After 6 to 8 weeks, the intermediate restorative material was removed. The caries in the base of the cavity appeared arrested and dry. **E,** The remaining caries has been removed. After the placement of a base, the tooth may be restored. **F,** The primary second molar has been restored with amalgam.

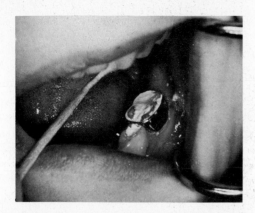

Fig. 8-5. Preformed steel band has been cemented to the tooth to support the indirect pulp treatment material.

the layer of calcium hydroxide offers some advantages to the dentist. The material lasts for several months, and it provides an excellent initial seal along the cavity walls. Furthermore, it is available in color-coded red, which will indicate to the dentist that dental caries remains.

If insufficient tooth structure remains after the caries removal to maintain the dressing, it is often helpful to adapt and cement a preformed stainless steel band to the tooth to support the material during the observation period (Fig. 8-5).

King, Crawford, and Lindahl have carried on an extensive investigation to determine whether the soft residual layer of carious dentin in teeth treated with the indirect pulp-capping material is contaminated with cultivatable microorganisms before treatment and whether this layer, if contaminated, can be rendered sterile by capping with either calcium hydroxide or zinc oxide–eugenol. Their study in young children indicated that the layer of residual carious dentin can be sterilized or the number of organisms can be greatly reduced when this layer is covered with either calcium hydroxide or zinc oxide–eugenol. Their findings further support the recommendation that only the necrotic layers of dentin be removed at the first visit and that the cavity be sealed as previously described, thereby allowing sclerosis of the dentin and the formation of reparative dentin to occur.

Minor routine operative procedures can be performed at subsequent visits. However, the treated teeth should not be reentered to complete the removal of caries for at least 6 or 8 weeks. During this time the caries process in the deeper layer is arrested, and many of the remaining microorganisms are destroyed by the germicidal action of the calcium hydroxide and the zinc oxide–eugenol.

If the pulp has not already been exposed by the caries process, it will have an opportunity to form a protective layer of secondary dentin during the waiting period. If the caries process has already invaded the pulp and has caused inflammation, the calcium hydroxide and the zinc oxide–eugenol will aid in neutralizing the irritants and will reduce the pulpal inflammation.

Studies carried out at the Indiana University School of Dentistry by Traubman, who used television linear and density measurement instrumentation, indicate that a calcium hydroxide–methylcellulose treatment increases secondary dentin deposition (sclerosis). The rate of regular dentin formation observed during the indirect pulp treatment technique was highest during the first month but continued during the year of experimental observation. At the end of the 1-year observation period, some teeth had formed as much as 390 μm of new dentin on the pulpal floor. This observation lends justification to leaving the calcium hydroxide dressing in place for a longer period before reentering the tooth for final caries excavation. The placement of an amalgam restoration over the indirect pulp treatment material will be a definite aid in retaining the treatment material during longer observation periods.

At the conclusion of the minimum 6- to 8-week waiting period, the tooth is anesthetized and isolated with the rubber dam, and the temporary restorative material and calcium hydroxide dressing are removed. Careful removal of the remaining carious material, now somewhat hardened and arrested, may reveal a sound base of dentin without an exposure of the pulp. If a sound layer of dentin covers the pulp, a liner material containing calcium hydroxide is applied, the cavity preparation is com-

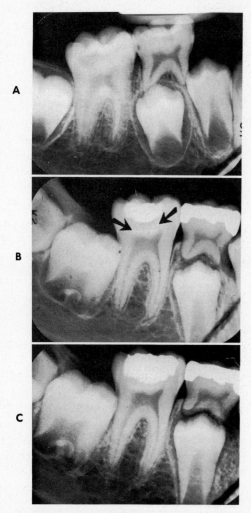

Fig. 8-6. A, Radiograph of the first permanent molar revealed a deep carious lesion. Gross caries was removed and calcium hydroxide placed over the remaining caries. The tooth was restored with amalgam and was not reentered for complete caries removal for a period of 3 months. **B,** Sclerotic dentin can be seen beneath the remaining caries and the covering of calcium hydroxide *(arrows).* **C,** The tooth was reentered and the remaining caries removed. A sound dentin barrier was observed at the base of the cavity. The amalgam restoration was replaced after complete caries removal.

pleted, and the tooth is restored in a conventional manner (Fig. 8-6). If a small pulp exposure is encountered, a different type of treatment, based on the clinical signs and symptoms and local conditions, must be used.

Nirschl and Avery performed indirect pulp therapy on 38 selected primary and young permanent teeth. Caries removal under rubber dam isolation was accomplished in the manner just described. One of two slightly different calcium hydroxide preparations* was used in each tooth as a sedative base, and the teeth were restored with amalgam.

The teeth selected for the study had to have deep carious lesions and had to fulfill the following criteria:

1. No history of spontaneous, unprovoked toothache (The tooth may have had a history of toothache associated with eating, as long as pain subsided immediately after removal of the stimulus.)
2. No tenderness to percussion
3. No abnormal mobility
4. No radiographic evidence of radicular disease
5. No radiographic evidence of abnormal internal or external root resorption

The pulpal status of the treated teeth was evaluated clinically and radiographically 3 and 6 months after treatment. At the 6-month postoperative visit the teeth were reentered to evaluate the base material, the residual carious dentin, and the dentinal base. Treatment was judged successful if:

1. The restoration was intact
2. The tooth had normal mobility
3. The tooth was not sensitive to percussion
4. The tooth had no history of pain following treatment
5. There was no radiographic evidence of abnormal root resorption
6. There was no radiographic evidence of radicular disease
7. There was no clinical evidence of direct pulp

*Dycal and Dycal Improved, L.D. Caulk Co., Milford, Del. 19963.

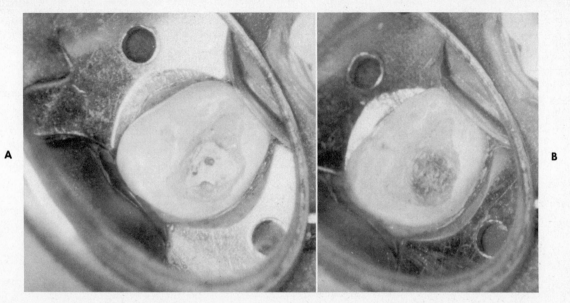

Fig. 8-7. A, This mandibular first primary molar had been treated by gross caries removal 6 months earlier. The calcium hydroxide base was dry and firm when the cavity was reopened. (The dark spots on the surface of the base material are amalgam particles that became embedded during the removal of the restoration.) **B,** The dark, residual, once-carious dentin in the cavity floor was soft and moist initially but was observed to be dry and hard at this 6-month evaluation.

exposure when the tooth was reentered and the residual carious dentin was examined or excavated

Successful treatment occurred in 32 (94.1%) of the 34 teeth that were available for the 6-month evaluation procedure. In all cases of successful treatment the base material and the residual carious dentin were observed to be "dry" on reentry and clinical examination. Of the successfully treated teeth, only four had residual carious dentin that felt somewhat soft when probed with an explorer; the rest felt hard (Fig. 8-7).

The results of this study and many previous studies demonstrate that indirect pulp therapy is a valuable therapeutic procedure in treating asymptomatic teeth with deep carious lesions. The procedure reduces the risk of direct pulp exposure and preserves pulp vitality. One may question the need to reenter the tooth if it has been properly selected and monitored, if a durable restoration is placed initially, and if no adverse symptoms develop. Long-term clinical and histologic studies are now under way to determine if reentry of treated teeth is necessary.

Vital pulp exposure

Although the routine practice of indirect pulp therapy in properly selected teeth will significantly reduce the number of direct pulp exposures encountered, all dentists who treat severe caries in children will occasionally be faced with treatment decisions related to the management of vital pulp exposures.

There is a strong tendency to treat all vital pulp exposures in a similar manner by applying a favorite pulp-capping material. However, the preoperative diagnosis should be the most important consideration and should dictate the type of treatment. The procedure should be decided only after a careful evaluation of the patient's symptoms and a review of the results of the diagnostic tests. The state of health of the exposed dental pulp is difficult to determine, especially in children, and there is often lack of conformity between clinical symptoms and histopathologic condition.

Size of the exposure and pulpal hemorrhage. In addition to the diagnostic aids in evaluating pulpal status, which have already been mentioned in this chapter, an evaluation of the pulp tissue at the exposure site is also necessary when the dentist encounters a direct pulp exposure. The size of the exposure, the appearance of the pulp, and the amount of bleeding are valuable observations in diagnosing the condition of the primary pulp. For this reason the use of a rubber dam to isolate the tooth is extremely important; in addition, with the rubber dam the area can be kept clean and the work can be done more efficiently.

The most favorable condition for vital pulp therapy is the small pinpoint exposure surrounded by sound dentin. However, a true carious exposure, even of pinpoint size, will be accompanied by inflammation of the pulp, the degree of which is usually directly related to the size of the exposure (Fig. 8-8).

A large exposure—the type that is encountered when a mass of leathery dentin is removed—is often associated with a watery exudate or pus at the exposure site. This tooth is unsuited for vital pulp therapy, since these conditions are indicative of advanced pulp degeneration and often of internal resorption in the pulp canal. Excessive hemorrhage at the point of carious exposure or during pulp amputation is invariably associated with hyperemia and generalized inflammation of the pulp. When a generalized inflammation of the pulp is observed, endodontic therapy or extraction of the tooth is the treatment of choice.

Dental hemogram. Guthrie's findings have substantiated the previously mentioned observations. His study was designed to investigate the value of a white blood cell differential count (hemogram) of the dental pulp as a diagnostic aid in determining pathologic or degenerative changes in the pulp. The first drop of blood from an exposed pulp was used for making the hemogram. The teeth were subsequently extracted. On the basis of a his-

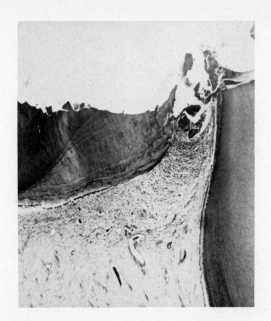

Fig. 8-8. Pulp exposed by caries will show inflammation at the exposure site. Fragments of necrotic dentin will be introduced into the pulp during the excavation of the caries.

tologic examination it was decided whether they would have been good candidates for a pulpotomy procedure. Those teeth in which the inflammatory process was localized to the coronal pulp area were classified as good candidates for a pulpotomy. If the inflammation extended into the pulp canal beyond the area of convenient amputation, the tooth was considered a poor candidate. Although there was no consistent blood picture throughout the group, the teeth considered to be poor risks all had an elevated neutrophil count and gave evidence of profuse bleeding and pain other than at mealtime. In the histologic examination, numerous teeth in the poor risk group showed evidence of internal resorption in the pulp canal.

The use of the dental hemogram is not a practical diagnostic method in the routine clinical management of vital pulp exposures. However, experimental use of the dental hemogram has confirmed that the history of spontaneous pain and the clinical evidence of profuse pulpal hemorrhage tend to cor-

relate well with significantly inflamed pulpal
tissue.

Vital pulp therapy techniques

Direct pulp capping (direct pulp therapy).
The pulp-capping procedure has been widely practiced for years and is still the favorite method of
many dentists treating vital pulp exposures. Although pulp capping has been condemned by
some, others report that if the teeth are carefully
selected, excellent results are obtained.

It is generally agreed that pulp-capping procedures should be limited to small exposures that
have been accidentally produced by trauma or during cavity preparation or to true pinpoint carious
exposures that are surrounded by sound dentin
(Fig. 8-9). Pulp capping should be considered only
for teeth in which there is an absence of pain, with
the possible exception of discomfort caused by the
intake of food. In addition, there should be either a
lack of bleeding at the exposure site, as is often the
case in a mechanical exposure, or an amount that
would be considered normal in the absence of a
hyperemic or an inflamed pulp.

The recommendation that the exposure site be
enlarged (pulp curettage) before the placement of
the capping material is not new. However, the
work of Kalins and Frisbie emphasized the need for
its consideration. When a pulp is exposed during
the preparation of a cavity or during the last stages
of caries removal, carious dentin chips will invariably be pushed into the pulp tissue. The presence of
pulpal inflammation of varying degrees, resorption, and encapsulation of dentin chips and fragments in exposed pulps after capping shows a
foreign body reaction, the severity of which is proportional to the total number of the chips present.
Necrotic material introduced with numerous small
chips of contaminated dentin will produce a diffuse
pulpitis or abscess. Enlarging the opening into the
pulp tissue allows the dentist to wash away the
debris, including the carious and noncarious fragments. When the exposure is of the pinpoint variety, it may be difficult to place the capping material
in contact with the exposed pulp. Enlargement of

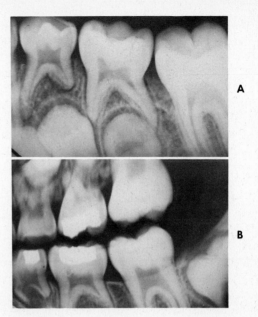

Fig. 8-9. A, Mesial pulp horn of the mandibular second
primary molar exposed during cavity preparation was
covered with calcium hydroxide. **B,** Dentinal bridge
across the mesial pulp horn is evidence of pulp healing.

the exposure site will facilitate this procedure.

All pulp treatment procedures should be carried
out under clean conditions using sterile instruments. The rubber dam should be used to isolate
the tooth to keep the pulp free of contamination.
All peripheral carious tissue should be excavated
before beginning to excavate the portion of the carious dentin most likely to result in pulp exposure.
Thus most of the bacterially infected tissue will
have been removed before actual pulp exposure
occurs. The work of Kakehashi, Stanley, and Fitzgerald and of Walshe, which is described later in
this chapter, supports the desirability of a surgically clean technique to minimize bacterial contamination of the pulpal tissue.

Caustic solutions should not be used to cauterize
or sterilize exposed pulp tissue before capping. The
delicate pulp tissue will be injured by these drugs,
reducing the healing potential. Only nonirritating
solutions, such as normal saline solution or chlora-

mine-T,* should be used to cleanse the region, flush the exposure site free of debris, and keep the pulp moist while the clot is forming before the placement of the capping material.

Calcium hydroxide is the material of choice for pulp capping (direct pulp therapy) of normal vital pulp tissue. The possibility of its stimulating the repair reaction is good. A commercially available calcium hydroxide capping material, such as Dycal, may be used. If the tooth is small (for example, a first primary molar), Dycal may also be used as the base for the amalgam restoration. In a long-term pulp-capping study in monkeys, McWalter, El-Kafrawy, and Mitchell observed that after 29 months all pulps capped with Dycal responded satisfactorily with complete bridging. There was no evidence of inflammation of the pulp or obliteration of the canal.

Pulpotomy. The removal of the coronal portion of the pulp has come to be an accepted procedure for treating both primary and permanent teeth with carious pulp exposures. The justification for this procedure is that the coronal pulp tissue, which is adjacent to the carious exposure, usually contains microorganisms and shows evidence of inflammation and degenerative change. The abnormal tissue can be removed and the healing can be allowed to take place at the entrance of the pulp canal in an area of essentially normal pulp. Even the pulpotomy procedure is likely to result in a high percentage of failures unless the teeth are carefully selected.

In the pulpotomy procedure the tooth should first be anesthetized and isolated with the rubber dam. A surgically clean technique should be used throughout the procedure. All remaining dental caries should be removed, and the overhanging enamel should be planed back to provide good access to coronal pulp. Pain during caries removal and instrumentation may be an indication of faulty anesthetic technique. More often, however, it indicates pulpal hyperemia and inflammation, making

*Chloramine solution: chloramine-T, 4 g; sodium chloride, 9 mg; distilled water, 100 ml.

the tooth a poor risk for vital pulpotomy. If the pulp at the exposure site bleeds excessively after complete removal of caries, the tooth is also a poor risk for vital pulpotomy.

The entire roof of the pulp chamber should be removed with a bur. No overhanging dentin from the roof of the pulp chamber or pulp horns should remain. No attempt is made to control the hemorrhage until the coronal pulp has been amputated. A No. 4 round bur may be used to remove the shelf of dentin around the periphery of the coronal chamber roof to produce a funnel-shaped access to the entrance of the root canals. A sharp discoid-type spoon excavator, large enough to extend across the entrance of the individual root canals, may be used to amputate the coronal pulp at its entrance into the canals. The pulp stumps should be cleanly excised with no tags of tissue extending across the floor of the pulp chamber. The pulp chamber should then be irrigated with a light flow of water from the water syringe and evacuated. Moist cotton pellets should be placed in the pulp chamber and allowed to remain over the pulp stumps until a clot forms. The formation of a blood clot is apparently essential for healing.

In recent years two general types of material have been used most often as dressings for the capping of the amputated pulp stumps. One material is calcium hydroxide; the other is zinc oxide–eugenol to which a small amount of formocresol may be added.

Laboratory and clinical observations indicate that a different technique and capping material are necessary in the treatment of primary teeth from those used for the permanent teeth. As a result of these observations, two specific pulpotomy techniques have evolved and are in general use today.

The *calcium hydroxide pulpotomy technique* is recommended in the treatment of permanent teeth with carious pulp exposures when there is a pathologic change in the pulp at the exposure site. This procedure is particularly indicated for permanent teeth with immature root development but with healthy pulp tissue in the root canals. It is also indi-

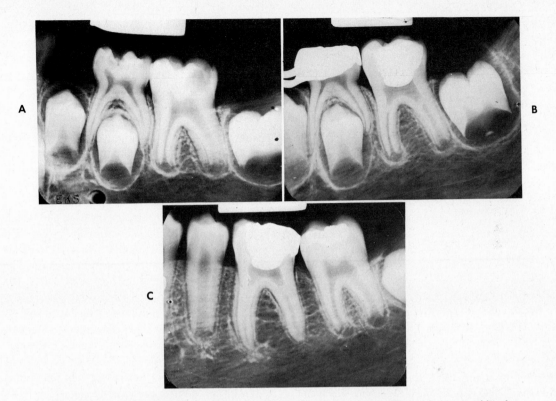

Fig. 8-10. A, Pulp of the first permanent molar was exposed by caries. The tooth was considered a candidate for the calcium hydroxide pulpotomy technique. **B,** Calcified bridge has formed over the vital pulp in the canals. **C,** Continued root development and pulpal recession are indicative of continuing pulpal vitality. The crown should be supported with a full-coverage restoration.

cated for a permanent tooth with a pulp exposure resulting from crown fracture when the trauma has also produced a root fracture of the same tooth. The technique is completed during a single appointment. Only teeth free of symptoms of painful pulpitis are considered for treatment. The procedure involves the amputation of the coronal portion of the pulp as described, the control of hemorrhage, and the placement of a calcium hydroxide capping material over the pulp tissue remaining in the canals (Fig. 8-10). A layer of zinc oxide–eugenol is placed over the calcium hydroxide to provide an adequate seal and then the tooth is prepared for full coverage. However, if the tissue in the pulp canals appears hyperemic after the amputation of the coronal tissue, a pulpotomy should no longer be con-

sidered. Endodontic treatment is indicated if the tooth is to be saved.

The *formocresol pulpotomy technique* is recommended in the treatment of primary teeth with carious exposures. The same diagnostic criteria recommended for the selection of permanent teeth for the calcium hydroxide pulpotomy should be used in the selection of primary teeth for the formocresol pulpotomy technique. The formocresol technique is also completed during a single appointment. A surgically clean technique should be used. The coronal portion of the pulp should be amputated as described previously, the debris should be removed from the chamber, and the hemorrhage should be controlled.

If there is evidence of hyperemia after the

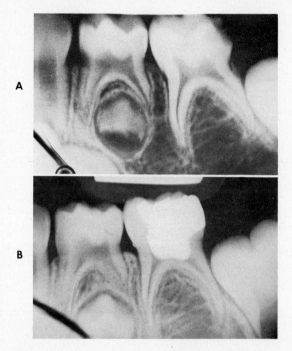

Fig. 8-11. A, Formocresol pulpotomy technique was completed. **B,** Normal appearance of the supporting tissues is indicative of a successful treatment. The tooth should now be restored with a chrome steel crown.

removal of the coronal pulp, indicating that inflammation is present in the tissue beyond the coronal portion of the pulp, the technique should be abandoned in favor of the partial pulpectomy, the complete pulpectomy, or even the removal of the tooth.

If the hemorrhage is controlled readily and the pulp stumps appear normal, it may be assumed that the pulp tissue in the canals is normal, and it is possible to proceed with the pulpotomy. The pulp chamber is dried with sterile cotton pellets. Next, a pellet of cotton moistened with a 1:5 concentration of Buckley's formocresol and lightly blotted on sterile gauze to remove the excess is placed in contact with the pulp stumps and is allowed to remain for 5 minutes. Since formocresol is caustic, care must be taken to avoid contact with the gingival tissues. The pellets are then removed and the pulp

chamber is dried with new pellets. A thick paste consisting of zinc oxide and eugenol is prepared and placed over the pulp stumps. A zinc phosphate cement or a second mix of zinc oxide–eugenol is placed over the paste, and the tooth is restored with a chrome steel crown (Fig. 8-11).

Some dentists prefer to make the pulp-capping material by mixing the zinc oxide powder with equal parts of eugenol and formocresol. There are no proven contraindications to adding formocresol to the mixture; however, there are no proven benefits. Ranly, Montgomery, and Pope have demonstrated in vitro that formaldehyde is not bound chemically in zinc oxide–eugenol cement and probably leaches out with time. However, García-Godoy has shown that incorporation of formocresol in zinc oxide–eugenol cement is apparently not necessary to obtain the characteristic and expected pulp reaction of the 5-minute formocresol pulpotomy technique. In view of the caustic nature of formocresol and the concern by some of the toxic and mutagenic potential from the excessive use of formocresol, its use in zinc oxide–eugenol paste is discouraged until some benefit can be demonstrated by future research.

A series of research studies by Loos and Han; Loos, Straffon, and Han; and Straffon and Han have led to the conclusion that a dilute (1:5 concentration) of Buckley's formocresol applied to tissue achieves the desired cellular response as effectively as the full-strength formocresol agent, yet allows a faster recovery of the affected cells. The researchers suggested that the 1:5 concentration is a safer medicament that would produce equally good results with fewer postoperative problems in pulpotomy procedures.

Morawa and associates have shown that in humans a dilute solution of a 1:5 concentration of Buckley's formocresol for the primary molar pulpotomy procedure is as successful as Buckley's formocresol full-strength. More recently, an in vitro study by Lazzari, Ranly, and Walker and an in vivo study in baboons by García-Godoy support the use of the 1:5 concentration of formocresol. Fuks and Bimstein have also demonstrated the effectiveness of the dilute formocresol pulpotomy technique in humans.

The original Buckley's formula for formocresol called for equal parts of formaldehyde and cresol. However, the formulation has been modified so that the commercial preparations currently available consist of 19% formaldehyde and 35% cresol in a solution of 15% glycerine and water.* The 1:5 concentration of this formula is prepared by first thoroughly mixing 3 parts of glycerine with 1 part of distilled water, then adding 4 parts of this diluent to 1 part of Buckley's formocresol and thoroughly mixing again.

Partial pulpectomy. A partial pulpectomy may be performed on primary teeth when coronal pulp tissue and the tissue entering the pulp canals are vital but show clinical evidence of hyperemia (Fig. 8-12). The tooth may or may not have a history of painful pulpitis, but the contents of the root canals should not show evidence of necrosis (suppuration). In addition, there should not be radiographic evidence of a thickened periodontal ligament or of radicular disease. If any of these conditions are present, a complete pulpectomy, which is described later, should be performed.

The partial pulpectomy technique, which may be completed in one appointment, involves the removal of the coronal pulp as described for the pulpotomy technique. The pulp filaments from the root canals are removed with a fine barbed broach; there will be considerable hemorrhage at this point. A Hedstrom file, placed in a porte polisher handle, will be helpful in the removal of remnants of the pulp tissue. The file removes tissue only as it is withdrawn and penetrates readily with a minimum of resistance. Care should be taken to avoid penetrating the apex of the tooth.

Many dentists are learning to effectively use root canal instruments placed in a special handpiece for root canal debridement. Root canal instrumentation may be facilitated with the judicious use of this mechanical technique, especially in canals that are difficult to negotiate with hand instruments. Cau-

*Young Dental Co., Maryland Heights, Mo. 63043.

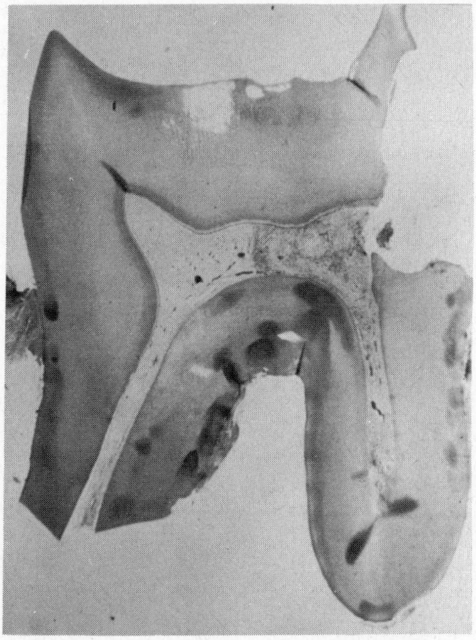

Fig. 8-12. Histologic section of a second primary molar with a carious pulp exposure. There was clinical evidence of hyperemia and inflammation of the pulp. Inflammation is evident in half the coronal pulp and into the pulp canal. This condition may be treated by the partial pulpectomy technique.

tious manipulation is important, however, to prevent overinstrumentation of the canal and apical tissues.

After the pulp tissue has been removed from the canals, a Luer-Lok syringe is used to irrigate them with 3% hydrogen peroxide followed by sodium hypochlorite. The canals should then be dried with sterile paper points. When hemorrhaging is controlled and the canals remain dry, a thin mix of zinc oxide–eugenol paste may be prepared, and paper points covered with the material are used to coat the root canal walls. Small Kerr files may be used to file the paste into the walls. The excess thin paste may be removed with paper points and Hedstrom files. A thick mix of the treatment paste should then be prepared, rolled into a point, and carried into the canal. Root canal pluggers may be used to condense the filling material into the canals. An x-ray film should be taken to evaluate

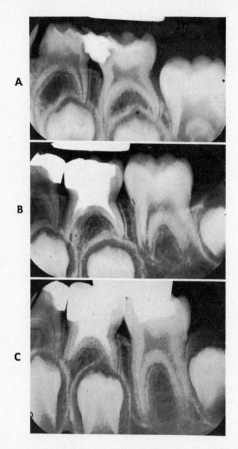

Fig. 8-13. A, Pulp in the second primary molar showed evidence of inflammation. The tooth was treated with the partial pulpectomy technique. **B,** Thirteen months after treatment, the second primary molar was asymptomatic and the supporting tissues appeared normal. **C,** Three years after the initial treatment, the radiograph of the second primary molar appears normal. The first permanent molar has erupted into a good position.

the success in completely filling the canals (Fig. 8-13). Further condensation may be carried out if necessary. The tooth should be restored with full coverage.

Nonvital pulp therapy technique

Complete pulpectomy. It is unwise to maintain untreated infected primary teeth in the mouth. They may be opened for drainage and often remain asymptomatic for an indefinite period of time. However, they are a source of infection and should be treated or removed. Cohen, Joress, and Calisti, in a bacteriologic study of infected primary molars, discovered that nine different strains of microorganisms having the potential of producing harmful effects could be found in the infected teeth. The morphology of the root canals in primary teeth makes endodontic treatment difficult and often impractical. The first primary molar canals are often so small that they are inaccessible even to the smallest barbed broach. If the canal cannot be properly cleansed of necrotic material, sterilized, and adequately filled, endodontic therapy will not be successful.

Hibbard and Ireland studied the primary root canal morphology by removing the pulp from extracted teeth, forcing acrylic resin into the pulp canals, and dissolving the covering of tooth structure in 10% nitric acid. It was apparent that initially there was only one root canal in each of the mandibular and maxillary molar roots. The subsequent deposition of secondary dentin throughout the life of the teeth caused a change in the morphologic pattern of the root canal, producing variations and eventual alterations in the number and size of the canals. The variations included lateral branching, connecting fibrils, apical ramifications, and partial fusion of the canals. These findings explain the complications often encountered in root canal therapy.

Endodontic procedures for the treatment of primary teeth with necrotic pulps are indicated if the canals are accessible and if there is evidence of essentially normal supporting bone (Fig. 8-14). If the second primary molar is lost before the eruption of the first permanent molar, the dentist is confronted with the difficult problem of preventing the first permanent molar from drifting mesially during its eruption. Special effort should be made to treat and retain the second primary molar even if it has a necrotic pulp.

Starkey (1981) developed the following *complete pulpectomy technique.* The rubber dam is applied, and the roof of the pulp chamber should be

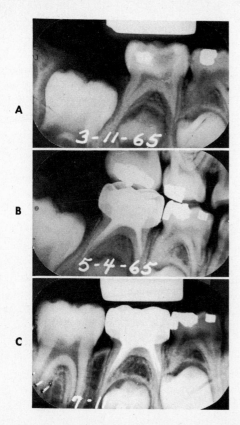

Fig. 8-14. A, Necrotic pulp resulted from a carious exposure of the pulp of the second primary molar. **B,** The pulp canals were treated and filled with zinc oxide–eugenol and formocresol. The tooth has been restored with a chrome steel crown. **C,** Two and a half years after treatment, the tooth is asymptomatic and the supporting bone appears normal. (Courtesy Dr. Paul E. Starkey.)

removed to gain access to the root canals as described previously in the pulpotomy technique. The contents of the pulp chamber and all debris from the occlusal third of the canals should be removed, with care taken to avoid forcing any of the infected contents through the apical foramen. A moistened pellet of camphorated monochlorophenol (CMCP) or 1:5 concentration of Buckley's formocresol, with excess moisture blotted, should be placed in the pulp chamber. The chamber may be sealed with zinc oxide–eugenol. At the second appointment, several days later, the tooth should

be isolated with a rubber dam and the treatment pellet removed. If the tooth has remained asymptomatic during the interval, the remaining contents of the canals should be removed using the technique described for the partial pulpectomy. The apex of each root should be penetrated slightly with the smallest file. (The dentist should experiment with dissociated primary molars to develop a "feel" for the instrument as it just penetrates the apex.) A treatment pellet should again be placed in the pulp chamber and the seal completed with zinc oxide–eugenol. After another interval of a few days, the treatment pellet should be removed. If the tooth has remained asymptomatic, the canals may be prepared and filled as described for the partial pulpectomy. However, if the tooth has been painful and there is evidence of moisture in the canals when the treatment pellet is removed, the canals should again be mechanically cleansed and the treatment repeated.

Erausquin and Muruzabal have shown that zinc oxide–eugenol is irritating to the periapical tissues and may produce necrosis of bone and cementum. For this reason, care should be taken not to force an excessive amount of canal-filling material past the apical end of the root canal.

Summary of pulp therapy philosophy

When one encounters clinical problems that will likely require pulp therapy to regain satisfactory oral health, treatment decisions are not always clear cut. Proper diagnosis of the pulpal problem is important to allow the dentist to select the most conservative treatment procedure that offers the best chance of long-term success with the least chance of subsequent complications. The dentist should think of the possible treatment options in a progressive manner that takes into account both treatment conservatism (for example, a pulpotomy is more conservative than a partial pulpectomy) and posttreatment problems (Fig. 8-15). The most conservative treatment possible may not always be the indicated procedure after the dentist also weighs the risks of posttreatment failure in a particular case.

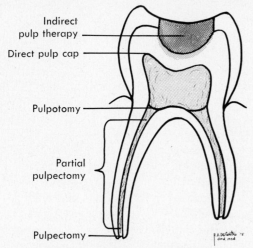

Fig. 8-15. Pulp therapy progression.

Labels on figure: Indirect pulp therapy, Direct pulp cap, Pulpotomy, Partial pulpectomy, Pulpectomy

Restoration of the pulpally involved tooth

It has been a common practice for some dentists to delay for weeks or months the permanent restoration of a tooth that has had vital pulp therapy. The purpose has been to allow time to determine whether the treatment procedure will be successful. However, failures in pulp therapy are usually not evident for many months. Rarely does a failure in pulp therapy or an endodontic procedure on a primary tooth cause the child to experience acute symptoms. Failures are usually made evident by pathologic root resorption or rarefied areas in the bone and discovered during regular recall appointments.

Primary and permanent molars that have been treated by the pulpotomy or pulpectomy technique will have a weak, unsupported crown that is liable to fracture. Often a fracture of the buccal or lingual plate occurs below the gingival attachment or even below the crest of the alveolar bone. This type of fracture makes subsequent restoration of the tooth impractical. Also, the delay in restoring the tooth with a material that will adequately seal the tooth and prevent an ingress of oral fluids is one cause for failure of the pulp to heal. A layer of zinc oxide–eugenol over the capping material and an amalgam restoration will adequately protect the pulp against contaminating oral fluids during the healing process.

An amalgam restoration may serve as the immediate restoration. However, as soon as it is practical the pulpally treated tooth should be prepared for a chrome steel or gold crown. Pulp treatment of a primary molar is often followed by placement of a chrome steel crown restoration during the same appointment.

Reaction of the pulp to various capping materials

Zinc oxide–eugenol. Before calcium hydroxide came into common use, zinc oxide–eugenol had been used more often than any other pulp-capping material. Many dentists have apparently had good clinical results with the use of zinc oxide–eugenol, but it is no longer recommended as a direct pulp-capping material.

Glass and Zander and also Seelig, Fowler, and Tanchester have reported that zinc oxide–eugenol in contact with vital tissue will produce chronic inflammation, abscess formation, and liquefaction necrosis. They reported that 24 hours after capping a pulp with zinc oxide–eugenol, the adjacent underlying tissue contains a mass of red blood cells and polymorphonuclear leukocytes. The hemorrhagic mass is demarcated from the underlying pulp tissue by a zone of fibrin and inflammatory cells. Two weeks after the capping with zinc oxide–eugenol, degeneration of the pulp is apparent at the capping site, and chronic inflammation extends into the apical portion of the pulp tissue. Lymphocytes, plasma cells, and polymorphonuclear leukocytes are seen around the site of the wound.

Zawawi used the subcutaneous connective tissue of the rat to determine the relative irritant and other effects of commonly used capping materials. Eleven commercial products containing zinc oxide–eugenol failed to stimulate osteogenesis. However, materials containing only calcium hydroxide did promote osteogenesis in as little as 2 days. The presence of zinc oxide possibly inactivated the ability of calcium salts to produce osteo-genesis.

Calcium hydroxide. Herman first introduced calcium hydroxide as a biologic dressing. Because of its alkalinity (pH of 12), it is so caustic that when placed in contact with vital pulp tissue, the reaction produces a superficial necrosis of the pulp. The irritant qualities seem to be related to its ability to stimulate development of a calcified barrier. The superficial necrotic area in the pulp that develops beneath the calcium hydroxide is demarcated from the healthy pulp tissue below by a new, deeply staining zone comprising basophilic elements of the calcium hydroxide dressing. The original pro-teinate zone is still present. However, against this zone is a new area of coarse fibrous tissue likened to a primitive type of bone. On the periphery of the new fibrous tissue, cells resembling odontoblasts appear to be lining up. One month after the capping procedure, a calcified bridge is evident radiograph-ically. This bridge continues to increase in thick-ness during the next 12-month period (Fig. 8-16). The pulp tissue beneath the calcified bridge re-mains vital and is essentially free of inflammatory cells.

Many research studies can be cited regarding calcium hydroxide as a pulp-capping material, and a few are included in the references for this chap-ter. Investigators who evaluate experimental pulp-capping agents commonly compare their results with the agent being tested with the results they can obtain with calcium hydroxide under similar condi-tions. Thus calcium hydroxide currently serves as the standard or control material for experimenta-tion related to pulp-capping agents. Calcium hydroxide is the material of choice for direct pulp-capping or vital pulpotomy techniques in perma-nent teeth.

Preparations containing formalin. The belief that the exposure of the pulp to formocresol or cap-ping it with materials that contain formocresol will promote pulp healing or even maintain the pulp in a healthy state has not been adequately substantiated. Although some recent studies have suggested that the formocresol pulpotomy technique can be ap-

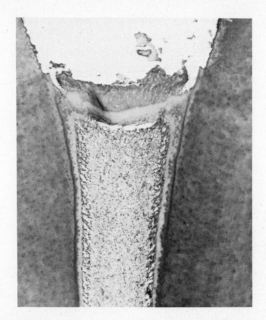

Fig. 8-16. Calcified bridge covering an amputated pulp that was capped with calcium hydroxide.

plied to permanent teeth, its use in permanent teeth remains questionable unless a subsequent pulpec-tomy and a root canal filling are also planned. The clinical success experienced in the treatment of pri-mary pulps with these materials is possibly related to the drug's germicidal action and fixation quali-ties rather than to its ability to promote healing.

Mansukhani reported a histologic study of 43 primary and permanent teeth that had been treated with the formocresol pulpotomy technique. She observed that the surface of the pulp immediately under the formocresol became fibrous and acido-philic within a few minutes after the application of formocresol. This reaction was interpreted as one of fixation of the living pulp tissue. After exposure of the pulp to formocresol for periods of 7 to 14 days, three distinct zones became evident: a broad acidophilic zone (fixation); a broad, pale-staining zone, wherein the cells and fibers were greatly diminished (atrophy); and a broad zone of inflam-matory cells concentrated at the junction with the pale-staining zone and diffusing deeply into the underlying tissue to the apex. No tendency to wall off the inflammatory zone by either a fibrous layer or a calcific barrier was seen. No reparative dentin formation was evident laterally, centrally, or peripherally. Rather, a progressive fixation of the pulpal tissue with ultimate fibrosis of the entire pulp occurred.

Doyle, McDonald, and Mitchell compared the success of the formocresol pulpotomy technique with the success of the calcium hydroxide pulpotomy technique. Experimental pulpotomies were performed on 65 normal human primary teeth, many of which could later be extracted for histologic examination. The formocresol technique was used on 33 teeth, and the calcium hydroxide technique was used in the treatment of the other 32. Under the conditions of this study the formocresol pulpotomy technique was superior to the calcium hydroxide technique for at least the first 18 months after the treatment. The results of the combined methods of evaluation indicated that the calcium hydroxide pulpotomy technique for primary teeth was successful in 61% of the cases. The formocresol pulpotomy resulted in 95% success at the end of 1 year.

Formocresol did not stimulate the healing response of the remaining pulp tissue but rather tended to fix essentially all of the remaining tissue (Figs. 8-17 and 8-18). Calcium hydroxide was associated with the formation of a dentin bridge and the complete healing of the amputated primary pulp in 50% of the cases that were available for histologic study.

Berger has also studied histologically the pri-

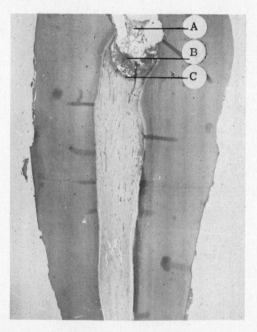

Fig. 8-17. Histologic section of a primary pulp exposed to formocresol for 4 days. The medicament contacted the pulp at *A*, the debris and blood clot are evident at *B*, and a markedly eosinophilic, compressed line is evident at *C*. The underlying pulp was a pale, homogeneously stained tissue with the loss of basophilic nuclei. (Courtesy Dr. Walter A. Doyle.)

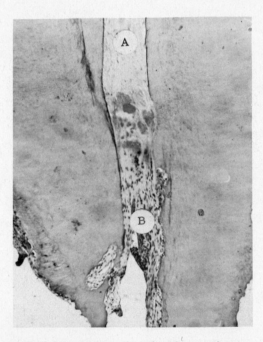

Fig. 8-18. Histologic section of a primary pulp exposed to formocresol for 41 days. The pulp, *A*, appeared pale and pink and there was a loss of cellular definition. Vital tissue can be seen in the apical portion, *B*. (Courtesy Dr. Walter A. Doyle.)

mary pulp tissue reaction to formocresol. He observed that, commencing 7 weeks after the formocresol pulpotomy, there was an ingrowth of granulation tissue through the apical foramen, replacing the necrotic tissue in the pulp canal. At later intervals the granulation tissue appeared progressively more coronal, until at 35 weeks after treatment it was close to, and in some instances at the site of, amputation. Osteodentin was present, repairing small areas of internal resorption and slightly narrowing the lumen of the canal.

Research on the use of formocresol as a pulp-capping agent has continued. Some of the more recent studies were cited earlier in this chapter. The 1:5 concentration of Buckley's formocresol is currently recommended for initial treatment of the pulps of primary teeth in the vital pulpotomy technique.

Glutaraldehyde. Glutaraldehyde has received attention recently as a potential pulp-capping agent for pulpotomy techniques. It is an excellent bactericidal agent and seems to offer some advantages when compared to formocresol.

Berson and Good have reported that glutaraldehyde seems to be superior to formaldehyde preparations for pulp therapy in the following ways:

1. Formaldehyde reactions are reversible but glutaraldehyde reactions are not.
2. Formaldehyde is a small molecule that penetrates the apical foramen, whereas glutaraldehyde is a larger molecule that does not.
3. Formaldehyde requires a long reaction time and an excess of solution to fix tissue, whereas glutaraldehyde fixes tissue instantly and an excess of solution is unnecessary.

Dilley and Courts compared the immunologic responses to four pulpal medicaments injected subcutaneously into rabbits. Two of the medicaments were 19% formaldehyde and 5% glutaraldehyde. The authors observed that glutaraldehyde and formaldehyde demonstrated low levels of antigenicity in the rabbits. They found that formaldehyde produced a greater humoral immunologic response than glutaraldehyde and that both agents elicited weak cell-mediated immune responses. They con-

cluded that glutaraldehyde may prove to be an efficacious pulpotomy medicament but that further research is needed.

Kopel and associates have used 2% glutaraldehyde as a pulpotomy medicament in human primary teeth with encouraging results. Although the sample size was quite small in the 6-month and 1-year groups, the researchers made the following observations:

1. Two percent aqueous glutaraldehyde is biologically acceptable for maintaining pulp vitality following a pulpotomy procedure.
2. The remaining pulp tissue does not resemble pulp tissue treated with formocresol when observed histologically.
3. The glutaraldehyde dressing produces an initial zone of fixation that does not migrate apically. The tissue adjoining the fixed zone has the cellular detail found in normal pulp tissue and presumably remains vital in vivo.
4. The fixed zone of tissue is eventually replaced by dense collagenous tissue through macrophagic action, suggesting vitality of the entire root tissue.

Certainly glutaraldehyde deserves further investigation as a possible pulp medicament. It seems to offer some advantages over the currently recommended vital pulp therapy dressings.

Capping materials containing antibiotics. Considerable attention has been given to the use of antibiotics in dentistry. The interest and use have naturally extended into the field of vital pulp therapy. The effectiveness of antibiotics in reducing the number of microorganisms remaining in the pulp tissue after vital pulp therapy has not been adequately established.

A review of recent reports would indicate that antibiotics have often been used indiscriminately in vital pulp therapy and many times without regard for the possible antagonistic activity between the capping material and the antibiotic. Kutscher and Yigdall found that the antibacterial activity of penicillin is almost entirely destroyed when it is used in combination with calcium hydroxide. Observations at Indiana University indicated that chlortet-

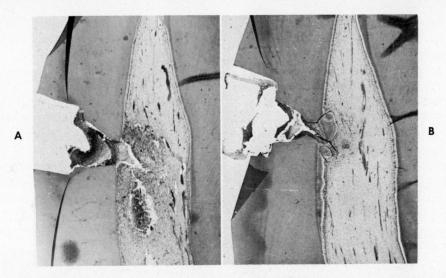

Fig. 8-19. Experimental pulp capping in monkey teeth. **A,** Surgical exposure of the pulp was capped with starch. At the 90-day observation period extensive inflammation of the pulp is evident. **B,** Pulp capped with the antibiotic material demonstrates minimum inflammation with incomplete calcific repair. (Courtesy Dr. G.R. Baker.)

racycline (Aureomycin), streptomycin, and oxytetracycline (Terramycin) retain some antibacterial activity for as long as 48 hours when incorporated in calcium hydroxide. However, chlortetracycline retards the proliferation of fibroblasts and consequently may interfere with pulp healing. Seltzer and Bender observed that pulpal necrosis and the development of an apical granuloma occurred when an aqueous solution of 250,000 units of penicillin was used on the vital pulpal tissue of dogs.

The findings of Baker indicate that antibiotic compounds may eventually be found effective in overcoming localized infection in the pulp at the site of a carious exposure. In Baker's experiment the pulps of 26 monkey teeth were surgically exposed and were allowed to remain open for 24 hours. They were then capped with an antibiotic compound consisting of 10% erythromycin estolate, 10% streptomycin sulfate, and starch as the vehicle. An equal number of teeth were capped with pure starch. A histologic examination of teeth

extracted at 30- and 90-day intervals revealed varying degrees of inflammation in all the teeth treated with either the antibiotic preparation or the starch control. However, the teeth treated with the antibiotic capping material exhibited much less inflammation than did the teeth treated with the starch control (Fig. 8-19). The pulps capped with starch often demonstrated abscess formation and necrosis. Calcific repair, which is considered important in the successful treatment of vital exposures, was not observed to be complete in any of the teeth.

A report by Gardner, Mitchell, and McDonald provides additional positive evidence of the value of an antibiotic and calcium hydroxide in treating infected dental pulps. Surgically exposed and infected permanent teeth in monkeys were treated with a pulp-capping compound containing 5% vancomycin (Vancocin) in combination with calcium hydroxide. The vancomycin had previously been shown to be effective against gram-positive microorganisms. Also, subcutaneous implants of the material in rats produced only a moderate inflam-

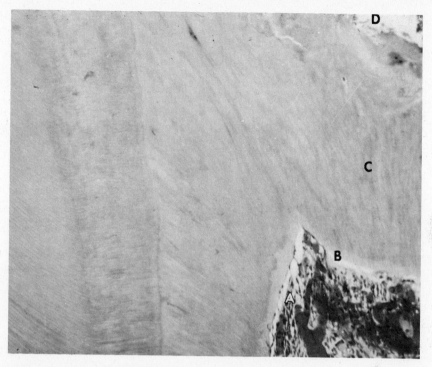

Fig. 8-20. Treatment of a carious exposure with vancomycin and calcium hydroxide. A dentin bridge displays an odontoblastic layer, *A,* predentin layer, *B,* and a complete dentin bridge, *C,* across the exposure site, *D.* (Courtesy Dr. Donald E. Gardner.)

matory reaction. The study demonstrated that vancomycin and calcium hydroxide were compatible and effective when used in combination in vitro against certain gram-positive and gram-negative bacteria. Although calcium hydroxide alone was an effective capping agent, the combination with vancomycin was somewhat more successful in stimulating regular reparative dentin bridges. Complete dentin bridging occurred as early as 30 days postoperatively when a combination of vancomycin, calcium hydroxide, methylcellulose, and water was used as a pulp-capping agent (Fig. 8-20).

Capping materials containing corticosteroids. Corticosteroids in combination with antibiotics have been used in the treatment of carious pulp exposure, including exposure in teeth with symptoms of painful pulpitis. A critical evaluation of the success of such treatment leads the dentist to agree with the findings of Fiore-Donno and Baume. They caution against the use of cortisone, antibiotics, and calcium hydroxide. Although this combination seems to produce clinical success, when the pulp is evaluated microscopically a degenerative condition is evident, including fibrous metaplasia, chronic inflammation, and inhibition of dentinogenesis.

Other new experimental capping materials. A variety of new experimental materials have attracted attention lately as potential pulp-capping materials. Tricalcium phosphate has been evaluated by several investigators including Boone and El-Kafrawy and Heys and associates. Dickey, El-Kafrawy, and Phillips have evaluated a crystalline form of pure calcium hydroxyapatite, and Ibarra has evaluated an experimental synthetic hydroxyapatite used in combination with both a chlorhexidine gluconate solution and distilled water as vehi-

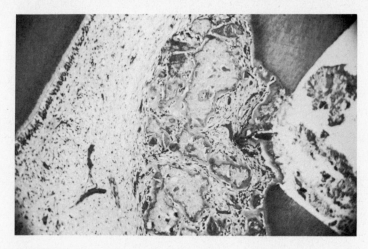

Fig. 8-21. Surgical exposure of the pulp of a monkey was capped with powdered bovine dentin. Atubular dentin bridging the exposure site was evident 42 days postoperatively.

cles. None of these proved to be as satisfactory as calcium hydroxide as a pulp-capping material. In addition, they are somewhat difficult to manipulate in their present forms.

Failures after vital pulp therapy

Failure in the formation of a calcified bridge across the vital pulp has often been related to the age of the patient, degree of surgical trauma, sealing pressure, improper choice of capping material, low threshold of host resistance, and presence of microorganisms with subsequent infection. Kakehashi, Stanley, and Fitzgerald studied the effect of surgical exposures of dental pulps in germ-free and conventional laboratory rats. The injured pulpal tissue, contaminated with microorganisms, failed to show evidence of repair; especially lacking were matrix formation and attempted dentinal bridging. In the germ-free animals, bridging began in 14 days and was complete in 28 days regardless of the severity of the exposure. The major determinant in the healing of exposed rodent pulps appeared to be the presence or absence of microorganisms.

Walshe provided further evidence that the success of vital pulp therapy depends on the adherence to a surgically aseptic technique. In his experiment

the teeth of monkeys were capped with bovine dentin mixed with methylcellulose, and histologic observations were made 42 days postoperatively. Approximately half the teeth capped with the experimental material were successfully repaired with atubular dentin (Fig. 8-21). The remaining teeth showed varying degrees of inflammation and repair. The Brown and Bren staining technique demonstrated the presence of microorganisms in the pulp of the teeth that failed to repair (Figs. 8-22 and 8-23). The stain also demonstrated microorganisms between the dentin walls and the filling material. The microorganisms were apparently introduced at the time of the pulp-capping procedure, or leakage of the restoration allowed them to gain entrance to the pulp chamber. This study likewise supports the need for a good surgical technique and the placement of a restoration that will provide the best possible seal.

A tooth that has been treated successfully with a pulpotomy technique should have, after 1 year, a normal periodontal ligament and lamina dura, radiographic evidence of a calcified bridge if calcium hydroxide was used as the capping material, and no radiographic evidence of internal resorption or pathologic resorption. Via used these criteria in an

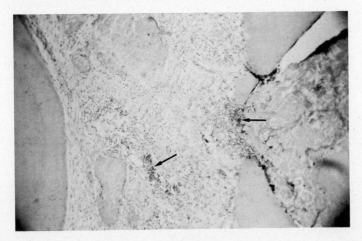

Fig. 8-22. Pulps capped with bovine dentin failed to undergo calcific repair and demonstrated microorganisms in the pulp. (Courtesy Dr. Martin Walshe.)

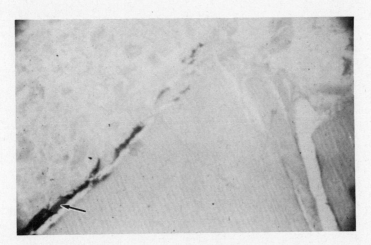

Fig. 8-23. Microorganisms may be seen between the dentin walls and the filling material. (Courtesy Dr. Martin Walshe.)

evaluation of 107 primary molars treated by the calcium hydroxide pulpotomy technique. The observation period was approximately 24 months, and results in only 31% of the teeth could be classified as successful at the end of that period. Sixty-nine percent of the treated teeth that failed showed evidence of internal resorption. Law's findings (1956) were similar in that 54% of 227 primary teeth treated by the calcium hydroxide method failed.

The treatment of permanent teeth by the calcium hydroxide method has resulted in a higher percentage of success when the teeth were selected carefully on the basis of existing knowledge of diagnostic techniques.

Internal resorption. Radiographic evidence of internal resorption occurring within the pulp canal several months after the pulpotomy procedure is the most frequently seen evidence of an abnormal response in primary teeth (Fig. 8-24). Internal resorption is a destructive process generally believed to be caused by osteoclastic activity, and it

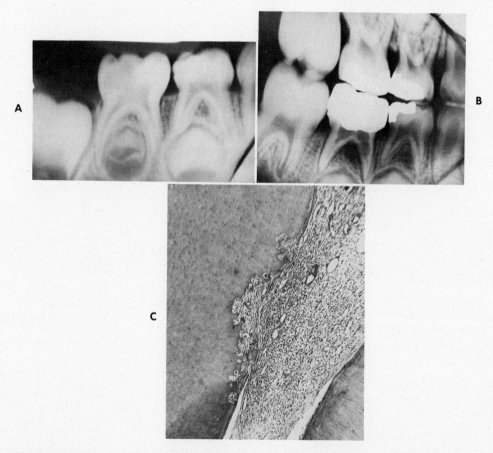

Fig. 8-24. A, Preoperative radiograph of a second primary molar treated with the calcium hydroxide pulpotomy technique. **B,** Two years after treatment, internal resorption and bone rarefaction are evident. **C,** There may have been inflammation of the pulp apical to the amputation site and beginning internal resorption at the time of the initial treatment.

may progress slowly or rapidly. Occasionally secondary repair of the resorbed dentinal area occurs.

No satisfactory explanation for the post-pulpotomy type of internal resorption has been given. It has been demonstrated, however, that with a true carious exposure of the pulp there will be an inflammatory process of some degree. The inflammation may be limited to the exposure site, or it may be diffuse and become evident throughout the coronal portion of the pulp. Amputation of all the pulp that shows the inflammatory change is often difficult or impossible, and abnormal pulp tissue is allowed to remain. If the inflammation extended to the entrance of the pulp canal, osteoclasts may have been attracted to the area; if it were

possible to examine the tooth histologically, small bays of resorption would be evident. This condition may often exist at the time of pulp therapy, although there is no way to detect it. The only indication would be the clinical evidence of a hyperemic pulp.

All the pulp-capping materials in use today are irritating to some extent and produce at least some degree of inflammation. Inflammatory cells attracted to the area as a result of the placement of an irritating capping material might well attract the osteoclastic cells and initiate the internal resorption. This may explain the occurrence of internal resorption even though the pulp is normal at the time of treatment.

Because the roots of primary teeth are undergo-

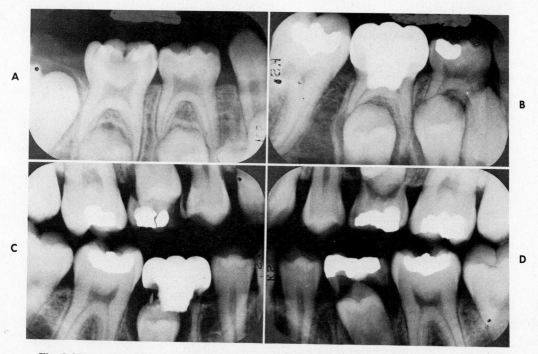

Fig. 8-25. A, A pulpally involved second primary molar was successfully treated with a formocresol pulpotomy and restored with a chrome steel crown. **B,** This 4-year posttreatment radiograph reveals long-term successful management. **C** and **D,** Bilateral bite-wing radiographs of the same patient 7 years after the pulpotomy reveal that the resorption of the pulpotomized molar is falling behind when compared with its antimere. The eruption of the permanent second premolar is also being delayed. The pulpally treated tooth should be extracted at this time. (Courtesy Wayne A. Moldenhauer.)

ing normal physiologic resorption, vascularity of the apical region is increased. There is osteoclastic activity in the area. This may predispose the tooth to internal resorption when an irritant in the form of a pulp-capping material is placed on the pulp.

Alveolar abscess. An alveolar abscess occasionally develops some months after pulp therapy has been completed. The tooth usually remains asymptomatic and the child is unaware of the infection, which may be present in the bone surrounding the root apices or in the area of the root bifurcation. A fistulous opening may be present, indicating the chronic condition of the infection. Primary teeth that show evidence of an alveolar abscess should be removed. Permanent teeth that have previously been treated by pulp capping or by pulpotomy and later show evidence of pulpal necrosis and apical infection may be considered for endodontic treatment if the pulp canals are accessible and if the root end morphology is favorable for this type of treatment.

Early exfoliation or overretention of primary teeth with pulp treatments

Occasionally a pulpally treated tooth previously thought to be successfully managed will loosen and exfoliate (or require extraction) prematurely for no apparent reason. It is thought that such a condition results from low-grade, chronic, asymptomatic localized infection. Usually abnormal and incomplete root resorption patterns of the affected teeth are also observed. When this occurs, space management must be considered.

Another sequela requiring close observation is the tendency for primary teeth having successful pulpotomies or pulpectomies to be overretained. This situation may have the untoward result of interfering with the normal eruption of permanent teeth and adversely affecting the developing occlusion. Close periodic observation of pulpally treated teeth is necessary to intercept such a developing problem at the proper time. Extraction of the primary tooth is usually sufficient. Starkey (1980) believes that this phenomenon occurs when normal physiologic exfoliation is delayed by the bulky

amount of cement contained in the pulp chamber. Even though the material is resorbable, its resorption is impaired significantly when large quantities are present (Fig. 8-25).

REFERENCES

American Dental Association: Accepted dental therapeutics, ed. 38, Chicago, 1979, The Association.

Baker, G.R.: Topical antibiotic treatment of infected dental pulps of monkeys, thesis, Indianapolis, 1966, Indiana University School of Dentistry.

Berger, J.S.: Pulp tissue reaction to formocresol and zinc oxide–eugenol, J. Dent. Child. **32:**13-28, 1965.

Berson, R.B., and Good, D.L.: Pulpotomy and pulpectomy for primary teeth. In Stewart, R.E., and others, editors: Pediatric dentistry: scientific foundations and clinical practice, St. Louis, 1981, The C.V. Mosby Co.

Boone, M.E., II, and El-Kafrawy, A.H.: Pulp reaction to a tricalcium phosphate ceramic capping agent, Oral Surg. **47:**369-371, 1979.

Buckley, J.: Practical therapeutics: a rational treatment for putrescent pulps, Dent. Rev. **18:**1193-1197, 1904.

Cohen, M.M., Joress, S.M., and Calisti, L.P.: Bacteriologic study of infected deciduous molars, Oral Surg. **13:**1382-1386, 1960.

Dickey, D.M., El-Kafrawy, A.H., and Phillips, R.W.: Pulp reactions to a calcium hydroxyapatite in monkeys, J. Dent. Res. **59** (special issue A)**:**360, abs. no. 371, 1980.

Dilley, G.J., and Courts, F.J.: Immunological response to four pulpal medicaments, Pediatr. Dent. **3:**179-183, 1981.

Dimaggio, J.J., and Hawes, R.R.: Evaluation of direct and indirect pulp capping, I.A.D.R. abs. no. 40, 1962, p. 24.

Dimaggio, J.J., and Hawes, R.R.: Continued evaluation of direct and indirect pulp capping, I.A.D.R. abs. no. 41, 1963, p. 380

Doyle, W.A., McDonald, R.E., and Mitchell, D.F.: Formocresol versus calcium hydroxide in pulpotomy, J. Dent. Child. **29:**86-97, 1962.

Erausquin, J., and Muruzabal, M.: Root canal fillings with zinc oxide–eugenol cement in the rat molar, Oral Surg. **22:**547-558, 1967.

Fiore-Donno, G., and Baume, L.J.: Effects of capping compounds containing corticosteriods on the human dental pulp, Helv. Odontol. Acta **6:**23-32, 1962.

Fuks, A.B., and Bimstein, E.: Clinical evaluation of diluted formocresol pulpotomies in primary teeth of school children, Pediatr. Dent. **3:**321-324, 1981.

Garciá-Godoy, F.: Penetration and pulpal response by two concentrations of formocresol using two methods of application, J. Pedod. **5:**102-135, 1981.

Gardner, D.E., Mitchell, D.F., and McDonald, R.E.: Treatment of pulps of monkeys with vancomycin and calcium hydroxide, J. Dent. Res. **50:**1273-1277, 1971.

Glass, R.L., and Zander, H.A.: Pulp healing, J. Dent. Res. **28:**97-107, 1949.

Glickman, I., and Shklar, G.: Effect of systemic disturbances on the pulp of experimental animals, Oral Surg. **7:**550-558, 1954.

Guthrie, T.J.: An investigation of the dental pulp hemogram as a diagnostic aid for vital pulp therapy, thesis, Indianapolis, 1959, Indiana University School of Dentistry.

Herman, B.: Biologische Wurzelbehandlung, Frankfurt, Germany, 1936, W. Kramer.

Heys, D.R., and others: Histologic considerations of direct pulp capping agents, J. Dent. Res. **60:**1371-1379, 1981.

Hibbard, E.D., and Ireland, R.L.: Morphology of the root canals of the primary molar teeth, J. Dent. Child. **24:**250-257, 1957.

Ibarra, A.J.: Pulp reactions to a synthetic hydroxyapatite and chlorhexidine in monkeys, thesis, Indianapolis, 1980, Indiana University School of Dentistry.

Kakehashi, S., Stanley, H.R., and Fitzgerald, R.J.: The effects of surgical exposure of dental pulps in germ-free and conventional laboratory rats. Oral Surg. **20:**340-349, 1965.

Kalins, V., and Frisbie, H.E.: The effect of dentin fragments on the healing of the exposed pulp, Arch. Oral Biol. **2:**96-103, 1960.

King, J.B., Crawford, J.J., and Lindahl, R.L.: Indirect pulp capping: a bacteriologic study of deep carious dentine in human teeth, Oral Surg. **20:**663-671, 1965.

Kopel, H.M., and others: The effects of glutaraldehyde on primary pulp tissue following coronal amputation: an in vivo histologic study, J. Dent. Child. **47:**425-430, 1980.

Kutscher, A.H., and Yigdall, I.: Bacteriologic evaluation of the compatibility of antibiotics and other therapeutic agents, Oral Surg. **5:**1096-1098, 1952.

Law, D.B.: An evaluation of vital pulpotomy technique, J. Dent. Child. **23:**40-44, 1956.

Law, D.B., and Lewis, T.M.: Effect of calcium hydroxide on deep carious lesions, Oral Surg. **14:**1130-1157, 1961.

Lazzari, E.P., Ranly, D.M., and Walker, W.A.: Biochemical effects of formocresol on bovine pulp tissue, Oral Surg. **45:**796-802, 1978.

Lewis, B.B., and Chestner, S.B.: Formaldehyde in dentistry: a review of mutagenic and carcinogenic potential, J.A.D.A. **103:**429-434, 1981.

Loos, P.J., and Han, S.S.: An enzyme histochemical study of the effect of various concentrations of formocresol on connective tissues, Oral Surg. **31:**571-585, 1971.

Loos, P.J., Straffon, L.H., and Han, S.S.: Biological effects of formocresol, J. Dent. Child. **40:**193-197, 1973.

Mansukhani, N.: Pulpal reactions to formocresol, thesis, Chicago, 1959, University of Illinois School of Dentistry.

McDonald, R.E.: Diagnostic aids and vital pulp therapy for deciduous teeth, J.A.D.A. **53:**14-22, 1956.

McWalter, G.M., El-Kafrawy, A.H., and Mitchell, D.F.: Long-term study of pulp capping in monkeys with three agents, J.A.D.A. **93:**105-110, 1976.

Mitchell, D.F., and Tarplee, R.E.: Painful pulpitis, Oral Surg. **13:**1360-1370, 1960.

Morawa, A.P., and others: Clinical evaluation of pulpotomies using dilute formocresol, J. Dent. Child. **42:**360-363, 1975.

Myers, D.R., and others: Distribution of ^{14}C-formaldehyde after pulpotomy with formocresol, J.A.D.A. **96:**805-813, 1978.

Myers, D.R., and others: The acute toxicity of high doses of systemically administered formocresol in dogs, Pediatr. Dent. **3:**37-41, 1981.

Nirschl, R.F., and Avery, D.R.: Evaluation of a new pulp capping agent: a clinical investigation, J. Dent. Res. **59**(special issue A):362, abs. no. 378, 1980.

Pfaff, P.: Abhandlung von den Zächnen des menschlichen Körpers und deren Krankheiten, Berlin, 1756.

Ranly, D.M., Montgomery, E.H., and Pope, H.O.: The loss of ^{3}H-formaldehyde from zinc oxide–eugenol cement: an in vitro study, J. Dent. Child. **42:**128-132, 1975.

Reeves, R., and Stanley, H.R.: The relationship of bacterial penetration and pulpal pathosis in carious teeth, Oral Surg. **22:**59-65, 1966.

Reynolds, R.L.: The determination of pulp vitality by means of thermal and electrical stimuli, Oral Surg. **22:**231-240, 1966.

Seelig, A., Fowler, R.C., and Tanchester, D.: Effect of penicillin C potassium plus calcium carbonate on surgically exposed dental pulps of the rhesus monkey, J.A.D.A. **48:**532-537; **49:**258, 1954.

Seltzer, S., and Bender, I.B.: Some influences affecting repair of the exposed pulps of dogs' teeth, J. Dent. Res. **37:**678-687, 1958.

Starkey, P.E.: Treatment of pulpally involved primary molars. In McDonald, R.E., and others, editors: Current therapy in dentistry, vol. 7, St. Louis, 1980, The C.V. Mosby Co.

Starkey, P.E.: Pulp therapy in dentistry for children, Indianapolis, 1981, The Indiana University Pedodontic Alumni Association.

Straffon, L.H., and Han, S.S.: Effects of varying concentrations of formocresol on RNA synthesis of connective tissues in sponge implants, Oral Surg. **29:**915-925, 1970.

Traubman, L., II: A critical clinical and television radiographic evaluation of indirect pulp capping, thesis, Indianapolis, 1967, Indiana University School of Dentistry.

Via, W.F.: Evaluation of deciduous molars treated by pulpotomy and calcium hydroxide, J.A.D.A. **50:**34-43, 1955.

Walshe, M.J.: Pulp reaction to anorganic bovine dentin, thesis, Indianapolis, 1967, Indiana University School of Dentistry.

Zander, H.A.: Rationale for diagnosis and treatment of pulp diseases, J. Fla. Dent. Soc. **18:**14-15, 1947.

Zawawi, H.: Rat connective tissue reactions to implants of certain pulp capping and cavity lining materials, thesis, Indianapolis, 1958, Indiana University School of Dentistry.

9   Local anesthesia for the child and adolescent

RALPH E. McDONALD
DAVID R. AVERY

It is generally agreed that one of the most important aspects of child behavior guidance is the control of pain. If children experience pain during restorative or surgical procedures, their future as dental patients may be damaged. Therefore it is important at each visit to reduce discomfort to a minimum and to control painful situations.

Since there is usually some discomfort associated with the procedure, a local anesthetic is almost always indicated when operative work is to be performed on the permanent teeth, and the same is true of cavity preparations in primary teeth. Dental procedures can be carried out more effectively if the child is comfortable and free of pain. The local anesthetic can prevent discomfort that may be associated with placing a rubber dam clamp, ligating teeth, and cutting tooth structure. Even the youngest child treated in the dental office normally presents no contraindications for the use of a local anesthetic.

Investigators have found that the injection is the dental procedure that produces the greatest negative response in children. Responses become increasingly negative over a series of four or five injections. Venham and Quatrocelli have reported that the series of dental visits sensitized the children to the stressful injection procedure while reducing their apprehension toward relatively nonstressful procedures. Thus dentists should antici-

pate the need for continued efforts to help the child cope with dental injections.

Topical anesthetics

The improved topical anesthetics that are available today greatly reduce the slight discomfort that may be associated with the insertion of the needle before the injection of the local anesthetic. Some topical anesthetics, however, present a disadvantage if they have a disagreeable taste to the child. Also, the additional time required to apply them may allow the child to become apprehensive concerning the approaching procedure.

Topical anesthetics are available in gel, liquid, ointment, and pressurized spray forms. However, the pleasant-tasting and quick-acting liquid, gel, or ointment preparations seem to be preferred by most dentists. These agents are applied to the oral mucous membranes with a cotton-tipped applicator. A variety of anesthetic agents have been used in topical anesthetic preparations, including ethyl aminobenzoate, butacaine sulfate, cocaine, dyclonine, lidocaine, and tetracaine.

Ethyl aminobenzoate (Benzocaine) liquid, ointment, or gel preparations are probably best suited for topical anesthesia in dentistry; they offer a more rapid onset and longer duration of anesthesia than other topical agents. They are not known to produce systemic toxicity as oral topical anesthet-

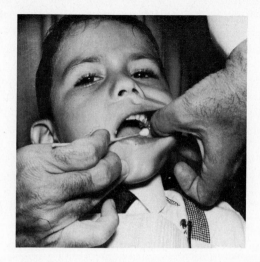

Fig. 9-1. Application of a topical anesthetic to the mucosa at the site of needle insertion will reduce discomfort associated with local anesthesia.

ics, but a few localized allergic reactions have been reported from prolonged or repeated use. Examples of the commercially available topical liquids are Topical Anesthetic (Blass),* Hurricaine,† and Topicale.‡ Hurricaine is also available in gel form, and Topicale is available in ointment form.

The mucosa at the site of the intended needle insertion is dried with gauze, and a small amount of the topical anesthetic agent is applied to the tissue with a cotton swab (Fig. 9-1). Topical anesthesia should be produced in approximately 30 seconds.

During the application of the topical anesthetic, the child should always be prepared for the injection. The explanation should not necessarily be a detailed description but simply an indication that the tooth is going to be put to sleep in order that decay can be removed without any discomfort.

Local anesthesia

In a survey of the use of local anesthesia for preschool children, McClure found that there is little factual information concerning injection procedures for young patients. He received considerable

interesting information from a questionnaire sent to 25 pedodontists, 25 oral surgeons, and 25 general practitioners. Many dentists responded that the local anesthetic should be warmed before injecting because it is more comfortable to the child, there is less tissue trauma and less postinjection pain, and the anesthetic seems to take effect more rapidly (Fig. 9-2).

Many dentists have recommended that aspiration be accomplished before injecting the local anesthetic solution (Fig. 9-3). It should be recognized, however, that aspiration is not always possible unless a large-gauge needle is used. Harris reported in a study of 8534 injections that 3.2% were positive to aspiration. As a result of his study, he advocates a needle no smaller than 25 gauge. Monheim believes that a 23-gauge needle is ideal for aspiration and that a needle smaller than 25 gauge is unwarranted and unsafe. He found that in 100 attempts in which aspiration of blood from a vein was attempted with 25-, 27-, and 29-gauge needles, aspiration was positive 3% of the time with the 29-gauge needle, 11% with the 27-gauge needle, and 98% with a 25-gauge needle.

Wittrock and Fischer and more recently Trapp and Davies have demonstrated that human blood

*Union Broach Co., Long Island City, N.Y. 11101.
†Beutlich, Inc., Chicago, Ill. 60645.
‡Premier Dental Products, Inc., Norristown, Pa. 19401.

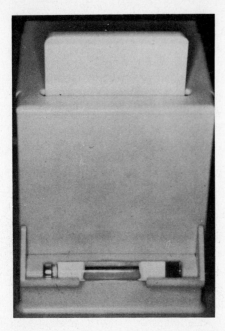

Fig. 9-2. Warming of the anesthetic solution will reduce postinjection discomfort.

can be readily aspirated with the smaller-gauge needles. Trapp and Davies reported positive aspiration through 23-, 25-, 27-, and 30-gauge needles without a clinically significant difference in resistance to flow. Regardless of the size of the needle used, it is generally agreed that the anesthetic solution should be injected slowly and the dentist should watch the patient closely for any evidence of an unexpected reaction.

The injections that are most commonly used in the treatment of children are described in the following sections.

Pressure injection ("jet" injection)

A technique of injecting local anesthetic by a pressure injection device rather than a needle has enjoyed renewed interest in recent years. This technique was introduced in 1947 by Figge and Scherer. A pressure injection instrument is based on the principle that small quantities of liquids forced through very small openings under high pressure (jets) can penetrate mucous membrane or

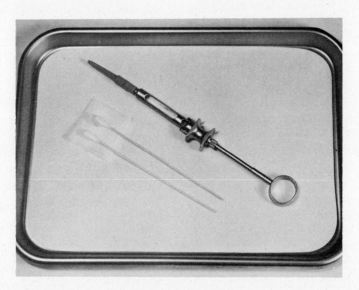

Fig. 9-3. Tray preparation for local anesthesia including a dry cotton applicator, a second applicator with a topical anesthetic ointment, and an aspirating syringe.

skin without causing excessive tissue trauma. One pressure injection device, the Syrijet Mark II,* holds a standard 1.8-ml Carpule of local anesthetic solution. It can be adjusted to expel 0.05 to 0.2 ml of solution under 2000 psi pressure.

Pressure injection produces surface anesthesia instantly and is used by some dentists instead of topical anesthetics. The method is quick and essentially painless, although the abruptness of the injection may produce momentary anxiety. The pressure injection technique is also useful for obtaining gingival anesthesia before placing a rubber dam clamp for isolation procedures that otherwise do not require local anesthetic, such as placing sealants in quadrants in which no operative procedures are planned. Similarly, soft tissue anesthesia may be obtained before band adaptation of partially erupted molars or for the removal of a very loose (soft tissue–retained) primary tooth. O'Toole has reported that the Syrijet may be employed in place of needle injections for nasopalatine, anterior palatine, and long buccal nerve blocks.

Anesthetizing mandibular teeth and soft tissue

Inferior alveolar nerve block (conventional mandibular block). When operative or surgical procedures are undertaken for the mandibular primary or permanent teeth, the inferior alveolar nerve must be blocked. The supraperiosteal injection technique may sometimes be useful in anesthetizing primary incisors, but it cannot be relied on for complete anesthesia of the mandibular primary or permanent molars.

Olsen reported that the mandibular foramen is situated at a lower level than the occlusal plane of the primary teeth of the child patient. Therefore the injection must be made slightly lower and more posteriorly than for an adult patient. An accepted technique is one in which the thumb is laid on the occlusal surface of the molars with the fingernail resting on the internal oblique ridge and the ball of the thumb resting in the retromolar fossa. Firm support during the injection procedure can be given

*Mizzy, Inc., Clifton Forge, Va. 24422.

by resting the ball of the middle finger on the posterior border of the mandible. The barrel of the syringe should be directed on a plane between the two primary molars on the opposite side of the arch. It is advisable to inject a small amount of the solution as soon as the tissue is penetrated and to continue to inject minute quantities as the needle is directed toward the mandibular foramen.

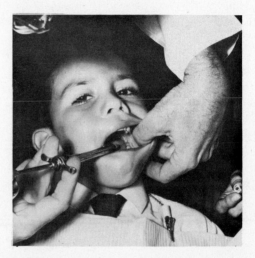

Fig. 9-4. The mandible is supported by the thumb and middle finger while the needle is directed toward the inferior alveolar nerve.

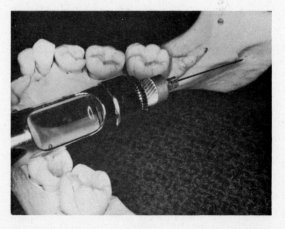

Fig. 9-5. Anesthetic solution is deposited around the inferior alveolar nerve.

The depth of insertion averages about 15 mm but will vary with the size of the mandible and its changing proportions depending on the age of the patient. Approximately 1 ml of the solution should be deposited around the inferior alveolar nerve (Figs. 9-4 and 9-5).

Lingual nerve block. The lingual nerve can be blocked by bringing the syringe to the opposite side with the injection of a small quantity of the solution as the needle is withdrawn. If small amounts of anesthetic are injected during insertion and withdrawal of the needle for the inferior alveolar nerve block, the lingual nerve will invariably be anesthetized as well.

Long buccal nerve block. For the removal of mandibular permanent molars or sometimes for the placement of a rubber dam clamp on these teeth, it is necessary to anesthetize the long buccal nerve. A small quantity of the solution may be deposited in the mucobuccal fold at a point distal and buccal to the indicated tooth (Fig. 9-6).

All the teeth on the side that has been injected will be anesthetized for operative procedures, with the possible exception of the central and lateral incisors, which may receive innervation from overlapping nerve fibers from the opposite side.

Infiltration for mandibular incisors. The terminal ends of the inferior alveolar nerves cross over the mandibular midline slightly and provide conjoined innervation of the mandibular incisors. Therefore a single inferior alveolar nerve block may not be adequate for operative or surgical procedures on the incisors, even on the side of the block anesthesia. The labial cortical bone overlying the mandibular incisors is usually thin enough for supraperiosteal anesthesia techniques to be effective.

If only superficial caries excavation of mandibular incisors is needed or if the removal of a partially exfoliated primary incisor is planned, infiltration anesthesia alone may be adequate. Incisor infiltration is most useful as an adjunct to an inferior alveolar nerve block when total anesthesia of the quadrant is desired. In this case the infiltration injection is made close to the midline on the side of

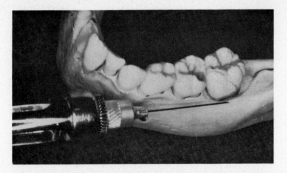

Fig. 9-6. In anesthetizing the long buccal nerve a small quantity of the solution may be deposited in the mucobuccal fold adjacent to the first permanent molar.

the block anesthesia, but the solution is deposited labial to the incisors on the opposite side of the midline. For example, if block anesthesia is used for the mandibular right quadrant, then anesthetic solution is infiltrated over the left mandibular incisors by inserting the needle just to the right of the midline diagonally toward the left incisors. Bilateral inferior alveolar nerve blocks are discouraged, especially in younger children, unless absolutely necessary.

Mandibular conduction anesthesia (Gow-Gates mandibular block technique). In 1973 Gow-Gates introduced a new method of obtaining mandibular anesthesia, which he referred to as "mandibular conduction anesthesia." This approach uses external anatomic landmarks to align the needle so that anesthetic solution is deposited at the base of the neck of the mandibular condyle. This technique is a nerve block procedure that anesthetizes virtually the entire distribution of the fifth cranial nerve in the mandibular area, including the inferior alveolar, lingual, buccal, mental, incisive, auriculotemporal, and mylohyoid nerves. Thus with a single injection the entire right or left half of the mandibular teeth and soft tissues can be anesthetized, with the possible exception of mandibular incisors, which may receive partial innervation from the incisive nerves of the opposite side. Gow-Gates suggested that once the technique

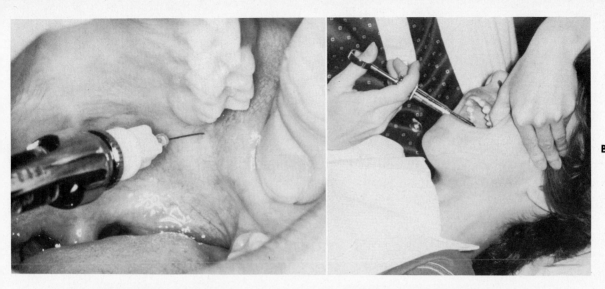

Fig. 9-7. A, Injection site for the Gow-Gates mandibular block technique. **B,** Barrel of the syringe is aligned parallel to a line from the corner of the mouth to the intertragic notch.

is learned properly, it rarely fails to produce good mandibular anesthesia. He had used the technique in practice more than 50,000 times. The technique has become increasingly popular and is often referred to as the ''Gow-Gates technique.''

The external landmarks to help align the needle for this injection are the tragus of the ear and the corner of the mouth. The needle is inserted just medial to the tendon of the temporal muscle and considerably superior to the insertion point for conventional mandibular block anesthesia. The needle is also inclined upward and parallel to a line from the corner of the patient's mouth to the lower border of the tragus (intertragic notch). The needle and the barrel of the syringe should be directed toward the injection site from the corner of the mouth on the opposite side (Fig. 9-7).

Anesthetizing maxillary primary and permanent incisors and canines

Supraperiosteal technique (local infiltration). Local infiltration (supraperiosteal technique) is used to anesthetize the primary anterior teeth. The injection should be made closer to the gingival margin than in the patient with permanent teeth, and the solution should be deposited close to the bone. After the needle tip has penetrated the soft tissue at the mucobuccal fold, it needs little advancement before the solution is deposited (2 mm at most), because the apices of the maxillary primary anterior teeth are essentially at the level of the mucobuccal fold. Some dentists prefer to ''pull'' the upper lip down over the needle tip to penetrate the tissue rather than advancing the needle upward. This approach works quite well for the maxillary anterior region (Figs. 9-8 to 9-10).

In anesthetizing the permanent central incisor teeth the puncture site is at the mucobuccal fold, so that the solution may be deposited slowly and slightly above and close to the apex of the tooth. Since there may be nerve fibers extending from the opposite side, it may be necessary to deposit a small amount of the anesthetic solution adjacent to the apex of the other central incisor to obtain adequate anesthesia in either primary or permanent teeth. If a rubber dam is to be applied, it is advisable to inject a drop or two of anesthetic solution into the lingual free marginal tissue to prevent the

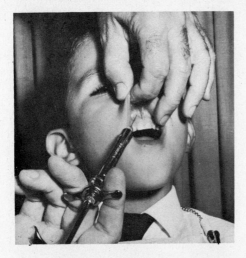

Fig. 9-8. Anesthetizing a primary central incisor. The supraperiosteal injection should be close to the bone and adjacent to the apex of the tooth.

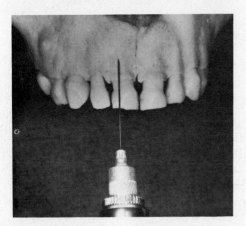

Fig. 9-9. Needle point is opposite the apex of the maxillary primary incisor.

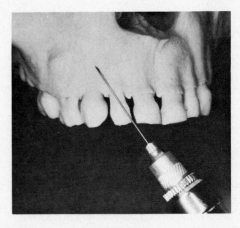

Fig. 9-10. Position of the needle for anesthetizing a maxillary primary canine.

discomfort associated with the placement of the rubber dam clamp and ligatures.

Before extraction of the incisors or canines in either the primary or permanent dentition, it will be necessary to anesthetize the palatal soft tissues. The nasopalatine injection will provide adequate anesthesia for the palatal tissues of all four incisors and at least partial anesthesia of the canine areas. Nerve fibers from the greater (anterior) palatine nerve usually extend to the canine area as well. If only a single anterior tooth is to be removed, adequate palatal anesthesia may also be obtained by depositing anesthetic solution in the attached palatal gingiva adjacent to the tooth to be removed. If it is observed that the patient does not have profound anesthesia of anterior teeth during the operative procedures with the supraperiosteal technique, a nasopalatine injection is advisable.

Anesthetizing maxillary primary molars and premolars

Traditionally dentists have been taught that the middle superior alveolar nerve supplies the maxillary primary molars, the premolars, and the mesio-

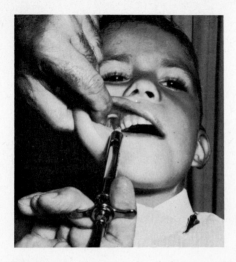

Fig. 9-11. Injecting the anesthetic solution to anesthetize the maxillary first primary molar for operative procedures.

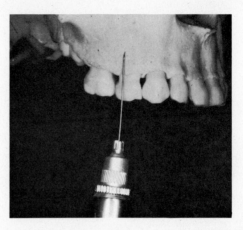

Fig. 9-12. Anesthetic solution is injected opposite the apices of the buccal roots of the first primary molar.

buccal root of the first permanent molar. There is no doubt that the middle superior alveolar nerve is at least partially responsible for the innervation of these teeth. However, Jorgensen and Hayden have demonstrated plexus formation of the middle and posterior superior alveolar nerves in the primary molar area on child cadaver dissections. The role of the posterior superior alveolar nerve in innervating the primary molar area has not previously received adequate attention. In addition, Jorgensen and Hayden have demonstrated maxillary bone thicknesses approaching 1 cm overlying the buccal roots of the first permanent and second primary molars in the skulls of children.

The bone overlying the first primary molar is thin, and this tooth can be adequately anesthetized by injecting anesthetic solution opposite the apices of the roots (Figs. 9-11 and 9-12). However, the thick zygomatic process overlies the buccal roots of the second primary and first permanent molars in the primary and early mixed dentition. This thickness of bone renders the supraperiosteal injection at the apices of the roots of the second primary molar much less effective; the injection should be supplemented with a second injection superior to the maxillary tuberosity area to block the posterior superior alveolar nerve as has been traditionally taught for permanent molars (Figs. 9-13 and 9-14). This supplemental injection will help compensate for the additional bone thickness and the posterior middle superior alveolar nerve plexus in the area of the second primary molar, which compromise the anesthesia obtained by injecting at the apices only.

To anesthetize the maxillary first or second premolar, a single injection is made at the mucobuccal fold to allow the solution to be deposited slightly above the apex of the tooth. Because of the horizontal and vertical growth of the maxilla that has occurred by the time the premolars erupt, the buccal cortical bone overlying their roots is thin enough to permit good anesthesia with this method. The injection should be made slowly, and the solution should be deposited close to the bone; these recommendations hold true for all supraperiosteal and block anesthesia techniques in dentistry.

Before operative procedures for maxillary primary molars and maxillary premolars, the appropriate injection technique(s) for the buccal tissues,

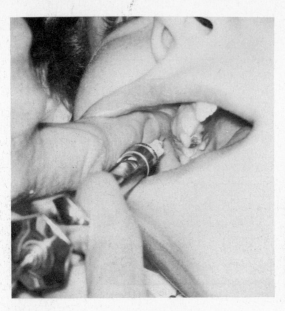

Fig. 9-13. Posterior superior alveolar injection for maxillary permanent molars and second primary molar. (Courtesy Dr. Paul E. Starkey.)

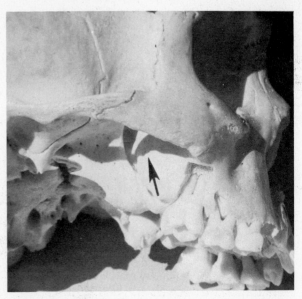

Fig. 9-14. Maxillary tuberosity target (*arrow*) area for posterior superior alveolar injection. (Courtesy Dr. Paul E. Starkey.)

as just described, should be performed. If the rubber dam clamp impinges on the palatal tissue, a drop or two of the anesthetic solution injected into the free marginal tissue lingual to the clamped tooth will alleviate the discomfort and will be less painful than the true greater (anterior) palatine injection. The greater palatine injection is indicated if maxillary primary molars or premolars are to be extracted or if palatal tissue surgery is planned.

Anesthetizing maxillary permanent molars

To anesthetize the maxillary first or second permanent molars, the child is instructed to partially close the mouth to allow the cheek and lips to be stretched laterally. The tip of the dentist's left forefinger (for a right-handed dentist) will rest in a concavity in the mucobuccal fold, being rotated to allow the fingernail to be adjacent to the mucosa. The bulbous portion of the finger is in contact with the posterior surface of the zygomatic process. Monheim suggests that the finger be on a plane at right angles to the occlusal surfaces of the maxillary teeth and at a 45-degree angle to the patient's sagittal plane. The index finger should point in the direction of the needle during the injection. The puncture point is in the mucobuccal fold above and distal to the distobuccal root of the first permanent molar. If the second molar has erupted, the injection should be made above the second molar. The needle is advanced upward and distally, depositing the solution over the apices of the teeth. The needle is inserted for a distance of approximately ¾ inch and in a posterior and upward direction; it should be positioned close to the bone with the bevel toward the bone (Figs. 9-13 and 9-14).

To complete the anesthesia of the first permanent molar for operative procedures, the supraperiosteal injection is made by inserting the needle in the mucobuccal fold and depositing the solution at the apex of the mesiobuccal root of the molar.

Anesthetizing the palatal tissues

Nasopalatine nerve block. Blocking the nasopalatine nerve will anesthetize the palatal tissues of

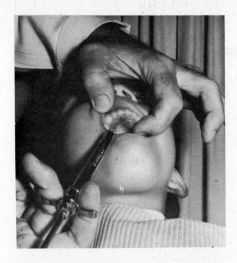

Fig. 9-15. Blocking of the nasopalatine nerve may be accomplished by injecting alongside the incisive papilla.

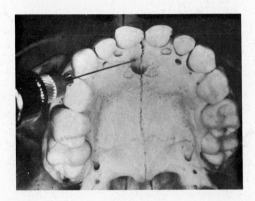

Fig. 9-16. The needle is directed upward into the incisive canal when anesthetizing the nasopalatine nerve.

the six anterior teeth. If the needle is carried into the canal, it is possible to anesthetize the six anterior teeth completely. However, this technique is painful and is not routinely used before operative procedures. If the patient experiences incomplete anesthesia after supraperiosteal injection above the apices of the anterior teeth on the labial side, it may be necessary to resort to the nasopalatine injection. The path of insertion of the needle is alongside the incisive papilla, just posterior to the central incisors. The needle is directed upward into the incisive canal (Figs. 9-15 and 9-16). Discomfort associated with the injection can be reduced by depositing the anesthetic solution in advance of the needle. When anesthesia of the canine area is required, it may be necessary to inject a small amount of anesthetic solution into the gingival tissue adjacent to the lingual aspect of the canine to anesthetize overlapping branches of the greater palatine nerve.

Greater (anterior) palatine injection. The greater palatine injection will anesthetize the mucoperiosteum of the palate from the tuberosity to the canine region and from the median line to the gingival crest on the injected side. This injection is used in conjunction with the middle or posterior alveolar nerve block before surgical procedures. The innervation of the soft tissues of the posterior two thirds of the palate is derived from the greater and lesser palatine nerves.

Before the injection is made, it is helpful to bisect an imaginary line drawn from the gingival

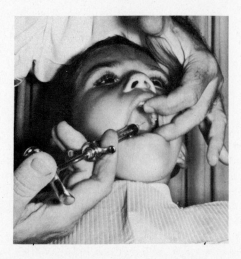

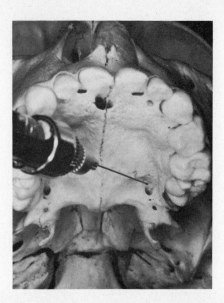

Fig. 9-17. Greater palatine injection is used in conjunction with the middle or posterior alveolar nerve block before removal of a maxillary primary molar.

Fig. 9-18. The needle is inserted approximately 10 mm posterior to the distal surface of the second primary molar.

border of the most posterior molar that has erupted to the midline. Approaching from the opposite side of the mouth, the dentist makes the injection along this imaginary line and distal to the last tooth (Figs. 9-17 and 9-18). In the child with only the primary dentition erupted, the injection should be made approximately 10 mm posterior to the distal surface of the second primary molar. It is not necessary to enter the greater palatine foramen. A few drops of the solution should be injected slowly at the point where the nerve emerges from the foramen.

Infraorbital nerve block and mental nerve block

The infraorbital nerve block and the mental nerve block are two additional local anesthetic techniques used by many dentists. The infraorbital nerve block anesthetizes the branches of the anterior and middle superior alveolar nerves. It also affects innervation of the soft tissues below the eye, half of the nose, and the oral musculature of the upper lip on the injected side of the face. This

leaves the child with a feeling of numbness above the mouth similar to that below the mouth when an inferior alveolar nerve is blocked. In addition there is temporary partial oral paralysis. These effects do not contraindicate the technique when it is truly needed. However, we find it difficult to justify in routine operative and extraction procedures for teeth innervated by the anterior and middle superior alveolar nerves, since the supraperiosteal techniques are more localized and just as effective. The infraorbital block technique is preferred for removal of impacted teeth (especially canines or first premolars) or large cysts, when moderate inflammation or infection contraindicates the supraperiosteal injection site, or when longer duration or a greater area of anesthesia is needed.

The mental nerve block leaves the patient with essentially the same feelings of numbness as the inferior alveolar nerve block. Blocking the mental nerve anesthetizes all mandibular teeth in the quadrant except the permanent molars. Thus the mental nerve block would make it possible to perform routine operative procedures on all primary teeth without discomfort to the patient. However, we believe that the inferior alveolar nerve block should be favored unless there is a specific contraindication at the inferior alveolar nerve injection site. The mental nerve block is no more comfortable for the patient, and the technique puts the syringe in clear view of the patient, whereas the inferior alveolar nerve block may be performed with the syringe out of the child's direct vision.

The reader is referred to Jorgensen and Hayden's *Sedation, Local and General Anesthesia in Dentistry* or Malamed's *Handbook of Local Anesthesia* for more detailed information concerning the infraorbital block, the mental block, or other local anesthetic techniques.

Periodontal ligament injection (intraligamentary injection)

The periodontal ligament injection has been used for many years as an adjunctive method of obtaining more complete anesthesia when supraperiosteal or block techniques failed to provide adequate anesthesia. Recently this technique has gained credibility as a good method of obtaining primary anesthesia for one or two teeth.

The technique is simple, requires only small quantities of anesthetic solution, and produces anesthesia almost instantly. The needle is placed in the gingival sulcus, usually on the mesial surface, and advanced along the root surface until resistance is met. Then approximately 0.2 ml of anesthetic is deposited into the periodontal ligament. For multirooted teeth, injections are made both mesially and distally. Considerable pressure is necessary to express the anesthetic solution.

A conventional dental syringe may be used for this technique. However, the great pressure required to express the anesthetic makes it desirable to use a syringe with a closed barrel to offer protection in the unlikely event that the anesthetic Carpule should break. Some syringes are equipped with a metal or Teflon sleeve that encloses the Carpule and provides the necessary protection should breakage occur.

Syringes designed specifically for the periodontal ligament injection technique have also been developed. One syringe, the Peri-Press,* is designed with a lever-action "trigger" that enables the dentist to deliver the necessary injection pressure conveniently. The Peri-Press syringe has a solid metal barrel and is calibrated to deliver 0.14 ml of anesthetic solution each time the trigger is completely activated (Fig. 9-19).

There are some possible psychologic disadvantages to the periodontal ligament injection technique, especially for the inexperienced pedodontic patient. The technique provides the patient with an opportunity to see the syringe and to watch the administration of the anesthetic. This may not be a significant problem for the experienced, well-adjusted dental patient, but it may contribute to the anxiety reaction of the new or anxiety-prone patient. In addition, the very design of the Peri-Press (resembling a handgun) probably has some adverse psychologic implication. Nevertheless, the periodontal ligament injection technique seems to offer a valuable adjunctive method of achieving dental anesthesia.

Malamed has reported a clinical study in which impressive results were obtained for certain procedures when the periodontal ligament injection technique was used. The sample size was extremely small for some procedures, and he pointed out that additional research was warranted. However, seven periodontal procedures (curettage and root planing) were performed with 100% effective anesthesia, and two teeth were extracted with 100% effective anesthesia (injections were administered to the mesial, distal, buccal, and lingual areas for these procedures). Seventy-one routine restorative procedures were performed under periodontal ligament anesthesia with 91.5% effectiveness. The technique proved 66.6% effective for crown preparations on 12 teeth, and eight endodontic procedures were adequately anesthetized only 50% of the time. Several different anesthetics were used, with and without vasoconstrictors, yet there

---

*University Dental Implements, Fanwood, N.J. 07023.

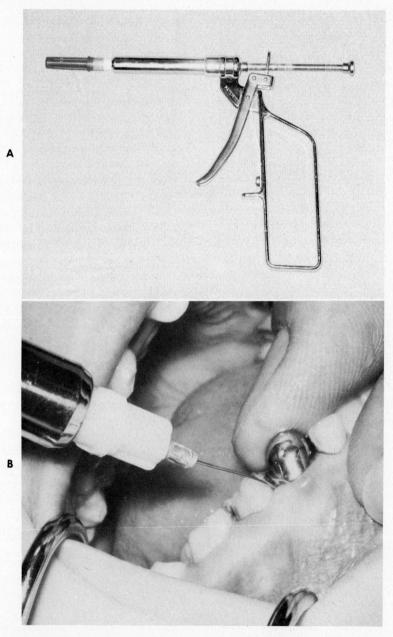

Fig. 9-19. A, Peri-Press syringe. **B,** Periodontal ligament injection of a mandibular first primary molar. (Courtesy Dr. John Bozic.)

seemed to be little difference in success rates or duration of pulpal anesthesia with the various agents. Because of the confined space and the limited blood circulation of the injection site for the periodontal ligament technique, vasoconstrictors may not be warranted as an additive to the anesthetic solution. In fact, vasoconstrictors might conceivably contribute to an ischemia of the periodontal ligament, which could at least contribute to localized postoperative discomfort or possibly cause more serious damage to the periodontal ligament. However, no serious postoperative problems have been reported with the technique. Walton and Abbott have also reported a clinical evaluation of the technique that showed a 92% success rate.

The periodontal ligament injection offers the following advantages for either primary or adjunctive anesthesia:

1. It provides reliable pain control rapidly and easily.
2. It provides pulpal anesthesia for 30 to 45 minutes, long enough for many single-tooth procedures without an extended period of postoperative anesthesia.
3. It is no more uncomfortable than other local anesthesia techniques and seems to be preferred by a large majority of patients.
4. It is completely painless if used adjunctively.
5. It requires very small quantities of anesthetic solution.
6. It does not require aspiration before injection.
7. It may be performed without removal of the rubber dam.
8. It may be useful in patients with bleeding disorders that contraindicate other injections.
9. It may be useful in young or handicapped patients in whom the problem of postoperative trauma to the lips or tongue is a concern.

Intraosseous injection, interseptal injection, and intrapulpal injection

Intraosseous, interseptal, and intrapulpal injection techniques have been known for many years,

but they have recently received renewed attention. The intrapulpal injection is an adjunctive anesthesia technique designed to obtain profound pulpal anesthesia during direct pulp therapy when other local anesthesia attempts have failed. The intrapulpal injection often provides the desired anesthesia, but the technique has the disadvantage of being painful initially although onset of anesthesia is usually rapid.

Intraosseous injection techniques (of which the interseptal injection is one type) require the deposition of local anesthetic solution in the porous alveolar bone. This may be done by forcing a needle through the cortical plate and into the cancellous alveolar bone, or a small round bur may be used to make an access in the bone for the needle. A small reinforced intraosseous needle may be used to penetrate the cortical plate more easily. This procedure is not particularly difficult in children because they have less dense cortical bone than adults. The intraosseous techniques have been advocated for both primary anesthesia and adjunctive anesthesia when other local injections have failed to produce adequate anesthesia. These techniques have been reported to produce profound pulpal anesthesia, but they do not seem to offer any advantages over the periodontal ligament injection except when the latter is contraindicated by infection in the periodontal ligament space.

Complications after a local anesthetic

True emergencies. Bennett identifies at least 16 possible complications of the psychologic effects of local anesthetic administration, the insertion of the needle, or the absorption of the anesthetic solution. This chapter is not intended to provide the reader with detailed information related to the management of these complications, some of which are life-threatening emergencies. Certainly all dentists should have and know how to use the basic life support equipment and drugs.

Anesthetic toxicity. Systemic toxicity from local dental anesthetics occurs only rarely because the quantity of anesthetic normally required to perform dental procedures does not approach toxic levels. Local anesthetic solutions are used so com-

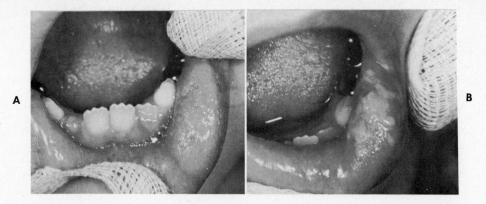

Fig. 9-20. A, Child who has ''chewed'' his lip after an inferior alveolar nerve block for operative procedures. **B,** Twenty-four hours after the initial trauma, a large ulcerated area is evident.

monly and so successfully by dentists that it is easy to forget that the drugs may be toxic if improperly used. It is most important for dentists who treat children to be acutely aware of the maximum recommended dosages of the anesthetic agents they use, since allowable dosages are based on the patient's weight. For example, according to the formula in *Accepted Dental Therapeutics* (Clark's rule), the toxic dose of lidocaine would be attained if hardly more than 1½ Carpules (3 ml) of 2% lidocaine with 1:100,000 epinephrine were injected at one time in a patient weighing 30 pounds (14 kg). Yet 5½ Carpules of the same anesthetic agent would be required to reach the toxic level in an adolescent patient weighing 100 pounds (46 kg). It is obvious that caution must be exercised when injecting local anesthetic agents in small children.

Trauma to soft tissue. Parents of children who receive regional local anesthesia in the dental office should be warned that the soft tissue in the area will be without sensation for a period of 1 hour or more. These children should be observed carefully so that they will not purposely or inadvertently bite the tissue. Children who receive an inferior alveolar injection for routine operative procedures may bite the lip, tongue, or inner surface of the cheek. Sometimes a parent calls the dentist's office an

hour or two after a dental appointment to report an injury to the child's oral mucous membrane. The parent may wonder if the accident occurred during the dental appointment; in all probability the child has chewed the area, and the result 24 hours later is an ulceration, often termed a ''traumatic ulcer'' (Fig. 9-20). Complications after a self-inflicted injury of this type are rare. However, the child should be seen in 24 hours, and a warm saline mouthrinse is helpful in keeping the area clean.

REFERENCES

American Dental Association: Accepted dental therapeutics, ed. 38, Chicago, 1979, The Association.

Bennett, C.R.: Monheim's local anesthesia and pain control in dental practice, ed. 6, St. Louis, 1978, The C.V. Mosby Co.

Figge, F.H.J., and Scherer, R.P.: Anatomical studies on jet penetration of human skin for subcutaneous medication without the use of needles, Anat. Rec. **97**(abs.):335, 1947.

Gow-Gates, G.A.E.: Mandibular conduction anesthesia: a new technique using extraoral landmarks, Oral Surg. **36**:321-328, 1973.

Harris, S.C.: Aspiration before injection of dental local anesthetics, Oral Surg. **15**:299-303, 1957.

Jorgensen, N.B., and Hayden, J., Jr.: Sedation, local and general anesthesia in dentistry, ed. 3, Philadelphia, 1980, Lea & Febiger.

Lilienthal, B.: A clinical appraisal of intraosseous dental anesthesia, Oral Surg. **39**:692-697, 1975.

Malamed, S.F.: Handbook of local anesthesia, St. Louis, 1980, The C.V. Mosby Co.

Malamed, S.F.: The periodontal ligament (PDL) injection: an alternative to inferior alveolar nerve block, Oral Surg. **53:**117-121, 1982.

McClure, D.B.: Local anesthesia for the preschool child, J. Dent. Child. **35:**441-448,1968.

Monheim, L.M.: Treatment and prevention of emergencies incidental to the use of anesthesia and the antibiotics, J. Oral Surg. **15:**289-298, 1957.

Olsen, N.H.: Anesthesia for the child patient, J.A.D.A. **53:**548-555, 1956.

O'Toole, T.J.: Administration of local anesthesia. In Snawder, K.D.: Handbook of clinical pedodontics, St. Louis, 1980, The C.V. Mosby Co.

Trapp, L.D., and Davies, R.O.: Aspiration as a function of hypodermic needle internal diameter in the in vivo human upper limb, Anesth. Prog. **27:**49-51, 1980.

Venham, L., and Quatrocelli, S.: The young child's response to repeated dental procedures, J. Dent. Res. **56:**734-738, 1977.

Walton, R.E., and Abbott, B.J.: Periodontal ligament injection: a clinical evaluation, J.A.D.A. **103:**571-575, 1981.

Wittrock, J.W., and Fischer, W.E.: The aspiration of blood through small-gauge needles, J.A.D.A. **76:**79-81, 1968.

10 Sedation and analgesia in pedodontics

JAMES A. WEDDELL
JAMES E. JONES

Behavior management for the child dental patient can be divided into three basic categories: psychologic, physical, and pharmacologic (the boxed material below illustrates a combination of the three). A personal approach by the dentist will reduce the child's apprehension and anxiety and promote rapport between the patient and dentist. The dentist should begin with tender loving care and maintain this atmosphere by consistent and firm management, positive reinforcement, and a pleasant manner to maintain the child's attention and cooperation. When pharmacologic aids are required, they should be used as adjuncts to rather than substitutes for the fundamental nonpharmaco-

logic approaches to behavior management. The dentist might combine the use of physical aids and extra assistance with mild tranquilizers, pharmacologic sedative agents, and inhalation sedative agents such as nitrous oxide and oxygen. A more extreme step is premedication with drug combinations that put the patient into a deeper state of sedation and analgesia. If these measures fail, general anesthesia can be used in the management of the dental patient. Whatever the combination, the safety of the child is of primary importance. Adequate preparation by the dentist, the assisting staff, the parents, and the patient allows the dentist to be efficient, effective, and well organized and promotes a reassuring air of confidence. Should a crisis arise, the dentist and staff are ready with appropriate emergency measures, including drug antidotes. As the child's knowledge of dental procedures increases, enhanced by a tell-show-do technique, he or she becomes gradually desensitized, and the dentist has less need for premedication agents.

Indications for use of premedication

Most children who have had proper guidance in the home, a happy home life, and satisfactory previous experience in the physician's or dentist's office will be satisfactory dental patients. However, there are always those few children who have behavioral problems or handicapping conditions or who are physically and mentally unable to cope with the situation. Such patients may be considered candidates for premedication. Results of a 1980

BASIC APPROACHES TO CHILD MANAGEMENT

1
Tender loving care and rapport
Consistently firm management
Positive reinforcement

2
Physical aids
Extra assistance
Tranquilizers and sedatives

3
Combinations of stronger premedications
General anesthesia

252

survey of attitudes and practices in behavior management by the American Academy of Pedodontics indicate that 80% of its members use premedication in certain cases, starting with children of 2 or younger and continuing with older patients. Behavior reactions cited as indications for premedication include fearfulness, hysteria, resistance, and aggression, and commonly used drugs include tranquilizers, chloral hydrate, and meperidine. Premedication has proved beneficial for long surgical or operative procedures for fearful and apprehensive children. To a limited degree, it may also be indicated for resistant and defiant children.

Parents' role in premedication

A consent from the parent or guardian regarding both premedication and dental treatment procedures for the child must be obtained in advance. Parents should be informed of procedures, medications, complications, and sequelae that might affect their child before, during, or after treatment. The parents should also be given a checklist to use in preparing the child for the appointment. The dentist's home telephone number should be on this checklist in case questions or problems arise. Information that should be made available to the parent before a premedication appointment includes the following:

1. The patient should have nothing by mouth (NPO) 3 to 4 hours before the appointment.
2. A parent must accompany the child.
3. Premedication does not usually eliminate the need for dental injections.
4. The child should never be left alone while under the effects of the medication.
5. The child will not be put to sleep, only "relaxed."
6. Because of a tendency toward drowsiness and clumsiness for several hours, the child should remain indoors and be watched closely after the appointment.
7. It is normal for the child to sleep after the appointment.
8. The parents should have the dentist's phone number and any other relevant information pertaining to their child.

Drug dosage

The following points should be considered when determining the dose of a premedicating drug for a child patient:

1. *Age of the child.* The younger the child, the *less* medication is required. The younger child may also exhibit a more atypical response to drug therapy. It should be kept in mind that allergenicity is greatest during childhood.
2. *Weight of the child.* The heavier child will require greater medication.
3. *Mental attitude of the child.* A nervous, excitable, or defiant child will usually require a larger dose of a drug.
4. *Physical activity of the child.* A child who appears to be hyperactive and hyperresponsive must be considered a candidate for increased drug dosage. Because children have a higher basal metabolic rate, their dosage in proportion to body weight must be greater than in adults (see boxed material below).
5. *Contents of the stomach.* The presence of food in the stomach can greatly alter drug absorption from the gastrointestinal tract following oral administration. To reduce nausea, the child should not take anything by mouth for 3 to 4 hours before the appointment when the use of premedication is anticipated.

METABOLIC RATE AT VARIOUS AGES

Rate	Cal/kg/hr
Premature	2.2
Full-term newborn	1.75
Infant	>2
Adult	1

From Levin, R.M.: Pediatric anesthesia handbook, Garden City, N.Y., 1973, Medical Examination Publishing Co., Inc.

6. *Time of day*. In general, a larger dose will be necessary at times other than normal rest periods. A young child patient, for instance, requires a greater amount during morning hours.

7. *Dosage formulas*. A therapeutic dose can cause unforeseeable problems in all age groups, especially in the very young or very old. The metric system is convenient in calculating drug dosages. Several commonly used rules to establish drug dosages for children between 2 and 10 years of age are given in the box below.

8. *Medical history*. Patients with a significant medical anomaly are the least predictable because of greater variability in physiologic and psychologic factors, which can influence the attainment of an effective concentration of the drug at the receptor.

9. *Level of sedation*. One dentist may consider sedation ideal when the patient makes no movements, whereas another prefers that the patient move or verbalize occasionally. Thus the amount of premedication varies according to the level of sedation desired.

10. *Route of administration*. Medication in young children can be given rectally, orally, intramuscularly, and by inhalation. In older children methods consist of oral, intramuscular, intravenous, and inhalation administration. Oral administration is the simplest and is associated with the fewest adverse effects. Furthermore, patients show less allergenicity with oral administration, although drug levels vary more because of absorption.

Routes of administration

Oral administration. Oral administration of premedication is most frequently used, and preparations are available in tablet, capsule, or liquid form. A child's ability to swallow tablets or capsules should be confirmed by the parent before such medications are prescribed. Tablets and capsules should be prescribed cautiously because aspiration of tablets may result in permanent brain damage from anoxia.

Since young children usually have difficulty swallowing tablets or capsules, a liquid form of the medication is preferred. However, some liquid

---

RULES FOR CALCULATING CHILDREN'S DOSAGES

Young's rule: $\dfrac{\text{Age of child (years)}}{\text{Age of child} + 12} \times \text{Adult dose} = \text{Child dose}$

Cowling's rule: $\dfrac{\text{Age of child at next birthday}}{24} \times \text{Adult dose} = \text{Child dose}$

Clark's rule: $\dfrac{\text{Weight of child (pounds)}}{150} \times \text{Adult dose} = \text{Child dose}$

Cassel's rule: Based on surface area and expressed as a percentage of the adult dose for patients weighing 145 pounds. (Since Cassel's rule uses the highest dose, it is not recommended for calculating local anesthetic dosages in children.)

Age	Pounds	Percentage of adult dosage
1	22	25%
3	33	33%
7	50	50%

Fried's rule: $\dfrac{\text{Age of child (months)}}{150} \times \text{Adult dose} = \text{Child dose}$

medications are not palatable, and having the child drink a carbonated beverage or juice immediately after the medication tends to minimize a negative reaction. The dosage of liquid medications should be prescribed in milliliters rather than teaspoons, since household teaspoons vary considerably (2.5 to 7.5 ml) and increase the likelihood of an underdose or overdose of medication. Although pharmacies provide devices for measurement of oral medications, the dentist may prefer to specify an oral syringe or medicine dropper for resistant patients.

Rectal or parenteral administration may be considered for the child who is unable to retain oral medication or who is not to be given anything orally. When the route of administration is changed, the dentist must also be aware of a possible need to change the dosage. For example, to obtain the same therapeutic blood level, the oral dosage of a medication must be larger than the intravenous dosage of the same drug.

Rectal administration. Rectal administration is infrequently used because of erratic absorption from the colon and absorption interference from fecal matter. Suppository drugs are most often used, and child restraint may be needed for proper insertion. For the child over 2 years of age, explanation is of particular importance to prevent extreme agitation. The child is usually placed in a Sims' or a knee-chest position. The suppository is lubricated with sterile, water-soluble jelly and gently inserted into the rectum beyond the internal sphincter. The child's buttocks are then held together for 5 to 10 minutes. If the child is prone to rectal abscesses, this route is contraindicated.

Parenteral administration. Parenteral administration of premedications includes intramuscular, intravenous, subcutaneous, and submucosal injections. We prefer and recommend the intramuscular and intravenous routes of administration. For an extremely small child, further dilution of the medication may be needed before administration. Injectable drugs should be properly labeled and stored, and expiration dates should be checked before use. The injection site should always be indicated on the dental record, and sites should be rotated for subsequent injections, thereby reducing the chance of tissue irritation. The child must always be restrained to avoid accidental injection in the wrong site or breaking the needle. Care must be taken to have a firm grasp on the lower portion of the syringe, since the child may move.

Intramuscular administration. The age of the child, the number of injections required, the muscle mass, the tissue integrity, and the amount of solution to be injected all influence the site selection for intramuscular administration. Table 10-1 illustrates the maximum amount of solution for a normally developing child.

A 27-gauge short needle is usually appropriate to penetrate the fat over the injection site and to deliver the medication into the muscle. The vastus lateralis muscle in the thigh is the site of choice because it is the largest muscle mass and is relatively free of major nerves and vessels. The injection site can be obtained by "pinching up" the

Table 10-1. Guidelines for maximum amounts of solutions to be injected into muscle tissues

Muscle group	Birth to 1½ yr (ml)	1½ to 3 yr (ml)	3 to 6 yr (ml)	6 to 15 yr (ml)	15 yr to adulthood (ml)
Deltoid	Not recommended	0.5*	0.5	0.5	1
Gluteus maximus	Not recommended	1*	1.5	1.5-2	2-2.5
Ventrogluteal	Not recommended	1*	1.5	1.5-2	2-2.5
Vastus lateralis	0.5-1	1	1.5	1.5-2	2-2.5

From Howry, L.B., Bindler, R.M., and Tso, Y.: Pediatric medications, Philadelphia, 1981, J.B. Lippincott Co.
*Not recommended unless other sites are not available.

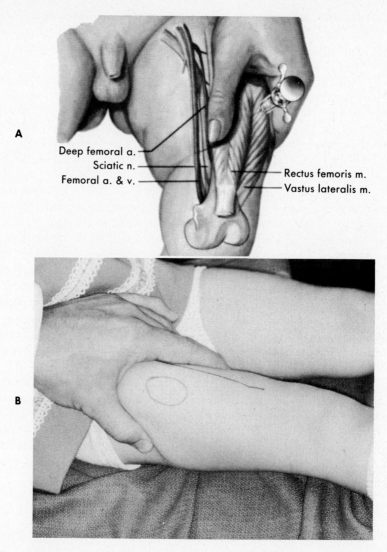

A

Deep femoral a.
Sciatic n.
Femoral a. & v.

Rectus femoris m.
Vastus lateralis m.

B

Fig, 10-1. A, Vastus lateralis region of child illustrating intramuscular injection site. **B,** Circle delineates the injection site on the thigh. (**A** courtesy Wyeth Laboratories, Philadelphia.)

muscle in the outer medial aspect of the center one third of the thigh (Fig. 10-1). For children from birth to 3 years, the dosage is 0.5 to 1 ml of solution. From 3 to 6 years, 1.5 ml can be used safely.

The gluteus maximus muscle in the buttock can also be considered an injection site after the age of 2½ or 3 years or after the child has walked for 1 year. The needle is inserted into the upper outer quadrant of the muscle mass to avoid the sciatic nerve, which is large and runs through the medial portion of the muscle. For patients less than 6 years of age, this site is recommended only if the vastus lateralis site is contraindicated (Fig. 10-2).

From 6 to 15 years, 1.5 to 2 ml can be used in either the thigh or buttock. Another site is the del-

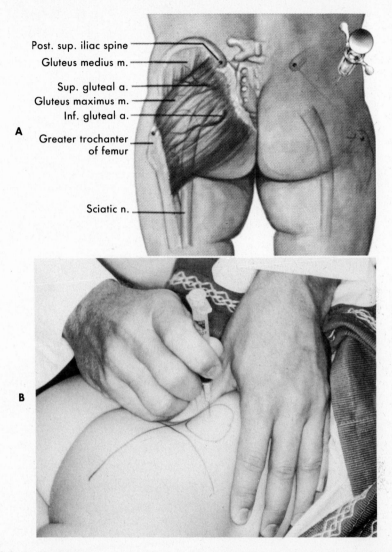

Post. sup. iliac spine
Gluteus medius m.
Sup. gluteal a.
Gluteus maximus m.
Inf. gluteal a.

A

Greater trochanter
of femur

Sciatic n.

B

Fig. 10-2. A, Gluteal region of child illustrating intramuscular injection site. **B,** Injection site on the buttock area. (**A** courtesy Wyeth Laboratories, Philadelphia.)

toid muscle, which is not used with children younger than 6 years because of their small muscle mass. This site also requires careful attention to positioning. To avoid nerves, the syringe should be placed in the center of the muscle mass at the junction of the lower and middle thirds (Fig. 10-3).

Intravenous administration. For premedication in young infants and toddlers, the intramuscular route is preferred over the intravenous route because of the difficulty and complications in starting intravenous infusions, the rapidity of adverse reactions, and the need for close rate-monitoring of fluids. However, when the child is receiving certain antibiotics intramuscularly for a prolonged period (7 to 14 days), the intravenous route is preferred because of the limited number of intramuscular

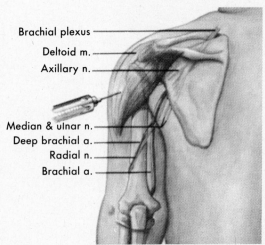

Brachial plexus

Deltoid m.

Axillary n.

Median & ulnar n.

Deep brachial a.

Radial n.

Brachial a.

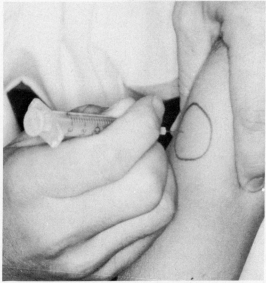

Fig. 10-3. A, Deltoid region illustrating intramuscular injection site. **B,** Injection site on the upper arm. (**A** courtesy of Wyeth Laboratories, Philadelphia.)

injection sites in the young child. Intravenous administration has the advantage of achieving therapeutic blood levels more quickly. In older patients, premedication involving the intravenous route can be very effective and safe, depending on the length of the procedure and the expertise of the clinician.

Monitoring patients receiving premedication

The patient's vital signs must be monitored every 10 minutes during a premedication appointment, since an individual's physiologic responses may vary. The heart rate can be monitored by palpation, by the Doppler* (ultrasonic flow detection), or by the Datascope,† which has multiple capacities (Fig. 10-4). Blood pressure can be carefully monitored by a cuff and stethoscope or the Doppler. Respiration can be observed and recorded, and temperature measurements can be monitored via a probe or a thermometer. Table 10-2 shows average pulse, blood pressure, and respiratory rates at various ages in children. Deviations from these recordings act as warning signals, and the dentist then makes proper adjustments to ensure the child's safety during the course of the appointment. An emergency kit with resuscitation equipment should be readily available during premedication appointments in case of respiratory or cardiovascular problems.

Drug selection

The ideal agent for safe premedication is efficient, rapidly absorbed, and nonirritating; it has minimal side effects and does not depress vital functions. The desired reactions of the dental patient to the pharmacologic agent are reduced anxiety and fear, an increased pain threshold, and improved coping with the dental visit. The dosage of the premedication must be considered because it greatly affects the characteristics of the premedication.

---

*Doppler -811, Parks Electronics Laboratory, Beaverton, Ore. 97005.
†Datascope Corp. 871-Monitor, Paramus, N.J. 07652.

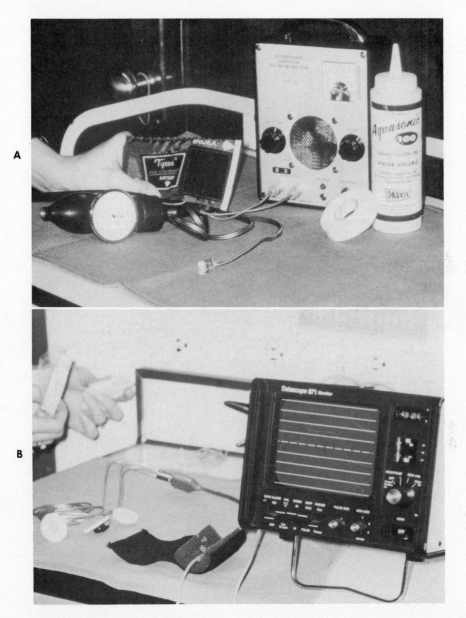

Fig. 10-4. A, Doppler and, **B,** Datascope instruments that facilitate monitoring the patient's vital signs during treatment under heavy sedation.

Table 10-2. Average pulse, blood pressure, and respiratory rates at various ages

Age	Average pulse rates at rest (beats/min)
Birth	140
1-6 mo	130
6-12 mo	115
1-2 yr	110
2-4 yr	105
4-6 yr	100
6-10 yr	95
10-14 yr	85
14-18 yr	82

	Average blood pressure (mm Hg)
Newborn	78/42
1 mo	86/54
6 mo	90/60
1 yr	96/65
2 yr	99/65
4 yr	99/65
6 yr	100/60
8 yr	105/60
10 yr	110/60
12 yr	115/60
14 yr	118/60
16 yr	120/65

	Average respiratory rates (breaths/min)
Premature	40-90
Newborn	30-80
1 yr	20-40
2 yr	20-30
3 yr	20-30
5 yr	20-25
10 yr	17-22
15 yr	15-20
20 yr	15-20

Modified and reproduced with permission from Lowrey, G.H.: Growth and development of children, 7th edition. Copyright 1978 by Year Book Medical Publishers, Inc., Chicago.

Although many drugs are available for premedication, relatively few are used. Aside from nitrous oxide, these drugs usually fall into one of the following categories: narcotics, barbiturates, antihistamines, or tranquilizers. A 1980 survey of the members of the Association of Pedodontic Diplomates identified the following premedications as the most commonly used:

Agent	Percent of members using
Tranquilizers	65
Chloral hydrates	50
Narcotics	46
Antihistamines	32
Barbiturates	15
Nitrous oxide–oxygen	
Used always or in selected cases	74
Never used	25

Compared to a 1971 survey of the same association, a significant increase in the amount of nitrous oxide analgesia is noted—with slight decrease in the use of other premedications. Ideally, dentists should limit themselves to the use of only a few drugs for managing the behavior of child patients, thereby gaining greater experience and expertise with these medications. Drug selections can be based on the behavior patterns exhibited by the child during the dentist's initial contact and the ability of the operator to achieve patient control using appropriate psychologic and physical management methods. Children with multiple handicaps (psychologic, physical, and medical) have a greater need for premedication than the general population, and they require more individual assessment so that drug selection will not interfere with their condition and yet will produce meaningful results. Selection usually falls into the following categories:

1. *Mild.* This category is useful for children who are tense, uncooperative, fearful, or outwardly apprehensive and who need some sort of preventive measure to get them past the first few appointments. As they mature into better dental patients, they usually do not need medication. For this category, drug selection is usually limited to:

a. Inhalation sedation with nitrous oxide–oxygen
b. An antianxiety drug such as hydroxyzine, administered orally
c. A phenothiazine derivative such as promethazine, administered orally
d. A benzodiazepine such as diazepam, administered orally
e. A sedative-hypnotic nonbarbiturate such as chloral hydrate, administered orally

2. *Moderate to severe.* This category is useful for children who are agitated and who obviously need some sort of pharmacologic aid, such as the following (some of which can be used either separately or in combination):
a. Inhalation sedation (with nitrous oxide–oxygen as an adjunct)
b. A benzodiazepine such as diazepam, administered orally, intramuscularly, or intravenously
c. A narcotic such as meperidine, administered intramuscularly or intravenously
d. Phenothiazines such as chlorpromazine and promethazine, administered intramuscularly as an adjunct
e. A sedative-hypnotic agent such as secobarbital, administered orally, intramuscularly, or intravenously

Highlights regarding many commonly used premedication agents in pedodontics are presented in the following discussion. However, the reader should recognize that the effects of these drugs are often multiple. For example, meperidine is classified as an analgesic agent, but it is also effective as a sedative-hypnotic.

Sedative-hypnotics. Barbiturates are effective sedative-hypnotics depending on the dose given, but they currently have limited use because of varying patient reactions, frequent side effects, and the availability of more effective premedications. This group of drugs has no analgesic effect.

Secobarbital (Seconal)

INDICATIONS: To help control anxiety, apprehension, and uncooperative attitudes in the pediatric dental patient

CHARACTERISTICS:
Mode of action:
1. Unknown—acts on all levels of the central nervous system (CNS), especially cortical regions
2. Onset—within 30 minutes when administered orally
3. Duration—3 to 4 hours
Properties:
1. Respiratory depression (especially with parenteral use)
2. CNS depression
3. Sleep-inducing
4. Slow elimination—slowly excreted by kidneys in 24 to 48 hours
5. Anticonvulsant potency
6. No analgesic action

SIDE REACTIONS:
1. Lassitude, restlessness
2. Vertigo, ataxia
3. Headache
4. Nausea, vomiting
5. Skin rash
6. Paradoxic hyperexcitability

PRECAUTIONS:
1. Lowers anticoagulant effects of coumarin
2. Has abuse potential
3. Has slow drug tolerance and cumulative effects
4. May precipitate excitement in patient with uncontrolled pain

CONTRAINDICATIONS:
1. Hepatic and/or renal dysfunction
2. Thyroid hypofunction
3. Barbiturate hypersensitivity
4. Concurrent use of other medications
5. Porphyria
6. Diabetes mellitus

FORMS AND DOSAGES COMMONLY USED IN CHILDREN:
Forms:
1. Capsules, 50 mg, 100 mg
2. Elixir, 20 mg/5 ml
3. Injectable, 50 mg/ml; 20-ml vial (more frequent complications with intramus-

cular administration requiring monitoring of vital signs for 30 minutes; intravenous infusion not recommended because of potent respiratory depression and lack of reversal agent)

Dosages:

0.50 to 1 mg/pound (children younger than 5 years), administered orally

1 to 3 mg/pound (children older than 5 years), administered orally

Not to exceed 200 mg/dose (with dosage adjusted to prevent excitement stage)

Chloral hydrate (Noctec, Kessodrate, Somnos, Aquachloral Supprettes)

INDICATIONS: To control and relieve mild to moderate anxiety by sedation and hypnotic action on the young child, especially the toddler

CHARACTERISTICS:

Mode of action:

1. Acts on CNS at cerebral hemispheres (exact mechanism unknown)
2. Onset—30 to 60 minutes when administered orally
3. Duration—6 to 8 hours but shorter effective working time for dental procedures (1 to 2 hours)

Properties:

1. Nonbarbiturate sedative
2. Safe and reliable
3. Rapidly effective
4. Sleep-inducing
5. Anxiety-alleviating
6. Absence of hangover
7. Unpleasant taste

SIDE REACTIONS:

1. Slight depression of respiration
2. Slight depression of blood pressure
3. Gastric irritation (nausea, vomiting)
4. Vertigo, ataxia

PRECAUTIONS:

1. Depresses contractility of myocardium and causes circulatory weakness
2. Potentiated with ethyl alcohol
3. Has chronic abuse potential

4. Causes warfarin-induced hypoprothrombinemia (if used for patient also taking warfarin)
5. Has no antidote; overdose treated by gastric lavage
6. Can cause coma, respiratory depression, hypotension, and hypothermia with toxic dose

CONTRAINDICATIONS:

1. Hepatic or renal impairment
2. Hypersensitivity
3. Gastritis, ulcers

FORMS AND DOSAGES COMMONLY USED IN CHILDREN:

Forms:

1. Capsules, 250 mg, 500 mg
2. Syrup, 500 mg/5 ml
3. Suppository, 650 mg, 1.3 g
4. Administered only orally, with full glass of water, juice, or milk to reduce gastrointestinal distress

Dosages:

25 to 50 mg/kg body weight (maximum of 1 g initially) for children over 60 pounds, less for sedation

ADJUNCT: May be used with other premedications and inhalation sedation

Antianxiety agents. Benzodiazepines are a group of antianxiety compounds that have depressant effects on the subcortical levels of the CNS. Diazepam is commonly used in pedodontic practice because of the wide margin of safety between therapeutic and toxic doses in children.

Diazepam (Valium)

INDICATIONS: For relief of mild to moderate tension and anxiety in the tense, cooperative child. Used intravenously to relieve moderate anxiety in the older child or teenager; also used in treatment of alcoholism and convulsive disorders

CHARACTERISTICS:

Mode of action:

1. Acts on parts of the limbic system (hypothalamus)

2. Oral administration preferred over intramuscular administration
3. Rapidly absorbed by gastrointestinal tract in 30 minutes
4. Duration—approximately 4 hours

Properties:
1. Benzodiazepine derivative
2. Tension and anxiety reliever
3. Skeletal muscle relaxant
4. Safety (difficult to administer overdose)

SIDE REACTIONS:
1. Drowsiness
2. Fatigue
3. Ataxia
4. Syncope
5. Hallucinations
6. Change in salivation
7. Amnesia produced when used intravenously
8. Skin rash, nausea

PRECAUTIONS:
1. Should not be mixed with other solutions
2. Depresses CNS
3. Potentiated by narcotics, monoamine oxidase inhibitors, barbiturates, and alcohol
4. Has abuse potential
5. Has prolonged effect (reduced clearance) with cimetidine

CONTRAINDICATIONS:
1. Pregnant women (hazardous to fetus, known to produce clefts in mice)
2. Children under 6 months of age
3. Patients with acute narrow-angle glaucoma
4. Known hypersensitivity
5. Hepatic or renal dysfunction

FORMS AND DOSAGES COMMONLY USED IN CHILDREN:

Forms:
1. Tablets, 2 mg, 5 mg, 10 mg
2. Injection, 5 mg/ml, 2-ml disposable syringe

Dosages:

Children over 2 years of age: 2 to 5 mg orally 1 hour before appointment

Teenagers: 5 to 10 mg orally 1 hour before appointment

Slow intravenous administration (not to exceed 1 ml [5 mg]/minute); dose, 0.25 mg/kg

ADJUNCT: When used with meperidine, may lower the blood pressure and potentiate the meperidine

Narcotic analgesics. Narcotic drugs are useful in dentistry for their analgesic properties as well as their sedative-hypnotic effect. Local anesthetics are still indicated as premedication agents for operative or surgical procedures.

Alphaprodine (Nisentil), fentanyl (Sublimaze), and meperidine (Demerol) are narcotics that have been used frequently as premedication agents in dentistry. Their actions are similar, but their dosages are quite different. Thus extreme caution is required if the dentist chooses to keep more than one of these drugs on hand for use. Meperidine is presented as a representative agent of this drug group.

Meperidine (Demerol)

INDICATIONS: Management of moderately to severely disruptive behavior in children; also relieves moderate pain

CHARACTERISTICS:

Mode of action:
1. Uncertain
2. Absorbed in 20 to 60 minutes from the gastrointestinal tract
3. Onset—10 to 15 minutes parenterally
4. Duration—3 to 4 hours

Properties:
1. Synthetic narcotic opiate
2. Analgesic
3. Sedative
4. Spasmolytic
5. Euphoria-producing

SIDE REACTIONS:
1. Itching nose
2. Nausea

3. Blushing of face
4. Dryness of mouth
5. Syncope
6. Profuse perspiration
7. Dizziness
8. Respiratory depression
9. Postural hypotension

PRECAUTIONS:

1. Causes severe depression if given with a monoamine oxidase inhibitor
2. Is metabolized in liver and excreted in urine (contraindicated for patients with liver damage)
3. May cause adverse reaction with alcohol and tricyclic antidepressants
4. May produce such reactions as respiratory depression, hypotension, profound sedation, and unconsciousness

CONTRAINDICATIONS:

1. Hypersensitivity
2. Severe hepatic dysfunction
3. Head injuries with increased intracranial pressure

FORMS AND DOSAGES COMMONLY USED IN CHILDREN:

Forms:

1. Elixir, 50 mg/5 ml
2. Tablets, 50 mg
3. Injection, 25 mg/ml, 75 mg/ml, in 1-ml or 2-ml disposable syringe
4. Injection, 50 mg/ml, 1 ml, in 2-ml disposable syringe or 30-ml vial
5. Injection (mepergan), 2-ml disposable syringe (meperidine, 25 mg; promethazine, 25 mg)

Dosages:

Orally or intramuscularly: 0.5 to 1 mg/pound or 2 mg/kg
Intravenously: 0.3 to 0.5 mg/kg

ADJUNCT: Used with promethazine, hydroxyzine, chlorpromazine, and diazepam (Note: when used in a combination, administer lower dose)

Narcotic antagonists. Antagonists (levallorphan and nalorphine, and more recently, naloxone) tend to reverse the harmful effects, including respiratory depression, of overdosages of natural and synthetic narcotics. Since none of these antidotes reverses respiratory depression resulting from barbiturates, basic resuscitation procedures are still used as essential adjuncts. Naloxone has fewer disadvantages and is the preferred narcotic antagonist.

Naloxone (Narcan)

INDICATIONS: Acts as antidote; reverses narcotic overdose; allows early discharge of ambulatory patients

CHARACTERISTICS:

Mode of action:

1. Onset rapid when given intravenously
2. Short duration
3. Intramuscular administration has longer duration than intravenous

Properties:

1. Pure narcotic antagonist
2. No pharmacologic activity
3. Also antidote to synthetic narcotics, propoxyphene, nalbuphine, pentazocine, and butorphanol
4. No known psychologic or physical dependence

SIDE REACTIONS:

1. Nausea and vomiting in excess dosages
2. Precipitates withdrawal symptoms in addicts

PRECAUTIONS: Cardiac irritability

CONTRAINDICATIONS: Hypersensitivity

FORMS AND DOSAGE:

Forms:

1. Intravenous, intramuscular, or subcutaneous injection: 0.01 mg/kg body weight
2. Injection (neonatal): 0.02 mg/ml, 2-ml ampules
3. Injection: 0.04 mg/ml, 1-ml ampules

Dosage:

Adult dose: 0.4 mg initially, repeated at 2- to 3-minute intervals as needed (dose may have to be repeated because duration of narcotics exceeds that of naloxone)

Anthistamines. Antihistamines are a heterogeneous group of therapeutic agents with multiple pharmacologic actions that antagonize histamines, thereby reversing smooth-muscle and nerve stimulation (that is, they are anticholinergic). Those commonly used in pediatric premedications include hydroxyzine (Vistaril, Atarax), diphenhydramine (Benadryl), and promethazine (Phenergan).

Hydroxyzine pamoate (Vistaril) and hydroxyzine hydrochloride (Atarax)

INDICATIONS: To alleviate manifestations of mild anxiety and tension in dental and other minor surgical procedures on the preschool or young school-age child; also useful in urticaria, pruritus, and enhancement of narcotics

CHARACTERISTICS:

Mode of action:
1. Rapidly absorbed by gastrointestinal tract in 15 to 30 minutes
2. Duration—approximately 3 to 4 hours
3. May suppress activity in certain key regions of subcortical areas of the CNS
4. Not a cortical depressant

Properties:
1. Rapid-acting ataractic with wide margin of safety (for example, absence of toxic effects on blood or liver—metabolized in liver and excreted in urine)
2. Antihistaminic
3. Antiemetic
4. Antispasmodic
5. Anticholinergic

SIDE REACTIONS:
1. Dryness of mouth
2. Drowsiness
3. No serious side effects reported and confirmed

PRECAUTIONS:
1. Potentiates CNS depressants (when used as adjunct, dosage decreased by 50%)
2. Causes drowsiness

CONTRAINDICATIONS:
1. Hypersensitivity
2. Parenteral form (never used subcutaneously or intravenously)

FORMS AND DOSAGES COMMONLY USED IN CHILDREN:

Forms:
1. Capsules (Vistaril), 25 mg, 50 mg
2. Intramusular injection (Vistaril), 10 mg/0.5 ml
3. Syrup (Atarax), 10 mg/5 ml

Dosages:
Depends on activity and behavior of the child; 25 to 50 mg 2 hours before treatment and 25 to 100 mg 1 hour preoperatively; over 6 years of age, 50 to 100 mg the night before treatment and 100 mg 1 hour preoperatively

ADJUNCT: Used with nitrous oxide–oxygen, meperidine, and chloral hydrate

Diphenhydramine (Benadryl)

INDICATIONS: For use in patient control of hypersensitivity reactions, local analgesia, motion sickness, and anxiety

CHARACTERISTICS:

Mode of action:
1. Competes with histamine for cell receptor sites on the cell's effector
2. Onset—30 to 60 minutes
3. Duration—4 to 6 hours

Properties:
1. Antihistaminic
2. Anticholinergic (drying)

SIDE REACTIONS:
1. Dryness of mouth
2. More drowsiness than caused by hydroxyzine
3. Tachycardia
4. Myocardial contraction
5. Excitation in the very young

PRECAUTIONS:
1. Hypertension
2. Heart disease
3. Glaucoma
4. Ulcer
5. Bladder obstruction, prostatic hypertrophy
6. Potentiator of alcohol and other CNS depressants

7. Overdose reactions include CNS depression, symptoms like those of atropine overdose, CNS stimulation in young children

CONTRAINDICATIONS:
1. Hypersensitivity
2. Newborn
3. Lower respiratory tract disease
4. Patients taking monoamine oxidase inhibitors

FORMS AND DOSAGES COMMONLY USED IN CHILDREN:

Forms:
1. Capsules, 25 mg, 50 mg
2. Elixir, 12.5 mg/5 ml
3. Both: 5 mg/kg/24 hr in four doses orally

Dosages:
Ampule, 1-ml and 10-ml vials
Parenteral dose: 5 mg/kg/24 hr—four doses not to exceed 300 mg; intravenous route is only recommended parenteral route

ADJUNCT: When used in combination with narcotics and other premedications, dosage decreased by 50%

Antipsychotic agents. Most of the phenothiazine derivatives may be classified as antipsychotic agents. The phenothiazines commonly used in dentistry include promethazine (Phenergan), chlorpromazine (Thorazine), and prochlorperazine (Compazine).

Extrapyramidal reactions can occur with phenothiazines. It is important to inform the patient of the possibility of these side effects to avoid fear and panic if they occur. Extrapyramidal reactions include dystonia and parkinsonism occurring early in therapy, which are manifested by spasms of neck muscles, spine and extremities, and eye muscles and facial grimacing. Parkinsonian symptoms are muscle rigidity and tremor. Other reactions include akathisia (constant moving of extremities) and restlessness. Management of these reactions includes discontinuation of medication, intravenous administration of antiparkinson medications such as diphenhydramine (Benadryl), or injection of intramuscular benztropine mesylate (Cogentin).

Promethazine (Phenergan). Promethazine, probably one of the most commonly administered mild pedodontic premedications, is often used in combination with meperidine.

INDICATIONS: To manage nausea, vomiting, preoperative and operative sedation, relief of apprehension and anxiety, and various allergic reactions (produces light sleep but patient is easily aroused)

CHARACTERISTICS:
Mode of action:
1. Acts on higher neural centers of diencephalon
2. Inhibits chemoreceptor trigger zone, the hypothalamus, and the reticular substance
3. Is well absorbed (15 to 30 minutes' onset)
4. Has 4- to 6-hour duration

Properties:
1. Phenothiazine derivative
2. Sedative and tranquilizer properties
3. Antiemetic
4. Antihistaminic

SIDE REACTIONS:
1. Dryness of mouth
2. More drowsiness than caused by diphenhydramine
3. Extrapyramidal reactions fairly unlikely
4. Mild hypotension (postural)
5. "Phenergan reaction"

PRECAUTIONS:
1. Potentiates CNS depressants
2. Causes chemical irritation at injection site
3. Is incompatible with alkaline drugs

CONTRAINDICATIONS:
1. Hypersensitivity
2. Blood dyscrasia or jaundice
3. Psychic or drug-induced depression
4. Severe asthma
5. Glaucoma
6. Children under 6 months of age

FORMS AND DOSAGES COMMONLY USED IN
  CHILDREN:
  Forms:
   1. Tablets, 12.5 mg, 25 mg orally
   2. Syrup (Phenergan Fortis), 25 mg/5 ml
      orally
   3. Suppository, 25 mg, 50 mg rectally
  Dosages:
   Oral: 0.5 to 1 mg/pound
   Injection: 25 mg/ml, 50 mg/ml, 1-ml am-
     pule
ADJUNCT: In combination: 0.25 to 0.5 mg/
  pound with meperidine, chloral hydrate, or
  barbiturates
Chlorpromazine (Thorazine)
INDICATIONS: To control severe anxiety and
  apprehension (used infrequently and only in
  combination because of undesirable side reactions)
CHARACTERISTICS:
  Mode of action:
   1. CNS dopaminergic receptor-blocking
   2. Inhibitory effects on chemoreceptor
      trigger zone in medulla
   3. Onset—1 hour when taken orally
   4. Duration—4 to 6 hours
  Properties:
   1. Sedation
   2. Anticholinergic effects
   3. Potentiator of barbiturates, antihista-
      mines, and narcotics
   4. Antiemetic
SIDE REACTIONS:
   1. Xerostomia, urinary retention, constipa-
      tion
   2. Blurred vision
   3. Nasal congestion
   4. Drowsiness
   5. Postural hypotension and tachycardia
   6. Agranulocytosis, increased susceptibility
      to infections, weight gain, edema, and
      photosensitivity with chronic use
PRECAUTIONS:
   1. CNS depression
   2. Possibility of hypotension with overdose

   3. Extrapyramidal reaction
   4. Antihistamine, barbiturate, and meperi-
      dine potentiator
   5. Cholestatic jaundice
   6. Antagonist—norepinephrine   (levartere-
      nol)
CONTRAINDICATIONS:
   1. Under 6 months of age
   2. Severe asthma
   3. Bone marrow depression, blood dyscra-
      sias, jaundice
   4. Glaucoma
   5. Hypersensitivity
   6. Convulsive disorders
FORMS AND DOSAGES COMMONLY USED IN
  CHILDREN:
  Forms:
   1. Suppository, 25 mg
   2. Tablets, 10 mg, 25 mg, 50 mg
   3. Concentrate, 30 mg/ml, 118-ml dropper
      bottle
   4. Concentrate, vial, 25 mg/5 ml, sensitive
      to light
  Dosages: Used primarily as adjunct: 0.25 to
   0.5 mg/pound of body weight orally or
   intramuscularly

Antiemetics. Many agents are available to control nausea and emesis in a dental patient after premedication or general anesthesia. These include
carbonated beverages, promethazine (Phenergan),
hydroxyzine (Vistaril), prochlorperazine (Compazine), and trimethobenzamide (Tigan). However,
antiemetics are not recommended for treatment of
uncomplicated vomiting in children, and their use
should be limited to prolonged vomiting of known
cause.

Reye syndrome, an acute, often fatal childhood
encephalopathy, has been associated with the use
of antiemetics. The cause and course of the disease
have not been established. This syndrome is characterized by an abrupt onset shortly after a nonspecific febrile illness, with persistent, severe vomiting; lethargy; irrational behavior; and progressive
encephalopathy leading to coma, convulsions,
and possibly death. Of course, the child should

be hospitalized and under the care of a physician.

The primary emphasis in the treatment of emesis should be directed toward the restoration of body fluids and electrolyte balance and the relief of fever and the causative disease process. Overhydration should be avoided because it may result in cerebral edema.

Prochlorperazine (Compazine)

INDICATIONS: To control moderate to severe nausea

CHARACTERISTICS: Antiemetic; general properties similar to those of other phenothiazines

SIDE REACTIONS:
1. Impairs mental alertness
2. Causes hypotension
3. Decreases leukocyte count and increases susceptibility to infections with long-term therapy

PRECAUTIONS:
1. Causes extrapyramidal reactions
2. Potentiates CNS depressants
3. May mask signs of overdose toxicity of other medications as a result of antiemetic action

CONTRAINDICATIONS:
1. Children under 2 years or under 20 pounds
2. Comatose or depressed states
3. Bone marrow depression
4. Hypersensitivity

FORMS AND DOSAGES COMMONLY USED IN CHILDREN:

Forms:
1. Tablets, 5 mg, 10 mg
2. Injection, 5 mg/ml in 2-ml ampule
3. Suppository, 2.5 mg, 5 mg, 25 mg
4. Syrup, 5 mg/5 ml

Dosages (oral or rectal):

Weight (pounds)	Dosage	Maximum (mg)
20-29	2.5 mg/day or b.i.d.	7.5
30-39	2.5 mg b.i.d. or t.i.d.	10
40-85	2.5 mg t.i.d. or 5 mg b.i.d.	15

Trimethobenzamide (Tigan)

INDICATIONS: For patients with moderate nausea and vomiting

CHARACTERISTICS:

Mode of action:
1. Depressant effect on chemoreceptor trigger zone of medulla
2. Onset—30 to 60 minutes rectally; 15 to 35 minutes intramuscularly
3. Duration—3 to 4 hours

Properties:
1. Antiemetic
2. Weaker than phenothiazines
3. Relatively free of side effects

SIDE REACTIONS:
1. Dizziness, drowsiness
2. Possible seizure

PRECAUTIONS:
1. Extrapyramidal reaction
2. Hepatotoxic potential

CONTRAINDICATIONS:
1. Hypersensitivity to benzocaine in rectal suppository
2. Hypersensitivity

FORMS AND DOSAGES COMMONLY USED IN CHILDREN:

Forms:
1. Capsules, 100 mg, 150 mg
2. Vials, 20 ml, 100 mg/ml
3. Suppository, 100 mg, 200 mg
4. Intramuscular injection not recommended for children

Dosages:

Weight (kg)	Oral dosage	Suppository dosage
Under 13	100 mg t.i.d.	100 mg t.i.d. or q.i.d.
13-40	100-200 mg t.i.d. or q.i.d.	100-200 mg t.i.d. or q.i.d.

Nitrous oxide–oxygen for analgesia and sedation

Nitrous oxide–oxygen has been useful as an analgesic and psychosedative agent. It has contributed to changing the attitudes of many children who initially exhibit anxiety toward dental treatment. Misunderstanding does exist because of misapplication and abuse of nitrous oxide in the dental environment. As a general anesthetic, it is a very weak agent, and surgical anesthesia can be obtained only by a dangerous deprivation of oxygen. When nitrous oxide is used as a relative analgesic agent, it produces a euphoric condition that modifies the pain threshhold without loss of consciousness. The use of nitrous oxide–oxygen is often misunderstood not only by the public but by other health-oriented professions.

Characteristics. Nitrous oxide–oxygen has the following characteristics:

1. Odorless and nonexplosive
2. Rapid onset and reversibility
3. Euphoria-producing
4. Mild analgesic or obtundent
5. Minimum side effects, if any (most commonly nausea)
6. No physical addiction
7. Sedation in higher concentration

It has been reported by Keller and confirmed by Baum and Tekavec that patients with cardiac defects experience a better arterial blood oxygen saturation level with nitrous oxide–oxygen than with local anesthetics and atmospheric air.

Drug interactions. There are no significant drug interactions; however, nitrous oxide is a CNS depressant, and its use with other CNS depressants should be avoided or the dosage of these drugs should be reduced. The clinical manifestations of oversedation usually include lack of response to sensory stimulation and respiratory depression. Management of oversedation includes decreasing the concentration of nitrous oxide, increasing the oxygen, and treating the patient's symptoms.

Precautions. Nitrous oxide should be administered only through machines equipped with ''failsafe'' controls. It should never be administered with less than 30% oxygen as an adjunct. However, the dentist must remember that all mechanical devices can malfunction. When administering nitrous oxide, the dentist should use careful technique and continuously observe the patient, who should never be left unattended.

References in the literature have called attention to the possibility of deleterious effects on the health of personnel exposed to trace amounts of residual inhalation anesthetics in hospital operating rooms. In a recent study by Cohen and others, the parallel between operating rooms and dental offices has been reported. However, potential adverse health problems are associated primarily with long-term occupational exposure of dental personnel to heavy use of nitrous oxide (greater than 8 hours in 1 week) and not with dental patients whose exposure is comparatively limited. Even so, it is desirable to use the lowest possible concentration of nitrous oxide.

Hazards

Increased spontaneous abortion rate. Cohen (1980) reported a 50% increase of spontaneous abortion among the wives of male dentists heavily exposed (greater than 8 hours a week) to nitrous oxide–oxygen during the year before conception. A 1.7- to 2.3-fold increase in the rate of spontaneous abortion was noted among female chairside assistants under similar conditions. No increased rate was observed among the wives of anesthesiologists, according to Cohen and associates and, in the United Kingdom, to Knill-Jones, Newman, and Spence. Higher concentrations of waste gases in the dental operatory would be a likely explanation.

Increased cancer. Cohen states that the rate of cancer among male dentists showed no increase, while female chairside assistants had a slight but not statistically significant increase. However, cancer of the cervix in female chairside assistants heavily exposed to nitrous oxide showed a 2.4-fold increase.

Congenital abnormalities in offspring of directly exposed women. No significant differences in congenital abnormalities are documented among children born to wives of men exposed to nitrous oxide–oxygen compared to wives of nonexposed dentists. However, the rate of musculoskeletal disorders among children of exposed female chairside assistants is increased twofold.

Liver disease. Cohen reports an increased incidence of liver disease in both male dentists (1.7-

fold increase) and female chairside assistants (1.6-fold increase) exposed to heavy use of nitrous oxide–oxygen in the dental operatory. This increase is similar to previous reports concerning personnel exposed to anesthetics in the operating room.

Kidney disease. Renal disease among personnel exposed to nitrous oxide–oxygen seems to be primarily renal lithiasis in males and urogenital infections in females. The incidence of kidney disease shows a slight (1.2-fold) increase in male dentists and a slightly higher (1.2- to 1.7-fold) increase in female chairside assistants exposed to nitrous oxide–oxygen.

General and nonspecific neurologic disease. Neurologic disease (generally numbness, tingling, and muscle weakness) has also been reported to occur among personnel exposed to nitrous oxide–oxygen. Cohen reports that the increase in neurologic disease is 1.2- to 1.9-fold among male dentists and 1.7- to 2.8-fold in female chairside assistants excessively exposed to inhalation anesthetics. With nonspecific neurologic disease, the exposed individuals, when they were compared to nonexposed control groups, showed a 1.8- to 3.8-fold increase among male dentists and a 2.1- to 4.4-fold increase among female chairside assistants. Myeloneuropathy associated with nitrous oxide–oxygen exposure or abuse (or both) has also been reported.

Loss of functional capabilities. Studies with children to investigate the psychomotor effects of nitrous oxide–oxygen show transient psychomotor impairment that affects coordination, dexterity, and audiovisual performance and lengthens reflex time. This is easily reversed with 100% oxygen administered for 3 to 5 minutes at the end of the child's appointment.

Recreational abuse. Recreational abuse of nitrous oxide–oxygen is highest among dentists and associated personnel. Eighteen cases of myeloneuropathy have been reported to result from nitrous oxide–oxygen abuse, with the symptoms beginning 5 to 7 months after the onset of abuse. Symptoms included paresthesia of the hands and legs,

loss of balance, and unsteady gait. Sixteen of the 18 cases were associated with self-administration of varying concentrations of nitrous oxide for 1 hour or more at least three times a week for more than 6 months. Two cases were caused by excessive secondary exposure as a result of faulty administration to patients. The treatment was discontinuation of nitrous oxide–oxygen exposure. Although symptoms lessened, numbness and paresthesia persisted several months before subsiding. The exact cause of this phenomenon is unknown, but Cohen and associates report that it may be related to an interaction of nitrous oxide with vitamin B_{12}.

Increased sexual phenomena and hallucinations. Jastak and Malamed report nine instances in which a male dentist was accused of sexually assaulting a female patient receiving greater than a 50% concentration of nitrous oxide without the presence of a female assistant. A majority of these cases involved formal hearings before state dental boards without loss of professional license. These incidents have resulted in recommendations that dentists not sedate a patient unless a dental assistant is in the room and that nitrous oxide concentrations greater than 50% not be routinely used.

• • •

This information is not intended to curtail the use of nitrous oxide–oxygen. Nitrous oxide inhalation is safe when used correctly and is an important adjunct to the practice of dentistry in many offices and clinics.

Sources of leakage of nitrous oxide. Nitrous oxide may leak from one of the following sources during administration:

1. From scavenging devices
   a. Low vacuum
   b. Improper design
2. Around exhalation valve
3. From the patient
   a. Around nasal mask
   b. Patient's mouth (talking, breathing, and so on)
   c. Absorption of gas (30 liters) in the blood

4. From the anesthesia machine (worn or loose parts)
   a. Valves
   b. Hoses
   c. Connections
   d. Tracking
5. From improper disposal of waste gases

In the absence of scavenging devices, after a 60-minute period the concentration of waste inhalation anesthetics in the dental operatory has been found to contain 500 to more than 6700 ppm of nitrous oxide. Over 200 ppm was found in all the other rooms of the dental suite. These particles are inhaled by all exposed personnel. Gas escapes into the room air through the relief valve and from the perimeter of the mask. Secondary leakage occurs from the approximately 30 liters of nitrous oxide that has been absorbed by the patient and is rapidly exhaled with oxygen administration. If no outside exhaust vent exists in the air-conditioning or heating system, gases are recirculated into all of the dental suite. Fresh air dilution via an air-conditioning system is an important factor in reducing the concentration of nitrous oxide, but an outside exhaust (nonrecirculation or one-pass system) is of equal importance. Studies show that room air contamination can be reduced from 900 ppm to 14 ppm by using appropriate control measures and scavenger systems.

Adverse reactions. Most adverse reactions result from the use of an excessive concentration of nitrous oxide. The major complications are nausea and vomiting. A study by Houck and Ripa concluded that the major cause of vomiting was related to a child's natural tendency to vomit and that it was unrelated to eating before therapy, nitrous oxide concentration, or duration of the sedative procedure. In evaluation of patients who are candidates for nitrous oxide–oxygen sedation, the tendency of the patient toward nausea and vomiting should be determined. Excessive concentrations of nitrous oxide can precipitate nausea and vomiting in anyone. If nausea begins, the concentration of nitrous oxide should be decreased by at least 10% until the symptoms disappear.

Contraindications. The following are contraindications to the use of nitrous oxide–oxygen:
1. Respiratory conditions such as the common cold, which prevents nasal breathing, and certain pulmonary conditions such as bronchitis and emphysema
2. Mentally handicapped individuals or those with psychiatric disorders
3. Children with a history of motion sickness
4. Children who in the past have had adverse reactions to administration of nitrous oxide–oxygen
5. Children suspected of drug abuse or who are taking CNS depressants

Dosages. Nitrous oxide is a compressed gas stored in blue gas cylinders at a pressure of approximately 760 psi. It is usually administered through inhalation at mixtures of between 20% and 50% nitrous oxide, with the remaining gas concentration being oxygen and room air. To prevent diffusion hypoxia, which produces signs and symptoms such as lethargy, headaches, nausea, and hangover, the administration of 100% oxygen for a minimum of 3 to 5 minutes is indicated after nitrous oxide–oxygen administration. Nitrous oxide can be used as an adjunct to other premedications; it can also be administered in conjunction with local anesthetics or used alone.

Equipment. It is imperative that procedures for a safe installation of nitrous oxide and oxygen gas lines, regulators, and valves be followed. There have been reports of explosions in dental offices, and in one instance an assistant was killed. The 1973 National Fire Protection Association's pamphlet (No. 56A, A311) contains a complete list of recommendations for safe installation.

Gases in the storage cylinders are under pressure—for example, a large (size D) cylinder of oxygen is under approximately 2400 psi. This pressure must be reduced by a regulator to a level slightly greater than atmospheric pressure before the gas can be used. The gas then travels by a flexible hose to a pipe system that delivers it to the individual operatory. In the operatory are outlets at the end of the pipe system, and the outlets attach to

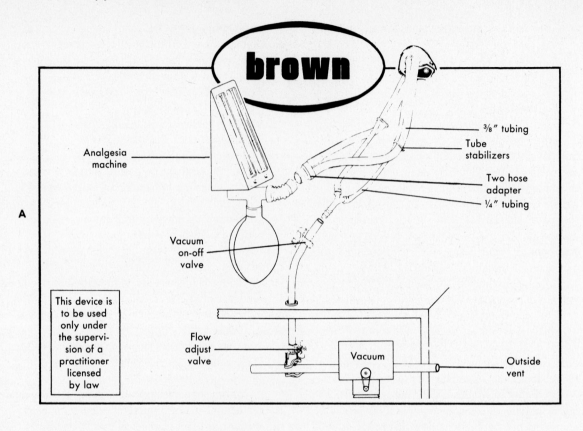

A

brown

Analgesia machine

³⁄₈″ tubing

Tube stabilizers

Two hose adapter

¹⁄₄″ tubing

Vacuum on-off valve

This device is to be used only under the supervision of a practitioner licensed by law

Flow adjust valve

Vacuum

Outside vent

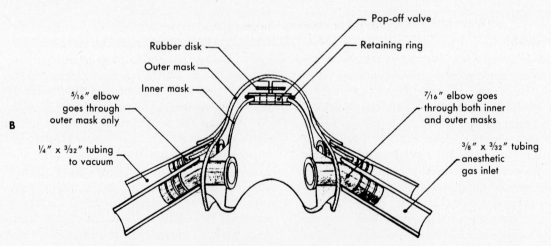

B

Rubber disk

Outer mask

Inner mask

Pop-off valve

Retaining ring

⁵⁄₁₆″ elbow goes through outer mask only

⁷⁄₁₆″ elbow goes through both inner and outer masks

¹⁄₄″ x ³⁄₃₂″ tubing to vacuum

³⁄₈″ x ³⁄₃₂″ tubing anesthetic gas inlet

Fig. 10-5. A, Schematic drawing illustrating how one scavenging system (Brown scavenging system, Summit Services, Inc., Campbell, Calif. 95008) is connected to the nitrous oxide–oxygen system. **B,** Schematic drawing of the scavenging mask. **C,** Nitrous oxide–oxygen machine (Quantiflex M.D.M., Fraser Sweatman Co., Lancaster, N.Y. 14086) and scavenging system (Brown, see above) ready for use.

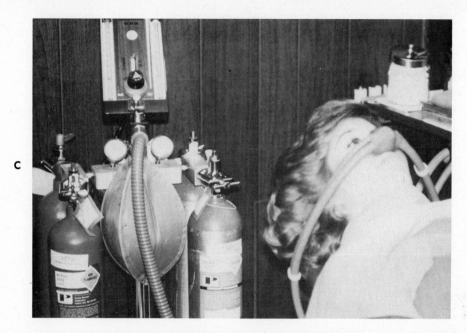

C

Fig. 10-5, cont'd. For legend see opposite page.

couplers via a flexible hose attached to the machine. The machine usually contains two flowmeters with valves to indicate the volume of gases delivered to the patient in liters per minute, an oxygen fail-safe system that will automatically shut off nitrous oxide flow if the oxygen flow should stop, an oxygen flush lever to deliver pure oxygen to the patient in great quantities, and a rebreathing bag that expands and contracts as the patient exhales and inhales and assures the dentist that the patient is breathing.

The nasal inhaler is the part of the delivery system that is in contact with the patient, and it should be attached to a scavenger system to remove the exhaled mixture. The scavenging equipment must meet or exceed guidelines of the American Dental Association's Council on Dental Materials, Instruments, and Equipment to ensure the safe use of nitrous oxide (Fig. 10-5).

The various scavenger systems vent the nitrous oxide–oxygen mixture into the mask via a one-way valve, while another one-way valve exhausts the gases. A reservoir usually holds the expired air before it is exhausted. The differences among scavenging systems in current use lie in mask and valve design and reservoir system.

As a safety precaution, color coding is used for the storage of the cylinders, hoses, flowmeters, and outlets. Green designates oxygen and blue designates nitrous oxide; the parts of one gas line are not interchangeable with the other. This helps prevent the error of attaching the nitrous oxide cylinder to the oxygen line or vice versa.

Administration. The importance of a thorough medical and social history to establish that there are no contraindications cannot be overemphasized. It is necessary to describe to the parents how the nitrous oxide–oxygen analgesia works, how it will affect the child, how it will benefit the child, and what problems might occur. It is also necessary to stress that the purpose of nitrous oxide–oxygen analgesia is to cause a tranquil, relaxed feeling without producing sleep or unconsciousness. Many dentists like to provide parents with a written state-

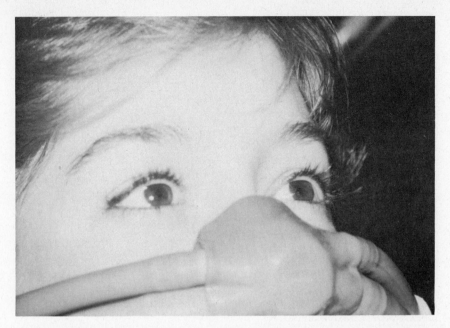

Fig. 10-6. The faraway stare of a patient under nitrous oxide–oxygen sedation.

ment about nitrous oxide–oxygen sedation to which they can refer at any time.

Introducing a young child patient to nitrous oxide–oxygen. The following procedure can be used to familiarize the patient with nitrous oxide–oxygen:

1. Show the child the equipment.
2. Explain the hoses, gauges, and mask in terms the child will understand. Comparing the equipment to that used by scuba divers or astronauts may be helpful in gaining the child's acceptance.
3. Ask the child to place the mask up to his or her nose, play a game of pretend, and breathe very slowly through the nose.
4. Suggest a positive, happy thought for the child to dwell on while the induction takes place.
5. Reassure the patient by describing the sensations that may be experienced, such as tingling of the toes and fingertips, buzzing or humming sensations, a state of relaxation,

heaviness in the arms and legs, and a happy safe feeling.

6. Assure the patient that breathing the gases will not produce sleep and that it is permissible to remove the mask if the patient feels the need to do so.

Maintaining the proper stage of analgesia and psychosedation. Children usually have a tidal volume of about 6 to 8 liters of air a minute, and it is important to maintain this volume during the administration of gases. The dentist begins with 8 liters of 100% oxygen and, as the patient becomes accustomed to the mask and equipment, lowers the level of oxygen and increases the nitrous oxide level until the patient is in the desired tranquil condition. For example, the patient might be receiving 2 liters of oxygen, 3 liters of nitrous oxide, and 2 liters of room air. The patient's clinical signs identify the proper stage of analgesia and sedation, which usually occurs in 3 to 5 minutes after nitrous oxide is introduced. The patient often smiles, the hands become more relaxed, and the mouth might open, but the patient will close it on request. The eyes assume a faraway stare (Fig. 10-6).

Advantages of nitrous oxide–oxygen analgesia and psychosedation. For some children, breathing the nitrous oxide–oxygen will be necessary only while receiving dental injections. Others may prefer to use it throughout the treatment time. Many times patients are sufficiently anesthetized to allow the dentist to complete simple restorations on the primary or permanent teeth without the use of a local anesthetic. This allows the child to leave the office without the danger of postoperative lip or tongue trauma. It also allows the dentist to restore teeth in both arches without fear of producing local anesthetic toxicity.

Some children have a low gag reflex threshold, making it difficult to obtain good radiographs or impressions. The use of nitrous oxide–oxygen tends to diminish this reflex.

It is advisable to use a rubber dam when employing nitrous oxide–oxygen, not only to help maintain a dry field, good visibility, and safety for the patient but also to provide a more closed system, which facilitates the maintenance of the proper stage of analgesia. As the treatment nears completion, administration of 100% oxygen for 3 minutes is required for the patient to leave the office fully recovered.

The Ad Hoc Committee on Trace Anesthetics and the Council on Dental Materials, Instruments, and Equipment of the American Dental Association, along with the National Institute for Occupational Safety and Health (NIOSH) of the Department of Health, Education and Welfare (now Health and Human Services), made the following recommendations on the use of inhalation and sedative agents*:

1. Attempt to maintain less than 50 ppm nitrous oxide in the dental office.
2. Follow NIOSH recommended guidelines.

---

*From American Dental Association: Dentist's desk reference: materials, instruments and equipment, Chicago, 1981, The Association, p. 25.

3. Monitor office for nitrous oxide at the time nitrous oxide equipment is installed and at four month intervals thereafter.
4. Institute a scavenging program. Select scavenging equipment that meets or exceeds the guidelines of the American Dental Association Council on Dental Materials, Instruments and Equipment. This will help ensure the effective and safe utilization of nitrous oxide sedation/anesthetic equipment. Each installation must be customized to meet the proposed standards and existing local and state codes.
5. Check nitrous oxide machine, lines, hoses, and mask for leakage.
6. Maintain adequate ventilation. The maximum circulation and venting to the outside should be achieved with a minimum of recirculation. The particulars of the situation can be worked out with local air conditioning engineers. Well functioning air conditioning and heating units that provide fresh air dilution will aid in the dispersal of the gas from the operatory and decrease the trace concentrations about the dentist and dental assistants.
7. Check to make sure air ventilation systems are functioning properly.
8. Use high speed evacuation systems vented to the outside.
9. Minimize talking with the patient and, if possible, use a rubber dam.
10. Use an air sweep fan which blows across the patient and increases mixing of air with nitrous oxide adjacent to operators.
11. Modify the air conditioning system to be of the non-recirculating type.
12. Exhaust waste gas away from windows, ventilators, air conditioning inlets, or other areas which might provide entrance back into the office. A roof exhaust, for example, might solve the problem.
13. Check the fit of the face mask.
14. Maintain and service equipment regularly.
15. Employ a method of nitrous oxide/oxygen administration which does not allow admixture of room air. Such a technique requires increased nitrous oxide concentrations and flow rates from the machine to reach the desired alveolar air concentration.

REFERENCES

A.D.A. ad hoc committee issues its report on trace gas hazards, A.D.A. News, Feb. 7, 1977, p. 3.

Album, M.M.: Sedative analgesics and belladonna derivatives in dentistry for children, J. Dent. Child. **26:**7-13, 1959.

Album, M.M.: Meperidine and promethazine hydrochloride for handicapped patients, J. Dent. Res. **40:**1036, 1961.

Album, M.M.: Use of anaesthesia for operative procedures on children, J.A.D.A. **67:**112-117, 1963.

Allen, G.E.: Council on Dental Materials and Devices: report on nitrous oxide–oxygen sedation machines and devices, J.A.D.A. **88:**611, 1974.

Aspes, T.: The effect of nitrous oxide sedation on the blood pressure of pediatric dental practice, J. Dent. Child. **42:**364, 1975.

Association of Pedodontic Diplomates: Survey of attitudes and practices in behavior management, Pediatr. Dent. **3:**246-250, 1981.

Bailson, G.: Sedative management. In Nowak, A.J., editor: Dentistry for the handicapped patient, St. Louis, 1976, The C.V. Mosby Co.

Baum, J.J., and Tekavec, M.M.: Blood-oxygen levels during the use of nitrous oxide–oxygen analgesia, Anesth. Prog. **16:**244-245, 1969.

Bennett, C.R.: Conscious sedation in dental practice, ed. 2, St. Louis, 1978, The C.V. Mosby Co.

Blitt, C.D., and Petty, W.C.: Reversal of lorazepam delirium by physostigmine, Anesth. Analg. **54:**607, 1975.

Cohen, E.N., and others: A survey of anesthetic health hazards among dentists, J.A.D.A. **90:**1291-1296, 1975.

Cohen, E.N., and others: Occupational disease in dentistry and chronic exposure to trace anesthetic gases, J.A.D.A. **101:**21, 1980.

Corbett, M.C.: Premedication for children, J. Dent. Child. **33:**125, 1966.

Council on Dental Materials and Devices: Guide to dental materials and devices, ed. 8, Chicago, 1976, American Dental Association.

Council on Dental Materials, Instruments and Equipment, American Dental Association: Council position on nitrous oxide scavenging and monitoring devices, J.A.D.A. **101:**62, 1980.

Council on Dental Therapeutics: Report on nitrous oxide–oxygen psychosedation, J.A.D.A. **84:**393, 1972.

Creedon, R.L.: Pharmacotherapeutic approaches to behavior management: alphaprodine. In Wright, G.Z., editor: Behavior management in dentistry for children, Philadelphia, 1975, W.B. Saunders Co.

Dentist's desk reference: materials, instruments and equipment, Chicago, 1981, American Dental Association.

Downes, J.J., Kemp, R.A., and Lambertsen, C.J.: The magnitude and duration of respiratory depression due to fentanyl and meperidine in man, J. Pharmacol. Exp. Ther. **158:**416, 1967.

Droter, J.A.: Meperidine hydrochloride as a dental premedication, Dent. Surv. **40:**53, 1964.

Everett, G.B., and Allen, G.D.: Simultaneous evaluation of cardiorespiratory and analgesic effects of nitrous oxide–oxygen inhalation analgesia, J.A.D.A. **83:**129, 1971.

Forbes, G.B.: Body surface area as a basis for dosage, Pediatrics **23:**3, 1959.

Freedman, D.X., and others: Report of the conference on the use of stimulant drugs in the treatment of behaviorally disturbed young school children, Psychopharmacol. Bull. **7:**23, 1971.

Gelmon, S.R., and Macko, D.J.: Sedation. In Castaldi, C.R., and Brass, G.A., editors: Dentistry for the adolescent, Philadelphia, 1980, W.B. Saunders Co.

Gradey, M.C.: Pharmacology in pediatric dentistry. In Forrester, D.J., Warpon, M.E., and Fleming, J., editors: Philadelphia, 1981, Lea & Febiger.

Greenfield, W.: Potential hazards of chronic exposure to trace anesthetic gases: implications for dentistry (commentary), J.A.D.A. **101:**158, 1980.

Gregg, J.M., Ryan, D.E., and Levin, K.H.: The amnesic actions of diazepam, J. Oral Surg. **32:**651, 1974.

Gutmann, L., and Johnsen, D.: Nitrous oxide–induced myeloneuropathy: report of cases, J.A.D.A. **103:**239, 1981.

Hargreaves, J.A.: Pharmacotherapeutic approaches to behavior management: diazepam. In Wright, G.Z., editor: Behavior management in dentistry for children, Philadelphia, 1975, W.B. Saunders Co.

Houck, W.R., and Ripa, L.W.: Vomiting frequency in children administered nitrous oxide–oxygen in analgesic doses, J. Dent. Child. **28:**404, 1971.

Houge, D.: The response to nitrous oxide analgesia in children, J. Dent. Child. **38:**129-133, 1971.

Howry, L.B., Bindler, R.M., and Tso, Y.: Pediatric medications, Philadelphia, 1981, J.B. Lippincott Co.

Jastak, J.T., and Greenfield, W.: Trace contamination of anesthetic gases: a brief review, J.A.D.A. **95:**758-762, 1977.

Jastak, J.T. and Malamed, S.F.: Nitrous oxide sedation and sexual phenomena, J.A.D.A. **101:**38-40, 1980.

Jones, T.W., and Greenfield, W.: Position paper of the ADA Ad Hoc Committee on trace anesthetics as a potential health hazard in dentistry, J.A.D.A. **95:**751, 1977.

Keller, M.J.: A comparative study of nitrous oxide–oxygen analgesia and local anesthetics in restorative dentistry, unpublished paper presented at the 22nd annual meeting of the American Academy of Pedodontics, Chicago, 1969.

Keller, M.J., and McDonald, R.E.: Local anesthesia sedation, relative analgesia and general anesthesia. In McDonald, R.E., and Avery, D.R.: Dentistry for the child and adolescent, ed. 3, St. Louis, 1978, The C.V. Mosby Co.

Knill-Jones, R.P., Newman, B.J., and Spence, A.A.: Anaesthetic practice and pregnancy: controlled survey of male anaesthetists in the United Kingdom, Lancet **2:**807-809, 1975.

Kopel, H.M.: The use of ataractics in dentistry for children, J. Dent. Child. **26:**14, 1959.

Lampshire, E.L.: Balanced medication, J. Dent. Child. **26:**25, 1959.

Lang, L.L.: An evaluation of the efficiency of hydroxyzine (Atarax-Vistaril) in controlling the behavior of child patients, J. Dent. Child. **32:**254-257, 1965.

Langa, H.: Relative analgesia in dental practice, ed. 2, Philadelphia, 1976, W.B. Saunders Co.

Langdon, D.E., Harlan, J.R., and Bailey, R.L.: Thrombophlebitis with diazepam used intravenously, J.A.M.A. **223:**184, 1973.

Levin, R.M.: Pediatric anesthesia handbook, Garden City, N.Y., 1973, Medical Examination Publishing Co., Inc.

Lowery, G.H.: Growth and development of children, ed. 7, Chicago, 1978, Year Book Medical Publishers, Inc.

Malamed, S.F.: Pharmacology and therapeutics of anxiety and pain control. In Braham, R.L., and Morris, M.E., editors: Textbook of pediatric dentistry, Baltimore, 1980, The Williams & Wilkins Co.

Marcy, J.H.: Anesthesia for dental procedures in the pediatric patient. In Bennett, C.R.: Monheim's general anesthesia in dental practice, ed. 4, St. Louis, 1974, The C.V. Mosby Co.

McCarthy, F.M., editor: Emergencies in dental practice, Philadelphia, 1979, W.B. Saunders Co., pp. 130-170.

Musselman, R.J., and McClure, D.B.: Promethazine. In Wright, G.Z., editor: Behavior management in dentistry for children, Philadelphia, 1975, W.B. Saunders Co.

Neu, C., DiMascio, A., and Demirgian, E.: Antiparkinsonian medication in the treatment of extrapyramidal side effects: single or multiple daily doses? Curr. Ther. Res. **14:**246, 1972.

Olsen, N.H.: Anesthesia for the child patient, J.A.D.A. **53:**548-555, 1956.

Physician's desk reference, ed. 31, Oradell, N.J., 1982, Medical Economics Co.

Robbins, M.B.: Chloral hydrate and promethazine as premedication for the apprehensive child, J. Dent. Child. **34:**526, 1967.

Shipper, P.E.: The mechanism of nitrous oxide analgesia, J. Am. Analg. Soc. **2:**4-6, 1964.

Sokoll, M.D., Hoyt, J.L., and Gergis, S.D.: Studies in muscle rigidity, nitrous oxide, and narcotic analgesic agents, Anesth. Analg. **51:**16, 1972.

Sonnenscheim, R.R.: A study of the mechanisms of nitrous oxide analgesia, J. Appl. Physiol. **1:**254-258, 1948.

Tobias, M., Lipschultz, D.H., and Album, M.M.: A study of three preoperative sedative combinations, J. Dent. Child. **42:**453, 1975.

Trapp, L.D.: Pharmacological management of pain and anxiety. In Stewart, R.E., and others, editors: Pediatric dentistry: scientific foundations and clinical practice, St. Louis, 1980, The C.V. Mosby Co.

Trieger, N.: Nitrous oxide: a study of physiological and psychomotor effects, J.A.D.A. **82:**142-150, 1971.

Upton, L.G., and Robert, R.C., Jr.: Hazard in administering nitrous oxide analgesia: report of a case, J.A.D.A. **94:**696-697, 1977.

Whitcher, C.E., Zimmerman, D.C., and Piziali, R.L.: Control of occupational exposure to N$_2$O in the dental operatory: final report, Contract No. CDC 210-75-0007, Cincinnati, 1977, National Institute for Occupational Safety and Health, Division of Field Studies and Clinical Investigation.

Whitcher, C.E., and others: Development and evaluation of methods for the elimination of waste anesthetic gases and vapors in hospitals, GPO Stock No. 1733-0071, Washington, D.C., 1975, U.S. Government Printing Office.

Whitcher, C.E., and others: Control of occupational exposure to nitrous oxide in the dental operatory, J.A.D.A. **95:**763, 1977.

Wright, G.Z., editor: Behavior management in dentistry for children, Philadelphia, 1975, W.B. Saunders Co.

Wright, G.Z., and McAulay, D.T.: Current premedicating trends in pedodontics, J. Dent. Child. **40:**185, 1973.

11 Hospital dental services for children and the use of general anesthesia

JAMES E. JONES
JAMES A. WEDDELL

The evolution of hospital dental services in the United States has been slow. In the early decades of this century, hospitals equipped with dental departments often limited dental treatment to relieving pain in ambulatory patients through the emergency room service. In 1938 the American Hospital Association, with representation from the American Dental Association, began development of the manual *Dental Care and Dental Internships in the Hospital,* which was published in 1941. In 1939 the Council on Medical Education and Hospitals of the American Medical Association stated that medical staff privileges should be extended to dentists who "are graduates of recognized dental colleges and whose professional ability and standing are known to the medical staff."

In 1944 a questionnaire circulated among the nation's dental schools found that undergraduate experience in hospitals was minimal and consisted mostly of random observations. The same minimal experience was found in 1971 when the dental school–hospital interrelationship was again evaluated. The average length of hospital experience during undergraduate dental education was 2½ weeks, although some schools provided a significantly longer time. Few students had the opportunity to perform general restorative procedures, and little attention was focused on specialty areas other than oral and maxillofacial surgery.

In recent years, with the increasing number of general practice residencies and postdoctoral spe-cialty programs, the qualified dentist finds that hospital staff privileges are available. Of the hospitals registered by the American Hospital Association, 52.9% have dental programs. Although, in the past, oral and maxillofacial surgeons assumed the major role of dentistry in hospitals, now fewer than 3000 of the approximately 40,000 dentists who hold hospital medical staff appointments are oral and maxillofacial surgeons. Active involvement in hospital dentistry has added a rewarding component to the practice of many dentists. Many hospitals have incorporated not only dental specialties but also general dental services, providing a comprehensive care facility in which to serve the community.

Obtaining hospital staff privileges

Requirements for obtaining hospital staff privileges vary among institutions. The dentist must fulfill two basic requirements to become a hospital staff member:

1. The applicant must have graduated from an accredited dental school.
2. The applicant must be licensed to practice dentistry in the state in which the facility is located.

Additional requirements may be needed for obtaining staff privileges. In a children's hospital, for example, dentists might be required to have adequate advanced training to treat and manage children in the hospital. The requirements may include a dental residency of 1 to 4 years in a teaching hospital in which the dentist (1) gains experience in recording and evaluating the medical history and current medical status of children, (2) receives instruction in physical examination techniques and in recognizing conditions that may influence dental treatment decisions, (3) learns to initiate appropriate medical consultations when a problem arises during treatment, (4) learns the procedure for admitting, monitoring, and discharging children, and (5) develops proficiency in operating room protocol. A rotation in which the dental resident was actively involved in administering general anesthetics to children is highly desirable. Current certification in basic cardiopulmonary resuscitation should be maintained by all members of the hospital's professional staff, including dentists.

As active members of the hospital staff, dentists should be aware of the hospital's bylaws, rules, and regulations. A copy of the bylaws should be obtained for easy reference. Fully understanding the responsibilities of staff membership will enable dentists to treat their patients within the established protocol of the institution. Most important, dentists should endeavor to provide the highest quality care within the specialty area for which they are trained.

Indications for general anesthesia in the treatment of children

General anesthesia for dental care in children should be only one component of the dentist's overall treatment regimen. It must be emphasized that all available management techniques, including acceptable restraints and premedication, should be attempted before the decision is made to use a general anesthetic. Situations in which general anesthesia has been the management technique of choice include the following:

1. Severe dental disease in physically or sensorially handicapped children
2. Severe dental disease in children with significant mental or psychologic deficiencies
3. Severe dental disease in uncontrollable children, regardless of age, who consistently resist conventional management procedures including restraints and premedication
4. Severe dental disease in children with a significant medical disease, such as cardiac disease, blood dyscrasias, or kidney disease, or with a documented allergy to local anesthetics
5. Sustained extensive trauma of the orofacial complex, which is usually managed in conjunction with consultants from the oral and maxillofacial surgery, neurosurgery, and orthopedic services

In all of these categories the severity of the child's dental disease is an important factor. Even under the most trying conditions, a few isolated carious lesions can usually be restored without resorting to the use of general anesthesia. It is the unfortunate child with dental disease throughout the oral cavity and an inability to cooperate in the dental chair who benefits from management with a general anesthetic.

Psychologic effects of hospitalization on children

Hospitalization is a frequent source of anxiety for children. From 20% to 50% of children demonstrate some degree of behavioral change after hospitalization. Separation of the child from the parent appears to be a significant factor in posthospitalization anxiety, although other causes are also documented. Allowing the parent to stay with the child during the hospitalization, and especially to be present when the child leaves for and returns from surgery, can reduce anxiety for the child and parent alike.

To limit the severity and duration of psychologic disturbances, the dentist should strive to reduce parental apprehension concerning the operative procedure. Because children often sense apprehension in their parents, effectively reducing the parents' anxiety will put the child more at ease. Thoroughly explaining the procedure, describing the normal postanesthetic side effects, and familiarizing the child and parents with the hospital can reduce postoperative anxiety.

Rev. 3-77	**CONSENT AND PRE-OPERATIVE NOTE**	M6316000	

I (we) hereby request and consent to the performance of the
following operation or procedure on the patient by

_____*John J. Doe, D.D.S.*_____

or members of the medical staff and personnel of the Indiana
University Hospitals, the administration of anesthetics
deemed advisable by the physician performing the operation
or procedure, the administration of blood or blood components
or derivatives, and extensions of the operation or procedure
if considered advisable by the physician performing the   [X] In-Patient [ ] Out-Patient
operation or procedure, and disposal of any tissue, organ or
body part, including scientific investigation excepting as
noted below:

— Operation or procedure _____*Dental restorations and extractions*_____

— Exceptions, if any:_____*None*_____

I acknowledge that I have had an opportunity to discuss with *John J. Doe, D.D.S.* the
operation or procedure, its purpose and nature, reasonable alternatives, possible consequences of remaining untreated, and risks and possible complications. I understand
that the practice of medicine is not an exact science, that it may involve the making
of medical judgments based upon the facts known to the physician at the time, that it
is not reasonable to expect the physician to be able to anticipate nor explain all
risks and complications, that an undesirable result does not necessarily indicate an
error in judgment, that no guarantee as to results has been made to nor relied upon
by me, and I wish to rely on the physician to exercise judgment during the course of
the procedure or operation which he feels at the time, based upon the facts then known,
are in my best interest.

WITNESSES:

_____   Patient's name:_____

_____   Patient's signature (See reverse side)

Date:_____

Relationship or authority if not signed by the patient

- -

PHYSICIAN'S NOTES

Possible complications of comprehensive dental care under general anesthesia as
explained to the parents:

1. Sore throat
2. Nausea and vomiting—possible aspiration
3. Respiratory congestion
4. Idiosyncratic drug reaction
5. Cardiac depression and arrest
6. Death—statistically remote, but a possible
    complication of general anesthesia

MEDICAL RECORD COPY	**CONSENT AND PRE-OPERATIVE NOTE**	**M-1**

B-CLIN. NOTES	E-LAB	G-X-RAY	K-DIAGNOSTIC	**M-SURGERY**	Q-THERAPY	T-ORDERS	W-NURSING	Y-MISC.

Fig. 11-1. Sample of form that may be used to obtain parental consent for dental treatment of a child
under general anesthesia.

A. Pediatric history

    1. Identification: age, sex, racial-ethnic profile
    2. Informant and estimate of reliability
    3. Problem leading to admittance
    4. History of present illness: date of onset, chronologic description of illness, presence or absence of previous similar episodes, treatment given prior to admittance
    5. Medical survey
        a. Immunization against diphtheria, pertussis, tetanus, polio, measles, mumps, rubella
        b. Previous hospitalizations, operations, major illnesses, or injuries
        c. Allergies, including food and drugs
        d. Dietary history—under 2 years of age
        e. Current medications
    6. Developmental status
        a. Infants less than 2 years: statement re: motor and language development
        b. Preschool children: general statement re: development
        c. Children in school: statement re: school performance
    7. Family history

B. Physical examination

    1. Vital signs: TRP, BP if more than 12 months of age
    2. Measurements: weight, height or length, head circumference if less than 12 months of age
    3. General observations: nutrition, color, distress
    4. Head: describe fontanel if present
    5. Eyes: pupils, extraocular movements
    6. Ears: tympanic membranes
    7. Nose: patency, secretions
    8. Mouth: teeth, pharynx, and tonsils
    9. Neck: masses
    10. Lungs: auscultation
    11. Cardiovascular: heart sounds, rate, rhythm, murmurs; femoral pulses
    12. Abdomen: masses, viscera
    13. Genitalia
        a. Male testes
        b. Female introitus
    14. Skin: eruption
    15. Lymph nodes
    16. Skeleton: joints, spine
    17. Nervous system: state of consciousness, gait if walking
    18. Summary list of problems on tentative diagnosis

Fig. 11-2. Components of the pediatric medical history and physical examination for admission to the hospital.

History and physical examination

Once the decision has been made to use a general anesthetic for a child patient, the dentist should evaluate the child's medical history, the current medical status, and the possibility of complications resulting from the procedure. The parents should be told of any potential complications, and their informed consent must be obtained (Fig. 11-1). The Joint Commission on Accreditation of Hospitals requires that all patients admitted to a hospital have a physical examination performed by a physician. The child's physician must therefore be consulted for the completion of a comprehensive history and physical examination (Fig. 11-2). If the

```
1.  Past dental history
2.  Head and neck physical examination
    a.  General
    b.  Head
    c.  Neck
    d.  Face
    e.  Lateral facial profile
3.  Intraoral examination
    a.  Lips
    b.  Tongue
    c.  Floor of mouth
    d.  Buccal mucosa
    e.  Hard and soft palate
    f.  Oropharynx
    g.  Periodontium
4.  Teeth
    a.  Caries
    b.  Eruption sequence
    c.  Occlusion molar, cuspid, overbite,
        overjet, and midline
5.  Oral habits
6.  Behavior
7.  Recommendations
```

Fig. 11-3. Components of the dental history and examination to be completed before hospitalization.

physician is not a member of the hospital staff, a staff physician should complete the history and physical examination before admission. The dentist should perform a thorough intraoral examination and submit a record of the findings together with a summary of the child's dental history and the reason for admission (Fig. 11-3). The hospital must be notified to reserve an appropriate surgical suite and a bed for the child. Two weeks before admission, a letter stating general instructions concerning the procedure, results of the dental examination, and pertinent dates and times should be mailed to the parents (Fig. 11-4).

Outpatient versus inpatient surgery

A young child or adolescent who requires a general anesthetic and who is free of any significant medical disorders and lives in the general area of the hospital can be considered for outpatient surgery. As an outpatient the child reports to the hospital on the morning of the surgery and is released several hours after the procedure is completed. This saves the parents the expense of a hospital room. If outpatient surgery is planned, the child must still undergo a complete preoperative evaluation including a comprehensive history and physical examination, hematologic evaluation, and urinalysis. The parents must have transportation available to return the child to the hospital should postoperative complications develop at home.

The child should be treated as an inpatient if a medical condition exists that requires close follow-up, if the child lives outside the general area of the hospital, or if the parents demonstrate questionable ability to comply fully with preoperative instructions.

If an outpatient procedure is planned, the parents should bring the child to the hospital at least 1½ hours before surgery. The nursing staff will verify that all preoperative instructions have been followed and that the appropriate laboratory tests have been completed.

Admission to the hospital

If the child is to be admitted as an inpatient, the child and parents should report to the hospital the day before the surgery. The parents must then complete the necessary forms for admission to the hospital. The dentist must write the child's admission orders, which give the nursing staff the preliminary information needed and outline the basic care procedures for the child (Fig. 11-5). The nursing staff will explain standard hospital procedures to the parents and make any recommendations needed to foster a comfortable experience for the patient.

The evening before surgery the dentist should visit the child in the ward. At this time the dentist can answer any questions the parents or the child might have. The dentist should also evaluate the preoperative laboratory data so that appropriate consultations can be initiated if any abnormal values are found. The dentist should record an admitting note in the medical chart to provide the supporting staff with a concise record of the child's medical history, current medical and oral status, diagnosis, and proposed treatment (Fig. 11-6). Abbreviations can be used when recording information in the medical chart (see pp. 285 and 286).

RE: William Smith

Dear Mr. and Mrs. Smith:

After an evaluation of William and discussing with you the extent of his dental disease, it has been decided to accomplish all necessary dental care in the hospital. A medical history and physical examination must be completed by your physician, Dr. Charles Brown, prior to William's admission to the hospital. It has been scheduled for him at 9:00 a.m. on March 9, 1983 at Dr. Brown's office. You should also bring your child to the hospital at 10:00 a.m. on March 10, 1983 for admission.

You are encouraged to remain with your child overnight if possible. Your child may bring his favorite toy or book. If any cold symptoms (runny nose or congestion) should develop before the scheduled admission, please contact our office immediately. It is better to postpone the general anesthetic if your child has a cold.

If you have any further questions concerning the procedure, please contact our office.

Sincerely,

John J. Doe, D.D.S.

Fig. 11-4. Sample letter to parents 2 weeks before their child's admission to the hospital.

1. Please admit (patient's name) to ward for comprehensive dental care under general anesthesia

2. CBC, PT, PTT (other if indicated)

3. UA

4. Lateral and PA chest films (if indicated)

5. History and physical examination by medical house officer (if not already completed)

6. Routine diet per age (special diet if indicated)

7. Weight of patient

8. Bedside privileges for parents

9. Restraints (if indicated)

10. Activity for patient (up ad lib, BRP with assistance, and so forth)

11. Continue present medications (list all normally taken, dosages, and times given), for example:

    | phenytoin | 50 mg | po | bid |
    | phenobarbitol | 60 mg | po | bid |

12. Notify Anesthesiology of admission for preoperative evaluation and medication

13. Medication for pain, infection, or sleep (if indicated)

14. Consultations (if indicated)

15. Arrange for transport to the operating room on (date) at (time)

16. Contact me if problems develop

Answering service phone number: 634-8567
Home phone number: 264-7886

Signature: *John J. Doe, DDS.*

Fig. 11-5. Dentist's admission orders for a patient.

1. Name, age, sex, race, chief complaint, and reason for admission

2. History of the present illness

3. Past medical history

4. Present medications (list all with dosages and times given)

5. Summary of intraoral examination and diagnosis

6. Plan for treatment

Signature: *John J. Doe, DDS.*

Fig. 11-6. Components of dentist's admitting note.

ABBREVIATIONS COMMONLY USED IN THE HOSPITAL

a.c.	Before meals	kg.	Kilogram
ad lib.	At liberty or at pleasure	L	Left
anom.	Anomalies	mand.	Mandible
aq	Aqueous, water	max.	Maxilla
B/F	Black female	MCH	Mean corpuscular hemoglobin
b.i.d.	Twice a day	MCHC	Mean corpuscular hemoglobin
B/M	Black male		concentration
B.P.	Blood pressure	MCV	Mean corpuscular volume
BRP	Bathroom privileges	meds.	Medication
B.S.S.	Black silk sutures	N	Normal
BUN	Blood urea nitrogen	N.C.	Noncontributory
bx	Biopsy	neg.	Negative
c̄	With	N_2O	Nitrous oxide
C.	Centigrade	NPO	Nothing by mouth
cap.	Capsule	NSA	No significant abnormality
CBC	Complete blood count	n/v	Nausea and vomiting
cc	Cubic centimeter	OOB	Out of bed
CC	Chief complaint	op	Operation
C.H.D.	Congenital heart disease	OPD	Outpatient department
CNS	Central nervous system	OR	Operating room
Cong.	Congenital	os	Mouth
CP	Cerebral palsy	PA	Posteroanterior
CR	Cardiorespiratory	p.c.	After meals
CV	Cardiovascular	P.E. (or Px)	Physical examination
d/c	Discontinue	Ped.	Pediatric
Dent.	Dental	PH	Past history
Diff.	Differential blood count	PI	Present illness
disch	Discharge	PMH	Past medical history
D5W	5% Dextrose in water	p.o.	By mouth
Dx	Diagnosis	Post. op	Postoperative
ECG	Electrocardiogram	Preop.	Preoperative
El	Elixir	prep.	Prepare
ER	Emergency room	p.r.n.	As occasion requires
FH	Family history	pro time	Prothrombin time
FUO	Fever of unknown origin	Pt.	Patient
Fx	Fracture	PT	Physical therapy
GA	General anesthesia	PTT	Partial thromboplastin time
ging.	Gingiva	Px	Physical examination
gtt.	Drops	q	Every
h	Hour	q.d.	Every day
Hct.	Hematocrit	q.h.	Every hour
HEENT	Head, eyes, ears, nose, and throat	q.i.d.	Four times a day
Hg	Mercury	q.n.	Every night
Hist.	History	q.o.d.	Every other day
HPI	History of present illness	q.s.	Sufficient quantity
h.s.	At bedtime	r	Rectal
I&D	Incision and drainage	R	Right
I.M.	Intramuscular	R.H.D.	Rheumatic heart disease
I&O	Intake and output	R.O. (or R/O)	Rule out
I.V.	Intravenous	ROS	Review of symptoms

Continued.

	ABBREVIATIONS COMMONLY USED IN THE HOSPITAL—cont'd			
RR	Respiratory rate		tbsp.	Tablespoon
R.R.	Recovery room		t.i.d.	Three times a day
RSR	Regular sinus rhythm		TPR	Temperature, pulse, and respiration
R̸	Take (or prescription)		Tx	Treatment
s̄	Without		UA	Urinalysis
SBE	Subacute bacterial endocarditis		WBC	White blood count
SH	Social history		WD	Well developed
S.H.	Serum hepatitis		W/F	White female
S/P	Status post		W/M	White male
stat	At once		WN	Well nourished
surg.	Surgery		WNL	Within normal limits
Sx	Signs and symptoms		w/o	Without

On the morning of the procedure the dentist and the staff should be in the operating room area 30 minutes before the start of the procedure. The dentist should evaluate how the child spent the evening, check that preanesthetic medications have been given, and determine that the child has been given nothing by mouth for the recommended time. An appropriate note should be made in the medical chart. If all information is found acceptable, the child is ready to be taken to the surgical suite.

Operating room protocol

All persons involved in the care of patients in the operating room must wear appropriate attire designed to prevent contamination of the surgical suite, hallways, and recovery room. This generally consists of a shirt, pants or skirt, and coverings for the face, head, and feet. A hood is used to cover all unshaven facial hair.

The dentist and the staff should be familiar with the standard 10-minute scrub technique for sterile procedures. Neither the medical nor the dental literature documents that a sterile technique is more advantageous than a modified sterile, or clean, technique for restorative dentistry. Therefore intraoral dental procedures are generally considered clean procedures rather than sterile procedures, and the use of sterile gloves during such procedures is at the discretion of the dentist. However, if a surgical dental procedure is anticipated, the dentist should wear sterile gloves and a sterile gown. It is important to remember that cross-contamination between patients in the hospital is always a possibility and that all necessary preventive precautions should be employed.

Anesthetic preparation of the child

After donning operating room attire, the dentist should report to the surgical suite and inform the anesthesiologist of any special requests concerning the procedure. Nasotracheal intubation is preferred to ensure good access to the oral cavity (Fig. 11-7). Special care is taken to protect the child's eyes (Fig. 11-8). The anesthesiologist is responsible for starting intravenous fluids, performing the intubation, stabilizing the tube, and securing the necessary monitoring equipment. The monitoring equipment should include (1) a precordial stethoscope, (2) a blood pressure cuff, (3) electrocardiographic leads, and (4) a temperature-monitoring device. The anesthesiologist must confirm that the child is in a stable condition for anesthesia and that the equipment is functioning properly (Fig. 11-9).

Before scrubbing, the dentist should obtain any needed preoperative x-ray studies (Fig. 11-10). All persons involved in the radiologic procedure should wear protective lead apparel. If adequate

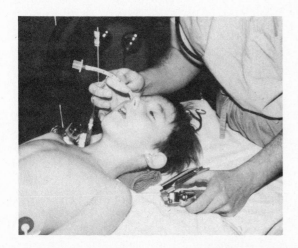

Fig. 11-7. Placement of the nasotracheal tube.

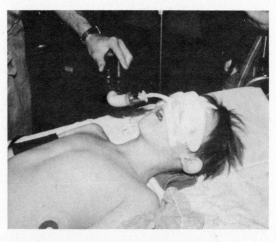

Fig. 11-8. Special eye guard protects the patient's eyes during the procedure.

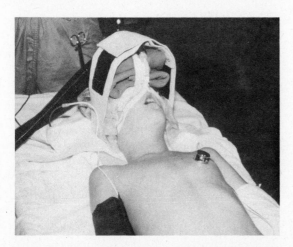

Fig. 11-9. Patient is in a stable anesthetic condition and ready for the dental procedure. Note the position of the precordial stethoscope, blood pressure cuff, and nasotracheal tube.

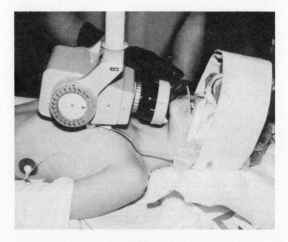

Fig. 11-10. Obtaining diagnostic radiographs. Note the use of protective lead gloves and gown.

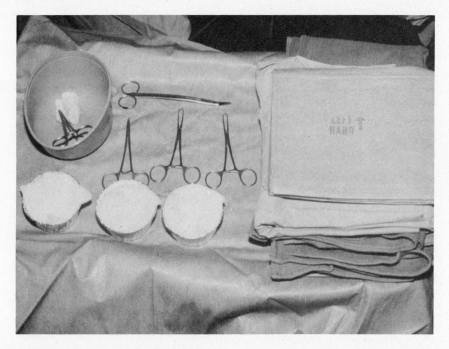

Fig. 11-11. Materials required for perioral cleaning. From upper left: pharyngeal throat pack, towel clamps, patient drapes, bacteriostatic cleaning agent, sterile water, and alcohol.

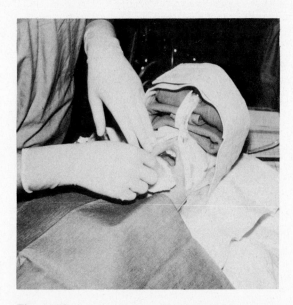

Fig. 11-12. Special care must be taken during perioral cleaning to prevent materials from entering the oral cavity.

preoperative x-ray studies have been previously obtained, the scrub procedure can be completed while the anesthesiologist intubates the patient.

Perioral cleaning, draping, and placement of pharyngeal throat pack

Before the dental procedure is begun, the perioral area is cleansed with three sterile 4 × 4 inch gauze pads. The first gauze pad is saturated with a bacteriostatic cleansing agent, the second with sterile water, and the third with alcohol (Fig. 11-11). This procedure is not intended to sterilize the area but only to remove gross debris (Fig. 11-12). A surgical sheet is then positioned over the remainder of the child's body. This helps to maintain body temperature and provides a clean field during the procedure (Fig. 11-13). The head is draped with three towels arranged to form a triangular access space for the mouth. The towels are secured in place with towel clamps or hemostats. The mouth should be fully exposed (Fig. 11-14). The anesthe-

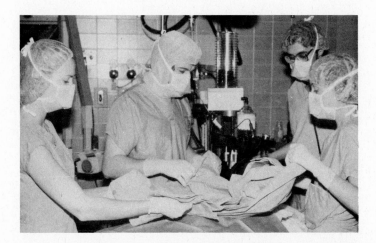

Fig. 11-13. Placing the surgical sheet.

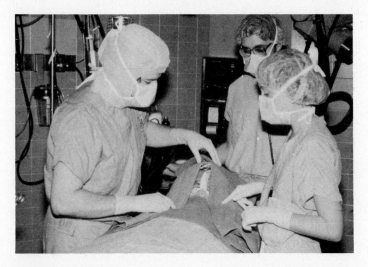

Fig. 11-14. Triangular draping of the oral cavity area. The endotracheal tube is exposed to allow easy monitoring of its connections.

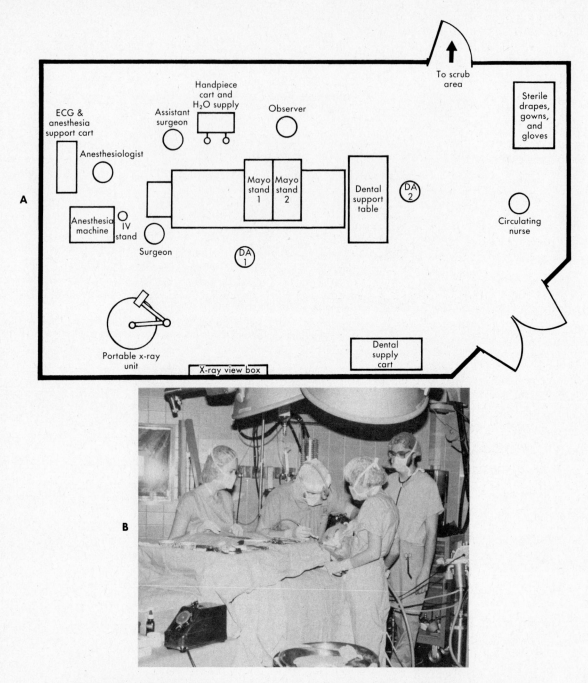

Fig. 11-15. A, Schematic drawing of the positions of personnel and equipment in the operating room. **B,** Operating room positions of the staff while performing the necessary dental procedures. From left: dental assistant, dental surgeon, assistant dental surgeon, and anesthesiologist.

siologist may request that part of the endotracheal tube remain exposed so that all connections can be easily monitored. The assistants then place all supporting carts and stands around the table in positions that the dentist finds comfortable and efficient (Fig. 11-15).

The patient's mouth is opened with the aid of a mouth prop. Care should be taken not to impinge on the lips or tongue with the prop (Fig. 11-16). The mouth is thoroughly aspirated. The pharyngopalatine area is sealed off with a strip of 3-inch sterile gauze approximately 18 inches long (Fig. 11-17). This packing reduces the escape of anesthetic agents and prevents any material from entering the pharynx. The gauze should be tightly packed around the tube, ensuring a good seal. Once the pack is in place, a thorough intraoral examination is performed, followed by a dental prophylaxis. The dentist should then evaluate any new x-ray studies that have been obtained and formulate a final treatment plan.

Restorative dentistry in the operating room

Instruments for restorative dental procedures in the operating room are the same as those for procedures in the dental operatory (Fig. 11-18). The use of quadrant isolation with a rubber dam is preferred (Fig. 11-19). After the completion of each quadrant, 10% stannous fluoride solution should be applied before the removal of the rubber dam.

The dentist should place restorations that will provide the greatest longevity with the least amount of maintenance, for example, full-coverage stainless steel crowns rather than large amalgam restorations on posterior primary teeth.

Completion of the procedure

The anesthesiologist should be notified 5 minutes before the completion of the procedure so the child can begin to be aroused and preparations can be made for extubation. The recovery room personnel are notified that the child will soon be arriving so they can begin preparations. On completion of the dental procedure, the oral cavity is thoroughly debrided and the throat pack is removed

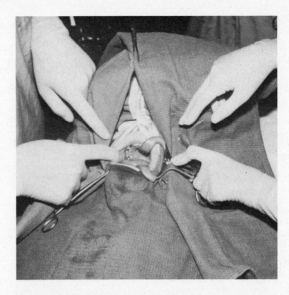

Fig. 11-16. Positioning of a mouth prop. Special care is taken not to impinge on the lips or tongue with the prop.

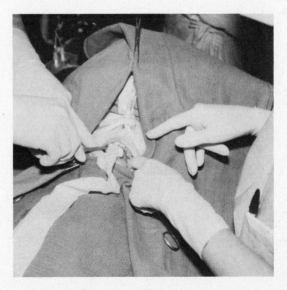

Fig. 11-17. Placement of the pharyngeal throat pack.

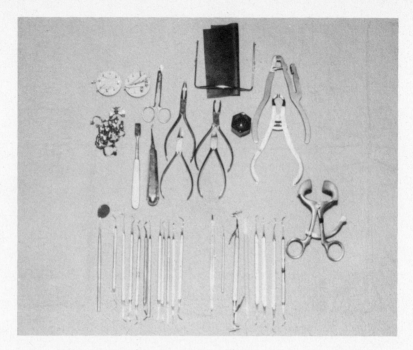

Fig. 11-18. Basic restorative dentistry equipment for the operating room.

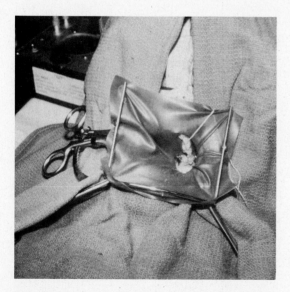

Fig. 11-19. Rubber dam isolation of the maxillary left quadrant.

carefully to prevent aspiration of any materials that might be lodged against it. At this time the anesthesiologist assumes responsibility for the child. The dentist should remain in the operating room during the extubation process to assist the anesthesiologist if necessary. When the child is transported to the recovery room, the dentist should accompany the anesthesiologist and provide assistance during the transportation.

Recovery room

When the child arrives in the recovery room, the dentist should inform the nursing staff of the procedures accomplished and of any special requests or instructions. If teeth have been removed, the nurse should be specifically instructed how and where to apply gauze packing for hemostasis. After confirming that the airway is patent, that the vital signs are stable, and that the anesthesiologist is confident the child is recovering well, the dentist

1. Maintain present IV and discontinue when the present bottle is empty or if it infiltrates (longer if indicated)

2. Vital signs q15 minutes until stable, then every 2 hours

3. Elevate head 30 degrees

4. For swelling: ice packs to area for 30 minutes on and 30 minutes off for 2 hours

5. For hemostasis: check oral hemorrhage q15 minutes for 1 hour; if needed, 4 X 4 inch sterile gauze to area with pressure

6. Restraints prn (if indicated)

7. Force fluids and encourage to void

8. Continue present antibiotic (if indicated)

9. Maintain present medications (list all normally taken, dosages, and times given)

10. Medication for nausea (if indicated)

11. Pain medication (if indicated)

12. Soft diet per age, as patient tolerates

13. Moist air with mist tent if patient suffers from croup

14. Call me if needed: Office phone number: 634-8567
Answering service phone number: 264-7886

Signature: *John J. Doe, DDS*

Fig. 11-20. Components of the dentist's postoperative orders for a patient.

1. Title of dental procedure

2. Type of intubation and anesthetic used

3. Number of teeth restored

4. Which teeth were extracted

5. Other procedures completed

6. Dental prophylaxis paste and topical fluoride used

7. Summary (length of procedure, how the child tolerated the procedure, and so forth)

Signature: *John J. Doe DDS*

Fig. 11-21. Components of the dentist's operative note.

1. Doctor's name and assistants' names

2. Patient's name and hospital number

3. Preoperative diagnosis

4. Postoperative diagnosis

5. Title of the operative procedure

6. Preparation for anesthesia (preoperative medications, type of intubation, and anesthetic agents used)

7. Surgical procedure
   a. Radiographs taken
   b. Description of scrub, draping procedure, and throat pack
   c. Number of teeth restored and type of restorations
   d. Number of teeth receiving pulp therapy
   e. Teeth extracted (name each)
   f. Gingival therapy procedures
   g. Band(s) for appliance(s) and impression(s)
   h. Dental prophylaxis and fluoride applied
   i. Other information (if indicated)

8. Estimated blood loss and hemostasis

9. Condition of patient at the conclusion of the surgical procedure

10. Condition of the patient on arrival in the recovery room

11. Prognosis

Fig. 11-22. Components of the dentist's dictated operative report.

should meet with the parents to give them a brief report of the child's condition and a review of the treatment. The parents should also be informed of the approximate time the child will be transported to the ward.

Postoperative care

Postoperative orders for the ward staff and an operative note should be completed by the dentist and recorded in the medical chart while the child is still in the recovery room (Figs. 11-20 and 11-21). The operative report should be dictated as soon

after the completion of the procedure as possible (Fig. 11-22).

After the child has been in the ward (or in the recovery holding room if treated as an outpatient) for several hours and has been closely monitored for stable vital signs, retention of liquids, and voiding, a decision is made whether to discharge the child or keep the child overnight for further evaluation. If the child is to be discharged, an appropriate note is recorded in the medical chart and a discharge summary is dictated (Fig. 11-23). Postoperative instructions and necessary prescriptions

```
1.  Patient's name and hospital number
    Date of admission
    Date of discharge
    Date of dictation
    Preoperative diagnosis
    Postoperative diagnosis

2.  Age, race, and sex of patient

    Reason for admission and treatment using a general
    anesthetic

3.  Results of preoperative history and physical
    examination (medical and dental) and present
    medications

    Name of the physician completing the history and
    physical examination

4.  Complete description of the surgical procedure
    (see no. 7 in Fig. 11-22)

5.  Patient's tolerance in the recovery room and ward

6.  Condition of the patient on discharge

7.  Individual whom patient is discharged to

8.  Home care instructions given to parents and
    medications prescribed (dosages and times
    to be given)

9.  Patient's next appointment

10. Copies of discharge summary sent to patient's
    physician and referring dentist or physician
```

Fig. 11-23. Components of the dentist's discharge summary statement.

are given to the parents, and an observation appointment for the child is arranged before the discharge. The dentist must be available that evening in case the parents need assistance in caring for their child after returning home.

Summary

There are several categories of dental problems in children that cannot be handled well in the office setting and are best managed in the hospital. The ability to manage children in the hospital environment and to provide comprehensive dental care using a general anesthetic for such children is a valuable part of the dentist's treatment regimen. Granting hospital staff privileges to qualified dentists has become routine at many hospitals seeking to provide comprehensive care for the community. The dentist who uses the hospital in the care of patients often finds it to be a rewarding component of practice.

REFERENCES

Album, M.M.: Operative dentistry under general anesthesia for difficult patients, J. Dent. Child. **20:**157-161, 1953.

Album, M.M.: Acquainting the dental student with general anesthesia procedures for handicapped children, J. Dent. Educ. **19:**197-210, 1955.

Album, M.M.: General anesthesia and premedication in dentistry for children, J. Dent. Child. **24:**215-223, 1957.

Album, M.M., Boyers, C.L., and Kaplan, R.I.: Hospital dentistry for the pedodontist: philosophy, J. Dent. Child. **35:**153-160, 1968.

Allen, G.D., and Sim, J.: Full mouth restoration under general anesthesia in pedodontic practice, J. Dent. Child. **34:**488-492, 1967.

American Academy of Pediatrics: Standards of child health care, Evanston, Ill., 1967, The Academy.

American Academy of Pedodontics: Hospital guidelines for pediatric dentistry, Pediatr. Dent. **2**(suppl.):1-17, 1979.

Archer, W.H.: American Dental Association and hospital dental service: a critical historical review 1920-1950, J. Hosp. Dent. Pract. **5:**53-66, 1971.

Asbell, M.B.: Hospital dental services in the United States: a historical review, J. Hosp. Dent. Pract. **3:**9-11, 34-36, 1969.

Atterbury, R.A.: Explaining hospital dentistry: preoperative procedures, Dent. Survey **45:**35-36, 1969.

Azevedo, A.B.: Pedodontics in hospital dentistry, J. Hosp. Dent. Pract. **4:**108-111, 1970.

Bachman, L., and Freeman, A.: General anesthesia for dental procedures in handicapped patients, Dent. Clin. North Am., pp. 443-453, July 1960.

Barr, C.E.: Dental schools and hospitals: a symbiotic relationship for dental education, J. Dent. Educ. **40:**284-286, 1976.

Boller, R.J., and Posnick, I.H.: Fifteen years of hospital dentistry, J. Dent. Child. **34:**55-64, 1967.

Brown, E., and Kopel, H.M.: A procedure of general anesthesia for operative dentistry, J. Dent. Child. **22:**184-187, 1955.

Council on Hospital Dental Service: Oral evaluation of hospitalized patients, J.A.D.A. **72:**911-912, 1966.

Davis, W.R., McConnell, B.A., and Oldenburg, T.R.: Dental procedures in the hospital operating room: placement of equipment and the efficient use of dental auxiliaries, J. Dent. Child. **35:**342-344, 1968.

Degan, B.J.: The hospital: a site for delivery of dental care, J. Hosp. Dent. Pract. **5:**67-74, 1971.

Emmertsen, E.: The treatment of children under general anesthesia, J. Dent. Child. **32:**123-124, 1965.

Gotowka, T., and Bailit, H.L.: Quality assurance systems for hospital outpatient dental programs: background, Special Care Dent. **1:**211-217, 1981.

Greene, N.M., and Falcetti, J.P.: A program of general anesthesia for dental care of mentally retarded patients, Oral Surg. **37:**329-336, 1974.

Gross, G.: General anesthesia for pedodontics, J. Dent. Child. **21:**25-29, 1954.

Harmelin, W.: Pediatric dentistry under general anesthesia, N.Y. State Dent. J. **32:**197-202, 1966.

Harmelin, W., and Cicero, J.: Systemic problem cases for dentistry under general anesthesia, N.Y. State Dent. J. **33:**209-215, 1967.

Holst, G.: The treatment of children under general anesthesia, J. Dent. Child. **32:**125-127, 1965.

Hooley, J.R.: Hospital dentistry, Philadelphia, 1970, Lea & Febiger.

Hooley, J.R., and Dwan, L.: Hospital dentistry, St. Louis, 1980, The C.V. Mosby Co.

Jackson, J.B.: Pediatric dental rehabilitation, J. Dent. Child. **33:**33-37, 1966.

Johnson, R.H.: Clinical laboratory tests of interest to the dentist, Dent. Clin. North Am., pp. 203-215, March 1968.

Kopel, H.M.: Writing orders for the hospitalization of dental patients, J. Dent. Child. **35:**405-409, 1968.

Mark, H.I.: In hospital dental services, Special Care Dent. **1:**61-64, 1981.

McDonald, R.E.: Treatment of children under a general anesthetic, Dent. Pract. **4:**7-12, 1966.

Monheim, L.M.: General anesthesia in dental practice, Dent. Clin. North Am., pp. 805-820, October 1970.

Musselman, R.J., and Roy, E.K.: Hospital management of the handicapped child, Dent. Clin. North Am., pp. 699-709, July 1974.

Olsen, N.H., Davis, W.B., and Sawusch, R.H.: The relationship of a pedodontic department to a teaching hospital, J. Dent. Child. **35:**491-494, 1968.

Ripa, L.W.: Hospital related activities in pedodontic specialty training program, J. Dent. Educ. **37:**9-12, 1973.

Rule, D.C., and others: Restorative treatment for children under general anesthesia: the treatment of apprehensive and handicapped children as clinic out-patients, Br. Dent. J. **123:**480-484, 1967.

Scott, J.G., and Allen, D.: Anesthesia for dentistry in children: a review of 101 surgical procedures, Can. Anesth. Soc. J. **17:**391-402, 1970.

Spiro, S.R.: Operative dentistry under general anesthesia, J. Dent. Child. **18:**38-45, 1951.

Thompson, R.: How to establish baselines for hospitalized dental patients, J. Hosp. Dent. Pract. **4:**74-80, 1970.

Tocchini, J.J.: The child patient and general anesthesia in the hospital, J. Dent. Child. **35:**198-207, 1968.

Tocchini, J.J., and Wycoff, C.C.: Hospital procedures in the care of the handicapped, Dent. Clin. North Am., pp. 261-280, July 1966.

Troutman, K.C., and Mayer, B.W.: Pedodontic oral rehabilitation: dental and anesthetic considerations, J.A.D.A. **82:**388-394, 1971.

Vincent, C.J.: Utilization of general anesthesia in the hospital: a pedodontic rationale, J.A.D.A. **67:**865-871, 1963.

Wenner, J.H., Greene, V.W., and King, J.L.: Monitoring microbial aerosols in an operating room during restorative dentistry, J. Dent. Child. **43:**25-29, 1977.

12 Restorative dentistry

RALPH E. McDONALD
DAVID R. AVERY

Recent advances in preventive dentistry and their application in the private dental office, the widespread acceptance of communal fluoridation, and greater emphasis on dental health education have resulted in a dramatic change in the nature of dental practice. Today the dentist devotes more time to preventive procedures and less time to the routine restoration of carious teeth.

Nevertheless, the restoration of carious lesions in primary and young permanent teeth continues to be one of the most valuable services that pedodontists and general practitioners provide for the children in their practices. Dentists are often judged by patients and fellow practitioners on the basis of the effectiveness of their preventive programs and of the degree of skill with which they can perform routine operative procedures.

Silver amalgam continues to be one of the most widely used materials in the restoration of children's teeth. The success of this filling material depends on the strict adherence to accepted procedures of cavity preparation and the manipulation and placement of the silver alloy. The basic principles related to the manipulation of restorative materials have been proved important through extensive research, and violation of these principles will result in a high percentage of clinical failures. This is true even with a time-proven material such as silver amalgam.

Maintenance of a dry field

The maintenance of a dry operating field during cavity preparation and placement of the restorative material will help ensure efficient operating and the development of a restoration that will be serviceable and that will maintain the tooth and the integrity of the developing occlusion.

It is generally agreed that the use of the rubber dam offers the following advantages:

1. *Saves time.* The dentist who has not routinely used the rubber dam need only follow the routine presented later in this chapter or a modification of it for a reasonable period to be convinced that operating time can be appreciably reduced. The time spent in placing the rubber dam is negligible, provided the dentist works out a definite routine and uses a chairside assistant. Heise reported an average time of 1 minute, 48 seconds to isolate an average of 2.8 teeth with the rubber dam in 302 cases. These applications of the rubber dam, placed with the aid of a capable dental assistant, were for routine operative dentistry procedures. The minimum time recorded for placing a rubber dam was 15 seconds (single tooth isolation), and the maximum time was 6 minutes. Many of the applications ranged from 25 to 50 seconds. Heise also observed that approximately 10 seconds is required to remove the rubber dam. The time required for the placement of the rubber dam will invariably be made up and additional time saved through the elimination of the rinsing, spitting, and talking routine of the child patient.

2. *Aids management.* The belief of a few dentists that the rubber dam technique is unacceptable for the young child patient cannot be substantiated. A few explanatory words and reference to the rubber

dam as a "raincoat" for the tooth or as a "Halloween mask" will invariably allay the child's fear. It has been found through experience that apprehensive or otherwise uncooperative children can often be controlled more easily with a rubber dam in place. Since the rubber dam efficiently controls the tongue and the lips, the dentist has greater freedom for completing the operative procedures.

3. *Controls saliva.* This is an extremely important consideration in completing an ideal cavity preparation for primary teeth. The margin of error is appreciably reduced when a cavity is prepared in a primary tooth that has a large pulp and often extensive carious involvement. Minute pulp exposures may be more easily detected when the tooth is isolated. It is equally important in instances of vital pulp exposure to observe the true extent of the exposure and the degree and type of hemorrhage from the pulp tissue. The rubber dam therefore can aid the dentist in observing teeth that are being considered for vital pulp therapy.

4. *Provides protection.* The use of the rubber dam will prevent foreign objects from coming into contact with oral structures. When small pieces of filling material, such as zinc cement, zinc oxide–eugenol, and silver amalgam, are dropped into the floor of the mouth or come into contact with the tongue, they stimulate salivary flow and interfere with the operative or restorative procedure. Medicaments used during the restorative procedure have a similar effect. A rubber dam also prevents the small child in a reclining position from swallowing or aspirating foreign objects and materials.

5. *Helps the dentist to educate parents.* Parents are always interested in the work that has been accomplished for their child. While the rubber dam is in place, the dentist can conveniently show parents the completed work after an operative procedure. The rubber dam creates the feeling that the dentist has complete control of the situation and that a conscientious effort has been made to provide the highest type of service.

Armamentarium for rubber dam placement. The armamentarium consists of 5 × 5 inch sheets of dark medium latex, a rubber dam punch, clamp forceps, a selection of clamps, and a Young's rub-

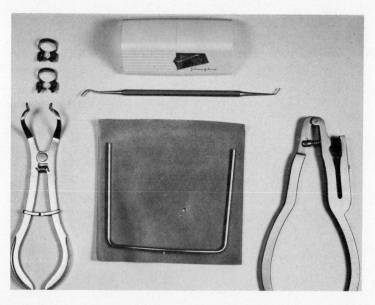

Fig. 12-1. Armamentarium recommended for the placement of the rubber dam for restorative procedures for children.

ber dam frame (Fig. 12-1). A piece of stiff cardboard with an opening 1¼ inch square in the center may be used as an aid in the proper placement of the holes in the rubber dam. The cardboard is placed on the piece of rubber dam, and each corner of the small square is marked with a ballpoint pen. These four points indicate where the punch holes for the clamp-bearing tooth are to be made, and their position depends on the quadrant of the mouth to be treated (Fig. 12-2). As experience is gained in applying the dam, the dentist will soon learn the proper position for punching the holes and the preceding step of marking the rubber at the four points will be unnecessary. If the holes are punched too far apart, the dam will not readily fit between the contact areas. In addition, when the proximal area is being operated on, a greater bulk of material between the teeth will greatly increase the possibility of tangling the bur in the rubber dam. In general, the holes should be punched the same distance apart as the holes on the cutting table of the rubber dam punch.

The large punch hole is always used for the clamp-bearing tooth and for most permanent molars. Generally speaking, the medium-sized punch hole is used for the premolars and primary molars. The second smallest hole is used for maxillary permanent incisors, whereas the smallest hole is adequate for the primary incisors and lower permanent incisors.

Selection of a clamp. The operator will soon develop a personal preference for clamps to secure the dam in isolating different areas in the mouth. It seems appropriate, however, to review a limited number of clamps that have been found effective.

The first choice of a clamp for a first permanent molar is the Ivory No. 7, which can be used for maxillary or mandibular teeth. In situations in which the clamp does not seem adequate, the S.S. White No. 201 may be considered. For the partially erupted permanent molar, an Ivory No. 14 or No. 14A is often the clamp of choice. If the tooth farthest distal is a second primary molar, the Ivory No. 3 clamp is adaptable to most maxillary and mandibular teeth. The S.S. White No. 209 clamp

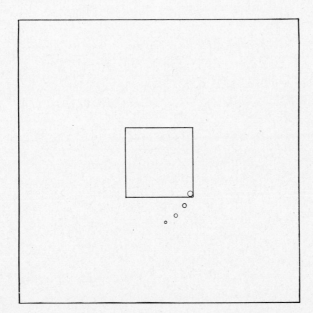

Fig. 12-2. A piece of cardboard may be used to assist in determining the position of the holes in the rubber dam. The corners of the square represent points where punch holes should be made for the clamp-bearing tooth.

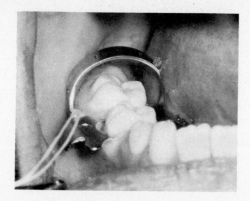

Fig. 12-3. An Ivory No. 3 clamp has been trial-fitted to the second primary molar. The clamp will be removed and placed in the rubber dam.

is usually adaptable to the primary canine and is helpful in securing the dam in the isolation of anterior teeth. The S.S. White No. 210 can be used on individual anterior teeth, or it may be placed on a first primary molar when that tooth is the farthest distal in the arch.

Unless the clamp is firmly anchored to the tooth, the tension of the stretched rubber will easily dislodge it. Therefore the proper selection of a clamp is of utmost importance. It is recommended that the clamp be tried on the tooth before the rubber dam is placed to ascertain that the clamp can be securely seated and will not be easily dislodged by the probing tongue, lip, or cheek musculature. An 18-inch length of dental floss should be doubled and securely fastened to the bow of the clamp. The floss will facilitate retrieval in the unlikely event that the clamp should slip and fall toward the patient's throat (Fig. 12-3).

The following procedure is recommended for a rubber dam application (Fig. 12-4). The previously selected and ligated clamp is placed in the rubber dam. The dentist grasps the clamp forceps with the clamp engaged. The assistant, seated to the left of the patient, grasps the upper corners of the dam with the right hand and the lower left corner between the left thumb and index finger while carrying the Young's frame over the left wrist. The

dam is moved toward the patient's face as the dentist carries the clamp to the tooth while holding the lower right portion of the dam. After securing the clamp on the tooth, the dentist transfers the clamp forceps to the assistant who receives it between the left index and middle fingers while continuing to hold the upper corners of the dam with the right hand. The dentist then removes the Young's frame from the assistant's left hand and places the frame under the rubber dam. The assistant may attach both upper corners while the dentist attaches both lower corners. The flat blade of a plastic instrument or a right-angle explorer may be used to remove the rubber dam material from the wings of the clamp and to complete the seal around the clamped tooth. If necessary, light finger pressure may be used to seat the clamp securely by moving it cervically on the tooth. If additional teeth are to be isolated, the rubber is stretched over them, and the excess rubber between the punched holes is placed between the contact areas with the aid of dental floss. The most anterior tooth and others if necessary are ligated to aid in the retention of the dam and the prevention of cervical leakage. The free ends of the floss are allowed to remain, since they may aid in the further retraction of the gingival tissue or of the patient's lip during the operative procedure. At the end of the operative procedure, the length of floss will also aid in removing the ligature (Fig. 12-4).

It is unwise to include more teeth in the rubber dam than are necessary to adequately isolate the working area. If the first or second permanent molar is the only tooth in the quadrant that is carious and if it requires only an occlusal preparation, it is often desirable to punch only one hole in the dam and to isolate the single tooth (Fig. 12-5). This procedure will require only seconds and will save many minutes.

Morphologic and histologic considerations

The crowns of the primary teeth are smaller but more bulbous than the corresponding permanent teeth, and the molars are bell shaped with a definite constriction in the cervical region. The characteris-

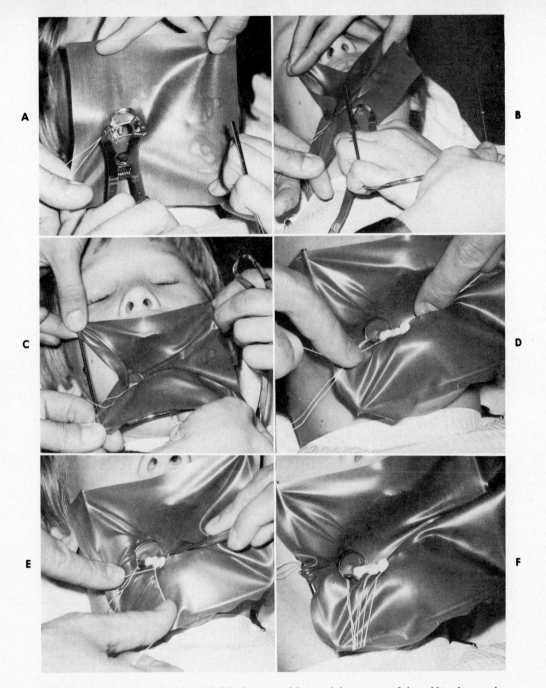

Fig. 12-4. A, The dental assistant holds the top and lower right corners of the rubber dam as the dentist holds the lower left corner and carries the clamp to the tooth. **B,** The dentist transfers clamp forceps to the assistant and receives the rubber dam frame. **C,** The assistant and dentist attach the corners of the rubber dam to the frame. **D,** Dental floss is used to carry the rubber dam between the teeth. **E,** The assistant supports the floss with a flat blade instrument while the dentist ties the knot. **F,** The teeth are isolated and ready for the operative procedure.

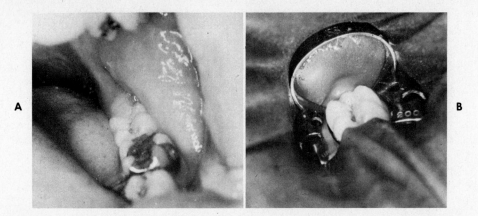

Fig. 12-5. A, The second permanent molar requires an occlusal restoration. It is not necessary to isolate more than a single tooth. **B,** A No. 200 clamp has been selected to hold the rubber dam in place. The rubber dam has retracted the tissue that extended over the distal marginal ridge.

tic sharp lingual inclination occlusally of the labial or buccal surfaces results in the formation of a distinct labiogingival or buccogingival ridge that ends abruptly at the cementoenamel junction. The sharp constriction at the neck of the primary tooth necessitates special care in the formation of the gingival floor during Class II cavity preparation. The buccal and lingual surfaces of the molars converging sharply occlusally form a narrow occlusal surface or food table, especially in the first primary molar. Therefore, since the isthmus of the cavity preparation must often be narrow, the restoration may fracture.

The pulpal outline of the primary teeth follows the dentinoenamel junction more closely than that of the permanent teeth. The pulpal horns are longer and more pointed than the cusps would suggest. Since there is less bulk or thickness of the dentin, the pulp is proportionately larger than that of the permanent teeth.

The development of the primary teeth begins during prenatal life, whereas the dentin and enamel of the permanent teeth develop during postnatal life. Calcification that has taken place during prenatal life is usually homogenous and is demarcated from the calcification that occurs during postnatal

life by a distinct neonatal line or series of rings. The lines indicate an interruption in the metabolic process during the newborn period. The dentin that forms during infancy usually appears granular and pebbly, and it is usually less dense than that of permanent teeth. Contrary to former opinion, the pulp of the primary teeth has the ability to form secondary dentin readily in response to external irritants. The secondary dentin, however, is more irregular than that formed in permanent teeth. The histologic characteristics of the primary teeth are essentially the same as those of the permanent teeth.

The enamel of the primary teeth is of uniform thickness. The enamel surface tends to be parallel to the dentinoenamel junction. Although it is generally agreed that the enamel rods in the gingival third of the primary teeth do not incline apically as they do in permanent teeth, Law and Shepard reported considerable variation in rod inclination, particularly in the occlusal portion of the primary teeth. After making a study of the histology of the primary teeth, Rowe and Ireland concluded that the enamel rods in the cervical third are inclined in an incisal or occlusal direction from the horizontal. They further observed that the enamel rod angles are different for the various primary teeth and that the rod angle increases gradually from the primary central incisor, with a 44-degree average, to the second primary molar, with an average of 32 degrees. The angles of enamel rods in the mandibular teeth were found to be greater than those in the maxillary teeth. There was no correlation observed between the enamel rod angle and the particular tooth surface.

Basic principles in the preparation of cavities in primary teeth

There is not complete agreement regarding the type of cavity preparation that should be made in a primary tooth. This lack of agreement becomes increasingly evident in the recommendations for the Class II cavity preparation in a primary tooth. There are, however, a number of basic principles related to the preparation of Class I and Class II cavities on which there should be agreement.

The cavity preparation should include areas that have carious involvement and, in addition, those that retain food and plaque material and may be considered areas of potential carious involvement.

Since a number of amalgam restorations in primary molars fail as a result of fracture in the area of the isthmus, this area should be of adequate width buccolingually without weakening the cuspal areas or endangering the pulp and it should be sufficiently deep to ensure adequate bulk. It has been suggested by Hartsook that the optimum average width of the isthmus is approximately half the intercuspal dimension of the tooth. This should certainly be the maximum width in teeth that are not extensively involved by caries. With the advent of improved amalgam alloys the tendency today is to reduce the width of the preparation at the isthmus even more, as is done in the permanent molar preparation (Fig. 12-6).

The depth of the occlusal portion of the preparation, including the isthmus, the dovetail, and the extension into the fissures, should be approximately 0.5 mm pulpally from the dentinoenamel junction.

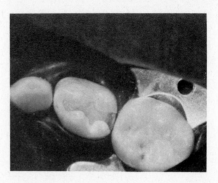

Fig. 12-6. Conservative but adequate extension of a Class II cavity preparation in a mandibular first primary molar. The isthmus of the preparation is approximately one-third the intercuspal dimension.

A flat pulpal floor is generally advocated. However, a sharp angle between the pulpal floor and the axial wall of the cavity should be avoided. The axiopulpal line angle should be beveled or grooved to reduce the concentration of stresses and to provide greater bulk of material in this area, which is vulnerable to fracture. Rounded angles throughout the preparation will result in less concentration of stresses and will permit more complete condensation of the amalgam restorative material into the extremities of the preparation.

In the Class II cavity the buccal and lingual extensions should be carried to self-cleansing areas. Consideration should be given in the cavity design to providing for greater buccal and lingual extension at the cervical area of the preparation to clear contact with the adjacent tooth. This divergent pattern, which is universally recommended for the proximal step, is necessary because of the broad, flat contact areas of the primary molars and because of the distinct buccal bulge in the gingival third.

Since many occlusal fractures of amalgam restorations result from sharp opposing cusps, it is advisable to identify these potentially damaging cusps with articulating paper before cavity preparation. The slight reduction and rounding of a sharp opposing cusp with a stone will reduce the number of fractures during the critical period of 6 to 8 hours after the placement of the amalgam.

Instruments needed for cavity preparation in primary teeth

With the use of the high-speed handpiece, the steps in the preparation of a cavity in a primary tooth are not difficult but do require precise operator control. Many authorities advocate the use of small, rounded-end carbide burs in the high-speed handpiece for establishing the cavity outline and performing the gross preparation. For efficiency and convenience, all necessary high-speed instrumentation for a given preparation may be completed with a single bur in most situations. Therefore the dentist should select the bur that is best designed to accomplish all the high-speed cutting required for the procedure being planned. Fig. 12-7 illustrates four high-speed carbide burs designed to cut efficiently and yet allow conservative cavity preparations with rounded line angles and point angles. Although the carious involvement of the occlusal grooves is less common in the primary teeth than in the permanent teeth, the cavity preparation is extended to include all the pits and fissures that are predisposed to caries.

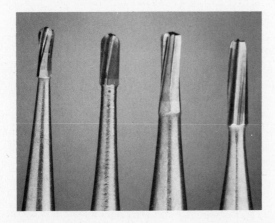

Fig. 12-7. High-speed carbide burs No. 329, No. 330, No. 245, and No. 256 that may be used for the gross cutting of cavity preparations.

Incipient Class I cavity in a very young child. During the routine examination of a child under 2 years of age, the dentist may occasionally discover an incipient carious lesion in the central fossa of one or more first primary molars, with all other teeth being sound. Thus restorative needs are present but minimal. Roche has suggested an expeditious approach to this problem. Because of the child's psychologic immaturity and because it is usually impossible to establish effective communication with the child, he advocates having the parent hold the child on his or her lap in the dental chair. This will help the child feel more secure and provide a better opportunity to restrain the child's movement during the operative procedure. The small cavity preparation may be made without the aid of the rubber dam or local anesthetic. A No. 331 bur is operated at low speed to open the decayed area to a depth just within the dentin and extend the cavosurface margin only to the extent of the carious lesion. Restoring the tooth with amalgam will arrest the decay and at least temporarily prevent further tooth destruction without a lengthy or involved dental appointment for the child. After the child has reached a manageable, communicative age, the preparation and restoration may be extended if necessary.

Pit or fissure Class I cavity. A small high-speed bur, such as a No. 329 or No. 330, may be used for the defective or carious areas on the occlusal surface. The bur is carried to a depth of approximately 0.5 mm beneath the dentinoenamel junction. With slight undermining and up and down motion, the preparation should be extended throughout the occlusal surface to include the pits and fissures. The marginal ridges should not be undermined unless caries extends into this area. Undermining the marginal ridges will weaken the tooth and will carry the margin of the restoration into an area of unsupported enamel rods. If carious material remains, it should next be removed with small round burs or spoon excavators. The walls of the cavity may be planed with a No. 256 bur at slow speed, and the overhanging enamel should be removed. The walls of the preparation should be almost parallel and perpendicular to a flat pulpal floor but with a slight convergence occlusally.

The need for extensive undercut areas at the base of the cavity for retentive purposes has not been substantiated. Distinct undercut or retentive areas, such as those produced by an inverted cone bur, may endanger the pulp and weaken the cusps of the teeth. The proper preparation and placement of amalgam will result in good adaptation of the amalgam to the cavity walls and adequate retention of the restoration.

If the pulpal floor contains a concavity resulting from the removal of deep caries, a suitable intermediate base should be placed before the insertion of the silver amalgam. A hard-setting calcium hydroxide material is recommended.

Deep-seated Class I cavity. The first step in the preparation of an extensive Class I cavity is to plane back the enamel that overhangs the extensive carious lesion. Then the cavity preparation should be extended throughout the remaining grooves and anatomic occlusal defects. The carious dentin should next be removed with large round burs or spoon excavators. If a carious exposure is not encountered, the cavity walls should be paralleled and finished as previously described.

In teeth with deep carious lesions and near pulp exposures, the depth of the cavity should be covered with a hard-setting calcium hydroxide material. A base of zinc phosphate cement or rapid-setting zinc oxide–eugenol may then be placed over the calcium hydroxide material to provide adequate thermal protection for the pulp.

Class II cavity. Approximately 70% to 80% of the cavity preparations in primary teeth are of the Class II variety. This fact has been attributed to the broad, flat, elliptical proximal contact of these teeth, the indifferent proximal contact that is often seen in children 3 to 4 years of age, and the relative thinness of the enamel in this region. If one proximal lesion is found during the radiographic examination, others are likely to be present. These lesions must be restored as soon as they are evident radiographically. Unless effective preventive procedures are initiated, the smallest "etching" can

progress to extensive involvement of the dentin within a 4- to 6-month period. Proximal lesions in a preschool child indicate excessive caries activity; a preventive and restorative program should be undertaken immediately.

Very small incipient proximal lesions may be "chemically restored" with topical fluoride therapy provided by the dentist, along with the use of home fluoride rinses. If this treatment regimen is accompanied by improved diet and improved oral hygiene, some incipient proximal lesions may remain in an arrested state indefinitely. However, the parents should be informed of the incipient lesions and emphasis should be placed on the need to continue practicing the recommended procedures and the need for periodic examinations. If the parents and the patient do not follow the instructions properly, conventional restorative procedures should be initiated before the incipient lesions become extensive carious lesions.

The first step in the preparation of a Class II cavity in a primary tooth involves opening the marginal ridge area with a bur. At a depth of approximately 0.5 mm pulpal to the dentinoenamel junction, the marginal ridge can be penetrated with an undermining action. Extreme care must be taken when breaking through the marginal ridge to prevent damage to the adjacent proximal surface, especially when the bur is revolving at high speed.

Unless there is extensive caries that might endanger the pulp, the carious material should not be removed until the establishment of a gingival seat, which can be done with the same bur. The bur is used in a pendulum-swinging fashion to undermine the marginal ridge and at the same time to establish the gingival depth. The gingival seat should be of sufficient depth to break contact with the adjacent tooth.

The bur that was used to prepare the gingival seat can then be used to prepare the occlusal portion of the cavity, which should be extended throughout the grooves and anatomic defects. The walls of the preparation should then be finished with the bur to remove unsupported enamel rods.

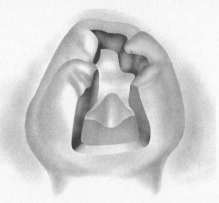

Fig. 12-8. Class II cavity preparation for a primary molar. The preparation includes diverging proximal walls and a beveled and grooved axiopulpal line angle.

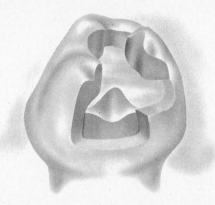

Fig. 12-9. Modified Class II preparation recommended for primary teeth with extensive proximal lesions in which excessive flaring of the proximal surfaces would result in fragile unsupported tooth structure. One or both of the cusps may be capped, depending on the amount of carious involvement.

After the development of the occlusal outline form, the proximal walls may be finished with small hatchets or chisels. The angle formed by the axial wall and the buccal and lingual walls of the proximal box should approach a right angle. The buccal and lingual walls that must necessarily diverge toward the cervical region, following the general contour of the tooth, should be carried into a self-cleansing area. If there is remaining carious material, it should be removed with round burs or spoon excavators and the necessary liner or intermediate base should be placed before the insertion of the silver amalgam.

The rounded-end cutting burs (No. 329, No. 330, No. 245, or No. 256) can be used for the gross cutting of the Class II cavity preparation. Burs of this type can be used to form both the occlusal and the proximal aspects of the cavity. Since they have rounded cutting ends, they will aid in the formation of a preparation in which rounded angles are recommended (Fig. 12-8).

Approximately 30% of the 1009 amalgam restorations in primary teeth observed by Castaldi were classified as failures because of defects at the proximal margins. These defects were found most often on the buccal proximal margin of the mandibular first primary molars. Such defects probably occur because the marginal enamel is poorly supported and is thus liable to fracture. Therefore, if the proximal cavity, particularly one involving the distal surface of the first primary molar, is larger than the incipient type, a modification of the Class II cavity preparation should be considered (Fig. 12-9). Capping of one or both of the cusps will result in a more serviceable amalgam restoration and will overcome the "ditching" effect that often occurs on the buccal and lingual proximal margins of the restoration.

Although many pedodontists advocate restoring most primary molars with extensive carious lesions, especially first primary molars, with chrome steel crowns, we urge the use of amalgam restorations whenever possible. Superior contour and better periodontal health can generally be achieved with amalgam restorations. The dentist's sound professional judgment is the key to selecting the restoration that will best serve the patient in each situation. An amalgam restoration capping the cusp of a first primary molar may be appropriate for a 7½-year-old child, whereas a chrome steel crown may be the restoration of choice for a similar cari-

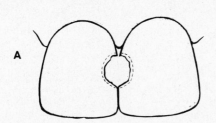 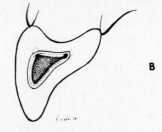

Fig. 12-10. A, Schematic drawing of carious lesions on the mesial surfaces of maxillary primary central incisors that do not undermine the mesial-incisal angles of the teeth. The dotted line indicates the proposed labial outline of the Class III cavity preparation. **B,** Proximal view illustrates that the Class III preparation is limited to the cervical two thirds of the primary incisor. (From Goldman, H.M., and others, editors: Current therapy in dentistry, vol. 4, St. Louis, 1970, The C.V. Mosby Co.)

ous lesion in the first primary molar of a 3-year-old child. Similarly, an MOD amalgam restoration has a better chance for success in a second primary molar than in a first primary molar.

Class III cavity. Carious lesions on the proximal surfaces of anterior primary teeth are not uncommon in children whose teeth are in contact and in those children who have evidence of arch inadequacy or crowding. Carious involvement of the anterior primary teeth, however, may be interpreted as evidence of excessive caries activity requiring comprehensive preventive program.

If the carious lesion has not advanced appreciably into the dentin and if removal of the caries will not involve or weaken the incisal angle, a small conventional Class III cavity may be prepared and the tooth may be restored with composite resin. This procedure will preserve the tooth structure and will maintain an esthetic quality that may not be found in other procedures.

The cavity is opened using slow speed and a No. 329 or No. 330 bur, which can be used to establish the cavity outline and the cervical seat. The same basic principles that have been accepted for permanent anterior teeth should be considered in the Class III preparation in a primary tooth— modified, of course, by the size of the pulp and the relative thinness of the enamel. The cervical seat should be carried gingivally to the extent that contact will be broken with the adjacent tooth. The

extent to which the preparation is carried incisally is governed by the position and size of the lesion and the amount of supporting tooth structure in the area. It should be remembered that abrasion and reduction of the clinical height of the anterior tooth usually continue until exfoliation. This fact is important in selecting the type of cavity preparation and filling material.

The labial and lingual surfaces of the preparation should be trimmed to supported enamel with small chisels or hatchets. Retentive angles or so-called retentive points should be placed in the preparation with a No. ½ bur, one at the incisal angle and one each at the labiogingival and the linguogingival angles (Fig. 12-10).

Modified Class III cavity preparation. The distal surface of the primary canine is a frequent site of caries attack. The position of the tooth in the arch, the characteristically broad contact between the distal surface of the canine and the mesial surface of the primary molar, and the height of the gingival tissue make it essentially impossible to prepare a typical Class III cavity and to restore it adequately. The modified Class III preparation uses a dovetail on the lingual or occasionally on the labial surfaces of the tooth. A lingual lock is normally considered for the maxillary canine, whereas the labial lock may be more conveniently cut on the mandibular teeth where the esthetic requirement is not so important. The preparation allows for addi-

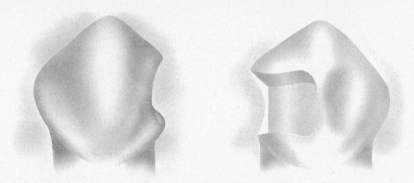

Fig. 12-11. Modified Class III preparation for a primary canine. The dovetail allows access for condensing of the silver amalgam to ensure adequate contact with the adjacent tooth.

tional retention and access necessary to insert the restorative material properly. The modified Class III preparation is often considered essentially a Class II preparation laid on its side or modified for an anterior tooth (Fig. 12-11). Silver amalgam is generally the restorative material of choice for this type of preparation. An amalgam restoration on the distal surface of a maxillary primary canine does not usually present an esthetic problem.

In the initial preparation of the cavity and the establishment of the outline form, small chisels or a No. 330 bur may be used. The labial wall of the cavity is carried to a self-cleansing area and is beveled toward the cavity. The bur can be inserted into the interproximal portion of the cavity from the lingual surface (labial on the lower teeth) to establish the boxing, which is approximately 1 mm in depth at the incisal and gingival areas. The bur is then used to prepare the dovetail, which should be carried 1 mm in depth or just below the dentinoenamel junction. The same principles regarding the width of the neck of the dovetail that apply to the development of a Class II cavity preparation are equally important in the modified Class III preparation. The walls of the dovetail should be finished with a fissure bur to remove unsupported enamel. Small retentive points are placed in the labiogingival and linguogingival angles and in the incisal angle.

Restoration of proximal-incisal caries in primary anterior teeth

Preformed stainless steel bands. The use of preformed stainless steel bands has been advocated by McConville and Tonn for the restoration of anterior primary teeth with deep mesial or distal caries involving the incisal angle. The band is fitted before caries removal. After caries removal with a bur or excavators, an appropriate base is placed in the deep portion of the cavity. The cavity and the band are filled with a creamy mix of cement, and the band is seated to place. After the cement has hardened, the excess cement is removed.

This cemented band technique may be the restoration of choice in the very young child with nursing bottle caries. With the use of accepted methods of restraining the child's movements, this procedure can be carried out quickly and yet provide a satisfactory long-term restoration. After the child has gained more maturity and has become a cooperative patient, the bands may be removed and more esthetic restorations provided.

If the carious involvement of an anterior tooth endangers the pulp, the cemented band is excellent for supporting the intermediate dressing in indirect pulp therapy. Only the gross caries is removed at the initial appointment; calcium hydroxide is

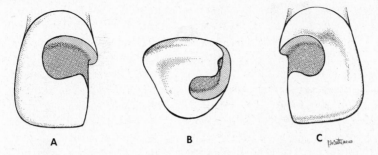

Fig. 12-12. Preparation for an esthetic resin restoration. **A,** Caries has been removed and the proximal slice and labial lock have been completed. **B,** Incisal view shows a shallow groove in the proximal surface. **C,** Lingual view demonstrates the establishment of a cervical seat and lingual lock.

placed on the remaining carious dentin and the previously fitted band is cemented on the tooth to seal the cavity and arrest the caries process. A waiting period of at least 6 weeks is indicated to allow adequate reparative dentin formation before the band is taken off the tooth and the remaining caries removed. If there is no evidence of a pulp exposure, the final restorative procedure is carried out.

Esthetic resin restoration. Doyle (1967) introduced a technique for the restoration of primary incisors in which dental caries approximates or involves the incisal edge of the teeth (Fig. 12-12). As with other operative procedures for the child patient, the use of the rubber dam facilitates maintenance of a dry field, better vision, and control of the lips and tongue.

The No. 69L bur is used to make a proximal slice in a labiolingual direction on the proximal portion of the carious tooth. A No. 330 bur is used to complete the preparation, including the establishment of a cervical seat similar to that described for the preparation of a Class III cavity (Fig. 12-13). Labial and lingual locks are then prepared in the cervical third of the tooth, carrying the base of the preparation into sound dentin. The remaining caries is removed, and a calcium hydroxide base is placed in the depth of the cavity.

The tooth may be restored with unfilled resin or

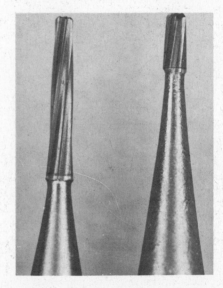

Fig. 12-13. No. 69L bur and No. 330 bur for the completion of the proximal portion of the Doyle preparation and the labial and lingual locks.

composite resin. If unfilled resin is used, incremental buildup of the material with a small brush is the recommended technique. With the composite resin restoration, a bulk pack technique would be appropriate. In either case a properly placed matrix tightly wedged at the cervical seat will aid the oper-

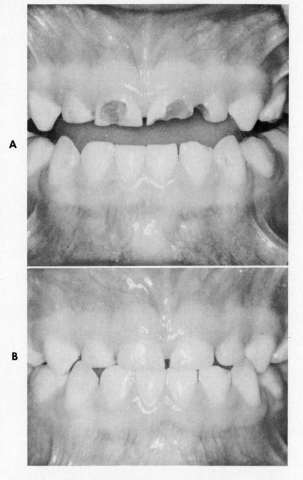

A

B

Fig. 12-14. A, Extensive carious lesions of the maxillary right central, left central, and left lateral incisors of a 3½-year-old patient. **B,** Postoperative view of the restored teeth. The restorations are retained with labial and lingual locks incorporated in the preparations. None of the restorations are full coverage, and the maxillary lateral preparation was designed as illustrated in Fig. 12-12.

ator in placing, shaping, and holding the material while polymerization occurs. A good matrix will also simplify the finishing procedures.

Initial finishing of the restoration may be accomplished with a No. 69L or similar type of bur. The excess resin is removed, and the contour of the restoration is established. The gingival margins

may be finished with a sharp scalpel blade. Final polishing may be accomplished with the rubber cup and a fine moist abrasive material (Fig. 12-14).

Chrome steel crowns. Primary incisors or canines that have extensive proximal lesions involving the incisal portion of the tooth may be restored with chrome steel crowns.

A steel crown of appropriate size is selected, contoured at the cervical margin, polished, and cemented into place. The crown technique is discussed in detail later in this chapter. The dentin exposed by caries removal should be covered with a calcium hydroxide–containing liner before the crown is cemented into place to reduce the possibility of pulpal irritation and postoperative discomfort. Although the crown will be retained well even on teeth that require removal of extensive portions of carious tooth structure, the esthetic requirement of some children may not be met by this type of restoration.

Fig. 12-15 illustrates a primary canine that had an extensive carious lesion involving the labial and mesial surfaces and the incisal portion of the tooth. The carious material was removed from the tooth, and the undercut areas, including the lingual surface, were reduced to allow the steel crown to be placed without interfering with proper occlusion. After proper contouring of the crown at the cervical margin, the labial portion of the metal was removed. Following cementation of the crown, the labial portion of the restoration was completed by the addition of resin.

Direct resin crowns. In 1979 Doyle introduced a new preparation technique for primary incisor jacket crowns that uses an undercut area around the gingival shoulder, retains as much enamel as possible for etching, and preserves the midportion of the natural incisal edge, whenever possible, to help retard incisal abrasion and improve retention. After excavating the caries, protecting the exposed dentin, and etching the enamel, the dentist restores the prepared incisor with a preformed acrylic jacket crown lined with self-curing restorative resin. After polymerization the cervical margins and the incisal edge of the restoration are finished and pol-

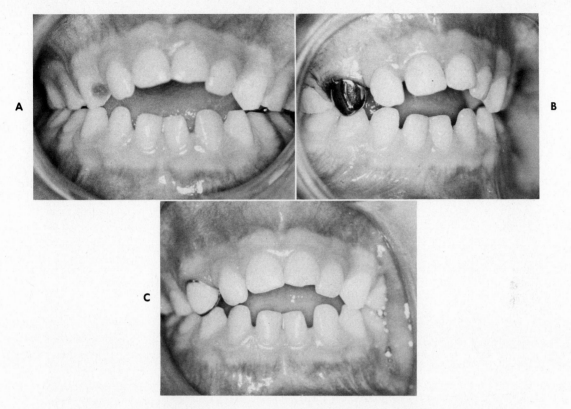

Fig. 12-15. A, An extensive carious lesion is evident in the maxillary right primary canine. **B,** After the removal of caries and preparation of the tooth, a chrome steel crown was fitted to the tooth. **C,** The labial portion of the steel crown was removed and the restoration cemented to the tooth. The labial portion of the restoration consists of resin. (Courtesy Dr. Lionel Traubman.)

ished so that there is no cervically overextended restorative material and so that the tooth's preserved natural incisal edge is exposed.

Webber and associates have described a resin crown technique very similar to Doyle's except that the tooth is restored with composite resin using a celluloid crown form as a matrix. They do not advocate preserving a portion of the incisal edge. They point out that very little finishing of the restoration is required when the celluloid crown has been properly fitted.

The restorations produced with Doyle's technique are quite satisfactory but require considerable finishing after polymerization. However, his idea of preserving a portion of the tooth's natural

incisal edge whenever possible seems valid. The natural incisal edge of the tooth should resist wear better than the resin restorative material. In addition, preserving the incisal area of the tooth preserves a greater surface area of etched enamel and greater length in the preparation, which will improve the retentive quality of the restoration.

The jacket crown technique illustrated in Fig. 12-16 incorporates the use of a celluloid crown form and composite resin as advocated by Webber and associates. Fig. 12-16 also illustrates the preservation of the tooth's natural incisal edge as advocated by Doyle. Either self-curing or light-curing composite resin materials may be used. The light-curing materials make it possible to carefully re-

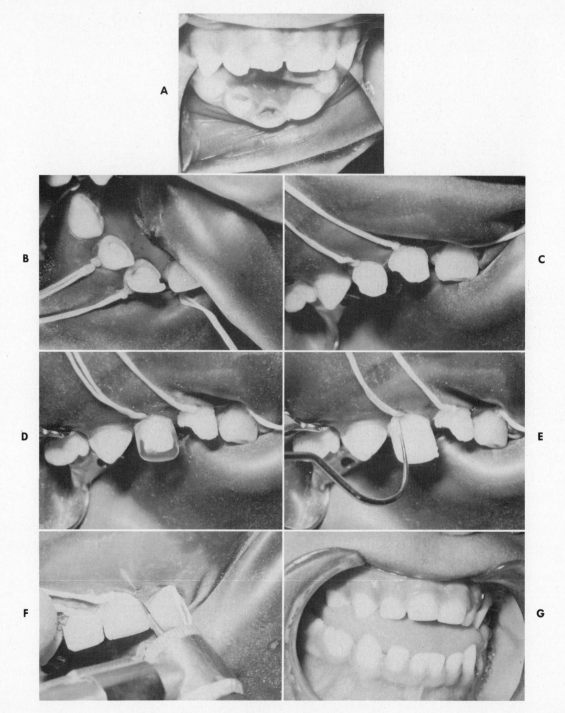

Fig. 12-16. For legend see opposite page.

move all excess material at the cervical margin before any polymerization takes place.

Polycarbonate jacket crowns. Another technique for jacket crown restorations on primary anterior teeth uses preformed, tooth-colored, polycarbonate crowns. The tooth that is to be restored is prepared in the conventional manner for a jacket crown, including a 1- to 2-mm reduction of the incisal edge. The proximal walls of the preparation should be essentially parallel with a slight tendency to converge cervically to provide some "undercut" retention. A shoulder is produced circumferentially to establish the cervical extension of the crown. The dentist selects a crown with the proper mesiodistal dimension and then trims the cervical portion of the crown to establish the correct incisocervical height and to fit the preparation shoulder (Fig. 12-17).

The crown may be luted into place with a polycarboxylate cement or an unfilled resin. Unfilled resin may require more finishing at the cervical margin, but it will also result in better marginal adaptation and retention of the restoration, especially if some enamel has been preserved in the preparation for etching. The unfilled resin will bond to the polycarbonate crown, resulting in a single unit that is well adapted to the preparation.

It is not unusual for the dentist to find that the

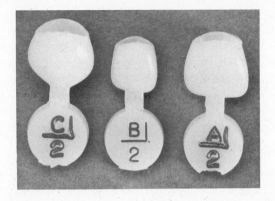

Fig. 12-17. Representative preformed polycarbonate anterior crowns as supplied by the manufacturer.

crown size selected to have the proper mesiodistal width has an inside dimension that is too small for the preparation. When this happens, it is best to select a larger crown that will cover the preparation and to reduce the outside dimension of the crown to the proper size. The proximal and incisal thicknesses of the preformed crowns are designed to allow adjustment in this manner. It may also be necessary to modify the tooth preparation to better fit the inside dimensions of the crown.

Only minor modifications of the inside of the crown should be made if the crown is to be ce-

Fig. 12-16. A, Extensive caries on the lingual surfaces of the maxillary right primary central and lateral incisors in a 2½-year-old patient. The maxillary left central incisor had been previously restored. **B,** The carious lesions have been excavated and the exposed dentin is covered with calcium hydroxide. **C,** Completed jacket preparations with cervical shoulders, slightly undercut walls at the cervical areas, and preservation of as much enamel and incisal tooth structure as possible. The enamel has been etched. **D,** Fitted celluloid crown form on the lateral incisor. The crown form should be trimmed to fit snugly and to just cover all cervical margins of the preparation. A snug fit at the cervical margin is very desirable, even if the incisal is too long, to minimize cervical finishing of the restoration. **E,** The crown form filled with composite resin has been seated, and the excess material is being carefully removed at the cervical with an explorer. Note excess material exuding from the vent hole placed on the mesial incisal of the crown form. **F,** The central incisor was restored in a similar fashion. The incisal edges of the restorations have been trimmed back to the natural tooth structure with the No. 7901 finishing bur, which is also being used to trim the cervical margins. The restorations are polished with flour of pumice followed by composite polishing paste in a rubber cup. **G,** The resin jacket crown restorations 2 months postoperatively. (Courtesy Dr. Robert Rust.)

mented with polycarboxylate cement. The inside of the crown is designed to "fit" a tooth preparation with good retentive qualities. Too much modification will compromise the crown's retentive capabilities. If the luting material is unfilled resin, more modification of the inside of the crown is possible because the resin will bond to the crown. Although polycarbonate crowns offer good esthetic results initially, they do not seem to provide long-term durability. They do not resist wear well, and in time they may chip or crack. If they are used to restore carious or fractured incisors in a 2-year-old child, it is likely that they will need repair or replacement before the normal exfoliation of the teeth.

Basic principles in the preparation of Class II cavities in permanent molars

The principles of cavity preparation for permanent molars, as presented many years ago by Black, are generally still advocated today. In recent years, however, as the result of extensive laboratory and clinical research, Gilmore and associates have recommended modifications of the original Black preparation. The most obvious difference is a reduction in the dimensions of the cavity preparation, made possible by the smaller burs available today and the precision methods of cutting tooth structure.

The following basic principles will serve as guides in the preparation of Class II cavities in permanent molars. All fissured grooves in the occlusal surface that appear caries susceptible should be extended and included in the preparation to prevent caries recurrence. However, they should be kept at a minimum width. The proximal portion of the restoration should be self-retentive. The proximal outline will be determined by the extent of the lesion and by the morphology of the adjacent tooth; the preparation is carried buccolingually to an area not quite touching the adjacent tooth to allow cleansing by the patient. The proximal outline should converge occlusally to a slight degree in the form of a mortise, generally following the buccal and lingual contour of the tooth. The gingival margin should be extended cervically to break contact with the adjacent tooth. Thus the outline of the cavity for the amalgam restoration is determined by the size of the carious lesion, the need for extension for prevention, and the occlusal anatomy of the tooth. Extensive cutting of the natural sound tooth structure will only weaken the tooth and the final restoration.

For detailed information about the various cavity preparation designs for permanent teeth, the reader should consult a standard textbook of operative dentistry listed in the references, such as those by Baum, Phillips, and Lund and by Gilmore and associates.

Protection of the pulp during cavity preparation

There has been considerable controversy regarding the necessity of using a water coolant when cavities are cut with carbide burs at ultrahigh speed (250,000 rpm). The cutting of the cavity preparation in a dry field with the tooth isolated by a rubber dam has the advantage of allowing a considerably better view of the tooth and cavity preparation. However, the concern has been that the elevation of pulpal temperature and the dehydration of the dentin could produce irreversible damage to the odontoblastic layer and the underlying pulpal tissues.

The "burning" of dentin and the buildup of heat sufficient to damage the pulp are possible if there is other than intermittent application of the bur to the tooth structure during the preparation of a cavity without the application of a water spray to the revolving bur. However, sufficient evidence has been presented (Bhaskar and Lilly; Bouschour and Matthews) to allow the conclusion that high-speed cavity preparation with only air as a coolant is acceptable if a light and intermittent bur pressure is used. Evidence indicates that when operating in a dry field at 3000 rpm with a large bur, the operator may produce more pulpal damage than with careful intermittent application of a small carbide bur revolving at a speed in excess of 200,000 rpm.

Cavity bases and liners

The base material is placed before the restoration of the cavity to provide thermal insulation for the dental pulp. There is also evidence that the use of a calcium hydroxide–containing material will favorably influence the formation of secondary dentin.

Bases are seldom required in primary teeth. However, deep cavities resulting from the removal of extensive caries should receive a base before the placement of a restoration. Zinc phosphate cement bases are used less frequently today because the cement is irritating to the pulp and because the acid in the liquid does not reach neutrality for many hours.

If a minute pulp exposure may be present, one of the rapid-setting calcium hydroxide–containing bases should be used. Only the deepest portion of the cavity should be filled, allowing the restoration to be supported by sound dentin.

Zinc oxide–eugenol bases containing an accelerator to promote rapid setting are acceptable when there is no danger of a pulp exposure. The addition of zinc acetate crystals (approximately 4%) to zinc oxide–eugenol produces a base material that sets rapidly.

It is important to avoid carrying the base onto the cavity wall margin of the preparation, since this would result in deterioration of the material and marginal leakage. The base selected should be sufficiently strong to resist displacement and fracture during the condensing of an amalgam restoration.

The routine use of a cavity varnish before placing an amalgam restoration will reduce the possibility of discoloration of the dentin and will help prevent marginal leakage. The application of two or three thin layers of quick-drying varnish to freshly cut dentin will also reduce sensitivity after the placement of the restoration.

Going has reported that a fresh Copalite varnish applied in a thin uniform coating over zinc oxide–eugenol or calcium hydroxide fulfills all the requirements of a good liner. A cavity liner should protect the pulp from thermal shock, insulate against the galvanic action inherent in all amalgam restorations, inhibit mercury penetration, provide an anodyne effect on the pulp, produce antibacterial activity, neutralize the acid of zinc phosphate and silicate cements, and reduce marginal leakage. The use of cavity varnishes is discussed in greater detail in Chapter 13.

Matrix retainers and bands

The selection of a matrix has long been recognized as an important step in the placement of an amalgam restoration. The matrix should be rigid enough to allow adequate packing pressure, ensuring a well-condensed restoration free from an excess of residual mercury. Numerous mechanical devices have been used in the past with apparent success. However, mechanical retainers, although convenient to use, may not produce the most desirable finished restoration.

The use of an uncontoured band will result in an amalgam restoration with a flat proximal surface and a high contact area that will favor food impaction and subsequent periodontal changes (Fig. 12-18). Phillips and associates (1956) evaluated eight matrix band techniques, including five different mechanical retainers, for their effectiveness in restoring the proximal contour of the amalgam restorations. Although none of the techniques perfectly reproduced the proximal surface, there were only

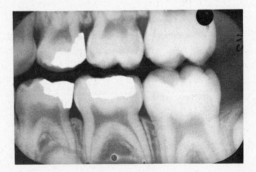

Fig. 12-18. Amalgam restorations with flat proximal surfaces, high contact area, and cervical overhang. An unsatisfactory restoration of this type will often result from the use of an uncontoured and improperly wedged matrix band.

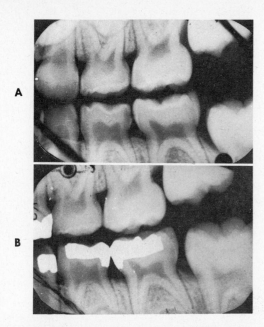

Fig. 12-19. A, Preoperative bite-wing radiograph demonstrates proximal mandibular molar caries and a lesion on the distal surface of the canine. **B,** Teeth have been restored to their normal proximal contour.

slight deviations when the band material was contoured, wedged, and supported. The results of the study clearly indicated that, regardless of the type of retainer or matrix used, wedging was imperative to eliminate a cervical flash of amalgam. Tocchini also believes that wedging and contouring the matrix band are essential in producing a multiple-surface amalgam restoration that has a normal proximal contour and is free of cervical overhang.

The isolation of the teeth with the rubber dam not only offers the advantages previously discussed in this chapter but also allows the use of the preformed or sectional matrix band technique. With the latter technique the contoured band can be easily retained and a restoration with the original proximal contour can be placed with consistency (Fig. 12-19).

Preformed band technique. In the preformed band technique a steel band material (0.0015 or 0.0020) is cut into strips 1½ inches in length. If a primary tooth is to be restored, band material ³⁄₁₆ inch wide is usually adequate. For permanent teeth, ¼-inch material is more desirable. The material is formed into a loop, placed around the prepared tooth, and pinched on the buccal surface. The free ends of the band may be riveted with a No. 141 pliers to secure the band to the tooth or the band may be removed and spot welded. The excess material should be trimmed from the free ends, and the proximal surface of the band should be contoured with the No. 114 pliers. The band is then replaced on the tooth and the cervical edge is tightly wedged.

Preformed stainless steel custom bands in assorted sizes are available from several manufacturers. It is often possible to select a band that will fit the prepared tooth snugly. It is necessary only to contour the proximal surface before its final placement and wedging at the cervical margin.

T-band matrix. Although it is incorrect to assume that one particular type of matrix retainer or band technique can be universally recommended for the placement of an amalgam restoration, the T-band matrix seems to approach the ideal. It can be easily placed, contoured, and removed, and it can be used in the placement of proximal surface restorations in primary or permanent teeth.

The T-band is available in two types—a narrow width and a wide width—with a choice of stainless steel or brass material. The steel material can be more adequately contoured and becomes work hardened and sturdy. The loop may be prepared in advance and slipped over the tooth and tightened, reducing the operating time. The band may be removed from the tooth, and the proximal surface may be contoured before wedging.

Hardwood wedges, which are available in a variety of sizes, are the choice of many dentists, particularly when they are wedging bands for permanent teeth. The custom wedge, however, is often more adaptable to the small interproximal areas between primary teeth (Figs. 12-20 and 12-21).

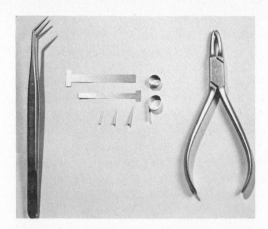

Fig. 12-20. The T-band will be an adequate matrix for most primary and permanent teeth if properly contoured, wedged, and on occasion supported with compound.

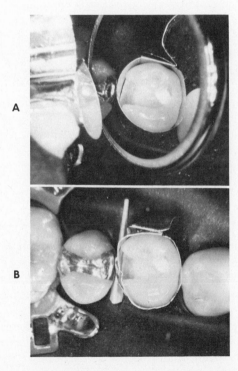

Fig. 12-21. A, Initial fitting of a T-band matrix to a maxillary first premolar. **B,** The properly fitted matrix after it has been contoured and wedged.

Condensation of the alloy

Gilmore and associates recommend that small increments of amalgam be used in building the restoration. Even when proper condensation techniques are employed, it is impossible to secure good adaptation of large increments of amalgam to the walls of the cavity.

The physical properties of an amalgam condensed with a proper hand technique are comparable to those of an amalgam condensed by a mechanical device.

When nonspherical alloys are employed, heavy pressure on the condenser is required to eliminate as much residual mercury as possible. The greater the condensation pressure, the lower is the residual mercury and the higher the strength. Condensation pressure of approximately 6 pounds is adequate. It must be remembered that the smaller the condenser point, the greater the pressure applied to the amalgam in terms of pounds per square inch. Thus the use of smaller condensing points results in higher condensation pressures than if larger points were used.

The use of amalgam that has been permitted to harden for longer than 3 or 3½ minutes makes it impossible to eliminate the mercury during condensation. Such amalgam, increments that are too dry, or inadequate condensation pressure leads to internal voids in the restoration and marginal chipping.

Burnishing the alloy

Burnishing by rubbing the carved amalgam surface with a smooth instrument is the last step in the manipulation of an amalgam restoration before the complete setting of the material. It is important if high-copper amalgam is used. Gilmore and associates point out that burnishing diminishes the surface microporosity by compaction. It also reduces the residual mercury content on the surface and at the margins. Burnishing can be started 2 to 3 minutes after carving. It produces a shiny surface and shortens the polishing time at a subsequent appointment.

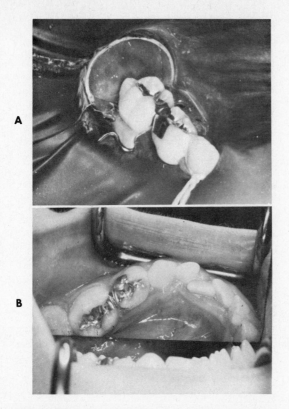

Fig. 12-22. Polished amalgam restorations. **A,** The rubber dam has been replaced for the polishing procedure. It is the practice of some dentists to invite the parents into the operatory to view the finished restorations before the removal of the rubber dam. **B,** A mirror view of the approximating restorations.

Polishing amalgam restorations

An amalgam restoration should be in place for at least 24 hours (preferably for 1 week) before polishing. A smooth, polished amalgam restoration will retain its color longer and will resist corrosion and tarnish (Fig. 12-22). The greatest advantage derived from polishing an amalgam restoration, however, lies in the opportunity for the dentist to remove the flash or amalgam that is inadvertently allowed to cover the cavosurface of the preparation after the carving of the restoration. The eventual breaking away of the excess material will result in a marginal defect and unsightly discoloration of the tooth. The marginal defect is often the site for recurrence of dental decay.

The initial contouring of amalgam restorations and the reduction of areas of excessive height, as evidenced by burnished facets in the amalgam, may be accomplished with small round diamond stones comparable in size to No. 2, No. 4, and No. 6 round burs. Care should be taken to minimize contact with the enamel. Excessive contact between the enamel margin and the diamond stone will fracture away any irregularly positioned enamel rods and will produce a roughened surface favoring plaque formation. Fine cuttle disks may be used to finish buccal and lingual proximal margins, avoiding the contact area. Gold-finishing burs may be used to shape and polish the occlusal surface. The final luster may be added by the application of moist tin oxide with a soft wheel brush and a rubber cup. Throughout the polishing procedure, care should be taken to avoid excessive heat production and the resultant drawing of mercury to the surface.

Cavity margin deterioration

Horwitz, Klein, and McDonald have used the intraoral television microscope for the micromeasurement of cavity margin deterioration. The buccoproximal margins of 51 mesio-occlusal silver amalgam alloy restorations were serially and periodically measured and evaluated throughout 1 year. Because all teeth had incipient proximal lesions, it was possible to complete an ideal type of cavity preparation under a rubber dam.

There was progressive gingival margin deterioration, ranging from 4.9 μm at 1 week to 54.8 μm at 1 year. On the occlusal margin the deterioration ranged from an average of 5.4 μm at 1 week to 77.7 μm at 1 year.

The gingival area of proximal margin deteriorated at a faster rate during the first 12 weeks than did the occlusal area. However, the occlusal area deteriorated faster during the last 24 weeks.

Although all the restorations were carefully carved and polished, microscopic flash was observed more frequently in the gingival area. The

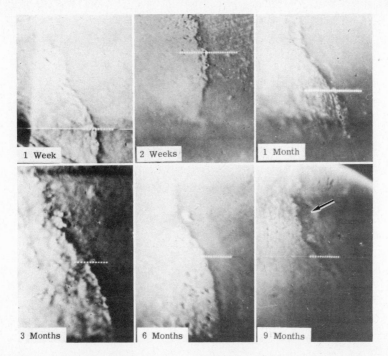

Fig. 12-23. Serial television micromeasurement (original magnification × 250) photographs indicate the line of measurement as a series of dots, calibrated to be 10 μm apart. Marginal defects representing sites for recurrent decay may be easily seen.

findings support the belief that it is more difficult to adequately carve and polish the gingival areas of amalgam restorations. Occlusal forces were perhaps responsible for the greater deterioration of the occlusal margins during the later periods of observation.

The micromeasurement photographs emphasized the importance of careful finishing of all margins of the amalgam to reduce the marginal deterioration resulting from fracturing away of excess material. Marginal defects such as those shown in Fig. 12-23 will often provide the site for recurrent decay. Although the newer, high-copper amalgam alloys have not been evaluated for marginal integrity by the television micromeasurement technique, many other types of evaluation have been done. The high-copper amalgams consistently give superior performance when compared with conventional alloys. Marginal deterioration seems to

be less significant when the materials are placed in adequate cavity preparations and handled properly.

Composite resin restorations for posterior teeth

The improvement in the properties of the composite resins has led many dentists to consider their use for Class I and Class II restorations (Fig. 12-24). In pedodontics the material has also proved useful in restoring badly damaged tooth crowns before making preparation for a steel crown or a full cast gold crown. The physical properties of restorative resins are discussed in Chapter 13.

Class II restorations. Phillips and associates (1972) made a critical observation of Class II composite resin restorations over a 2-year period and compared them with amalgam restorations. No recurrent marginal caries was detected in the 124

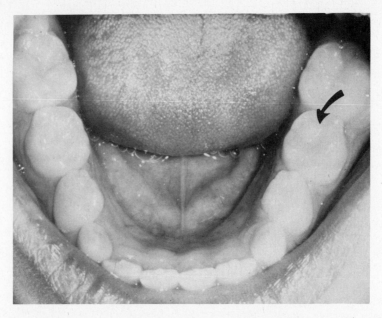

Fig. 12-24. A distal occlusal composite resin restoration was placed in the lower left second primary molar 6 months before the photograph. Note the esthetic result.

paired restorations during the 2-year observation period. At the end of 2 years a number of restorations of each material exhibited some degree of marginal breakdown; however, no gross fractures occurred among the composite restorations. Amalgam restorations exhibited little or no change in anatomic form, whereas a moderate change was observed in approximately half the composite resins. The change in anatomic form appeared to be the result of occlusal wear. A change in color match was observed in approximately 60% of the composite resins during the 2-year period. However, the change appeared to result from a surface stain rather than from a color shift of the material. Many of the restorations were reevaluated after a 3-year period, but the findings did not differ significantly from the 2-year results. The researchers concluded that until formulations are improved, the use of composite systems in Class II restorations should be limited to situations in which the esthetic result is the major consideration and the cavity preparation is conservative.

As the research and development of composite materials continue, the materials continue to improve. Evaluating the durability of improved composite restorative materials in posterior teeth is an ongoing process. Since the initial clinical research by Phillips and associates, Nelson and associates completed a similar 3-year study that compared the performance of an improved composite material with a high-copper amalgam in posterior primary teeth. Their study incorporated the use of etched enamel margins and a resin bonding agent on the teeth that were restored with the improved composite material. They observed that amalgam and composite resin restorations showed little difference in performance in the posterior primary dentition over the 3-year period. They concluded that a dentist would be justified in using composite restorations with acid etch and bonding agents in the late primary dentititon where the projected life span of the tooth is 3 years or less.

If an esthetic restorative material can be produced that will be durable and provide perfect (chemical) bonding to tooth structure, it will significantly affect the current principles of restorative dentistry. It would then be necessary only to remove carious material and restore the tooth without regard for the basic principles of cavity preparation outlined in this chapter. Some have suggested that such a restorative approach, using composite restoratives and etching techniques, may already be appropriate for primary teeth. Leifler and Varpio used a modified Class II cavity preparation for shallow proximal caries in primary molars. Caries excavation was performed in the conventional manner, but other cavity preparation was minimal. Retention of the restorative material was dependent on etched enamel on the occlusal surface and along the proximal box. After 2 years, 41% of the restorations were graded excellent and 25% were observed to have minor defects but were still clinically acceptable. Occlusal wear was not a problem during the period of the study.

Leinfelder and Vann recently reported on a somewhat similar approach to composite restorations in primary molars that is being evaluated by clinical research. The modified preparations simply involve the removal of carious enamel and dentin with extension only for visual and mechanical access. The preparation margins are beveled to enhance the bonding of the restorative material to the etched enamel and to reduce the incidence of enamel fractures at the margins.

At this writing these deviations from the accepted principles of restorative dentistry are experimental and are not yet recommended for routine use. We believe that a significantly improved restorative technique will be developed in the foreseeable future. Research and development of materials and techniques should continue. However, for the time being, high-copper amalgam materials placed in conventional cavity preparations are recommended to the practitioner who routinely provides restorative services to patients. Whenever composite restorative materials are employed (even for routine anterior restorations), the use of enamel etching and resin bonding agents is also recommended.

Interim restoration for hypoplastic permanent molars. The dentist who routinely treats children occasionally faces a difficult restorative problem when severely hypoplastic first permanent molars erupt. Often the teeth are so defective that they require restoration at a very early stage of eruption. Many of these teeth have been saved by early restoration with chrome steel crowns as an interim procedure. However, this is a difficult procedure that sometimes requires sacrificing sound tooth surfaces to provide adequate space for the crown. Such full-coverage restorations are difficult to fit, and the best results one can achieve are often disappointing.

The newer composite materials have proved to be a more satisfactory interim restoration for many of these teeth. Such a resin "buildup" restoration allows preservation of all sound tooth structure and is dependent on some enamel surfaces to provide retention and marginal seal for the restorative material, which is bonded to the available etched enamel. The defective areas are excavated and any exposed dentin is protected with calcium hydroxide in the conventional manner, but little or no additional tooth preparation is done. Usually even undermined enamel surfaces are preserved for additional retention and support of the restorative material. In some cases a gingivectomy around the erupting tooth may first be necessary to allow adequate access to and isolation of the defective areas. Even if the restoration requires occasional repair, it still often provides a more satisfactory interim result than the chrome steel crown. In addition, a more satisfactory preparation for a later cast restoration can usually be made following the interim resin restoration than can be achieved after the tooth has been prepared for a chrome steel crown.

Chrome steel crowns

The chrome steel crown, as introduced by Humphrey, has proved to be a serviceable restoration in selected cases. Unless it is properly handled, however, the restoration will be inadequate.

There are a number of indications for the chrome

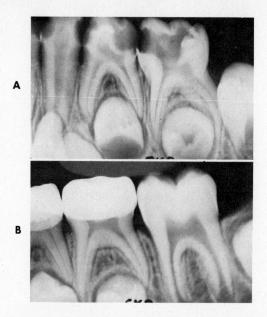

Fig. 12-25. A, Primary molars with extensive carious lesions and inadequate tooth structure to support an amalgam restoration. **B,** Adequately contoured chrome steel crowns have maintained the relationship of the primary teeth in the arch.

steel crown in dentistry for children, including the following:

1. A restoration for a primary or young permanent tooth with extensive carious lesions
2. A restoration for a hypoplastic primary or permanent tooth that cannot be adequately restored with silver amalgam or a composite resin interior restoration
3. A restoration for a tooth with a hereditary anomaly, such as dentinogenesis imperfecta or amelogenesis imperfecta
4. A restoration after a pulpotomy in a primary or permanent tooth in which there is increased danger of fracture of the remaining coronal tooth structure
5. An attachment when there is an indication for a crown and loop space maintainer
6. An attachment for habit-breaking appliances.
7. A restoration for a fractured tooth

8. A restoration for a first primary molar when it is to be the abutment for a distal extension appliance

The chrome steel crown is most often used to restore teeth with extensive carious lesions when there is inadequate support for the retention of an amalgam restoration (Fig. 12-25).

Preparation of the tooth. A local anesthetic should be administered and a rubber dam placed as for other restorative procedures. The proximal surfaces are reduced with a No. 69L bur at high speed (Fig. 12-26). Care must be taken not to damage adjacent tooth surfaces during the proximal reductions. A wooden wedge placed tightly between the surface being reduced and the adjacent surface may be used to provide a slight separation between the teeth for better access. Near-vertical reductions are made on the proximal surfaces and carried gingivally to the extent that the contact with the adjacent tooth is broken and an explorer can be passed freely between the prepared tooth and the adjacent tooth. The gingival margin of the preparation on the proximal surface should be a smooth featheredge with no ledge or shoulder present. The cusps and the occlusal portion of the tooth may then be reduced with the No. 69L bur revolving at high speed. The general contour of the occlusal surface is followed, and approximately 1 mm of clearance with the opposing teeth is provided (Fig. 12-27).

The No. 69L bur at high speed may also be used to remove all sharp line and point angles. It is usually not necessary to reduce the buccal or lingual surfaces; in fact, it is desirable to have an undercut on these surfaces to aid in the retention of the contoured crown. In some cases, however, it may be necessary to reduce the distinct buccal bulge, particularly on the first primary molar.

If any carious dentin remains after these steps in crown preparation are completed, it is excavated next. In the event that a vital pulp exposure is encountered, the 5-minute formocresol pulpotomy procedure is usually carried out. The dentist may begin the process of selecting and fitting the crown during the time the formocresol treatment is being applied to the amputated pulp tissue.

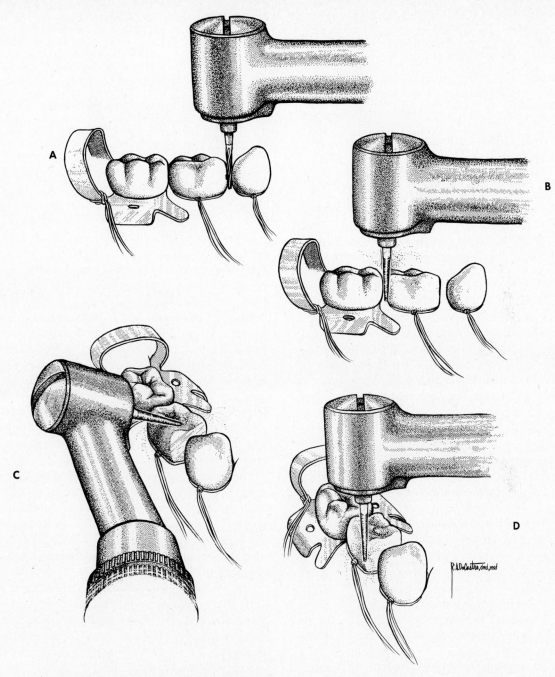

Fig. 12-26. Steps in the preparation of a primary molar for a chrome steel crown restoration using a No. 69L bur in the high-speed handpiece. **A,** Mesial reduction. **B,** Distal reduction. **C,** Occlusal reduction. **D,** Rounding the line angles.

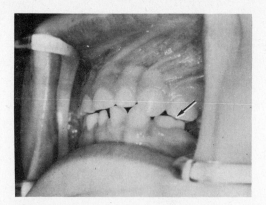

Fig. 12-27. Approximately 1 mm of tooth structure has been removed from the occlusal surface to allow clearance with the opposing teeth and to prevent traumatic occlusion after the placement of the crown.

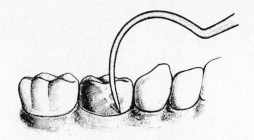

Fig. 12-28. A scratch if made at the level of the free margin of the gingival tissue as an aid in determining where additional metal must be removed.

Selection of crown size. The smallest crown that completely covers the preparation should be chosen. The crown should be reduced in height with contouring scissors until it clears the occlusion and is approximately 0.5 to 1 mm beneath the free margin of the gingival tissue. The patient can force the crown over the preparation by biting an orangewood stick or a tongue blade. After making a scratch mark on the crown at the level of the free margin of the gingival tissue, the dentist can remove the crown and determine where additional metal must be cut away with a No. 11B curved shears to prevent damage to the gingival attachment (Fig. 12-28).

With a No. 137 pliers, the cut edges of the chrome crown are redirected cervically and the crown is replaced on the preparation. The child is again directed to bite on tongue blades to forcibly seat the crown so that the gingival margins may be checked for proper extension.

In selected situations the newer precontoured and shorter crowns require very little modification.

Contouring the crown. The No. 112 or No. 114 ball-and-socket pliers used only at the cervical third of the buccal and lingual surfaces will help to closely adapt the margins of the crown to the cer-

vical portion of the tooth. The handles of the pliers are tipped toward the center of the crown, thereby stretching the metal and curling it inward as the crown is moved toward the pliers from the opposite side. The No. 137 pliers is used to improve the contour on the buccal and lingual surfaces (Fig. 12-29). This pliers may also be used to contour the proximal areas of the crown and develop desirable contact with adjacent teeth. Trimming and contouring are continued until the crown fits the preparation snugly and extends under the free margin of the gingival tissue. For final close adaptation of the cervical margin when abrupt inward curling of the metal is needed, the No. 800-417 pliers is effective (Fig. 12-30).

The crown should be replaced on the preparation after the contouring procedure to see that it snaps securely into place. The occlusion should be checked at this stage to make sure that the crown is not opening the bite or causing a shifting of the mandible into an undesirable relationship with the opposing teeth (Fig. 12-31).

The final step before cementation is to produce a knife-edged gingival margin that may be polished and well tolerated by the gingival tissue. A rubber abrasive wheel can be used to produce the smooth margin.

Although the manufacturers of chrome steel crowns have increased the selection of sizes for molar teeth, there may be an occasion to modify the best-fitting crown to produce a more desirable

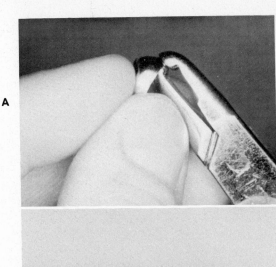

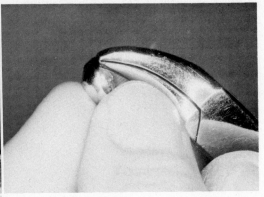

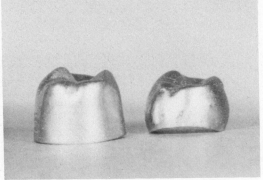

Fig. 12-29. A, The No. 112 or No. 114 pliers is used to contour the buccal and lingual surfaces. The crown is held firmly with the pliers, and pressure is exerted with the finger from the opposite side of the crown to bend the surface inward. **B,** The No. 137 pliers is "walked" completely around the cervical margins of the crown to direct all margins inward with smooth flowing contour. **C,** The crown on the right was the same size and shape as the crown on the left before it was trimmed and contoured. This illustrates the effectiveness of the contouring procedures with the pliers as described.

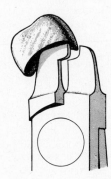

Fig. 12-30. Final close adaptation of the crown to the cervical margin of the preparation may be accomplished with the aid of No. 800-417 pliers.

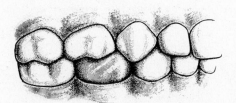

Fig. 12-31. Final adaptation of the crown should result in good occlusion before cementation.

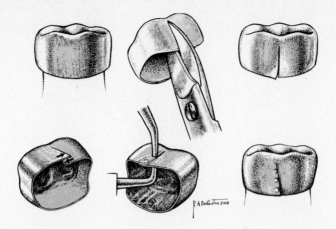

Fig. 12-32. Technique for adapting an oversize crown to a prepared tooth.

adaptability to the prepared cervical margin. Mink and Hill have referred to methods of modifying steel crowns for primary and permanent teeth.

The oversize crown may be cut as illustrated in Fig. 12-32 and the cut edges overlapped. The crown is replaced on the tooth to ensure that it now fits snugly at the cervical region, and a scratch is made at the overlapped margin. The crown is removed from the tooth and the overlapped material repositioned and welded. A small amount of solder is flowed over the outside margin. The crown is finished in the previously recommended manner and cemented to the prepared tooth.

If the dentist encounters a tooth that is too large for the largest crown, a similar technique may be helpful. The crown may be cut on the buccal or lingual surface. After the crown has been adapted to the prepared tooth, an additional piece of 0.004-inch stainless steel band material may be welded into place. A small amount of solder should be added to the outer surface of the margins. The crown may then be contoured in the usual manner, polished, and cemented into place.

REFERENCES

Baum, L., Phillips, R.W., and Lund, M.R.: Textbook of operative dentistry, Philadelphia, 1981, W.B. Saunders Co.

Bhaskar, S.N., and Lilly, G.E.: Intrapulpal temperature during cavity preparation, J. Dent. Res. **44:**644-647, 1965.

Black, G.V.: A work on operative dentistry, vol. 2, ed. 5, Chicago, 1924, Medico-Dental Publishing Co.

Bouschour, C.F., and Matthews, J.L.: A four-year clinical study of teeth restored after preparation with an air turbine handpiece with an air coolant, J. Prosthet. Dent. **16:**306-309, 1966.

Castaldi, C.R.: Analysis of some operative procedures currently being used in pedodontics, J. Can. Dent. Assoc. **23:**377-384, 1957.

Doyle, W.A.: Esthetic restoration of deciduous incisors: a new Class IV preparation, J.A.D.A. **74:**82-84, 1967.

Doyle, W.A.: A new preparation for primary incisor jackets, Pediatr. Dent. **1:**38-40, 1979.

Gilmore, H.W., and others: Operative dentistry, ed. 4, St. Louis, 1982, The C.V. Mosby Co.

Going, R.E.: The best cavity liner: Copalite varnish over zinc oxide–eugenol or calcium hydroxide, J.A.D.A. **69:**415-422, 1964.

Hartsook, J.T.: Principles involved in preparing proximo-occlusal cavities in deciduous teeth, J.A.D.A. **51:**649-654, 1955.

Heise, A.L.: Time required in rubber dam placement, J. Dent. Child. **38:**116-117, 1971.

Horwitz, B.A., Klein, A.I., and McDonald, R.E.: Intraoral television micromeasurement of cavity margin deterioration, J. Dent. Res. **46:**700-707, 1967.

Humphrey, W.P.: Uses of chrome steel in children's dentistry, Dent. Surv. **26:**945-949, 1950.

Law, D.B., and Shepard, S.L.: A method for determination of enamel rod direction in primary teeth, Proc. Am. Acad. Pedod. **8:**21, 1955.

Leifler, E., and Varpio, M.: Proximoclusal composite restorations in primary molars: a two-year follow-up, J. Dent. Child. **48:**411-416, 1981.

Leinfelder, K.F., and Vann, W.F., Jr.: The use of composite resins in primary molars, Pediatr. Dent. **4:**27-31, 1982.

McConville, R.E., and Tonn, E.M.: A method of restoring deciduous anterior teeth, J.A.D.A. **75:**617-620, 1967.

Mink, J.R., and Hill, C.J.: Modification of the stainless steel crown for primary teeth, J. Dent. Child. **38:**61-69, 1971.

Nelson, G.V., and others: A three-year clinical evaluation of composite resin and a high-copper amalgam in posterior primary teeth, J. Dent. Child. **47:**414-418, 1980.

Phillips, R.W., and others: Proximal contour of Class II amalgam restorations made with various matrix band techniques, J.A.D.A. **53:**391-402, 1956.

Phillips, R.W., and others: Observations on a composite resin for Class II restorations: two-year report, J. Prosthet. Dent. **28:**164-169, 1972.

Phillips, R.W., and others: Observations on a composite resin for Class II restorations: three-year report, J. Prosthet. Dent. **30:**891-897, 1973.

Roche, J.R.: Restorative dentistry. In Goldman, H.M., and others, editors: Current therapy in dentistry, vol. 4, St. Louis, 1970, The C.V. Mosby Co.

Rowe, W., and Ireland, R.L.: Enamel rod direction in the cervical third of primary teeth, Proc. Am. Acad. Pedod. **9:**24-25, 1956.

Tocchini, J.: Preformed multiple matrix bands, J. Calif. Dent. Assoc. Nev. Dent. Soc. **35:**22-24, 1959.

Webber, D.L., and others: A method of restoring primary anterior teeth with the aid of a celluloid crown form and composite resins, Pediatr. Dent. **1:**244-246, 1979.

13 Dental materials in pedodontics

RALPH W. PHILLIPS

Approximately one third of the current dental research effort is directly concerned with the development of better materials and improved techniques for their manipulation. This research has resulted in an ever-increasing body of knowledge related to the behavior of dental materials and has brought forth an avalanche of new products. These developments place an increasing responsibility on the dentist, who must critically analyze the literature and the claims of the manufacturer to determine the materials and techniques that will provide maximum service to the patient. So that an intelligent and correct decision may be made, an appreciation of the clinical significance of the chemical, physical, and biologic properties of dental materials is essential. It is from this concept that the modern science of dental materials has evolved, and this philosophy provides the framework of reference for the subject matter presented in this chapter.

The oral cavity is a formidable obstacle to the maintenance of the integrity of tooth structure and the materials used in its restoration or replacement. Biting stress on the cusp of a molar tooth may be as great as 207 MPa (30,000 psi). The pH of the dental plaque, foods, and beverages fluctuates daily from ranges of low acidity to high alkalinity. The temperature during the course of a normal meal may vary as much as 150° F (66° C). The warm, moist oral cavity contains a variety of enzymes and debris, providing optimum conditions for the accumulation of surface deposits that can tarnish or corrode metallic restorations. For these and other reasons restorative materials are readily subject to

fracture, solubility, dimensional change, and discoloration. If these dyscrasias are to be minimized, the dental material must possess certain minimum chemical and physical properties. Furthermore, those properties must be maintained during the manipulation and placement of the restoration.

The American Dental Association specification program has contributed greatly to providing the dentist with high-quality dental materials that have been carefully compounded to resist the rigors of the oral cavity. Thirty-seven of the most commonly used restorative materials are now encompassed by the specification program. Whenever a material is covered by the respective specification, only those on the certified list of approved products should be used. From that list the dentist may select the brand that provides the desired manipulative characteristics.

The *Federation Dentaire Internationale* (International Dental Federation) has been instrumental in the development of specifications on an international basis. That activity has been formalized under the auspices of the *International Standards Organization* (ISO). The ISO is a body composed of national standards organizations from 84 countries. Approximately 30 specifications for dental materials and devices have so far been adopted under that program.

The Medical Devices Amendments of 1976 gave the U.S. Food and Drug Administration (FDA) the regulatory authority to protect the public from hazardous or ineffective medical devices. That legislation was the culmination of a series of attempts to provide safe and effective products, beginning with the passage of the Food and Drug Act of 1906, which did not include any provision to regulate medical device safety or the claims made for devices. The 1976 legislation requires the classification and regulation of all noncustom medical devices intended for human use. The term "device" includes "any instrument, apparatus, implement, machine, contrivance, implant, or in vitro reagent used in the diagnosis, cure, mitigation, treatment or prevention of disease in man or animals." Some dental products (such as fluoride products) are considered drugs, but most products used in the operatory are considered devices and are thus subject to control by the FDA Bureau of Medical Devices. Also included are over-the-counter products sold to the public, such as floss and denture adhesives.

To date 242 dental items have been classified. This activity, in conjunction with the American Dental Association specification program for dental materials and devices, is providing a crucial framework for standards development and for better assurance to dentists and patients that the product is safe and effective as claimed. A number of other countries have government agencies comparable to the FDA that include at least some dental materials and devices under the umbrella of their regulatory authority.

Microleakage and biologic considerations

Possibly the greatest deterrent to the development of an "ideal" restorative material is the leakage that occurs along the restoration-tooth interface. There is as yet no truly adhesive dental material. Overwhelming evidence shows that all materials permit ingress of deleterious agents, such as acid, food debris, and microorganisms, between the walls of the prepared cavity and the restoration. A certain incidence of the clinical failure of materials can be associated with this phenomenon. In some cases the microleakage may be the precursor of secondary caries, marginal deterioration, postoperative sensitivity, and pulp pathology. Microleakage poses a particular problem in the child patient in whom the floor of the cavity preparation

may be close to the pulp. The added insult to the pulp caused by the seepage of irritants that may penetrate around the restoration and through the thin layer of dentin, or a microscopic exposure, may produce irreversible pulpal reactions.

This phenomenon is frequently referred to in other chapters in this book, since the selection of the proper restorative material for a given situation is based to a certain extent on the capability of the material to minimize microleakage. In this chapter attention is given to the various parameters involved in attaining maximum bonding to the tooth to reduce the potential problems associated with the microleakage phenomenon.

It is appropriate at this time to describe the two mechanisms for bonding materials together, in this case the restorative material to tooth structure. This is particularly important now because an increasing number of manufacturers are claiming "adhesion" of a cement or resin to tooth structure. The dentist should assume a critical posture in analyzing such claims before making a change in established restorative procedures.

One method of bonding substances together is entirely mechanical, such as attaching a bolt into two pieces of wood to hold them together. In dentistry, acid etching is commonly used to improve the bonding of a restorative resin to enamel via the formation of resin tags into the etched enamel, as will be discussed here and elsewhere in the text.

However, for true adhesion to occur, the bonding is at a molecular level and involves an interaction between the molecules of the adhesive and the adherend. For example, in dyed fabric the molecules of the dye are held to the molecules of the fabric by true chemical adhesion. The only dental material currently in use that has the potential for truly adhering to tooth structure is that based on polyacrylic acid, that is, the polycarboxylate and glass ionomer cements.

With the advancements that have been made in surface chemistry and the development of adhesives for all types of unusual application, the dentist is often mystified as to why truly adhesive dental materials have not been developed. Certainly the advent of an adhesive restorative material would markedly alter many phases of dental practice. The need for the typical cavity preparation would no longer be a prime consideration, because adhesion would eliminate the need for retention via the cavity preparation. In many situations it would no longer be necessary to use auxiliary aids, such as cavity varnishes and etching techniques, to compensate for the microleakage that is a potential hazard around the amalgam or resin restorations.

Unfortunately, tooth structure inherently possesses very undesirable characteristics from the standpoint of a substance that would promote bonding of a potential adhesive. It is rough, unhomogeneous in composition, covered with a tenacious layer of surface debris, and wet. All of these factors discourage adhesion. Furthermore, the reactivity (surface energy) of enamel is low, and therefore the surface does not easily attract other molecules to it.

Incidentally, it has been shown that topical fluorides tend to reduce even further the surface energy of enamel. It is further postulated that the result is a reduction in plaque accumulation. This observation suggests another explanation for the mechanism of topical fluoride therapy in the reduction of caries, namely that a fluoride-treated tooth stays cleaner longer.

To carry this line of thinking one step further, the surface energy of all restorative materials, particularly metallic ones, is higher than that of normal intact tooth structure. Therefore there is a greater tendency of debris to accumulate on the surface of restorations than on the adjoining enamel. This could, in part, account for the surprisingly high incidence of secondary caries associated with all restorative materials with the exception of silicate cement. The higher surface energy of the restorative material tends to attract debris, and that accumulation is the precursor to marginal deterioration.

Cavity varnishes

The role of a cavity varnish is of particular interest. Cavity varnishes have been used empirically for many years as a liner for the cavity preparation, but only recently has their effect in protecting the underlying tooth structure been established. An intelligent decision on whether a base alone is sufficient or whether both varnish and base are necessary requires a knowledge of the specific effects of each type of material.

The typical dental cavity varnish is principally a natural rosin or a synthetic resin that has been dissolved in a solvent such as chloroform, ether, or acetone. When painted onto the cavity preparation, the solvent evaporates and leaves a thin film. This film is commonly believed to be an effective thermal insulator.

Teeth that have been restored with metallic restorations appear to be less sensitive to hot and cold beverages and foods when a cavity varnish has been used. Although cavity varnishes do have a low thermal conductivity, they are not applied in a sufficient thickness to serve as a thermal insulator. The thickness of the layer of cavity varnish that is present after the amalgam restoration has been condensed into the preparation is approximately 4 μm. Since thermal diffusion through a substance is controlled by the thermal conductivity and thickness of the material, a layer of only 4 μm is not adequate to provide insulation against heat or cold. It is necessary to remember that cavity varnishes do not protect the pulp against thermal shock. This is one of the functions of the cement base.

However, postoperative sensitivity to thermal shock does seem to be reduced when a cavity varnish is used. The reason is that the varnish tends to minimize microleakage when it is used in conjunction with many restorative materials. This effect is of particular importance in the case of the amalgam restoration, since gross leakage occurs around this material during the first few days and weeks. One reason for continuing sensitivity may be the irritation caused by fluids and debris that penetrate around the restoration. Although this leakage decreases with time as corrosion products accumulate between the restoration and the tooth, the initial leakage is a matter of concern. The cavity varnish serves as an effective sealer against this initial microleakage around amalgam and other restorative materials, such as direct gold.

Another common problem associated with the amalgam restoration is the discoloration of the adjoining tooth structure caused by the penetration of metallic ions from the amalgam into enamel and dentin. These ions, particularly tin, can in time react with sulfur, chlorine, or oxygen to form dark compounds. The cavity varnish provides an inhibitory barrier to this metallic migration and lessens the likelihood of unsightly color change.

The layer of varnish is also beneficial in preventing acid from zinc phosphate or silicate cement from penetrating into dentin. The pH of these cements remains low for an extended period. Under certain circumstances this acid can penetrate thicknesses of dentin of 0.5 mm or greater, producing the pulpal irritation associated with these materials. Although the penetration of acid is not entirely precluded by the cavity varnish, it is retarded. Thus it is important that a cavity varnish be employed in the deep cavity whenever acid-containing materials are to be inserted subsequently.

Since an appropriate therapeutic cement base is also generally recommended in the deep cavity preparation, the question arises as to the need for a varnish in such a case. It can be argued that a base of calcium hydroxide or zinc oxide–eugenol cement would either neutralize the acid or serve as a barrier to its penetration into dentin. Such bases, even when used in minimal thicknesses of only 0.1 mm, are effective inhibitors to acid penetration. Therefore, when a base is used under a silicate or zinc phosphate cement, a cavity varnish is probably unnecessary. However, there are situations in pedodontics in which the cavity preparation cannot be made sufficiently large to contain both a base and the cement restoration. In those situations a varnish is essential.

There are various methods for applying the varnish, for example, a camel's hair brush or a wire loop. A small cotton applicator formed on the end of a root canal reamer is a particularly convenient means of placing the varnish into all the areas of the cavity preparation or into pinholes.

The varnish must be thin, not viscous. Thick layers of varnish do not wet the tooth and will not effectively seal the margins. To prevent evaporation of the solvent and thickening of the varnish, the top should be placed on the bottle immediately after use. When the varnish becomes thick as it ages, it should be thinned with an appropriate solvent or discarded.

The varnish is put on in several applications. Each layer is permitted to dry for approximately 20 seconds before placement of the next layer. The purpose of the two or three applications is not to build up the thickness of the layer but to provide a more continuous coating. As the varnish dries, it tends to form small pinholes, and the second and third applications help to fill these voids. To serve effectively as a sealant or acid inhibitor, the coating must be as nonporous as possible.

It is unnecessary to remove the varnish from the margins of the amalgam cavity preparation. In the normal oral environment no deterioration occurs if the varnish is present in a thin layer at the margin. When used in conjunction with silicate cement, however, the varnish should be removed from enamel. If possible, the varnish should be applied only to dentin. The reason for this will be explained subsequently.

Cavity varnishes are not generally used in conjunction with the acrylic resin restoration. The conventional acrylic resin is softened by or will react with the solvent.

Cavity varnishes can be used with some of the popular composite resins. However, with the acrylic resins, in certain cases the resin may soften at its interface with the varnish. Thus, the safety of using a varnish in conjunction with a composite depends on the exact resin chemistry involved. The same effect may also occur between the eugenol in a zinc oxide–eugenol cement base and certain commercial composites. Thus, whenever possible, a calcium hydroxide base is the protective material of choice.

It must be remembered that if a varnish is used with a composite, the purpose is not to improve the seal to tooth structure. Rather, the varnish serves as an aid to protecting the underlying dentin and pulp against the irritation of the resin itself. However, if one is concerned about the effect of the resin on the pulp, a cement base is probably indicated.

Table 13-1. Effects of cavity varnishes and cement bases in providing protection to the pulp from various types of insult

Varnish	Base
Inhibits microleakage	Provides thermal insulation
Prevents penetration from amalgam into tooth structure	Has a therapeutic effect on the pulp
Inhibits acid penetration	Inhibits acid penetration
	Supports condensation of amalgam

Cement bases

The function of the cement base is to promote recovery of the injured pulp and to protect it against further insult. In addition to providing a barrier against acid, the base serves as an effective thermal insulator when it is employed under the metallic restoration. As is true for cavity varnishes, the base must be of sufficient thickness to provide insulation. Approximately 0.5 mm is adequate for this purpose.

The base must also support the condensation of the amalgam. If the strength of the base is inadequate, the cement will distort or fracture, permitting the amalgam to penetrate and come in contact with the dentin floor and thereby eliminating the thermal protection afforded by the base. In the past it was generally believed that only zinc phosphate cement possessed sufficient strength to withstand the condensation pressures of amalgam. There is now evidence that several of the commercial fast-setting calcium hydroxide or zinc oxide–eugenol base materials have sufficient strength to serve effectively without the need for an additional layer of zinc phosphate cement. In certain cases, such as a Class II preparation that involves the restoration of an angle or of a deep depression, it may be necessary to cover the more biologically acceptable calcium hydroxide or zinc oxide–eugenol cement base with a layer of the stronger zinc phosphate cement.

A cavity varnish and a cement base serve somewhat different functions; yet in other ways they complement each other. The purposes of each material are summarized in Table 13-1. Thus it is apparent that in certain situations, such as the deep cavity preparation restored with amalgam, both a varnish and a base are required to provide protection against all the types of insult that may occur. If the base is a biologically acceptable material, such as calcium hydroxide or a zinc oxide–eugenol cement, it is applied first, followed by the varnish. If a phosphoric acid cement were being used, the varnish would be inserted initially to provide protection against the acid of the cement.

Amalgam

Amalgam is still the most commonly employed material for restoring the carious lesion, comprising approximately 80% of all restorations. Its popularity for the simple restoration will no doubt continue until the wear resistance of composite resins can be documented and their suitability in replacing amalgam as a permanent restorative material in the permanent dentition can be determined. The unique clinical success of amalgam through 150 years of use has been associated with many characteristics, one of which is the germicidal or antibacterial properties of metallic ions, such as silver, mercury, or copper, that constitute the material. It is more likely that its excellent clinical service, even under adverse conditions, is due to the tendency for the microleakage to decrease as the restoration ages in the oral cavity. Even though the margins of the amalgam restoration may often appear wide open, the restoration-tooth interface immediately below the exposed margin is filled with corrosion products that inhibit leakage. Amalgam is unusual from this standpoint. The microleakage around other restorative materials either remains constant or tends to become progressively worse.

Nevertheless, failures of amalgam restorations are commonly observed. These may occur in the form of recurrent caries, fracture (either gross or severe marginal breakdown), dimensional change, or involvement of the pulp or periodontal membrane. More significant than the type of failure is its cause. It has generally been recognized that two factors lead to such clinical failures—improper design of the prepared cavity and faulty manipulation. In other words, the deterioration of amalgam restorations can be readily associated with neglect in observing the fundamental principles of cavity design or abuse in preparing and inserting the material.

There is yet one other factor involved, and that is the commercial alloy used. It is now appreciated that there are differences in the performance of certain products, irrespective of cavity design or manipulative technique. With this knowledge, some decided changes have occurred in alloy formulation, and a host of new products have been introduced. The following section deals with alloy selection.

Selection of the alloy. Certain criteria are involved in the selection of an alloy. The importance of each will vary with the individual dentist. The first criterion is that the alloy meets the requirements of the American Dental Association Specification No. 1 or a similar specification.

The manipulative characteristics are extremely important and a matter of subjective preference. Rate of hardening, smoothness of the mix, and ease of condensation and finishing vary with the alloy and the working speed and choice of the operator. For example, the "feel" of lathe-cut amalgams during condensation is entirely different from that of spherical amalgams. It is essential that the alloy selected be one with which the dentist and assistant feel comfortable, since the operator variable is a major factor entering into the clinical lifetime of the restoration. Use of alloys and techniques that will encourage standardization in the manipulation and placement of the amalgam will enhance the quality of the service rendered. Coincident with this is the delivery system provided by the manufacturer—its convenience, expediency, and ability to reduce human variables. The alloy may be purchased in the form of either a powder or a pellet. Many manufacturers offer preproportioned alloy and mercury in disposable capsules. There are certain advantages and disadvantages to this form, as will be discussed shortly.

Obviously, the physical properties should be reviewed in the light of claims made for superiority of one alloy over competing products. Such an analysis of properties must be accompanied by a documented review of clinical performance in the form of well-controlled clinical studies. This is especially necessary for alloy formulations that depart from traditional compositions and in which an exact correlation between properties and performance has not yet been established.

Alloys of conventional composition are still available, and acceptable amalgam restorations can be obtained with many of these. However, the newer high-copper system is now the alloy of choice. Improved physical properties, the elimination of the gamma-two phase, and the better corrosion resistance associated with the high-copper alloys generally lead to superior clinical performance.

Lastly, owing to the escalation in the price of silver, the cost of the alloy has assumed new importance. This criterion should not be given too much weight when balanced against the alloy's ability to render maximum clinical service. However, if all other factors are equal, it is sensible to purchase the less expensive brand.

Traditionally, amalgam alloys have been prepared by cutting small particles from a cast ingot by means of a lathe. These filings are often referred to as *lathe-cut* alloys. Small particles are preferred over larger-grained alloys, since they provide greater strength, superior manipulation, and a smoother surface that better resists corrosion.

The alloy may be supplied either in the form of a powder of cut filings or as pellets. The pellet form offers the convenience of a preweighed quantity of alloy, thus eliminating the need for an alloy dispenser. The failure to attain a proper mix with the pellet is probably due to inadequate trituration or to use of an improperly designed capsule and pestle relationship. The pestle should be considerably shorter and smaller than the corresponding dimensions of the capsule. Otherwise the pellet will be wedged in the end or side of the capsule and will never be broken up into the individual alloy particles. Longer trituration time is generally required to break down the pellet than that needed to amalgamate the filings.

A wide variety of mercury and alloy dispensers, or proportioners, are available to the dental profession. They are of two general types. The most common type is the dispenser based on volumetric proportioning; the other measures by weight.

Most dispensers for alloy in powder form are relatively accurate if properly used. The chief objection to the volumetric devices is that the alloy tends to cling to the walls and corners of the dispensing well. Also, the powder tends to pack in the container, making the weight inaccurate from one measurement to the next. Furthermore, any volumetric measurement for a specified weight of alloy depends on the particle size of the alloy; the larger particle size requires a larger volume than does a small particle size to obtain the same weight. Consequently, the volume of the dispenser must be gauged for a given alloy and cannot be used for any other brand.

Because mercury is a liquid, it can be measured by volume without appreciable loss of accuracy. Standard deviations in weight of mercury as low as ±0.5% may be attained with a number of commercial mercury dispensers. However, even though the mercury dispenser may be well designed to provide reproducible spills of mercury, caution must be exercised in its use. The dispenser should be held almost vertical to ensure consistent spills of mercury. Tilting the bottle to a 45-degree angle results in unreliable mercury/alloy ratios. The dispenser should be at least half full when used. If the dispenser is one-fourth full or less, the weight of mercury dispensed may be erratic. Finally, use of dirty mercury leads to entrapment of the contaminants in the reservoir and orifice of the device, preventing accurate delivery of the mercury.

If such variables are not controlled, variation in individual spills of mercury may be 3% or 4%. With low mercury/alloy ratios, variations of this magnitude result in an unusable mix.

In the case of pellets, if the amalgam alloy and mercury dispensers are not from the same manufacturer, the directions for use of the dispenser may not indicate the setting required to obtain the proper ratio for another product. Then it is necessary to weigh a pellet (for example, on a pharmaceutical balance) and calculate the amount of mercury required for the desired ratio. Increments of mercury may then be dispensed and weighed and the desired adjustment of the dispenser established.

Disposable capsules containing preproportioned aliquots of mercury and alloy are now available. They contain alloy either in pellet form or as a preweighed portion of powder in conjunction with the appropriate quantity of mercury. To prevent amalgamation from occurring during storage, the mercury and alloy are separated from each other by a plastic membrane. Before trituration, the membrane is ruptured and the mercury falls into the compartment with the alloy. Although more expensive, the preproportioned material is convenient and eliminates the chance of inaccurate mercury spills during proportioning.

There are some disadvantages of preproportioned capsules other than expense. There is no opportunity to make minor adjustments in the mercury/alloy ratio to accommodate personal preference for a slightly drier or wetter mix. Likewise, there is no latitude in varying the size of the mix supplied by the manufacturer.

Regardless of the method used, the proper amount of mercury and alloy must always be gauged before the start of trituration. The addition of mercury after trituration is contraindicated.

By use of an atomizing technique, amalgam alloys may be produced in the form of small spheres rather than filings. The primary merit of the *spherical* alloys is that the strength properties do not seem to be influenced as greatly by condensation as for the conventional alloys. Other than that, the properties are comparable. The manipulative characteristics are somewhat different in that the amalgam does not tend to have the "body" of a lathe-cut alloy and thus does not resist condensation as readily. The technique must be adjusted accordingly.

High-copper alloys. The newest advancement in alloy formulation is the introduction of the high-copper alloys. The concept behind these products centers on the setting reaction that occurs during the hardening of the amalgam. The hardened amalgam from a traditional silver-tin alloy is composed of three principal components: (1) remnants of the original alloy particles (the gamma phase), (2) particles of a silver-mercury compound (the gamma-one phase), and (3) particles of a tin-mercury compound (the gamma-two phase). There is now good evidence that the weak, corrosion-prone component is the gamma-two phase. Therefore, alloys are being designed to eliminate the formation of this phase in the setting reaction, thereby producing an amalgam that would be stronger and less susceptible to marginal breakdown. This is being accomplished by the judicious addition of copper at levels higher than have been used previously.

The first such alloy of this type was the *dispersion* system. In such an alloy dispersed spherical particles of a silver-copper eutectic are added to filings of a conventional silver-tin alloy. Such alloys are also referred to as *admix* alloys. The result is that the copper preferentially combines with the tin to form the eta phase (a copper-tin reactant compound) and thereby eliminates virtually all of the weak, corrosion-prone gamma-two phase. High-copper alloys can also be made by use of a *single composition* particle. Unlike the admix alloy, each of these alloy particles has the same chemical composition, usually silver, copper, and tin. The copper content of these newer alloys ranges from 12% to 30%.

The alloys from the high-copper system also tend to have low creep. Creep is the tendency of a material to deform under stress and is somewhat synonymous with the property of flow. This property has been associated with the marginal breakdown (ditching) so commonly noted with the amalgam restoration. An example of the clinical performance of low- and high-creep alloys can be seen in Fig. 13-1.

However, factors other than the creep properties of the alloy may be involved in this type of dyscra-

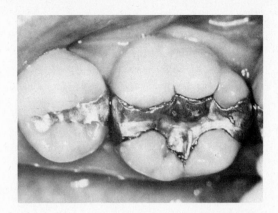

Fig. 13-1. Three-year-old amalgam restorations. The one at left was placed with a low-creep alloy, whereas the one at right was a high-creep alloy. (Courtesy J. Osborne.)

sia. Unsupported enamel at the marginal areas may in time fracture, as will thin ledges of amalgam left over the enamel following carving. Corrosion has also been suggested as the precursor to this phenomenon, as have various strength properties. Thus it is obvious that several mechanisms, working separately or synergistically, may be identified with marginal breakdown. Although creep is one of several properties used to determine the potential in vivo performance of an alloy, there is no substitute for well-controlled clinical studies. The high-copper alloy system is the preferred one for the reasons cited.

However, regardless of the alloy used, manipulation plays a vital role in controlling the properties and the behavior of the restoration. The clinical success of the restoration is dependent on meticulous attention to the principles of manipulation.

Mercury/alloy ratio. One of the three variables that control the final mercury content of the restoration is the original mercury/alloy ratio. Under a given set of conditions, the more mercury used in the original mix, the more will be the residual mercury. To minimize the residual mercury, low mercury/alloy ratios are commonly employed (the ''Eames technique''). Ratios of 50% mercury or less may be used with certain alloys, whereas other brands may require 52% or 53% to achieve a mix with proper working consistency. It must be remembered that too little mercury is as dangerous as too much. Each alloy particle must be wetted by the mercury to ensure a homogeneous structure and a smooth surface.

At these low mercury levels in the original mix, the weighing of the alloy and mercury must be accurately controlled. Deviations of as little as 0.5% mercury may result in unusable mixes.

Trituration. The second manipulative variable that controls the residual mercury content is trituration. The longer the trituration time, the less will be the amount of mercury left in the condensed restoration. If the mix is underamalgamated, the setting time is decreased, and less mercury will be eliminated during condensation. As is discussed later in the chapter, since the residual mercury controls the strength of the restoration, thorough trituration is imperative. The danger in amalgamation generally is undertrituration, *not* overtrituration.

The correct trituration time varies depending on the composition of the alloy, the mercury/alloy ratio, the size of mix, and other factors. The best guide is to acquire an appreciation for the appearance of a proper mix and then to adjust the trituration time accordingly for the prevailing office conditions. The recognition of a proper consistency can be readily gained through experience. An example of an undertriturated mix may be seen in Fig. 13-2, *A*. Such an amalgam will set unduly rapidly, resulting in a high residual mercury content. The strength will thereby be reduced, and the likelihood of fracture or marginal breakdown will be enhanced. The granular texture will produce a rougher surface that will accelerate corrosion. If trituration is carried to the consistency shown in Fig. 13-2, *B*, maximal properties and clinical behavior may be anticipated.

Condensation. The specific technique employed in condensing the individual increments is described in Chapter 12. It is sufficient to say that the purpose of condensation is to adapt the amalgam to the walls of the cavity preparation as closely as possible, to minimize the formation of internal

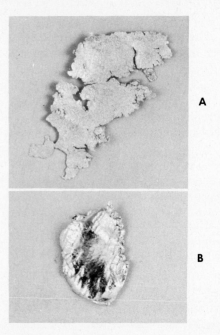

Fig. 13-2. A, Undertriturated mix of amalgam. **B,** Properly triturated mix. (From Phillips, R.W.: Science of dental materials, ed. 8, Philadelphia, 1982, W.B. Saunders Co.)

voids, and to express excess mercury from the amalgam. The greater the condensation pressure, the less will be the residual mercury left in the restoration and the greater will be the strength. The selection of the condenser and the technique of ''building'' the amalgam should be designed to achieve those objectives.

Although a mechanical condenser is not superior to *proper* hand condensation, it offers the advantage of reducing fatigue of the operator. Since the human variable is minimized, the procedure is more standardized.

Residual mercury. The residual mercury content of amalgam is controlled by three variables: (1) the original mercury/alloy ratio, (2) the amount of trituration, and (3) the condensation pressure. For this reason excess mercury should be minimized in the original ratio, the amalgam must be thoroughly triturated, and maximum condensation

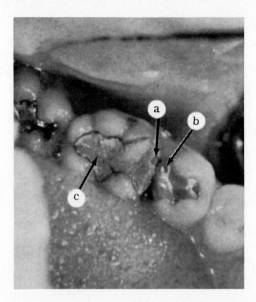

Fig. 13-3. Amalgam restorations after 1 year in the mouth. The condition of the restoration in the first molar with high mercury content is in contrast to that in the second premolar with a lower mercury content. Facets *a* and *b* show the effect of traumatic occlusion. A fracture is seen at *c*. (From Phillips, R.W.: The science of dental materials, ed. 7, Philadelphia, 1973, W.B. Saunders Co.)

pressure must be used. Furthermore, increments of amalgam that have been permitted to harden longer than 3 minutes should be discarded, and a fresh mix should be made. Amalgam that has set too long will invariably retain more mercury during its condensation.

Mercury is very important to the physical behavior of the amalgam restoration. An analysis of clinical restorations indicates a wide variation in their mercury content. It is of particular interest that the mercury concentration is characteristically higher in the marginal areas. This observation is true regardless of the method of condensation or the "dryness" of the increments used to build the restoration. Whether hand or mechanical condensation is used, mercury analysis of a large number of restorations reveals that the mercury content of the marginal areas averages 2% to 3% higher than that of the bulk of the restorations. The higher mercury content at the margins is important because these areas are critical in terms of corrosion, fracture, and secondary caries.

Restorations that have an unduly high mercury content have been judged by visual examination to be clinically unsatisfactory. This is to be expected because a marked decrease in the strength of traditional silver-tin amalgams occurs at a mercury content of approximately 55%. When clinical restorations with a low-copper alloy containing various quantities of mercury were placed, those containing mercury in excess of 55% showed an appreciably higher incidence of marginal fracture and surface deterioration than did those containing mercury in the 50% range, as shown in Fig. 13-3. The higher the mercury content, the greater was the incidence and severity of dyscrasia that occurred as the restorations aged.

Since high mercury content has the same effect on the strength and creep of high-copper alloys as on these properties in the older, low-copper amalgams, high-copper amalgam restorations with an excessive mercury content would also be expected to exhibit a greater incidence of marginal degradation. If the mercury content is too high, the weaker and corrosion-susceptible gamma-two phase will be formed.

The loss in strength caused by excess mercury also invites fracture through the bulk of the restoration. However, a more frequent cause of such fractures—for example, at the isthmus of the cavity preparation—is trauma. A sharp, plunger-occluding cusp produces a small concentrated point of stress on the restoration that the brittle amalgam cannot survive. Occlusion should always be suspected and adjusted in this type of failure. Often a slight rounding of the opposing cusp will prevent a recurrence when the restoration is replaced. Likewise, the patient, particularly the child, should be warned about accidental or intentional stress during the first few hours after the restoration has been inserted. Amalgam may appear strong, but it gains its strength relatively slowly. Biting on the amalgam for the first 2 or 3 hours should be avoided.

Moisture. Moisture contamination of a conventional amalgam alloy will invariably invite a failure. The zinc that may be present in the alloy will react with the water, and hydrogen gas will be formed. As this gas builds up within the amalgam, a marked expansion will be produced. The expansion may be as great as 500 μm in certain alloys. This delayed expansion causes a protrusion of the amalgam from the cavity preparation, enhancing the possibility of debris being trapped at the overhanging margins. Recurrent caries often results. The voids produced by the gas markedly reduce the strength and produce a rougher surface that invites corrosion.

Such moisture contamination can result from failure to maintain a dry field during the placement of the restoration or from perspiration. Amalgam should never be mulled in the palm of the hand or touched with the fingers. This is unnecessary and is always dangerous, since traces of moisture are invariably present on the surface of the skin. Exposure to saliva immediately after the amalgam has been completely condensed is not harmful. It is only moisture within the amalgam as it is being prepared or inserted that is to be avoided.

Alloys are now available that contain no zinc, and apparently their physical properties are comparable to those of their counterparts that contain zinc. However, there is no excuse for moisture contamination, regardless of the composition of the alloy. Moisture incorporated in a nonzinc alloy will lead to reduced strength and an inferior surface.

In those rare instances in which saliva contamination appears to be unavoidable, there are two alternatives. A nonzinc alloy may be preferred to avoid delayed expansion in case traces of saliva come into contact with the amalgam during condensation. If a conventional zinc-containing alloy is used, the condensation procedure must be sacrificed for speed. It is better to condense the amalgam rapidly in three or four increments before it becomes contaminated than to employ the more exacting but longer condensation procedure of using smaller and more increments.

Polishing. The amalgam restoration is not finished until it has been polished. The final amalgam structure is composed of particles of the original alloy surrounded by a matrix of silver-mercury and tin-mercury compounds. During carving the alloy particles are pulled out, leaving voids. These surface roughnesses are reduced by polishing, and the smoother surface will better resist corrosion. There is also some evidence that polishing may reduce the amount of the gamma-two phase that is present on the surface of some restorations following carving. The elimination of that phase would also reduce the tendency for corrosion.

The generation of heat should be avoided during polishing. Mercury will be drawn to the amalgam surface whenever the temperature of the amalgam exceeds 140° F (60° C). This mercury will in time diffuse back into the bulk of the amalgam to leave a porous, weak structure. Only wet pastes should be used, and polishing should be delayed for at least 48 hours or even for a week. Premature polishing will disturb the hardening amalgam and will produce an outer layer that is mercury rich. Subsequently the surface becomes dull or rough.

It has generally been believed that burnishing of the surface or margins of the restoration is contraindicated. However, if done carefully, avoiding the generation of heat, burnishing may actually improve the adaptation, hardness, and corrosion resistance of the margins of the restoration.

Mercury toxicity. From the earliest use of mercury, it has been asked whether this material can produce local or systemic effects in humans. It is still occasionally conjectured that mercury toxicity from dental restorations is the cause for certain undiagnosed illnesses. It has been further suggested that a real hazard may exist for the dentist or dental assistant when mercury vapor inhaled during mixing produces an accumulative toxic effect. The matter has once again come to the foreground with the recent concern over mercury pollution of the environment.

Mercury from the restoration undoubtedly penetrates the tooth structure. An analysis of dentin underlying amalgam restorations reveals the presence of mercury, which may account in part for subsequent discoloration of the tooth. Use of radioactive mercury in silver amalgam has also revealed that some mercury may even reach the pulp.

However, the possibility of toxic effects on the patient from these traces of mercury penetrating the tooth or sensitization caused by mercury salts dissolving from the surface of the amalgam is most remote. The danger has been evaluated in numerous studies. The patient's encounter with mercury vapor during insertion of the restoration is too brief and the total amount of mercury vapor too small to be injurious. Furthermore, mercury leached from the amalgam is apparently not converted to the lethal form of methyl or ethyl mercury and is excreted rapidly by the body. The problem has been reviewed in detail, and the reader is referred to the literature.

Dentists and their auxiliaries are exposed daily to the risk of mercury intoxication. Although metallic mercury can be absorbed through the skin or by ingestion, the primary risk to dental personnel is from inhalation. The American Dental Association estimates that one dental office in 10 exceeds the maximum safe exposure level for mercury. However, only a few cases of serious mercury intoxication resulting from dental exposure have been reported, and the potential hazard can be greatly reduced if not eliminated by attention to a few precautionary measures.

Obviously the operatory should be well ventilated. All excess mercury, including waste and amalgam removed during condensation, should be collected and stored in well-sealed containers. If spilled, it must be cleaned up as soon as possible. It is extremely difficult to remove mercury from carpeting. Ordinary vacuum cleaners merely disperse the mercury further through the exhaust. Mercury suppressant powders are helpful but should be considered temporary measures. If mercury comes in contact with the skin, the skin should be washed with soap and water.

As noted previously, the capsule used with a mechanical amalgamator should have a tight-fitting cap to avoid mercury leakage. When grinding amalgam a water spray and suction should be used; eye protection and a disposable mask are recommended.

Periodic monitoring of exposure levels is an important part of a hygiene program for handling toxic materials. Current recommendations suggest that this procedure be conducted at least once a year. Several techniques are available. Instruments can sample the air in the operatory and yield a time-weighted average for mercury exposure. Film badges can be worn by office personnel in a manner similar to radiation exposure badges. Biologic determinations of mercury levels in blood or urine can be performed on office staff.

The risk to dental personnel of mercury exposure cannot be ignored. However, close adherence to simple hygiene procedures will help ensure a safe working environment.

Silicate cement

As with any restorative material, silicate cement has certain characteristics that are desirable but others that limit its usefulness. Under oral conditions it tends to stain and disintegrate. The strength is inadequate to permit its use as a permanent restoration whenever it may be subject to stress. These deficiencies place particular demands on the dentist or the assistant in maintaining, by proper manipulation, the essential properties at as high a level as possible. The average lifetime of a silicate restoration is approximately 4 years. Because of the lack of permanence, silicate cement is seldom used as an anterior restorative material and has been largely replaced by the composite resins. However, because of its ability to resist secondary caries, silicate cement could well remain a part of the armamentarium of the pedodontist for restorations in the mouths of child patients who have a high caries index. For this reason, silicate cement warrants discussion. In addition, the new glass ionomer system, to be discussed later in the chapter, is based to a certain extent on that of silicate cement.

Anticariogenic effect. The anticariogenic characteristics of silicate cement are unique. Recurrent or secondary caries is seldom encountered around the silicate cement restoration even when gross disintegration has occurred. No other material has such an ability to resist caries.

This beneficial effect may be attributed to the effect of the fluoride present in the cement powder.

A fluoride flux such as calcium fluoride is usually employed during manufacture in sintering the other ingredients. The typical silicate cement powder contains approximately 15% fluoride. During and after the placement of the cement, the fluoride reacts with the adjoining tooth structure in much the same manner as does a topically applied aqueous fluoride solution. The enamel solubility is markedly reduced, thus building up the resistance to acid attack and to caries.

Recent research suggests that fluoride, even in small quantities, may act as an enzyme inhibitor and thus prevent the metabolism of carbohydrates. This finding indicates a second viable mechanism through which silicate could function as an anticariogenic agent. In fact, chemical analyses of plaque collected at the margins of resin, amalgam, and cast gold restorations reveal a difference in composition, as compared with the plaque accumulated at the margins of silicate cement restorations. Plaque associated with silicate cement has an appreciably higher carbohydrate/nitrogen ratio than does the plaque taken from the margins of all other types of restorations. Since protein nitrogen serves as an index to the bacterial content of the plaque, these data imply either that the metabolism of carbohydrate present in the plaque associated with silicate restorations is inhibited to a certain extent or that fewer microorganisms are present. When comparable tests were conducted on plaque taken from restorations of a silicate prepared with a nonfluoride flux, the plaque composition was similar to that found at the margins of other types of restorations.

Thus it appears that silicate cement may inhibit caries via at least two mechanisms, both of which are related to the presence and release of fluoride from the cement. Since there is evidence that the fluoride ions are slowly released throughout the life of the restoration, the protective mechanism is undoubtedly a continuous one.

Manipulation. The set silicate cement is composed of particles of the original cement powder surrounded by a matrix that is essentially a gel. The vulnerable portion of the structure is this gel matrix, which is highly soluble, weak, and easily stained. A cardinal principle in the manipulation of silicate cement is to minimize the gel. The greater the amount of powder per given amount of liquid, the less will be the quantity of gel. In turn, the physical properties are directly related to the powder/liquid ratio. A low ratio produces a mix of low strength and high solubility, invariably resulting in a rapid disintegration of the clinical restoration. Only by the use of a cool slab can the maximum quantity of powder be incorporated, the percent of gel matrix minimized, and optimum physical properties attained. However, the slab temperature should never be below the dew point; a film of water on the glass surface will contaminate the mix.

The mixing of the cement powder is done rapidly, initially incorporating larger amounts of powder into the liquid as compared with zinc phosphate cement. Although the mixing time may not be as critical as formerly believed, the mix should be completed in approximately 1 minute to prevent the gel from being distributed as it forms.

Proper care of the powder and liquid is essential. The cement liquid contains orthophosphoric acid and approximately 30% to 35% water, depending on the brand of cement. The water has a marked effect on the setting time. As little a 0.1% change in water concentration may produce an erratic setting time. If the liquid loses water by undue exposure to the office environment, the cement will set more slowly. The reverse is also true. To preserve the proper acid/water ratio, the top should always be placed on the bottle immediately after dispensing. Likewise, the liquid should never be placed on the mixing slab until just before the mix is to be made.

These fundamental rules for the manipulation of silicate cement apply equally to a zinc phosphate or a silicophosphate cement.

Even when such manipulative factors are rigidly controlled, there is considerable variation in the behavior of a silicate cement from one mouth to another. In some patients a silicate restoration may last 10 years, whereas in others replacement may be required in only 1 year. This difference is probably associated with acid. Silicate cements are highly soluble in organic acids, such as lactic, acetic, and especially citric acid. For this reason disintegration of a silicate restoration is generally greater in the cervical area where the pH is apt to be lower owing to retention of plaque. It would be expected that a child patient with unusual dietary habits, such as a high intake of citrus fruits or beverages, might exhibit rapid deterioration of a silicate cement regardless of the brand or the manipulative technique employed. Unhygienic conditions would also contribute to plaque accumulation that would harbor deleterious acids.

Dental cements

There are a number of types of cements that may be used as luting agents. Each has inherent desirable and undesirable characteristics. Thus the selection of a particular class of cement is governed by the individual situation presented by the patient.

Until recently, zinc phosphate cement was the most commonly used luting agent, and it still enjoys wide use. Composed essentially of a liquid of phosphoric acid that is mixed with zinc oxide powder, the cement has excellent handling characteristics in terms of setting time, fluidity, and film thickness. Furthermore, this type of cement has a long history. The dentist can anticipate a certain longevity if the cement is handled properly and the casting fits precisely.

On the other hand, because of the acid liquid, zinc phosphate cement is an irritant, and proper pulp protection by means of a cavity varnish or cement base is essential. In those situations where past experience clearly indicates that sensitivity and pulp response are likely to be problems, a cement that is more biologically compatible is indicated, such as a reinforced zinc oxide–eugenol or a polycarboxylate cement. Because the latter type is now used extensively, and because it is a delicate cement in terms of manipulation, additional attention is given to it in the following section.

Polycarboxylate cements. None of the classic cements used in dentistry actually adheres to tooth structure. The retention of a cast restoration or an orthodontic band with a zinc phosphate cement, for example, is entirely mechanical in nature. The exception to this is the polycarboxylate, or polyacrylate, cement.

The powder is primarily zinc oxide, and the liquid is polyacrylic acid or a copolymer of that acid. Although the pH of the cement is comparable to that of zinc phosphate cement, the biologic properties are excellent. Apparently the larger acid molecule cannot penetrate dentin as readily as can phosphoric acid. Because of its good biologic properties, this type of cement is useful as a base or as a luting agent, particularly when the cavity preparation is deep.

In addition, as the cement sets against the tooth structure, a chemical adhesive bond is formed between the cement liquid and primarily the calcium in the apatite present in enamel and dentin. The adhesive mechanism is of use for the cementation of gold restorations or chrome steel crowns and for the attachment of orthodontic brackets directly to enamel. (Various resins, in conjunction with acid etch techniques, are also used for "direct bonding.")

When the cement is used as a luting agent, several manipulative factors influence the wetting of the tooth by the cement and thereby retention of the restoration. First, it is essential that any debris left in the cavity preparation be removed so that the setting cement can bond to the clean tooth. Water or a dilute solution of hydrogen peroxide (1% to 3%) is a biologically acceptable cleansing agent. As with all types of cement, the powder and liquid should not be dispensed until just before the mix is to be made. To slow down the setting reaction and provide longer working time, a chilled slab may be used. The powder, but *not* the liquid, may be stored in a refrigerator until ready for use. Polyacrylic acid liquid has poor stability at either high or low temperature. The powder and liquid should be mixed rapidly; the mix should be completed within 30 seconds.

An excessive concentration of powder should be

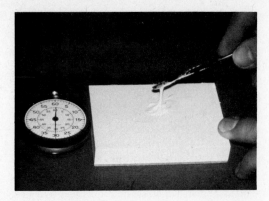

Fig. 13-4. Proper mix of polycarboxylate cement showing glossy surface.

avoided. If the mix is too thick, insufficient acid is present to produce bonding to the tooth. A workable powder/liquid ratio is approximately 2:1. One manufacturer supplies a calibrated syringe for dispensing the liquid. When properly prepared, the mix has a glossy appearance, as shown in Fig. 13-4, and extrudes into a thin film. It is important that minimal time be involved between completion of the mix and placement of the cement.

When polycarboxylate cement is used in conjunction with a gold restoration, it is essential that the inside surface of the casting be cleaned. The common laboratory technique used in the fabrication of a small casting employs a pickling solution to remove any oxides from the alloy. These solutions are acids or salts of acids, such as hydrochloric or sulfuric. They leave a microscopic film on the surface of the metal, and a polycarboxylate cement will not bond to that chemically dirty surface. In time leakage and loss of retention occur along the cement-restoration interface. Therefore the cavity side of the casting must be mechanically abraded to expose the clean metal for bonding to the cement. Various types of Airbrasive devices are available for this purpose, or a fine stone can be used to carefully abrade the metal.

Glass ionomer cements. The newest luting cement is the glass ionomer. The powder is an aluminosilicate glass similar to that of silicate ce-

ments. The liquid is basically an aqueous solution of a copolymer of polyacrylic acid, analogous to the liquid of the polycarboxylate cement just discussed. In addition, the glass ionomer cement liquid generally contains small amounts of other acids, such as itaconic or tartaric, added to improve working and setting characteristics.

The glass ionomer cements adhere to tooth structure by virtue of the polyacrylic acid in the liquid. The chemical adhesion to tooth structure is the same as that described for the polycarboxylate cements. As with polycarboxylate cements, the adhesion to enamel is superior to the bond to dentin.

The glass ionomer cement is nonirritating to the pulp, eliciting a response comparable to that of polycarboxylate cement, as would be anticipated on the basis of composition. In addition, the glass ionomer cement possesses the potential for inhibiting or reducing secondary caries because of the release of the fluoride that is a constituent of the silicate glass powder.

The prepared tooth structure should be meticulously cleaned and dried to promote adhesion of the cement. The retention of the casting can be improved if the inside surface is cleaned, as described for the polycarboxylate cement. The mixing procedure is similar to that described for zinc polycarboxylate cement. The powder is introduced into the liquid in large increments and spatulated rapidly for 45 seconds. As with all cements, the properties of a glass ionomer cement are markedly influenced by manipulative factors. The recommended powder/liquid ratio varies with different brands, but it is in the range of 1.25 to 1.5 g of powder per 1 g of liquid.

Cementation should be done before the cement loses its shiny appearance. Glass ionomer cement, like zinc phosphate cement, becomes brittle once it has set. When the cement hardens, the excess or "flash" can be removed by flicking or breaking the cement away at the margins.

Glass ionomer cement is particularly susceptible to attack by water during setting. Therefore it is necessary to coat all the accessible margins of the restoration to protect the cement from premature exposure to moisture. Newer formulations may be more resistant to the aqueous environment.

Temporary restorations

The temporary restoration should possess unusually good biologic characteristics, have minimal solubility, and be rigid, strong, and resistant to abrasion. The relative importance of each of these properties depends on the degree of permanence desired. For example, in the carious mouth it is often desirable to remove all of the caries immediately and place temporary restorations. These restorations may subsequently be replaced with more permanent restorative materials. In such situations it may be necessary for the temporary restoration to serve for several months or longer. Strength and abrasion resistance are of paramount importance in these cases, whereas usually the restoration need remain in place only for days. In the latter instance more emphasis must be placed on the biologic properties when the material is selected.

In an older technique for the temporary restoration, amalgam alloy filings were added to the mix of zinc phosphate cement. This increased the tensile strength and improved the resistance to abrasion. Silicophosphate cements also possess excellent durability. Since this type of cement is based on a silicate cement powder, it has the added advantage of being somewhat anticariogenic by virtue of the fluoride present. As discussed, the underlying dentin must be protected by a base or a varnish, or both, when these cements are used.

Because of its excellent tissue tolerance and ability to minimize initial microleakage patterns, zinc oxide–eugenol cement systems have become the material of choice for the long-term, or holding, type of restoration. The main problem has been to improve the strength, rigidity, and resistance to abrasion of the conventional zinc oxide–eugenol mixture. This has been accomplished in a number of ways, such as by the addition of polymers and by the surface treatment of the zinc oxide powder. The result is a much tougher material that has surprising durability. These products are particularly useful in the indirect pulp-capping therapy discussed in Chapters 7 and 8.

Reinforced zinc oxide–eugenol cements are also available for use as luting agents. Some of these are referred to as EBA cements because they contain orthoethoxybenzoic acid as a strengthening agent in the eugenol. The new glass ionomer cement has potential as a temporary restorative. For example, it is useful for restoring eroded areas in adult patients when exposed areas of cementum and dentin are present. Because of its desirable biologic and adhesive characteristics, the cement can be used to restore these lesions without the necessity of retention via a cavity preparation. However, the use of current formulations in stress-bearing restorations, such as the Class II, is not indicated because of the low ductility of the cement.

For many years red copper cement was a commonly used temporary restorative material, but it is no longer popular. Because of its low pH, it ranks high on the list of pulpal irritants. Furthermore, there is no evidence that the copper ion present has any lasting germicidal or antibacterial effect.

Restorative resins

Resins have certain qualities that justify their use as a dental restorative material. The first resin systems used in dentistry were primarily poly(methyl methacrylate) and are usually referred to as *acrylic* resins. Initially they have excellent esthetic characteristics, are insoluble in oral fluids, and have low thermal conductivity. However, they have a high coefficient of thermal expansion, low strength, and poor resistance to abrasion, and they are not anticariogenic.

The unfilled acrylic resins are still available but have largely been superseded by the *composite* resins, usually supplied as a paste rather than as a powder and liquid. A composite structure is one in which a filler has been added to a matrix material to improve the physical properties. Enamel and bone are excellent examples of composite structures. In dental composites the goal is to improve the strength and hardness and to lower the coefficient of thermal expansion, as compared with the older acrylic resins. Dentists appear to prefer the composite resins because of their esthetic appearance, more rapid polymerization, and paste form.

Various fillers are used, such as quartz and boron silicate glass, present in concentrations as high as 80%.

In addition, a somewhat different resin is generally employed, being a reaction product between an epoxy resin and methacrylic acid. This molecule is often referred to as BIS-GMA and is probably best termed a thermosetting acrylic resin. Most of the conventional commercial composites are chemically activated via the peroxide-amine induction system. The two pastes are identical except that one contains the benzoyl peroxide initiator and the other the tertiary amine activator or accelerator. When the two pastes are mixed, the material polymerizes.

Light-curing conventional composite resins are now being marketed. Although photocuring has had extensive use in industry, it has only recently been applied to dental restoratives. The first system used in dentistry employed *ultraviolet light*. In the ultraviolet light–curing system, benzoin methyl ether or higher alkyl benzoin ethers are employed as the activator for the peroxide curing system. On exposure to light waves in the ultraviolet range, the ether decomposes to form free radicals that trigger polymerization.

Some products make use of *visible light* activation, using radiation greater than 400 nm. The activating compounds for visible light are commonly diketones and aromatic ketones used in conjunction with reducing agents.

An advantage of the visible light–curing system, as compared to ultraviolet light systems, is that a greater depth of resin can be cured by visible light. Also, the resin can be polymerized through enamel, which is particularly advantageous in Class III restorations. Furthermore, the intensity of ultraviolet light tends to decrease with time. Thus the light must be tested continually to ensure that the resin is being properly polymerized. The intensity of visible light remains relatively constant until the bulb fails completely.

An advantage of light-curing systems is that the dentist has complete control over the working time and is not confined to the standard curing cycle of the self-cure. This is particularly beneficial when large restorations such as Class IV are placed. There are still some difficulties with light curing. With certain light-curing systems there is a lower percentage of conversion of the monomer, a lower degree of polymerization, and a limited depth of cure. However, when the light-curing composite resins are properly cured, their properties are similar to those of chemically cured materials.

A new series of restorative resin composites is based on the use of an extremely small filler particle; hence these are called *microfilled* or *microfine* resins. They have also been called ''polishable'' composites, although the term is not very exact. They differ from the traditional composite principally in the nature and size of the filler.

In the microfilled resin the particle size of the filler, precipitated silica, is approximately 0.04 μm, which is below the wavelength of visible light. These particles of microfine silica may be dispensed directly into the paste, but usually they are predispensed in a monomer and chloroform. The chloroform is removed and the monomer is then polymerized by the manufacturer, after which it is pulverized and used as all or part of the filler in a traditional resin paste matrix. A small amount of colloidal silica may also be added to the matrix resin. This type of dispersion is often called an ''organic filler,'' but obviously this term is misleading because inorganic colloidal silica is the filler used in the ''organic'' polymerized particle. The structure of the microfilled resin is shown in Fig. 13-5.

The interesting and appealing characteristic of the microfilled resins is that they can be finished to an extremely smooth surface, which has always been a major problem with the traditional composites. The filler particles in the composites have a hardness and an abrasion resistance that are entirely different from those of the resin matrix. This leads to a rough surface, since during finishing particles are plucked out or left protruding from the

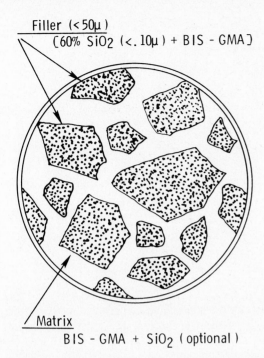

Filler (<50μ)
(60% SiO₂ (<.10μ) + BIS - GMA)

Matrix
BIS - GMA + SiO₂ (optional)

Fig. 13-5. Structure of a microfilled resin. (From Phillips, R.W.: The science of dental materials, ed. 8, Philadelphia, 1982, W.B. Saunders Co.)

matrix. With the microfilled resins, during finishing the polymerized resin filler particles wear at the same rate as the matrix and a markedly smoother surface results. Even if some of the very small colloidal silica particles are dislodged, the surface irregularities cannot be detected by the eye.

However, as with all dental materials, when formulations are changed to enhance one property, there is the risk that other desirable characteristics may be altered or sacrificed. In the case of the microfilled resins, the problem centers on the fact that because of the particle size of the silica, and thus the very high surface area, less filler can be incorporated, at least with current formulations. The filler load is generally only approximately 40% as compared with a filler load of 75% to 80% for the classic composite. Thus, the microfilled composite has a higher resin matrix content. Certain properties are altered accordingly. Such resins are softer, have a slightly higher coefficient of thermal expansion and polymerization shrinkage, and may have higher water sorption.

Whether this tradeoff in properties will lead to less satisfactory clinical performance will be determined only through well-controlled clinical studies. Because the microfilled resin system has been on the market for only a few years, a valid comparison with the traditional composites in terms of long-term behavior in the oral cavity cannot be made at this time. Certainly the microfilled resin has the advantage of eliminating one of the real difficulties with the previous type of composite, namely the inferior surface that is left after polishing.

Regardless of whether one of the newer composites or one of the older poly(methyl methacrylate) products is employed, the use of resin should be confined to Class III, Class V, and Class IV restorations. In the latter case, wires have traditionally been employed to assist in retention. However, the use of acid etch techniques has largely eliminated the need for the auxiliary retention as provided by the pins (see Figs. 17-23 to 17-26). As yet the properties of the dental resins that are available do not indicate that their routine use is warranted where the restoration is subject to masticatory stress. Their greatest deficiency in this regard is lack of adequate resistance to wear, resulting in a change in anatomic contour when used in Class II restorations. Because of the wear problem, use of any resin in Class I or Class II preparations should be limited to restorations in which esthetics is the primary consideration (the premolar), and a conservative cavity preparation should be used whenever possible. It must be emphasized that there is a tremendous amount of activity in this field. It is possible that in the near future a truly wear-resistant composite may be developed. In the meantime a critical posture should be taken in regard to the use of currently available composites in the Class II preparation in the permanent dentition. There is evidence that such materials may be satisfactory for restorations in the primary dentition.

Resin is not an easy material to master; the dentist who is not willing to gain experience in its use and to understand the relationship of the inherent properties to the oral cavity should use other restorative materials.

The greatest problem associated with restorative resins is microleakage. Research is now in progress toward the creation of resins that will adhere to tooth tissue. These efforts may eventually lead to systems that will alter current methods for restoring the carious lesion. As yet, however, no truly adhesive resins have been developed, and the phenomenon of microleakage is of particular consequence in the use of this material. Since resin has no caries-inhibitory or antibacterial effect, leakage at the tooth-resin interface is of greater consequence in producing pulpal reactions or in contributing to the loss of the physical integrity of the restoration than it is with any other dental material. The coefficient of thermal expansion of any dental resin is considerably higher than tooth structure, thus tending to further increase the possibility of leakage. For this reason the operative procedure must be designed to achieve maximum initial adaptation of the resin to the cavity preparation.

Luting agents, referred to as "primers" or "sealers," are often supplied by manufacturers of unfilled acrylic resins. These liners do not produce adhesion between the resin and the tooth, but they tend to clean the surface of the cavity preparation and provide better wetting of the resin.

The most satisfactory method for improving the mechanical bonding of the resin to the enamel is by the use of acid etch techniques. The dentin is protected against the acid by a calcium hydroxide base or a varnish, and then the enamel is etched with a solution of phosphoric acid for approximately 1 to 2 minutes, depending on the rate of decalcification for that particular tooth. Various concentrations of acid are supplied, but one between 35% and 50% is satisfactory.

The next critical step in the technique is the use of a stream of water to remove the precipitants produced during etching. If this debris is not flushed off the enamel surface, the resin tags cannot form.

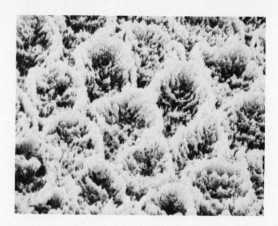

Fig. 13-6. Surface of enamel etched for 2 minutes with 50% phosphoric acid ($\times 3000$).

The resin-enamel bond strength is directly related to the wash time. For example, it has been shown that the mean tensile bond strength of one resin to enamel doubled when the wash time was extended from 15 seconds to 1 minute. A minimum wash time of 45 seconds is recommended. The surface must then be dried for at least 15 seconds.

Any film of moisture on this cleaned surface will inhibit resin penetration into the etched area. If the surface should be contaminated by saliva, the saliva film cannot be completely removed by washing. Rather the surface should be dried, re-etched for 10 seconds, rewashed, and dried.

An etched enamel surface can be seen in Fig. 13-6. The acid cleans the enamel to provide better wetting of the resin. It also creates pores into which the resin flows to produce tags that increase retention markedly. Furthermore, the better bond should reduce the possibility of marginal stain, which is the invariable result of microleakage.

In addition to acid etch solutions, some manufacturers also supply "enamel bond" agents. These usually consist of the unfilled resin matrix used in the composite itself. According to the manufacturers, the low-viscosity resin will ensure good wetting of the tooth and maximum resin tag formation. Although the use of such agents may provide a more foolproof system, the acid etch part of the technique is the main factor involved in ensuring maximum bonding.

Dental resins are no more irritating to the pulp than are a number of other commonly used restorative materials. Whenever the cavity preparation is deep, the same precautions are taken as with those materials.

Pit and fissure sealants

Through the years various materials and techniques have been advocated for preventing caries in the susceptible pit and fissure areas of molar teeth in child patients. The most recent technique makes use of resin systems that can be applied to the occlusal surfaces of the teeth. The objective is for the resin to penetrate the pits and fissures to polymerize and seal these areas against the oral flora. Several types of resin, filled and unfilled, have been employed as pit and fissure sealants. Light-cured systems and glass ionomer cement are also used for this purpose. However, with most of the latter products the viscosity limits the use to fissures where the access is at least 100 μm.

The success of this technique, as for any resin, is dependent on obtaining and maintaining an intimate adaptation of the sealant to the tooth surface and thereby sealing it. Therefore the sealants must be of relatively low viscosity so that they will flow readily into the depths of the pits and fissures and wet the tooth. To enhance wetting and mechanical retention of the sealant, the tooth surface is first conditioned by etching with acid.

The physical properties of these sealants have not yet been well defined. However, it is assumed that they resemble the counterpart systems used in restorative dentistry. Undoubtedly the sealants would be susceptible to occlusal wear. However, this might not pose a serious problem as long as the material is retained in the pit or fissure and the seal is maintained at the periphery.

Reported reductions in occlusal caries resulting from the careful use of pit and fissure sealants have been impressive. However, it must be recognized that these materials are in the developmental stage.

Much remains to be determined with respect to their effectiveness and the parameters governing their use. For example, most studies reported thus far involve careful case selection and meticulous application of the material to surfaces that appear to be caries free. If the surface is noncarious and reasonably accessible, apparently it can be cleaned and etched with sufficient adequacy to provide intimate adaptation of the material and an effective seal, at least for a limited time. (The frequency at which the material should be reapplied has not been established.)

If the pit or fissure is carious or not reasonably accessible, it is unlikely that the surface can be cleansed sufficiently to obtain the necessary mechanical bonding of the resin to the tooth. In such a situation the subsequent leakage might actually enhance the progression of caries.

Until further research resolves these and other questions, the sealant materials should be used under carefully controlled conditions. For the present they are probably best suited to community dentistry projects and offices in which the emphasis is on preventive dentistry.

Impression materials

All three of the elastic impression materials are used in dentistry for children, although irreversible hydrocolloid (alginate) and the rubber base materials are more frequently employed than reversible hydrocolloid. The inherent accuracy of reversible hydrocolloid and the rubber base materials (the polysulfide polymers, silicone, or polyether types) is comparable, and selection should be based on ease of manipulation, armamentarium required, and other subjective factors. Alginate is satisfactory when meticulous reproduction of detail is not essential. The alginate impression will not provide the sharpness of detail or the density in the stone model that can be attained with the other materials.

A discussion of the properties and manipulation of these materials is beyond the scope of this chapter, and the techniques for use are outlined elsewhere. However, because of their popularity, it is appropriate to emphasize that the success of the rubber base materials is dependent on matters such as (1) use of a custom-made tray to minimize the bulk of material, (2) bonding of the rubber to the tray by means of a rubber cement, (3) a minimum curing time of 8 minutes in the oral cavity, and (4) pouring the stone die as soon as possible.

REFERENCES

Composites

Buonocore, M.G.: The use of adhesives in dentistry, Springfield, Ill., 1975, Charles C Thomas, Publisher.

Jordan, R.E., and others: Restoration of fractured and hypoplastic incisors by the acid etch technique: a three-year report, J.A.D.A. **95**:795, 1977.

Leinfelder, K.F. and Taylor, D.F.: Current status of composite resins, N.C. Dent. J. **61**:17, 1978.

Ortiz, R.F., and others: Effect of composite resin bond agent on microleakage and bond strength, J. Prosthet. Dent. **41**:51, 1979.

Raptis, C.N., Fan, P.L., and Powers, J.M.: Properties of microfilled and visible light cured composites, J.A.D.A. **99**:631, 1979.

Simonsen, R.J.: Clinical application of the acid etch technique, Chicago, 1978, Quintessence Publishing Co.

Amalgam

Greener, E.H.: Amalgam: yesterday, today, and tomorrow, Oper. Dent. **4**:24, 1979.

Leinfelder, K.F.: Clinical performance of amalgams with high content of copper, Oper. Dent. **5**:125, 1980.

Mahler, D.B.: Dental amalgam. In Craig, R., editor: Dental materials review, Ann Arbor, 1977, University of Michigan Press.

Report of Council on Dental Materials, Instruments and Devices: Recommendations in dental mercury hygiene, March, 1978, J.A.D.A. **96**:487, 1978.

Wrijhoef, M.M.A., Vermeersch, A.G., and Spaunauf, A.J.: Dental amalgam, Chicago, 1980, Quintessence Publishing Co.

Cements

Harper, R.H., and others: In vivo measurements of thermal diffusion through restorations of various materials, J. Prosthet. Dent. **43**:180, 1980.

Maldonado, A., Swartz, M.L., and Phillips, R.W.: An in vitro study of certain properties of a glass ionomer cement, J.A.D.A. **96**:785, 1978.

Mitchem, J.C., and Gronas, D.G.: Clinical evaluation of cement solubility, J. Prosthet. Dent. **40**:453, 1978.

Mount, G.J., and Makinson, O.F.: Clinical characteristics of a glass ionomer cement, Br. Dent. J. **145**:67, 1978.

Norman, R.D., and others: Effects of restorative materials on plaque composition, J. Dent. Res. **51**:1596, 1972.

Smith, D.C.: A review of the zinc polycarboxylate cements, J. Can. Dent. Assoc. **37**:22, 1971.

Wilson, A.D., and Crisp, S.: Ionomer cements, Br. Poly. J. **7**:279, 1975.

Adhesion

Beech, D.R.: Adhesion and adhesives in the oral environment, Austral. Coll. Dent. Surg. **5**:128, 1977.

Buonocore, M.G.: Principles of adhesive restorative materials, J.A.D.A. **67**:382, 1963.

Glantz, P.: On wettability and adhesiveness, Odontol. Rev. **20**(suppl. 17):1, 1969.

von Fraunhofer, J.A.: Adhesion and adhesives. In Scientific aspects of dental materials, London, 1975, Butterworth & Co., pp. 49-95.

General

Baum, L., Phillips, R.W., and Lund, M.R.: Textbook of operative dentistry, Philadelphia, 1981, W.B. Saunders Co.

Phillips, R.W.: Skinner's science of dental materials, ed. 8, Philadelphia, 1982, W.B. Saunders Co.

14 Gingivitis and periodontal disease

RALPH E. McDONALD
DAVID R. AVERY

The gingiva, as described by Goldman and Cohen, is the mucous membrane that extends from the cervical portion of the tooth to the mucobuccal fold. The gingiva is divided into the papillary portion, which occupies the interdental space; the marginal portion, which forms the collar of free gingiva around the neck of the tooth; and the attached gingiva, which is the portion attached by dense fibrous tissue to the underlying alveolar bone.

The gingival tissues are normally light pink, although the color may be related to the complexion of the individual, the thickness of the tissue, and the degree of keratinization. The surface of the gingiva has a stippled appearance, varying from fine to coarsely grained. Zappler described the tone of the gingiva in the child as frequently flabbier than that in the adult; he also described the connective tissue of the lamina propria as less dense. In the healthy adult the marginal gingiva has a sharp knifelike edge; during the period of eruption in the child, however, the gingivae are thicker and have rounded margins.

Gingivitis is an inflammation involving only the gingival tissues next to the tooth. Microscopically, it is characterized by the presence of an inflammatory exudate and edema, some destruction of collagenous gingival fibers, and ulceration and proliferation of the epithelium facing the tooth and attaching the gingiva to it.

Voluminous data show that inflammatory periodontal disease is a major health problem. The insidious nature of the disease is indicated by the documented occurrence of slight gingival inflammation in children, increasing severity in youths and young adults, and frequent progression to partial or complete loss of the dentition in middle or later life. The major etiologic factors associated with the disease are uncalcified and calcified bacterial plaque.

Bacterial plaque is composed of soft bacterial deposits that firmly adhere to the teeth. Plaque is considered to be a complex, metabolically interconnected, highly organized bacterial system consisting of dense masses of microorganisms embedded in an intermicrobial matrix. In sufficient concentration it can disturb the host-parasite relationship and cause dental caries and periodontal disease.

Eastcott and Stallard have observed that plaque begins to form within 2 hours after the teeth are brushed. Coccal-shaped bacteria form first on a thin fenestrated *pellicle* (organic bacteria-free film deposited on the tooth surface). The surface is completely covered with a smooth material 3 hours after brushing. Within 5 hours plaque microcolonies develop, apparently by cell division. Between 6 and 12 hours, the covering material becomes thinner and is reduced to discontinuous small scattered areas. About 30% of the coccal-shaped bacteria are in various stages of division by 24 hours. Rod-shaped bacteria appear for the first time in 24-hour-old plaque. Within 48 hours the surface of the plaque is covered with a mass of rods and filaments.

Dental calculus, which is considered to be calcified dental plaque, is discussed again later in the chapter. It is classified as supragingival or subgingival, depending on its location on the tooth. *Supragingival calculus* occurs as hard, firmly adherent masses on the crowns of teeth. *Subgingival calculus* is found as a concretion on the tooth in the confines of the periodontal pocket. The surface of dental calculus is always covered by uncalcified plaque. Calculus is an important factor in the development of gingival and periodontal disease.

Severe gingivitis is relatively uncommon in children, although numerous surveys have shown that a large portion of the child population has a mild, reversible type of gingivitis.

Weddell and Klein recently conducted a study to determine the prevalence of gingivitis in a group of children between the ages of 6 and 36 months. The children, patients of pediatricians in the Indianapolis area, had been born in the area, which has a fluoridated water supply. In 299 white children, gingivitis was present in 13% of those 6 to 17 months of age, 34% of those in the 18- to 23-month age group, and 39% of those in the 24- to 36-month age group. Black children were not included because of the inconsistency of their gingival colors. The gingivitis observed by Weddell and Klein was for the most part eruption gingivitis. Nevertheless, their findings support the fact that an oral hygiene program should be initiated by parents when the child is very young.

Carter and Wells observed in an examination of 29,500 Kansas City, Missouri, children ranging in age from 6 to 12 years that the average incidence of gingivitis was about 50%. The incidence of gingivitis ranged from 37% in 6-year-old boys to 57% in 10-year-old boys. The papillae and margins were the most commonly involved gingival units. In independent studies by Massler, Schour, and Chopra and by Rosenzweig, the incidence of gingivitis was observed to be highest in boys in the 9- to 17-year age group, whereas girls had the highest incidence in the age range of 5 to 8 years.

In a study including 1123 children from age 7 to 13 years in three Indiana communities, Moore found the incidence of gingivitis to be higher than in previously reported studies. The papillary-marginal-attached (PMA) index was used to determine the prevalence and severity of gingivitis. Duncan's occupational socioeconomic index was used to determine the socioeconomic status of each child. Gingivitis was considered present when one or more papillae, margins, or attached gingival units were affected. Ninety-three percent of the children manifested some degree of gingivitis, whereas only 7% had mouths that appeared to be completely free of evidence of gingivitis. The severity of gingivitis and the accumulation of oral debris were inversely related to socioeconomic status, whereas toothbrushing habits appeared to be directly related to socioeconomic status.

In a study of approximately 1700 children 9 to 14 years of age by Suomi and associates, it was found that a relatively high percentage of children of all racial-ethnic groups had calculus (both supragingival and subgingival). From 56% to 85% of the children in the various age, sex, and racial-ethnic groups had supragingival calculus. The findings of this study indicate that most children 9 to 14 years of age who are of low socioeconomic status would benefit from inclusion in a preventive periodontal disease program based on improving oral hygiene.

In a study of 2876 children residing in a naturally fluoridated area, Murray confirms the high prevalence of gingivitis in the young population. He observed that inflammation of one or more papillae or margins associated with the incisor and canine teeth occurred in 90% of children aged 8 to 18 years. He, too, points to the importance of a good standard of oral cleanliness in reducing gingivitis and, ideally, preventing the progression of the disease in later life.

Simple gingivitis

Eruption gingivitis. A temporary type of gingivitis is often observed in young children when the primary teeth are erupting. This gingivitis, often associated with "difficult eruption," subsides after the teeth emerge into the oral cavity.

The greatest increase in the incidence of gingivitis in children is often seen in the 6- to 7-year age

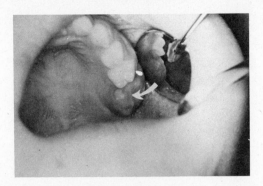

Fig. 14-1. Mild inflammation *(arrow)* is evident in the tissue partially covering the crown of the erupting first permanent molar.

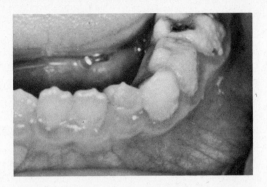

Fig. 14-2. Gingivitis resulting from poor oral hygiene and reduced function in the area. A painful second primary molar has interfered with normal function on this side of the mouth.

group when the permanent teeth begin to erupt. Goldman and Cohen have suggested that this increase in gingivitis occurs because the gingival margin receives no protection from the coronal contour of the tooth during the early stage of active eruption, and the continual impingement of food on the gingivae causes the inflammatory process.

Food debris, materia alba, and bacterial plaque often collect around and beneath the free tissue, partially cover the crown of the erupting tooth, and cause the development of an inflammatory process (Fig. 14-1). This inflammation is most commonly associated with the eruption of the first and second permanent molars, and the condition can be painful and can develop into a pericoronitis or a pericoronal abscess. Mild eruption gingivitis requires no treatment other than improved oral hygiene. Painful pericoronitis may be helped by irrigating the area with a counterirritant such as 4-point solution.* Pericoronitis accompanied by swelling and lymph node involvement should be treated with antibiotic therapy.

Gingivitis associated with poor oral hygiene. The degree of dental cleanliness and the healthy condition of the gingival tissues in children are definitely related. Horowitz and associates observed

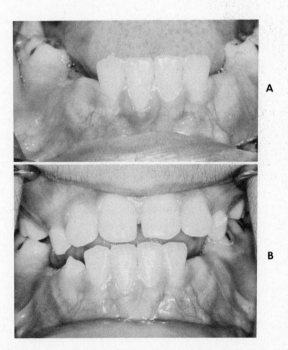

Fig. 14-3. A, Localized gingival inflammation and recession associated with minimal plaque accumulation on mandibular right central incisor. **B,** Gingival health was markedly improved after a thorough plaque removal regimen was initiated at home.

---

*Phenol (5%), 5 ml; tincture aconite, 10 ml; tincture iodine, 15 ml; glycerin, 20 ml.

significant reductions in gingivitis scores of schoolchildren after the initiation of a supervised daily plaque removal program. Children in grades 5 to 8 participated in the program, and successful results were maintained during 3 school years. The mean gingivitis scores were reduced 40% among girls and 17% among boys during the program period, while the children in the control group maintained essentially the same gingivitis scores for the period of the study. Adequate mouth hygiene and cleanliness of the teeth are related to frequency of brushing and the thoroughness with which bacterial plaque is removed from the teeth. Favorable occlusion and the chewing of coarse detergent-type foods have a beneficial effect on oral cleanliness.

Gingivitis associated with poor oral hygiene is usually classified as a mild type in which the papillae and marginal tissues are inflamed. This mild gingivitis is reversible and can be treated with a good oral prophylaxis, the removal of calcareous deposits and accumulated food debris, and teaching good toothbrushing and flossing techniques to keep the teeth free of bacterial plaque (Figs. 14-2 and 14-3).

Acute gingival disease

Herpes simplex virus infection. Herpesvirus causes one of the most widespread viral infections. The primary infection usually occurs in a child under 5 years of age who has had no contact with the type 1 herpes simplex virus (HSV-1) and who therefore has no neutralizing antibodies. It is believed that 99% of all primary infections are of the subclinical type. The infection may also occur in susceptible adults who have not had the primary infection (Fig. 14-4).

Silverman and Beumer have reported 25 patients with primary herpetic gingivostomatitis of adult onset. The individuals, ranging in age from 18 to 41 years, were studied with respect to clinical features and confirmatory laboratory findings. All subjects had fever, malaise, cervical lymphadenopathy, and erythema and ulcers of the gingiva and other mucosal sites. They had no history of

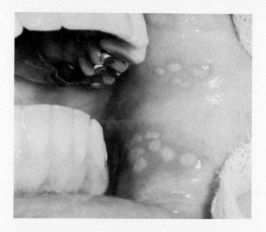

Fig. 14-4. Ulcerated stage of primary herpes in a young adult. Note the circumscribed confluent areas of inflammation.

similar attack. Sources of infection or contagious factors were not apparent.

In some preschool children the primary infection may be characterized by only one or two mild sores on the oral mucous membranes, which may be of little concern to the child or may go unnoticed by the parents. In other children the primary infection may be manifested by acute symptoms (*acute herpetic gingivostomatitis*). The active symptoms of the acute disease usually occur between the ages of 2 and 6 years, even in children with clean mouths and healthy oral tissues. In fact, these children seem to be as susceptible as those with poor oral hygiene. The symptoms of the disease develop suddenly and include, in addition to the fiery red gingival tissues, malaise, irritability, headache, and pain associated with the intake of food and liquids of acid content. A characteristic oral finding in the acute primary disease is the presence of yellow or white liquid-filled vesicles. In a few days the vesicles rupture and form painful ulcers, 1 to 3 mm in diameter, which are covered with a whitish gray membrane and have a circumscribed area of inflammation (Figs. 14-5 and 14-6). The ulcers may be observed on any area of the mucous membrane, including buccal mucosa, tongue, lips, hard

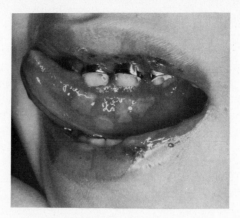

Fig. 14-6. Several large painful ulcers are evident on the tongue of a preschool child with acute herpetic gingivostomatitis.

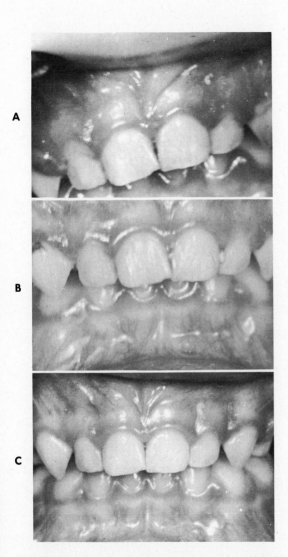

Fig. 14-5. A, Acute herpetic gingivostomatitis in an 18-month-old child. The fiery red gingival tissues and the presence of ulcers on the mucous membrane are characteristic findings. **B,** Marked improvement is evident within a week after the occurrence of the acute symptoms. **C,** Symptoms of the disease have subsided in 2 weeks. Mild inflammation of isolated gingival papillae is still evident.

and soft palate, and the tonsillar areas. Large ulcerated lesions may occasionally be observed on the palate or gingival tissues or in the region of the mucobuccal fold. This distribution makes the differential diagnosis more difficult. An additional diagnostic criterion is a fourfold rise of serum antibodies to HSV-1. The lesion culture will also be positive to HSV-1.

The primary infection is often incorrectly diagnosed as Vincent infection and may be incorrectly treated with penicillin, which fixes the virus and greatly prolongs the clinical course of the disease. It is only during the primary attack that the lesions and inflammatory involvement occur over such a widespread area in the mouth.

Treatment of acute herpetic gingivostomatitis in children should be directed toward the relief of the acute symptoms in order that fluid and nutritional intake be maintained. The application of a mild topical anesthetic such as dyclonine (Dyclone) before mealtime will temporarily relieve the pain and allow the child to take a soft diet. Since fruit juices are usually irritating to the ulcerated area, a vitamin supplement is indicated during the course of the disease. Bed rest and isolation from other children in the family are recommended. Hale and associates reported an outbreak of herpes simplex infection in a group of 13 children occupying one floor in an orphanage. The children ranged in age from 11 to 35 months. In three of the children a mild fever of brief duration and small oral lesions were the only signs of infection, and these might easily have been unobserved in a situation different from that of an institutional study. The remaining children had symptoms of acute infection.

The topical application of tetracyclines to the ulcerated areas will aid in the control of a secondary infection, and this treatment has been observed to favorably alter the course of the infection. The antibiotic powder from the capsules may be applied to the lesions with a moistened cotton applicator after each meal. There is little or no risk of causing intrinsic staining of the developing teeth when the drug is used in this manner for a few days. The minimum effective dose of an antihistaminic drug will often make the child more comfortable and may produce drowsiness, which will encourage rest. The treatment of less severe primary infections may be concerned only with keeping the mouth clean and maintaining an adequate dietary intake and symptomatic treatment.

The herpes simplex infection runs a 10- to 14-day course, and little can be done to shorten the recovery period. Suggested treatment methods for the virus infection include the topical application of corticosteroids, the injection of trypsin, oral and topical use of antihistamines, and the use of gamma globulin. Since the results of these treatments have been inconclusive and often contradictory, the treatment should be supportive and symptomatic.

After the initial primary attack during the early childhood period, the herpes simplex virus remains inactive for periods of time. The inactive virus resides in sensory nerve ganglia but will often reappear later as the familiar *cold sore,* usually on the outside of the lips (Fig. 14-7). Thus the disease has been commonly referred to as "recurrent herpes labialis" (RHL). With the recurring attacks, the sores develop in essentially the same area on the lip. The recurrent form of the disease has often been related to conditions of emotional stress and

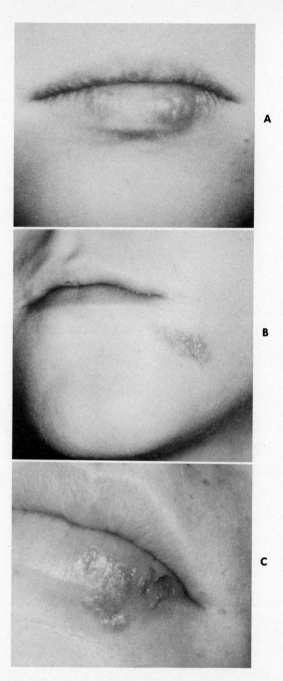

Fig. 14-7. Recurrent herpes labialis (RHL). **A,** Early vesicular lesions. **B,** Mature vesicular lesion. **C,** Appearance of herpes labialis after rupture of vesicles and crusting of the lesion.

lowered tissue resistance resulting from various types of trauma. Excessive exposure to sunlight may be responsible for the appearance of the recurrent herpetic lesions on the lip. Lesions on the lip may also appear after dental treatment and may be related to irritation from rubber dam material or even routine daily procedures.

The treatment of RHL continues to be empirical and experimental. The symptomatic use of bland emollient creams or ointments is sometimes helpful. The use of idoxuridine (Herplex and Stoxil) remains controversial. The manufacturers of the ointments, which may be applied topically at the first symptom of the lesion, claim that the active ingredient inhibits replication of herpes simplex virus by irreversibly inhibiting the incorporation of thymidine into the viral DNA.

The long list of proposed remedies for herpes simplex infection now includes the amino acid lysine. The oral therapy is based on lysine's antagonistic effect on another amino acid, arginine. Griffith, Norins, and Kagan conducted an initial study in which 250 patients were given daily lysine doses of 1000 mg and were told to avoid eating arginine-rich foods such as chocolate and nuts. The lysine therapy was continued until the patients had been lesion free for 6 months. L-Lysine monohydrochloride is available commercially in capsule form or tablets containing 100 or 312 mg of L-lysine.* The patients reported that pain disappeared overnight in virtually every instance. New vesicles failed to appear, and a majority considered the resolution of the lesions to be more rapid than in the past. There was also a reduction in frequency of occurrences. The authors conclude that improper food selection may make adequate lysine intake precarious for some individuals. Ingestion of cereals, seeds, nuts, and chocolate would produce a high arginine/lysine ratio and favor herpetic lesions; similar results are obtained by adding arginine to the medium in the laboratory to induce herpes proliferation. The avoidance of these foods, coupled with the selection of foods with adequate

lysine, such as dairy products and yeast, should discourage herpes infection. The authors postulate this may explain the low incidence of herpes in infants before they are weaned from a predominantly milk diet.

Terezhalmy, Bottomley, and Pellen have reported that the use of water-soluble bioflavonoid–ascorbic acid complex is effective in the treatment of recurrent herpes labialis. The daily incremental dose administered in several clinical studies varied from 300 to 4800 mg each of bioflavonoid and ascorbic acid. The authors indicate that since the toxicity of the ascorbic acid is relatively low, daily doses of up to 5000 mg may be prescribed without fear of toxic effects. The therapeutic regimen was found to be most effective when instituted in the early prodromal stage of the disease process and was observed to shorten the duration of the subjective symptom of pain and to reduce the incidence of the objective symptoms of vesiculation and disruption of the vesicular membrane. Optimum remission of symptoms was obtained in approximately 4 days with the therapeutic dosage of 600 mg of water-soluble bioflavonoid–ascorbic acid complex.

Brooks and associates have reported that dentists are frequently exposed to HSV-1. They evaluated the risk of infection by the virus through assessing disease experience, comparing the individual's history with the results of complement fixation or antibody titration tests or both. Their study group consisted of 525 dental students, 94 dental faculty members, and 23 staff members. Although almost all of those with a history of herpetic infection showed antibodies to HSV-1, only 57% of those lacking such a history had neutralizing antibody titers of 1:10 or higher. This finding suggests that a significant portion of practicing dentists risk primary herpetic infection. Consequently, dentists and dental auxiliaries without a history of herpetic lesions might benefit from serologic testing. Considering the occupational disability that often accompanies HSV-1 infection of the finger or eye, health professionals who lack HSV-1 antibodies should protect themselves with surgical gloves and

---

*General Nutrition Corp., Pittsburgh, Pa. 15222.

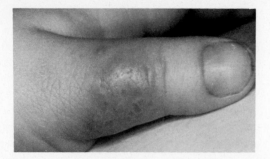

Fig. 14-8. Primary herpetic infection involving the dorsal surface of the thumb of a 3-year-old child. An acute primary infection was present in the mouth.

safety glasses while treating patients with active herpetic lesions.

Primary herpetic infection has been observed on the dorsal surface of the thumb of a child patient (Fig. 14-8). The child was a thumb-sucker, and the acute primary infection was present in the mouth. The dorsal surface of the thumb, which rested on the lower incisor teeth, apparently became irritated, and there was an inoculation of the virus. The oral condition and the lesions on the thumb subsided in 2 weeks.

Recurrent aphthous ulcer (canker sore). The recurrent aphthous ulcer (RAU)—also referred to as recurrent aphthous stomatitis (RAS)—is a painful ulceration on the mucous membrane that occurs in school-age children and in adults. The ulcers are most prevalent in individuals in the 10- to 20-year age range and are seen in males and females in the ratio of 1:2. These ulcers, according to definitions adopted in the epidemiologic literature, are characterized by recurrent ulcerations on the moist mucous membranes of the mouth, in which both discrete and confluent lesions form rapidly in certain sites and feature a round to oval crateriform base, raised reddened margins, and pain. They may appear in the form of attacks of single or multiple lesions, but they can be clearly distinguished from primary or secondary viral infections, bacterial infections (necrotizing ulcerative gingivitis), dermatologic conditions (lichen planus, pemphigus), and

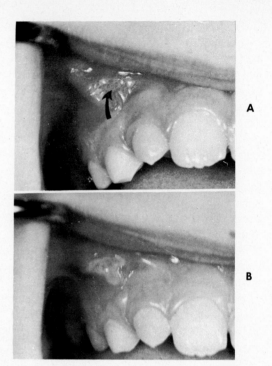

Fig. 14-9. A, Evidence of the development of a recurrent aphthous ulcer (RAU) in the mucobuccal fold above the primary canine. An area of inflammation and vesicle formation is apparent *(arrow)*. **B,** Five days later the lesion is a well-developed ulcer with a circumscribed area of inflammation.

traumatic episodes (contusions, lacerations, burns) by the healthy appearance of adjacent tissues and the lack of distinguishing systemic features. They may or may not be associated with ulcerative lesions elsewhere. Lesions persist for intervals of 4 to 12 days and heal uneventfully, leaving scars only rarely and only in unusually large lesions. The description of RAU frequently includes the term ''canker sores'' (Fig. 14-9).

The cause of the RAU is unknown. The condition may be caused by a delayed-type hypersensitivity to the L form of *Streptococcus sanguis,* which is a common inhabitant of the normal oral microbiota of humans. It is also possible that the lesions are caused by an autoimmune reaction of the oral epithelium. Epidemiologic studies by Ship

(1972) have provided evidence for this. These data suggest that both RHL and RAU may be produced by the same mechanism, despite the known infectious agent of RHL and the absence of any known virus for RAU.

Graykowski, Barile, and Stanley have isolated the L form of bacteria from patients with aphthous lesions. Blood culture from patients with lesions in the acute stage was positive for the organisms, whereas blood examined during quiescence was sterile.

Ship (1966) attempted to relate the occurrence of the aphthous ulcers to allergy, inheritance, food intake, and socioeconomic status. Although all these conditions seem to be related to the recurrence of the ulcers in some patients, the findings are still inconclusive. In 1972 Ship applied epidemiologic precepts to studies of RAU of the mouth and related previous disorders. These data have served to distinguish RAU-susceptible persons from RAU-resistant persons on the basis of group analysis and have identified the persons most likely to have this syndrome. The evidence indicates that the highest disease rates occur in middle- and upper-class students in professional schools; intermediate rates have been observed in hospital and clinic outpatient visitors in the middle classes; and the lowest rates have been reported among indigent hospital patients. These prevalence data have ranged from a high of 60% (student nurses) to a low of 5% (indigent male hospital patients), both having been reported from the same institution by the same investigators and thus ruling out geographic factors.

Although bacterial agents are undoubtedly important to the development of RAU, the susceptibility of certain persons to aphthae, as shown in clinical studies, gives reason to suspect some precipitating factors. In a recent review of the clinical problem, Antoon and Miller suggested that minor trauma is a common precipitating factor accountable for as much as 75% of the episodes. Injuries caused by cheek biting and minor facial irritations are probably the most common precipitating factors. Nutritional deficiencies are found in 20% of individuals with aphthous ulcers. The clinically detectable deficiencies include iron, vitamin B_{12}, and folic acid. While screening patients with aphthous ulcers, Wray observed a history of unusually high incidence of gastrointestinal disorders. Stress may prove to be an important precipitating factor, particularly in stress-prone groups such as students in professional schools and military personnel.

In September 1977 the National Institute of Dental Research sponsored a 2-day workshop devoted to aphthous stomatitis and Behçet syndrome. The papers presented at the workshop were published in the December 1978 issue of the *Journal of Oral Pathology* (vol. 7, no. 6). The participants concluded that studies dealing with the etiologies of these diseases should be intensified and that attempts to identify the roles of viruses, autoimmunity, and folic acid levels should be increased. Current evidence tends to favor an immunologic disorder and suggests that bacterial infections are probably secondary.

A variety of treatments have been recommended for RAU, but a completely successful treatment has not been found. The topical application of tetracyclines to the ulcers is often helpful in reducing the pain and in shortening the course of the disease. A mouthwash containing a suspension of one of the tetracyclines has been helpful to some, but the mouthwash should not be swallowed. The application of triamcinolone acetonide (Kenalog in Orabase) to the surface of the lesions before meals and on retiring may also be helpful.

Necrotizing ulcerative gingivitis (Vincent infection). The infectious but not contagious disease commonly referred to as "Vincent infection" is rare in preschool-age children in the United States, occasionally occurs in children 6 to 12 years old, and is common in young adults. Reade has reported one instance of the typical picture of ulcerative gingivitis in a 15-month-old infant. *Treponema vincentii* and gram-negative fusiform bacilli were demonstrated in a smear. Recovery occurred within 36 hours after penicillin therapy and the application of hydrogen peroxide.

Pindborg and associates have reported that

2.36% of the children examined at the dental college at Bangalore, India, had acute necrotizing gingivitis.

Vincent infection can be easily diagnosed because of the involvement of the interproximal papillae and the presence of a pseudomembranous necrotic covering of the marginal tissue (Fig. 14-10). Two microorganisms, *Borrelia vincentii* and fusiform bacilli, referred to as ''spirochetal organisms,'' are generally believed to be responsible for the disease. The clinical manifestations of the disease include inflamed, painful, bleeding gingival tissue, poor appetite, fever as high as 104° F (40° C), general malaise, and a fetid odor.

The disease responds dramatically within 24 to

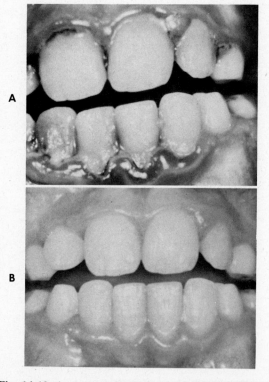

Fig. 14-10. A, A rare example of necrotizing ulcerative gingivitis in an 8-year-old boy. **B,** Local treatment and improved oral hygiene produced a dramatic recovery from the infection.

48 hours to subgingival curettage, debridement, and the use of mild oxidizing solutions. If the gingival tissues are acutely and extensively inflamed when the patient is first seen, antibiotic therapy is indicated. Improved oral hygiene and the use of mild oxidizing mouthrinses after each meal will aid in overcoming the infection.

Collins and Hood have reported that applying vancomycin dental ointment to the involved area with the finger three times a day is a valuable adjunct to therapy.

There should be no difficulty in distinguishing Vincent infection from acute herpetic gingivostomatitis, although, as previously mentioned, the two are frequently confused. Round ulcers with red areolae on the lips and cheeks are characteristic of herpetic gingivostomatitis. Therapeutic trial ''cleaning'' will bring about a favorable response in Vincent infection but not in acute herpetic gingivostomatitis. Therapeutic trial antibiotics will reduce the acute symptoms in Vincent infection but not in the virus infection. Acute herpetic gingivostomatitis is most frequently seen in preschool-age children, and its onset is rapid. Vincent infection rarely occurs in the preschool age group and develops over a longer period of time, usually in a mouth in which irritants and poor oral hygiene are present. On the other hand, acute oral infections initially diagnosed as Vincent infection have frequently been found later to be an oral manifestation of one of the xanthomatoses. The early stages of conditions such as Hand-Schüller-Christian disease or Letterer-Siwe disease are associated with many of the symptoms of Vincent infection.

Acute candidiasis (thrush). *Candida (Monilia) albicans* is a common inhabitant of the oral cavity but may multiply rapidly and cause a pathogenic state when tissue resistance is lowered. Young children in a hospital clinic sometimes develop thrush after local antibiotic therapy, which allows the fungus to proliferate. The lesions of the oral disease appear as raised, furry, white patches, which can be removed easily to produce a bleeding underlying surface. Graham reported the successful treatment of thrush with an antifungal antibiotic, nystatin (Mycostatin). A suspension of 1 ml (100,000 units) may be dropped into the mouth for local action four times a day. The drug is nonirritating and nontoxic and is more effective than the older treatment of applying gentian violet.

Neonatal candidiasis, contracted during passage through the vagina and erupting clinically during the first 2 weeks of life, is a commonplace occurrence. Sonnenschien and Clark believe, however, that candidiasis contracted in utero and clinically manifested at birth is extremely rare.

Acute bacterial infections. The prevalence of acute bacterial infection in the oral cavity is unknown. Blake and Trott reported acute streptococcal gingivitis with painful, vivid red gingivae that bled easily. The papillae had enlarged, and gingival abscesses had developed. Cultures showed a predominance of hemolytic streptococci. Acute infections of this type may be more common than was previously realized. Littner and associates recently reported five cases, all in adults between the ages of 20 and 27. However, the diagnosis is difficult to make without extensive laboratory tests. Broad-spectrum antibiotics are recommended if the infection is thought to be bacterial in origin. Improved oral hygiene is important in treating the infection. The placement of dental restorations to restore adequate function after the reduction of acute symptoms is equally important.

Chronic nonspecific gingivitis

A type of gingivitis commonly seen during the preteenage and teenage period is often referred to as "chronic nonspecific gingivitis." The chronic gingival inflammation may be localized to the anterior region, or it may be more generalized. Although it is rarely painful, it may persist for long periods of time without much improvement (Fig. 14-11).

Glauser and associates have observed an unusual gingivitis in Navajo Indians between the ages of 12 and 18 years, similar to that seen in Fig. 14-12, in which the fiery red gingival lesion is not accompanied by enlarged interdental labial papillae or closely associated with local irritants. The gingivi-

tis showed little improvement after a prophylaxis. The age of the patients involved and the prevalence of the disease in girls suggested a hormonal imbalance as a possible factor. Histologic examination of tissue sections and the use of special stains ruled out a bacterial infection. Inadequate oral hygiene, which allows food impaction and the accumulation of materia alba and bacterial plaque, is undoubtedly the major cause of this chronic type of gingivitis.

The etiology of gingivitis is complex and is considered to be based on a multitude of local and systemic factors. Since dietary inadequacies are often found in the preteenage and teenage groups,

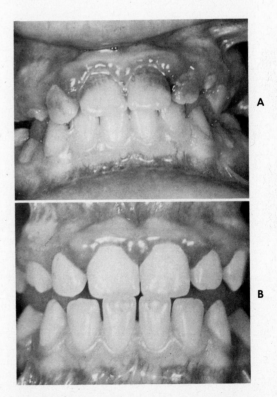

Fig. 14-11. A, Chronic nonspecific gingivitis. The cause of this type of gingivitis is complex, and it often persists for prolonged periods of time without significant improvement. **B,** After 9 months of treatment, hyperplastic gingival tissue is still evident in the anterior maxillary region.

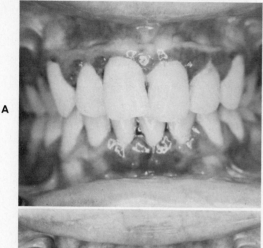

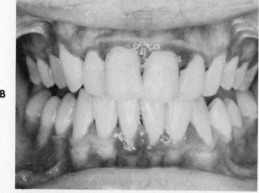

Fig. 14-12. A, Fiery red gingival lesions essentially limited to the anterior labial tissues. Only minimum local deposits were evident. The gingivitis was classified as the chronic nonspecific type. **B,** Limited improvement was evident after 6 months of local treatment. A hormonal imbalance and vitamin deficiency were suspected as contributing etiologic factors.

the 7-day diet survey described in Chapter 7 is an important diagnostic aid. Insufficient quantities of fruits and vegetables in the diet, leading to a subclinical vitamin deficiency, may be an important predisposing factor. An improved dietary intake of vitamins and the use of multiple-vitamin supplements will improve the gingival condition in many children.

McCombie and Stothard, after examining 1500 Vancouver schoolchildren, concluded that there is a positive relationship between poor oral hygiene and gingivitis. They also observed that children with regular dental care had less gingivitis. Ash, Gitlin, and Smith have also observed a high positive correlation between the degree of plaque and the degree of gingivitis.

Malocclusion, which prevents adequate function, and crowded teeth, which make oral hygiene and plaque removal more difficult, are also important predisposing factors in gingivitis. Carious lesions with irritating sharp margins, as well as faulty restorations with overhanging margins (both of which cause food accumulation), also favor the development of the chronic type of gingivitis.

A wide variety of local irritants can produce a hyperplastic type of gingivitis in children and young adults. The irritation to the gingival tissue produced by mouth breathing is often responsible for the development of a chronic hyperplastic form of gingivitis, particularly in the maxillary arch. All these factors should be considered contributory to chronic nonspecific gingivitis and should be corrected in the treatment of the condition.

Conditioned gingival enlargement

Puberty gingivitis. A distinctive type of gingivitis occasionally develops in children in the prepubertal and pubertal period. Cohen, in a study of 270 boys and girls in the 11- to 14-year age group, observed that gingival enlargement in the anterior segment occurred with regularity in the prepubertal and the premenarchial period, as well as in pubescence. The gingival enlargement was marginal in distribution and, in the presence of local irritants, was characterized by prominent bulbous interproximal papillae far greater than gingival enlargements associated with local factors.

Sutcliffe's survey of a group of children between the ages of 11 and 17 years revealed an initial high prevalence of gingivitis that tended to decline with age. In both sexes the prevalence of gingivitis tended to decrease with age. Initially, 89% of 11-year-olds and 92% of 12-year-olds were affected. It should be recalled, however, that with increasing age there is increased evidence of more adequate

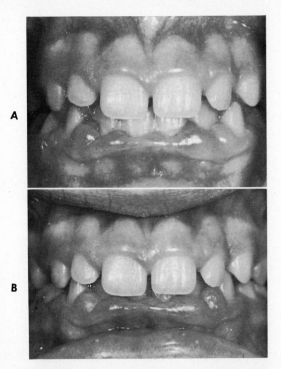

Fig. 14-13. A, Puberty gingivitis. The enlargement of the gingival tissues was limited to the mandibular anterior region. B, Local treatment resulted in only a slight improvement of the condition. A persistence of the hyperplastic enlargement would suggest the need for gingivoplasty.

brushing. Girls tended to reach their maximum gingivitis experience earlier than did boys.

The enlargement of the gingival tissues in puberty gingivitis is confined to the anterior segment and may be present in only one arch. The lingual gingival tissue generally remains unaffected (Fig. 14-13). Treatment of puberty gingivitis should be directed toward improved oral hygiene, removal of all local irritants by thorough root planing, restoration of carious teeth, and dietary recommendations necessary to ensure an adequate nutritional status. Cohen observed a marked improvement in the gingival inflammation and enlargement after the oral administration of 500 mg ascorbic acid. However, the improvement did not occur until the vitamin had been taken for approximately 4 weeks.

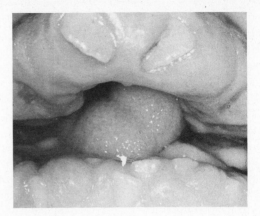

Fig. 14-14. Fibromatosis in a 14-year-old girl. The gingival tissues have enlarged to the extent that they almost cover the crowns of the teeth.

Severe cases of hyperplastic gingivitis that do not respond to local or systemic therapy should be treated by gingivoplasty. Surgical removal of the thickened fibrotic marginal and interproximal tissue has been found effective. Recurrence of any hyperplastic tissue will be minimal if adequate oral hygiene is maintained.

Fibromatosis. Gingival fibromatosis may be idiopathic; however, it generally follows a familial pattern. Jorgenson and Cocker's observations led to the conclusion that gingival fibromatosis may be inherited as a dominant or recessive trait, with the generalized and local forms being manifestations of the same genetic defect. This rare type of gingivitis has been referred to as "elephantiasis gingivae" and also as "hereditary hyperplasia of the gums." The gingival tissues appear normal at birth but begin to enlarge with the eruption of the primary teeth. Although mild cases are observed, the gingival tissues usually continue to enlarge with eruption of the permanent teeth until the tissues essentially cover the clinical crowns of the teeth (Fig. 14-14). The dense fibrous tissue often causes displacement of the teeth and malocclusion. The condition is not painful until the tissue enlarges to the extent that it partially covers the occlusal surface of the molars and becomes traumatized during mastication.

Zackin and Weisberger described fibromatosis histologically as a moderate hyperplasia of the epithelium, with hyperkeratosis and elongation of the rete pegs. The increase in tissue mass is primarily the result of an increase and thickening of the collagenous bundles in the connective tissue stroma. The tissue shows a high degree of differentiation, and a few young fibroblasts are present.

Surgical removal of the hyperplastic tissue has frequently been the treatment of choice. However, hyperplasia can recur within a few months after the surgical procedure and can return to the original condition within a few years. Although the tissue usually appears pale and firm, the surgical procedure is accompanied by excessive hemorrhage. Therefore quadrant surgery rather than removal of all the excess tissue at one time is usually recommended. In adults, recurrence has not been observed after the removal of teeth and the construction of dentures.

Dilantin gingivitis. Many children who receive phenytoin (Dilantin) over a prolonged period of time develop a painless hyperplasia of the gingivae. The exact mechanism of action of the drug has not been established. Baer (1974) refers to several theories of action, such as the creation of a vitamin C deficiency, a reduction in salivary flow, or an allergic mechanism. He believes that the most logical explanation is an exaggerated connective tissue response resulting from an alteration of the adrenocortical function.

The hyperplasia is of the generalized type, affecting the interproximal, labial, and lingual tissues. Inflammation of the tissues precedes the hyperplastic stage, which is followed by fibroblastic proliferation and collagen deposition.

A mild form of gingival enlargement occurs in some, whereas in others the tissue may cover essentially all the crowns of the teeth (Figs. 14-15 and 14-16). The degree of involvement is often related to the amount of local irritants present. Excellent oral hygiene is necessary to keep the condition under control. Antihistaminic drugs have been used in an effort to control the gingival enlargement, but the results have been undramatic.

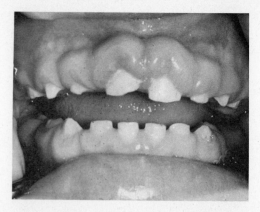

Fig. 14-15. Dilantin gingivitis in a preschool-age child. The enlarged gingival tissue covers two thirds of the maxillary primary lateral incisors and canines.

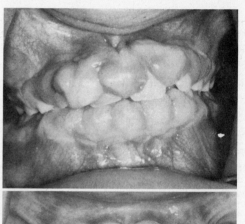

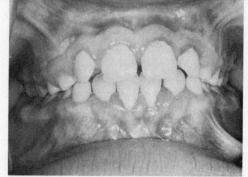

Fig. 14-16. A, Dilantin gingivitis of the severe generalized type. **B,** Surgical removal of the overgrowth of hyperplastic gingival tissue results in temporary improvement of the condition. Excellent oral hygiene is essential in controlling the gingival enlargement.

Strean and Leoni reported the use of an anti-inflammatory corticosteroid, 0.1% dexamethasone 21-phosphate-neomycin sulfate (Neodecadron), to massage the gingivae. This was effective before the gingivae reached the overgrowth stage.

Stambaugh, Morgan, and Enwonwa have observed the occurrence of a marked ascorbic acid deficiency associated with Dilantin hyperplasia. They reported that the daily intake of 1000 mg ascorbic acid resulted in improvement in both appetite and the patient's gingival condition, even without the elimination of local factors.

The use of a plaque-reducing agent, such as vancomycin, has the potential of inhibiting plaque growth and thus reducing gingival inflammation in individuals with Dilantin gingivitis. The drug in ointment form, although not readily available for routine use, has been found by Mitchell and also by Kaslick, Tuckman, and Chasens to be a very effective plaque-preventive drug and ideal for topical application to the teeth and gingival tissues of severely handicapped persons (Fig. 14-17). The ointment can be applied by the patient, who places an amount on the finger and smears it buccally and lingually over each quadrant of the mouth.

The surgical removal of severely overgrown tissue in Dilantin gingivitis and good oral hygiene after surgery are generally considered to be the most effective treatment. However, even these procedures have often been followed by a gradual recurrence of the fibrous tissue.

A preliminary study of a pressure appliance for Dilantin gingival hyperplasia has been reported by Davis, Baer, and Palmer. Immediately after the surgical removal of hyperplastic tissue, an impression was taken and a positive pressure splint was constructed. Periodontal dressings were removed at the end of 1 week and the positive pressure appliance was inserted. Seven of the nine members of the experimental group had no recurrence of gingival hyperplasia, one had a slight recurrence, and one had a moderate recurrence. The natural rubber, mouth-protector type of appliance and the cast chrome–cobalt framework type that is lined with soft plastic were equally effective. The appliance,

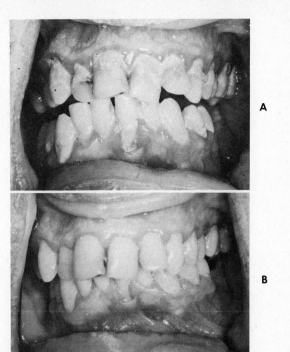

Fig. 14-17. A, Gross accumulation of plaque covers the gingival portion of the teeth with resultant advanced gingivitis. **B,** Vancomycin ointment was applied daily to the teeth and gingival tissues. In 1 week, with no additional therapy, there was a marked improvement in the cleanliness of the teeth and an improvement in gingival health. (Courtesy Dr. S. Miles Standish.)

usually used only at night, may be worn night and day if such a schedule is required. Babcock as well as Sheridan and Reeve have also reported success in controlling the gingival overgrowth with positive pressure appliances.

Steinberg suggested that a series of pressure appliances may help reduce the size of the gingival overgrowth without surgery. He reported one case in which existing systemic conditions contraindicated surgical removal of the gingival tissue. After oral hygiene was improved, pressure appliances were made on stone casts of the patient's upper and lower arches after trimming away 2 mm of the stone in the gingival overgrowth areas. The patient

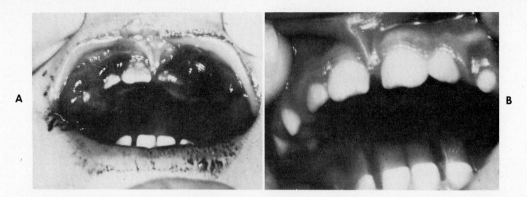

Fig. 14-18. A, Severe scorbutic gingivitis in a 16-month-old child. Large hematomas were evident in the maxillary arch. The condition was initially incorrectly diagnosed as Vincent infection. **B,** Daily administration of 400 mg of ascorbic acid resulted in a dramatic recovery.

wore the appliance about 12 hours each day for 4 weeks; then a new pressure device was made. Steinberg observed a marked decrease in the size of the gingival lesions after 8 weeks of therapy. He suggested that a series of such appliances could succeed in gradually reducing gingival overgrowth to clinically tolerable limits. He also pointed out that this therapeutic approach is not practical for the average patient but that it may prove valuable for patients with contraindications to oral surgery.

Whatever the treatment, excellent oral hygiene should be stressed for children receiving Dilantin therapy.

Scorbutic gingivitis

Gingivitis associated with vitamin C deficiency differs from the type of gingivitis related to poor oral hygiene. The involvement is usually limited to the marginal tissues and papillae. The child with scorbutic gingivitis may complain of severe pain, and spontaneous hemorrhage will be evident. Miller and Roth described scorbutic gingivitis as primarily a capillary disease in which the endothelium swells and degenerates. The vessel walls become weakened and porous, resulting in hemorrhage. The capillaries supplying the gingivae are terminal and anastomose freely. Infarcts are created in the interdental papillae, causing necrosis.

Severe clinical scorbutic gingivitis is rare in children. However, it may occur in children allergic to fruit juices when an adequate dietary supplement of vitamin C is neglected (Fig. 14-18). When blood studies indicate a vitamin C deficiency to the exclusion of other possible systemic conditions, the gingivitis will respond dramatically to the daily administration of 250 to 500 mg of ascorbic acid.

A less severe type of gingivitis resulting from vitamin C deficiency is probably much more common than most dentists realize. Inflammation and enlargement of the marginal gingival tissue and papillae in the absence of local predisposing factors are possible evidence of scorbutic gingivitis (Figs. 14-19 and 14-20). Questioning the child and parents regarding eating habits and using the 7-day diet survey will frequently reveal that the child is receiving inadequate amounts of foods containing vitamin C. Complete dental care, improved oral hygiene, and vitamin C supplement with other water-soluble vitamins will greatly improve the gingival condition.

Periodontal diseases in children

Periodontitis. Periodontitis is an inflammatory disease of the gingiva and deeper tissues of the periodontium. It is characterized by pocket formation and destruction of the supporting alveolar

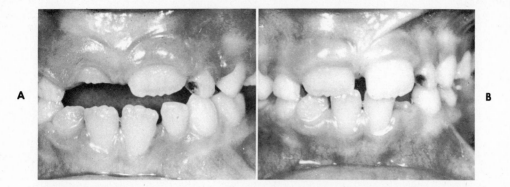

Fig. 14-19. A, Mild gingivitis caused by a vitamin C deficiency. The marginal tissue and papillae were painfully enlarged. A dietary history revealed that the child's diet was grossly deficient in fruits and vegetables. **B,** Improvement in diet and greater emphasis on oral hygiene resulted in a marked improvement in the oral health.

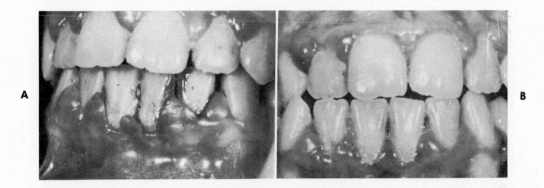

Fig. 14-20. A, Scorbutic gingivitis in a 13-year-old girl. The diet was almost entirely lacking in foods containing vitamin C. **B,** An improved diet, supplemental amounts of fresh fruit juices, and toothbrushing instruction resulted in an improved gingival condition in 2 weeks.

bone. Periodontitis is considered a direct result of gingivitis that has advanced and has been neglected, and it ultimately causes loss of a tooth or teeth. Initially, cuplike resorption and marginal translucency of the alveolar crests are observed in the radiograph. The presence of alveolar resorption in the child or young adult may cause confusion between juvenile periodontitis (periodontosis) and periodontitis. The local environmental factors, type and pattern of the resorption, and mobility and migration of the teeth must be carefully evaluated before making a differential diagnosis. Treatment

of these lesions necessitates curettage and debridement as illustrated in Fig. 14-21. The procedure removes the ulcerated and hypoplastic pocket epithelium and in the case of osseous lesions includes the debridement of the diseased (bony) area. The mechanical procedure also removes the enzymes that originate from the accumulated bacterial flora and those derived from degenerating tissue cells.

Juvenile periodontitis or periodontosis. One of the least understood of the destructive processes affecting the periodontium of children and young adults is juvenile periodontitis or periodontosis.

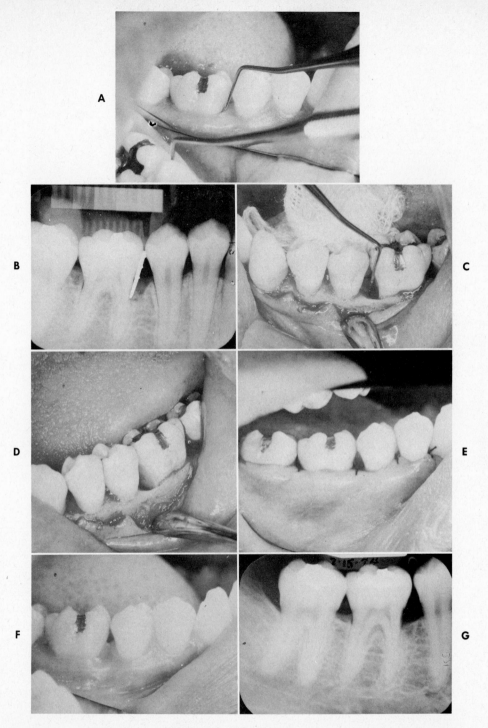

Fig. 14-21. A, Probe in a mesial defect on the mandibular left first molar of a 16-year-old boy (mirror view). **B,** Radiograph showing depth of osseous defect. **C,** Periodontal probe showing depth of osseous defect. **D,** Defect completely debrided. **E,** Area sutured (mirror view). **F,** Area 6 months after surgery (mirror view). **G,** Radiograph 15 months after surgery. (Courtesy Dr. Timothy J. O'Leary.)

The condition is rare in preschool children. At the World Workshop in Periodontics, the committee on periodontal pathology reported that:

Evidence to support the conventional concept of periodontosis is unsubstantiated. It was the consensus of the section that the term periodontosis is ambiguous and that the term should be eliminated from periodontal nomenclature. Nevertheless, the committee is aware that some evidence exists to indicate that a clinical entity different from adult periodontitis may occur in adolescents and young adults.*

---

*From Baer, P.N.: J. Periodontol. **42:**516-520, 1971.

Baer has reported that there is sufficient evidence to warrant considering the condition as an entity different from the disease periodontitis, which normally occurs in the adult patient. He has suggested the following definition:

Periodontosis is a disease of the periodontium occurring in an otherwise healthy adolescent, which is characterized by a rapid loss of alveolar bone about more than one tooth of the permanent dentition. There are two basic forms in which it occurs. In one form of the disease, the only teeth affected are the first molars and incisors. In the other, more generalized form, it may affect most of the dentition. The amount of destruction manifested is

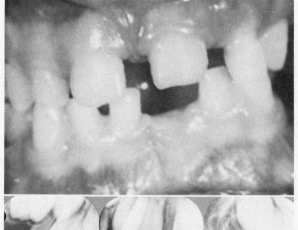

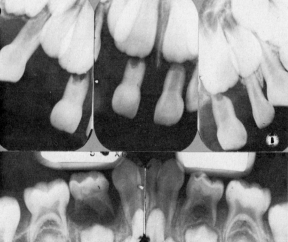

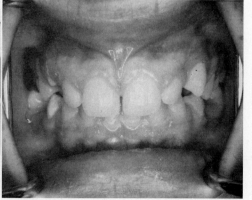

Fig. 14-22. **A,** Juvenile periodontitis in a 4½-year-old girl. Loosening, migration, and spontaneous loss of the primary teeth occurred. **B,** A generalized loss of alveolar bone can be seen in the radiographs. **C,** Eight years after the initial observation of an involvement of the supporting tissues, there is evidence of normal gingival tissues. It is believed that dietary counseling and excellent oral hygiene contributed to the success of the treatment.

Continued.

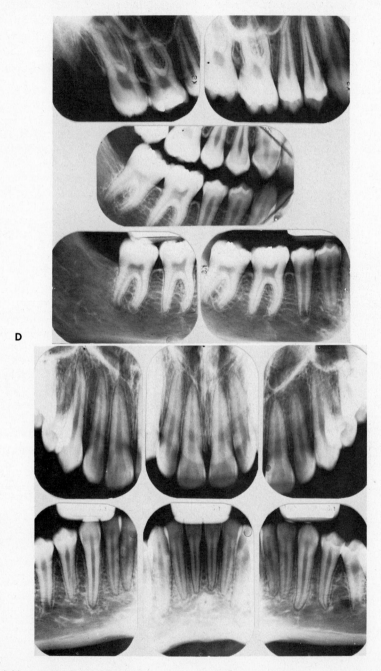

D

Fig. 14-22, cont'd. D, Radiographs made after the eruption of the permanent teeth demonstrate normal alveolar structures.

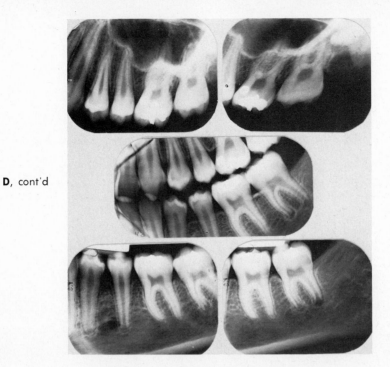

D, cont'd

Fig. 14-22, cont'd. For legend see opposite page.

not commensurate with the amount of local irritants present.*

Although Baer in his definition restricts the disease to alveoloclasia about the permanent teeth, juvenile periodontitis can involve both the primary and the permanent teeth with greater involvement of the anterior teeth, causing their loosening and migration (Figs. 14-22 and 14-23). Melnick, Shields, and Bixler also confirm the finding in the primary dentition of young children. They presented data from two families with histories of decreased serum alkaline phosphatase levels, absence of liver isozyme fractions, decreased overall width of the tubular bone, and decreased medullary space with relatively increased cortical area. In one child there was primary dentition alveoloclasia without involvement of the permanent dentition.

*From Baer, P.N.: J. Periodontol. **42:**516-520, 1971.

They concluded that periodontosis is probably inherited as an X-linked dominant trait, with decreased penetrance but relatively consistent gene expressivity. Sonis has also reported the disease involving primary molars in two siblings.

Since gingival inflammation is not one of the early features, the condition may be detected first in the routine radiographic examination. A symptom of periodontosis in a child is a spontaneous loss of the primary teeth several years before normal exfoliation. Although nutritional deficiencies, debilitating disease, hormonal disturbance, and metabolic imbalances have been suggested as possible etiologic factors, it is rarely possible, even with hospitalization and complete laboratory studies, to determine the cause. Cohen has suggested that failure in attempts to find a systemic influence may be due to the lack of a precise laboratory test, or it may be that the primary etiologic factors were

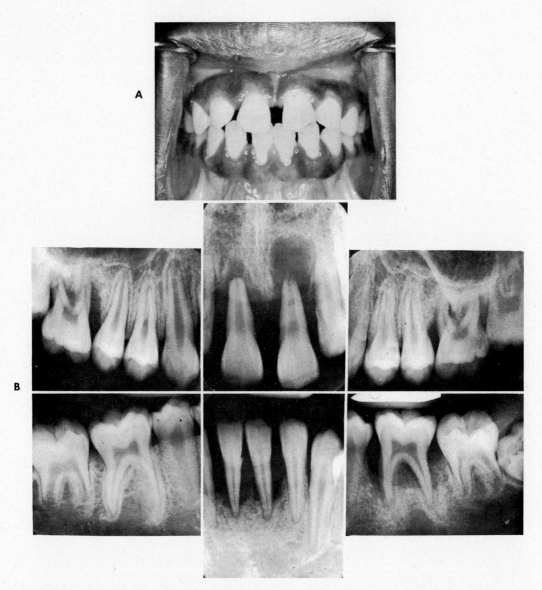

Fig. 14-23. A, Evidence of mild gingivitis in a 12-year-old boy. Clinical examination revealed extensive mobility of the anterior teeth. **B,** Radiographs revealed loss of support in the incisor and first permanent molar areas. The maxillary central incisors, mandibular incisors, and first permanent molars were removed. Partial dentures were constructed.

not present at the time of the metabolic evaluation.

In the permanent dentition a classic pattern of bone destruction has been described as an arc-shaped loss extending from the distal surface of the second premolar to the mesial surface of the second molar. In the posterior regions in this classic pattern, the loss occurs bilaterally and is similar or identical on both sides. Clinically, however, the patterns of bone loss may vary markedly. In rare instances only the molars are affected; however, only one proximal surface of a molar may be affected. Usually the mesial, but occasionally the distal, aspect may show involvement. The amount and distribution of bone loss depend on whether the patient has the localized or generalized form of the disease and whether the disease is diagnosed at an early or a late stage.

Local factors, including calculus deposits and traumatic occlusion, although often related to the condition in adults, are rarely evident as important predisposing factors in children. Hawes reported three patients with juvenile periodontosis and early loss of teeth in whom skin disease was present. However, he could find no typical association of systemic factors in children with periodontosis.

The treatment of juvenile periodontitis has been for the most part unsuccessful. The removal of deciduous teeth that have lost their bony support has been recommended in an attempt to rid the mouth of infection and delay the involvement of the permanent teeth. In the permanent dentition the elimination of pockets, improved oral hygiene, and dietary counseling are the treatment of choice.

An 8-year follow-up of the successful treatment of the patient seen in Fig. 14-22 would support the conclusion that the factors that contributed initially to the destructive changes in the supporting tissues of the primary teeth are no longer present.

Papillon-Lefèvre syndrome (precocious periodontosis). Coccia, McDonald, and Mitchell have observed Papillon-Lefèvre syndrome in a 2½-year-old child. The syndrome is rare and the cause unknown. However, the affected children displaying a familial disposition to the disorder demonstrate an autosomal recessive mode of inheritance.

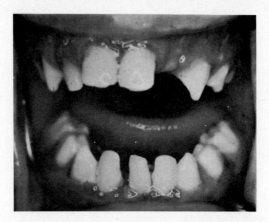

Fig. 14-24. Intraoral condition of a 2½-year-old child who had Papillon-Lefèvre syndrome. There were inflammatory gingival engorgement and accumulated accretions, especially in the mandibular incisor area.

The observations made of the young child in Fig. 14-24 are typical of those reported by Gorlin, Sedans, and Anderson. The primary teeth erupted at the normal time. However, as early as 2 years of age the child rubbed the gingival tissues and acted as if they were painful. There was a tendency toward gingival bleeding when the teeth were brushed. Hyperkeratosis of the palms and soles was present (Fig. 14-25); the first evidence was erythema and scaliness noted initially at 8 months of age. Repeated laboratory tests, including complete blood count, urinalysis, and microserum calcium and phosphorus determinations, were essentially normal.

At 2½ years of age there was a looseness of all the primary teeth, and full-mouth radiographs revealed severe horizontal bone resorption (Fig. 14-26). Because of gingival inflammation, patient discomfort, and infected periodontal pockets, all the primary teeth were removed by age 3 years. Histologic sections of the teeth displayed a premature resorption pattern with essentially normal pulp tissue. Cementum was apparently normal and covered the root structure. An accumulation of adherent basophilic plaque, made up of a mass of filamentous microorganisms, was noted on almost the entire length of the root surface.

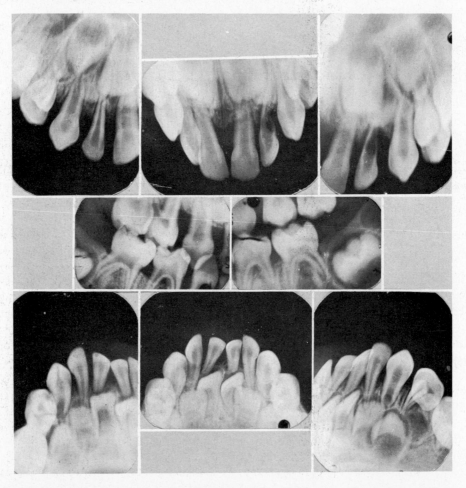

Fig. 14-25. A, Hyperkeratosis of the palmar surfaces of the hands *(arrow).* Erythema and scaliness were noted initially at 8 months of age. **B,** Hyperkeratosis of the plantar surfaces of the feet *(arrow).*

Fig. 14-26. Full-mouth and bite-wing radiographs of the child with Papillon-Lefèvre syndrome. Severe horizontal bone resorption is readily detected in all four quadrants. The incisor areas display extreme alveolar bone loss to the extent that only the apical third of the root remains supported.

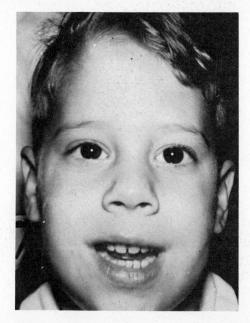

Fig. 14-27. Three-year-old child with complete dentures.

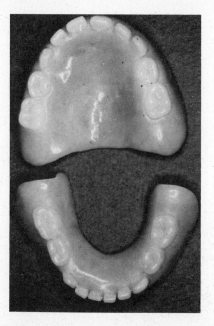

Fig. 14-28. Constructed complete dentures, which were later modified to allow the eruption of the mandibular incisors and the first permanent molars.

Complete dentures were constructed 3 months after the removal of the primary teeth. The child tolerated the dentures well, both functionally and psychologically (Figs. 14-27 and 14-28). The first permanent molars and the mandibular central incisors erupted at the expected time, and the denture base was adjusted to allow for the emergence of the teeth.

Although previous reports have indicated that the permanent dentition will also be affected, the child whose history is reported here has been followed into young adulthood, and the dentition, including the supporting tissues, appears normal (Fig. 14-29). The patient has successfully undergone orthodontic treatment.

Recent reports of the effectiveness of tetracycline therapy as an adjunct to meticulous subgingival debridement in the management of periodontal disease prompted McDonald to reinvestigate the history in the reported Papillon-Lefèvre case. The father, a physician, reported that tetracylines were given repeatedly for ear infections between the ages of 3 and 6 years. This regimen may have been responsible for eliminating pathogens and preventing the destructive process from being carried into the permanent dentition.

Abnormal mandibular labial frenum

A mandibular anterior frenum occasionally inserts into the free or marginal gingival tissue and causes subsequent recession and pocket formation. The abnormal frenum attachment is most often observed in the central incisor area (Fig. 14-30), although it may involve the labial tissue in the canine areas. The abnormal attachment is frequently associated with a vestibular trough throughout the anterior region that is more shallow than normal.

Movements of the lip cause the abnormal frenum to pull on the fibers inserting into the free marginal

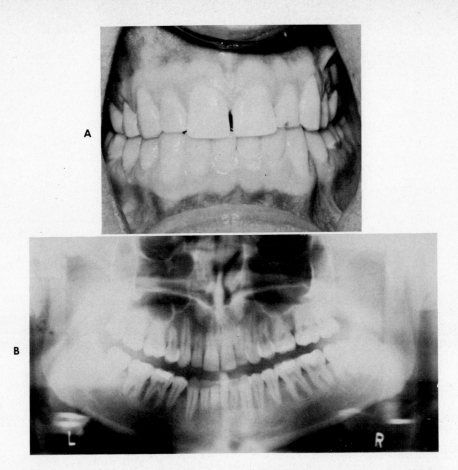

Fig. 14-29. Photographs 15 years after initial diagnosis of Papillon-Lefèvre syndrome at age 2½. **A,** Functional occlusion is noted following 18 months of orthodontic treatment. The clinical examination revealed good oral hygiene and normal gingival tissues. **B,** Panoramic radiographic survey revealed normal alveolar bone. Some apical root resorption related to orthodontic treatment can be seen in the mandibular incisors.

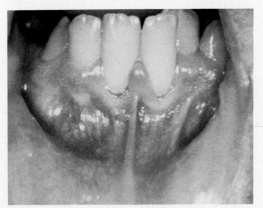

Fig. 14-30. Abnormal attachment of the frenum. The fibers can be seen extending to the papilla between the central incisors with branching auxiliary fibers inserting in the marginal tissue.

tissue. Food accumulates and causes inflammation and eventually the development of a pocket between the labial surface of the tooth and the vestibular mucosa. Early treatment of the abnormal frenum attachment is indicated to prevent continued stripping of the labial tissue, subsequent loss of alveolar bone, and possible eventual loss of the tooth. Although traumatic occlusion and poor oral hygiene are occasionally associated with the gingival stripping condition, the abnormal frenum attachment is more often the offender.

Techniques for mandibular frenectomy and increasing vestibular depth. Bohannan has published a series of reports of his studies in the alteration of vestibular depth and frenectomy. Three different surgical procedures, which he refers to as *complete denudation, periosteum retention,* and *vestibular incision,* have been studied as methods to produce increased vestibular depth and frenum alteration.

The complete denudation procedure is preceded by a routine gingivectomy extending laterally to the first premolars. By blunt dissection, the periosteum and adherent fibrous tissue are detached apically, and the labial plate is exposed to a depth of approximately 12 mm. The resulting soft tissue flap is removed by excision. A rapid-setting zinc oxide–eugenol dressing is placed directly over the osseous tissue and is changed at 7-day intervals for 4 weeks.

The periosteum retention procedure, as carried out by Bohannan, does not always result in maintenance of the desirable amount of vestibular depth. The procedure is essentially the same as that previously described, except that the periosteum is allowed to remain.

The vestibular incision method (mandibular frenectomy) is a surgical procedure that we have used with success. The elimination of the abnormal frenum should remain the objective of the procedure, although it is often desirable also to alter the vestibular depth. However, the frenum is the primary etiologic factor in the stripping of the gingival tissue and labial pocket formation.

A preliminary prophylaxis should be performed to remove hard deposits, debris, and plaque material from the teeth. The surgical procedure should be more extensive than a conservative incision of the frenum. Such a procedure would allow the muscle fibers to reattach, with resultant scar tissue formation, and would perhaps make the condition more severe (Fig. 14-31).

A local anesthetic is given before the surgical procedure. A right and left inferior alveolar injection is the one of choice. Some dentists prefer to inject the local anesthetic solution throughout the operative field. However, caution should be exercised because the anesthetic may distend the tissue, making it more difficult to find landmarks during the surgical procedure.

The lower lip should be stretched outward and downward, and an incision approximately 1 cm in depth beyond the level of the vestibular trough should be made at a right angle to the underlying bone. The incision is made at the junction of the mucobuccal attached gingiva and should extend at least two teeth on either side of the attachment. If the abnormal attachment is in the incisor area, an incision is often made from an area opposite one canine to the canine on the other side of the mouth. The connective tissue and muscle attachments are then freed by blunt dissection with a periosteal elevator. No attempt is made to strip the underlying periosteum.

A periodontal pack or some type of splint must be used to prevent reattachment of the tissue and to allow granulation to occur at a greater depth. A piece of rubber tubing 2 to 3 mm in diameter and the exact length of the incision can be coated with surgical paste and sutured in the trough. The patient is seen 24 hours postoperatively, and any granulation tissue that has developed over the ends of the tubing is removed. The pack is normally removed after 4 to 5 days, and the wound is irrigated as necessary until healing takes place.

As an alternate method of encouraging healing at a new depth, the entire surgical wound is filled with a stiff periodontal dressing of the zinc oxide–eugenol type. The pack, which extends over the labial surface of the anterior teeth, may be covered

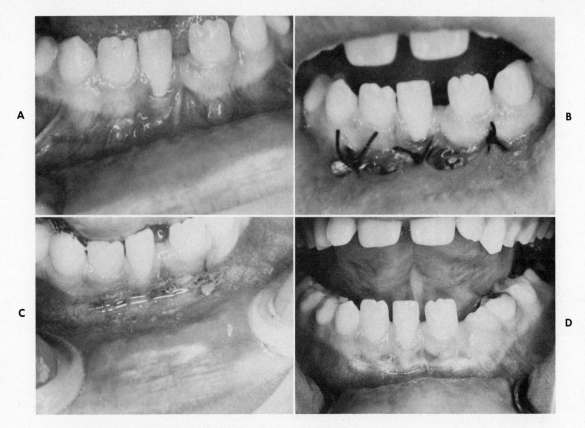

Fig. 14-31. A, Tissue has been stripped and a pocket formed on the labial surface of the right central incisor. Frenectomy and increasing the depth of the vestibular trough are indicated. **B,** An incision has been made and a pack has been placed and secured with three sutures. **C,** Five days after the operation the pack was removed. Granulation tissue has formed and normal healing is taking place. **D,** Three months after the operation, improvement in the health of the gingival tissue in the mandibular anterior region is evident.

with dry foil and allowed to remain for 3 to 4 weeks with only weekly changes (Fig. 14-32). Some dentists ligate an acrylic splint to the teeth after surgery to aid in the reestablishment of the new depth of the sulcus.

Free gingival autograft procedure. The free gingival autograft procedure may be considered for children and young adults when there is a prominent tooth position that is complicated by absence of attached gingiva, a shallow vestibular fornix, and a high midline frenum attachment (Fig. 14-33).

As advocated by O'Leary, in the free gingival graft procedure the receptor site is first prepared. When a high frenum attachment has contributed to the mucogingival problem, tension is placed on the lower lip to activate the frenum and trace its insertion into the marginal tissue. With the use of a Bard-Parker No. 15 scalpel blade, a horizontal incision is made at the mucogingival junction including the attachment of the frenum into the gingiva. The mucosa is displaced apically by blunt dissection, leaving a nonmovable receptor site consisting of periosteum and a thin covering of firm

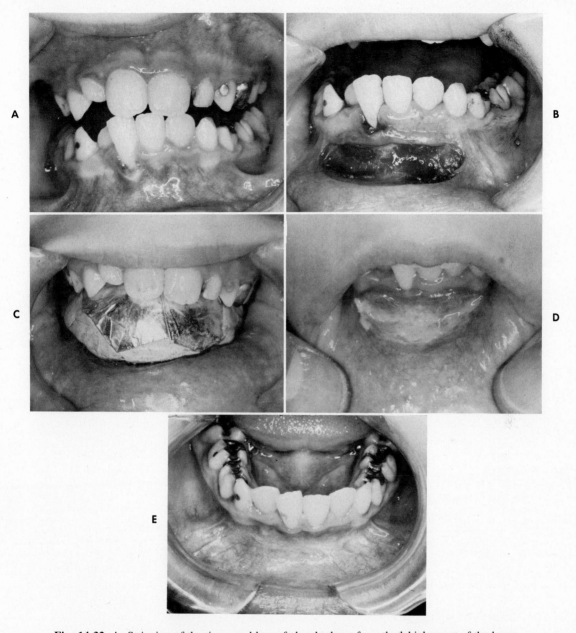

Fig. 14-32. A, Stripping of the tissue and loss of alveolar bone from the labial aspect of the lower right central incisor are related to an abnormal frenum attachment and shallow vestibule. **B,** An incision has been made and the connective tissue and muscle attachments have been freed by blunt dissection. **C,** A periodontal pack has been placed and covered with dry foil. **D,** One week after the operation there is evidence of granulation tissue. **E,** An improvement is evident in the gingival contour of the tissue surrounding the right central incisor.

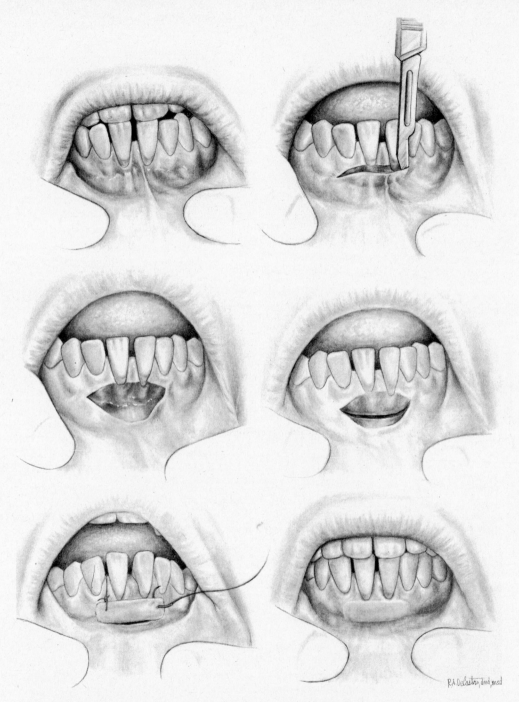

Fig. 14-33. The free gingival graft procedure may be considered for children and adults when there is a shallow vestibular fornix and a high midline frenum attachment.

connective tissue. Any gingival epithelium coronal to the primary incision is trimmed away, leaving a receptor bed of connective tissue with an adequate blood supply.

The next step is to fenestrate the periosteum to help prevent mobility of the graft after healing. To do this, two horizontal incisions, 1 mm apart, are made through the periosteum at the apical boundary of the displaced mucosa. The isolated periosteum between the two horizontal incisions is peeled away, exposing the facial cortical plate of bone. A template of adhesive foil slightly larger than the mandibular receptor site is made, and the palatal donor site is anesthetized. The template is placed on the anesthetized tissue and is outlined with a shallow incision using a Bard-Parker No. 15 scalpel blade or an Orban gingivectomy knife. The graft is freed from the underlying submucosa by sharp dissection. The operator should strive to secure an intermediate thickness graft (approximately 1 mm thick).

After the graft is removed from the palate, the connective tissue side is inspected to make sure that no fatty tissue remains on it (adherent fatty tissue would prevent revascularization of the graft from the connective tissue of the receptor site). If present, the fatty tissue is cut away with small surgical scissors or a Bard-Parker No. 15 scalpel blade. The graft is carried to the receptor site, and any final trimming is done to secure a close approximation of the donor tissue to the receptor site. The graft is sutured into position using 5-0 Dacron suture and an atraumatic needle. Normally a suture at the coronal aspect of each end of the graft is enough to secure it. The graft is covered with adhesive foil, which in turn is covered with a hard-setting periodontal dressing. When the patient returns 7 to 10 days after surgery, the dressing is removed, the area is debrided and irrigated, and the sutures are removed. A second dressing is usually placed for another 5 to 7 days.

When the second dressing is removed, the area is again debrided, and the teeth are polished. At this time the graft should be firmly fixed to the underlying receptor site, and the epithelial covering should be continuous with that of the contiguous gingiva and oral mucosa. The patient is instructed to gently clean away any debris from the area with a cotton ball soaked in warm water and to continue the interdental flossing routine. Normal brushing can usually be reintroduced between the twenty-first and twenty-fifth days.

Clinical assessment of oral cleanliness, gingivitis, and periodontal disease

Plaque control record. O'Leary, Drake, and Naylor developed the plaque control record to give the dentist, hygienist, and dental educator a simple method of recording the presence of plaque on individual tooth surfaces (mesial, distal, facial, and lingual).

At the initial appointment a suitable disclosing solution, such as Bismarck brown, is painted on all exposed tooth surfaces. After the patient has rinsed, the operator, using an explorer, examines each stained surface for soft accumulations at the dentogingival junction. When found, these accumulations are recorded by making a dash in the appropriate spaces on the record form. Fig. 14-34, *A,* shows a form completed at the patient's first appointment for learning plaque control. No attempt is made to differentiate between varying amounts of plaque on tooth surfaces.

After all teeth are examined and scored, an index can be derived by dividing the number of plaque-containing surfaces by the total number of available surfaces. The same procedure is carried out at subsequent appointments to determine the patient's progress in learning and carrying out the prescribed oral hygiene procedures. Fig. 14-34, *B,* shows a patient's progress from the initial assessment to the point (fifth session) at which plaque control is deemed satisfactory.

A detailed approach to teaching toothbrushing, flossing, and plaque control is described in Chapter 15.

Simplified Oral Hygiene Index. Greene and Vermillion have described a method of scoring tooth surfaces in determining the Simplified Oral Hygiene Index (OHI-S). The six surfaces exam-

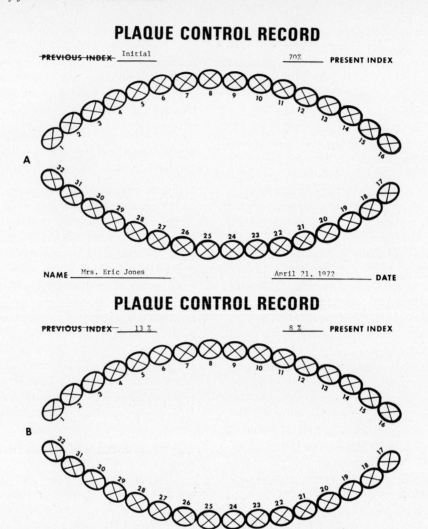

Fig. 14-34. A, Plaque accumulations recorded at the initial control appointment. B, Plaque accumulations recorded at the fifth session.

ined for the OHI-S are selected from four posterior and two anterior teeth. In the posterior portion of the dentition, the first fully erupted tooth distal to the second premolar, usually the first molar but sometimes the second molar, is examined on each side of the arch. The buccal surfaces of the selected maxillary molars and the lingual surfaces of the selected mandibular molars are inspected.

In the anterior portion of the mouth, the labial surface of the maxillary right central incisor and the labial surface of the mandibular left central incisor are scored. To obtain the scores for debris and calculus, each of the six preselected tooth surfaces is examined first for debris, then for calculus. The following criteria are applied to determine the scores for each surface examined (Fig. 14-35):

DEBRIS SCORING CALCULUS SCORING

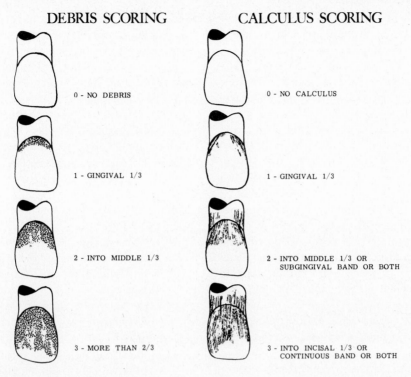

DEBRIS SCORING

0 - NO DEBRIS

1 - GINGIVAL 1/3

2 - INTO MIDDLE 1/3

3 - MORE THAN 2/3

CALCULUS SCORING

0 - NO CALCULUS

1 - GINGIVAL 1/3

2 - INTO MIDDLE 1/3 OR
    SUBGINGIVAL BAND OR BOTH

3 - INTO INCISAL 1/3 OR
    CONTINUOUS BAND OR BOTH

Fig. 14-35. A method of recording the debris and calculus in scoring tooth surfaces for determining the Simplified Oral Hygiene Index.

0—No debris or stain present

1—Soft debris covering not more than one third of the tooth surface or the presence of extrinsic stains without debris regardless of the surface area covered

2—Soft debris covering more than one third but not more than two thirds of the exposed tooth surface

3—Soft debris covering more than two thirds of the exposed tooth surface

The surface area covered by debris is estimated by running the side of a No. 5 explorer over the tooth surface being examined and noting the extent of the debris.

The amount of supragingival calculus is determined in a similar manner and scores are assigned according to the following criteria:

0—No calculus present

1—Supragingival calculus covering not more than one third of the exposed tooth surface being examined

2—Supragingival calculus covering more than one third but not more than two thirds of the exposed tooth surface, or the presence of individual flecks of subgingival calculus

3—Supragingival calculus covering more than two thirds of the exposed tooth surface or a continuous heavy band of subgingival calculus around the cervical portion of the tooth

After the scores for the debris and calculus are recorded, the index values are calculated. For each individual the debris scores are totaled and divided by the number of surfaces scored. A score for a group of individuals is obtained by computing the average of the individual scores. The average individual or group score is known as the Simplified Debris Index (DI-S).

The same methods are used to obtain the calculus scores or the Simplified Calculus Index (CI-S). The average individual or group debris and calculus scores are combined to obtain the OHI-S.

PMA Index. Massler and Schour have developed the PMA Index, based on the extension of the inflammation to surrounding tissues as an objective method of assessing gingivitis. The gingival tissues surrounding the buccal aspect or the labial aspect are divided into three anatomically well-defined units: the papillae (P), the marginal gingivae (M), and the attached gingivae (A) (Fig. 14-36). Each gingival unit is examined and recorded as affected when there is clinical evidence of inflammatory changes. The involved papillae, margins, and attached gingival units are totaled to provide the PMA Index for each child. When the gingival status of groups of children is compared, the units are totaled and divided by the number of children in each observation group.

Massler and Schour have also suggested that since gingivitis in children occurs most often in the anterior segments of both arches, the sum of those involved gingival units surrounding the six anterior teeth will provide a reliable index of the extent of gingivitis. The index may be further modified to include observation of only the anterior labial surfaces.

Moore has used the PMA Index to determine the severity of gingivitis in 1123 children. His study indicated that the socioeconomic status of the family and the severity of gingivitis are inversely proportional. Further investigation showed that accumulation of oral debris and toothbrushing habits are affected by socioeconomic status. Less accumulated oral debris and better toothbrushing habits were found at the high socioeconomic level.

Russell Periodontal Index. A system of classification and scoring for prevalence of periodontal disease has been developed by Russell. The condition of the investing tissues is estimated individually for each tooth in the mouth.

The following criteria are applied in determining the Russell Periodontal Index (Fig. 14-37):

0—*Negative.* There is no evidence of inflammation of the investing tissues or loss of function resulting from destruction of supporting tissues.

1—*Mild gingivitis.* There is inflammation of the free gingiva, but it does not circumscribe the tooth.

2—*Gingivitis.* Inflammation completely circumscribes the tooth, but there is no apparent break in the epithelial attachment.

6—*Gingivitis with pocket formation.* The epithelial attachment has been broken, and there is a definite periodontal pocket. The tooth is firm in its socket and has not drifted.

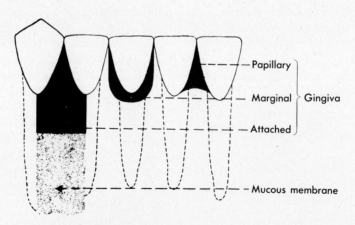

Fig. 14-36. Anatomic units referred to in the PMA Index.

8—*Advanced destruction with loss of masticatory function.* The tooth may be loose, may have drifted, or may even be depressible in its socket.

The score for the patient is the average of scores for all the teeth in the mouth.

The greatest difficulty in using this method is distinguishing between normal gingivae and gingivae with mild inflammation.

Stains and deposits on teeth

Previous work regarding the staining of teeth of children has been related primarily to studies of orange and green stain of the extrinsic type. It has been generally accepted that the stain has a microbial origin, although some reports have suggested that oral iron preparations or tonics may be responsible for an additional type of extrinsic staining.

Staining is generally believed to be caused by extrinsic agents, which can be readily removed from the surface of the teeth with an abrasive material. The agents that are responsible for staining are deposited in enamel defects or become attached to the enamel without bringing about a change in its surface.

Pigmentation, in contrast to extrinsic staining, is associated with an active chemical change in the tooth structure, and the resultant pigment cannot be removed without altering the tooth structure.

Green stain. The cause of green stain, which is most often seen on the teeth of young individuals, is unknown, although it is thought to be the result of the action of chromogenic bacteria on the enamel cuticle. The color of the stain varies from dark green to light yellowish green. The deposit is seen most often in the gingival third of the labial surface of the maxillary anterior teeth. The stain collects more readily on the labial surface of the maxillary anterior teeth in mouth breathers. It tends to recur even after careful and complete removal. The enamel beneath the stain may be roughened or may have undergone initial demineralization. The roughened surface is thought to be related to the frequency of recurrence of the stain (Fig. 14-38).

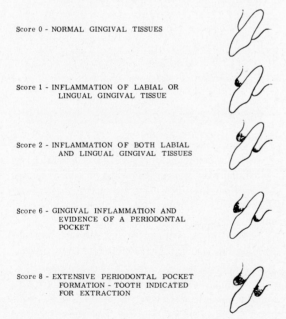

Score 0 - NORMAL GINGIVAL TISSUES

Score 1 - INFLAMMATION OF LABIAL OR LINGUAL GINGIVAL TISSUE

Score 2 - INFLAMMATION OF BOTH LABIAL AND LINGUAL GINGIVAL TISSUES

Score 6 - GINGIVAL INFLAMMATION AND EVIDENCE OF A PERIODONTAL POCKET

Score 8 - EXTENSIVE PERIODONTAL POCKET FORMATION - TOOTH INDICATED FOR EXTRACTION

Fig. 14-37. Scoring and determining the Russell Periodontal Index.

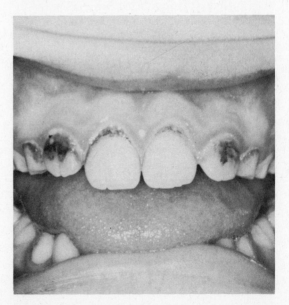

Fig. 14-38. Dark green stain is evident on maxillary anterior teeth. Papillary and marginal gingivitis is also present. The patient had poor oral hygiene and was a mouth breather.

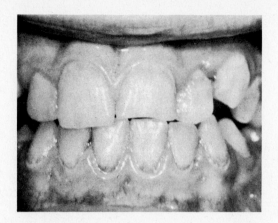

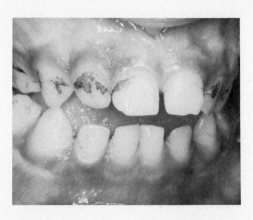

Fig. 14-39. Orange stain is evident in the gingival third of the mandibular anterior teeth. An unusual feature is the presence of a light green stain on the maxillary anterior teeth.

Fig. 14-40. Black stain is evident on the primary teeth. The stain is difficult to remove, particularly when it collects in roughened areas of the tooth.

Orange stain. The cause of orange stain is likewise unknown. Orange stain occurs less frequently and is more easily removed than green stain. The stain is most often seen in the gingival third of the tooth and is associated with poor oral hygiene (Fig. 14-39).

Black stain. A black stain occasionally develops on the primary or permanent teeth of children, but it is much less common than the orange or green type (Fig. 14-40). The stain may be seen as a line following the gingival contour, or it may be apparent in a more generalized pattern on the clinical crown, particularly if there are roughened or pitted areas. The black type of stain is difficult to remove, especially if it collects in pitted areas. Many children who have black stain are relatively free from dental caries.

Removal of stains. The extrinsic type of stains can be removed by polishing with a rubber cup and flour pumice. If the stain is resistant and difficult to remove, the excess water should be blotted from the pumice and the teeth should be dried before the polishing procedure. Since stains are most often seen in a mouth in which there is poor oral hygiene, improving the oral hygiene will minimize the recurrence of the stain.

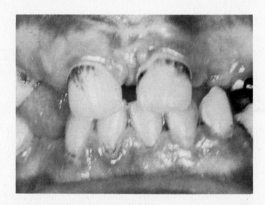

Fig. 14-41. Pigmentation of carious and precarious enamel. The color ranges from light brown to black, the darker pigmentation being evident in the area of greatest caries involvement. The pigmentation is evidence of caries arrest.

Pigmentation caused by stannous flouride application. During the first clinical trials involving the topical application of an 8% stannous fluoride solution, certain areas of the tooth became discolored. A characteristic pigmentation of both carious and precarious lesions has been found to be associated with exposure to stannous fluoride (Fig. 14-41).

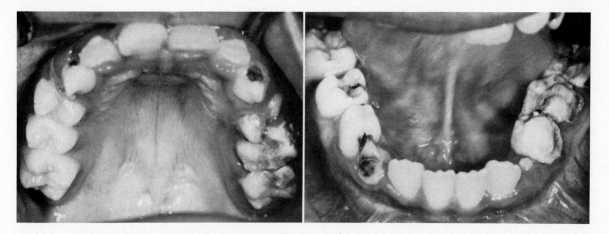

Fig. 14-42. Gross accumulations of calculus are seen on the clinical crowns of the posterior teeth on the left side of the mouth. The fact that the child chewed mostly on his right side accounts partially for the greater cleanliness on that side.

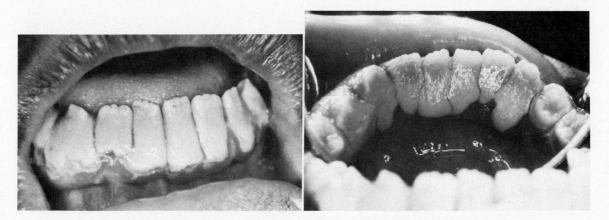

Fig. 14-43. Young adult with calculus covering the labial and lingual surfaces of the mandibular anterior teeth. After the calculus was removed, amelogenesis imperfecta was apparent. The rough surface of the crown favorably influenced the deposition of calculus.

Hyde studied a group of 105 children between the ages of 9 and 19 years who had had one application of 8% stannous fluoride each 6 months for 3 years and, in addition, had used a stannous fluoride dentifrice. The amount of pigmentation was observed to be greater in the patients with a high caries incidence as measured by the DMFT and DMFS indexes. The only portion of the enamel that became pigmented was that previously affected by the caries process. Black pigmentation in particular was seen in patients with a lower than average oral hygiene rating. The surfaces most commonly affected by pigmentation were the occlusal surfaces of molars and premolars. The labial surfaces of the anterior teeth were next most frequently pigmented.

Calculus

Calculus is not often seen in preschool children, and even in children of grade school age it occurs with much less frequency than in adult patients. A low caries incidence is related to high calculus incidence.

MacNeill observed that 53% of 226 children in an institutional environment had calculus. He related the high incidence of calculus formation to the high-protein diet.

Mentally retarded children often have accumulations of calculus on their teeth. This accumulation may be related to abnormal muscular function, a soft diet, poor oral hygiene, and stagnation of saliva.

Turesky, Renstrup, and Glickman's observations regarding early calculus formation in children and adults substantiate those of others, indicating that calculus begins as a soft, adherent, bacteria-laden plaque that undergoes progressive calcification. They observed calculus formation on cellulose acetate strips that were fixed in children's mouths. Plaque material that accumulated on the strips underwent progressive hardening. A soft plaque material consisted for the most part of bacteria appearing as a dense meshwork of diffusely distributed gram-negative cocci with occasional rod forms. Filamentous or thread-shaped organisms were scarce. Leukocytes and epithelial cells were also scattered within the amorphous matrix.

Gross accumulations of calculus are occasionally seen in teenage and preteenage children (Figs. 14-42 and 14-43). Traiger reported a 14-year-old girl who had excessive deposits of supragingival and subgingival calculus. The calculus covered the labial surfaces of the anterior teeth, extended into the mucobuccal fold, and covered the attached gingiva.

Supragingival deposits of calculus occur most frequently and in greater quantity on the buccal surfaces of the maxillary molars and the lingual surfaces of the mandibular anterior teeth. These areas are near the openings of the major salivary glands. The local factors are unquestionably important in the initiation of calculus formation.

REFERENCES

Antoon, J.W., and Miller, R.L.: Apththous ulcers—a review of the literature on etiology, pathogenesis, diagnosis, and treatment, J.A.D.A. **101**:803-808, 1980.

Ash, M.M., Jr., Gitlin, B.N., and Smith, W.A.: Correlation between plaque and gingivitis, J. Periodontol. **35**:428, 1964.

Babcock, J.R.: The successful use of a new technique for Dilantin gingival hyperplasia, Periodontics **3**:196-200, 1965.

Baer, P.N.: The case for periodontosis as a clinical entity, J. Periodontol. **42**:516-520, 1971.

Baer, P.N.: Periodontal disease, Philadelphia, 1974, J.B. Lippincott Co., p. 233.

Blake, G.C., and Trott, J.R.: Acute streptococcal gingivitis, Dent. Pract. **10**:43-45, 1959.

Bohannan, H.M.: Studies in the alteration of vestibular depth. I. Complete denudation, J. Periodontol. **33**:120-128, 1962.

Bohannan, H.M.: Studies in the alteration of vestibular depth. II. Periosteum retention, J. Periodontol. **33**:354-359, 1962.

Bohannan, H.M.: Studies in the alteration of vestibular depth. III. Vestibular incision, J. Periodontol. **34**:209-215, 1963.

Brooks, S.L., and others: Prevalence of herpes simplex virus disease in a professional population, J.A.D.A. **102**:31-34, 1981.

Carter, W.J., and Wells, J.E.: Epidemiology of gingival disease in Kansas City, Missouri school children, Midwest. Dent. **36**:21-24, 1960.

Coccia, C.T., McDonald, R.E., and Mitchell, D.F.: Papillon-Lefevre syndrome: precocious periodontosis with palmar-plantar hyperkeratosis, J. Periodontol. **37**:408-414, 1966.

Cohen, L.: Etiology, pathogenesis and classification of aphthous stomatitis and Behcet's syndrome, J. Oral Pathol. **7**:347-352, 1978.

Cohen, M.M.: The effect of large doses of ascorbic acid on gingival tissue at puberty, J. Dent. Res. (abs.) **34**:750-751, 1955.

Cohen, M.M.: The gingiva at puberty, J. Dent. Res. (abs.) **34**:679, 1955.

Cohen, W.D., and Goldman, H.M.: Periodontal disease in children, P.D.M., July 1962.

Collins, F.J., and Hood, H.M.: Topical antibiotic treatment of acute necrotizing ulcerative gingivitis, J. Dent. Med. **22**:59-64, 1967.

Davis, R.K., Baer, P.N., and Palmer, J.H.: A preliminary report on a new therapy for Dilantin gingival hyperplasia, J. Periodontol. **34**:17-22, 1963.

Duncan, O.D.: A socioeconomic index for all occupations. In Reiss, A.J., Jr.: Occupational and social status, New York, 1961, The Free Press.

Eastcott, A.D., and Stallard, R.E.: Sequential changes in developing human dental plaque as visualized by scanning electron microscope, J. Periodontol. **44**:218-224, 1973.

Glauser, R.O., and others: An unusual gingivitis among Navajo Indians, Periodontics **1**:255-259, 1963.

Goldman, H.M., and Cohen, D.W.: Periodontal therapy, ed. 6, St. Louis, 1979, The C.V. Mosby Co.

Gorlin, R.J., Sedans, H., and Anderson, V.E.: The syndrome of palmar-plantar hyperkeratosis and premature periodontal destruction of the teeth, J. Pediatr. **65:**895-908, 1964.

Graham, R.: Oral thrush in infancy treated with nystatin, Lancet **2:**600-601, 1959.

Graykowski, S.A., Barile, M.F., and Stanley, H.R.: Periadenitis aphthae: clinical and histopathologic aspects of lesions in a patient and of lesions produced in rabbit skin, J.A.D.A. **69:**118-126, 1964.

Greene, J.C., and Vermillion, J.R.: The simplified oral hygiene index, J.A.D.A. **68:**7-13, 1964.

Griffith, R.S., Norins, A.L., and Kagan, C.: A multicentered study of lysine therapy in herpes simplex infection, Dermatologica **156:**257-267, 1978.

Hale, B.D., and others: Epidemic herpetic stomatitis in orphanage children, Dent. Abs. **8:**556, 1963.

Hawes, R.R.: Report of three patients experiencing juvenile periodontosis and early loss of teeth, J. Dent. Child. **27:**169-177, 1960.

Hooks, J.J.: Possibility of a viral etiology in recurrent aphthous ulcers and Behcet's syndrome, J. Oral Pathol. **7:**353-364, 1978.

Horowitz, A.M., and others: Effects of supervised daily dental plaque removal by children after 3 years, Community Dent. Oral Epidemiol. **8:**171-176, 1980.

Hyde, E.J.: A study of pigmentation in incipient and advanced carious lesions of teeth exposed to stannous fluoride: its association with caries incidence and oral hygiene, thesis, Indianapolis, 1960, Indiana University School of Dentistry.

Jorgenson, R.J., and Cocker, M.E.: Variation in the inheritance and expression of gingival fibromatosis, J. Periodontol. **45:**472-477, 1974.

Kaslick, R.S., Tuckman, M.A., and Chasens, A.I.: Effect of topical vancomycin on plaque and chronic gingival inflammation, J. Periodontol. **44:**366-368, 1973.

Littner, M.M., and others: Acute streptococcal gingivostomatitis, Oral Surg. **53:**144-147, 1982.

MacNeill, S.: Dental calculus disposition and the institutional environment, Dent. Abs. **2:**123, 1957.

Massler, M., and Schour, I.: The P-M-A index of gingivitis, J. Dent. Res. (abs.) **28:**634, 1949.

Massler, M., Schour, I., and Chopra, B.: Relations of malnutrition, endemic dental fluorosis and oral hygiene to the prevalence and severity of gingivitis, J. Periodontol. **22:**205-211, 1951.

McCombie, F., and Stothard, D.: Relationships between gingivitis and other dental conditions, J. Can. Dent. Assoc. **30:**506-513, 1964.

Melnick, M., Shields, S.D., and Bixler, D.: Periodontosis: a phenotype and genetic analysis, Oral Surg. **42:**32-41, 1976.

Miller, S.C., and Roth, H.: The present state of knowledge of scorbutic gingivitis, N.Y. State Dent. J. **23:**208-212, 1957.

Mitchell, D.F.: Personal communication, 1966.

Moore, R.M.: A study of the effect of water fluoride content and socioeconomic status on the occurrence of gingivitis in school children, thesis, Indianapolis, 1963, Indiana University School of Dentistry.

Munford, A.G.: Papillon-Lefevre syndrome: report of two cases in the same family, J.A.D.A. **93:**121-124, 1976.

Murray, J.J.: The prevalence of gingivitis in children continuously resident in a high fluoride area, J. Dent. Child. **41:**133-139, 1974.

O'Leary, T.J.: Personal communication, 1982.

O'Leary, T.J., Drake, R.B., and Naylor, J.E.: The plaque control record, J. Periodontol. **43:**38, 1972.

Olson, J.A., and Silverman, S.: Management of recurrent aphthous stomatitis. In McDonald, R.E., and others, editors: Current therapy in dentistry, vol. 7, St. Louis, 1980, The C.V. Mosby Co.

Pindborg, J.J., and others: Acute necrotizing gingivitis in children in South India, Dent. Abs. **11:**584-585, 1966.

Reade, P.C.: Infantile acute ulcerative gingivitis: a case report, J. Periodontol. **34:**387-390, 1963.

Robinson, R.E.: Mucogingival junction surgery, J. Calif. and Nev. Dent. Soc. **33:**379-385, 1957.

Rosenzweig, K.A.: Gingivitis in children of Israel, J. Periodontol. **31:**404-408, 1960.

Russell, A.L.: A system of classification and scoring for prevalence surveys of periodontal disease, J. Dent. Res. **35:**350-359, 1956.

Shafer, W.G.: Personal communication, 1982.

Sheridan, P.J., and Reeve, C.M.: Effective treatment of Dilantin gingival hyperplasia, Oral Surg. **35:**42-46, 1973.

Shillitoe, E.J., and Silverman, S.: Oral cancer and herpes simplex virus—a review, Oral Surg. **48:**216-224, 1979.

Ship, I.I.: Socioeconomic status and recurrent aphthous ulcers, J.A.D.A. **73:**120-123, 1966.

Ship, I.I.: Epidemiologic aspects of recurrent aphthous ulcerations, Oral Surg. **33:**400-406, 1972.

Silverman, S., Jr., and Beumer, J., III: Primary herpetic gingivostomatitis of adult onset, Oral Surg. **36:**496-503, 1973.

Sonis, A.L.: Periodontosis of the primary dentition: a case report, Pediatr. Dent. **2:**53-55, 1980.

Sonnenschien, H., and Clark, D.H.: Congenital cutaneous candidiasis, Am. J. Dis. Child. **107:**260-266, 1964.

Stambaugh, R.V., Morgan, A.F., and Enwonwa, C.O.: Ascorbic acid deficiency associated with Dilantin hyperplasia, J. Periodontol. **44:**244-247, 1973.

Steinberg, A.D.: Clinical management of phenytoin-induced gingival overgrowth in handicapped children, Pediatr. Dent. **3**(special issue)**:**130-136, May 1981.

Strean, L.R., and Leoni, E.: Dilantin gingival hyperplasia: newer concepts related to etiology and treatment, N.Y. State Dent. J. **25:**339-347, 1959.

Suomi, J.D., and others: Oral calculus in children, J. Periodontol. **42:**341-345, 1971.

Sutcliffe, P.: A longitudinal study of gingivitis and puberty, J. Periodontol. Res. **7:**52-58, 1972.

Terezhalmy, G.T., Bottomley, W.K., and Pellen, G.B.: The use of water-soluble bioflavonoid–ascorbic acid complex in the treatment of recurrent herpes labialis, Oral Surg. **45:**56-62, 1978.

Traiger, J.: Unusual deposition of calculus: report of a case, Oral Surg. **14:**623-624, 1961.

Turesky, S., Renstrup, G., and Glickman, I.: Histologic and histochemical observations regarding early calculus formation in children and adults, J. Periodontol. **32:**7-14, 1961.

Weddell, J.A., and Klein, A.I.: Socioeconomic correlation of oral disease in six-to-thirty-six month children, Pediatr. Dent. **3:**306-310, 1981.

Wray, D., and others: Recurrent aphthae: treatment with vitamin B_{12}, folic acid and iron, Br. Med. J. **2:**490-493, 1975.

Zackin, S.J., and Weisberger, D.: Hereditary gingival fibromatosis: report of a family, Oral Surg. **14:**825-835, 1961.

Zappler, S.E.: Periodontal disease in children, J.A.D.A. **37:**333-345, 1948.

15 Toothbrushing, flossing, and oral hygiene instruction

PAUL E. STARKEY

Every dentist has a distinct responsibility to properly advise young patients and their parents of the importance of cleaning the teeth and to recommend and demonstrate a method that will be effective in maintaining cleanliness in the oral cavity. It is well documented that there is a direct relationship between dental disease and the state of cleanliness of the oral cavity. Chapters 7 and 12 have discussed the cause of dental caries and periodontal disease. Proper oral hygiene is extremely important in preventing initial episodes or the recurrence of caries and periodontal disease.

The most practical way to prevent oral disease is to develop a method that will allow each patient to maintain the best possible oral hygiene. This means maintaining oral cleanliness by the mechanical dispersion and removal of adherent microorganisms from the oral cavity. Such an approach implies brushing and flossing. However, even daily brushing and flossing do not necessarily mean that cleanliness of the oral cavity is being maintained. Parents and children alike must be convinced that, while the teeth should be brushed after meals to remove large particles of food, stimulate the tissues, and give a feeling of well-being, a thorough cleaning, including staining, brushing, flossing, and inspection, must be done at least once a day and preferably before bed. This chapter discusses these acts and their impact on the control of dental disease.

Toothbrushing

Brush design. It is likely that some form of brush has been used by humans since their primitive state. Anthropoids no doubt removed debris from around their teeth by using splinters of wood or twigs. Evidence exists that people originally chewed a stick of special wood until it became something like a brush on one end, which they then used to clean debris from around their teeth. From this crude beginning has evolved the modern brush, which generally has a cellulose or resinous handle and nylon bristles.

Harris pointed out in 1839 that there existed a great difference in opinion among dentists as to what kind of brush was best to use. Some preferred ''hard'' brushes, some ''medium,'' and some ''soft.''

In a study of the relative abrasiveness of natural and synthetic bristles on cementum and dentin, Manly and Brudevold found that the toothbrush itself, whether it has synthetic or natural bristles, has little or no abrasive effect on enamel and dentin. Abrasion of tooth structure is independent of the stiffness or composition of the bristles but depends almost entirely on the properties of the dentifrice used in conjunction with the toothbrush. For example, a medium-abrasive tooth powder will increase the abrasive action of any toothbrush by several hundred percent.

Swartz and Phillips (1953) studied the effects of

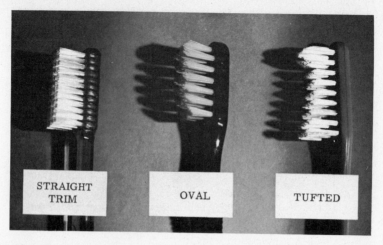

STRAIGHT
TRIM

OVAL

TUFTED

Fig. 15-1. Three toothbrush designs displayed by retailers and most easily available.

the diameter of nylon bristles on enamel surfaces. They found no significant difference in the final luster attained with various diameters of nylon bristle in toothbrushes. In a 1956 study these same investigators found that, when immersed in water, nylon bristles tended to retain their stiffness much better than the natural bristles and that they also regained their original values more rapidly.

Before World War II, toothbrush bristles were made from the hides of animals. When the war interfered with the source of supply of natural bristles, the nylon bristle was developed. At first these were heavy and stiff and the nylon brush was not popular. However, they have since been greatly improved and have been found to have distinct advantages. They last longer and are more easily cleaned. They do not become soggy or soft and do not easily split or fray. In addition, methods have been devised for easily standardizing the diameters of the bristles.

There is little agreement about the best brush to recommend from the standpoint of hardness. Most likely there will never be agreement. Too stiff a brush, however, can lacerate delicate gingival tissues.

The recent upsurge in interest in teaching good home care has probably brought about a greater

unanimity of opinion regarding the type of brush to use. The three designs most prominently displayed by retailers and most easily available today are the straight trim, oval, and tufted (Fig. 15-1). The most commonly advocated brushing techniques use a soft-bristle brush. I recommend a soft nylon brush with an overall length of about 5 inches for the primary dentition and a soft nylon brush with an overall length of about 6 inches for the mixed and permanent dentitions.

Brushing techniques. The method of toothbrushing that should be recommended and taught to a patient depends on the dentist's evaluation of the patient's needs.

Suomi reviewed the literature on the preventive aspects of periodontal diseases for the Council on Dental Research and concluded that sufficient evidence has accumulated to indicate that keeping the teeth clean is effective in controlling periodontal disease and that toothbrushing is the method most commonly recommended for removing deposits of oral debris and plaque from the teeth. However, he found that no one method of toothbrushing has been shown to be clearly superior to others; the thoroughness of plaque and debris removal by the careful and correct application of any brushing method is more important to the maintenance of periodontal health than the method itself. He judged that dentifrices are useful for cleansing the teeth but that the overzealous use of dentifrices with strong abrasives is contraindicated, especially if softer portions of the teeth are exposed. As a result of his review of the literature, Suomi concluded that that no one kind of toothbrush should be recommended for use by all persons but that the dentist should tailor the instructions and the selection of a brush to the individual patient.

The seven predominant toothbrushing techniques are described in the following paragraphs.

"Scrub brush" method. The brush is held firmly in the hand and the teeth are brushed in a back-and-forth motion similar to a scrubbing motion used on a floor. The direction of the motions may change and may even be haphazard.

Fones' method. The teeth are held in occlusion and the brush is pressed firmly against the teeth and gingival tissues and revolved in circles with as large a diameter as possible.

Roll method. The bristles of the brush are placed as high in the vestibule as possible in the buccal region, with the sides of the bristles touching the gingival tissues. The patient exerts as much lateral pressure as the tissues can tolerate with the sides of the bristles and moves the brush occlusally. The tissue blanches under pressure as the blood is forced out of the capillaries. As the brush approaches the plane of occlusion, it is turned slowly so that the ends of the bristles touch the enamel of the tooth. Release of the pressure allows the blood to rush into the capillaries again. The brush is then placed as high in the vestibule as possible, and the rolling motion is repeated. Patients are instructed to give each area eight definite strokes toward the occlusal surface of the teeth; the brush is then moved to a new area.

Charters' method. The ends of the bristles are placed in contact with the enamel of the teeth and the gingival tissue with the bristles pointed at about a 45-degree angle toward the plane of occlusion. Strong lateral and downward pressure is then placed on the brush and the brush is vibrated gently back and forth 1 mm or so. This gentle vibratory procedure forces the ends of the bristles between the teeth and cleans the interproximal tooth surfaces well. This technique also massages the interproximal tissues well.

Stillman's method. The brush is placed in approximately the same position as required for the beginning stroke of the roll method, except that it is nearer the crowns of the teeth. The handle is vibrated or "shimmied" gently in a rapid but slight mesiodistal movement. This technique forces the bristles into the interproximal spaces and hence cleans the teeth in that area well. It also adequately massages the gingival tissues.

Physiologic method. This technique is advocated by some who believe that because food is deflected apically during mastication, the gingival tissues and teeth should be brushed in the same direction. With a soft brush, the gingival tissues are brushed from the crown toward the root in a gentle sweeping motion. Although the technique can be effective, caution must be used in this method.

Bass method. In brushing the buccal, labial, and lingual surfaces, the bristles are forced directly into the gingival crevices and into the sulci between the teeth at about a 45-degree angle to the long axis of the tooth. With the bristles forced into the crevices as far as possible, short, back-and-forth movements of the brush dislodge all soft material that the bristles reach on the teeth within the crevices. At the same time the teeth are cleaned above the gingival tissue in the sulci and between the teeth as far as the bristles can go. The occlusal surfaces are brushed by applying the bristles to the surface, pressing down firmly, and moving the brush back and forth with short strokes. The anterior teeth are brushed on the lingual side by directing the bristles of the heel or the side of the brush into the gingival crevices and sulci between the teeth at about the same 45-degree angle as at all other places.

Infant tooth cleaning. Pedodontists are becoming more acutely aware of the need for the child's first nonemergency dental visit to be much earlier than recommended in past years. Shortly after the first primary teeth erupt and as soon as is conve-

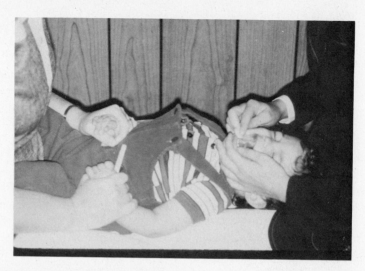

Fig. 15-2. Two people sitting and facing each other with knees touching form a table to restrain a very young child for efficient brushing. The child's arms and legs are restrained by the one while the other does the brushing.

nient for both the dentist and the parent, the infant should be brought to the dental office. This provides the opportunity to explain to the parents the importance of certain preventive concepts, for example, weaning the child around 1 year of age and avoiding nursing caries by refraining from using a propped bottle for feeding or allowing the infant to go to sleep with a bottle. This first visit also provides the opportunity to explain to the parent the importance of allowing a dentist to examine the child after any trauma to the primary dentition, which most often occurs during the toddler stage. Furthermore, the parent can be given instructions in cleaning the primary teeth shortly after they have erupted.

Carlsson, Grahnen, and Jonsoon have documented the presence of bacteria that can initiate dental disease on newly erupted teeth. It is the parents' responsibility to clean the infant's teeth. The technique for accomplishing this is illustrated in Fig. 15-2.

If both parents are available, they may sit in a straight chair, facing each other with their knees touching. This forms a table where the father, for

example, may restrain the child's legs by allowing them to extend between his arms and body while using his hands to restrain the child's arms. The mother, with the child's head on her lap, can do the brushing. This is particularly effective with the very young child who finds it difficult to cooperate.

The teeth should be wiped or brushed with a gentle scrubbing action using a soft, multitufted small brush without any dentifrice. Even though the infant may be uncooperative at first, with repetition and distraction, cooperation and relaxation usually occur. Initially the cleaning sessions are very short, but as more primary teeth erupt, the sessions become longer and eventually the transition is made to the technique of brushing the primary dentition (Fig. 15-3).

Method for brushing the primary dentition. Only in recent years has attention been given to the differences in the anatomy of the primary teeth and the permanent teeth as they relate to toothbrushing. In the past, dentists taught brushing for the preschool child just as they did for the adult, or else they simply did not mention the difference.

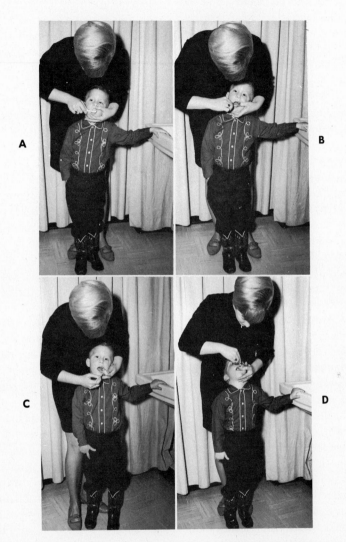

Fig. 15-3. A, Proper stance. The child's head is cradled in left arm of parent as he leans back against her. The fingers of the parent's left hand retract the lips as the right hand brushes. **B,** Brushing lingual surfaces of mandibular teeth. The back of the brush head displaces the tongue as the buccal musculature is retracted by the parent's left hand. **C,** Brushing buccal surfaces of mandibular teeth. **D,** The child's head tipped far back for brushing of maxillary teeth. Note good vision and access.

The "scrub brush" method for some time was generally condemned or at least was not considered acceptable, primarily because of the irritation to the gingival tissues at the neck of the tooth and the abrasion often seen at the gingival margin as a result of vigorous toothbrushing using that method. In addition, the scrub brush method was believed to be ineffective in removing debris from between the teeth.

Kimmelman and Tassman pointed out that the scrubbing action best dislodges debris on the tooth surfaces of primary teeth. Primary tooth and arch anatomy, particularly the presence of the cervical ridges or bulges on the buccal and labial surfaces of primary teeth, permits far more thorough cleaning by horizontal strokes. In addition, the presence of these cervical bulges protects the gingival tissue and provides safety from this standpoint.

Parents' role in toothbrushing. Parents should continue to assist their children in toothbrushing for several years after infancy. One study of toothbrushing habits of children has shown that those age 5 years and under brush less than 20 seconds. In the same study, about 35% of the children in this age group were unable to control the brush. Also, it was found that the toothbrushing performance of children under 7 years of age was much briefer and more haphazard than that of older children. Preschool-age children or those in the primary dentition stage usually have not yet developed their skills to the degree that they can perform efficient toothbrushing.

McClure included 175 preschool children in a study to observe the effectiveness of toothbrushing by the child, as compared with the results when parents brushed the child's teeth. At the same time, he compared the efficiency of the horizontal scrubbing technique with the roll technique, when performed by the child and by the parent.

One group of children brushed their own teeth without any instruction, one group brushed their teeth with instructions in the roll method, and a third group brushed their teeth with instructions in the scrub brush method.

Three other groups had their teeth brushed by a parent. The parents in one group were given instructions in the roll method, another group was given instructions in the scrub brush method, and the third group was given no instruction.

In all instances the parents brushed significantly better than the children. Scrubbing horizontally proved to be more effective than the roll method for the primary dentition when either the child or parent brushed. The parents who had been given instructions brushed more effectively than those who had not been instructed. It is interesting to note, however, that the children who brushed their teeth without instruction did a more effective job of brushing than the group of children who brushed their own teeth after receiving instruction in the roll method. It was observed that the group who brushed without instruction used the scrub brush method, which seems to be more natural for children.

More recently Sangnes, Zachrisson, and Gjermo reported a study in which they compared the plaque-removing ability of the vertical (roll) brushing technique with the horizontal (scrub) technique in 41 children 5 years of age. Brushing with the scrub technique gave significantly lower plaque values on buccal and lingual surfaces than the roll technique. This result supports the work of McClure.

Hall and Conroy support McClure's findings that parents brush their children's teeth significantly more effectively than do the children themselves. Therefore the preschool child's parent should be instructed to brush the child's teeth and to use the scrub brush method. A technique for the parent brushing the teeth is illustrated in Fig. 15-3.

The child stands in front of the parent and leans back. The parent uses the left arm to cradle the child's head. In this manner, if there is movement of the child or parent, their movements are together. When brushing the lower anterior teeth, the parent uses the fingers of the left hand to retract the child's lip. The right hand is free to brush. In this manner all of the lower teeth can be brushed on all surfaces. The fingers of the parent's left hand can be used to retract the cheek when brushing the posterior teeth and the back of the brush head can be used to hold back the tongue as the lingual surfaces of the lower teeth are being brushed.

When the maxillary teeth are being brushed, the child is asked to tip the head back. Looking directly into the mouth, the parent has adequate vision and access while brushing the tooth surfaces. Again, the fingers of the left hand can be used to retract the child's lips and cheek.

Nowak describes several other methods particularly useful in brushing the handicapped child's teeth. The parent may be seated in a straight chair and have the child seated on the floor in front of the chair. The child leans back between the parent's legs and the teeth are brushed in the same manner as previously described when the child is standing.

The child may be seated in a straight chair with the parent standing behind the chair (Fig. 15-4). Again, the child leans the head back against the parent while the parent brushes. If the child is confined to a wheelchair, this same technique may be employed.

Another technique particularly effective for the handicapped child is with the parent sitting on one edge and at the end of the bed. The child lies perpendicular to the parent with the child's head in the parent's lap as the teeth are brushed.

It has been my experience that when parents are given specific instruction in a detailed approach to brushing the child's teeth, they are more motivated to follow through with the recommendations given.

It was recommended earlier that the roll method or Bass method should be employed for the mixed dentition. A question then arises regarding what to teach the preschool child about toothbrushing. Parents are advised to brush for the child and, after completing the cleaning, to encourage the child to brush also. However, no specific instructions are given to the child. The child will usually scrub brush, but no attempt should be made to indoctrinate the child into this method. When the anterior permanent teeth begin to erupt, the child should

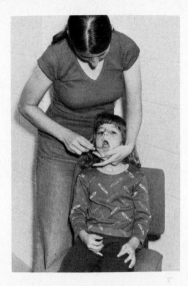

Fig. 15-4. The child sits in a straight chair and leans head back against the parent for efficient brushing by the parent.

then be instructed in the roll or Bass method. Parents should continue to brush until the child has demonstrated efficiency and interest in carrying out the procedure. This is often as late as 9 or 10 years of age. When parents continue to brush the teeth for the child into the period of mixed dentition, they should use a combination of the scrub brush method and the roll or Bass method.

Method for brushing the mixed and young adult dentition. The roll method is an acceptable technique for brushing the mixed dentition and the young adult dentition. It is a method that is not excessively complicated or difficult, and it will do an adequate job of stimulating the gingival tissues as well as removing debris from the teeth. If periodontitis is present, the patient can be taught Stillman's vibratory technique as an adjunct to the roll method. As the brush is carried occlusally and rolled slightly, the handle can be gently vibrated to force the bristles between the teeth.

Another popular method for brushing the mixed and young adult dentition is based on the Bass method and is illustrated in Fig. 15-5. The handle

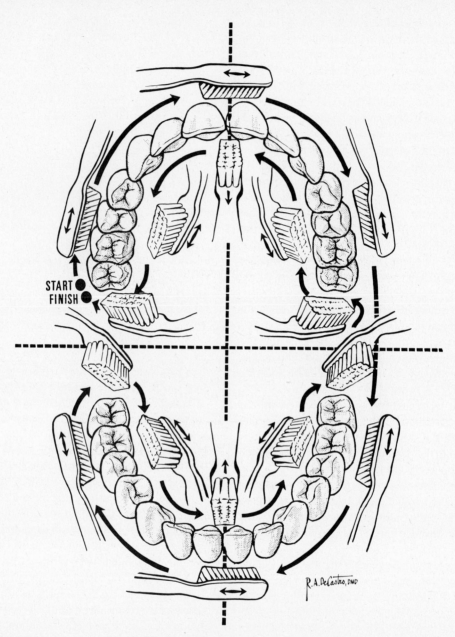

START ●
FINISH ●

R. A. DeCastro, DMD

Fig. 15-5. Systematic approach to brushing the teeth begins with the buccal aspects of the teeth in the maxillary right quadrant and follows the arrows. Bristles are held at a 45-degree angle to the long axis of the teeth and are directed to the gum line. Short back-and-forth strokes are used, allowing bristles to remain in the same place. The handle of the brush is placed parallel to the biting surfaces except when brushing the lingual aspects of the anterior teeth and the posterior aspects of the last tooth in each quadrant, when a heel-toe direction of brushing is used.

of the toothbrush is placed parallel to the biting surfaces of the teeth. The bristles are angled approximately 45 degrees to the long axis of the teeth and directed toward the gumline. Short, back-and-forth (not up-and-down) strokes are used in brushing, allowing the bristles to remain in the same place. A systematic approach is used by brushing only two or three teeth at a time, beginning with the buccal aspects of the teeth in the maxillary right quadrant, moving to the labial aspects of the maxillary anterior teeth, then to the buccal aspects of the maxillary left quadrant, then down to the buccal aspects of the teeth in the mandibular left quadrant, the labial aspects of the mandibular anterior teeth, and the buccal aspects of the mandibular right quadrant, then to the lingual aspects of the mandibular right quadrant, the lower anterior teeth, and the mandibular left quadrant, then up to the lingual aspects of the maxillary left quadrant, the maxillary anterior teeth, and the maxillary right quadrant. The occlusal surface is brushed by placing the bristles against the surface, pressing down firmly, and moving the brush back and forth with short strokes. The distal aspects of the most posterior teeth in each quadrant are cleaned with the toe of the brush as the teeth are systematically brushed, moving from one quadrant to another. When the lingual aspects of the anterior teeth are brushed, the handle of the brush is held parallel to the long axis of the teeth, and the action of the brush is in a heel-and-toe direction.

The length of time that should be used in brushing the teeth depends largely on the patient's skill and needs. The minimum time recommended is about 3 minutes. There is a wide difference in the time people take to brush their teeth, even when they are using an efficient procedure.

The electric toothbrush. Many studies have reported the comparative effectiveness of the electric toothbrush. Most of these reports are favorable. Several studies have recently been done with children in comparing the effectiveness of the electric and the manual toothbrush.

Hall and Conroy compared toothbrushing efficiency for preschool children when the child used both the electric and the manual brush and when the parent brushed the child's teeth using both types of brushes. They found that the electric toothbrush removed significantly more debris and plaque than the hand brush when used by the child or by the parent. They also found, as mentioned previously, that the parent brushed better with both brushes than did the children.

Conroy and Melfi compared the electric and manual toothbrushing methods for cleaning effectiveness in a group of children 5 to 12 years of age. They concluded that two reciprocating electric toothbrushes, one a modified arcuate type and the other a short-stroke type, were more effective for the removal of dental plaque and debris for schoolchildren than the manual brushes. In addition, they found that this could be done more rapidly with the electric brush than with the manual type. Huff and Taylor have also reported finding an electric toothbrush to be more effective than the manual brushes in cleaning children's teeth.

Certainly, efficient toothbrushing can be done for the preschool child by the parent using a manual brush just as efficient brushing can be done by older children with a manual brush if properly motivated. However, the electric toothbrush can be recommended in both instances if parents are willing to purchase the instrument. There is often increased interest in cleaning the teeth when the electric brush is purchased, which usually decreases in time. Its use with handicapped children has long been advocated and is certainly justified.

The dentifrice. Over the years, dozens of dentifrices have been offered to the public and have been heavily promoted on radio and television, through advertisements in newspapers and magazines, and through direct mail advertising. However, in the last three decades, serious efforts have been made to investigate claims for the effectiveness of some of these dentifrices.

There are two purposes of a dentifrice—to assist the toothbrushing by freeing the accessible surface of the teeth of newly deposited debris and stain and to act as a caries-preventive agent.

In the 1930s the ammoniated dentifrices were popular, and many believed they were effective as caries-preventive agents. However, well-controlled studies failed to support the belief. The penicillin dentifrices were also studied and found to be effective with closely controlled supervision but not without this supervision. However, concern for the dentifrices' production of penicillin-resistant bacteria in the mouth and the possibility of their induction of penicillin sensitivity caused the interest in them to subside.

Other types of dentifrices have also been studied, such as the chlorophyll and sarcosinate dentifrices, but the fluoride dentifrices have been given the greatest attention during recent years and have received considerable support as a result of documentation of their effectiveness. A fluoride dentifrice should be recommended to the patient. The following are those that are approved by the American Dental Association or documented by the Food and Drug Administration:

Improved Crest (NaF)	Approved, 1981
Colgate (MFP)	Approved, 1969
Gleem (NaF)	Documented, 1973
Macleans Fluoride (MFP)	Approved, 1976
Aqua-Fresh (MFP)	Approved, 1978
Aim (MFP)	Approved, 1980

"Swish and swallow." In 1963 the American Dental Association began promoting the "swish and swallow" method of eliminating retained material from the mouth immediately after eating when brushing is impractical.

Coykendall reported a study describing a simple and colorful test to demonstrate the benefit of the "swish and swallow" method. This is done by having the patient eat a candy orange slice and then rinse for 15 seconds with 15 ml distilled water. The rinse water is collected, and the procedure is repeated three or four times with no time interval between rinses. Approximately 0.2 ml from each rinse plus 1 drop of $3N$ hydrochloric acid is then put into a test tube and heated for 1 minute in a boiling water bath. This is necessary to hydrolize sucrose to glucose and fructose, since the indicator is sensitive only to reducing sugars. After the rinse

water is heated, the sample is diluted with 9 drops (0.4 ml) distilled water. A urine sugar test tablet* is dropped into each tube. These tablets test for reducing sugars by providing all necessary reagents for a Fehling's test. A 2% sugar solution produces an orange color, and lower concentrations provide varying shades of brown and green. After the reactions have stopped, the colors in the tubes are compared with the color chart supplied with the tablets. Coykendall's study revealed that after one candy orange slice had been eaten, most individuals' first rinse contained 0.13 to 0.3 sucrose, which is equivalent to a 1% to 2% solution; however, the second and third rinse showed greatly reduced sugar concentration. By the fourth and fifth rinses, most of his subjects had no detectable sugar in their rinse water. Only half as much sugar was eliminated if the first rinse was delayed for as little as 2 minutes. It is interesting to note that with no rinse at all, sugar was detected in the saliva 20 minutes after one piece of this candy had been eaten.

This rather simple test might be used effectively to demonstrate to a patient or groups of people the effectiveness of the "swish and swallow" method.

Patients should be encouraged, if they are unable to brush immediately after each time they eat, to thoroughly rinse the mouth with water and swallow. They should repeat the "swish and swallow" procedure four or five times immediately after eating.

The effectiveness of this procedure will be directly related to how well the dentist or auxiliary personnel have motivated the patient to practice this additional method of prevention. It seems likely that demonstration of this test to the patient will produce greater motivation.

Flossing

After describing his method of toothbrushing, Bass wrote in 1954 that when his method is followed, the bristles of the brush reach between the teeth and into the gingival crevices as far as they

---

*Ames Co., Inc., Elkhart, Ind. 46514.

will go, from the buccal or labial side and from the lingual side, but there is a place along the middle between the teeth where the bristles do not reach from either side. The proximal surfaces not reached by the bristles and those within the gingival crevices have not been cleaned. He emphatically stated that the only way to clean these important areas is by the proper use of the right kind of dental floss.

In the study by Sangnes, Zachrisson, and Gjermo mentioned previously, in which they found the horizontal (scrub) technique to be more effective in plaque removal on the buccal and lingual surfaces of the primary dentition than the vertical (roll) technique, they also reported that the plaque scores were consistently higher on proximal than on buccal and lingual surfaces. The difference between the two techniques on the proximal surfaces was not statistically significant. Most dentists agree that to remove all plaque from the teeth, the combination of toothbrushing and dental flossing must be used. No doubt the major lack in most oral hygiene programs is the inadequate use of dental floss.

Most researchers seem to agree with Bass that the right kind of dental floss consists of a large number of microscopic nylon filaments, unwaxed and untwisted except just enough to hold it together when in use.

A number of different techniques have been proposed and diagrammed for flossing the teeth. I prefer the following:

1. Using 2 or 3 feet of unwaxed floss, wrap all but about 9 inches around the middle finger of the right hand.
2. Wrap enough of the loose end around the left middle finger to hold it (Fig. 15-6, *A*).
3. Pass the floss over the tips of the thumbs, or of the thumb and forefinger, or of both forefingers, keeping them about 1 inch apart (Fig. 15-6, *B*).
4. Pass the floss between each pair of teeth. This is done by drawing it gently in a sawing motion through the contact points. Do not snap it through.

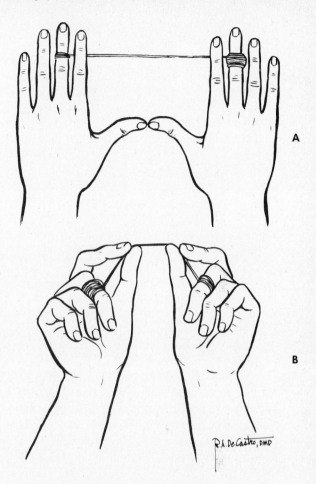

Fig. 15-6. A, All but about 9 inches of a 2- or 3-foot length of floss is wrapped around the middle finger of the right hand. The rest is used to secure the floss to the left middle finger. **B,** The floss is passed over the tips of the thumbs or of thumb and forefinger, or of both forefingers, keeping them about 1 inch apart.

5. After passing the floss between the contact points, curve it around the anterior tooth and carry it beneath the gingival tissue until resistance is felt. Polish that tooth surface by rubbing the floss up and down. Do the same for the mesial surface of the posterior tooth of the pair.

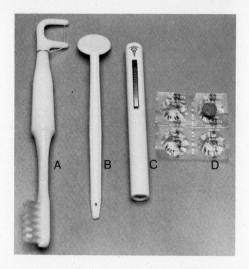

Fig. 15-7. A, Floss holder and toothbrush. **B,** Disposable mirror. **C,** Penlight. **D,** Disclosing tablets.

6. As the floss becomes frayed or soiled, wind it from the right finger to the left, much as a take-up reel would do on a tape recorder.

Some parents and children may find it difficult to manipulate dental floss as described above and prefer to use a floss holder (Fig. 15-7, *A*). Properly applied, it can be a good adjunct to cleaning the teeth and removing plaque from the proximal areas.

Oral hygiene instruction

Rationale for giving home care instruction. An organized routine for instructing patients in toothbrushing and flossing is necessary if the dentist expects to be effective in motivating patients to give themselves good home care. Each dentist must decide how much time and effort will be expended in the office in giving home care instructions. The time and effort will be related to the dentist's own individual conviction as to the importance of home care.

For some time dentists generally believed that gingival disturbances were relatively rare in the child patient. However, a number of studies have shown that mild gingivitis is common in children. Moore examined 1123 children, ages 7 to 13 years, and found at least one gingival unit exhibiting inflammation in 93%. He concluded that the severity of gingivitis and the accumulation of oral debris are directly related to toothbrushing habits. He also found a relationship between the severity of gingivitis and different socioeconomic levels of children. Children in lower socioeconomic levels have a greater amount and severity of gingivitis than those in the higher socioeconomic levels, probably because children in the higher socioeconomic levels have been exposed to more routine and regular dental care, involving instruction and motivation in good oral hygiene. Although the relationship between gingivitis in the primary and mixed dentition and periodontal disease in the permanent dentition is not clear, many dentists are concerned about this possibility.

Weddell and Klein conducted a study of oral disease in 441 children between 6 and 36 months of age who were born and reared in an area with a fluoridated water supply. They found no dental caries in children 6 to 11 months of age but at least one carious lesion in 4.2% of the children 12 to 17 months of age. Dental caries was identified in 19.8% of the children in the 24- to 29-month age group and in 36.4% of the 30- to 36-month age group. Among the 299 white children examined, gingivitis was present in 13.2% of those 6 to 17 months of age, 33.9% of those 18 to 23 months of age, and 38.5% of those 24 to 36 months of age. The authors observed that dental caries prevalence and severity of gingivitis in children 6 to 36 months of age are independent of sex and socioeconomic status. They also found an increased prevalence of gingivitis in young children with dental caries compared with children without dental caries. They concluded that parental guidance and treatment for the prevention of dental disease are indicated very early in a child's life.

Regular use of the toothbrush after eating and thorough cleaning of the teeth before retiring are essential to maintain good health of the soft tissues surrounding the teeth. This type of care is certainly to be encouraged and should be taught to child dental patients.

There is also considerable evidence that toothbrushing contributes to limiting dental caries. To be effective in this respect, the toothbrushing must be done immediately after eating. Independent studies by Stephan and by Fosdick (1950) demonstrated that acid production occurs almost immediately after the food has reached the bacterial plaque. In one investigation by Fosdick (1950), 702 individuals were studied over a 2-year period. Of those, 273 served as controls and 429 were test subjects. Those in the experimental group brushed their teeth within 10 minutes after the ingestion of food or sweets and rinsed their mouths immediately thereafter. The control group continued with their customary brushing procedures, providing that this did not include toothbrushing immediately after food ingestion. The majority of those in the control group brushed their teeth only on arising and retiring. The findings of this study seem to indicate that brushing immediately after meals reduces tooth decay by approximately 50%.

McDonald conducted a dentifrice study involving 44 children and observed a ''significant reduction in the positive reactions to the Snyder test when the children had oral hygiene instruction and followed supervised toothbrushing routine immediately following each meal.'' He also reported that the toothbrushing routine was beneficial in the correction of gingivitis, particularly the type resulting from poor oral hygiene.

Wright, Banting, and Feasby reported that a 52% to 55% reduction in the number of new proximal caries resulted from frequent flossing. Lindhe, Axelsson, and Tollskog, as well as Badersten, Egelberg, and Koch, noted a 54% to 95% decrease in proximal dental caries when flossing, interdental tips, prophylaxis, and topical fluorides were used. However, Horowitz and associates and Silverstein and associates failed to show significant proximal caries reductions following supervised flossing each school day.

Wright, Feasby, and Banting reported a study indicating that frequent interdental flossing by trained auxiliaries can significantly reduce proximal caries. In this study the subjects were first-grade students. Trained auxiliaries flossed the children's teeth each school day for the 20-month study period. It would seem that if the dental staff properly instructs a parent in the flossing technique and if the instructions are carried out in the routine home program, flossing is helpful in reducing caries.

In addition to other studies with human subjects that tend to support the belief that toothbrushing and flossing can limit caries, there are good animal studies of toothbrushing that add support. Volker and Klapper, working with Syrian hamsters, found that the ability of high-sugar diets to produce severe caries in these animals can be reduced by toothbrushing. This emphasizes the importance of the protective action of mechanical cleansing.

The results of some studies seriously question the benefits of toothbrushing from the standpoint of caries control. However, the evidence that supports the role of toothbrushing in limiting caries, in improving the condition of the soft tissues, and in carrying therapeutic pastes daily to the teeth certainly should motivate the dentist to teach toothbrushing.

Ideally, then, the teeth should be brushed immediately after each time a person eats. In addition, the teeth should be thoroughly cleaned by brushing and flossing each evening. There is a long time between the last eating in the evening and the morning, during which there is a decrease in the flow of saliva and movements of the mouth that would clear debris from the teeth. Thus the thorough removal of all plaque once a day is best timed after the last time the individual eats before retiring, as this act will tend to inhibit any caries activity during the night.

Dudding and Muhler, in a study involving 374 children, classified them as having ''good'' or ''poor'' oral hygiene. Sixty-one percent of those whose oral hygiene was classified as ''good'' said they learned their toothbrushing practices from their dentist. Only 33% of those whose oral hygiene was classified as ''poor'' gave the same information. Certainly the dentist and the auxiliary personnel play an important role in the establishment of good oral hygiene practices.

Home care instruction in the office. For any preventive program to be effective, those instructing in preventive measures must understand the fundamental facts in the course of dental caries and periodontal disease to communicate this information to patients as a basis for motivating them to good home care. In the past several years many dentists have developed enthusiasm for promoting good preventive programs for their patients. There is no reliable evidence, however, that most patients can discipline themselves so that personal requirements for the success of the program can be satisfied over a long period of time. There are many who continue to use tobacco even though they are aware of the potential adverse results; there are many who continue to overeat who are acutely aware of the potential adverse results; there are many who have been well informed of the personal requirements necessary to control dental disease yet fail to satisfy these requirements. We must learn much more about the psychologic and emotional aspects of motivating patients to carry out preventive programs on a sustained basis.

An excellent self-instructional course in preventive dentistry techniques, entitled "Developing a Plaque Control Program," has been developed by the University of California School of Dentistry under a National Institutes of Health training grant from the Division of Dental Health, United States Public Health Service.* Although primarily designed for the continuing education of dentists, it is appropriate for training dental auxiliaries and is a fresh approach to learning to motivate patients to practice good home care using sound psychologic principles.

During the past several years, despite the fact that we are still in an era of insufficient knowledge and frustration in our efforts to motivate patients to good preventive programs, successes in preventive care have been experienced. We should continue our efforts with the knowledge that we have much yet to learn in order to significantly increase our effectiveness.

A good preventive practice incorporates an organized program of preventive home care for pa-

tients. This practice begins with the use of methods to teach patients the causes of dental caries and periodontal disease.

After the role of plaque in dental caries and periodontal disease is explained to the patients, they should be told that the teeth should be brushed after eating to remove particles of food, to help avoid offensive breath, and to enjoy the feeling of a clean mouth. After the last time they eat and before they retire, they should thoroughly clean the oral cavity. The procedure for thoroughly cleaning the oral cavity involves four steps: staining, brushing, flossing, and inspection. These should be discussed in detail and demonstrated to patients and parents as a part of their home care instruction.

Staining. Because plaque is not apparent to the patient, a disclosing agent should be used to stain the plaque so that it may be identified for removal. A variety of disclosing agents are available, most of which are solutions of erythrosine. One of these solutions prepared commercially is Trace. The active ingredient is erythrosine. Instructions for several different methods of applying the stain are included on the dispenser bottle and are common methods used. Three of these methods are as follows:

1. Place 3 to 4 drops under the patient's tongue and have the patient wipe the teeth with the tongue for a few seconds.
2. Place 10 drops in 1 to 2 tablespoons of water and ask the patient to swish the solution around in the mouth.
3. Paint the solution on the tooth surfaces with a cotton applicator. After the application, ask the patient to rinse.

The bacterial plaque will be stained a dramatic red. The third method is the one that I generally use and recommend.

Disclosing tablets or wafers are also available. One of these, Butler's Red Coat (Fig. 15-7, *D*), carries the following instructions on the package:

Crush one tablet between the teeth and swish around in the mouth for at least ½ minute. Expectorate into bowl of running water. The red-colored areas remaining on the teeth indicate the presence of overlooked areas in your

---

*Praxis Publishing Co., Berkeley, Calif. 94701.

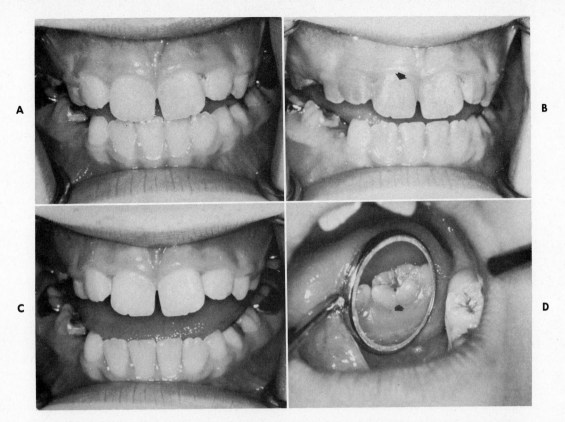

Fig. 15-8. A, Unstained teeth before cleaning. **B,** Plaque *(arrow)* identified with disclosing agent. **C,** Same mouth after teeth have been cleaned. **D,** Plaque *(arrow)* identified by staining on lingual cervical third of mandibular molar.

brushing and may contain harmful dental plaque. A thorough removal of these areas can avoid an accelerated accumulation of this plaque. For best results, follow the instructions of your dentist.

Fig. 15-8, *A,* demonstrates the need for the use of disclosing agents to stain the teeth in order to identify the plaque. Fig. 15-8, *B,* shows the same mouth following identification of the plaque with the disclosing agent. Fig. 15-8, *C,* shows the mouth again after the patient has removed the stained plaque with the toothbrush and dental floss. Note in Fig. 15-8, *D,* the plaque identified by staining on the cervical third of the lingual surface of a lower first permanent molar.

Toothbrushing. As indicated previously, the horizontal scrub technique should be used for the primary dentition. Depending on the child's age and ability to cooperate, the parent should be instructed in the method to use for brushing the child's teeth. I have found the technique illustrated in Fig. 15-2 to be effective in most instances.

For the older child the dentist or the auxiliaries should offer instruction in the method of brushing to be used, tailoring it to the child's individual needs. Nevertheless, parents should be present and attempts should be made to motivate them to accept the responsibility to see that home care and instructions are carried out. Nowak believes that a dentifrice should not be used during the process of

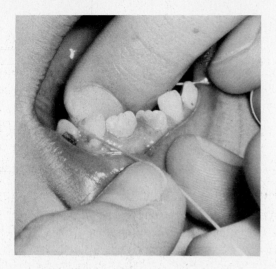

Fig. 15-9. Stained plaque being removed with dental floss.

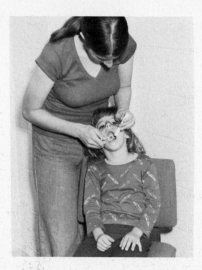

Fig. 15-10. Parent inspecting after cleaning by using disposable mirror and penlight.

cleaning the teeth, because it is not really necessary for that purpose. He believes that the foaming action that covers the teeth when a dentifrice is used makes the inspection of the teeth difficult. He recommends that a wet, soft toothbrush be used to scrub the teeth. After staining, brushing, and flossing and after inspection to see that the teeth are clean, he instructs the parents that fluoridated dentifrice be placed on the brush and that the child again scrub the teeth so that they will have the effect of the fluoride as well as the deodorizing of the tissue and breath. I concur with this recommendation. Having the child brush after the inspection and removal of any remaining plaque allows the child to be an active participant in the routine and also allows the young child to develop the habit of regular brushing. The fluoridated dentifrice should also be used routinely when the teeth are brushed after each meal.

Flossing. After the teeth have been thoroughly brushed and all plaque has been removed from the surfaces that can be reached with the brush, the parent or patient must remove the plaque from the areas of the teeth inaccessible to the brush with dental floss (Fig. 15-9).

Inspection. After an attempt has been made to remove all the stained plaque with the brush and dental floss, the parent should inspect the teeth to ascertain that all plaque has been removed (Fig. 15-10). This requires good lighting. The patient can be provided with a disposable dental mirror for this purpose (Fig. 15-7, *B*). A good pen flashlight is very useful for this inspection (Fig. 15-7, *C*). A variety of other lighting aids are available for enhancing this inspection.

A very useful lamp is the one shown in Fig. 15-11. It has a magnifying mirror with the lamp below, which is directed into the mouth. Many dentists use this lamp or a similar one in their office when providing instructions for home care. This lamp can be purchased by the patient and is also excellent for home care.

Instruction cards. Fig. 15-12 is an example of a printed outline of instructions for home care that may be given to the parent or to the child. This card summarizes the home care instructions and serves as a guide for the parent in carrying out the routine. A blank space can be left for the child's name on the card, giving it a personal touch. Blanks are also left for the parent or child to mark each day the

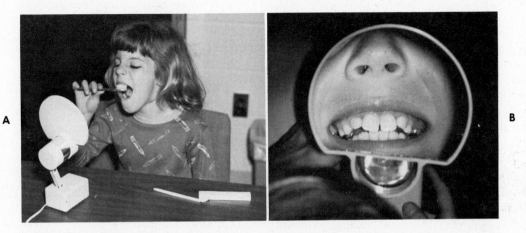

Fig. 15-11. A, Child brushing teeth using an electric lamp mirror. **B,** The electric lamp mirror efficiently illuminates the mouth for plaque identification and inspection.

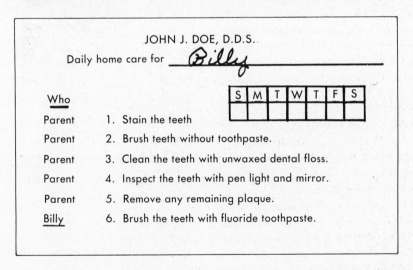

Fig. 15-12. Card that may be given to child or parent lists step-by-step instructions for daily cleaning of the teeth. Note that the child's name (Billy) has been placed in the blank spaces at the top and adjacent to step 6. The card may be taped to the bathroom mirror or wherever the teeth are cleaned.

instructions have been followed. Some dentists provide stars to be placed in the blocks as a motivating factor. Each card is good for 1 week. During active treatment the child may return the card to the office at each visit for the dentist or staff to see. This provides the opportunity for reinforcement.

For the older child a modification of the card may be used. Under the column "Who," blanks may be filled in by the dentist or the dental staff regarding who will do the steps.

Dental auxiliaries. A good preventive practice uses dental auxiliaries for the instruction program. Many dental hygienists and dental assistants are highly motivated and effective in their instructional programs with patients. However, dentists, hygienists, and assistants experience some degree of boredom or fatigue after instructing patients in home care day in and day out and may lose some enthusiasm and effectiveness. Some dentists have found that rotating the assignments for giving these instructions among the staff often reduces this problem.

Some dentists have also discovered that certain parents and older teenagers become highly motivated to good home care. Occasionally these individuals may be recruited to part-time employment as members of the staff to help instruct patients in home care. For example, a highly motivated teenager might be employed to teach home care for 2 hours a day after school hours. Patients scheduled for this purpose would be seen during this time. This is an especially useful arrangement if the dentist includes a reinforcement program.

Films. Many dentists find the use of dental health education films effective in teaching patients the causes of dental caries and periodontal disease.

The American Society of Dentistry for Children, the American Dental Association, and many commercial firms have made available a wide variety of films and brochures for use in instructing patients in good home care, including the use of disclosing tablets and solutions, toothbrushing techniques, and dental flossing techniques.

Individualized instruction. In the control of den-

tal disease for the individual patient the dentist must use knowledge of the prevention of dental disease and individualize the preventive program for the patient. If the patient has already had dental caries, the dentist should analyze the patient's diet and instruct the patient to correct the dietary intake (Chapter 16). The dentist may use a variety of caries activity tests to evaluate the problems of oral disease for each patient (Chapter 7).

• • •

Above all, if dentists and auxiliaries expect to be effective in the preventive program of their practice, they must be convinced of the importance of their program and must "practice what they preach."

REFERENCES

Badersten, A., Egelberg, J., and Koch, G.: Effect of monthly prophylaxis on caries and gingivitis in school children, Comm. Dent. Oral Epidemiol. **3:**1-4, 1975.

Bass, C.C.: The optimum characteristics of dental floss for personal oral hygiene, Dent. Items Int. **70:**921-934, 1948.

Bass, C.C.: The optimum characteristics of toothbrushes for personal oral hygiene, Dent. Items Int. **70:**697-718, 1948.

Bass, C.C.: An effective method of personal oral hygiene. II., J. La. State Med. Soc. **106:**100-112, 1954.

Bell, D.G.: Teaching home care to the patient, J. Periodontol. **19:**140-143, 1948.

Bennett, C.G.: Disclosing solutions for pedodontics, J. Dent. Child. **31:**131-134, 1964.

Blass, J.L.: Toothbrush instructions by a controlled method, N.Y. J. Dent. **19:**242-245, 1949.

Carlsson, J., Grahnen, H., and Jonsoon, G.: Lactobacilli and streptococci in the mouths of children, Caries Res. **9:**333, 1975.

Charters, W.J.: Eliminating mouth infections with the toothbrush and other stimulating instruments, Dent. Dig. **38:**130-136, 1932.

Conroy, C.W., and Melfi, R.C.: Comparison of automatic and hand toothbrushes: cleaning effectiveness for children, J. Dent. Child. **33:**219-225, 1966.

Coykendall, A.L.: "Swish and swallow" is effective, J. Dent. Child. **33:**162-163, 1966.

Curtis, G.H., McCall, C.M., Jr., and Overaa, H.I.: A clinical study of the effectiveness of the roll and Charters' method of brushing teeth, J. Periodontol. **28:**277-280, 1957.

Dudding, N.J., and Muhler, J.C.: What motivates children to practice good oral hygiene? J. Periodontol. **31:**141-142, 1960.

Fones, A.C.: Mouth hygiene, ed. 4, Philadelphia, 1934, Lea & Febiger.

Fosdick, L.S.: The etiology and control of dental caries, J.A.D.A. **29**:2132-2139, 1942.

Fosdick, L.S.: The reduction of the incidence of dental caries. I. Immediate toothbrushing with a neutral dentifrice, J.A.D.A. **40**:133-143, 1950.

Hall, A.W., and Conroy, C.W.: Comparison of automatic and hand toothbrushes: toothbrushing effectiveness for preschool children, J. Dent. Child. **38**:309-313, 1971.

Harris, C.A.: Cleanliness of the teeth, Am. J. Dent. Sci. **1**:9-12, ser. 1, No. 2, 1839-1841.

Hine, M.K.: Prophylaxis, toothbrushing, and home care of the mouth as caries control measures, J. Dent. Res. **27**:223-229, 1948.

Hine, M.K.: The use of the toothbrush in the treatment of periodontitis, J.A.D.A. **41**:158-168, 1950.

Hoover, D.R., and Robinson, H.B.G.: Effect of automatic and hand toothbrushing on gingivitis, J.A.D.A. **65**:361-367, 1962.

Horowitz, A.M., and others: Effect of supervised daily plaque removal by children: results after third and final year, J. Dent. Res. **56A**:85, 1977.

Huff, G.C., and Taylor, P.P.: Clinical evaluation of toothbrushes used in pedodontics, Tex. Dent. J. **83**:6-11, 1965.

Jordan, W.A., and Peterson, J.K.: Caries inhibiting value of a dentifrice containing stannous fluoride: final report of a two-year study, J.A.D.A. **58**:42-44, 1959.

Keller, M.J.: Personal communication, 1968.

Kimmelman, B., and Tassman, G.C.: Research in designs of children's toothbrushes, J. Dent. Child. **27**:60-64, 1960.

Klein, H.R.: Personal communication, 1968.

Lindhe, J., Axelsson, P., and Tollskog, G.: Effect of proper oral hygiene on gingivitis and dental caries in Swedish school-children, Comm. Dent. Oral Epidemiol. **3**:150-155, 1975.

Manly, R.S., and Brudevold, F.: Relative abrasiveness of natural and synthetic toothbrush bristles on cementum and dentin, J.A.D.A. **55**:779-780, 1957.

McCauley, H.B.: Toothbrushes, toothbrush materials and design, J.A.D.A. **33**:283-293, 1946.

McClure, D.B.: A comparison of toothbrushing technics for the preschool child, J. Dent. Child. **33**:205-210, 1966.

McDonald, R.E.: Effectiveness of a penicillin-containing dentifrice in the control of gingivitis and oral acid-producing microorganisms, J. Dent. Child. **20**:47-51, 1953.

Moore, R.M.: A study of the effect of water fluoride content and socioeconomic status on the occurrence of gingivitis in school children, thesis, Indianapolis, 1963, Indiana University School of Dentistry.

Muhler, J.C., and others: The effect of a stannous fluoride-containing dentifrice on caries reduction in children, J. Dent. Res. **33**:606-612, 1954.

Muhler, J.C., and others: The effect of a stannous fluoride-containing dentifrice on caries reduction in children. II. Caries experience after one year, J.A.D.A. **50**:163-166, 1955.

Nowak, A.J.: Dentistry for the handicapped patient, St. Louis, 1976, The C.V. Mosby Co., pp. 167-192.

Oldenberg, T.R., and Wells, H.B.: The effectiveness of the electric toothbrush in reducing oral debris in handicapped children, I.A.D.R. (abs.) **41**:86, 1963.

Peffley, G., and Muhler, J.C.: Effect of a commercial stannous fluoride dentifrice with controlled brushing on caries in children, J. Dent. Res. (abs.) **38**:670-671, 1959.

Peterson, J.K., and Jordan, W.A.: Caries-inhibiting value of a dentifrice containing stannous fluoride: first year report of a supervised toothbrushing study, J.A.D.A. **54**:589-594, 1957.

Quigley, G.A., and Hein, J.W.: Comparative cleansing efficiency of manual and power brushing, J.A.D.A. **65**:26-29, 1962.

Sangnes, G., Zachrisson, B., and Gjermo, P.: Effectiveness of vertical and horizontal brushing techniques in plaque removal, J. Dent. Child. **39**:94-97, 1972.

Shick, R.A., and Ash, M.M., Jr.: Evaluation of the vertical method of toothbrushing, J. Periodontol. **32**:346-353, 1961.

Silverstein, S., and others: Effect of supervised deplaquing on dental caries, gingivitis and plaque, J. Dent. Res. **56A**:85, 1977.

Smith, T.S.: Anatomic and physiologic conditions governing the use of the toothbrush, J.A.D.A. **27**:874-878, 1940.

Starkey, P.E.: Instructions to parents for brushing the child's teeth, J. Dent. Child. **28**:42-47, 1961.

Stephan, R.M.: Changes in hydrogen-ion concentration on tooth surfaces and in carious lesions, J.A.D.A. **27**:718-723, 1940.

Stillman, P.R.: A philosophy of the treatment of periodontal disease, Dent. Dig. **38**:314-319, 1932.

Suomi, J.D.: Prevention and control of periodontal disease, J.A.D.A. **83**:1271-1287, 1971.

Swartz, M.L., and Phillips, R.W.: Effects of diameter of nylon bristles on enamel surface, J.A.D.A. **47**:20-26, 1953.

Swartz, M.L., and Phillips, R.W.: Effect of certain factors upon toothbrush bristle stiffness, J. Periodontol. **27**:96-101, 1956.

University of California School of Dentistry: Developing a plaque control program, Berkeley, Calif., 1972, Praxis Publishing Co.

Volker J.F., and Klapper, C.E.: Some observations on dental caries in Syrian hamsters, Oral Surg. **7**:207-212, 1954.

Weddell, J.A., and Klein, A.I.: Socioeconomic correlation of oral disease in six to thirty-six month children, Pediatr. Dent. **3**:306-310, 1981.

Wright, G.Z., Banting, D.W., and Feasby, W.H.: Effect of interdental flossing in the incidence of proximal caries in children, J. Dent. Res. **56**:574-578, 1977.

Wright, G.Z., Feasby, W.H., and Banting, D.B.: The effectiveness of interdental flossing with and without a fluoride dentifrice, Pediatr. Dent. **2**:105-109, 1980.

16 Nutrition and dental health

DAVID K. HENNON

In many of the medical and dental specialties, nutrition still is not receiving enough emphasis. Perhaps this is because some practitioners think nutrition is too elementary to be considered an important part of a professional practice or because nutritional counseling has shown little or no success. In the latter instance this is understandable because improvement in the nutritional status of the individual often is not readily obvious. In the former instance those who regard nutrition as elementary perhaps have not considered the complicated and intricate role of macronutrients and micronutrients in intermediary cellular metabolism.

A general definition of nutrition is the science that deals with food and nutrients and their role in attaining and maintaining health. Nutrition is certainly a basic science, as well as an applied science, and it embraces many other scientific disciplines, such as biochemistry, physiology, endocrinology, enzymology, microbiology, animal husbandry, and food technology.

It is the purpose of this chapter to relate certain aspects of nutrition to the dental practice. Less emphasis is placed on the mechanics of dietary surveys, counseling, and education because this material is discussed in Chapter 7. Attention is devoted instead to the role of nutrients in growth and development, methods of judging nutritional status, and factors affecting the intake of recommended nutrients.

Importance of nutrition

How is the question, "Why do you consider nutrition an important part of your practice?" answered by dental practitioners? An answer often given is, "Because of the role of proper food selection and intake in controlling dental caries." This aspect of nutrition is of course important, but in light of present knowledge the practitioner should consider the importance of nutrition not only to the oral cavity but to the health and happiness of the individual, family, community, and nation.

The dentist can no longer regard the scope of nutrition to be only a matter of selective dietary counseling for individual patients. The world situation in regard to food supply is such that in the future long-established food habits or preferences and subsequently dietary counseling may require significant modification because of the increasing demand for foodstuffs.

Malnutrition is widespread in most Third World countries. There is an ever-increasing prevalence of protein-calorie malnutrition, which primarily affects infants and young children. Current evidence shows that a significant number of women of reproductive age are also undernourished. With the present rate of increase in the world population, all nations will ultimately be faced with providing subsistence levels of nutrition for their citizens. A global nutrition crisis will result if new food sources are not found and if improved agricultural techniques and methods of food preservation and distribution are not developed.

In areas where the food supply is abundant the threat of a dwindling food supply seems remote. However, even in these areas not all individuals enjoy the proper food nutrients that are available. There are many causes for this, such as socioeconomic status, poor food habits, and religious and social customs. Even in the midst of plenty many people may be malnourished.

The report of the Ten State Nutritional Survey in the United States indicates that iron-deficiency anemia is a major nutritional problem in most of the groups studied. Blood levels of vitamin A, ascorbic acid, and riboflavin were below normal in poverty groups, minority groups, and children under 10 years of age.

It is claimed that adolescents have the poorest dietary intake of the general population, yet their nutritional health is reasonably good. However, recent surveys continue to show that teenage diets are usually deficient in iron, calcium, riboflavin, and vitamin A. Over 50% of the female teenagers surveyed ate less than two thirds of the recommended dietary allowances for iron, calcium, and vitamin A. This is of concern because of the trend toward earlier marriages and teenage pregnancies.

Obesity is another nutritional problem in the United States. This is especially serious when the relationship of obesity to cardiovascular disease, hypertension, and diabetes is considered. Adolescent obesity is of particular concern because the risks to health and longevity are similar to those of the adult. The psychologic and social aspects of obesity are also serious. Adolescent obesity may lead to body image disturbances, poor self-concepts, and cases of disturbed personality.

Osteoporosis is common in the elderly, particularly women. Several studies have suggested that a low calcium intake over many years may be a significant etiologic factor in this condition.

How does the preceding discussion relate to dentistry? First, researchers are attempting to find other sources of food; therefore our concepts of what constitutes a food may change drastically in the next several years. High-protein flours have been developed from plant seeds and from ground fish. Algae have been tried as food, primarily for animals but also for humans. Second, because many people have poor food habits, counseling the young dental patient in what constitutes an ade-

quate diet and how to achieve it should materially improve the public's awareness of the importance of good nutrition.

Role of nutrition in growth and development

Some pedodontists and general practitioners who treat children suggest that a child's first routine dental visit occur as soon as convenient for the parents but no later than 12 to 18 months of age. At this time the dentist has an excellent opportunity to observe the child during one of the most dynamic growth periods. The practitioner's influence may help the parents establish good nutrition and oral hygiene practices for the child. A discussion of nursing caries would be appropriate during the counseling session.

Sound dietary counseling at this point is important, since proper eating habits, started early in life, greatly influence the health of the individual in later years. For example, a nutritional study in adolescent boys showed that a modification of dietary fats and cholesterol lowered blood cholesterol levels. Thus one of the important risk factors in atherosclerotic disease was partially controlled. It is also recognized that early malnutrition causes retarded physical growth and may impair learning and negatively influence behavior.

A basic understanding of the growth process is vital in the clinical evaluation of the child patient. A discussion of growth of the face and dental arches is presented in Chapters 18 and 20.

When the pattern of growth as determined by the rate of increase in body weight is graphed, a growth curve is obtained, as shown in Fig. 16-1. The most rapid rate of growth occurs in the prenatal and early infancy period. From about 2 to 5 years of age the rate of growth diminishes; then there is a slight acceleration of growth around 6 to 8 years of age. This acceleration is known as the prepubertal growth spurt. At the time of puberty, which occurs around 9 to 12 years of age in girls and 12 to 15 years of age in boys, the last major period of growth and development takes place.

During the period of decreasing growth rate (from 2 to 5 years of age) the appetite of many

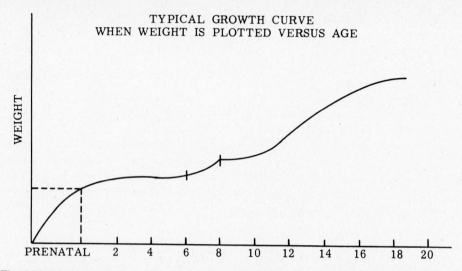

Fig. 16-1. The most rapid rate of growth occurs in the prenatal and early infancy period. From about 2 to 5 years of age, the rate of growth diminishes; then there is a slight acceleration of growth between 6 and 8 years of age. This acceleration is known as the "prepubertal growth spurt." At the time of puberty, which occurs around 9 to 12 years of age in girls and 12 to 15 years of age in boys, the last major period of growth and development takes place.

children may be decreased because of the lowered physiologic demands for food. Often, because of parental pressure, feeding problems develop in these children. How effective, then, is a nutrition counseling session with the parent during which an attempt is made to explain that a decrease in the refined carbohydrate intake is desirable for the dental health of the child? The parent is happy when the child can be induced to eat any food at all. A more detailed discussion concerning feeding problems in children is presented later in the chapter.

If a child is provided with adequate nutrients for growth, within normal limits a general trend of growth can be expected in that child. If the expected growth pattern does not occur, some factor has disturbed the growth process. Numerous factors, such as decreased food intake, disease, genetic factors, and emotional problems, may disrupt the normal growth pattern. Any deviation from the normal growth pattern can be detected more readily when a child is observed, weighed, and measured at regular intervals. In infants and young children, mea-

surements of weight and height are excellent parameters for the assessment of growth and the judgment of nutritional status.

Judging nutritional status

Even though the dentist's responsibility primarily concerns the oral health of the patient, the practitioner should be aware that the systemic condition of the child is partially reflected in the oral condition. Therefore some background in appraising the total health and nutritional status of the child will aid immeasurably in the overall assessment.

There are several ways to judge nutritional status, none of which would alone be completely adequate. However, two methods that are available to all practitioners are the clinical evaluation and the diet survey.

Clinical evaluation. Although a complete physical examination of the patient is not within the scope of the dentist, many things can be learned about the patient by observing the physical appearance and asking the parent a few well-chosen questions concerning eating, sleeping, and hygiene habits. Healthy, normal children should have a fairly regular pattern of eating, sleeping, and other physiologic functions. If a parent mentions that the child does not rest well or is nervous and emotional, the dentist could suspect that the child may have a feeding problem as well. Observation of the skin, hair, nails, and muscle tone can provide clues as to whether the child is well nourished. During the routine oral examination, observation of the mucous membranes can give an indication of the child's level of nutrition. For example, anemic conditions may cause the buccal mucosa to be paler than normal. Deficiencies of vitamins, such as thiamin, riboflavin, or niacin, may result in a reddened, angry-looking mucosa.

Diet survey. The use of a diet survey not only is valuable from the standpoint of providing information regarding eating habits and their relation to dental caries but also may show deficiencies of nutrient intake that result in a substandard level of nutrition. When the diet survey is used, however, it must be remembered that this type of subjective acquisition of information is of little value if the patient or parent ''pads'' the survey to make it look good.

When the diet survey is analyzed, it is helpful to assess the adequacy of the total diet by comparing it with the recommended dietary allowances and the basic four food groups. However, these references are for average groups and not necessarily for individuals. Therefore they should not be used as an absolute standard. If a patient's survey does not attain these standards, it does not necessarily mean that the child is malnourished. A deficient intake accompanied by clinical signs of malnutrition would be more positive evidence that a state of poor nutrition exists.

The practitioner who believes that the diet survey analysis is too time consuming to use in a busy practice may wish to consider one of the commercially available computer-analyzed diet surveys. The same pitfalls exist as with any other form of diet survey that depends on the patient to supply accurate information. However, if the diet survey presented for computer analysis is reasonably accurate, different aspects of the patient's dietary habits can be easily compared. For example: How frequently is between-meal food eaten? How many solid and liquid cariogenic foods are eaten? How does the patient's intake of the basic four food groups compare with the recommended levels?

Other ways of judging nutritional status are biochemical tests and growth charts and graphs. These methods are generally not well adapted for use in the dental office.

Factors affecting the intake of recommended nutrients

There are several reasons why people do not have a well-balanced diet. In children, one major reason is a feeding problem that has been induced at home or that has been caused by misconceptions about child feeding practices.

Rust has written an excellent article on this subject. He believes that all aspects of an adequate diet are important when considering feeding habits of children. It is during childhood that the greatest good or evil, nutritionally speaking, is accomplished. Rust has stated that more eventual health benefits can be provided for the United States as a whole through proper nutrition of infants and young children than by any other combined efforts of the medical and dental professions.

An adequate supply of food is not a problem in the United States—there is an overabundance of food. The problem is *how* food is fed and not *what* is fed. Many parents complain, ''My child just doesn't eat.'' This remark can be interpreted to mean that the child's intake is not sufficient to satisfy the adults in the family. Often some of the most malnourished children are to be found in families of higher socioeconomic levels. A feeding problem in an orphanage is the exception rather than the rule.

If there is emotional conflict at mealtime, the children sit sullenly awaiting the end of the ordeal so that they may leave the table and satisfy their hunger peacefully with crackers and cookies, away from the stress and strain of parental influence.

Many beliefs concerning child nutrition are incorrect and may do appreciable harm. For instance, it is widely believed that children should be given increasing amounts of food as they become older and more active. However, the child's growth rate rather than activity largely determines the appetite. When the growth rate decreases, the appetite also decreases. It is frequently believed that all that is needed for a child to be well nourished is a quart of milk daily, regardless of the child's age, likes or dislikes, or capacity. This much milk during the preschool years may interfere with the eating of solid foods. Also, it encourages the eating of excessive amounts of starch foods and sweets, which are "washed down" so conveniently. One to 1½ pints of milk a day is sufficient for most children until adolescence, provided the diet is balanced in other respects.

Many people think that children need vegetables in large quantities to get vitamins and minerals. Although a variety of vegetables should be included in a well-chosen diet, children frequently refuse vegetables at certain ages. When this occurs, fruit may be substituted, since some children find it more palatable than vegetables.

Minerals, especially calcium, and vitamins have received so much emphasis that many people think they serve as substitutes for food. These are essential food factors, but they are not substitutes for a well-balanced diet, which usually contains most of the required minerals and vitamins.

At one time the lack of emphasis on adequate protein intake made it seem unimportant in childhood nutrition. However, protein is very important because only protein provides the nutrients necessary for growth, for protection against infection, for building of red blood cells, enzymes, and hormones, and for many other important functions. Milk is probably the most important food in infancy, but with the beginning of the second year it becomes less important. The toddler who drinks milk and eats no solid protein foods frequently has an insufficient intake of protein and other necessary nutrients. Because milk is bulky, it satisfies hunger and decreases the desire for solid protein foods.

Many parents are concerned about their child's eating habits and are convinced the child will starve and lose weight unless forced to eat. However, no child of normal intelligence will starve when food is available. If a child is forced to eat, a true dislike for eating at mealtime may develop and the child will fill up on soft drinks, cookies, crackers, sandwiches, and confections between meals.

Some parents do not like their child to go hungry and believe the child should be kept full of food of one kind or another at all times. Actually, the satisfaction of hunger at mealtime is a pleasure, but many parents who would like nothing better than to see their children sit down and eat a hearty meal do not permit them to become hungry enough to do so.

Many think that children will choose a sound diet of their own accord, regardless of what foods are made available. Rust has pointed out that many children, particularly those who have developed a dislike for eating at mealtime because of forcing, will consume unbalanced, harmful diets if permitted to eat what and when they choose. In these children true cases of malnutrition may develop.

Rust has listed the following basic rules that, if properly understood and practiced, should eliminate most feeding difficulties in healthy children:

1. Avoid forced feedings that may result in the development of hatred for foods and a decreased food intake.
2. Discourage between-meal eating so that good eating habits will be established and dental caries will be prevented and controlled.
3. Avoid discussion that attaches undue importance to a particular food. Using dessert as a bribe to have the child eat vegetables is as ineffectual as using bribes for good behavior in other activities.
4. Avoid excessive milk intake, which only serves to reduce the hunger and natural desire for other basic foods.
5. Avoid excessive intake of refined carbohydrates, which are too often permitted to merely satisfy the child's hunger.
6. Make mealtime a pleasant family social event, with food incidental. This approach will bring

about many benefits, not only in better nutritional results but often in relaxed tensions and improved behavior patterns of the child as well.

From a practical point of view the education of parents in the correct psychologic approach to solving nutritional problems of children is the most important consideration. Medical and dental practitioners must understand the basic principles of nutrition in order that they may guide and correctly advise the parents with whom they have contact.

Other factors affecting the intake of recommended nutrients are food faddism and nutritional misinformation. The multibillion dollar "health foods" business is supported by persons who buy food supplements, special foods, or special cooking implements purported to be essential in maintaining a safe nutrient intake. Extravagant claims are made for the magical properties of certain foods or food combinations in preventing or curing diseases or abnormal conditions, such as cancer, arthritis, heart disease, diabetes, dandruff, and flat feet. Some diet reducing plans are poorly designed and may induce nutrient deficiencies if followed for prolonged periods.

Poor eating habits are deterrents to obtaining a satisfactory nutrient intake. Many habits are learned at home and are perpetuated from generation to generation. Children tend to imitate the food likes or dislikes of their parents. Therefore a child will be unreceptive to suggestions to modify eating habits if the parent does not set an example.

Food customs and taboos based on religious or ethnic beliefs may be a factor in preventing the ingestion of the necessary nutrients. Successful dietary counseling of a person of any culture or subculture requires an understanding of the food habits of the group. Often the method of cooking is a significant factor in decreasing the nutrient value of foods and thus the adequacy of the diet. For example, minerals and vitamins are lost if the water used to cook vegetables is discarded. The use of copper-lined (not copper-clad) pots and pans causes the destruction of several nutrients.

Persons living alone may develop poor eating habits and fail to follow a well-balanced diet. This results from the lack of social contact during mealtime and the bother of "fixing a meal just for one."

Constituents of an adequate diet

The nutrients have been classified into six major groups: proteins, carbohydrates, lipids, vitamins, minerals, and water. All of these are required daily to promote optimum growth, to maintain body tissues, and to regulate metabolic function.

Early research in nutrition was directed toward determining the factors necessary for health and the quantity of each nutrient required. Although much progress has been made in this regard, nutritional researchers have not yet determined the level of some nutrients required for daily maintenance. However, from the information that has been obtained, certain standards have been established.

Since 1940 the Food and Nutrition Board of the National Research Council has developed formulations of nutrient intake judged to be sufficient to maintain good nutrition in the U.S. population. The efforts of the Board resulted in the establishment of the "National Research Council Recommended Dietary Allowances" (Table 16-1), which was first published in 1943. The allowances are intended to aid in planning for food supplies and to guide the interpretation of food intake records of population groups. The nutritional status of groups or individuals must be judged on the basis of physical, biochemical, and clinical observations along with evaluations of food or nutrient intake.

The allowances are only recommendations for the amounts of nutrients that should be ingested each day. They are not estimates of quantities needed per capita in the national or local food supply or in food purchased, and they should not be confused with nutrient requirements. Also, the recommended allowances do not apply to special nutrient needs that result from infections, metabolic disorders, chronic diseases, or other conditions requiring specific dietary treatment.

Proteins. Proteins are nutrients specifically required by the body for growth, tissue repair, and synthesis of many constituents of the body, such as antibodies, hormones, and enzymes. The signifi-

Table 16-1. Food and Nutrition Board, National Academy of Sciences–National Research Council Recommended Daily Dietary Allowances,* Revised 1980.

Designed for the maintenance of good nutrition of practically all healthy people in the U.S.A.

	Age (years)	Weight (kg)	Weight (lb)	Height (cm)	Height (in)	Protein (g)	Fat-Soluble Vitamins Vitamin A (µg RE)†	Fat-Soluble Vitamins Vitamin D (µg)‡	Fat-Soluble Vitamins Vitamin E (mg α-TE)§	Vitamin C (mg)	Thiamin (mg)	
Infants	0.0-0.5	6	13	60	24	kg × 2.2	420	10	3	35	0.3	
	0.5-1.0	9	20	71	28	kg × 2.0	400	10	4	35	0.5	
Children	1-3	13	29	90	35	23	400	10	5	45	0.7	
	4-6	20	44	112	44	30	500	10	6	45	0.9	
	7-10	28	62	132	52	34	700	10	7	45	1.2	
Males	11-14	45	99	157	62	45	1000	10	8	50	1.4	
	15-18	66	145	176	69	56	1000	10	10	60	1.4	
	19-22	70	154	177	70	56	1000	7.5	10	60	1.5	
	23-50	70	154	178	70	56	1000	5	10	60	1.4	
	51+	70	154	178	70	56	1000	5	10	60	1.2	
Females	11-14	46	101	157	62	46	800	10	8	50	1.1	
	15-18	55	120	163	64	46	800	10	8	60	1.1	
	19-22	55	120	163	64	44	800	7.5	8	60	1.1	
	23-50	55	120	163	64	44	800	5	8	60	1.0	
	51+	55	120	163	64	44	800	5	8	60	1.0	
Pregnant						+30	+200	+5	+2	+20	+0.4	
Lactating						+20	+400	+5	+3	+40	+0.5	

From Food and Nutrition Board, National Academy of Sciences–National Research Council: Recommended dietary allowances, ed. 9, Washington, D.C., 1980.

*The allowances are intended to provide for individual variations among most normal persons as they live in the United States under usual environmental stresses. Diets should be based on a variety of common foods in order to provide other nutrients for which human requirements have been less well defined.

†Retinol equivalents. 1 retinol equivalent = 1 µg retinol or 6 µg β carotene.

‡As cholecalciferol. 10 µg cholecalciferol = 400 IU of vitamin D.

§α-tocopherol equivalents. 1 mg d-α tocopherol = 1 α-TE.

||1 NE (niacin equivalent) is equal to 1 mg of niacin or 60 mg of dietary tryptophan.

cance of proteins is reflected in the name, which, derived from the Greek, means "of first importance." Biochemically, proteins are chains of amino acids joined together in a characteristic bonding known as the "peptide linkage." The individual characteristics of each protein are determined by the number, sequence, and spatial arrangement of the amino acids comprising the protein.

Proteins are classified according to their biologic value, which is determined by the "completeness" of the amino acids and the degree of utilization. Proteins that are absent or deficient in certain amino acids are said to be incomplete and thus are lower in biologic value than proteins that have all the amino acids present in a proportion favorable for best utilization.

There are 22 amino acids that, in varying proportions and combinations, form the proteins. Those that cannot be synthesized in the body to meet daily requirements are termed "indispensable." Those that can be formed by the degradation of an indispensable amino acid, such as tyrosine from phenylalanine, are labeled "semidispensable." Those that are synthesized in the body in amounts sufficient to meet daily requirements

Water-Soluble Vitamins					Minerals					
Ribo-flavin (mg)	Niacin (mg NE)‖	Vita-min B_6 (mg)	Fola-cin¶ (μg)	Vitamin B_{12} (μg)	Cal-cium (mg)	Phos-phorus (mg)	Mag-nesium (mg)	Iron (mg)	Zinc (mg)	Iodine (μg)
0.4	6	0.3	30	0.5**	360	240	50	10	3	40
0.6	8	0.6	45	1.5	540	360	70	15	5	50
0.8	9	0.9	100	2.0	800	800	150	15	10	70
1.0	11	1.3	200	2.5	800	800	200	10	10	90
1.4	16	1.6	300	3.0	800	800	250	10	10	120
1.6	18	1.8	400	3.0	1200	1200	350	18	15	150
1.7	18	2.0	400	3.0	1200	1200	400	18	15	150
1.7	19	2.2	400	3.0	800	800	350	10	15	150
1.6	18	2.2	400	3.0	800	800	350	10	15	150
1.4	16	2.2	400	3.0	800	800	350	10	15	150
1.3	15	1.8	400	3.0	1200	1200	300	18	15	150
1.3	14	2.0	400	3.0	1200	1200	300	18	15	150
1.3	14	2.0	400	3.0	800	800	300	18	15	150
1.2	13	2.0	400	3.0	800	800	300	18	15	150
1.2	13	2.0	400	3.0	800	800	300	10	15	150
+0.3	+2	+0.6	+400	+1.0	+400	+400	+150	*h*††	+5	+25
+0.5	+5	+0.5	+100	+1.0	+400	+400	+150	*h*††	+10	+50

¶The folacin allowances refer to dietary sources as determined by *Lactobacillus casei* assay after treatment with enzymes (conjugases) to make polyglutamyl forms of the vitamin available to the test organism.

**The recommended dietary allowance for vitamin B_{12} in infants is based on average concentration of the vitamin in human milk. The allowances after weaning are based on energy intake (as recommended by the American Academy of Pediatrics) and consideration of other factors, such as intestinal absorption.

††The increased requirement during pregnancy cannot be met by the iron content of habitual American diets nor by the existing iron stores of many women; therefore the use of 30-60 mg of supplemental iron is recommended. Iron needs during lactation are not substantially different from those of nonpregnant women, but continued supplementation of the mother for 2-3 months after parturition is advisable in order to replenish stores depleted by pregnancy.

are called ''dispensable.'' This term is misleading, however, since it implies that there is no need to obtain these amino acids from a well-selected, adequate diet. To promote optimum protein synthesis, all amino acids should be present in favorable ratios. To accomplish this, it is much more efficient to obtain the amino acids through a well-chosen, adequate diet than to depend on the synthesis of the missing semidispensable or dispensable amino acid from the indispensable amino acids within the body.

In general, animal proteins are more complete and of higher biologic value than plant proteins.

Typical examples of good sources of animal proteins are meats, eggs, fish, milk, and other dairy products. Examples of plant protein sources are the grains, such as wheat, rye, corn, and oats, and the legumes, such as soybeans or other types of dried beans. Although these latter sources of proteins are often deficient in one or more of the indispensable amino acids such as lysine, tryptophan, or methionine, the ingestion of these foods along with some form of animal protein or with other carefully selected types of plant protein provides adequate amounts of all the amino acids. It is easier to obtain the necessary amount of protein by including some type of animal protein in the diet each day than by relying solely on plant sources.

The need for protein varies according to the conditions present. During the first month of life, 2.2 g/kg of body weight/day is the estimated amount required to provide a satisfactory growth rate. This level decreases to 2 g/kg/day by the sixth month. The recommended intake for the normal adult is about 0.8 g/kg/day. During pregnancy and lactation the daily protein need is greater. The allowances suggest increasing the recommended daily intake an additional 30 g during pregnancy and 20 g during lactation. During periods of convalescence from a condition that has caused nitrogen loss, the needs for both protein and energy are increased, just as they are during periods of rapid growth.

Carbohydrates. Regardless of the role of some carbohydrates in causing dental caries, the importance of carbohydrates in nutrition is great.

The carbohydrates include the starches, sugars, gums, and dextrins. On hydrolysis, the more complex carbohydrates yield the simple sugars. These sugars are the monosaccharides (glucose, fructose, galactose), the disaccharides (sucrose, maltose, lactose), and the polysaccharides (starches, celluloses). The carbohydrates of major nutritional significance are the disaccharides and starches. The disaccharides are readily hydrolyzed to the constituent monosaccharides. The starches are hydrolyzed to the simple sugars but require a longer period of time for this conversion.

The major function of carbohydrates is to provide energy for the chemical work of the body. In addition, the carbohydrates, especially the dextrins, provide an environment for the promotion of a favorable intestinal flora. Psychologically, the carbohydrates play an important role. They are needed to provide ''something sweet'' or ''something filling,'' cravings that have been experienced by everyone. However, it is this function of carbohydrates that is so detrimental to dental health. It is difficult to convince young patients or their parents that the constant craving for ''something sweet'' will result in a deleterious dental condition that will affect their health.

Every effort should be made to have the patient completely cease between-meal eating of refined carbohydrates. However, not all carbohydrates should be removed from the diet. Growing children have a need for energy that is great in comparison with that of adults. To suggest that a child refrain from eating carbohydrates would be detrimental. Nutritional counseling ideally should be directed toward finding suitable substitutes for the refined carbohydrates so that energy needs can be met.

The need for energy is also a good reason to discourage the excessive use of low-calorie beverages by young people in an attempt to control dental caries. These beverages have no food value, and an adequate diet may not be eaten at mealtime.

Carbohydrates are present in all foods in varying amounts, but the major sources are the grains and the products made from them (such as cereals, bread, crackers, spaghetti, and macaroni) and the starchy plants (such as potatoes, corn, peas, and beans). A considerable amount of carbohydrate in the form of lactose is obtained from milk.

Lipids. Lipids or fats, when considered as foodstuffs, are neutral fats (esters of fatty acids with glycerol). The whole family of compounds called lipids, however, includes the fats and other compounds that resemble them in physical properties. Simple lipids are neutral fats and waxes; however, cholesterol, vitamin A esters, and vitamin D esters are also classified as waxes. Compound lipids include the phospholipids, the glycolipids, and the sulfolipids. There are also derived lipids (from the simple and compound lipids), certain types of alcohols (such as sterols and carotenols), and certain hydrocarbons (such as squalene, carotenoids, and vitamins D, E, and K) that belong to the class of compounds known as the lipids.

The main function of dietary fat is to supply energy in a fairly condensed form. One gram of fat furnishes about 9 calories to the body, whereas 1 g of protein or carbohydrate furnishes only about 4 calories. In addition, fats supply the essential fatty acids that are needed by the body for optimum growth and maintenance of tissue. Fats also serve as vehicles for the fat-soluble vitamins that are obtained naturally in foods.

Like the carbohydrates, fats fulfill a psychologic role in nutrition. Meals without fat are tasteless or unappealing and lack satiety value. Although excess fat should be avoided, some fat, either naturally present in foods, such as meats, or in the form of spreads or salad dressings, adds much to the satisfaction of a meal.

The relationship of dietary fats to atherosclerosis is important, since heart disease is the leading cause of death in the United States and some other countries. The cause of atherosclerosis has not been determined conclusively. The available information does suggest that it is desirable to reduce the percentage of fat in the diet to about 30%, and, of this amount, to increase the ratio of polyunsaturated fatty acids to the saturated fatty acids. In practical terms this means being more conservative with the use of fats and using more vegetable oils than animal fats.

A person who is consuming a balanced diet, maintaining a desirable weight, and getting adequate exercise does not need to worry about a normal intake of foods with high cholesterol or saturated fat content. These foods are not risk factors in balanced diets.

Vitamins. Perhaps no other area of nutrition is as intriguing as the vitamins. This is primarily because of the relatively recent discovery of many of the vitamins and because the results of solitary deficiencies of some vitamins are so vividly demonstrated in experimental animals and in humans.

Vitamins can be defined as accessory food factors, necessary daily in trace amounts to maintain the cellular integrity of the body. What is implied in the definition is that these accessory food factors must be ingested from exogenous sources. Generally, the body does not synthesize the vitamins in amounts sufficient to meet the daily needs. Some vitamins, however, can be synthesized in the body in amounts that significantly augment the levels ingested in food. For example, vitamin K is synthesized in the intestines by the bacterial flora; about half the vitamin K in humans is estimated to be of intestinal origin. Vitamin D can be easily synthesized by the action of sunlight on a vitamin

D precursor in the skin, but many variables cause the amount formed to be inadequate to fulfill daily needs. For example, heavily pigmented skin stops about 95% of ultraviolet radiation from reaching the deeper layers where vitamin D is synthesized. Seasonal variations in the amount of sunlight and areas of atmospheric pollution also affect the amount of ultraviolet energy available for this conversion.

The vitamins are classified according to their extraction with ether or water into the fat-soluble vitamins (A, D, E, and K) and the water-soluble vitamins (B complex and C).

Fat-soluble vitamins. The health of the tissues of epithelial origin, such as the skin, hair, eyes, and mucosal epithelium, is associated with *vitamin A*. It is sometimes known as the anti-infection vitamin, probably because of its role in maintaining the integrity of the ciliated epithelium in the respiratory tract rather than any special property in preventing infection. It is important in tooth formation because of the epithelial origin of the enamel organ. Vitamin A deficiency has been shown to cause cleft palate in rats and swine.

Deficiencies of vitamin A cause changes in the skin and eyes as well as internal changes in organ systems. Nyctalopia, xerophthalmia, and keratomalacia are eye changes associated with vitamin A deficiency. The skin becomes dry and scaly with follicular hyperkeratosis.

Since vitamin A is stored in the liver, production of a deficiency requires several months. Vitamin A occurs naturally or as a precursor in many foods. Therefore, except in severe malnutrition or prolonged dietary inadequacy, a vitamin A deficiency is unlikely to occur. Vitamin A occurs in milk, eggs, and meat, especially liver. Precursors in the form of carotene and other carotenoids are found in the yellow pigmented vegetables, such as carrots, pumpkin, squash, and cantaloupe, and in the dark green leafy vegetables, such as broccoli, kale, and spinach.

Vitamin D is known as the antirachitic vitamin. It is related chemically to cholesterol, and one precursor, 7-dehydrocholesterol, is found in the skin. The action of sunlight changes the 7-dehydrocholesterol to an active form of vitamin D that in adults may provide adequate amounts of the vitamin (as long as there is no interference with the ultraviolet radiation needed to reach the skin precursor).

Vitamin D is necessary for normal calcification of osseous tissues and is important in the development of healthy bones and teeth. A deficiency of vitamin D in children is one of the causes of rickets. A vitamin D deficiency in adults results in osteomalacia. The primary defect in vitamin D deficiency is a failure of calcification of bone matrix.

The sources of vitamin D are not as many or as varied as those of vitamin A. Before the fortification of milk and other foods with irradiated ergosterol (vitamin D_2 or calciferol), rickets was a common disease. The use of vitamin D–fortified milk was a major factor in reducing the prevalence. Today, except in isolated cases of malnutrition, the disease is virtually nonexistent.

The widespread fortification of infant foods with vitamin D is not without its hazards, however. Although most of the B-complex vitamins and ascorbic acid are relatively nontoxic in extremely high doses, the fat-soluble vitamins, especially vitamins A and D, do cause toxic symptoms if ingested in great amounts for a period of several weeks. Compared with vitamin A, the margin of safety between the recommended daily intake and the toxic level is much less for vitamin D. In Great Britain many infant foods are fortified with vitamin D. A few years ago, during a 2-year period, more than 200 cases of idiopathic hypercalcemia of infancy were observed. This condition was associated with vitamin D intakes of as much as 4000 IU daily, mainly as calciferol added to infant foods.

Vitamin E is sometimes referred to as the antisterility vitamin because it prevents atrophy of the gonads and spontaneous abortions in rats. However, its role in human reproduction has not been determined.

Vitamin E is important as an antioxidant. It thus protects vitamin A, which is easily destroyed by oxidation. The antioxidant properties of vitamin E may also prevent the hemolysis of erythrocytes by tissue peroxides. This function of vitamin E is regarded as the first clearly demonstrated role of the essentiality of vitamin E in human nutrition.

Vitamin E deficiency has been observed only in adults with chronic failure to absorb fat. No specific clinical symptoms were noticed. However, laboratory tests showed increased fragility of red blood cells, increased urinary excretion of creatine, indicative of muscle loss, and deposition of ceroid pigment in the muscle of the small intestine.

Some nutrients achieve widespread popularity because of uncorroborated reports showing them to be effective in curing certain abnormal conditions. Vitamin E is one of these. The number of maladies that vitamin E is supposed to cure is limited only by the imagination. Vitamin E is purported to relieve menstrual problems, soften and remove old scars, increase stamina and energy, prevent angina pectoris, protect the lungs from air contaminants, treat cystic fibrosis and muscular dystrophy, and be an effective topical agent in cosmetics. However, the only valid therapeutic uses for vitamin E are in the treatment of hemolytic anemia in premature babies and deficiencies caused by malabsorption of fats and oils. Otherwise, vitamin E is not responsible for any of the miracle cures that are ascribed to it. Because the diet provides adequate levels of vitamin E, a normal, healthy individual need not resort to vitamin E supplements.

The best sources of vitamin E are the seed grain oils, such as wheat germ oil; oysters and eggs are also good sources of this vitamin.

Vitamin K is known as the antihemorrhagic vitamin. Because of its role in the blood-clotting mechanism, its discoverer, Dam, called it vitamin K to indicate "Koagulating vitamin." In a deficiency of vitamin K, plasma prothrombin activity is decreased, which in turn increases the clotting time of the blood. Therefore serious hemorrhages may occur in vitamin K deficiency.

Newborn infants often have decreased prothrombin levels. To prevent a condition known as hemorrhagic disease of the newborn, vitamin K is given to the mother during labor or to the infant soon after delivery. Vitamin K given to infants with hemorrhagic tendencies causes an increase in prothrombin concentration to the normal level within 48 hours.

Conditions such as prolonged oral antibiotic therapy, severe diarrhea, or obstructive jaundice cause a decrease in the prothrombin concentration of the blood. Supplemental vitamin K will restore the concentration to normal. In obstructive jaundice, bile salts alone or with vitamin K are effective in restoring the prothrombin level. In cases of severe liver damage, such as hepatitis, cirrhosis, or malignancy, vitamin K given by any route may not affect the prothrombin level. This lack of response has been used as a test for liver function.

Vitamin K is of no value in treating hemorrhagic conditions unless a deficiency or inadequate utilization of the vitamin exists or unless a lowered prothrombin level is present.

Vitamin K is obtained naturally in several ways. Bacterial synthesis in the intestine normally supplies an adequate amount in humans. Vitamin K is also obtained from green leafy vegetables. Liver is an excellent source. Except for the abnormal conditions mentioned previously, a deficiency of vitamin K is unlikely to occur if the diet is adequate and if the bacterial synthesis in the intestine is unimpaired.

Water-soluble vitamins. The B-complex vitamins and ascorbic acid (vitamin C) comprise the important water-soluble group of vitamins. As a general rule, the B-complex vitamins function as the active sites of coenzymes in intermediary metabolism. Many clinical signs and symptoms in vitamin-deficient conditions can now be explained on the basis of altered biochemical function.

Although many signs and symptoms may be characteristic of a deficiency of a single vitamin, it is rare that only one B-complex vitamin is deficient.

Thiamin (B₁) was one of the first B vitamins discovered. The symptoms of a deficiency (beri-beri) were known long before the vitamin was isolated. In 1882 it was observed that increasing the use of barley, vegetables, meat, and condensed milk and decreasing the amount of polished rice in the diets

of the sailors in the Japanese navy cured and prevented beri-beri, a common disease in Asia at that time.

The disorder is characterized by degenerative changes in the nervous system. At first there is an ascending peripheral neuritis of the legs and then development of a multiple peripheral neuritis. Edema with subsequent hypertrophy of the heart may be present. Clinically, three different types of thiamin deficiency may be recognized: (1) "dry beri-beri," in which a multiple peripheral neuritis is the main feature; (2) "wet beri-beri," in which edema, changes in tendon reflexes, paresthesia, and muscle cramps are common; and (3) the "cardiac" type, which rapidly progresses to acute heart failure.

Thiamin deficiency is more common in areas where the diet is mainly unenriched white rice and white flour. In the United States thiamin deficiency is rare because of the enrichment of rice and flour. However, thiamin deficiency is common in alcoholics because of decreased consumption, increased need, and decreased absorption of this vitamin. Other persons at risk are patients undergoing long-term dialysis, patients who are being fed intravenously for long periods of time, and persons with chronic febrile infections. Persons consuming large amounts of tea or raw fish may also have an increased risk of thiamin deficiency, since tea contains a thiamin antagonist and raw fish contains a thiamin-destroying enzyme.

In carbohydrate metabolism, thiamin in the coenzyme thiamin pyrophosphate is essential to convert pyruvate to acetaldehyde and carbon dioxide. A thiamin deficiency causes lactic and pyruvic acids to accumulate in the tissues, primarily the blood and brain. It has been observed that fat, which does not require thiamin for metabolism, will ameliorate the effects of thiamin deficiency, since energy can be obtained from fat metabolism rather than carbohydrate metabolism.

Because of thiamin's important role in carbohydrate metabolism, excessive use of highly refined carbohydrates in the absence of an adequate thiamin intake is a health hazard and is detrimental to the dentition. Good sources of thiamin are pork, liver, yeast, whole grains, enriched flours and cereals, and fresh green vegetables. Since thiamin is destroyed by heat, care should be taken during food preparation to minimize thiamin losses.

Riboflavin (B₂) is a vitamin found in several coenzymes, the flavoproteins, which are essential in oxidation-reduction reactions in intermediary metabolism. Cellular activity cannot occur if the oxidation-reduction reactions are suppressed because of a deficiency of riboflavin.

Clinical signs of riboflavin deficiency were observed 20 years before the vitamin was discovered. The lesions observed were generally accepted as being caused by a dietary deficiency and could be cured with doses of B-complex vitamins.

The clinical signs of riboflavin deficiency are varied but can include eye lesions, especially vascularization of the cornea, angular stomatitis, glossitis, and seborrheic dermatitis around the nose and scrotum. It should be emphasized that glossitis and skin lesions are present with deficiencies of other B-complex vitamins; therefore a positive diagnosis of riboflavin deficiency must be based on biochemical tests.

Several investigators have reported low urinary riboflavin levels in women taking oral contraceptives. These findings may indicate a possible increased need for riboflavin during oral contraceptive usage, but at this time the data are insufficient to recommend an increased allowance of the vitamin.

The best sources of riboflavin are dairy products and meat. If these food items are routinely included in the normal mixed diet, it is unlikely that riboflavin deficiency will occur. Because the vitamin is destroyed by light, milk in clear glass containers should not be exposed to sunlight. Fortunately, riboflavin is heat stable and is not destroyed in ordinary cooking procedures.

Niacin is known as the antipellagra vitamin. Pellagra is a deficiency syndrome that has been recognized for over 200 years as endemic in areas of the world where corn is a major part of the diet. In the 1930s the Public Health Service was still reporting the prevalence of pellagra in the United States, especially in the southern states. The syndrome is characterized in the early stages by weakness, lassitude, anorexia, and gastric upset. Later this is followed by the classic "three D's"—dermatitis, diarrhea, and dementia. In addition, glossitis and stomatitis are common features. The dermatitis occurs in areas of the body that are exposed to heat, light, or trauma, such as the face, hands, knees, elbows, and feet, or in parts of the body in contact with body secretions.

Biochemically, niacin functions as a constituent of two important coenzymes, nicotinamide adenine dinucleotide (NAD) and nicotinamide adenine dinucleotide phosphate (NADP). NAD and NADP function in the series of reactions involved in the intracellular respiratory mechanism of all cells. They aid in the transfer of hydrogen atoms that are by-products of various biochemical reactions. The hydrogen atoms are eventually transferred to oxygen to form water.

Tryptophan, one of the essential amino acids, is a precursor to niacin. Therefore the recommended allowances are stated in terms of the preformed vitamin or as niacin equivalents. Generally, 60 mg of tryptophan will be equivalent to 1 mg of niacin. This ratio cannot be held as inflexible, but for practical purposes it is convenient to have some estimation of the amount of tryptophan in the diet in order to evaluate niacin requirements.

Good sources of niacin or niacin equivalents are all types of high-quality protein, such as meat, fish, eggs, and milk, and flours and cereals enriched with niacin. Peanuts and peanut butter are also high in niacin content.

Pyridoxine (B₆) is a vitamin that functions as a coenzyme in reactions involving decarboxylation and transamination of amino acids. A deficiency in humans commonly produces a seborrheic dermatitis about the eyes, in the eyebrows, and at the angles of the mouth. Glossitis indistinguishable from that caused by niacin deficiency may occur, as well as conjunctivitis, cheilosis, and angular stomatitis that resembles riboflavin deficiency.

Pregnant women given 6.6 mg of pyridoxine

three times daily in the form of lozenges or 20 mg in a single oral dose were observed to have fewer DMFT than controls who were given a placebo. There is, however, insufficient information regarding the relationship of pyridoxine to dental caries to recommend pyridoxine supplements for control of dental caries.

An increased pyridoxine requirement has been linked to the use of oral contraceptives. However, whether a true deficiency is produced or not remains equivocal. The present data do not seem to justify routine supplementation with pyridoxine. If the use of oral contraceptives does change the requirement for vitamin B_6, the change appears minor and of doubtful clinical significance.

Because pyridoxine is distributed widely among various foodstuffs, a deficiency of this vitamin is unlikely unless the diet is extremely poor.

Pantothenic acid is widely distributed in natural foodstuffs and has been found in all forms of living things. The name of the vitamin itself reflects this property—the Greek word *pantothenos* means "universal occurrence."

Pantothenic acid is vitally important in intermediary metabolism where it functions as a part of coenzyme A, which is involved in the release of energy from carbohydrates and is needed for the synthesis and degradation of fatty acids, sterols, and steroid hormones. It also functions in the acetylation of choline and sulfonamide drugs and is involved in the synthesis of porphyrins and many other compounds of prime importance to the body.

In experimental animals a deficiency of this vitamin causes neuromuscular degeneration, adrenocortical insufficiency, and death. Because of its wide distribution, pantothenic acid deficiency in humans is rare. It can be produced experimentally by feeding semisynthetic diets and a pantothenic acid antagonist. The resulting syndrome consists of fatigue, malaise, headache, disturbances of sleep, nausea, cramps, epigastric distress, occasional vomiting, and flatulence. Subjects complain of paresthesia of the extremities, muscle cramps, and impaired coordination.

In the United States the customary daily dietary intake of pantothenic acid is approximately 7 mg and may vary from 5 to 20 mg. A daily intake of 4 to 7 mg is usually adequate for adults; a higher intake may be needed during pregnancy and lactation and for children.

Folacin is essential in the metabolism of one-carbon units in the intracellular synthesis of purines, pyrimidines, methionine, and serine. Folacin is the generic name for compounds having nutritional properties and chemical structures similar to those of folic acid (pteroylglutamic acid, PGA).

A deficiency of this vitamin causes maturation arrest of bone marrow, glossitis, and gastrointestinal disturbances. Megaloblastic anemia during pregnancy may occur because of a dietary lack of folic acid, insufficient absorption caused by vomiting, the increased demand for folic acid by the fetus, or some unknown defect in the synthesis of folic acid coenzymes. Persons with sprue or with other malabsorption syndromes may exhibit megaloblastic anemia; an extremely poor diet may also result in megaloblastic anemia. This type of anemia may develop in persons with scurvy or in infants on an unsupplemented milk diet because of the combined deficiencies of ascorbic acid and folic acid.

Because folic acid in excess of 0.1 mg each day may prevent the hematologic signs of anemia but at the same time allow the neurologic symptoms to progress in persons with pernicious anemia, the sale of preparations containing more than 0.1 mg per daily dose is prohibited except by prescription (Federal Register, July 20, 1963).

Vitamin B_{12} (cyanocobalamin) is essential for the normal function of all cells, especially those of the marrow, nervous system, and gastrointestinal tract. In cells, vitamin B_{12} acts in the transfer of methyl groups that occur in the synthesis of a number of compounds, and it is involved in the synthesis of purine and pyrimidine nucleosides. The vitamin may also maintain sulfhydryl (SH) groups in the reduced state. Since SH groups are present in many enzyme systems, this property may be a major metabolic role for the vitamin. There is evidence indicating that vitamin B_{12} is linked with protein, carbohydrate, and fat metabolism, but its major role is probably in nucleic acid and folic acid metabolic processes.

Vitamin B_{12} is bound to protein in foods of animal origin. There is little vitamin B_{12} in vegetables. Intrinsic factor, a glycoprotein enzyme secreted by the stomach, is necessary to facilitate absorption of vitamin B_{12} by removing it from its protein combination. A deficiency of vitamin B_{12} results in pernicious anemia. The deficiency can occur for several reasons. In some persons intrinsic factor may be lacking because of genetic factors or because of total or subtotal gastrectomy. In vegetarians a sore tongue, paresthesias, amenorrhea, and signs of spinal degeneration may develop, although anemia is rare in deficiency resulting from vegetarianism. Other causes of deficiency are parasitic infections, as with fish tapeworms, or anatomic malformations, such as blind intestinal loops, pouches, or diverticula. Sprue and malabsorption syndromes can cause a deficiency of vitamin B_{12}. Many of these deficiency states are complicated by deficiencies of other essential nutrients.

Biotin is necessary in the enzyme systems of bacteria, animals, and probably humans. It is a required component in reactions involving the carboxylation and decarboxylation of various compounds associated with carbohydrate, lipid, and protein synthesis.

Biotin is found in a wide variety of foods. Intestinal synthesis by bacteria is also an important source of this vitamin. In humans, deficiency states of biotin are observed only when the diet contains large amounts of raw egg white. This occurs because a protein (avidin) in raw egg white combines with biotin and prevents absorption of the vitamin by the intestine.

The required daily intake of biotin is estimated to be 100 to 300 μg. The average American diet provides ample amounts to fulfill this need.

Ascorbic acid (vitamin C) is classed as a water-soluble vitamin, but it is different chemically from the B-complex vitamins. Ascorbic acid is a compound of six carbon atoms; its structural formula resembles the hexoses, which are precursors to ascorbic acid. Most animals can synthesize ascorbic acid in their own bodies, but in guinea pigs and in humans and other primates the metabolic pathway leading to the formation of ascorbic acid is blocked. Therefore the ascorbic acid needed for daily requirements must be ingested from exogenous sources.

Scurvy, the deleterious effect of ascorbic acid deficiency, has been recognized for centuries. It was described as early as 1500 BC in Egyptian writings. An account of the occurrence, symptoms, and treatment of scurvy in British sailors was given in a comprehensive treatise by Lind in the 1750s. It was not until 1928, however, that ascorbic acid was isolated and identified as the antiscorbutic substance.

Ascorbic acid is essential for tissues of mesenchymal origin: fibrous tissue, teeth, developing bone, and blood vessels. Changes in these tissues are responsible for the clinical signs seen in scurvy. Fortunately, scurvy is now a rare disease in the United States. It still may be observed occasionally in infants whose milk formula is unfortified and who refuse fruit juice. In adults, scurvy is usually seen only in those who have grossly deficient diets resulting from poverty, alcoholism, nutritional misinformation, food faddism, or chronic illness.

Although clinical scurvy is rare, it is probable that many cases of ascorbic acid deficiencies exist on a subclinical basis. The term "scurvy" refers to ascorbic acid deficiency associated with the classic signs of the deficiency: weakness; easy fatigue; shortness of breath; pain in bone, joints, and muscles; dry rough skin; purpura; petechial hemorrhages or ecchymoses; swollen, spongy, inflamed gingiva; and extremely mobile teeth. A person may be deficient in ascorbic acid but not exhibit any of the clinical signs of scurvy. In this case biochemical tests are required to determine levels of ascorbic acid in the tissues.

Ascorbic acid has many metabolic functions: (1) oxidation of phenylalanine and tryosine, (2) hydroxylation of aromatic compounds, (3) conversion of folacin (folic acid) to folinic acid (active form of folic acid), (4) development of odontoblasts and other specialized cells (collagen and cartilage), and (5) maintenance of strength of blood vessels.

The amount of ascorbic acid recommended as the daily allowance is about three to six times as great as the level of intake necessary to protect against scurvy. The recommended daily intake (35 to 50 mg for infants and growing children and 60 mg for adults) allows a margin of safety and ensures enough ascorbic acid to promote optimum health for long periods of time or when the body is subjected to situations of stress.

Ascorbic acid has been widely publicized as a cure for the common cold when given in amounts of 2 to 10 g daily. Although single large doses are probably harmless, regular ingestion may cause systemic conditioning. Several investigators have reported the development of scurvy in individuals who had consumed large amounts of ascorbic acid for long periods of time and then resumed a normal diet. Under normal dietary conditions, those who had habitually ingested large amounts of ascorbic acid may become deficient in ascorbic acid some time after stopping the regimen. For this reason and because the relationship of ascorbic acid to the common cold is still vague, it is perhaps best not to use massive doses of ascorbic acid over long periods of time.

Most people recognize that citrus fruits are excellent sources of ascorbic acid. However, fresh vegetables such as broccoli, cabbage, Brussels sprouts, cauliflower, spinach, and tomatoes are also good sources of ascorbic acid. Liver is an excellent source of this vitamin. Ascorbic acid is destroyed by heat and oxidation. Cooking fresh vegetables just to the point of palatability conserves about 50% of the original ascorbic acid content. Canned fruits and vegetables also contain about 50% of the original ascorbic acid content. To minimize ascorbic acid losses in cooking, pans should be covered and copper pots should not be used. After preparation, steam warming should be avoided because it will quickly destroy all remaining ascorbic acid.

Minerals. The fifth class of nutrients is the minerals. Of all the elements, about 35 are recognized as being important in human nutrition and 19 of these are considered essential. Some minerals, such as calcium and phosphorus, are needed in fairly large amounts, whereas others, such as iodine, fluorine, and zinc, are required only in trace amounts.

Minerals fulfill various functions in the body, are interrelated and balanced against each other, and cannot be considered as single elements with circumscribed functions. Calcium, phosphorus, fluorine, and some of the trace minerals are constituents of the ossified tissues. Sodium, potassium, calcium, and chlorine function in the maintenance of acid-base balance and the physiologic regulation of the basic ions. Iron, copper, and cobalt are essential in blood formation. Other ions such as magnesium, zinc, manganese, molybdenum, and other trace minerals function as constituents of various enzyme systems.

Since the trace elements are probably present in sufficient amounts in an adequate diet, there is little chance that deficiencies of these nutrients would occur. Green leafy vegetables, fruits, whole grains, seafoods, organ meats, and lean meats are all good sources of the trace elements.

Because of their special importance in nutrition, several minerals are discussed in more detail in the following paragraphs.

Calcium. The skeletal tissues of the body contain over 99% of the total body calcium and 70% to 80% of the total body phosphorus. The composition of the bone mineral is basically a hydroxyapatite that varies in composition because other ions, such as lead, strontium, and magnesium, are incorporated during formation. When fluoride is available during bone or tooth formation, the resulting crystal is called "fluorapatite."

In addition to its vital role in skeletal tissues, calcium is necessary to maintain acid-base equilibrium and to help control muscle tone. Its essential role in regulation of the heartbeat is well known.

Calcium is also necessary for the normal blood-clotting mechanism.

Calcium is absorbed against a concentration gradient in the stomach and by passive diffusion throughout the remainder of the small intestine. It is incompletely absorbed, the amount depending on various modifying factors. Calcium is absorbed more efficiently during times of increased need, when adequate vitamin D is available, and when the gastric acidity is low. Calcium absorption is decreased or impaired by phytates, oxalate, and fatty acids that form insoluble or poorly soluble complexes.

Calcium is excreted in the feces and urine. The amount in feces is primarily unabsorbed calcium and averages from 300 mg to 1 g a day. The kidney threshold for calcium is about 7 mg/100 ml, but the level of urinary calcium is largely dependent on endogenous factors characteristic of the individual.

Calcium intakes of 800 mg daily are recommended for adults and for children between 1 and 9 years of age. The allowance for boys and girls between 10 and 18 years of age and during pregnancy and lactation is 1200 mg daily.

Phosphorus. It is generally agreed that diets supplying adequate amounts of calcium also contain sufficient amounts of phosphorus. Therefore a phosphorus deficiency is unlikely unless the diet is grossly inadequate.

Phosphorus is vital to health because of its role in all body processes. Phosphorus not only is an important bone mineral but also occupies a primary role in energy transformations. Phosphate compounds in the form of adenosine diphosphates and triphosphates (ADP and ATP) plus other compounds containing a high-energy phosphate bond are essential to provide energy for biochemical reactions. Many coenzymes have phosphate radicals—for example, thiamin pyrophosphate, coenzyme A, NAD, and NADP. Many compounds that are absorbed by active transport mechanisms require phosphorylation.

Phosphates have received considerable attention in dental health since it was discovered that various soluble phosphates are effective in preventing den-

tal caries in animals and humans. Stookey, Carroll, and Muhler reported that significant reductions in dental caries were observed after the use of presweetened breakfast cereals to which 0.5% NaH_2PO_4 and 0.5% Na_2HPO_4 had been added. More recently, Rowe and associates added 0.2% soluble phosphate to ready-to-eat cereals but found no anticariogenic benefits after a 3-year clinical trial. To date, all the clinical trials of the cariostatic effect of phosphates have been equivocal. Because of the stringency of the Food and Drug Administration regulations pertaining to demonstrated effectiveness of new drugs and because of the increased number of uncontrollable variables in human clinical studies, the addition of phosphates to foodstuffs specifically to prevent dental caries will probably not be approved for many years, if at all.

Iron. Iron is an essential mineral for the body. It is present in hemoglobin and myoglobin; in several enzymes such as catalases, peroxidases, and the cytochromes; and in storage compounds (ferritin and hemosiderin). Over 70% of the iron is in hemoglobin; 26% is stored; about 3% is in myoglobin; and the remainder, about 0.3%, is in the iron-containing enzymes and the iron transport mechanism.

Iron is usually absorbed in the ferrous form by way of the lymphatics, with the greatest uptake in the duodenum. Evidence suggests that absorption is related to physiologic demand. The absorption rate is increased during periods of increased demand such as in growth, pregnancy, or hemorrhage. In the normal adult less than 10% of food iron is absorbed if the body stores are adequate. In infants and young children, however, 10% or more is usually absorbed.

Iron is normally lost from the body in the feces, urine, and sweat and from the growth and removal of skin, hair, and nails. The average amount lost is about 1 mg daily in the adult male and postmenopausal female. The body preserves its iron supply by reusing the iron that is released from hemoglobin catabolism and from the normal death and replacement of tissue cells.

A deficiency of iron results in hypochromic microcytic anemia. The frequency of occurrence is greatest among infants and children and among women during the years of menstruation and child-bearing. In adult males, iron-deficiency anemia is rare unless some cause for abnormal blood loss is present, such as ulcers or hemorrhoids.

Studies of iron balance indicate that a daily iron intake of 10 mg for men and postmenopausal women is sufficient to maintain iron equilibrium. However, the recommended intake is increased to 18 mg daily for boys and girls 11 to 18 years of age and for women in the childbearing years because of the critical need for iron in these individuals. Since this quantity of iron is difficult to obtain from the usual diet, additional supplementation with iron-containing foods may be desirable.

As recorded in the Federal Register (December 3, 1971), the Commissioner of the Food and Drug Administration proposed increases in the required level of iron in flour and wheat products (40 mg per pound of flour or enriched farina, and 25 mg per pound of enriched bread, buns, or rolls). This proposal touched off a controversy. Public health nutritionists, the Council on Foods and Nutrition of the American Medical Association, and the Food and Nutrition Board of the National Academy of Sciences–National Research Council endorsed the proposal. Some physicians objected, however, because they believed an increase in dietary iron might be harmful to persons with a rare condition known as hemochromatosis. The question is still unresolved.

Good sources of iron are meats, shellfish, egg yolk, and legumes. Fair sources are green leafy vegetables, whole grain, and enriched cereal products.

Fluorine. Fluorine is of particular interest because of its role in dental health and because of its possible value in the prevention of osteoporosis. In nature fluorine is never found in the free state but occurs as fluoride salts in various compounds. Fluoride is abundant and is widely distributed in nature. Over 95% of the absorption of orally ingested fluoride occurs rapidly in the stomach and upper part of the small intestine. It is absorbed as the fluoride ion by a process of diffusion. There is no evidence of an active transport mechanism. The absorption is modified by various factors, such as age, sex, and amount of prior exposure to fluoride. Interference of ions such as aluminum, magnesium, and calcium tends to decrease fluoride absorption, as does the presence of food in the stomach.

After fluoride is absorbed, it is distributed to the extracellular fluids. The body has two mechanisms to metabolize fluoride: deposition in the skeleton and urinary excretion. The major part of the fluoride retained is deposited in bones and teeth, but trace amounts may be found in soft tissues, such as the heart, liver, and kidneys. The amount of fluoride retained is also influenced by age, sex, and prior exposure to fluoride. In young children as much as 30% to 50% of an ingested dose of fluoride may be retained in the skeletal tissues. In adults, however, only about 2% to 10% of fluoride is retained.

When fluoride is incorporated into bones or teeth, the hydroxyapatite structure is changed to fluorapatite by the replacement of the hydroxyl groups with fluorine atoms. Some fluoride is also incorporated in the adsorption layer of the apatite crystal. Fluoride continues to accumulate at a slow rate in the skeletal tissues throughout life. There is no evidence that this has any deleterious physiologic effects.

Fluoride excretion occurs almost entirely through the kidney. There is some fecal excretion of fluoride, part of which has been secreted into the colon but most of which is unabsorbed fluoride. Small amounts of fluoride are found in saliva, milk, and perspiration. In hot weather appreciable amounts of fluoride may be excreted in perspiration. This manner of fluoride excretion must be considered when fluoride balance studies are conducted in hot weather. Urinary excretion is rapid; within 1 hour after oral ingestion of fluoride the urinary concentration of fluoride is significantly elevated. Within limits, the urinary excretion of fluoride will be increased if the intake of fluoride is increased so that the physiologic balance can be maintained.

Fluoride is not bound permanently in bone.

When decreased intake occurs, the urinary level, which is a reliable index of fluoride exposure, remains elevated. This indicates that fluoride is being mobilized from the bone. There are two phases by which fluoride can be lost from the skeleton. The first is rapid and lasts about 1 month. In this phase fluoride is lost by exchange of fluoride ions on the surface of the apatite crystals with hydroxyl ions of the extracellular fluid. In children a second phase of fluoride mobilization occurs, which may last for several years. This phase is the normal resorption-deposition cycle of developing bones that releases the bound fluoride to the extracellular fluid. Part of this fluoride, however, can be redeposited in the newly forming bone.

The most effective, safe, and economical method of obtaining systemic fluoride during the period of tooth formation is through the water supply, either naturally or mechanically fluoridated to the optimum level. The effectiveness of communally fluoridated water in preventing dental caries has been demonstrated repeatedly. For those who do not have access to a fluoridated water supply, alternative methods of providing fluoride systemically have been proposed. These alternatives, such as fluoride in tablets or solutions with or without vitamins or in milk, salt, or cereal, all have one serious disadvantage: they must be used regularly during the period of tooth development to obtain the maximum benefit. The most commonly used supplemental fluoride preparations are the solutions and tablets. Recently reported studies have shown that a vitamin-fluoride preparation is effective in preventing dental caries in the primary and permanent dentitions. The results also confirmed that the effectiveness is the result of both a systemic and a topical action of the fluoride.

Fluoride supplements are available to the patient only by prescription, and several factors must be considered before prescribing them. What is the fluoride content of the patient's drinking water? If it is a private water supply, it must be analyzed for fluoride. Fluoride concentrations in communal water systems are listed in state or federal publications. The American Dental Association's Council

on Dental Therapeutics suggests limiting the use of fluoride supplements to children whose drinking water has a fluoride concentration no greater than 70% of the optimum concentration for their geographic area.

Are the parents sufficiently motivated and cooperative to continue the fluoride therapy as long as needed to achieve optimum results? Tablet distribution programs and clinical studies have shown that only a small number of parents maintain the required dosage schedule. Some parents also think that doubling the daily dose will double the benefits. Therefore with fluoride supplements the possibility of underdosage and overdosage is always present.

Should a vitamin-fluoride product be used, or should fluoride alone be prescribed? Both types are equally effective. In a combination product the fluoride and vitamins are both metabolically active and do not interfere with each other's utilization. The fluoride-vitamin product should be prescribed if the child is already taking vitamins or is going to start taking vitamins because it is more convenient for the parent to administer a single dose. Also, the fluoride is probably ingested more regularly in a combination product than in a plain fluoride supplement. If the child is old enough to ingest a tablet, the fluoride supplement, with or without vitamins, should be in chewable tablet form. Several studies have shown that a significant topical effect occurs when the tablet is chewed and the resulting saliva mixture is swished around the teeth before swallowing.

What dosage should be used? According to the American Dental Association's Council on Dental Therapeutics, when the drinking water is deficient in fluoride, 1 mg fluoride ion can be given to children 3 years of age and older. Children between 2 and 3 years of age are given 0.5 mg fluoride. For children under 2 years of age it is recommended that drinking water be prepared to a 1 ppm fluoride level by adding a 1-mg fluoride tablet or 5 ml of a liquid (containing 1 mg flouride/5 ml) to a quart of water. Since many parents are not highly motivated to prepare the water to be used for the child's food

Table 16-2. Supplemental fluoride dosage schedule (in mg F/day*) according to fluoride concentration of drinking water

Age (yr)	Concentration of flouride in water (ppm)		
	<0.3	**0.3-0.7**	**>0.7**
Birth to 2	0.25	0	0
2-3	0.50	0.25	0
3-13	1.00	0.50	0

From American Dental Association: Accepted dental therapeutics, ed. 38, Chicago, 1979, The Association.
*2.2 mg sodium fluoride contains 1 mg fluoride.

or formula, the Council suggests that a daily dose of 0.25 mg fluoride may be a satisfactory alternative. A liquid product should be used for children less than 3 years of age to prevent possible tablet aspiration. However, a child younger than 3 may be given a chewable tablet if the parents supervise and the child has sufficient motor development.

What quantity of product should be dispensed? Table 16-2 shows the current recommendations from the American Dental Association's Council on Dental Therapeutics for supplemental fluoride dosages at various levels of fluoride concentration in drinking water. The Council suggests that no more than 264 mg of a sodium fluoride preparation be dispensed for home use. This amount provides 120 mg fluoride and is enough for 4 months (1 mg fluoride daily). If the prescription is marked for two or three refills, the supply will be sufficient until the patient can be reevaluated and a new prescription written.

Is there any danger of causing fluorosis? During tooth formation the chance of fluorosis is present whenever fluoride is ingested. However, cosmetically objectionable fluorosis is generally not a problem. In one study conducted long enough to observe fluorosis, no objectionable fluorosis was reported with daily dosages ranging from 0.5 to 1 mg fluoride. The 0.5-mg fluoride supplement was started after birth and continued until 3 years of age, at which time the dosage was increased to 1 mg fluoride daily. In another study, 0.5 to 1 mg

additional fluoride was given to children who lived in areas with nearly adequate (suboptimum) levels of fluoride in their drinking water. The average age of the children when starting to receive 0.5 mg fluoride daily was 5½ months. Even under these conditions, no objectionable fluorosis was detected.

Water. No discussion of inorganic nutrients would be complete without mention of water. Its importance is second only to that of oxygen. When the water supply is inadequate, adverse effects promptly occur in the body. Water not only serves as an essential nutrient but also forms the major component of the body. It is a means of chemical transport and the medium in which the metabolic reactions occur.

The water intake includes that ingested as fluids or in food and the water produced by the metabolism of foodstuffs in the body. The major route of water excretion is by way of the kidneys. However, water in the feces, sweat, and expired air accounts for about half the loss of body water. Physical activity and environmental temperature affect the amount of water lost through lungs and skin.

The National Research Council indicates the minimum water requirements for adults under the most favorable conditions to be about 1 to 1.5 liters daily as supplied from food, drink, and water of metabolism. A reasonable standard for calculating water allowances is 1 ml/calorie of food for adults. The value for infants is 1.5 ml/calorie of food. The sensation of thirst usually serves as an adequate guide to water intake. However, in infants, sick people, or persons exposed to extreme heat or sweating, this thirst sensation may not be adequate to ensure sufficient water intake.

REFERENCES

Admed, F., Bamji, M.S., and Iyengar, L.: Effect of oral contraceptive agents on vitamin nutrition status, Am. J. Clin. Nutr. **28:**606-615, 1975.

American Dental Association: Accepted dental therapeutics, ed. 38, Chicago, 1979, The Association.

Beal, V.A.: Nutrition in the life span, New York, 1980, John Wiley & Sons, Inc.

Briggs, M., and Briggs, M.: Oral contraceptives and vitamin nutrition, Lancet **1:**1234-1235, 1974.

Council on Foods and Nutrition: Western Hemisphere Nutrition Congress, Proceedings, Chicago, 1966, American Medical Association.

Follis, R.H., Jr.: Deficiency disease, Springfield, Ill., 1958, Charles C Thomas, Publisher.

Food and Nutrition Board, National Academy of Sciences–National Research Council: Recommended dietary allowances, ed. 9, Washington, D.C., 1980.

Goodhart, R.S., and Shils, M.E., editors: Modern nutrition in health and disease, ed. 5, Philadelphia, 1973, Lea & Febiger.

Hennon, D.K., Stookey, G.K., and Beiswanger, B.B.: Fluoride-vitamin supplements: effects on dental caries and fluorosis when used in areas with sub-optimum fluoride in the water supply, J.A.D.A. 95:965-971, 1977.

Hennon, D.K., Stookey, G.K., and Muhler, J.C.: The clinical anticariogenic effectiveness of supplementary fluoride-vitamin preparations: results at the end of three years, J. Dent. Child. 33:3-12, 1966.

Hennon, D.K., Stookey, G.K., and Muhler, J.C.: The clinical anticariogenic effectiveness of supplementary fluoride-vitamin preparations: results at the end of five and a half years, J. Pharmacol. Ther. Dent. 1:1-6, 1970.

Hennon, D.K., Stookey, G.K., and Muhler, J.C.: Prophylaxis of dental caries: relative effectiveness of chewable fluoride preparations with and without added vitamins, J. Pediatr. 80:1018-1021, 1972.

Marino, D.D., and King, J.C.: Nutritional concerns during adolescence, Pediatr. Clin. North Am. 27:125-139, 1980.

McGandy, R.B., and others: Dietary regulation of blood cholesterol in adolescent males: a pilot study, Am. J. Clin. Nutr. 25:61-66, 1972.

Nizel, A.E.: The science of nutrition and its application in clinical dentistry, ed. 2, Philadelphia, 1966, W.B. Saunders Co.

Present knowledge in nutrition, ed. 4, New York, 1976, The Nutrition Foundation, Inc.

Rowe, N.H., and others: Effect of phosphate-enriched ready-to-eat breakfast cereals on dental caries experience in adolescents: a three-year study, J.A.D.A. 90:412-417, 1975.

Rust, B.K.: Special problems of nutrition for children, J. Indiana State Dent. Assoc. 42:7-11, 1963.

Sanpitak, N., and Chayutimonkul, L.: Oral contraceptives and riboflavin nutrition, Lancet 1:836-837, 1974.

Stookey, G.K., Carroll, R.A., and Muhler, J.C.: The clinical effectiveness of phosphate-enriched breakfast cereals on the incidence of dental caries in children: results after two years, J.A.D.A. 74:752-758, 1967.

U.S. Department of Health, Education and Welfare: Ten state nutrition survey, 1968-1970, DHEW Pub. No. (HSM)72-8133, Atlanta, 1972, Health Services and Mental Health Administration, Center for Disease Control.

17 Management of traumatic injuries to the teeth and supporting tissues

RALPH E. McDONALD
DAVID R. AVERY
THEODORE R. LYNCH

A traumatic injury with accompanying fracture of a permanent incisor is a tragic experience for the young patient and is a problem that requires experience, judgment, and skill perhaps unequaled by any other portion of the dentist's practice. The dentist whose counsel and treatment are sought after a traumatic injury is obligated either to treat the patient with all possible means or to immediately refer the patient to a specialist. The dental health of the young patient is involved, and the child's appearance, marred by an unsightly fracture, must be restored to normal as soon as possible to relieve the consciousness of being different from other children. Slack and Jones observed that progress of children in school and their behavior elsewhere, as well as their psychologic well-being, can be adversely influenced by an injury to the teeth that causes an unsightly fracture.

Traumatic injuries to the teeth of children or adults present unique problems in diagnosis and treatment. The diagnosis of the extent of the injury after a blow to a tooth, regardless of loss of tooth structure, is difficult and often inconclusive. Trauma to a tooth is invariably followed by pulpal hyperemia, the extent of which cannot always be determined by available diagnostic methods. Congestion and alteration in the blood flow in the pulp may be sufficient to initiate irreversible degenerative changes, which over a period of time can cause pulpal necrosis. In addition, the apical vessels may

have been severed or damaged enough to interfere with the normal reparative process. Treatment of traumatic injury causing pulp exposure is particularly challenging, since the prognosis of the involved tooth is often uncertain for an indefinite period of time.

The treatment of fractured teeth, particularly in young patients, is further complicated by the often difficult but extremely important restorative procedure. Although the dentist may prefer to delay the restoration because of a questionable prognosis for the pulp, often a malocclusion can develop within a matter of days as a result of a break in the normal proximal contact with adjacent teeth. Adjacent teeth may tip into the area created by the loss of tooth structure (Fig. 17-1). This loss of space will create a problem when the final restoration is contemplated. There must often be a compromise with an ideal esthetic appearance, at least in the initial restoration, because of the questionable prognosis or because the tooth is young and has a large pulp or is still in the stage of active eruption.

Often the prognosis for success depends on the rapidity with which the tooth is treated after the injury, regardless of whether the procedure involves protecting a large area of exposed dentin or treating a vital pulp exposure. A number of factors can be considered common to all types of traumatic injury to the anterior teeth. These important considerations should become a checklist invariably

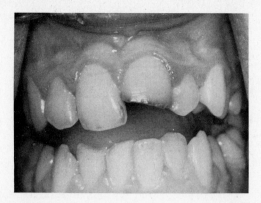

Fig. 17-1. Loss of the incisal third of the maxillary left central incisor has allowed the right central incisor to tip into the area. Satisfactory restoration of the fractured tooth cannot be accomplished until the space is regained. Major orthodontic treatment will be required.

used by the dentist in the diagnosis of and treatment planning for traumatic injury.

History and examination

The routine use of a clinical evaluation sheet for injured anterior teeth has been helpful during the initial examination and subsequent examinations of an injured tooth (Fig. 17-2). The form, which becomes a part of the patient's record, serves as a checklist of important questions and observations that must be made by the dentist and the auxiliary personnel during the examination of the child.

History of the injury. The time of the injury should first be established. Unfortunately, many patients do not seek professional advice and treatment immediately after an injury. Occasionally the accident is so severe that dental treatment cannot be started immediately because other injuries have higher priority. The dental prognosis is logically dependent, often to a great extent, on the time that has elapsed between the accident and the time that emergency treatment is provided. This situation is particularly true in pulp exposures, for which pulp capping or pulpotomy would be the procedure of choice.

Only by taking a complete history can the dentist

learn of previous injuries to the teeth in the area. Repeated traumatic injuries to the teeth are not uncommon in children with protruding anterior teeth and in those who are active in athletics. In these patients the prognosis may be less favorable. The dentist must rule out the possibility of a degenerative pulp or adverse reaction of the supporting tissues as a result of previous trauma.

The patient's complaints and experiences after the injury are often valuable in determining the extent of the injury and in estimating the ability of the injured pulp and supporting tissues to overcome the effects of the injury. Pain caused by thermal change is indicative of pulpal hyperemia and is an indication that the immediate treatment should be directed toward relieving this condition and preventing further injury to the pulp by external irritants. Pain occurring when the teeth are brought into normal occlusion may indicate that the tooth has been displaced. Such pain could likewise indicate an injury to the periodontal and supporting tissues. The likelihood of eventual pulpal necrosis increases if the tooth is mobile at the time of the first examination; the greater the mobility, the greater the chance of pulp death.

Trauma to the supporting tissues may cause inflammation and the initiation of peripheral root resorption. In instances of severe injury, teeth can be lost as a result of pathologic root resorption and pulpal degeneration.

Clinical examination. The clinical examination should be conducted after the teeth in the area of injury have been carefully cleaned of debris. A pledget of cotton moistened with warm water or hydrogen peroxide can be used to clean the tooth and the surrounding area. When the injury has resulted in a fracture of the crown, the dentist should observe the amount of tooth structure that has been lost and should look for evidence of a pulp exposure. With the aid of a good light, the clinical crown should be examined carefully for cracks and craze lines, the presence of which could influence the type of "permanent" restoration for the tooth. With light transmitted through the teeth in the area, the color of the injured tooth should be carefully

CLINICAL EVALUATION SHEET FOR INJURED ANTERIOR TEETH

History

Patient's name

1. Date of this examination

_____

Mo.   Date   Yr.

2. Date (and time) of injury

_____

3. Time elapsed (days or hours) since injury

_____

4. How injury occurred _____

_____

_____

_____

5. Where injury occurred _____

_____

_____

6. Previous history of injury

Yes _____ No _____

a. If yes, date of previous injuries_____

_____

_____

b. Previous fracture, mobility or

displacement? _____

_____

_____

c. Previous pain, discomfort or

sensitivity? _____

_____

_____

_____

Age _____ Injured
tooth no. _____
Yrs.   Mos.

7. Patient's complaints (current)

a. Pain on mastication

Yes _____ No _____

If yes, describe _____

_____

_____

b. Reaction to thermal change

Yes _____ No _____

If yes, describe _____

_____

_____

c. Other complaints (describe)

_____

_____

8. Soft tissue observation

Laceration   Yes _____ No _____

Swelling   Yes _____ No _____

If yes, describe _____

_____

9. Occlusion (Angle classification)

_____

Fig. 17-2. Clinical evaluation sheet for injured anterior teeth.

Continued.

Patient _____ Date _____

CLINICAL EVALUATION SHEET FOR INJURED ANTERIOR TEETH

I. Diagrammatic chart

1. Draw pulp outline in red.

Tooth no. _____

2. Draw injury in black.

3. Indicate displacement with arrow.

II. Initial clinical examination

1. Classification (Ellis) _____

2. Color (trans. light) _____

3. Response to percussion _____

4. Mobility (degree) _____

5. Pulp response—electric _____

```
7   8  |  9   10
□   □  |  □   □      Heat _____
_____|_____
□   □  |  □   □      Cold _____
26  25 |  24  23
```

III. Initial radiographic examination

1. Pulp size
2. Root development
3. Root fracture

4. Periapical pathology
5. Alveolar fracture
6. Other

IV. Initial treatment

1. Pulp: _____

_____

2. Coverage: _____

_____ 3. Splint _____

4. Rx _____

V. Subsequent visit no. 1 Date _____

1. Pulpal resp.
```
7   8  |  9   10
□   □  |  □   □
```

2. Radiographic Exam.
```
□   □  |  □   □
26  25 |  24  23
```

3. Treatment and comments: _____

_____

VI. Subsequent visit no. 2 Date _____

1. Pulpal resp.
```
7   8  |  9   10
□   □  |  □   □
```

2. Radiographic exam.
```
□   □  |  □   □
26  25 |  24  23
```

3. Treatment and comments _____

_____

VII. Subsequent visit no. 3 Date _____

1. Pulpal resp.
```
7   8  |  9   10
□   □  |  □   □
```

2. Radiographic exam.
```
□   □  |  □   □
26  25 |  24  23
```

3. Treatment and comments _____

_____

VIII. Subsequent visit no. 4 Date _____

1. Pulpal resp.
```
7   8  |  9   10
□   □  |  □   □
```

2. Radiographic exam.
```
□   □  |  □   □
26  25 |  24  23
```

3. Treatment and comments _____

_____

Fig. 17-2, cont'd. Clinical evaluation sheet for injured anterior teeth.

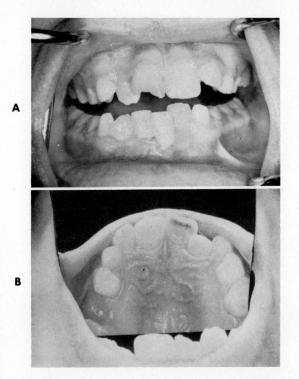

A,

B,

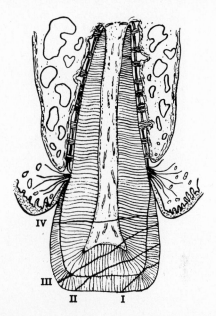

Fig. 17-4. Classification of fractures of the crown of anterior teeth.

Fig. 17-3. A, Fractured central incisor appeared darker than the adjacent teeth 3 days after the injury. The pulp was not exposed, but it was in a "state of shock" and did not respond to pulp tests. **B,** The reddish appearance of the dentin is evidence of severe hyperemia and congestion within the pulp tissue. The prognosis for retaining vitality of the pulp is poor.

compared with that of adjacent uninjured teeth. Severely traumatized teeth often appear darker and reddish, although not actually discolored, indicating pulpal hyperemia and congestion (Fig. 17-3). This appearance indicates that the pulp at some later time may undergo degenerative change terminating in pulpal necrosis.

Ellis' classification of crown fracture is widely accepted and is useful in recording the extent of damage to the tooth (Fig. 17-4). The following is a modification of Ellis' classification:

Class I—Simple fracture of the crown involving little or no dentin

Class II—Extensive fracture of the crown in-

volving considerable dentin but not the dental pulp

Class III—Extensive fracture of the crown with an exposure of the dental pulp

Class IV—Loss of the entire crown

The vitality test should be made in all cases (Fig. 17-5), and the teeth in the immediate area, as well as those in the opposing arch, should be tested. The best prediction of continued vitality of the pulp of a damaged or traumatized tooth is the vital response to electric pulp testing at the time of the initial examination. A negative response, however, is not always reliable evidence of pulp death because some teeth that give such a response soon after the injury may recover vitality after a time. This fact has been substantiated by Rock and associates after taking complete records of 500 children who suffered injuries to incisor teeth. When the electric pulp tester is used, the normal reading should first be determined by testing an uninjured tooth on the opposite side of the mouth and recording the lowest number at which the tooth responds. If the injured

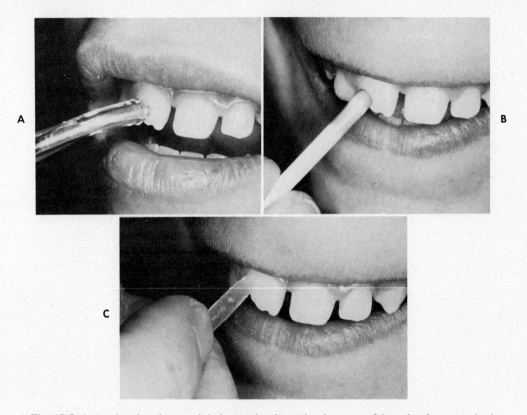

Fig. 17-5. A, An electric pulp tester is being used to determine the status of the pulp of a traumatized tooth. The adjacent and opposing teeth should also be tested. **B,** A piece of heated gutta-percha is used for the thermal test. **C,** Cold is applied to a tooth with an ice cone.

tooth requires more current than that for a normal tooth, the pulp is undergoing degenerative change. If less current is needed to elicit a response from a traumatized tooth, it is usually an indication of pulpal hyperemia.

Many practitioners question the need for the electric vitality test immediately after the injury. Since the electrical stimulus has been shown to produce negligible additional pulpal irritation, its use is not contraindicated because of additional trauma. However, the patient's measured responses to the test may be almost meaningless. This occurs when the patient does not feel the stimulus and gives no response to the test. The reliability of the electric pulp test depends on valid responses from the patient. The mere presence of this new, ''unknown'' instrument may create anxiety in children that hampers their ability to respond accurately to the test. Since an unscheduled emergency appointment for treatment of an injury is a new experience, it seems reasonable to introduce the child to the instrument during the first emergency visit when the child does not know what to expect. This gives the dentist an opportunity to allay the child's anxiety about the instrument during a time when the responses are not as important as they will be on subsequent visits. It should also be remembered that the electric pulp test is frequently unreliable even on normal teeth with incompletely formed apices.

The thermal test is also helpful in determining the degree of pulpal injury after trauma. It is definitely the most reliable in testing primary incisors in young children. Failure of a tooth to respond to heat is indicative of pulpal necrosis. The response of a tooth to a lower degree of heat than is necessary to elicit a response in adjacent teeth is an indication of pulpal hyperemia or inflammation.

Pain occurring when ice is applied to a normal tooth will subside when the ice is removed. A more painful reaction to cold indicates a pathologic change within the pulp, the nature of which can be determined by correlating the reaction with other clinical observations.

Failure of a recently traumatized tooth to respond to the pulp test is not uncommon and may indicate a previous injury with a resulting necrotic pulp. However, the traumatized tooth may be in a "state of shock" and as a result may fail to respond to the accepted methods of determining pulp vitality. The failure of a pulp to respond immediately after an accident is not an indication for endodontic therapy. Instead, emergency treatment should be completed and the tooth should be retested in a week or 10 days. If at the end of 2 weeks the pulp does not respond to the vitality test, it can be assumed that the apical vessels have been severed or that the pulp has undergone degenerative change and further treatment is necessary.

Radiographic examination. The examination of traumatized teeth cannot be considered complete without a radiograph of the injured tooth, the adjacent teeth, and the teeth in the opposing arch. The relative size of the pulp chamber and canal should be carefully examined. Irregularities or an inconsistency in the size of the chamber or canal as compared with adjacent teeth may be evidence of a previous injury. This observation is important in determining the immediate course of treatment. In young patients the stage of apical development often indicates the type of treatment, just as the size of the coronal pulp and its proximity to the area of fracture influence the type of restoration that can be used. A root fracture as a result of the injury or one previously sustained can be detected by a careful examination of the radiograph. However, the presence of a root fracture may not influence the course of treatment, particularly if the fracture line is in the region of the apical third. Teeth with root fractures in this area rarely need stabilization, and a fibrous or calcified union will usually result. If teeth have been discernibly dislocated, with or without root fracture, two or three radiographs of the area at different angles may be needed to clearly define the defect and aid the dentist in deciding on a course of treatment.

The greatest value of the radiograph is that it provides a record of the tooth immediately after the injury. Frequent, periodic radiographs reveal evidence of continued pulp vitality or adverse changes that take place within the pulp or the supporting tissues. In young teeth in which the pulp recovers from the initial trauma, the pulp chamber and canal will decrease in size coincident with the normal formation of secondary dentin. After a period of time an inconsistency in the true size or contour of the pulp chamber or canal in comparison with that of adjacent teeth may indicate a developing pathologic condition.

In cases in which more complex facial injuries have occurred or jaw fractures are suspected, extraoral films may also be necessary to help identify the extent and location of all injury sequelae. Oblique lateral jaw radiographs and panoramic films are often useful adjuncts to this diagnostic process.

Emergency treatment of soft tissue injury

Traumatic injury to the teeth of children is often accompanied by abrasion of the facial tissues and even puncture wounds. The dentist must recognize the possibility of the development of tetanus after the injury and must carry out adequate first aid measures.

Children with up-to-date protection of active immunization are protected by the level of antibodies in their circulation produced by a series of injections of tetanus toxoid. Primary immunization is usually a part of medical care during the first 2 years of life. However, in 1966 Convery reported that more than 20% of first-grade children entered school in Indiana without tetanus immunization.

When the child who has had the primary immunization receives an injury from an object that is likely to have been contaminated, the antibody-forming mechanism may be activated with a booster injection of *toxoid*. An unimmunized child can be protected through "passive" immunizations with tetanus *antitoxin*.

The dentist examining the child after a traumatic injury should determine the child's immunization status, carry out adequate debridement of the wound, and, when indicated, refer the child to the family physician. Convery has emphasized that even a trivial injury can have a fatal outcome. The mortality in reported cases of tetanus has been between 50% and 60%.

Emergency treatment and temporary restoration of fractured teeth without pulp exposure

A traumatic injury to a tooth that causes a loss of only a small portion of enamel should be treated as carefully as one in which greater tooth structure is lost. The emergency treatment of minor injuries in which only the enamel is fractured may consist only of smoothing the rough, jagged tooth structure. However, without exception a thorough examination should be conducted as previously described. The patient should be reexamined at 2 weeks and again at 1 month after the injury. If the tooth appears to have recovered at that time, continued observation should be the rule at the patient's regular recall appointments.

Traumatic injuries with a resultant extensive loss of tooth structure and exposed dentin require an immediate temporary restoration or protective covering, in addition to the complete diagnostic procedure. In this type of injury, initial pulpal hyperemia and the possibility of further trauma to the pulp by pressure or by thermal or chemical irritants must be reduced. In addition, if normal contact with adjacent or opposing teeth has been lost, the temporary restoration or protective covering can be designed to maintain the integrity of the arch. Since an adequate permanent restoration may depend on maintaining the normal alignment and position of teeth in the area, this part of the treatment is as important as maintaining the vitality of the teeth. A number of restorations that will satisfy these requirements can easily be fabricated.

Reattachment of tooth fragment (fragment restoration). Occasionally the dentist may have the opportunity to reattach the fragment of a fractured tooth using resin and etching techniques. Tennery has reported the successful reattachment of tooth fragments for eight teeth in five patients. One reattached fragment was subsequently lost as the result of a second traumatic episode. Starkey (1979) has reported successful reattachment of one tooth fragment on a lower central incisor 2 days after the injury.

This procedure is atraumatic and seems to be the ideal method of restoring the fractured crown. Sealing the injured tooth and esthetically restoring its natural contour and color are accomplished simply and constitute an excellent service to the patient. The procedure provides an essentially perfect temporary restoration that may be retained a long time in some cases.

It is not often that the fractured tooth fragment remains intact and is recovered after an injury, but when this happens, the dentist may consider the reattachment procedure. The tooth requires no mechanical preparation because retention is provided by enamel etching. If little or no dentin is exposed, the fragment and the fractured tooth are etched and reattached with a sealant resin material. If only a small amount of dentin is exposed, it should be protected with calcium hydroxide before etching, but the dressing is removed before reattaching the fragment.

If considerable dentin is exposed or if a direct pulp cap is indicated, a thin protective dressing of calcium hydroxide should remain over the exposed dentin of the tooth. In this case the inside portion of the fragment must be modified with a bur to allow for the thickness of the calcium hydroxide dressing when the fragment is repositioned on the tooth. The removal of a small amount of the remaining

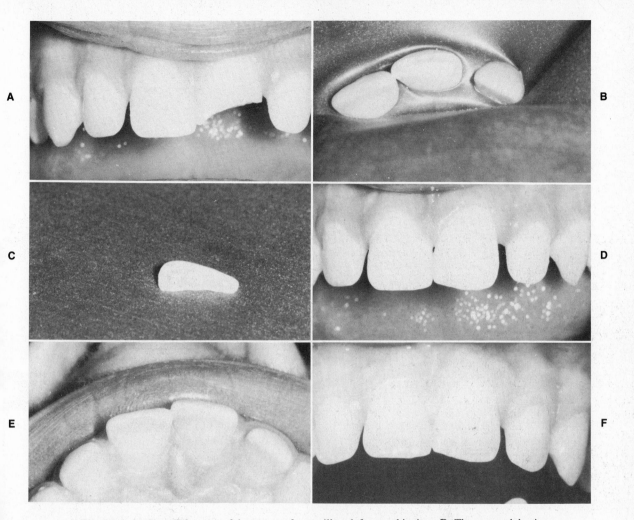

Fig. 17-6. A, Class II fracture of the crown of a maxillary left central incisor. **B,** The exposed dentin of the tooth is covered with hard-setting calcium hydroxide; all fractured enamel remains exposed. **C,** Part of the dentin is removed from the tooth fragment with a high-speed bur; the enamel is not disturbed. **D,** ''Fragment restoration'' immediately after removing the rubber dam. **E,** Incisal view of the restored tooth illustrates the tooth's natural susceptibility to fracture because of its labial position. **F,** Restored tooth 22 months after injury. No additional treatment has been required.

dentin on the inner surface of the fragment must be done carefully so that the outer enamel margins are undisturbed. The outer enamel is important to provide guidance for the exact repositioning of the fragment on the fractured tooth.

Fig. 17-6 illustrates the successful management of a Class II fracture of the maxillary left central incisor in a 15-year-old boy who was treated approximately 2 hours after the injury. At this writing the reattached fragment has been a successful restoration for more than 2 years. The natural labial position of the tooth made it more susceptible to injury. After the fragment was trial seated to confirm a perfect fit, the exposed dentin of the fractured tooth was covered with a thin layer of hard-setting calcium hydroxide that was allowed to remain as a sedative dressing between the tooth and the restored fragment. A portion of the dentin in the fragment was removed with a bur to provide space for the calcium hydroxide dressing. The fragment was then soaked in etchant and the fractured area of the tooth was also etched well beyond the fracture site. After thorough rinsing and drying of all etched enamel, the fragment and the etched portion of the tooth were painted with a light-curing sealant material. The fragment was carefully seated to its correct position and held firmly while the material was cured with the light. A small amount of enamel had been lost, leaving a defect about 1 mm in diameter on the labial surface. This defect was filled with composite resin. Subsequent radiographs and vitality tests suggested that the tooth had responded favorably. The restoration could have also been accomplished with self-curing materials.

Temporary acid etch resin. The excellent marginal seal and retention derived from applying esthetic restorative resin materials to etched enamel surfaces have revolutionized the approach to restoring fractured anterior teeth in recent years. The acid etch resin technique has been shown to be highly successful and versatile in many situations involving anterior trauma.

It may not be advisable to restore an extensive crown fracture with a finished esthetic resin restoration on the day of the injury, since it is usually best not to manipulate the tooth more than is absolutely necessary to make a diagnosis and provide emergency treatment. Also, such emergencies are usually treated in unscheduled appointments, and this should be carried out as efficiently as possible to prevent significant disruption to the dentist's scheduled appointments. A temporary restorative resin restoration can be placed in an efficient manner and is often the treatment of choice.

After the exposed dentin is protected with calcium hydroxide and the enamel adjacent to the fracture is etched, the restorative resin material is applied as a protective covering at the fracture site. As a short-term temporary restoration, it requires little or no finishing and does not need to restore the tooth to normal contour. However, the restoration should cover the fractured surfaces and maintain any natural proximal contacts the patient may have had before the injury. After an adequate recovery period (at least 4 weeks), the esthetic resin restoration may be completed, often without removing all of the temporary resin material. The surfaces of the temporary restoration should be "freshened" with a bur, however, before applying the new material. The margins of the new restoration should extend beyond the margins of the temporary restoration and onto newly etched enamel (Fig. 17-7). The esthetic acid etch resin restoration is discussed and illustrated later in this chapter.

Orthodontic band. Although the orthodontic band is only a temporary restoration, it will serve adequately as a retainer for a therapeutic dressing on the exposed dentin and will maintain contact with the adjacent teeth (Fig. 17-8). However, it does not meet the esthetic requirements of an anterior restoration and should be replaced after an adequate recovery period.

A preformed orthodontic band can be adapted directly to the injured tooth. If extensive loss of tooth structure or tooth mobility makes this procedure difficult, however, the band can be adapted to a corresponding intact tooth. After the tooth has been washed free of debris and has been dried, a dressing of calcium hydroxide paste should be applied to the exposed dentin. The protective band may then be cemented in place. This type of protective covering has the advantage of being easily and quickly prepared for the fractured tooth. In addition, the clinical crown is usually sufficiently exposed to enable the dentist to make periodic pulp tests during the initial period of observation. The band is generally allowed to remain undisturbed for 4 to 6 weeks or until recovery of the dental pulp is reasonably evident.

Chrome steel crown. The chrome steel crown is one of the most stable restorations for the temporary protection of a fractured tooth. If the coronal fracture is extensive with a vital pulp exposure (especially Class IV), this crown may be the tempo-

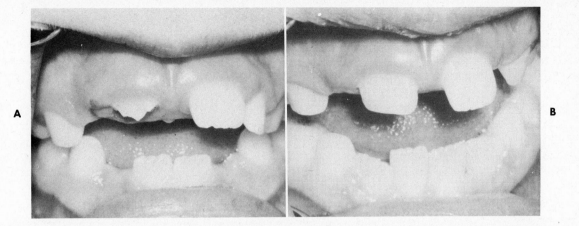

Fig. 17-7. A, Extensive crown fracture of the partially erupted maxillary right central incisor. The area was isolated with cotton rolls, a calcium hydroxide dressing was placed over the exposed dentin, and a temporary acid etch resin restoration was placed. **B,** A few months later the temporary restoration is still satisfactory and the tooth has recovered from the injury. Further eruption of the tooth now makes it convenient to restore the tooth with an esthetic acid etch resin restoration.

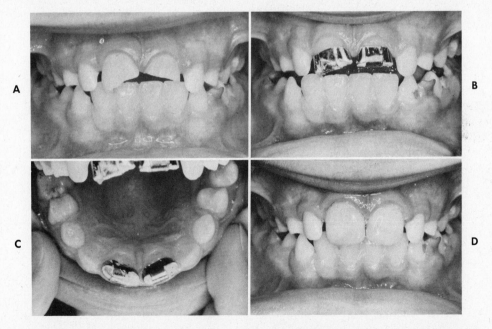

Fig. 17-8. A, Class II fractures of the maxillary central incisors. The exposed dentin must be covered to protect the pulps from thermal and chemical irritation. **B,** A band has been cemented to each tooth to support a dressing of calcium hydroxide. An additional piece of band material has been welded to the labial and lingual aspects of the bands. **C,** Mirror image of the protective coverings. **D,** Two months after the injury the teeth have been restored with resin restorations.

rary restoration of choice to provide the protection required to maintain pulpal vitality and enhance pulpal recovery.

The chrome steel crown may also be indicated when emergency dental services are required away from the dental operatory. For example, the dentist may be called to a hospital or a private home to alleviate pain associated with a fractured tooth in a patient recovering from other multiple injuries sustained in an accident. The patient may be confined to a bed and completely immobilized. In such a situation the dentist may need to provide stable coverage of the fractured tooth under compromised conditions. A steel crown restoration may be the most practical choice until the patient is in a better position to receive more complete dental care.

The principal disadvantages of this restoration include its completely unsatisfactory esthetic appearance and the inability to accurately evaluate pulpal responses during the recovery period without removing and usually ruining the crown. If skillfully placed, however, this restoration will protect the fractured tooth from contact with the adjacent and opposing teeth and will adequately support a protective dressing on the exposed dentin and pulp tissues.

The chrome steel crown temporary restoration is not indicated for most routine crown fractures, since the esthetic restorative resin techniques have been improved so much. However, adequate protection of a fractured lower anterior tooth may still present a special problem. The retention of an acid etch resin may not always be adequate on a lower incisor, and the esthetic needs are not usually as important as for a maxillary incisor. Therefore the chrome steel crown is still a viable temporary solution to such problems (Fig. 17-9).

A crown that is essentially the same mesiodistal width as the natural tooth crown is adjusted with contouring scissors to extend approximately 0.5 mm beneath the free gingival margin. To help in adapting the crown to the fractured tooth, an orangewood stick can be placed on the incisal edge of the metal crown and tapped lightly with a mallet. When the crown has been fully seated on the tooth, the occlusion should be checked to make certain there will be no premature contact. In some instances a slight reduction of the remaining incisal tooth structure may be necessary. The gingival margin can be contoured with No. 114 pliers to help ensure a snug fit at the cervical area of the tooth and thus prevent irritation of the gingival tissues as a result of overhanging margins.

Treatment of vital pulp exposures

Traumatic injury resulting in an exposure of the pulp in young patients often presents a challenge in diagnosis and treatment even greater than that presented by a pulp exposed by caries. In addition to treating the pulp at the exposure site, the dentist must keep in mind that as a result of the blow, conditions may be present for many unpredictable reactions in the pulp or supporting tissues. The immediate objective in treatment, however, should

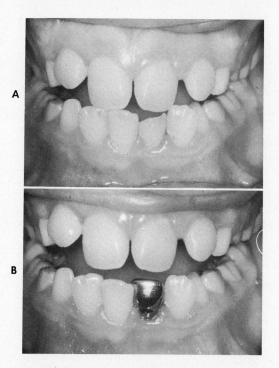

Fig. 17-9. A, Class II fracture of a permanent lower central incisor. **B,** A chrome steel crown has been prepared to cover the injured tooth. The crown, which must not be in traumatic occlusion, will support a calcium hydroxide dressing on the exposed dentin.

be the selection of a procedure designed to maintain the vitality of the pulp. In the treatment of vital pulp exposure there are at least three choices of treatment—direct pulp therapy (pulp capping), pulpotomy, and pulpectomy with endodontic therapy.

Direct pulp therapy (pulp capping). If the patient is seen within an hour or two after the injury, if the vital exposure is small, and if sufficient crown remains to retain a temporary restoration to

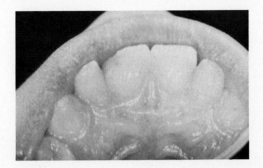

Fig. 17-10. Class III type of injury to a permanent central incisor. A small pulp exposure is evident that should be covered with a calcium hydroxide capping material and protected with an orthodontic band or acid etch restoration.

support the capping material and prevent the ingress of oral fluids, the treatment of choice is direct pulp therapy (Fig. 17-10). If the final restoration of the tooth will require the utilization of the pulp chamber or the pulp canal for a post, a pulpotomy or a pulpectomy is the treatment of choice.

Even though the pulp at the exposure site has been exposed to oral fluids for a period of time, the tooth should be isolated with a rubber dam, and the treatment procedure should be completed in a surgically clean environment. It has long been assumed that the healthy pulp will survive and will repair small injuries even in the presence of a few bacteria, the same as any other connective tissue. The crown and the area of the actual exposure should be washed free of debris with nonirritating solutions, such as saline or chloramine-T. The pulp should be kept moist before the placement of the pulp-capping material.

A dressing of calcium hydroxide is currently the material of choice as a pulp-capping agent. The prime requisite of pulpal healing is an adequate seal against oral fluids. Therefore a restoration should be placed immediately that will protect the pulp-capping material until the healing process is well advanced (Fig. 17-11). A thin layer of dentin-

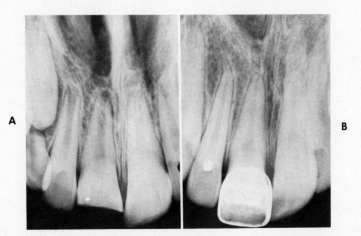

Fig. 17-11. A, The pulp of a permanent central incisor has been exposed as a result of a traumatic injury. The pulp was capped with calcium hydroxide. **B,** Radiograph of a successful pulp capping. Continued root end development indicates pulp vitality. The tooth was restored with an esthetic resin–faced chrome steel crown, but an acid etch resin restoration is currently recommended.

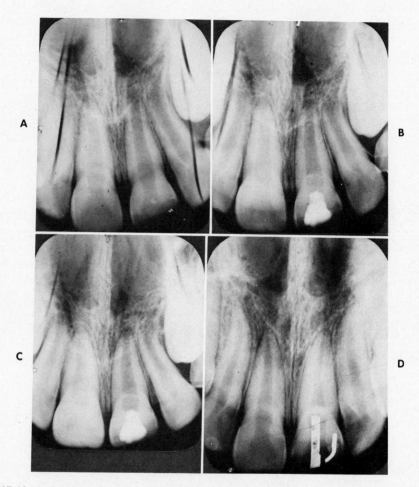

Fig. 17-12. A, Central incisor with pulp exposure. Since the patient was not seen until several days after the accident, a pulpotomy was the treatment of choice. **B,** One month after the pulpotomy, evidence of a calcified bridge is seen at the cervical level of the pulp chamber. **C,** Three months postoperatively the bridge is clearly visible. **D,** The fractured tooth was restored with a post, pin, and unfilled resin; this radiograph taken 3½ years postoperatively demonstrates normal root end completion and root canal anatomy of the pulpotomized tooth. With the current use of acid etch and composite resin, the post and pin would be unnecessary because sufficient tooth structure remains to support the resin.

like material should cover the vital pulp tissue within 2 months.

If the injured tooth presents a good indication for direct pulp therapy, there is a definite advantage in providing this treatment. The pulp will remain reparative and secondary dentin will develop and allow the tooth to be restored without loss of normal pulp vitality.

Pulpotomy. If the pulp exposure in a traumatized immature permanent (open apex) tooth is large, if the patient did not seek treatment until several hours or days after the injury, or if there is insufficient crown remaining to hold a temporary restoration, the immediate treatment of choice is a calcium hydroxide pulpotomy (Fig. 17-12). This treatment is also indicated in immature permanent teeth if necrotic pulp tissue is evident at the exposure site with inflammation of the underlying coronal tissue. Yet another indication is in the mature permanent (closed apex) tooth when the trauma has caused both a pulp exposure and a root fracture.

The procedure is essentially the same as that for a pulpotomy on a tooth with carious pulp exposure as described in Chapter 8. The exposure site should be conservatively enlarged with a fissure bur, and the tooth structure should be removed sufficiently to expose the entire top of the pulp chamber. The coronal pulp is then amputated with a small, sharp spoon excavator. Since the vasoconstrictor in the anesthetic solution often reduces the amount of pulpal bleeding, little hemorrhage will occur. The pulp chamber should be thoroughly and carefully cleaned of particles of dentin, remnants of pulp tissue, and blood clots with the small spoon excavator; it should be irrigated with normal saline or chloramine-T solution. When the pulp chamber is clean, a pledget of moist cotton should be placed over the amputated pulp stumps and allowed to remain there until a clot forms. A dressing of hard-setting calcium hydroxide is then gently placed in the pulp chamber over the vital pulp tissue. If sufficient tooth structure remains, the tooth may be restored with a temporary resin restoration. A composite resin is placed in the remaining portion of the pulp chamber, and all fractured areas are also restored with composite resin after the enamel has been etched. The temporary resin may then be "built up" to an esthetic resin restoration a few weeks later. If little or no coronal tooth structure remains, the resin may need to be reinforced with a steel tube, or a resin and steel tube post and core followed by a jacket restoration may be indicated as described later in this chapter.

Some experts on pulp therapy recommend conventional pulpectomy and root canal fillings for all teeth treated with calcium hydroxide pulpotomies soon after the root apices close. They view the calcium hydroxide pulpotomy as an interim procedure solely to achieve normal root development and apical closure. They justify the pulpectomy and root canal filling after apical closure as necessary to prevent an exaggerated calcific response that may result in total obliteration of the root canal (calcific metamorphosis or calcific degeneration).

We have observed this calcific degenerative response and agree that it should be intercepted with root canal therapy if it occurs after apical closure. However, long-term successes following calcium hydroxide pulpotomy can be documented in which no calcific metamorphosis has been observed. We have followed such successful cases for more than 10 years without seeing any adverse results. McCormick has reported one case of a tooth successfully treated with a calcium hydroxide pulpotomy that was observed for more than 19 years and never required further pulp therapy.

If healthy pulp tissue remains in the root canal, if the coronal pulp tissue is cleanly excised without excessive tissue laceration and tearing, if the calcium hydroxide is placed gently on the pulp tissue at the amputation site without undue pressure, and if the tooth is adequately sealed, there is a high probability that long-term success can be achieved without follow-up root canal therapy.

Some dentists advocate the formocresol pulpotomy technique in permanent teeth rather than the calcium hydroxide treatment. The procedures are similar, but in the former technique the amputated pulp is treated with formocresol on a cotton pellet and then capped with zinc oxide–eugenol cement in which a drop of formocresol has been incorporated (see "Pulpotomy technique for primary teeth" in Chapter 8). Most advocates of the formocresol pulpotomy for permanent teeth believe that the procedure should always be followed by a pulpectomy and root canal filling after root end closure. For those who adopt the philosophy that pulpotomies should be routinely followed by conventional root canal therapy, the formocresol technique is an acceptable approach because gaining access to the root canal is generally easier after a formocresol pulpotomy than after a calcium hydroxide pulpotomy. With few exceptions, the goal of a permanent tooth pulpotomy is to achieve normal root end closure of an immature tooth (apexigenesis). Either technique will achieve this goal in properly selected cases.

Pulpectomy with endodontic treatment. One of the most challenging endodontic procedures is the treatment and subsequent filling of the root canal of a tooth with an open or a funnel-shaped apex. The lumen of the root canal of such an immature tooth is largest at the apex and smallest in the cervical area and is often referred to as a "blunderbuss" canal. Hermetic sealing of the apex with conventional endodontic techniques is usually impossible without apical surgery. The surgical procedure is traumatic for the young child and should be avoided if possible.

In instances of Class III or Class IV fractures of young permanent teeth with incomplete root growth and a vital pulp, the pulpotomy technique (as just described) is the procedure of choice. The successful pulpotomy allows the pulp in the root canal to maintain its vitality and allows the apical portion to continue to develop. For Class IV fractures the eventual restoration may require a post in the root canal. Before the completion of this type of restoration, the dentinal bridge that has formed after the pulpotomy can be perforated and routine endodontic procedures can be undertaken in a now completely developed root canal.

Occasionally a patient has an acute periodontal abscess associated with a traumatized tooth. The trauma may have caused a very small pulp exposure that was overlooked, or the pulp may have been devitalized as a result of injury or actual severing of the apical vessels. A loss of pulp vitality may have caused interrupted growth of the root canal, and the dentist is faced with the task of treating a canal with an open apex.

If an abscess is present, it must be treated first. If there is acute pain and evidence of swelling of the soft tissues, drainage through the pulp canal will give the child almost immediate relief. An opening the size of a No. 6 round bur should be made into the pulp chamber. If pain is caused by the pressure required to make the opening into the pulp, the tooth should be supported by the fingers or with a compound splint shaped to cover the labial surface of the tooth and adjacent teeth. Drainage should be allowed to continue for several days or until the acute symptoms subside. Antibiotic therapy is generally indicated in addition to the treatment described. Warm saline mouthrinses every hour will also relieve the symptoms and will help keep the opening to the canal free of debris.

Therapy to stimulate root growth and apical repair subsequent to pulpal necrosis in anterior permanent teeth (apexification). The conventional treatment of pulpless anterior teeth usually requires apical surgery if the teeth have open apices. Many young teeth have been saved in this manner. However, a less traumatic endodontic therapy called apexification has been found to be highly effective in the management of immature necrotic permanent teeth. The apexification procedure should precede conventional root canal therapy in the management of teeth with irreversibly diseased pulps and open apices.

Frank has described a technique based on the normal physiologic pattern of root development that brings about the resumption of apical development so that the root canal can be obliterated by conventional canal filling techniques. The procedure described by Frank and demonstrated in repeated clinical trials at Indiana University School of Dentistry stimulates the process of root end development, which was interrupted by pulpal necrosis, to continue to the point of apical closure (Fig. 17-13). Often a calcific bridge develops just coronal to the apex. When the closure occurs, or

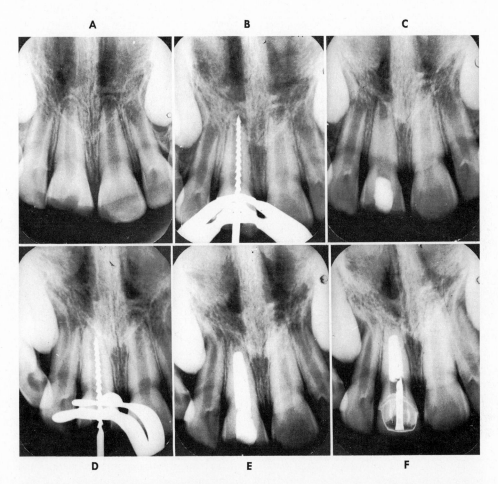

Fig. 17-13. Series of radiographs demonstrating treatment to stimulate root end development of a pulpless young anterior permanent central incisor. **A,** An injury several months before the first appointment had resulted in a pulp exposure. An acute abscess was present at the beginning of treatment. An opening to the pulp chamber was made to allow drainage. **B,** Four days after the initial treatment the canal length was established. Files were used to clean the canal. Hydrogen peroxide and chloramine-T solutions were used for irrigation and cleansing of the canal. Calcium hydroxide and CMCP were used to fill the canal. **C,** One month after initial treatment. **D,** Six months after initial treatment a definite calcified "stop" is encountered when the file is introduced. The canal was cleansed thoroughly with hydrogen peroxide and chloramine-T solution. Gutta-percha was used to fill the canal. **E,** Five months after the placement of the gutta-percha canal filling. **F,** A 6-month postoperative radiograph. A tube and resin core have been placed and the tooth has been restored with a jacket crown. (Courtesy Drs. Paul E. Starkey and Joe Camp.)

when the calcific "plug" is observed in the apical portion, routine endodontic procedures may be completed, thus preventing the possibility of recurrent periapical pathosis.

The following steps are included in the technique:

1. The affected tooth is isolated with a rubber dam, and an access opening is made into the pulp chamber.
2. A file is placed in the root canal, and a radiograph is taken to establish the accurate root length. It is important to avoid placing the instrument through the apex, which would injure or destroy the epithelial diaphragm.
3. After the removal of the remnants of the pulp with barbed broaches and files, the canal is flooded with hydrogen peroxide to aid in the removal of debris. The canal is then irrigated with chloramine-T solution.
4. The canal is dried with large paper points and loose cotton.
5. A thick paste of calcium hydroxide and camphorated monoparachlorophenol (CMCP) is transferred to the canal with the aid of an amalgam carrier. An endodontic plugger may be used to push the material to the apical end, but an excess of material should not be forced beyond the apex of the tooth.
6. A cotton pledget is placed over the calcium hydroxide, and the seal is completed with a layer of zinc oxide–eugenol covered with zinc phosphate cement.

If the child has painful symptoms during the immediate postoperative period, the dressing should be removed, the canal should be irrigated and dried, and a cotton pellet dampened with CMCP should be sealed in the pulp chamber. The filling procedure should then be repeated in 1 or 2 weeks.

Weine recommends that the apexification procedure be completed in two appointments. After instrumentation, irrigation, and drying of the canal during the first appointment, he advises sealing a cotton pellet lightly dampened with CMCP in the pulp chamber for 1 to 2 weeks. During the second appointment the debridement procedures are repeated before filling the canal with a thick paste of calcium hydroxide and CMCP or calcium hydroxide in a methylcellulose paste.

Whether the tooth is filled in one or two appointments (or more) should be determined to a large extent by the clinical signs and symptoms present and to a lesser extent by operator convenience. The signs and symptoms of active infection should be eliminated before filling the canal with the treatment paste. Absence of tenderness to percussion is an especially good sign before filling the canal. Because of the wide-open communication to periapical tissues, it is not always possible to maintain complete dryness in the root canal. If the canal continues to weep but other signs of infection seem to be controlled after two or three appointments, the dentist may elect to proceed with the calcium hydroxide paste treatment.

As a general rule the treatment paste is allowed to remain 6 months. The root canal is then reopened to determine if the tooth is ready for a conventional gutta-percha filling as determined by a "positive stop" when the apical area is probed with a file. Often there is also radiographic evidence of apical closure. Frank has described four successful results of apexification treatment: (1) continued closure of the canal and apex to a normal appearance, (2) a dome-shaped apical closure with the canal retaining a "blunderbuss" appearance, (3) no apparent radiographic change but a positive stop in the apical area, and (4) a positive stop and radiographic evidence of a barrier coronal to the anatomic apex of the tooth.

If apical closure has not occurred in 6 months, the root canal is retreated with the calcium hydroxide paste. If weeping in the canal was not controlled before filling, retreatment is recommended 2 or 3 months after the first treatment.

Although apical closure often occurs in a 6-month period, Avery has monitored retreatment for over 2½ years before favorable results were achieved. Retreatment of the canal at 6-month intervals for an extended period seems justified as long as the patient remains free of adverse signs and symptoms, since apical closure is likely to occur eventually.

Ideally the postoperative radiographs should demonstrate continued apical growth and closure as in a normal tooth. However, any of the other three previously described results are considered successful. When closure has been achieved, the canal is obliterated in the conventional manner with gutta-percha.

Controversy exists concerning the best vehicle to add to the calcium hydroxide powder. Cvek believes that the addition of toxic antibacterial drugs, such as CMCP, is not justified. However, Camp (1968) demonstrated a higher success rate in infected teeth in immature dogs with calcium hydroxide and CMCP than in similar teeth treated with calcium hydroxide and sterile distilled water. Both Weine and Cvek recommend commercially available preparations packaged for use in a syringe to facilitate filling the canal to the apical area. Arens prefers to mix chemically pure calcium hydroxide powder with a small amount of local anesthetic solution. He states that only enough anesthetic solution is used to control the powdery nature of the calcium hydroxide but that the mixture still appears dry; it is densely packed in the canal with root canal pluggers.

Currently there seems to be a trend away from incorporating antibacterial agents such as CMCP in the calcium hydroxide treatment paste. It is generally agreed that calcium hydroxide is the major ingredient responsible for stimulating the desired calcific closure of the apical area. Calcium hydroxide is also an antibacterial agent. It may be that CMCP does not enhance the repair; on the other hand, its use as described here has not been shown to be detrimental. The members of the pedodontic and endodontic faculties at Indiana University School of Dentistry have observed many successful apexification treatments during a 15-year period with the calcium hydroxide and CMCP combination. Of course, we cannot determine if the cases were successfully treated in spite of the treatment regimen or because of it and if there is a better treatment regimen. Only additional research and clinical experience can answer these questions; certainly more than one treatment paste has been employed with success.

It should be recognized that teeth treated by the apexification method are susceptible to fracture.

Reaction of the tooth to trauma

Pulpal hyperemia. The dentist must be cognizant of the inadequacies of present methods of determining the initial pulpal reaction to an injury and of the difficulty in predicting the long-range reaction of the pulp and supporting tissues to the insult.

A traumatic injury of even a so-called minor nature is immediately followed by a condition of pulpal hyperemia. In a consideration of the problem, Box emphasized that collateral circulation does not exist in the dental pulp and that a hyperemic condition can lead to infarction and pulpal necrosis. The hyperemic condition with a single outlet of veins leads to an increased danger of strangulation of the vessels.

Congestion of blood within the pulp chamber a short time after the injury can often be detected in the clinical examination. If a strong light is directed on the labial surface of the injured tooth and the lingual surface is viewed in a mirror, the coronal portion of the tooth will often appear reddish as compared with the adjacent teeth. The color change may be evident for several weeks after the accident and is often indicative of a poor prognosis.

Internal hemorrhage. The dentist will occasionally observe temporary discoloration of a tooth after injury. Hyperemia and increased pressure may cause the rupture of capillaries and the escape of red blood cells with subsequent breakdown and pigment formation. The extravasated blood may be reabsorbed before gaining access to the dentinal tubules, in which case little if any color change is noticeable and it is temporary in nature (Fig. 17-14). In more severe cases there is pigment formation in the dentinal tubules. The change in color is evident within 2 to 3 weeks after the injury, and although the reaction is reversible to a degree, the

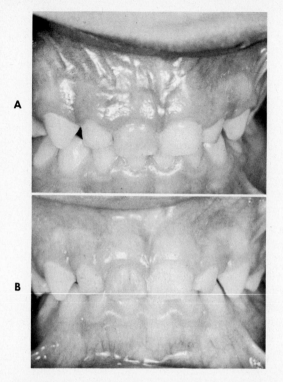

Fig. 17-14. A, Left central incisor became discolored within 2 weeks after a traumatic injury. A pulp test indicated that the pulp was vital. **B,** Six months after the traumatic injury, the tooth responded to the vitality test and there was less discoloration of the crown.

crown of the injured tooth retains some of the discoloration for an indefinite period of time. In cases of this type there is a fair chance that the pulp will retain its vitality. Discoloration that becomes evident for the first time months or years after an accident, however, is evidence of a necrotic pulp.

Calcific metamorphosis of the dental pulp. A frequently observed reaction to trauma is the partial or complete obliteration of the pulp chamber and canal (Fig. 17-15). Even though the radiograph may give the illusion of complete obliteration, an extremely fine root canal and remnants of the pulp will persist. The reaction until recently was considered to be a physiologic repair response of the pulp and an accelerated reaction that, once initiated,

may continue until the pulp is completely replaced with a dentinlike calcified tissue. There is acceptance of the report by Patterson and Mitchell that this form of calcific metamorphosis is a pathologic deviation from the normal pulp and surrounding dentin.

The crowns of teeth that have undergone this reaction may have a yellowish, opaque color. The response to the electric pulp test diminishes from nearly normal in the early stages of calcific metamorphosis to an absence of electric stimulation at the time of near obliteration. Primary teeth demonstrating calcific metamorphosis will usually undergo normal root resorption, and permanent teeth will often be retained indefinitely. However, a permanent tooth showing signs of calcific changes as a result of trauma should be regarded as a potential focus of infection. A small percentage demonstrate pathologic change many years after the traumatic injury (Fig. 17-16). For this reason endodontists recommend that root canal therapy be instituted as soon as marked diminution of the pulp canal becomes apparent.

Internal resorption. Internal resorption is a destructive process generally believed to be caused by odontoclastic action; it may be observed radiographically in the pulp chamber or canal within a few weeks or months after a traumatic injury. The destructive process may progress slowly or rapidly and may cause a perforation of the crown or root within a few weeks (Fig. 17-17). Mummery described this condition as "pink spot" because when the crown is affected, the vascular tissue of the pulp shines through the remaining thin shell of the tooth. If a perforation occurred, he referred to it as "perforating hyperplasia of the pulp."

If evidence of internal resorption is detected early, before it becomes extensive with resulting perforation, the tooth may possibly be retained by instituting endodontic procedures.

Peripheral root resorption. Traumatic injury with damage to the periodontal structures may cause peripheral root resorption (Fig. 17-18). This reaction starts from without, and the pulp may not become involved. Usually the resorption continues

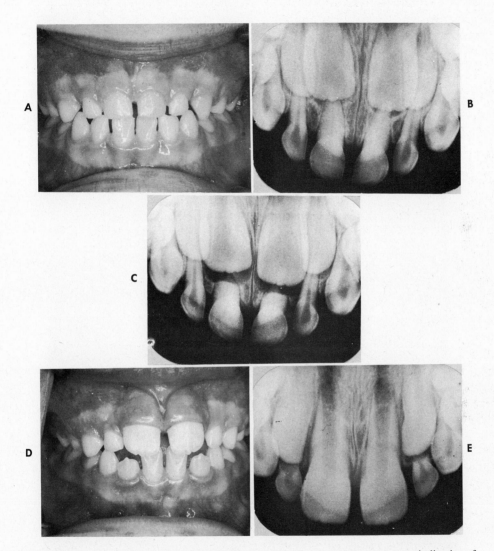

Fig. 17-15. A, Maxillary primary central incisors have a yellow, opaque appearance, indicative of a previous traumatic injury. **B,** The radiograph demonstrates almost complete obliteration of the pulp chambers and canals. **C,** Normal root resorption of the primary central incisors has occurred. **D** and **E,** The permanent incisors have erupted. White opaque areas appear on the labial surface of the maxillary central incisors, indicative of the initial injury.

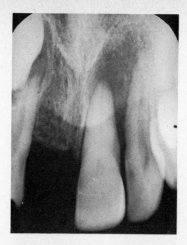

Fig. 17-16. A traumatic injury occurred 10 years before acute symptoms developed in the left central incisor. An area of apical pathology may be seen. The right central incisor was lost at the time of the injury.

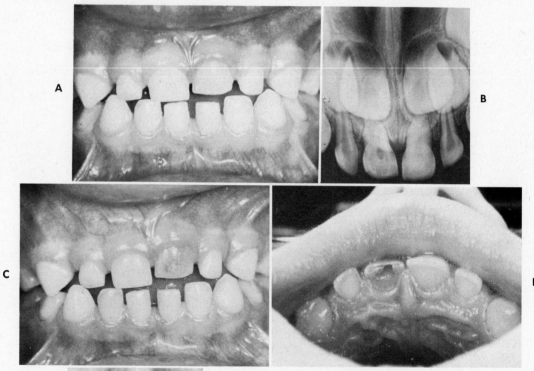

A

B

C

D

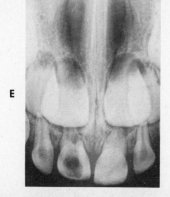

E

Fig. 17-17. Internal resorption in a traumatized primary incisor. **A,** The tooth 6 months after the injury. The crown had a slight pinkish color. **B,** The radiograph shows internal resorption in the pulp chamber and canal and some evidence of attempted repair. **C,** There was subsequent deep discoloration of the crown as the destructive process continued, accompanied by proliferation of the pulp tissue. **D,** A perforation can be seen on the lingual surface of the primary incisor. **E,** The radiograph shows the degree of the resorption. The tooth was extracted.

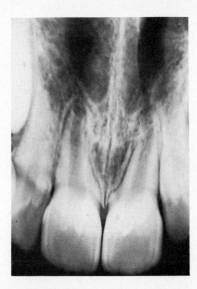

Fig. 17-18. Radiographic evidence of peripheral root resorption. In these teeth the pulpal vitality was retained, and root resorption did not continue.

unabated until gross areas of the root have been destroyed. In exceptional cases the resorption may become arrested, and the tooth may be retained. Peripheral root resorption is most often observed in severe traumatic injuries in which there has been some degree of displacement of the tooth.

Pulpal necrosis. Little relationship exists between the type of injury to the tooth and the reaction of the pulp and supporting tissues. A severe blow to a tooth causing displacement often results in pulpal necrosis. The blow may cause a severance of the apical vessels, in which case the pulp undergoes autolysis and necrosis. In a less severe type of injury the hyperemia and slowing of blood flow through the pulpal tissue may cause eventual necrosis of the pulp. In some cases the necrosis may not occur until several months after the injury.

A tooth receiving a traumatic injury that causes coronal fracture may have a better prognosis than a tooth that sustains a severe blow without fracturing the crown. Part of the energy of the blow dissipates as the crown fractures rather than all the energy

being absorbed by the tooth's supporting tissues. Thus the periodontium and the pulp of the injured tooth sustain less trauma when the crown fractures. The prognosis for long-term retention of the tooth and for maintaining pulp vitality may then improve. However, because some teeth do not recover from traumatic blows that seem relatively minor, all injured teeth should be closely monitored.

Traumatically injured teeth with subsequent pulpal necrosis are commonly asymptomatic, and the radiograph is essentially normal. It should be realized, however, that these teeth are probably infected and that acute symptoms and clinical evidence of infection will inevitably develop at a later date. The tooth with the necrotic pulp should therefore be extracted or treated with endodontic procedures, whichever is indicated.

Chirnside conducted excellent bacteriologic and histologic studies of intact teeth found to be pulpless after trauma. Aerobic and anaerobic microorganisms similar to the types normally found in the mouth were found in 50% to 75% of the canals opened. In other canals only remnants of the pulp could be detected, or the pulps had varying degrees of autolysis.

As a result of the work by Macdonald, Hare, and Wood, it may be theorized that the microorganisms in the pulp canal contribute to pulp death. The presence of bacteria in pulp already inflamed might compound the injury and lead to eventual pulp necrosis.

Grossman has investigated the origin of microorganisms in the root canal of traumatized pulpless teeth with associated acute or chronic abscess. The pathway by which the microorganisms reached the pulp was through severed blood vessels in the periodontium, the source of the microorganisms being the gingival sulcus or the bloodstream, or both. In dog experiments *Serratia marcescens* was able to reach the pulp tissue or pulp canals of traumatized teeth from the gingival sulcus.

A necrotic pulp in an anterior primary tooth may be successfully treated if no extensive root resorption or bone loss has occurred (Fig. 17-19). The

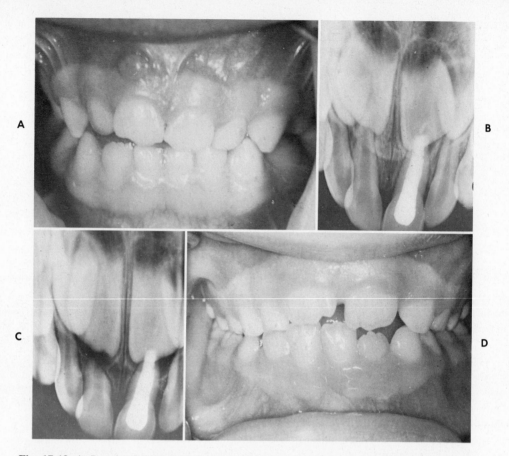

Fig. 17-19. A, Preschool child with evidence of a chronic alveolar abscess. The tooth was considered suitable for endodontic treatment. **B,** Radiograph of the tooth after endodontic treatment and the filling of the canal with zinc oxide–eugenol. **C,** The treated tooth is undergoing normal root resorption. The root canal filling material is also being resorbed. **D,** The primary incisor was retained for an adequate period of time to allow the normal eruption of the permanent successor.

treatment technique is essentially the same as that for permanent teeth. However, trauma to the periapical tissues during canal instrumentation must be carefully avoided. After the canal has been properly prepared and a negative culture has been obtained, the canal is filled with zinc oxide–eugenol. The canal walls are first lined with a thin mix of the canal filling material. A thicker mix should then be placed in the pulp chamber. Over this is placed a pledget of cotton, and the material is forced into the canal with a small amalgam plugger.

Ankylosis. One of the more infrequent reactions observed after trauma to anterior primary or permanent teeth is ankylosis. The condition is caused by injury to the periodontal membrane and subsequent inflammation, which is associated with invasion by osteoclastic cells. The result is irregularly resorbed areas on the peripheral root surface. In histologic sections repair can be seen that may cause a mechanical lock or fusion between alveolar bone and root surface. Clinical evidence of ankylosis is a difference in the incisal plane of the ankylosed tooth and adjacent teeth. The adjacent teeth con-

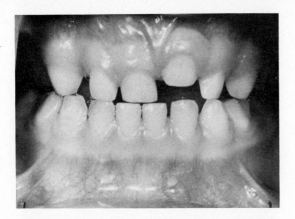

Fig. 17-20. Left primary central incisor received a blow 1 year before this photograph. The tooth was not depressed at the time of the injury. However, it became ankylosed and failed to continue to erupt.

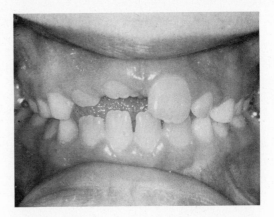

Fig. 17-21. Permanent central incisor that became ankylosed after a traumatic injury. The incisor failed to erupt and had to be removed surgically.

tinue to erupt, whereas the ankylosed tooth remains fixed in relation to surrounding structures (Figs. 17-20 and 17-21). The radiograph shows an interruption in the periodontal membrane of the ankylosed tooth, and the continuous dentin and alveolar bone can often be seen.

The ankylosed anterior primary tooth should be removed surgically if there is evidence of its causing delayed or ectopic eruption of the permanent successor. If ankylosis of a permanent tooth occurs during active eruption, eventually a discrepancy between the position of this tooth and its adjacent ones will be obvious. The uninjured teeth will continue to erupt and may drift mesially with a loss of arch length. Therefore the removal of a permanent tooth that becomes ankylosed is often necessary, especially if the ankylosis occurs during the preteenage or early teenage years.

Restoration of fractured teeth

The restoration of a fractured tooth is as important as the emergency treatment designed to aid in the recovery of the pulp after the trauma. A number of restorations have been advocated, and although the dentist has a wide choice of techniques and types of restorations, the circumstances surrounding the case often dictate the type of restoration for the patient. The prognosis of pulp healing, the amount of tooth structure remaining, the stage of eruption of the tooth, the size of the dental pulp and degree of root closure, the normalcy of the occlusion, and the wishes of the patient must all be considered in the selection of a temporary restoration, an intermediate restoration, or the "permanent" restoration. In the young patient, although it is often desirable to wait for continued eruption of the tooth or to determine the outcome of a vital pulp procedure, a delay of even a few weeks is often sufficient to allow the tipping of adjacent teeth, overeruption of opposing teeth, or other undesirable changes in the occlusion.

Esthetic acid etch resin restoration. With an improvement in the resin restorative materials and the advent of enamel etching techniques, interest in the tooth-colored resin restorations has been renewed. Investigations involving laboratory experiments and extensive clinical trials have demonstrated that acid etching of enamel prepared for an angle or incisal restoration will result in retention of the restoration equally as well as when pin support is used. Ayers found that the acid etch technique, when employed with a shoulder preparation that extended 1.7 mm or greater onto the labial and lingual surfaces of the enamel, offered a higher resistance to lingual force than double pin–retained restorations.

Before the use of acid etch techniques it was important to establish well-defined margins for resin restorations. Resin flash or featheredge margins permitted marginal leakage, resulting in staining or possibly recurrent caries. A butt joint margin at the tooth-resin interface was necessary to reduce the incidence of staining and recurrent caries. Resin restorations with featheredge margins have proved to be quite satisfactory, however, when placed on etched enamel.

Some dentists still prefer to restore fractured anterior teeth with resin restorations that have well-defined margins. A short shoulder or chamfer preparation cut circumferentially around the fracture site but maintained in enamel will satisfy the requirement of well-defined margins in the preparation when desired. Such a preparation allows the dentist to place a restoration that accurately reproduces the anatomy of the lost tooth structure. Although the featheredge restorative technique requires excessive contour in the restoration, it offers the advantage of creating less irritation to the pulp, since little or no tooth cutting is required. In some cases the excess contour is relatively insignificant, but it may be more significant if the restoration is large (50% or more of the crown) or if the fracture extends near or below gingival tissue. Excessive contour on the lingual surface of a maxillary anterior tooth may interfere with normal occlusion. Because of these factors, the dentist may elect to use a shoulder preparation for some fractured teeth and a featheredge technique for others. The dentist may also find some cases in which the featheredge technique is desirable on the labial surface to achieve better esthetic blending of the resin with the tooth but a shoulder preparation is needed on the lingual surface to accomodate the occlusion. Both techniques are presented in the following discussion.

The preparation of the tooth and the placement of the restoration should be accomplished while the teeth are isolated with a rubber dam. The shade of the resin should be determined *before* placing the rubber dam because dehydration of the tooth

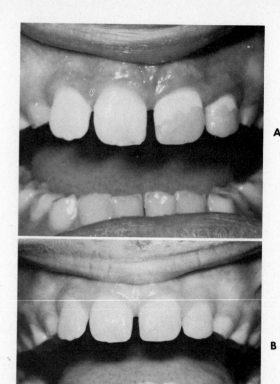

Fig. 17-22. A, Resin restorations on maxillary left central and lateral incisors immediately after completing the restorations and removing the rubber dam. The initial impression is that the shade of resin was improperly selected. However, the shades of the previously isolated teeth are considerably lighter than normal because of dehydration of the enamel. **B,** The proper shade selection is confirmed after hydration of the affected teeth returned to normal, as seen in this photograph taken 1 week postoperatively.

causes it to appear lighter than normal (Fig. 17-22).

When a shoulder preparation is desired, a No. 556 or No. 256 bur in a high-speed handpiece is used to produce the shoulder *in the enamel* around the entire circumference of the fracture (Figs. 17-23 and 17-24). The shoulder should be about 1

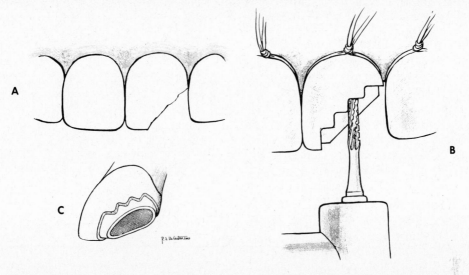

Fig. 17-23. A, Class II fracture of a permanent incisor. **B,** No. 556 or No. 256 bur is used to prepare a shoulder in the enamel. **C,** Preparation in the enamel includes the entire fracture area.

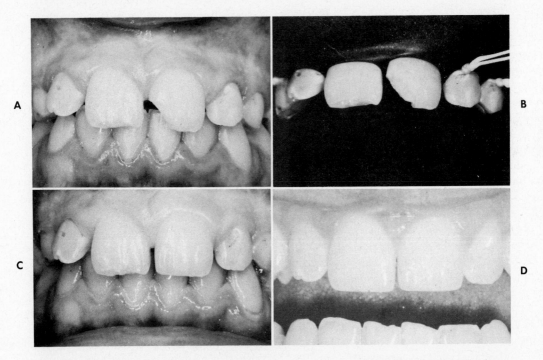

Fig. 17-24. A, Class II fracture of maxillary left central incisor. **B,** Fractured incisor has been prepared and etched before application of the sealer and resin. **C,** Nine-month postoperative photograph of the resin restoration. **D,** This 7½-year postoperative photograph still shows an acceptable esthetic and functional restoration, although close examination reveals loss of material along the incisal edge as a result of functional wear.

mm in depth cervically and a little more than half-way through the thickness of the enamel. Sharp cavosurfaces should be developed around the entire cavity outline. The labial cavosurface margin should be irregular to provide a better esthetic blending of the resin with the tooth structure.

The exposed dentin should be protected from acid penetration by covering it with a calcium hydroxide liner. A dilute phosphoric acid solution (etchant or tooth conditioner) is applied to the enamel surface of the preparation for 60 seconds with a fine camel's hair brush or a saturated cotton pellet. The tooth is then flushed with water and dried with air. Ideally, the etched area should appear frosty and opaque.

A celluloid matrix may be placed interproximally and wedged for close adaptation at the gingival margin. In large restorations an open-faced stainless steel crown or celluloid crown matrix may be used to help contour the restoration.

If the unfilled resin is used, the resin cavity sealer (primer) is applied with a fine camel's hair brush. The resin restoration is built to contour by dipping a fine brush in the liquid monomer, then in the polymer powder, and applying it to the acid etched preparation (incremental buildup technique). When the resin has been built to adequate contour to allow for finishing, the material is covered with a protective film to avoid evaporation of the monomer during polymerization. Both Starkey and Jordan and their associates have reported good clinical success after 3 years with several different resin restorative systems and techniques.

The composite resin materials are frequently used for the featheredge technique in the restoration of fractured anterior teeth. Often, little or no instrument preparation of the fractured incisor is necessary with the featheredge technique. Instead the resin margins are allowed to overlap the fractured edges to become featheredge margins on the etched sound enamel cervical to the fracture (Figs. 17-25 to 17-27). This procedure requires a slightly overcontoured restoration and therefore has limitations. The dentist should be alert to resultant potential undesirable changes in gingival health or the

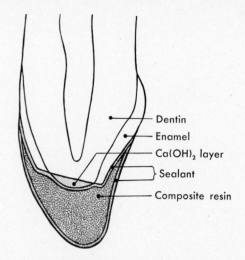

Fig. 17-25. This sagittal drawing illustrates the application of a featheredge restoration on a fractured incisor. Little or no tooth preparation is required before placing calcium hydroxide on the exposed dentin and etching the enamel. Slight beveling of the fractured enamel margins is suggested. The drawing also illustrates the need to overcontour the labial and lingual surfaces with the featheredge restoration.

creation of traumatic occlusion. Slight beveling of the fractured enamel margins with a stone or diamond is usually recommended with the featheredge technique to remove loose enamel rods and ensure a fresh surface for etching. The exposed dentin should be protected with a layer of hard-setting calcium hydroxide, and etching should extend 2 or 3 mm beyond the fracture to allow an adequate surface for featheredging the resin restorative materials. Most manufacturers supply an etching kit, which usually includes an etchant, a sealant-type material, the composite resin materials, and a shade guide. The sealant-type resin is applied to the etched enamel surface as the enamel bonding agent and also to the finished surface of the composite restoration as a glaze. The autopolymerizing materials require a bulk pack technique and usually a crown form matrix. The light-polymerized materials offer the advantages of allowing the clinician to build or sculpt the restoration in small

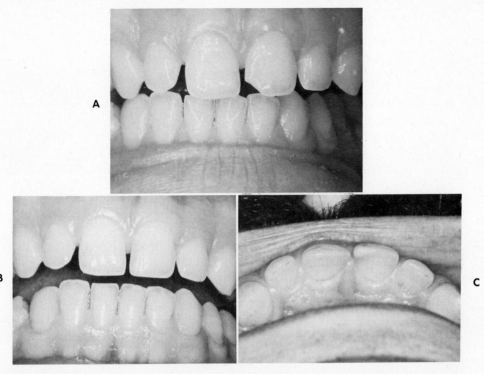

Fig. 17-26. A, Fractured central incisor that is indicated for the featheredge acid etch resin restoration. **B** and **C,** One-year postoperative photographs of the restoration. The incisal view exhibits the amount of overcontouring that naturally occurs with this technique. In this situation the overcontouring does not have adverse effects on esthetic appearance, occlusion, or gingival health.

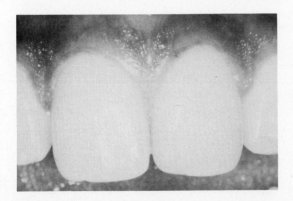

Fig. 17-27. Mesial-incisal composite restoration on the maxillary left central incisor is over 6 years old. No additional treatment or repair has been required since the restoration was placed.

increments and minimizing finishing time, but they usually require more time for placement than do the autopolymerizing materials. Clinical studies at Indiana University have confirmed that excellent and durable restorations may be obtained with either the unfilled or composite resin materials and with either the butt joint or featheredge margins (Figs. 17-28 to 17-30). Composite resin restorative materials may also be used with the shoulder preparation technique.

Finishing disks and large round burs may be used to contour the labial and lingual surfaces. A sharp scalpel blade may be used to remove flash from the margins of the restoration.

Resin post and core reinforced with steel tube. A jacket restoration may be the restoration of

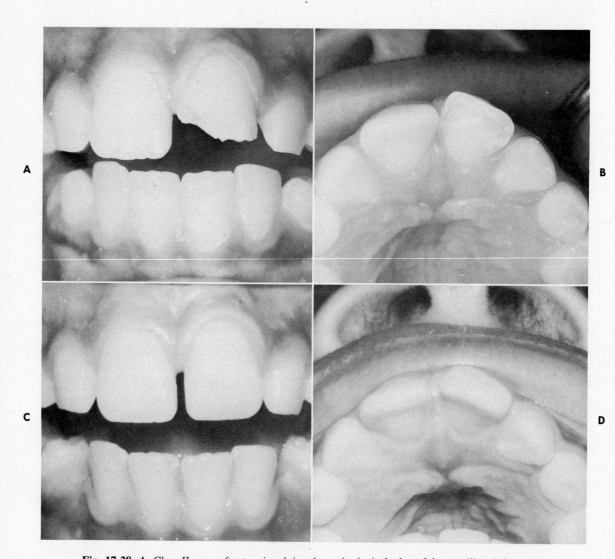

Fig. 17-28. A, Class II crown fracture involving the entire incisal edge of the maxillary left central incisor. **B,** Incisal view illustrates rotation and labial position of the tooth, making it more susceptible to trauma. **C** and **D,** Six-month postoperative views of the tooth restored with an esthetic acid etch composite resin restoration using the featheredge technique. Incisal view illustrates how an illusion of better tooth alignment was achieved by leaving the mesial half of the labial surface undercontoured.

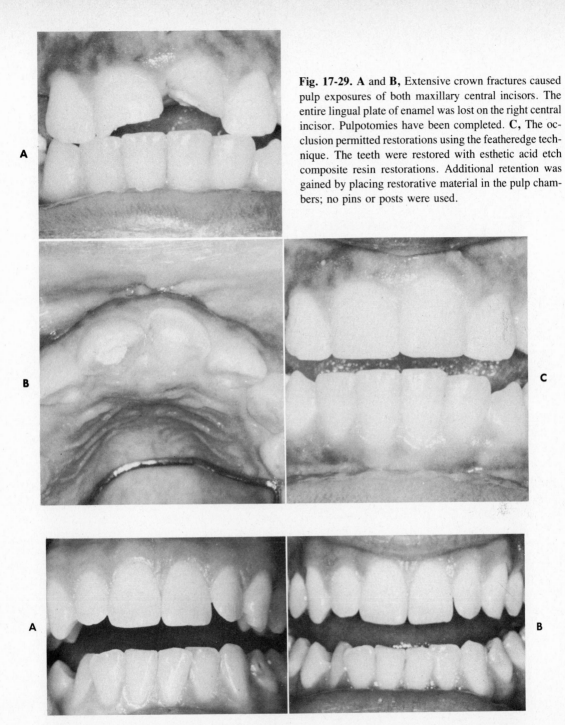

Fig. 17-29. **A** and **B,** Extensive crown fractures caused pulp exposures of both maxillary central incisors. The entire lingual plate of enamel was lost on the right central incisor. Pulpotomies have been completed. **C,** The occlusion permitted restorations using the featheredge technique. The teeth were restored with esthetic acid etch composite resin restorations. Additional retention was gained by placing restorative material in the pulp chambers; no pins or posts were used.

Fig. 17-30. **A,** Two large mesial-incisal acid etch resin restorations on the maxillary central incisors placed 2 weeks previously. The right central incisor was restored with ultraviolet light–polymerized sealant and composite resin materials using the acid etch featheredge technique. The left central incisor was restored with an unfilled self-curing resin after making a circumferential shoulder preparation in enamel and etching the preparation. **B,** Same restorations 3 years postoperatively. Both restorations are still comparable and quite satisfactory. The unfilled resin restoration on the left central incisor shows slight evidence of incisal edge wear.

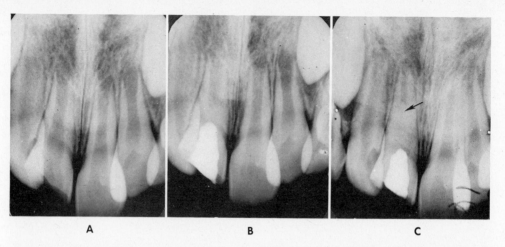

Fig. 17-31. A, Pulp exposure was treated by the pulpotomy technique. **B,** A wider than normal dentin bridge has formed, suggesting calcific metamorphosis. **C,** Evidence of continued apical development. Two thirds of the pulp canal is filled with calcified material *(arrow)*.

choice for extensive crown fracture (Class IV) after the pulpotomy procedure. Often there is insufficient crown structure remaining to support the jacket restoration without reinforcement.

The pulpotomy procedure for a fractured anterior tooth with an incompletely developed root end is sometimes considered an interim treatment. When root end closure occurs, some dentists prefer to reenter the tooth, perforate the calcified bridge, extirpate the pulp, and obliterate the pulp canal with gutta-percha. The rationale for this treatment is that occasionally, many months after the pulpotomy procedure, the pulp canal becomes partially obliterated or shows evidence of calcific metamorphosis (Fig. 17-31). If the conventional cast gold post and core are used, it is virtually impossible to remove the post and institute endodontic treatment. The resin post and core described by Starkey meet the requirement of providing sufficient support for a jacket restoration. The post, made of steel tubing and resin, may be easily removed.

The following technique is carried out after there is radiographic evidence of a calcified bridge covering the amputated pulp in the root canal (Fig. 17-32):

1. The pulp canal is reentered, and the old dressing of calcium hydroxide is removed. The bridge should be inspected with a sterile instrument to make certain there is a complete covering of the pulp. The canal is irrigated first with hydrogen peroxide and then with sodium hypochlorite.

2. The shoulder of the jacket crown preparation is completed. The walls of the preparation should be as parallel as possible for maximum retention.

3. A piece of 0.036-inch steel tubing is selected and cut to proper length. The tubing, when placed in the canal, should extend from the bridge to several millimeters beyond the crown preparation. The tube is perforated in several areas with a No. 1 or No. 2 round bur. The incisal edge will need to be flattened to keep it within the incisal portion of the resin core.

4. A thin layer of calcium hydroxide is replaced over the dentin bridge. An appropriate cementing material is placed on the apical end of the tubing, and it is carried to the canal adjacent to the bridge.

5. Self-curing unfilled resin is placed in the chamber around the tubing by means of the

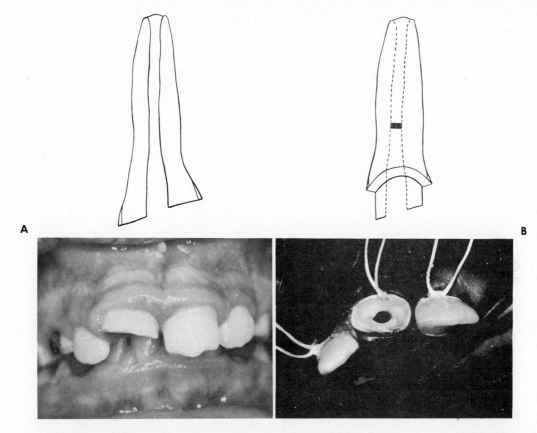

Fig. 17-32. Acrylic jacket crown in combination with the resin post and core reinforced with a steel tube. **A,** A large pulp exposure resulted from a traumatic injury, necessitating a calcium hydroxide pulpotomy procedure. **B,** After there is radiographic evidence of a dentin bridge, the pulp chamber is reentered and cleansed of debris. (Courtesy Dr. Paul E. Starkey)   *Continued.*

brush technique, and the core is built up to excess in the same manner.

6. After polymerization has occurred, the jacket preparation is completed.
7. The rubber base impression is taken, and the jacket crown technique is carried to completion.

Reaction of permanent tooth buds to injury

The dentist who provides emergency care for a child after a traumatic injury to the anterior primary teeth must be aware of the possibility of damage to the underlying developing permanent teeth.

Andreasen, Sundstrom, and Ravn have reported the effect of traumatic injuries to primary teeth on their permanent successors. In a clinical and radiographic study of 213 teeth, these investigators demonstrated that more than 40% of the young patients had changes in the permanent teeth that could be traced to traumatic injury to the primary dentition. The close anatomic relationship between the apices of primary teeth and their developing permanent successors explains why injuries to primary teeth may involve the permanent dentition (Fig. 17-33).

The dentist and the physician should also be

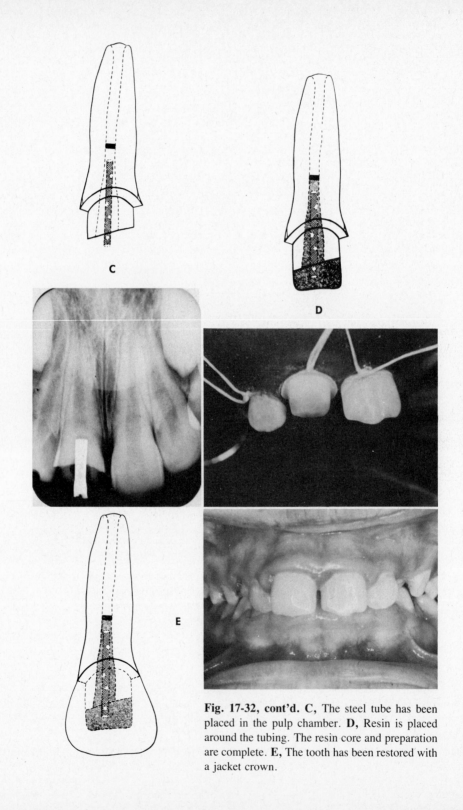

Fig. 17-32, cont'd. C, The steel tube has been placed in the pulp chamber. **D,** Resin is placed around the tubing. The resin core and preparation are complete. **E,** The tooth has been restored with a jacket crown.

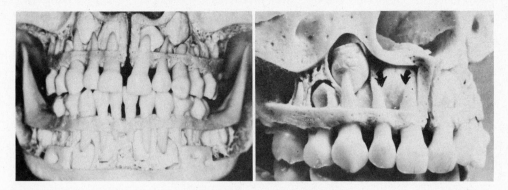

Fig. 17-33. Skull of a 5-year-old child, revealing the relationship between primary and permanent teeth. Note that both the central and lateral primary incisors are in close relationship to the permanent incisors *(arrows)*. (From Andreasen, J.O.: Scand. J. Dent. Res. **79**:219-283, 1971.)

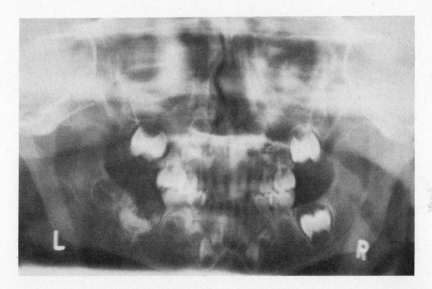

Fig. 17-34. This radiograph of a 4-year-old child reveals improper formation of the mandibular left first permanent molar. At 18 months, the child had been viciously attacked by a dog. There had been a severe puncture wound of the lower left jaw from the dog's canines, although it was not known then that the injury involved the permanent molar tooth bud. The calcified lesion was removed and microscopically diagnosed as a developing tooth with displaced enamel matrix into follicular tissue. Early removal enhances the potential of the normal developing second permanent molar to eventually acquire an acceptable first permanent molar position.

aware of the possibility of trauma to permanent tooth buds from other unusual injuries so that the parents may be informed of the possibility of defective permanent tooth development. Some injuries to the face and jaws may not appear to have caused any dental injuries initially, but the problem may be noticed several months or years later (Fig. 17-34).

Hypocalcification and hypoplasia. Cutright's experiments with miniature pigs have shown many lesions similar to those seen in permanent human teeth as a result of trauma, infection, or both. He observed small areas that showed destruction of the ameloblasts and a pitted area where a thin layer of enamel had been laid down before the injury. In other teeth there was evidence of destruction of the ameloblasts before any enamel had been laid down, resulting in hypoplasia that clinically appeared as deep pitting.

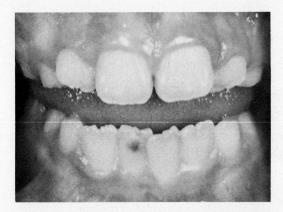

Fig. 17-35. Isolated hypoplastic area on the labial surface of the mandibular right permanent central incisor. There was a history of a traumatic injury to the primary tooth when the child was less than 2 years old.

In later years, erupted permanent teeth in the human may show a variety of these defects including gross malformations of the crown (Figs. 17-35 and 17-36). Small pigmented hypoplastic areas have been referred to as "Turner tooth." Small hypoplastic defects may be restored by the acid etch technique.

Reparative dentin. If the injury to the developing permanent tooth is severe enough to remove the thin covering of developing enamel or cause destruction of the ameloblasts, the subjacent odontoblasts have been observed to produce a reparative type of dentin. The irregular dentin bridges the gap where there is no enamel covering to aid in protecting the pulp from further injury.

Displacement of primary and permanent anterior teeth (luxation)

Intrusion and extrusion of teeth. The displacement of anterior primary and permanent teeth is a frequent occurrence and presents a challenge in diagnosis and treatment for the dentist (Figs. 17-37 to 17-39). Relatively few studies have been reported that can be used as a guide in treating traumatic injuries of this type.

The intrusion by forceful impaction of maxillary anterior primary teeth is a common occurrence in

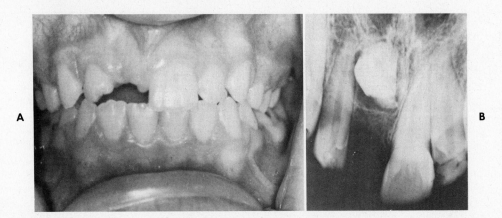

Fig. 17-36. A, Hypoplastic areas on the permanent lateral incisors. The right central incisor has not erupted. **B,** Malformed central incisor. This condition can be traced to a severe traumatic injury to the primary teeth.

children during the first 3 years of life. Frequent falls and striking the teeth on hard objects may force the teeth into the alveolar process to the extent that the entire clinical crown becomes buried in bone and soft tissue. Although there is a difference of opinion regarding treatment of injuries of this type, it is generally agreed that immediate attention should be given to soft tissue damage. The intruded teeth should be observed; with few exceptions, no attempt should be made to reposi-

tion them after the accident. Most injuries of this type occur at an age when it would be difficult to construct a splint or a retaining appliance to stabilize the repositioned teeth.

Normally the developing permanent incisor tooth buds lie lingual to the roots of the primary central incisors. Therefore, when an intrusive displacement occurs, the primary tooth usually remains labial to the developing permanent tooth. If the intruded primary tooth is found to be in a lin-

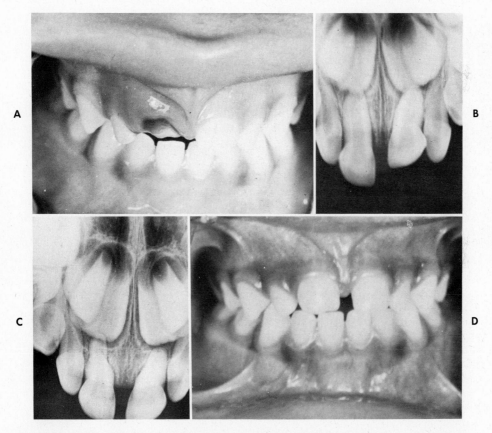

Fig. 17-37. A, Intrusion of the maxillary right primary central incisor. **B,** The degree of intrusion of the primary tooth. Damage to the permanent teeth often results from an injury of this type. **C,** A radiograph 8 months after the injury shows that the injured tooth has reerupted. The pulp has retained its vitality, although there is evidence of partial obliteration of the pulp canal. External root resorption has occurred on the adjacent central incisor. (Radiographs are reversed compared to the others in this chapter.) **D,** The injured central incisor has assumed its normal place in the arch and probably will be retained until its normal exfoliation time.

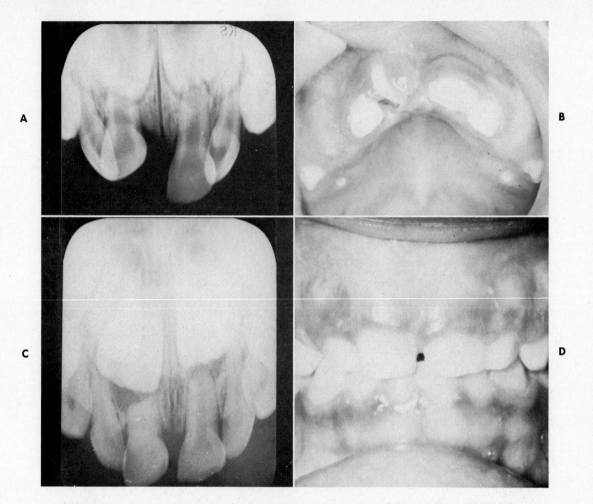

Fig. 17-38. A, Radiograph made shortly after the total intrusion of the maxillary right primary central incisor of a child 22 months of age. The tooth was rotated approximately 90 degrees, and it appears that there may also be a partial midroot fracture. **B,** Appearance of tooth and healing soft tissues 2 weeks after the initial injury. No definitive treatment of the tooth was rendered. **C and D,** The same patient at 6 years, 5 months of age (4 years, 7 months after injury). The intruded tooth has undergone advanced root resorption and calcific metamorphosis, but the area is asymptomatic and the soft tissues appear healthy. The improved position of the tooth occurred spontaneously as the tooth reerupted. One year after this photograph was made, the tooth exfoliated normally.

gual or encroaching relationship to the developing permanent tooth, it should be removed. Such a relationship may be confirmed with a lateral radiograph of the anterior segment.

The examination should be carried out as previously described, and radiographs should be made to detect evidence of root fracture, fracture of the alveolar bone, and evidence of damage to permanent teeth. However, predicting whether the permanent successors will show evidence of interrupted growth and development is impossible unless actual encroachment of their space can be seen radiographically.

Schreiber observed 42 cases of intruded primary

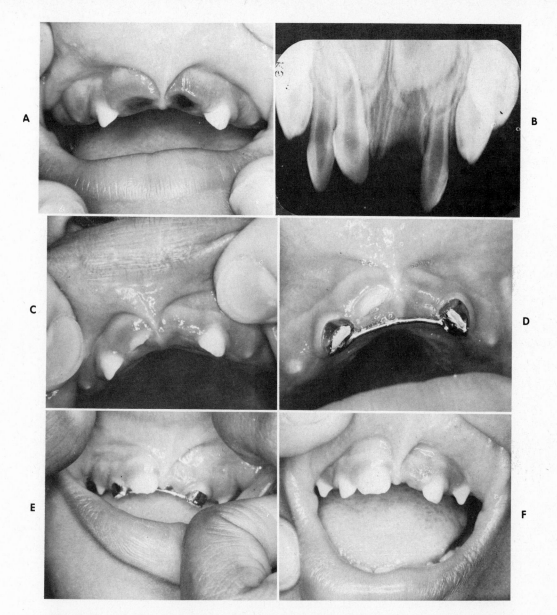

Fig. 17-39. A, A 14-month-old child with a partially intruded maxillary right primary lateral incisor, a totally intruded right central incisor, an avulsed left central incisor, and a loosened left lateral incisor. **B,** Radiograph of injured area taken the same day as the trauma. **C,** Area 2 weeks after injury; the right central incisor shows evidence of reeruption. Space loss was a special concern, since the canines were actively erupting. **D,** Cemented space maintainer in position. **E,** Eruption of right central incisors is continuing 2 months after the injury. **F,** Four months after the injury the response is favorable. The space maintainer should be recemented and should remain in place at least until the canines and the central incisor are fully erupted. A more esthetically pleasing space maintainer may be considered later.

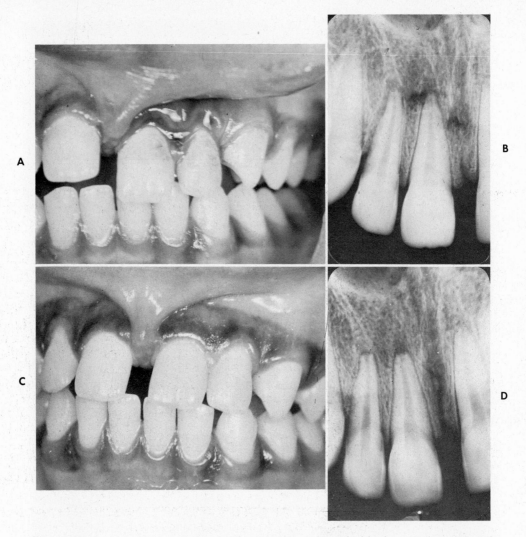

Fig. 17-40. A, A severe blow to the maxillary anterior teeth resulted in the extrusion of the left central and lateral incisors. **B,** A radiograph demonstrates a fracture of alveolar bone. **C,** One month after the repositioning and stabilization of the teeth, they are firmly attached and the gingival tissues appear normal. **D,** A radiograph demonstrates healing of the fractured alveolar bone, but there is evidence of apical root resorption. Endodontic treatment was recommended.

teeth, 26 of which were retained after reeruption. Primary anterior teeth intruded as the result of a blow may be expected to reerupt within 3 to 4 weeks after the injury. In a later study of the results of 248 traumatic episodes to primary incisors, Ravn reported 88 cases of intrusion. Of these teeth,

four were extracted within 2 weeks because of infection and four did not reerupt and were extracted several months later, but the remaining 80 teeth fully reerupted within 6 months. Incipient reeruption was observed 14 days after the injury in a few instances. Occasionally these teeth will retain their vitality and later undergo normal resorption and be replaced on schedule by their permanent successor. During the first 6 months after the injury, however, the dentist often observes one or more of the reactions of the pulp and supporting tissues that have been mentioned previously in this chapter, the most common of which is pulpal necrosis. Even after reeruption a necrotic pulp can be treated if the tooth is sound in the alveolus and no pathologic root resorption is evident.

Primary teeth that are displaced but not intruded should be repositioned by the dentist or parent as soon as possible after the accident to prevent interference with occlusion. The prognosis for severely loosened primary teeth is poor. Frequently the teeth remain mobile and undergo rapid root resorption.

Skieller observed 60 children treated for looseness of one or more young teeth. Loosened teeth were divided into three groups: simple looseness, dislocation with impaction, and dislocation with extrusion. He concluded that the immediate and future prognosis for the pulp was more favorable if root formation was still incomplete at the time of the accident. Root resorption, which was observed in all three groups of loosened teeth, was most common in impaction. Teeth with complete root formation seemed to undergo resorption more frequently than those with incomplete root formation. However, when resorption did occur, it was more extensive and progressed more rapidly in teeth with incomplete root development.

Intruded permanent teeth apparently have a poorer prognosis than do similarly injured primary teeth. The tendency for the injury to be followed by rapid root resorption, pulpal necrosis, or ankylosis is greater. The treatment preferred by Andreasen consists of gradually repositioning the tooth orthodontically over a 3- or 4-week period and then continuing to stabilize the tooth for 3 or 4 more weeks. If the tooth is completely intruded, he recommends immediate surgical positioning of the tooth so that approximately half of the intruded crown is exposed to affix the orthodontic bracket.

The extrusion of permanent teeth usually results in the teeth becoming pulpless. The immediate treatment involves the careful repositioning of the teeth and stabilization following the technique, which is described later in the chapter (Fig. 17-40). If the repositioned teeth do not respond to the pulp test within 2 to 3 weeks after repositioning, endodontic treatment should be undertaken before there is evidence of root resorption, which often follows severe injuries of this type.

Dilaceration. The condition referred to as "dilaceration" occasionally occurs after the intrusion or displacement of an anterior primary tooth. The developed portion of the permanent tooth is twisted or bent on itself, and in this new position growth of the tooth progresses. Cases have been observed in which the crown of a permanent tooth or a portion of it develops at an acute angle to the remainder of the tooth (Fig. 17-41).

Rushton reported that an injury during development may cause the subsequent appearance of an additional cusp, crown, or denticle. Partial duplication of the affected teeth may occur, with the appearance of gemination in the part of the tooth formed after the injury.

Replantation. Replantation is the technique in which a tooth, usually one in the anterior region, is reinserted into the alveolus within a reasonably short time after its loss or displacement by accidental means. There are few reports in the literature of this technique proving successful for indefinite periods of time. Slow or even rapid root resorption usually occurs with even the most precise and careful technique. Replantation continues to be practiced and recommended, however, because prolonged retention is occasionally achieved. The replanted tooth serves as a space maintainer and often guides adjacent teeth into their proper position in the arch, a function that is important during the transitional dentition period. The replantation procedure also has a psychologic value. It gives the unfortunate child and parents hope for success; even though they are told of the possibility of eventual loss of the tooth, it softens the blow of the accident (Fig. 17-42).

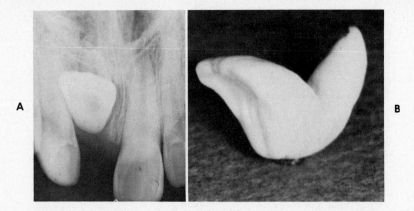

Fig. 17-41. A, Dilacerated unerupted permanent central incisor. There was a history of a traumatic injury at the age of 3 years. **B,** Dilacerated tooth after its surgical removal.

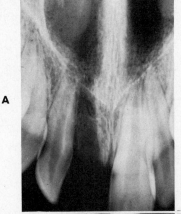

Fig. 17-42. A, Patient who lost a central incisor as the result of a traumatic injury. Since the patient was treated within 2 hours after the accident, replantation was recommended. **B,** After the replantation procedure, peripheral root resorption is evident along the mesial surface. **C,** The relationship of the replanted tooth in the arch and the normalcy of the gingival tissue.

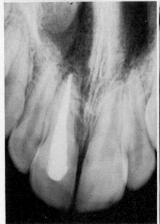

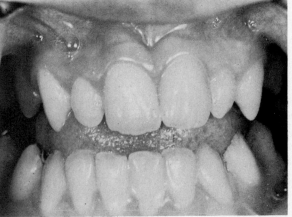

The success of the replantation procedure is undoubtedly related to the length of time that elapses between the loss of the tooth and its replacement in the socket. There have been reports that immediate replacement of a permanent tooth occasionally results in maintaining vitality and indefinite retention. However, replantation should be generally viewed as a temporary measure. Under favorable conditions, many replanted teeth are retained for 5 or 10 years and a few for a lifetime. Others, however, fail soon after replantation.

Camp reports that the tooth most commonly avulsed in both the primary and the permanent dentition is a maxillary central incisor. Most often an avulsion injury involves only a single tooth. Avulsion injuries are three times more frequent in boys than in girls and occur most commonly in children 7 to 11 years of age when permanent incisors are erupting. Andreasen suggests that the loosely structured periodontal ligament surrounding the erupting teeth favors complete avulsion.

The sooner a tooth can be replanted in its socket after avulsion, the better the prognosis will be for retention without root resorption (Figs. 17-43 and 17-44). Andreasen and Hjørting-Hansen reported a follow-up study of 110 replanted teeth. Of those replanted within 30 minutes, 90% showed no discernible evidence of resorption 2 or more years later. However, 95% of the teeth replanted more than 2 hours after the injury showed root resorption. If the tooth has been out of the mouth for less than 30 minutes, the prognosis is therefore more favorable. Also, if the apical end of the tooth is incompletely developed at the time of the injury, there is a greater chance of regaining pulp vitality following replantation. If the apex is closed, the dentist should proceed with a pulpectomy a few days after the replantation, even if the extraoral time for the tooth was brief.

If a parent calls to report that a tooth has been avulsed, the dentist should instruct the parent to replace it in the socket immediately and to hold it in place with light finger pressure while the patient is brought to the dental office. If the avulsion occurred in a clean environment, nothing should be done to the tooth before the parent replants it. If the tooth is dirty, an attempt should be made to clean the root surface, but it is very important to preserve any remnants of the periodontal ligament that are still attached to the root. Therefore the root should not be scrubbed or cleaned with chemical agents. Probably the best way to clean the tooth is for the parent to gently suck or lick it. A second, less desirable alternative is to hold the tooth under cold running tap water. Normal saline is better than tap water if it is available.

The tooth should be kept moist during the trip to the dental office if the parent cannot or will not replant it. Camp recommends that the tooth be carried to the office in the patient's mouth if possible. It may be placed in the buccal vestibule or under the tongue. If the patient is unable to store the tooth in this manner reliably (consider the nature of the injury and the age and anxiety level of the patient), the tooth may be transported held in the parent's mouth. If neither of these alternatives is possible, the tooth may be carried in a small cup into which the patient drools to bathe the tooth with saliva (and blood) while being brought to the office. Recent work by Blomlöf, Otteskog, and Hammarström suggests that milk may also be a good storage medium for avulsed teeth.

The patient should receive immediate attention after arriving at the dental office. If the tooth has not already been replanted, the dentist should make every effort to minimize the additional time that the tooth is out of the socket. The patient's general status should be quickly assessed to confirm that there are no higher-priority injuries.

If an evaluation of the socket area shows no evidence of alveolar fracture or severe soft tissue injury, if the tooth is intact, and if only a few minutes have elapsed since the injury, the dentist should replant the tooth immediately. Under the conditions just described, every effort should be directed toward preserving a viable periodontal ligament. If the tooth was cleanly avulsed, it can probably be replanted without local anesthetic (at least the dentist should try) and the initial radiograph can also be delayed until the tooth is replaced in the socket

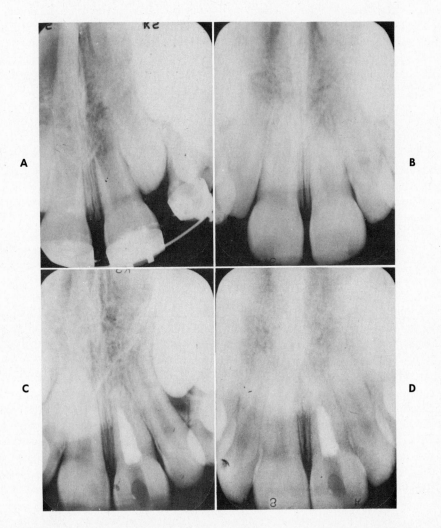

Fig. 17-43. A, An immature permanent left central incisor soon after replantation and stabilization. The tooth was replanted by the mother within 15 minutes after avulsion. The dentist instructed her by phone before the child was brought to the dental office. The tooth had erupted only about 3 mm when it was avulsed. **B,** Replanted tooth 11 months after injury shows continued but blunted root development and thickened apical calcification. The tooth was then treated with a paste of calcium hydroxide and CMCP for several months. **C,** Two years after the injury, soon after the root canal was obliterated with gutta-percha. **D,** A favorable response can be seen 5½ years after the injury. (Courtesy Dr. Guthrie E. Carr.)

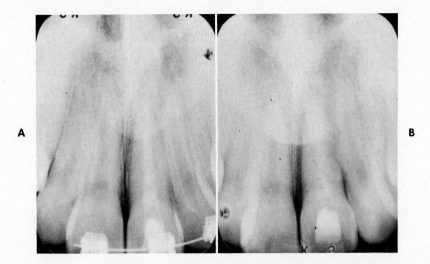

Fig. 17-44. A, Maxillary left central incisor immediately after replantation and root canal filling with calcium hydroxide and CMCP. The tooth had been avulsed 2½ days earlier and had been stored in a dresser drawer and allowed to dry since that time. **B,** Radiograph 15 months after the injury shows evidence of external root resorption along the mid-distal portion of the root and to a lesser degree along the mesial root surface. This resorptive process will continue and the tooth will be lost in time. The response of the replanted tooth is still more favorable than might be expected in view of the dry storage and the long period of time between avulsion and replantation. (Courtesy Dr. Guthrie E. Carr.)

and held with finger pressure. The minutes saved may contribute to a more successful replant. If a clot is present in the socket, it will be displaced as the tooth is repositioned; the socket walls should not be scraped with an instrument. If the tooth does not slip back into position with relative ease when finger pressure is used, local anesthetic and a radiographic evaluation are indicated. Local anesthetic should also be administered when fractured and displaced alveolar bone must be repositioned before replanting the tooth. Soft tissue suturing may be delayed until the tooth has been replaced in the socket; however, the suturing should be done to control hemorrhage before stabilizing the tooth with the acid etch resin and wire splint. Splinting techniques are discussed in the next section of this chapter.

Sherman studied the mechanism by which the replanted tooth becomes secured in the alveolus. Intentional replantation was performed on 25 incisors in dogs and monkeys. The root canals were hermetically sealed with gutta-percha, and the teeth were splinted for 1 month. Subsequent microscopic examination under fluorescent and incandescent light revealed deposition of secondary cementum and new alveolar bone, which entrapped the periodontal fibers (Fig. 17-45).

In the past, few attempts were made to replant avulsed primary teeth; however, there are a few recent reports of success with the procedure. Camp recommends extirpating the pulp and filling the primary tooth canal with zinc oxide–eugenol. He reports that it may be necessary to suture the tooth in place, placing the suture material around the tooth, over the incisal edge, and through the soft tissues. The acid etch resin and wire method of splinting may also be used. Replantation should not be considered if there is evidence of advanced root resorption or if the child has a sucking habit. In fact, the replantation of primary teeth should be

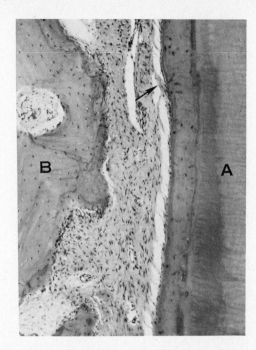

Fig. 17-45. Microscopic section of a tooth replanted with the periodontal ligament intact. The reattachment of the periodontal fibers is illustrated by their crossing the tear in the periodontal ligament. **A,** Tooth. **B,** Alveolar bone. (Courtesy Dr. Philip Sherman, Jr.)

attempted only when very favorable conditions exist (a clean injury without other injury or significant behavior complications) and when the tooth can be replanted within approximately 30 minutes after the avulsion.

Andreasen has emphasized that the preservation of an intact and viable periodontal ligament is the most important factor in achieving healing without root resorption. Delicate handling of the tooth, storage in an appropriate moist environment, quick replantation, and appropriate stabilization are all important in preserving the periodontal ligament. Undesirable periodontal ligament reactions may result in replacement resorption (ankylosis) or inflammatory resorption of the root. Either reaction may cause eventual loss of the tooth unless the resorption can be controlled.

Stabilization of replanted teeth. After replantation of a tooth that has been avulsed, a splint is required to stabilize the tooth during at least the first week of healing. Camp has stated that an acceptable splint should meet the following criteria:

1. Is easy to fabricate directly in the mouth without lengthy laboratory procedures
2. Can be placed passively without causing forces on the teeth
3. Does not touch the gingival tissues, causing gingival irritation
4. Does not interfere with normal occlusion
5. Is easily cleaned and allows for proper oral hygiene
6. Does not traumatize the teeth or gingiva during application
7. Allows approach for endodontic therapy
8. Is easily removed

The splint should also allow mobility of the replanted tooth that is comparable to the normal mobility of a tooth. Rigid stabilization seems to stimulate replacement resorption of the root. Hurst has demonstrated that rigid stabilization of a replanted tooth is detrimental to proper healing of the periodontal ligament.

The acid etch resin and wire splint satisfies all the criteria just described. It can be used in most situations requiring the stabilization of one or more teeth if sufficient sound teeth remain for anchorage (see Fig. 17-48). Rectangular or round orthodontic wire is bent to approximate the arch configuration along the midportion of the labial surfaces of the teeth to be incorporated in the splint. At least one sound tooth on each side of the tooth to be stabilized is included. The size of the wire is not critical, but rectangular wire should be at least 0.016 × 0.022 inch and round wire at least 0.020 inch. If three or four teeth need to be stabilized, a stiffer wire (such as 0.032-inch round wire) would be required. If round wire is used, a right-angle bend should be made near each end of the wire to prevent rotation of the wire in the resin.

If the labial enamel surfaces to be etched are not plaque free, they should be cleaned with a pumice slurry, rinsed, thoroughly dried, and isolated with cotton rolls. The enamel surfaces are etched for 1 minute with a phosphoric acid etchant; the gel form is convenient. The enamel surfaces are thoroughly washed and dried again. The wire is then attached to the abutment tooth by placing increments of the resin material over the wire and onto the etched enamel. The resin should completely surround a segment of the wire, but it should not encroach on the proximal contacts or embrasures. The replanted tooth is then held in position while resin is used to bond it to the wire. The resin may be lightly finished if necessary after polymerization. The splint is easily removed (usually 7 to 14 days later) by cutting through the resin with a bur to uncover the wire. The remaining resin may be smoothed temporarily and removed several weeks later after more complete healing has occurred. If the splint is used to stabilize lower teeth, it may be necessary to affix the wire to the lingual surfaces if placing it on the labial surfaces will interfere with natural occlusion. However, because lingual surfaces are more likely to be contaminated with saliva during the procedure, labial placement is preferred whenever possible.

Direct bonded orthodontic brackets may also be placed on the teeth, and a light labial arch wire bent to accurately conform to the natural curvature of the arch is then ligated to the brackets. If properly done this technique results in an excellent splint. However, it requires much more accurate and precise wire bending than the acid etch resin and wire technique (without brackets) to achieve a passive appliance.

If the patient is mentally retarded or very young and does not tolerate foreign objects in the mouth well, or if there are insufficient abutment teeth available for the acid etch resin and wire splint, the suture and acid etch resin splint advocated by Camp may be an acceptable alternative (Fig. 17-46).

In general, stabilization for replanted teeth without other complications is required for 7 to 14 days. The periodontal ligament fibers should have healed sufficiently after the first week to remove the splint. However, the patient should be advised not to bite directly on the replanted tooth for 3 to 4 weeks after the injury and then gradually to begin to function normally. During this time, food may be cut into bite-size pieces and chewed carefully with unaffected teeth. The patient should maintain good oral hygiene by brushing and flossing normally and using saline or mouthwash rinses. Antibiotics are not generally required after avulsion injuries unless there has been known contamination that may foster infection. The dentist should consult the patient's physician to be certain that the tetanus immunization level is adequate.

The development of acid etch techniques has revolutionized splinting procedures. Other stabilization methods are no longer routinely indicated for uncomplicated tooth splinting. Resin or metal splints that cover the teeth, removable appliances, interdental wiring, and ligated arch bars all have significant disadvantages when compared with the other splints described in this chapter. They should be used only when the preferred splints are not applicable because of severe mutilation.

Endodontic management of replanted teeth. All replanted permanent teeth with complete apical root development should have a pulpectomy soon after replantation regardless of the length of time the tooth was out of the mouth. Even though a few reports of revitalization exist, the chances for revitalization are remote at best. Moreover, adverse reactions are virtually certain if degenerating pulp tissue is allowed to remain in the canals for more than a few days. The risk/benefit ratio for the patient favors pulpal extirpation.

Since replantation should be done as soon as possible after the injury, the dentist should not take time to extirpate the pulp before replantation unless the injury is several hours old or the avulsed tooth has been allowed to dry. However, the pulp should be extirpated before the splint is removed and preferably during the first week after the injury. A cotton pellet dampened with CMCP may be sealed in the pulp chamber after debridement and irrigation. However, the canal should not be filled for at least 2 weeks after the injury. When the canal is filled,

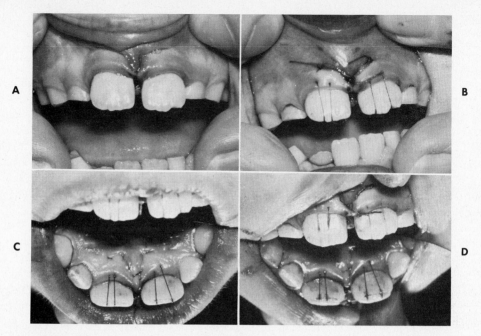

Fig. 17-46. Suture and acid etch resin splint. **A,** The maxillary central incisors have been replanted. Proper stability of an acid etch resin and wire splint may be difficult to obtain, since two permanent teeth need to be supported and only smaller primary teeth are readily available as abutments. The labial surfaces of the replanted teeth are etched. **B** and **C,** A suture in place over each tooth. Starting in the labial tissue, each suture crosses the incisal edge, enters the lingual tissue, recrosses the incisal edge, and reenters the labial tissue, and the ends are tied. **D,** Resin is placed over a small portion of the suture and the etched enamel to retain the suture in proper position. (From Camp, J.H.: Replantation of teeth following trauma. In McDonald, R.E., and others, editors: Current therapy in dentistry, vol. 7, St. Louis, 1980, The C.V. Mosby Co.)

calcium hydroxide paste is the material of choice.

Research by Andreasen (1981) suggests that early extirpation of the pulp helps to control the early onset of inflammatory root resorption. Filling the root canal with calcium hydroxide also controls and may even arrest inflammatory root resorption. However, if the calcium hydroxide is placed in the canal too soon (before adequate healing of the periodontal ligament), it may stimulate replacement root resorption. Andreasen suggests that 2 weeks after the replantation is the ideal time to fill the canal with calcium hydroxide. The use of calcium hydroxide as a root canal filling material was described previously in the discussion of apexification.

If the avulsed permanent tooth has immature root formation with an open apex, the chances of pulpal revitalization after replantation improve considerably, especially if replantation occurs less than 30 minutes after avulsion. If the avulsed tooth has been cared for properly, there is a reasonable chance for revitalization even if the tooth is replanted 2 hours after the injury. However, many do not revitalize. Those that do respond favorably may still require root canal treatment several months later. During the time the pulp tissue is allowed to remain beyond 1 week, evaluation of the tooth is recommended at 3- or 4-day intervals until favorable signs of healing without pulp pathosis are conclusive (vitality tests are unreliable) or until a decision is made to extirpate the pulp. The pulp should be extirpated when the first signs of degeneration appear.

Rubber dam isolation is always desirable when performing pulp therapy. It can usually be employed even during the pulp extirpation procedure while several teeth are splinted together. Instead of separate holes in the rubber dam for each tooth, a slit is made so the rubber can be placed over all teeth in the splinted segment. This does not afford perfect isolation, but it is generally better than cotton rolls. In addition, the rubber dam helps prevent the swallowing or aspiration of foreign objects during treatment. If small endodontic instruments are used without rubber dam protection, they should be secured with a length of dental floss to facilitate retrieval in the unlikely event they are dropped in the patient's mouth.

The calcium hydroxide material used to fill the root canal should be replaced every 3 to 6 months until a decision is made to fill the canal with guttapercha. The optimum duration of the calcium hydroxide treatment is unknown, but generally calcium hydroxide should be kept in the canal for at least 1 year or until root end closure (apical plug) occurs beyond 1 year. If an adjacent tooth is still unerupted, Camp recommends continuing the calcium hydroxide treatment until after the eruption of the adjacent tooth. It is believed that eruption may stimulate or accelerate the resorptive process of a nearby replanted root.

Management of root fractures. Root fracture of primary teeth is relatively uncommon because the more pliable alveolar bone allows displacement of the tooth. When root fracture does occur, it should be treated in the same manner as that recommended for permanent teeth; however, the prognosis is less favorable. The pulp in a permanent tooth with a fractured root has a better chance to recover, since the fracture allows immediate decompression and circulation is more likely to be maintained.

Root fractures that occur in the apical half of the tooth are more likely to undergo repair. Fractures in the apical third are often repaired without treatment. In fact, many apparently are undetected until evidence of a calcified repair is seen radiographically some time after the injury (Fig. 17-47).

Andreasen has described four modalities of healing after root fractures: (1) healing with calcified tissue, which is characterized by a uniting callus of hard tissue that may consist of dentin, osteodentin, or cementum; (2) healing with interposition of connective tissue, which results from the fractured root surfaces being covered by cementum with connective tissue fibers joining the two fragments; (3) healing with interposition of bone and connective tissue, which shows a bony bridge and connective tissue positioned between the fragments; and (4) healing with interposition of granulation tissue. The last is the least favorable form of attempted repair. The teeth usually present unfavorable symptoms that are sometimes accompanied by fistulas resulting from necrosis of the coronal portion of the pulp. These teeth require follow-up treatment or extraction.

Gross separation of the root fragments invariably causes inflammation in the area and subsequent resorption of the approximating fractured surfaces (Fig. 17-48). In order for repair to take place, the fragments must be maintained in apposition. Therefore a splint is usually necessary, particularly if the coronal fragment is mobile.

Both Andreasen and Camp recommend a relatively long stabilization period for teeth with fractured roots. Andreasen suggests 2 to 3 months, and Camp recommends 10 to 12 months. Over the past few years the recommended stabilization period for fractured roots has increased. A longer stabilization seems to encourage the more favorable type of healing with calcified tissue. If teeth with root fractures are stabilized soon after the injury, and if the coronal portion of the tooth was not completely avulsed, replacement root resorption is not a common sequela. Thus a longer stabilization period is acceptable.

The occlusion should be adjusted so that the

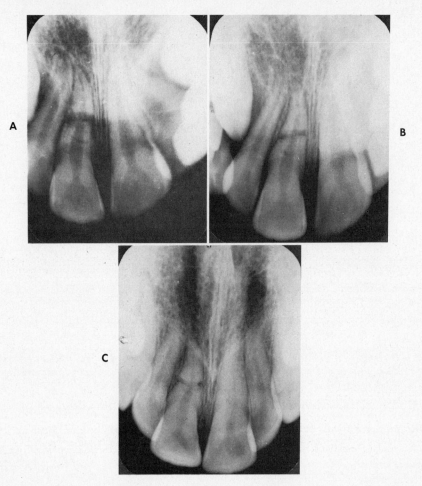

Fig. 17-47. A, Root fracture is evident in the apical half of the central incisor, but parent did not seek treatment until 2 weeks after the injury. The tooth was stabilized with a splint for 4 weeks. (Stabilization for 10 to 12 weeks is now recommended.) **B,** The tooth responded favorably to pulp testing and had this radiographic appearance 1 month later. **C,** More than 2 years had elapsed when this radiograph revealed a normal periapical appearance. The tooth responded normally to vitality tests, and there was slight mobility but no sensitivity to percussion.

injured tooth is not traumatized during normal masticatory function. Follow-up radiographs and pulp tests should be made at frequent intervals during the 6-month period after the injury.

Other displacement injuries of teeth requiring stabilization. Teeth subjected to less severe luxation injuries may also benefit from stabilization with an acid etch resin and wire splint during the recovery period. The severity of the injury will help determine the length of time the splint should remain in place. Splinting time may vary from 1 to 2 weeks for teeth that have been discernibly loosened (subluxation) to 6 to 8 weeks for teeth that have been laterally displaced, fracturing the alveolar process. As with all tooth injuries, periodic evaluation is required for at least 6 months to afford

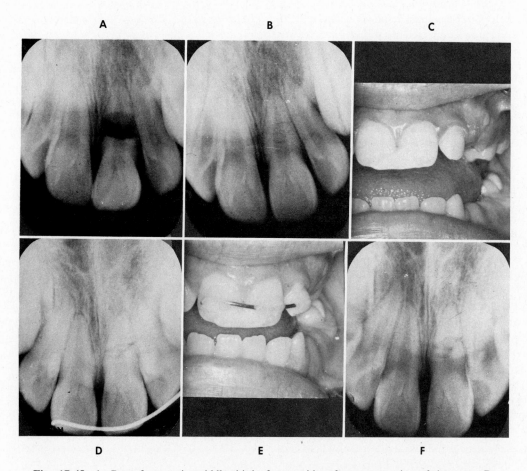

Fig. 17-48. A, Root fracture in middle third of root with a 3-mm separation of the parts. **B,** Approximately 1 hour after the injury the coronal portion of the tooth had been repositioned under local anesthesia with finger pressure. The mesial-incisal-labial areas of both central incisors were etched and self-curing resin was applied to hold tooth in position while this radiograph was made to confirm proper reapproximation of the fractured root surfaces. **C,** Appearance of stabilized left central incisor at the time radiograph was made to confirm good reapproximation. After satisfactory repositioning was confirmed, the tooth was further stabilized with the acid etch labial wire technique. This injury did not result in significant soft tissue trauma, and hemorrhage was controlled easily. **D** and **E,** Radiograph and photograph reveal satisfactory progress 2 weeks after the injury. The wire splint was removed at that time, but the resin attachment to the mesial labial of both central incisors was allowed to remain 1 more week. (Stabilization for 10 to 12 weeks is now recommended.) **F,** Nine months after the injury the tooth was vital, sound in the alveolus, and asymptomatic.

the dentist the opportunity for early intervention if adverse sequelae develop, after which evaluation at regular recall appointments should continue. The following are recommended stabilization times for various injuries as suggested by Andreasen.

Type of Injury	Time of Stabilization
Replantation	1 week
Subluxation	2 weeks
Extrusion	2 or 3 weeks
Intrusion	6 to 8 weeks
Lateral luxation	6 to 8 weeks
Root fracture	2 to 3 months

The reader is referred to Andreasen's text for an excellent and more comprehensive presentation of dental injuries.

Management of oral burns

As a result of secondary wound-healing and scar contracture, burns involving the perioral and intraoral tissues can cause varying degrees of microstomia. A common cause of oral burns is electrical trauma. The most frequently encountered electrical injury to children is a burn about the mouth. Electrical burns to the mouth occur most frequently in children between the ages of 6 months and 3 years and are equally common among boys and girls.

Oral electrical burns most commonly occur when (1) the child places the female end of a "live" extension cord into the mouth, (2) the child places the female end of a live appliance cord into the mouth, or (3) the child sucks or chews on exposed or poorly insulated live wires.

The pathogenesis of a burn resulting from electrical trauma can only be surmised. One plausible theory is that an electric arc is produced between a source of the current, such as the female end of an extension cord, and oral tissues. The electrolyte-rich saliva provides a short circuit between the cord terminals and mouth, resulting in the arc phenomenon. This type of burn characteristically involves intense heat, causing coagulation tissue necrosis.

Nature of the injury. The nature of electrical burns is variable. The clinical manifestations depend on several factors, such as the degree and duration of contact, the source and magnitude of

electric current, the state of grounding, and the relative degree of resistance at the point of contact. The wound may be superficial, involving only the vermilion border of one or both lips, or it may be a very destructive, full-thickness, third-degree burn. The more serious burns to the mouth generally involve not only a portion of the upper and lower lips, but the commissure as well. Damage associated with the more serious burns may extend intraorally to the tongue, the labial vestibule, the floor of the mouth, or the buccal mucosa. There have also been reports of damage to hard tissue, such as the mandible and the primary and permanent teeth.

With third-degree burns, subcutaneous tissues may be damaged. The tissue destruction may be much more extensive than is initially evident. Since nerves are frequently damaged, the patient will probably have paresthesia or anesthesia. Therefore pain is generally not a significant problem. Likewise, hemorrhage is usually inconsequential because blood vessels are cauterized when the injury is sustained. Nevertheless, it is important to be aware of the potential for spontaneous arterial bleeding, which may occur anytime during the first 3 weeks of healing. Spontaneous hemorrhage may be associated with the rupture of blood vessel walls that have been weakened by the passage of current. Bleeding can also occur with sloughing of necrotic tissue that overlies regenerating granulation tissue.

The clinical appearance of an electrical burn involving the lips and commissures reflects the fact that the wound is caused by intense, localized heat, as much as 3000° C. The wound is characteristic of coagulation necrosis, in which there has been heat-induced coagulation of protein, liquefaction of fats, and vaporization of tissue fluids.

During the first few days after the accident, the center of the lesion is generally comprised of grayish or yellowish tissue that may be depressed relative to a slightly elevated, narrow, erythematous margin of tissue that surrounds it (Fig. 17-49).

Within a few hours after the injury there may be a marked increase in edema. The margins of the

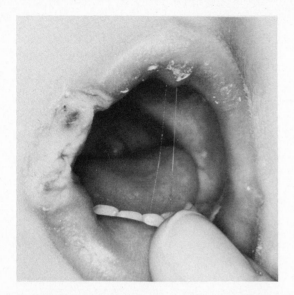

Fig. 17-49. Appearance of injury to the upper lip and commissure 5 days after electrical burn.

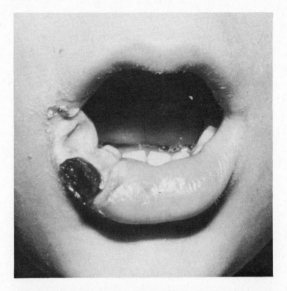

Fig. 17-50. Appearance of injury to the lower lip and commissure 10 days after electrical burn. The dark lesion on the lower lip is an eschar.

wound may become ill defined and the lips protuberant. The patient may drool uncontrollably because of the loss of sensation. In 7 to 10 days the edema begins to subside. The delineation between the central nonviable tissue and the surrounding viable tissue becomes more apparent. The necrotic tissue, known as ''eschar,'' becomes charred or crusty in appearance and begins to separate from the surrounding viable tissue (Fig. 17-50). The eschar sloughs off 1 to 3 weeks after the burn. Healing occurs by secondary intention as granulation tissue proliferates and matures. Two or 3 months after the accident the wound becomes indurated as a result of fibrous tissue formation. For an additional 6 months there is a propensity for the immature scar tissue to bind the lips, alveolar ridges, and other involved structures. If not treated during this time, contraction of the fibrotic scar tissue results in unesthetic and functionally debilitating microstomia. The scar tissue softens as it matures, and by 9 months to 1 year after the injury the potential for tissue contraction is markedly decreased. The duration of the healing process and

the selected course of treatment depend on the extent and severity of tissue destruction. Because of the variable nature of burn injuries, the treatment implemented may be surgery or appliance therapy, or no treatment may be given.

Treatment. Assessing the general physical status of a patient who has sustained an electrical burn to the mouth is the first treatment priority. Subsequently, the extent of the burn is carefully evaluated and local measures are initiated, such as control of minor hemorrhage or conservative debridement of nonviable tissue.

The immunization status of the patient must be ascertained, and tetanus toxoid or depot triple antigen (DPT) administered when appropriate. Many physicians prescribe a broad-spectrum antibiotic as prophylaxis. However, we have not found it necessary or prudent to prescribe antibiotics in the absence of infection.

The parents need to be made aware of the possibility of spontaneous arterial hemorrhage during the first 3 weeks. We instruct them to place firm pressure, with gauze, to the bleeding area for 10

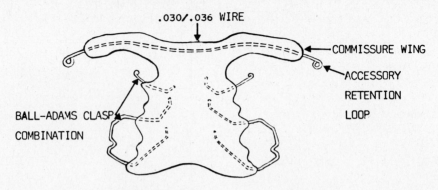

Fig. 17-51. Major components of the burn appliance. (Courtesy Dr. Mark I. Thompson.)

minutes. If bleeding persists, they are to bring the child to the emergency room. In our experience hemorrhage has not been a significant problem and does not warrant prophylactic hospitalization except for the most severe and extensive injuries.

There is considerable diversity of opinion as to the surgical management of burn injuries to the mouth, especially with regard to the time when such surgery should be performed. We believe that no initial surgical intervention is warranted. Instead, the treatment of choice is the use of an acrylic prosthetic appliance. The primary functions of such an appliance are to prevent contracture of healing tissue and to serve as a framework on which a more normal-appearing commissure may be created and preserved after completion of the healing process. Many patients at James Whitcomb Riley Hospital for Children have benefited greatly from the use of prosthetic appliances in the management of oral burns. Moreover, surgical procedures have been circumvented in cases where good patient compliance prevailed.

The major components of the burn appliance are illustrated in Fig. 17-51. The appliance can be removed when the patient eats, when the teeth and appliance are cleansed, or when modifications of the wings are necessary. When in place the appliance is a static base from which the wings extend laterally to provide contact with both commissures. If symmetry relative to the midline is to be main-

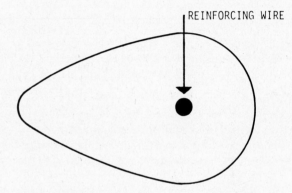

Fig. 17-52. Cross-sectional view of the commissure wing of the burn appliance. (Courtesy Dr. Mark I. Thompson.)

tained during the healing process, it is imperative that the wings make contact with the commissures equidistant from the midline, with essentially equal pressure being exerted at these points.

The shape and location of the wings are important, not only in preventing contracture or cohesion of the lips during healing but also in shaping the affected commissure so as to duplicate the unaffected commissure. The wing is contoured so it is thickest in its occlusocervical dimension on the labial aspect. It is tapered to nearly a knife-edge at the point of contact with the commissure. In a cross-sectional view (Fig. 17-52), the commissure wing appears similar to the wing of an airplane. The wings should be large enough only to maintain the correct shape of the commissure. The proper size of the wings will keep any esthetic liability to a minimum and enhance acceptance and compliance by the child and parent.

Ideally the patient who has sustained an electrical burn to the mouth should be seen by the dentist between the fifth and tenth days after the burn. The initial appointment is probably the most crucial to the success or failure of the burn appliance. Parental apprehension and feelings of guilt are often high, and the trust and confidence of both the parents and the child must be acquired as soon as possible. They should be told in detail what they can expect from the dental services offered and what is expected of them. We show the parents and the child slides from previous cases, not only to demonstrate the appearance and purpose of the appliance but also to show them that they are not the only ones who have experienced the physical and psychologic trauma associated with such an accident. We also show slides of patients who did not have an appliance after sustaining their injury or who did not wear their appliance as instructed. The impact of such illustrative materials can be dramatic.

After the consultation session, the initial data are recorded, photographs are taken, and alginate impressions are obtained for fabrication of the appliance. The appliance is generally delivered between the tenth and fourteenth days after the injury. At the delivery appointment and at each subsequent appointment the statements made in the initial consultation session should be reinforced. Constant encouragement and positive reinforcement are important psychologic aids in enhancing compliance.

After delivery of the appliance the patient is usually seen at 2 days, 1 week, 3 weeks, and 7 weeks. During this period most of the major modifications of the wings and other components of the appliance are made. The patient's compliance is closely monitored during this period. Once the appliance is properly modified and the patient is wearing the appliance as instructed, the appointments can be spaced out over 4- to 6-week intervals. The appliance should be worn 24 hours a day for 12 months except for eating and cleaning (Fig. 17-53).

The burn appliance may not eliminate the need for minor surgical revisions of the lips or surrounding cutaneous tissues. Its purpose is to obviate more difficult surgical procedures, since good results are hard to attain and maintain when surgically restoring the shape and location of the oral commissure. The appliance can prevent asymmetry of the commissures resulting from tissue cohesion and scar contracture. It can provide a more normal-appearing commissure after healing. The successful use of this appliance ultimately depends on patient compliance (Fig. 17-54).

Infants or toddlers who do not have primary molars that can be used for intraoral anchorage will not be able to retain the burn appliance without extraoral stabilization. Fig. 17-55 illustrates a "headgear" type of extraoral anchorage apparatus. It is made of durable cloth, such as denim lined with gingham, and provides a static base from which elastic material extends to the wings of the burn appliance.

Patients who have sustained a burn injury to the mouth but who did not have access to burn appliance therapy or were noncompliant in wearing their burn appliance may have tissue cohesion, contraction, and deformation as a result of healing. Such patients may require a commissurotomy to reestablish the original dimensions and symmetry of the mouth. Unfortunately, with healing, there is again a tendency for wound contraction and distortion. Therefore it may be necessary for the patient to undergo more than one such surgical procedure unless surgery is followed by appliance therapy.

The use of the burn appliance after a commissurotomy differs from the utilization after a burn injury in two respects: (1) the appliance must be delivered by the time the sutures are removed, since by the second week after surgery there may already be a decrease in the lateral extension of the primary incision as a result of wound healing, and (2) the total time that the patient needs to wear the

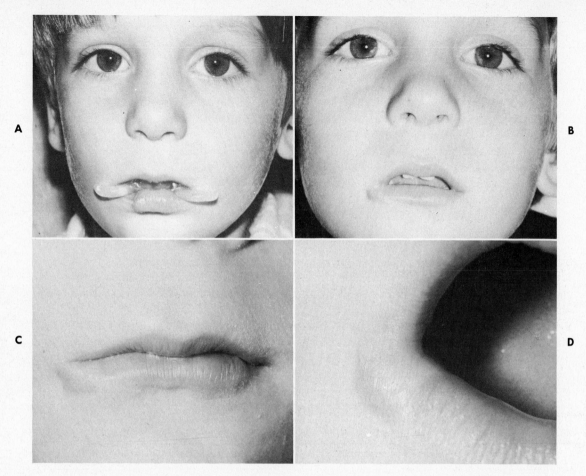

Fig. 17-53. A, Properly fitted burn appliance in the mouth. **B,** Nine-month result. **C,** One-year result showing properly shaped commissure and symmetry of the lips. **D,** Patient has good function. This is the same patient shown in Fig. 17-50.

appliance may be less than 1 year. The patient wears the appliance 24 hours a day except for eating and cleaning.

Trauma prevention

Dental practitioners should be proud of the fact that we are a "prevention-oriented" profession. Prevention is especially predominant in dentistry for children. We strive to prevent dental caries, periodontal disease, and malocclusion. If disease is present, our treatment becomes part of an overall prevention plan designed to halt the progress of disease and prevent its recurrence. The success of the prevention plan, provided there is parent and patient cooperation, is reasonably predictable.

Unfortunately, our ability to prevent traumatic injuries to oral structures is limited. Living and growing carry a high risk of trauma. A child will not learn to walk without falling, and few children reach the age of 4 years without having received a blow to the mouth. We cannot totally prevent trauma. Moreover, the results of treatment of trau-

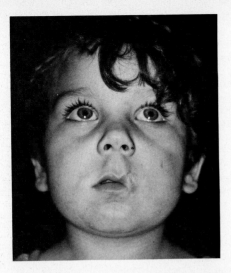

Fig. 17-54. Burn patient who did not wear the appliance as recommended, shown 10 months after the injury. Surgical correction will be considerably more difficult in this patient. (Courtesy Drs. Roger Wood, Richard Quinn, and Joe Forgey.)

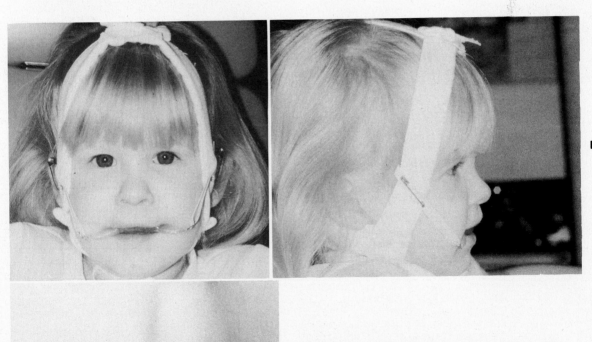

Fig. 17-55. A and **B,** Properly fitted burn appliance with headgear to enhance stability and retention of the appliance. **C,** Nine-month result with appliance therapy. This is the same patient shown in Fig. 17-49.

matic injuries are often less predictable than those of other types of dental treatment.

On the brighter side, there are preventive measures that have been proved to reduce the prevalence of traumatic episodes in certain environmental situations. For example, because the prevalence of fractured incisors is higher among those with protrusive anterior teeth, many dentists are recommending early reduction of excessive protrusion to reduce the susceptibility of such teeth to injury. The use of safety car seats and restraining belts has prevented many injuries to infants and young children. The protective mouth guard described in Chapter 26 has prevented or reduced the severity of countless injuries to the teeth of youngsters participating in organized athletic activities; active youngsters should be encouraged to wear their mouth guards during high-risk unsupervised athletic activities as well. Parents should be reminded that accessible "live" electric cords are potentially dangerous, especially to small children who still use their mouths to evaluate their environment. When we have the opportunity to save a child from pain and suffering, an ounce of prevention is worth a pound of cure.

REFERENCES

Andreasen, J.O.: Traumatic injuries of the teeth, ed. 2, Philadelphia, 1981, W.B. Saunders Co.

Andreasen, J.O., and Hjørting-Hansen, E.: Replantation of teeth. I. Radiographic and clinical study of 110 human teeth replanted after accidental loss, Acta Odontol. Scand. **24:**263-286, 1966.

Andreasen, J.O., Sundstrom, B., and Ravn, J.J.: The effect of traumatic injuries to the primary teeth on their permanent successors, Scand. J. Dent. Res. **79:**219-283, 1971.

Arens, D.E.: Personal communication, 1982.

Ayers, A.J.: Retention of resin restorations by means of enamel etching and by pins, thesis, Indianapolis, 1971, Indiana University School of Dentistry.

Barry, G.N.: Replanted teeth still functioning after 42 years: report of a case, J.A.D.A. **92:**412-413, 1976.

Blomlöf, L., and Otteskog, P.: Viability of human peridontal ligament cells after storage in milk or saliva, Scand. J. Dent. Res. **88:**436-440, 1980.

Blomlöf, L., Lindskog, S., and Hammarström, L.: Periodontal healing of exarticulated monkey teeth stored in milk or saliva, Scand. J. Dent. Res. **89:**251-259, 1981.

Blomlöf, L., Otteskog, P., and Hammarström, L.: Effect of storage in media with different ion strengths and osmolalities on human periodontal ligament cells, Scand. J. Dent. Res. **89:**180-187, 1981.

Box, H.K.: Histological and histopathological studies of the dental pulp, Oral Health **12:**223-252, 265-293, 1922.

Camp, J.H.: Continued apical development of pulpless permanent teeth following endodontic therapy, thesis, Indianapolis, 1968, Indiana University School of Dentistry.

Camp, J.H.: Replantation of teeth following trauma. In McDonald, R.E., and others, editors: Current therapy in dentistry, vol. 7, St. Louis, 1980, The C.V. Mosby Co.

Camp, J.H.: Personal communication, 1982.

Chirnside, I.M.: A bacteriological and histological study of traumatized teeth, N.Z. Dent. J. **53:**176-191, 1957.

Convery, L.P.: Tetanus prophylaxis for the child with soft tissue injury: the dentist's responsibility, J. Indianap. Dist. Dent. Soc. **21:**11-13, 1966.

Cutright, D.E.: The reaction of permanent tooth buds to injury, Oral Surg. **32:**832-839, 1971.

Cvek, M.: Endodontic treatment of traumatized teeth. In Andreasen, J.O.: Traumatic injuries of the teeth, ed. 2, Philadelphia, 1981, W.B. Saunders Co.

Ellis, R.G., and Davey, K.W.: The classification and treatment of injuries to the teeth of children, ed. 5, Chicago, 1970, Year Book Medical Publishers, Inc.

Fountain, S.B., and Camp, J.H.: Traumatic injuries. In Cohen, S., and Burns, R.C.: Pathways of the pulp, ed. 3, St. Louis, The C.V. Mosby Co. In press.

Frank, A.L.: Therapy for the divergent pulpless tooth by continued apical formation, J.A.D.A. **72:**87-93, 1966.

Grossman, L.I.: Origin of microorganisms in traumatized pulpless sound teeth, J. Dent. Res. **46:**551-553, 1967.

Hurst, R.V.: Regeneration of periodontal and transeptal fibers after autografts in rhesus monkeys: a qualitative approach, J. Dent. Res. **51:**1183-1192, 1972.

Jordan, R.E., and others: Restoration of fractured and hypoplastic incisors by the acid etch resin technique: a three-year report, J.A.D.A. **95:**795-803, 1977.

Larson, T.H.: Splinting oral electrical burns in children: report of two cases, J. Dent. Child. **44:**382-384, 1977.

Macdonald, J.B., Hare, G.C., and Wood, A.W.S.: Bacteriologic status of the pulp chambers in intact teeth found to be nonvital following trauma, Oral Surg. **10:**318-322, 1957.

McCormick, F.E.: Calcium-hydroxide pulpotomy: report of a case observed for nineteen years, J. Dent. Child. **48:**222-225, 1981.

Mummery, J.H.: Some further cases of chronic perforating hyperplasia of the pulp, the so-called "pink spot," Br. Dent. J. **47:**801-811, 1926.

Needleman, H.L. and Berkowitz, R.J.: Electric trauma to the oral tissues of children, J. Dent. Child. **41:**19-22, 1974.

Oeconomopoulos, C.T.: Electrical burns in infancy and early childhood, Am. J. Dis. Child. **103:**35-38, 1962.

Patterson, S.S., and Mitchell, D.F.: Calcific metamorphosis of the dental pulp, Oral Surg. **20:**94-101, 1965.

Ravn, J.J.: Sequelae of acute mechanical traumata in the primary dentition, J. Dent. Child. **35:**281-289, 1968.

Rock, W.P., and others: The relationship between trauma and pulp death in incisor teeth, Br. Dent. J. **136:**236-239, 1974.

Rushton, M.A.: Partial duplication following injury to developing incisors, Br. Dent. J. **104:**12, 1958.

Schreiber, C.K.: The effect of trauma on the anterior deciduous teeth, Br. Dent. J. **106:**340-343, 1959.

Sherman, P., Jr.: A histologic study of intentional replantation of teeth in dogs and monkeys, thesis, Indianapolis, 1967, Indiana University School of Dentistry.

Skieller, V.: The prognosis for young teeth loosened after mechanical injuries, Acta Odontol. Scand. **18:**171-181, 1960.

Slack, G.L., and Jones, J.M.: Psychological effect of fractured incisors, Br. Dent. J. **99:**386-388, 1955.

Starkey, P.E.: The use of self-curing resin in the restoration of young fractured permanent anterior teeth, J. Dent. Child. **34:**15-29, 1967.

Starkey, P.E.: Reattachment of a fractured fragment to a tooth, J. Ind. Dent. Assoc. **58:**37-38, 1979.

Starkey, P.E., and others: A comparison of two resin systems in the restoration of fractured young anterior teeth, J. Ind. Dent. Assoc. **60:**9-14, 1981.

Tennery, T.N.: The fractured tooth reunited using the acid-etch bonding technique, Tex. Dent. J. **96:**16-17, 1978.

Weine, F.S.: Endodontic therapy, ed. 3, St. Louis, 1982, The C.V. Mosby Co.

Wood, R.S., Quinn, R.M., and Forgey, J.E.: Treating electrical burns of the mouths of children, J.A.D.A. **97:**206-208, 1978.

Wright, G.Z., Colcleigh, R.G., and Davidge, L.K.: Electrical burns to the commissure of the lips, J. Dent. Child. **44:**377-381, 1977.

18 Basic concepts of growth of the face and dental arches

W. BAILEY DAVIS

This chapter is intended to give students and dentists an outline to help organize their basic information for evaluating and planning treatment for the developing dentition. As students begin to use what they have learned about growth and development, they find the most prevalent problem is that of genetic variation. It becomes frustrating to apply knowledge of multiple longitudinal growth studies, graphs, and specific population information to the individual patient.

Cephalometric norms and standards have been established to compare individual patients with group populations, and current studies are programming these data to enable predictions of the growth of the face and dental structures. Cephalometric analysis is covered in detail in Chapter 19. For further information concerning the growth of the face and dental structures, the reader should consult the classic texts by Barnett, Enlow, Lowrey, Moyers, and Van der Linden and Duterloo, which are listed in the references for this chapter.

The dentist will always be confronted with unique or unusual growth problems that will not fit a specific classification. These cases will undoubtedly require consultation with other specialists to arrive at a final treatment plan.

The following eight topics or relationships are described to assist the student in arranging information about the developing occlusion. The topics should be evaluated independently and then collectively to determine the best plan and time for treatment. An appropriate record of each area evaluated should be made, and a summary of the occlusion should be reviewed at each recall appointment until treatment begins.

Skeletal relationship of the maxilla to the mandible in facial profile

The first and most important consideration in diagnosis and treatment of the developing occlusion is the relationship of the maxilla and the mandible to each other and to the anterior cranial base. Clinical examination of the patient's profile will demonstrate pronounced deviations in skeletal balance. The anteroposterior skeletal relationship of the maxilla and mandible can be determined clinically by the position of the maxillary and mandibular canines when the mandible is placed in centric position. The condyles must be placed in the most retruded position when the canine relationship is recorded to be sure that there are no occlusal interferences or shifts in the occlusion. The Angle classification of a straight or neutral profile, Class I; a convex or maxillary protrusion, Class II; and a concave or prognathic mandible profile, Class III, is still the most widely accepted skeletal and dental classification system.

The clinical examination can always be verified by a lateral-oriented cephalometric film taken with the patient in centric position. There are multiple cephalometric analyses that relate the maxilla, mandible, and cranial base (see Chapter 19 on cephalometrics). The two measurements illustrated

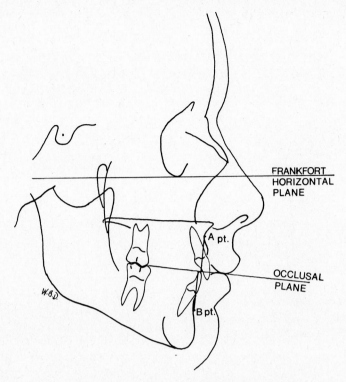

Fig. 18-1. Relationship of the maxillary basal bone *(A point)* to the mandibular basal *(B point)* to plane of occlusion. Perpendiculars are dropped from respective A and B points of plane of occlusion. Normally the B point will fall approximately 0.5 to 1.5 mm behind the A point.

in Fig. 18-1 relate the basal bone of the maxilla to the mandible along the plane of occlusion and give a clue to the functional relationship of the denture as well. The normal range of maxillary basal bone (A point) to mandibular basal bone (B point) is −0.5 to −1.5 mm. Fig. 18-2 indicates the types of imbalance that may occur between maxillary and mandibular skeletal bases as points A and B vary anteriorly and posteriorly. The mandible should normally be slightly behind the maxilla in profile to allow the normal overbite and overjet relationship of the maxillary and mandibular incisors. Longitudinal studies indicate that the A-B relationship to the occlusal plane is fairly constant during growth of the face, and therefore reasonable prediction of facial balance can be made by the time incisors or anterior segments have finished their eruption.

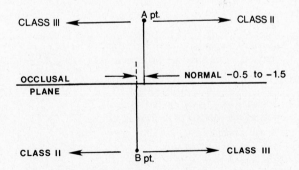

Fig. 18-2. As the B point moves anteriorly, a Class III relationship develops. As the B point moves inferiorly or posteriorly, a Class II skeletal relationship occurs if the A point remains constant. If the B point remains constant and the A point moves anteriorly, a Class II pattern develops. If the A point moves posteriorly, a Class III relationship develops.

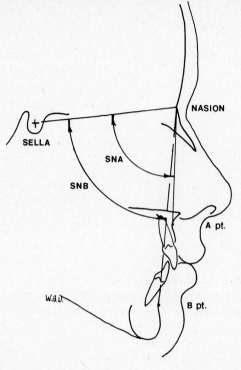

Fig. 18-3. Skeletal profile measurement of maxilla to cranial base and mandible to cranial base is made by measurement of the SNA and SNB angle (see text).

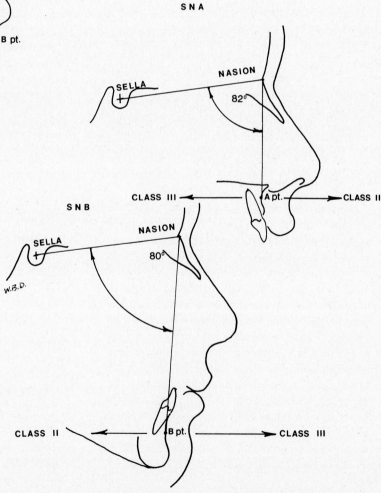

Fig. 18-4. SNA is normally 82 degrees. As the A point moves anteriorly, the angle increases, giving a Class II developmental pattern; as the angle decreases, the A point moves posteriorly, giving a Class III pattern. The sella-nasion B point reflecting the position of the mandible to the cranial base normally produces an angle of 80 degrees. As the B point moves anteriorly, a Class III pattern would be predicted. As the B point moves posteriorly or the angle decreases, a Class II skeletal pattern can be expected.

The relationships of the maxilla and the mandible to the anterior cranial base *(sella-nasion)* are illustrated in Fig. 18-3. This measurement employs an angle made by the anterior cranial base plane of sella-nasion and a line between A point and nasion and B point and nasion. As the angle increases or decreases, the respective changes in skeletal balance can be noted (Fig. 18-4). This relationship also remains quite stable during growth. Severe skeletal Class II and Class III conditions may be more difficult to predict and may produce wider variations. Patients with these conditions usually require orthodontic corrections and may even need surgical correction of the skeletal imbalance. Evaluation of the developing occlusion should always include the skeletal evaluation first. Enlow's textbook, which thoroughly describes the concepts of facial growth and development, may be used.

Position of the upper and lower lips in the lower facial profile

The dentist has little control over the facial form of the patient, with the exception of the upper and lower lip contour, which can be influenced by the anteroposterior position of the maxillary and mandibular incisors. The genetic variability in the U.S. population makes it difficult to define a range of facial normality. Burstone (1967) evaluated facial esthetics, combining the techniques of cephalometrics and those of the artist. In his discussion of the integumental profile, Burstone describes the variability of soft tissue thickness, facial height, length of the nose, and size of the chin. Emphasis is directed to the influence of the upper and lower lips in facial beauty and how the maxillary and mandibular incisors can alter the anteroposterior posture of the lips.

Evaluation of the lip thickness, length, and posture should be part of every occlusion evaluation. The clinical examination and history should indicate if oral habits, tongue thrusting, incisor flaring, or atypical facial or skeletal patterns exist. To further evaluate lip posture, the patient should be instructed to swallow, to allow the mandible to return to the rest position, and then to allow the upper and lower lips to relax and gently touch. A lateral headplate should be obtained in this posture and the following evaluations made.

Two lines are drawn on the cephalometric tracing, one from the junction of the nasal columella and the upper lip to the most prominent point of the soft tissue over the chin. The other line connects the tip of the nose and the same chin point. The triangle formed by these two lines and the inferior border of the nose is referred to as the "esthetic triangle." A well-balanced soft tissue pattern should place the upper and lower lips inside this triangle (Fig. 18-5, *B*).

As the lips approach the outer limits of the esthetic triangle (Fig. 18-5, *A*), bimaxillary protrusion or fullness of the lower face is noted. Retropositioning of the anterior denture with extractions or orthodontic treatment should improve the soft tissue profile.

If the upper and lower lips are retropositioned, a concave soft tissue pattern is recorded (Fig. 18-5, *C*). The dentist should make every effort during this child's development to allow the maxillary and mandibular denture to be held forward to support the lips. Extractions for these patients should be avoided if possible; if extractions are necessary, lingual arch or supportive therapy may be considered.

The dentist should always determine the posture of the soft tissue before treatment and weigh the consequences of either flattening the lower face profile and lips by extraction therapy or protruding the profile by flaring the incisor segments. Severely imbalanced facial patterns may require surgical correction in conjunction with conventional orthodontic care. The effect on facial appearance should always be a major point in treatment planning and consultations with the patient and parents.

Dental relationship

The clinician usually examines the occlusal relationship of the maxillary and mandibular teeth before taking a close look at the skeletal and soft tissue patterns. The relationship of the primary and

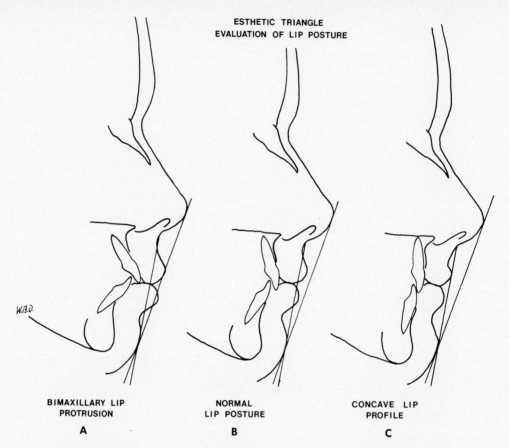

ESTHETIC TRIANGLE
EVALUATION OF LIP POSTURE

BIMAXILLARY LIP
PROTRUSION

A

NORMAL
LIP POSTURE

B

CONCAVE LIP
PROFILE

C

Fig. 18-5. A, Bimaxillary protrusion caused by flaring of maxillary and mandibular incisors, with the resultant lip posture. This profile can be improved by altering the position of the lower and upper incisors. This condition responds well to extraction therapy. **B,** Normal posture of the upper and lower lips, which fall evenly within the esthetic triangle. **C,** Concave soft tissue profile with drape of lips behind the esthetic triangle. An effort should be made to support the anteroposterior position of the maxillary and mandibular incisors. It is unwise to extract teeth without ensuring that the incisor position can be supported.

permanent maxillary and mandibular canines in centric occlusion and in centric position is the most accurate clinical measurement of the anteroposterior skeletal relationship of the maxilla to the mandible. Fig. 18-6 represents the variations in the canine relationships with the conventional Angle classification. It is important to evaluate the skeletal, soft tissue, and dental relationships independently. Frequently, a diagnosis of Class II or Class III dental relationships can be made in a reasonably normal or well-balanced skeletal and soft tissue

pattern. There is a definite distinction between a skeletal-dental Class II pattern, in which maxillary and mandibular basal bone is imbalanced, and a dental Class II pattern, in which the skeletal bases are Class I. The diagnosis and treatment timing may be quite different.

The occlusal-mesial-distal relationship of the maxillary and mandibular primary canines rarely changes after 4 to 6 years of age; therefore prediction of the skeletal-dental relationship at maturity can be made. The interarch relationship of the

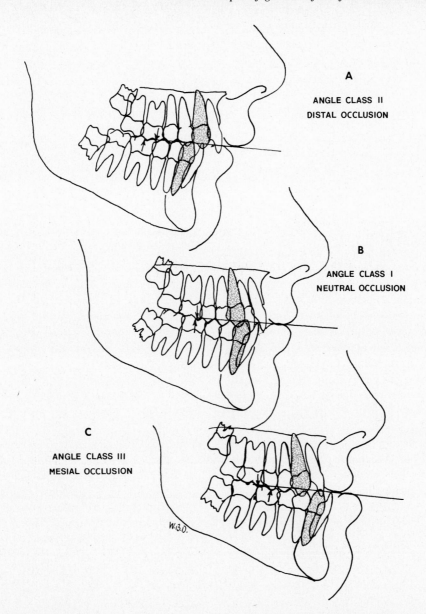

A
ANGLE CLASS II
DISTAL OCCLUSION

B
ANGLE CLASS I
NEUTRAL OCCLUSION

C
ANGLE CLASS III
MESIAL OCCLUSION

W.B.D.

Fig. 18-6. A, Angle Class II, or distal occlusion, illustrates the mesial relationship of the maxillary canine to the mandibular canine, with associated anterior position of maxillary incisors and upper lip. The maxillary first permanent molar may occlude on the marginal ridges of the mandibular second premolar and first permanent molar. **B,** Normal Angle Class I, or neutral occlusion, illustrating the maxillary canine occluding distal to the mandibular canine when the mandible is placed in centric position. The mesiobuccal cusp of the maxillary first permanent molar should occlude in the buccal groove of the mandibular first molar. **C,** Angle Class III, the retroposition of the maxillary canine and maxillary cross-bite of the central incisor, with retruded upper lip. The maxillary molar is distal in occlusion to the lower first molar. The mesiobuccal cusp occludes into the distal fossa of the lower first molar.

occlusion may be more severe in skeletal Class II and Class III relationships, in open bites, and in cases of oral habits and a variation in the mesiodistal width of the maxillary and mandibular permanent teeth.

Class III dental and skeletal relationships have the most unpredictable growth potentials and therefore discourage early orthodontic intervention. When treatment is planned for these children, the correction of the relationship of maxilla to mandible, anterior cross-bites, and intra-arch relationships should be postponed until late adolescence when the growth pattern has stabilized.

Class II skeletal patterns are best corrected during adolescent growth, when the clinician can take advantage of eruption and retropositional orthodontic forces on the maxillary teeth to correct the dental relationship. The position of the maxillary molars must be supported in full cusp dental Class II and skeletal Class II cases. If space is lost in the maxillary arch by early extractions, the maxillary anterior segment, central incisors, lateral incisors, and canines cannot be retropositioned into a normal Class I canine relationship with normal anterior overbite and overjet. It is also important that the clinician make every effort to support the anterior relationship of the lower incisors in Class II dental patterns to afford minimum overjet relationships between maxilla and mandible. The placement of a mandibular lingual arch is often necessary during the transition of the denture to ensure that the anterior segment is maintained in the most forward position.

The extreme variations in the Class II and Class III skeletal and dental patterns are best treated with a surgical approach, which enables the basal bone of the maxilla or the mandible to be repositioned in conjunction with the final correction of the occlusion. Surgical procedures on the maxilla and mandible should not be attempted until the growth of both arches is completed.

The Angle Class I skeletal and dental case should be considered for interceptive procedures to maintain normal dental relationships and tooth position throughout the stages of mixed dentition. A severely crowded Class I dental arch with 10 to 12 mm of arch length inadequacy will require the eventual removal of permanent teeth to accommodate a normal arch form. In these severe arch length cases, it is important for the dentist to observe the developmental sequence with adequate panoramic radiographs and to provide space for the developing occlusion through the selective removal of primary and permanent teeth as needed to minimize crowding. Serial extractions are discussed later in the chapter.

Evaluation of the anteroposterior position of the mandibular central incisors and anterior segment

Evaluation of the anteroposterior position of the mandibular central incisors should be considered before evaluation of the arch length, overbite, and overjet and in conjunction with the evaluation of the relationship of the lips and soft tissue profile of the lower face. The mandibular incisor segment position should always be determined first in the evaluation of disharmonies of the occlusion because it represents the anterior limits and arc formed by the incisor segment in the developing occlusion. The position of the lower incisor segment in relation to the skeletal base is determined from the lateral headplate. The axial inclination of the lower incisors to the mandibular plane or the body of the mandible and to the Frankfort horizontal plane is frequently used for this evaluation. A more important relationship is the labial position of the lower incisors to a line drawn from point A to pogonion (Fig. 18-7). The labial surface of the lower incisor in whites lies slightly anterior to the A-pogonion plane and should afford normal lip balance in this position. Bimaxillary protrusion of the incisors is also a normal, genetically determined relationship. In these cases there is a more pronounced labial flaring of the lower incisors with an associated lip protrusion or fullness. In planning changes for bimaxillary profiles the dentist should consult the patient and explain the soft tissue alterations.

The position of the lower incisor is an important

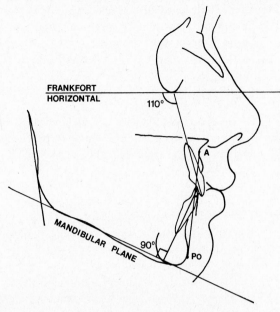

Fig. 18-7. Lower incisor position should be evaluated from a lateral headplate. The axial inclination of the lower incisor makes an approximate 90-degree angle with the mandibular plane. The maxillary incisor intersects the Frankfort horizontal plane at approximately 110 degrees. The lower incisors should fall slightly in front of the A-pogonion plane to adequately support the lips.

factor in accurately interpreting the overbite and overjet relationships of the anterior segments (Fig. 18-8). Premature loss of mandibular primary teeth allows the lower anterior teeth to migrate lingually, usually tipping distally right or left depending on the space available. This lingual migration creates an adverse overbite-overjet relationship and deviation of the dental midlines. If severe lingual version occurs, the occlusal plane will also be affected, producing supereruption of the mandibular incisors, and if not supported, the posterior teeth will be tipped mesially.

The dentist should always evaluate the lower incisor position before the eruption of the permanent mandibular canines and first premolars. If the anterior segment is not in proper position, consideration should be given to correcting the position of the lower anterior segment before the eruption of the permanent canines and premolars.

It is always necessary to consider the position of the lower incisors before determining the actual size and length of the dental arch. This is described further in the discussion of arch length evaluation.

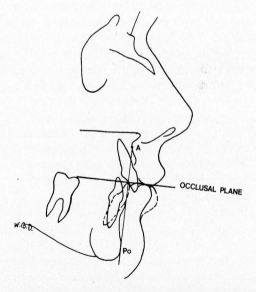

Fig. 18-8. Demonstration of lingual tipping and supereruption of lower incisor following premature extraction of primary or permanent teeth. This allows a lack of lip support for the lower lip, increases overbite and overjet, and allows a "V-ing" of the occlusal plane.

The relationship of the lower incisor segment to the maxillary and mandibular skeletal bases or the A-pogonion plane becomes an important point in the assessment of the developing occlusion.

Class I skeletal and dental pattern. It is important that the lower incisors be maintained in their normal arch and anteroposterior position to afford adequate lip support, maintain maximum lower arch length, minimize the degree of overbite and overjet, and provide the maxillary anterior segment a proper arc form for good occlusion and an esthetic appearance.

Class II skeletal and dental pattern. The initial problem in the Class II skeletal and dental pattern is the anteroposterior relationship of the maxilla to the mandible. Increased lingual version of the lower anterior segment dramatically increases the severity of the Class II relationship and ultimately makes treatment more difficult. The labial position of the mandibular-anterior segment *should always be supported*. Extraction in the mandibular arch in Class II malocclusion should be avoided.

Class III skeletal and dental pattern. A lingual inclination of the lower incisors improves the appearance of the soft tissue and the dental relationship and may afford a natural improvement for the less severe dental Class III relationships. In the more severe Class III skeletal patterns it is important to maintain the lower incisors in their normal position and axial inclination to the mandibular basal bone to ensure the arch length needed for the eruption of the remaining permanent teeth. The Class III relationship should then be considered for correction by a surgical procedure at a later age or after skeletal maturity.

Severe arch length discrepancies. In severe arch length discrepancies where teeth have been lost prematurely and lower incisors have collapsed lingually, compounding the arch length inadequacy, it may be necessary to prematurely remove primary or permanent teeth to allow a more favorable eruption pattern. It is important to first assess the soft tissue profile to determine if support of the anterior segment is necessary.

It has often been stated that the first permanent molar is the keystone in the dental arch. Even more important may be the position and support of the mandibular incisors. More attention must be given to the development of this portion of the dental arch.

Functional plane of occlusion

The functional plane of occlusion of the maxillary and mandibular arches is a constructed or imaginary plane representing the contact points of the maxillary and mandibular teeth in centric occlusion. The plane of occlusion has been described as formed by two lines drawn from the tips of the lower canines and incisal edges to the tips of the mesiobuccal cusps of the mandibular permanent first molar (Fig. 18-9). It is important that the occlusal plane be maintained in the transition from the primary to the permanent dentition to allow the permanent teeth to meet and function in good occlusion. The occlusal plane can be determined clinically by placing an intraoral photographic mirror or other flat surface on the mesiobuccal cusp of the first permanent molar and mandibular incisors and observing the relationship of the canines, premolars, or primary molars to this constructed plane. An assessment of the occlusal plane should always be made before any interceptive or treatment changes in the occlusion are considered.

Premature loss or early extraction of primary teeth usually has an adverse effect on the mandibular occlusal plane. Extractions may alleviate dental crowding in the developing dentition, but usually the mandibular first permanent molar will tip or drift mesially following removal of primary molars. The lower incisors will tip lingually and assume a supererupted position following premature extraction if unsupported from the lingual surface. The drifting of anterior and posterior dental segments allows a "V-ing" of the occlusal plane (Fig. 18-10) and prevents an adequate functional interdigitation with the maxillary arch at the extraction site. Early loss of teeth in the maxillary arch will sometimes allow supereruption of the antagonizing lower teeth. In cases where teeth are removed prematurely or where caries has caused

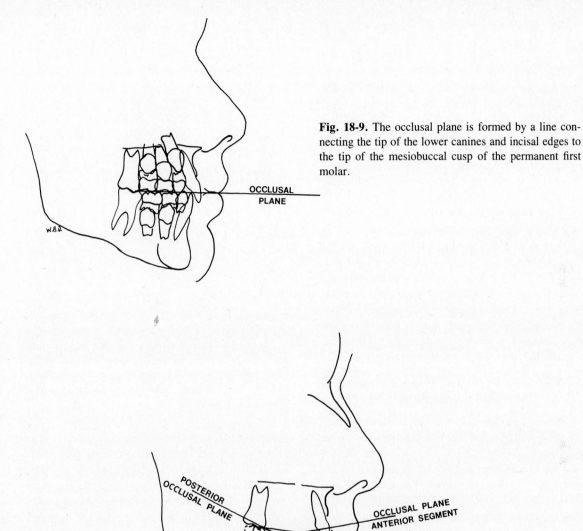

Fig. 18-9. The occlusal plane is formed by a line connecting the tip of the lower canines and incisal edges to the tip of the mesiobuccal cusp of the permanent first molar.

Fig. 18-10. Mesial tipping of mandibular first permanent molar and lingual tipping of lower incisors following premature extraction of primary molars or permanent first premolars. This procedure allows the posterior occlusal plane to tip mesially and the anterior occlusal plane to tip distally, forming a "V-ing" relationship and preventing the mandibular occlusal plane from providing good interdigitation with the maxilla. Note the increase in the supereruption of lower incisors and in overbite and overjet. The mandibular midline is usually also compromised with distal tipping.

severe changes in the occlusal plane, allowing the molars and incisors to tip adversely, the parents should be encouraged to have the occlusal plane reestablished. As the permanent teeth erupt, conventional orthodontic measures can be employed to reestablish a functional plane of occlusion.

Premature removal of permanent teeth to alleviate dental crowding is contraindicated if the patient will be unable to eventually have the occlusal plane reestablished with orthodontic care. In cases where there is minimal arch length discrepancy, it may be advisable to allow the teeth to erupt into malocclusion and recommend that treatment be carried out at a later date or even as an adult.

In pronounced arch length discrepancies in the maxilla, where the premature extraction of maxillary primary first molars and permanent first premolars may be considered to allow improved canine eruption and alleviate crowding, the development of the maxillary arch may be enhanced without adversely affecting the occlusal plane if the mandibular arch is left intact without extractions.

Overbite, overjet, and midline relationships of the maxillary and mandibular incisors

Almost every dental chart has a place to record overbite, overjet, and midline relationships of the maxillary and mandibular incisors. The vertical and horizontal relationships of the maxillary and mandibular incisors are referred to respectively as "overbite" and "overjet." Deviation of the midline of the maxillary and mandibular central incisors from the facial midline should be recorded and considered in arch length and incisor position evaluation. *Overbite* is that portion of the maxillary incisor that overlaps the mandibular incisor in centric occlusion and is usually measured from the incisal edge of the mandibular incisor to the incisal edge of the maxillary incisor (Fig. 18-11). The range of overbite in acceptable occlusion varies from 0.5 to 6 mm (3 mm is average). Overbite may also be expressed as a percentage representing the labial surface of the mandibular incisor in centric occlusion (Fig. 18-12). It may be more significant clinically to express the degree of overbite of the

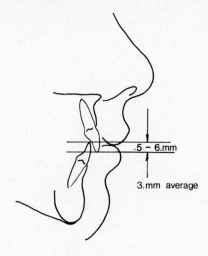

OVERBITE

Fig. 18-11. Overbite is measured from the tip of the mandibular incisor to the tip of the maxillary incisor as illustrated. Overbite ranges from 0.5 to 6 mm in acceptable occlusion with an average of 3 mm. Overbite can also be expressed as the percentage of the mandibular incisor covered by the maxillary incisor in centric occlusion. A range of 50% or less is normal in acceptable occlusions (Fig. 18-3).

maxillary incisor to the occlusal plane rather than to the mandibular central incisal edge. However, this is not widely accepted. *Overjet* is the distance from the labial surface of the mandibular incisor to the lingual or occluding surface of the maxillary central incisor (Fig. 18-13). The overjet may vary from 0 to 2 mm in acceptable occlusion.

The degree of overbite and overjet has little meaning in diagnosis until many other facts are known. The skeletal classification, soft tissue drape of the upper and lower lips, and dental classification must be considered first. In addition, the clinician should determine the axial inclinations of the maxillary and mandibular incisors, as well as the position of the lower incisor in relation to the A-pogonion plane. After these determinations are made, the overbite and overjet relationships can be measured and the results interpreted in the diagnosis and treatment plan.

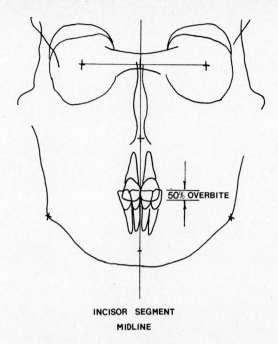

INCISOR SEGMENT
MIDLINE

Fig. 18-12. The facial midline can be constructed from a posteroanterior cephalometric film, dropping a perpendicular at the midpoint between the optic foramen, nasal septum, and angles of the ramus. The facial midline should also represent the contact point of the maxillary and mandibular central incisors.

Overbite can be decreased by intruding the maxillary and mandibular incisors or can be increased by erupting the incisors. Incisor intrusion is difficult and requires a well-controlled biomechanical orthodontic technique. Many orthodontic techniques correct or decrease overbite by overerupting permanent posterior teeth, causing a hinging open of the mandible and thus a relative change in incisor position. This method of correcting overbite is not recommended by most orthodontists because it may not always be a stable correction. The muscles of mastication will usually return the vertical dimension of the lower face to the original position after the orthodontic appliances are removed.

Overjet can be increased by skeletal and dental imbalance of the maxilla and mandible or by the ectopic position of the maxillary and mandibular incisors as a result of thumb-sucking, tongue thrusting, or lingual drifting of the mandibular incisors following the premature loss or extraction of teeth in the posterior segments. Lingual version of the mandibular incisor always increases the overjet and overbite relationship (see Fig. 18-10).

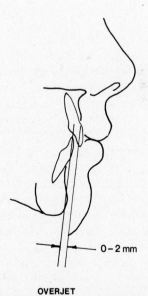

OVERJET

Fig. 18-13. Overjet measures the incisal edge of the lower incisor to the lingual occluding surface of the maxillary incisor. Overjet ranges from 0 to 2 mm in acceptable occlusion.

The midline relationship is evaluated along with facial esthetics and is a starting point for the dental arch length determination. It should also be evaluated with overbite and overjet to assess the mesial or distal relationship of the incisors. The loss of midline balance with tipping or drifting of maxillary and mandibular incisors will add to adverse relationships in the occlusion and an unesthetic appearance.

If optimum axial inclinations of the maxillary and mandibular incisors are maintained during the development of the occlusion, problems of overbite, overjet, and midline should not become major in the final occlusion and the final orthodontic correction of Class II and Class III malocclusions will be easier.

Arch length determination

The dental arch length should be determined after the eruption of the incisor segments. Several methods of arch length determination (analysis) are described in detail in Chapter 20. The following method is the one I routinely use. To properly determine the dental length of the mandibular and maxillary arch, it is necessary to first determine the position of the upper and lower lips in relation to the incisor segment of the denture. The proper incisor position should afford normal support of the lips within the esthetic triangle (see Fig. 18-5, *B*). The cephalometric film must be consulted to determine the anterior position of the lower incisors to the A-pogonion line (Fig. 18-14) and the axial inclination of the incisors to the alveolar base. The midline of the face must be determined; this point is referred to as the midline of the incisor segments. Finally, the overbite and overjet relationships should be evaluated to determine if the lower incisors are in normal occlusion, flared, or in lingual version. Once these assessments have been made and the correct anterior position of the mandibular incisors is determined, it is possible to proceed with a fairly accurate arch length determination.

From oral examination or a dental cast, an imaginary line should be drawn through the contact points of the four central incisors and continued

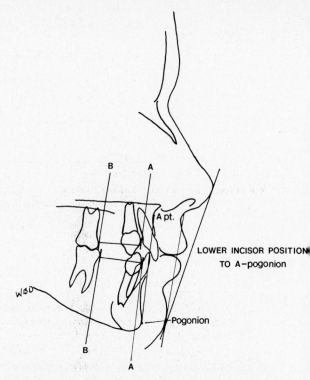

LOWER INCISOR POSITION TO A—pogonion

Fig. 18-14. Lateral cephalometric films should be referred to in conjunction with arch length determination to determine the anteroposterior position of the lower incisor segment to the skeletal bases (A-pogonion line).

posteriorly through the contact points of the canines, first premolars, or primary molars to the mesial contact of the first permanent molars. Fig. 18-15 illustrates the imaginary line connecting the contact points of the dental arch. The mesiodistal width of the central and lateral incisors is scribed appropriately from the facial-dental midline to determine the distal boundary of the incisor segment. Based on studies done by Moyers at the University of Michigan, the average mesiodistal width of the lower right and left posterior segments is approximately 21 mm (Figs. 18-16 and 18-17). Through measurement of the patient's incisor sizes and establishment of point B on Fig. 18-16, the amount of space available to the unerupted premolars and canines can be estimated. The arch length inade-

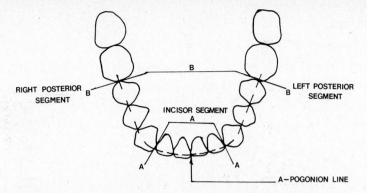

RIGHT POSTERIOR SEGMENT

B

B

LEFT POSTERIOR SEGMENT

B

INCISOR SEGMENT

A

A'

A'

A

A—POGONION LINE

Fig. 18-15. An imaginary line is drawn through the contact points of the incisor segment, canines, premolars, and contact of the 6-year molar to determine arch size. The mesiodistal widths of the central incisors and the lateral incisors are scribed on this arc representing point A. This illustrates the amount of space necessary for eruption and correct position of the incisor segment. The distance between the distal contact of the lateral incisor and the mesial contact of the first permanent molar represents space available for unerupted canines and premolars.

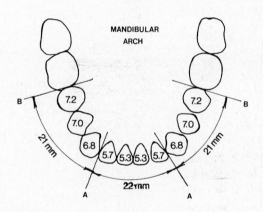

MANDIBULAR ARCH

B

B

7.2

7.2

7.0

7.0

21 mm

21 mm

6.8

6.8

5.7 5.3 5.3 5.7

22 mm

A

A

Fig. 18-16. The mesiodistal width of the average tooth size taken from the Michigan study. The mandibular incisor segment requires approximately 22 mm. Each posterior segment requires approximately 21 mm. Measure the mesiodistal width of each tooth in the incisor segment and right and left posterior segments and record them in the appropriate boxes on the charts in Fig. 18-18. This chart can be referred to during the patient's regular recall appointments in the developmental stages to monitor the space available.

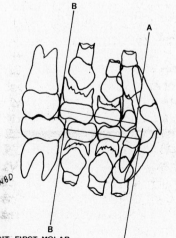

B

A

WBD

B

MESIAL PERMANENT FIRST MOLAR

A DISTAL LATERAL INCISOR

Fig. 18-17. A lateral view of mixed dentition. Points A and B correspond to the distal contact point of the lateral incisor and the mesial contact point of the first permanent molar, representing linear distance available for the developing canine and two premolars.

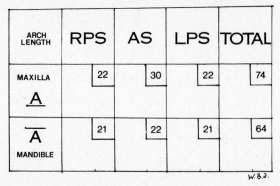

ARCH LENGTH	RPS	AS	LPS	TOTAL
MAXILLA A	22	30	22	74
A MANDIBLE	21	22	21	64

Fig. 18-18. Arch length analysis charts enable the clinician to record the space available in each of six segments as the dentition develops. A clinical arch length analysis should be completed at least once a year during the transition in the dentition. *RPS,* Right posterior segment; *AS,* anterior segment; *LPS,* left posterior segment.

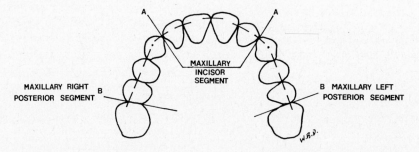

Fig. 18-19. The maxillary dental arch length is determined in the same way as the mandibular. The incisor segment extends through the distal contact point of both lateral incisors, with the A-B distance representing the amount of space available for the posterior segments.

quacy or redundancy should be recorded on the patient's chart. Fig. 18-18 illustrates a chart that can be used to record arch length for future reference.

The maxillary arch is determined in the same manner once the lower incisor position is determined. The position of the maxillary incisor segment should be an arc slightly larger and approximately 0.5 to 1 mm anterior to the mandibular arch form. The mesiodistal width of the maxillary incisors is approximately 30 mm (Fig. 18-19). Once point A is determined for the maxillary incisors and point B is established, the amount of space available for the unerupted canines and premolars can

be measured. The average sum of the mesiodistal width of the maxillary posterior segment is approximately 22 mm (Fig. 18-20).

Following the individual segment assessment of arch length, the measurements can be recorded in the chart and added to express arch redundancies or lack of space. This evaluation identifies individual segment problems where premature loss of teeth may have created arch length discrepancies.

When treatment is planned for an arch length discrepancy, it is important to determine if there is crowding in specific segments or if a generalized problem exists throughout the arch. The dentist should continue to assess arch length until the

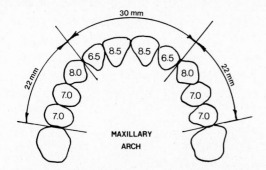

Fig. 18-20. The average mesiodistal width of individual teeth in the maxillary arch (from the Michigan study) and the average space necessary for both anterior incisor segments and right and left posterior segments.

approximate time that the canines and premolars are to erupt and plan treatment to ensure that space will be available. The sequence of eruption may vary among the quadrants.

Every effort should be made to prevent the first permanent molars from drifting forward until all teeth have erupted. Any redundancy created with the exfoliation of the second primary molar should be made available for the correction of minor incisor crowding or rotation before allowing mesial molar drifting. If primary teeth are lost, it is important to maintain the anterior segment in its correct position A-pogonion so that entrapment of the lower canines and premolars will not occur. It is often necessary to place a mandibular lingual or holding arch or correct the lower incisor segment before the eruption of the permanent canines and first premolars so that they will not erupt ectopically.

In severe arch length discrepancies (-10 to -12 mm) where soft tissue profile and the skeletal relationships of the maxilla and mandible are normal (Class I), it may be wise to prematurely remove primary teeth and sometimes permanent first premolars to allow all the teeth to erupt along the dental arch. This should not be attempted without considering space management for the first permanent molars and the incisor segment. Refer to the seven

conditions for selective extraction later in this chapter.

In skeletal and dental Class II patterns it is important to maintain the lower arch without extractions whenever possible. This enhances the eventual orthodontic correction of the Class II malocclusion by minimizing the anteroposterior overjet discrepancy.

The severe Class III skeletal and dental patterns normally require surgical retrusion of the mandibular skeletal base to accommodate the lateral width and the anteroposterior relationship of the maxilla and the mandible. Therefore it is important in the Class III skeletal and dental patterns to apply the same rules of space management and arch length development as in the Class I relationship. If a severe arch length inadequacy exists, extractions in the Class III malocclusion may be considered as in Class I cases. The final surgical-orthodontic correction of the skeletal imbalance should be delayed until skeletal and dental maturity.

Eruption sequence

The dentist assuming responsibility for the development of the child's occlusion should be familiar with the variation in eruption patterns and recognize the persistent problems of crowding. If one pays close attention to the repetition in the types of dental crowding, it becomes obvious that malocclusions can be easily predicted long before they develop into major problems. Through evaluation of the developing permanent teeth with the panoramic radiograph or the 45-degree lateral-oriented head film, the developmental paths or axial inclinations of the permanent teeth can be evaluated before the teeth erupt (Fig. 18-21).

Every child should have a radiographic examination of the unerupted developing dentition to determine eruption sequence by 7 or 8 years of age or shortly after the maxillary and mandibular incisor segments have erupted. Through evaluation of the dental arch length and the axial path of development of the unerupted teeth on the dental radiograph, ectopic eruptions can be predicted before they occur. Eruption of the permanent teeth into

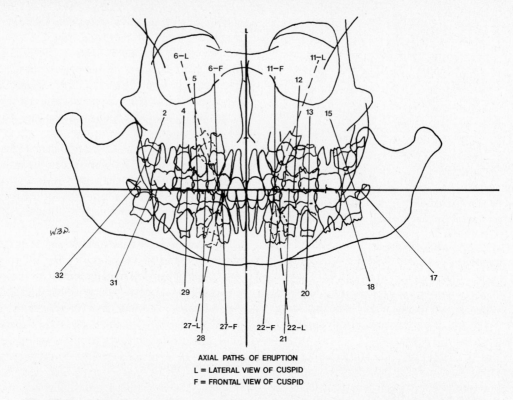

AXIAL PATHS OF ERUPTION
L = LATERAL VIEW OF CUSPID
F = FRONTAL VIEW OF CUSPID

Fig. 18-21. Axial paths of eruption. A panoramic radiograph should be made for each patient after the eruption of anterior segments to evaluate axial paths of development of the remaining permanent dentition. This radiographic illustration combines the frontal view, demonstrating central and lateral incisors in fully erupted normal occlusion, with the panoramic view of the posterior segment. Unerupted permanent canines in the frontal view are lettered F. Canines in the lateral view are lettered L. Lines drawn through the central axis of individual teeth indicate the normal path of eruption. If the long axis of the tooth appears ectopic before eruption, the clinician should be prepared to intercept or provide adequate corrective treatment. Once the tooth has attained two thirds to three fourths of its root development, it should begin to demonstrate active eruption.

the dental arch should be expected when the root development is two-thirds to three-fourths complete. Successive diagnostic radiographs should be made of the developing occlusion if the teeth are not erupting on time. The following stages of development should be carefully supervised.

First permanent molar, 5 to 6 years. At 6 years of age the first permanent molars should be erupting into occlusion. The maxillary first permanent molar may become lodged beneath the distal surface of the maxillary second primary molar, causing root resorption and partial impaction of the first permanent molar. Occasionally the maxillary molar will erupt to the buccal surface. If the child does not have normal eruption of the first permanent molars, treatment should be started to direct the permanent molar into its normal position (Chapter 20).

Mandibular incisor segment, 6 to 7 years. At approximately 6 to 7 years of age the mandibular lower incisors begin to erupt. The lower incisors can be evaluated before their eruption with an occlusal radiographic film, which will show the crown position and axial inclination. When arch length inadequacies exist in the incisor segment between the primary canines, ectopic eruption of the lower lateral incisors can be seen. The lower lateral incisors may exfoliate the primary canines and either erupt to the lingual surface or appear in severely rotated positions in the dental arch. The more severe the arch length discrepancy, the more severe the crowding of the lower incisors will be.

Maxillary incisor segment, 8 to 9 years. The maxillary incisors may exhibit ectopic axial inclinations resulting in lingual version of a cross-bite relationship with the lower incisors. They may also develop axial rotations as they erupt. Because the maxillary central incisors are the first teeth to erupt in the anterior segment, they should have a good chance for normal eruption. This may not be true, however, if there are supernumerary incisors, a heavy frenum attachment, oral habits, severe arch length inadequacy, retained primary teeth, or birth anomalies, such as a cleft lip and/or palate.

The maxillary lateral incisor frequently becomes locked to the lingual aspect between the maxillary central incisor and the maxillary canine. Usually the lateral incisors erupting to the lingual surface have a normal axial inclination and eventually require complete translation mechanics to reposition them correctly in the anterior segment. On occasion the maxillary lateral incisor erupts to the labial surface as in the Class II, Division 2 case. To correct ectopic lateral incisors, the permanent canines must first be moved distally to create space and then the lateral incisors can be moved into normal alignment with an appropriate orthodontic appliance. In many cases it is not wise to treat the ectopic lateral incisor problem before the eruption of the permanent canine or until adequate space is available to reposition the crown and root of the lateral incisor.

Mandibular canine, 9 to 11 years. The mandibular canines are frequently forced to the buccal surface as a result of inadequate arch length or ectopic development of the mandibular lateral inci-

sors. It is important to assess the position of the mandibular canines before their eruption and to be prepared to provide adequate space so that the canine will take its normal position in alveolar bone and will not be forced to the buccal surface, resulting in a poor buccal plate of supporting bone. On occasion the mandibular canines will develop to the lingual aspect and remain impacted, or eruption may progress toward the midline and roots of the lower incisors. The treatment of ectopic or malpositioned mandibular canines should be considered as soon as the root development is two-thirds to three-fourths complete and the tooth has started to erupt.

Maxillary canine, 10 to 12 years. If there is an arch length inadequacy, the maxillary canines will also be forced to either the labial or the lingual positions. Rarely do labially positioned maxillary canines become impacted. They usually erupt through the buccal plate of bone. The lingually directed canines, however, are more frequently impacted and, if untreated, proceed toward the roots of the lateral and central incisors. By the time the root of the maxillary canine is two-thirds developed, its path of eruption should be evaluated. If it is anticipated that there will be problems in its normal descent, treatment to intercept and guide the eruption is recommended.

First premolar, 9 to 11 years. The maxillary and mandibular second premolars are frequently blocked out of the dental arch when they are the last teeth to erupt in the individual quadrants. If there is an arch length discrepancy, these teeth are often impacted or erupt to the lingual surface. As they erupt, the force exerted on the contacts of the dental arch may cause other teeth to be displaced from normal contact and alignment. A decision should be reached before the malocclusion becomes compounded if adequate space for the developing premolars does not exist so that eventual removal of tooth mass or orthodontic correction of the occlusion can be recommended.

Second permanent molar, 12 to 14 years. The development of the second permanent molar may also become impacted or ectopic as a result of a short arch length or ectopic axial inclinations. In cases of vigorous mandibular lingual arch therapy or maxillary headgear therapy, the eruption of the second permanent molars may be affected.

Third molar, 19 to 25 years. The third molar, or wisdom tooth, more conventionally causes problems of impaction as a result of insufficient alveolar bone. It is wise to observe the development and position of the crowns in early adolescence and make a decision by the middle or late teens if removal of the third molars is to be considered.

• • •

By continually evaluating the young patient to determine dental and developmental age the dentist will be in a position to make an early diagnosis of ectopic development and malocclusions and to suggest a treatment plan that may shorten orthodontic treatment.

Davis' rules for serial extractions

The term "serial extraction" is often applied to the selective removal of primary and permanent teeth to alleviate severe arch length problems in Class I skeletal-dental cases. Cases of premature extraction to improve dental development should be followed up with adequate treatment to ensure proper occlusion. For successful serial extraction treatment, serial extractions should be considered only:

1. In skeletal Class I patients
2. When the soft tissue profile of the lips is convex (see Fig. 18-5, *A*) or when lips are supported in normal profile (see Fig. 18-5, *B*)
3. When the position of the lower incisor is well ahead of the A-pogonion line; the incisor segment must be supported if any lingual version is expected and in severe arch length inadequacy (greater than 12 mm) (see Fig. 18-7).
4. When the occlusal plain is relatively flat anterior to the mandibular first permanent molar
5. When the relationship of the overbite, over-

jet, and midline of the incisor segment is ideal (see Figs. 18-11 to 18-13)
6. When the dental arch length inadequacy is from 9 to 12 mm; when greater inadequacy exists, space management may also be needed
7. When a favorable eruption sequence of the first premolar and the canine can be produced to enable the first premolar to erupt before the permanent canine; tooth buds should never be enucleated before eruption, since this may cause severe damage to potential alveolar bone and periodontal attachments

Before the extractions, the parents must always be informed of the need for follow-up orthodontic care because selective extractions alone will rarely correct a developing malocclusion. The correction of axial inclinations, occlusal plane, individual tooth-to-tooth alignment, and proper interdigitation will always require some orthodontic management. However, if the management is properly timed and the sequence of development is carefully supervised, the need for major orthodontic treatment is minimized and the time required for orthodontic treatment may often be reduced by many months. There should also be less expense to the patient when a well-planned Class I serial extraction treatment is provided.

Summary

Following evaluation of all eight diagnostic points, the severity of the malocclusion and the optimum time for treatment should be determined. If the skeletal pattern is normal or Class I, every effort should be made to maintain the developing segments of the dental arches in ideal position. If a Class II dental-skeletal pattern is diagnosed, it is important to consider maintaining the integrity of the lower arch to accommodate all teeth without extractions, if possible. It is equally important to preserve the distal position of the maxillary permanent molars so all space can be used for correction of the Class II maxillary anterior segment. The patient should be prepared for orthodontic correction in the preadolescent or adolescent period. The maxillary and mandibular arches should be supervised independently in the skeletal Class III pattern until the permanent teeth erupt in their respective segments. The patient should then have orthodontic correction either with conventional appliances or through a surgical-orthodontic approach.

The relationship of upper and lower lips should advise the dentist of the need for supporting anterior teeth and correcting adverse axial inclinations. The dentist should be aware of the stages of dental development and should evaluate x-ray films carefully many months ahead of eruption so that ectopic development can be minimized.

The student and the dentist should continue to add their experience to this classification, making diagnosis and treatment planning for the developing occlusion one of the major considerations in their preventive dentistry program.

REFERENCES

Barnett, E.M.: Pediatric occlusal therapy, St. Louis, 1974, The C.V. Mosby Co.

Broadbent, H.B.: Bolton standards of dento-facial developmental growth, St. Louis, 1975, The C.V. Mosby Co.

Burstone, C.J.: The integumental profile, Am. J. Orthod. **44:**1-25, 1958.

Burstone, C.J.: Lip posture and its significance in treatment planning, Am. J. Orthod. **53:**262-284, 1967.

Enlow, D.H.: Handbook of facial growth, Philadelphia, 1975, W.B. Saunders Co.

Lowrey, G.H.: Growth and development of children, Chicago, 1973, Year Book Medical Publishers, Inc.

Moyers, R.E.: Handbook of orthodontics, ed. 3, Chicago, 1973, Year Book Medical Publishers, Inc.

Van der Linden, F.P.G., and Duterloo, H.S.: Development of the human dentition, ed. 3, New York, 1973, Harper & Row Publishers, Inc.

19   Cephalometrics

WILLIAM W. MEROW

As students of dentistry, we must in the beginning concentrate on the morphology and pathology of the human dentition and its supporting structures. Long hours spent in mastering restorative and replacement techniques further concentrates our thinking on the dentition. In the broader view, however, students and practitioners of dentistry must become students of the human face to more completely understand the relationship of the dentition to the development and function of the face. This concept is particularly important for those whose practices include children and adolescents because it is during these years that developmental and functional patterns are established. The dentist has a significant opportunity to guide these patterns. A study of cephalometric radiography is proposed as a means of furthering an understanding of the significance of craniofacial and dentofacial morphology to the study and practice of dentistry.

Cephalometric radiography, or "cephalometrics" as it is more frequently called, is a technique employing oriented radiographs for the purpose of making head measurements. It is the only method in current use permitting accurate quantitative assessment of the head in living subjects.

The purpose of this chapter is to provide a basic overview of the technique and principles of cephalometric radiography and the manner in which it is used. It is intended to offer a concept of the variations in facial morphology and a technique for evaluating them.

Use of cephalometric techniques

Before describing the various cephalometric measurements, it is appropriate to consider how and for what purposes this technique is used. Measurements made on oriented head films have been widely used in both research and clinical practice.

In the research application three primary efforts have been made: (1) the accumulation of data related to craniofacial growth changes, (2) the establishment of statistical norms for cranial and dentofacial dimensions, and (3) the evaluation of response to various treatment procedures.

In growth research much has been learned of the morphologic and dimensional patterns of skull growth. It must be emphasized, however, that the information is limited to changes in shape and size. Changes in rate, direction, and pattern of growth have been recorded, but the cephalometric technique does not locate the sites of growth or measure the contribution of growth sites. The single film does provide a static evaluation of the individual's size and shape at that point in time. Subsequent films of the same individual provide an evaluation of size and shape changes in the interval between films but do not show exactly where the growth occurred.

The use of established statistical norms for cranial and dentofacial dimensions must be approached cautiously. It is common clinical practice to make a number of prescribed measurements and compare these with established norms. When the word "normal" is used, the researcher and clinician may ask, "What is a normal face or a normal head?" or "Normal with reference to what?" Many thousands of cephalometric head films have been traced in an effort to find this "norm," and there appears to be a pattern in human physiognomy. However, because biologic, genetic, and environmental variables result in many individual variations within this pattern, reasonable judgment should be employed in evaluating individual measurements.

The clinician works with one patient at a time. When the individual's measurements are compared with statistically derived norms, the patient is being compared with a generalization drawn from a large group of individuals. The clinician may be attempting to forecast the pattern of facial growth of a young patient by comparing the static measurements with those of a large group of similar individuals whose patterns of facial growth have been statistically evaluated. Efforts to forecast facial growth, although meeting with increasing success, are occasionally victims of biologic variability.

In practice, the clinician compares the patient's measurements or pattern with the established norms and notes areas of deviation. The clinician must then use judgment to determine whether the noted deviation represents a deterrent to normal development or function. In this respect the severity of the deviation becomes significant. Measurements that are greater than 1 standard deviation away from the norm usually indicate the presence of a significant abnormality requiring special attention.

In general, cephalometrics provides assistance in diagnostic evaluation, assessment of growth pattern and growth change, and evaluation of response to treatment procedures. The extent to which deviations from the norms influence the evaluation of individual patients is a judgment made by the clinician, which is incorporated with all the other diagnostic information that has been accumulated.

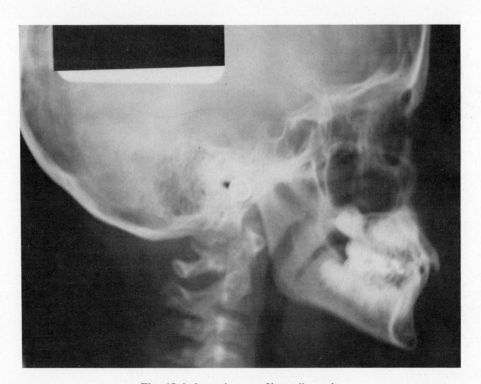

Fig. 19-1. Lateral, or profile, radiograph.

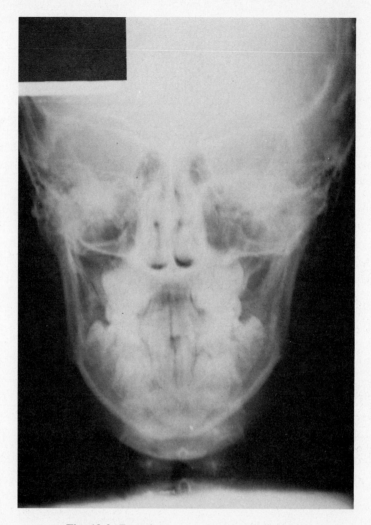

Fig. 19-2. Frontal, or anteroposterior, radiograph.

Technique

There are two basic principles necessary for the satisfactory use of cephalometric radiography. First, it is necessary that the patient be oriented to the x-ray beam in such a way that repeated exposures may be made on successive occasions under the same conditions and that all patients are similarly positioned during exposure. Second, it is necessary that these conditions be standardized so that research and clinical data may be exchanged throughout the world.

Two radiographic views are obtained, a lateral or profile view (Fig. 19-1) and a frontal or anteroposterior view (Fig. 19-2). The lateral view is normally taken with the left side of the face closest to the film cassette, and the AP view is taken with the face closest to the film.

The essential equipment includes a holder to position the x-ray tube and a cephalostat or a head-positioning device, which is located in a precise relationship to the tube head. The most common contemporary design features a horizontal bar with

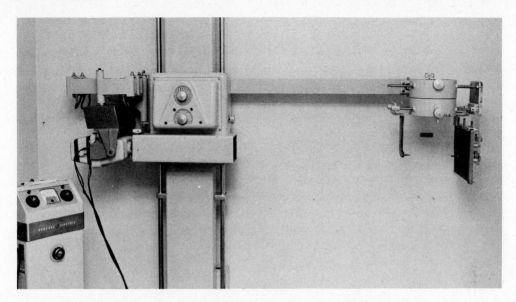

Fig. 19-3. Wall-mounted counterbalanced cephalometer.

the x-ray tube mounted on one end and the cephalostat on the other. The entire assembly is adjustable vertically in a counterbalanced system to allow for variation in patient height (Fig. 19-3).

The cephalostat positions the patient's head by means of laterally adjustable ear posts. Small metal rings imbedded in the ear posts assist in alignment of the cephalostat so that the ear post axis is centrally aligned to the source of radiation. When properly aligned, the upper edges of the ear post rings are superimposed on the film.

The linear distance from tube target to subject is standardized at 5 feet from target to the midsagittal plane of the patient's head. The film cassette is perpendicular to the ear post axis and positioned against the patient's head (Fig. 19-4).

To keep exposure at the lowest possible level consistent with high-quality radiographs, high-speed intensifying screens are built into the film cassettes. These screens function by fluorescing during radiation exposure. The effect of these screens is to reduce the amount of radiation necessary to produce a satisfactory image on the film. This principle also permits shorter exposure time,

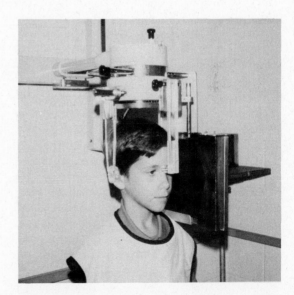

Fig. 19-4. Patient positioned in cephalostat with film cassette in position. (Courtesy Dr. Theodore R. Lynch.)

which reduces the possibility of patient movement causing a blurred image. The cone of radiation is collimated to cover just the area of the film (usually 8 × 10 inches).

Because the film range is inadequate to provide sharp skeletal contrast and soft tissue profile outline at the same time, it is usually necessary to employ additional means for the latter. The soft tissue profile outline may be obtained by placing an aluminum screen on the cassette over the profile area, outlining the profile with a radiopaque material, or employing a second film formulated for this purpose.

The lateral, or profile, film is exposed with the patient positioned in the cephalostat so that the right side of the face is toward the x-ray tube. The ear posts are located in the ear openings and moved together until the head is held firmly. A slight upward movement of the cephalostat enhances firm contact of the ear posts with the superior bony outline of the ear opening, which reduces error caused by variation in soft tissue thickness or patient posture. The head should be upright with the patient looking straight ahead. Exposure is usually made with the teeth in centric occlusion, although rest position or maximum open position may be necessary for certain special applications. The film cassette should be as close to the patient's face as possible to minimize the magnification effect of diverging rays. For the AP film the cephalostat is rotated 90 degrees and the patient is placed in the ear posts with the face toward the film cassette. It is necessary to apply more exposure for the AP film than for the lateral film.

Because x-rays emanate from a point source and are therefore divergent, a certain amount of magnification of image occurs. Also, this divergence of rays results in a double-image effect on bilateral structures, such as the orbits, the mandibular outlines, and the posterior teeth. This effect is most evident in peripheral areas of the film where the degree of ray divergence is most pronounced. When landmarks involving bilateral structures are selected, it is recommended that a midpoint between the right and left sides be used.

When students begin to study the oriented radiograph, they are confronted by a crowded assortment of overlapping lines, shadows, and contours of varying intensity that are difficult to interpret and identify. A clear knowledge of craniofacial anatomy is prerequisite to reading and tracing the film. It is helpful for beginners to have a skull and the dental casts at hand while tracing the film.

For purposes of facilitating a cephalometric analysis, a tracing of the film is made. Equipment and materials necessary for tracing and analysis include a viewbox, preferably with variable light intensity; 0.003-inch tracing acetate with one matte surface; a millimeter rule; a protractor; a compass; draftsman's triangles; and a sharp medium-hard (No. 3) pencil. To maintain accuracy, the matte acetate is taped to one edge of the film.

Some cephalometric landmarks are not always easily identified. It is helpful to mask the viewbox to block all peripheral light and at the same time to reduce the room illumination. These measures increase the contrast in the film. Accuracy and consistency in tracing techniques are essential and are developed only through practice.

Most diagnostic concern relates to anteroposterior and vertical relationships as seen in the profile view. Most malrelations occur in this plane. Thus the lateral film is the more widely used, and discussion in this chapter emphasizes this profile view. The AP film is useful for determining breadth and symmetry but is more difficult to interpret because of many superimposed structures.

An example of the lateral tracing showing the various landmarks used in most contemporary analyses is shown in Fig. 19-5. Definitions of the landmarks and points are provided in the glossary on p. 528. The lateral film tracing includes the soft tissue profile, bony profile, outline of the mandible, posterior outline of the brain case, odontoid process of the axis, anterior lip of the foramen magnum, clivus, sella turcica outline, roof of the orbit, cribriform plate, lateral and lower borders of the orbit, outline of the pterygomaxillary fissure, floor of the nose, roof of the palate, soft palate, root of the tongue, posterior pharyngeal wall, and

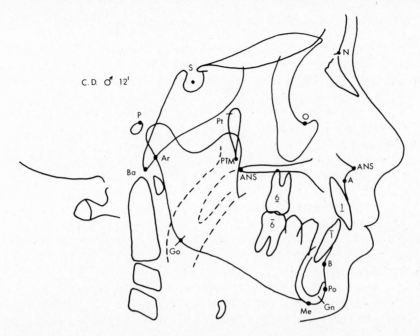

Fig. 19-5. Lateral tracing with standard cephalometric landmarks (see the glossary on p. 528).

body of the hyoid bone. As a minimum, the first permanent molars and the most anterior central incisor teeth should be traced.

All cephalometric analyses attempt to provide a means of evaluating the spatial relationship between various parts of the craniofacial and dental structures, horizontally and vertically in the sagittal plane. Basically, the evaluation of the lateral film includes the flexure of the cranial base, relation of the maxilla and mandible to each other and each to the cranial reference, and position and posture of the dentition in relation to facial structures. To evaluate these relationships, a system of anatomic points and landmarks has been developed. By connecting certain of these with lines to form reference planes, angular and linear measurements can be made. Norms have been established for these measurements and relationships that provide the clinician with a comparison between the individual patient and average values of similar measurements. It is not the purpose of this chapter to dis-

cuss the development or relative merits of any of the many cephalometric analyses that have been proposed. Rather, the chapter is intended to provide an overview of the clinical application of cephalometrics employing measurements that I have found useful for this type of evaluation.

Reference planes

Because cephalometric evaluation is a process of observing relationships, an initial description of several commonly used reference planes and lines is provided. Fig. 19-6 illustrates the most frequently used horizontal planes and lines.

The sella-nasion (SN) line is drawn from the selected point sella to nasion and represents the anteroposterior extent of the anterior cranial base. It serves as a cranial reference when relating facial structures to the cranial base.

The Frankfort horizontal plane (FHP) is drawn tangent to the superior outline of anatomic porion and extends anteriorly through orbitale. It is widely

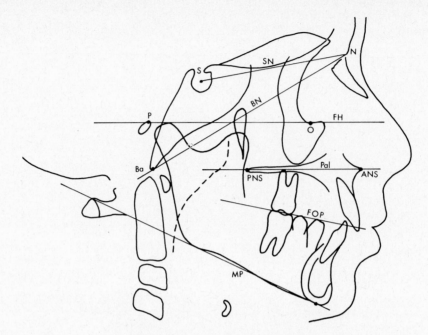

Fig. 19-6. Frequently used reference planes.

accepted as the horizontal reference plane of the head.

The basion-nasion (BN) plane is drawn tangent to the inferior outline of the anterior lip of the foramen magnum (basion) and extends anterosuperiorly through the nasion. It represents the cranial base and is roughly parallel to the "hafting zone" of the face. It is used in relating facial structure to the cranium in initial evaluation as well as changes occurring in growth or treatment.

The palatal plane is a line extending through and connecting the anterior nasal spine (ANS) and the posterior nasal spine (PNS). It is useful in determining postural tilt of the maxilla and treatment changes in the maxillary dentition.

The functional occlusal plane (FOP) passes over the distal cusps of the most posterior molars in occlusion and the cusp tips of the first premolars or first primary molars, whichever are present. The vertical relationship of the incisor teeth to the FOP provides an assessment of dental deep bite or open bite.

The mandibular plane (MP) is drawn tangent to the inferior border of the symphysis outline and is extended posteriorly tangent to the lower border of the mandible posterior to the antegonial notch. The mandibular plane may be related to the cranial reference for an assessment of facial divergence and vertical proportion in the lower face.

Skeletal assessment

An evaluation of the craniofacial skeleton in profile involves an assessment of both anteroposterior and vertical relationships. The clinician is concerned with the anteroposterior position of the chin, the maxilla, the anterior teeth, and the soft tissue. In the vertical dimension the ratio of posterior to anterior face height and vertical relationships in the dentition are of primary interest.

The facial angle may be used to determine anteroposterior chin position (Fig. 19-7). The measurement employed is the angular relationship between the FHP and the facial plane. The facial plane is a line drawn from nasion through pogonion. The

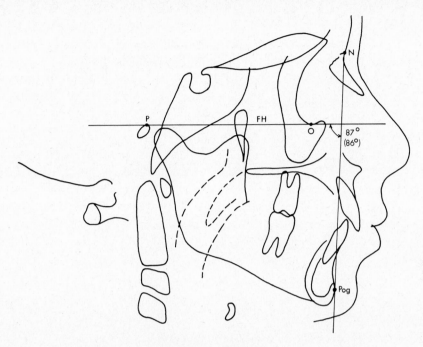

Fig. 19-7. Facial angle.

mean value for this angle is 86 degrees with a clinical variation of ±3 degrees. Values larger than the mean would indicate a tendency toward lower face prognathism and Class II malocclusion, whereas smaller values would be associated with a retrognathic mandible and possible Class II malocclusion. The mean value of 86 degrees is at age 9 years. The value increases with normal growth at the approximate rate of 1 degree every 3 years. The tracing used in Fig. 19-7 shows a facial angle of 87 degrees, which is essentially normal because this patient is 12 years of age.

Although not employed in the analysis discussed later in the chapter, the SNA-SNB angles are used frequently for relating the maxilla and mandible to each other and to the cranial reference. The angles are measured between the SN line and the nasion–point A (NA) and nasion–point B (NB) lines, respectively (Fig. 19-8). Some authors question the reliability of points A and B to represent maxillary and mandibular basal structure, pointing to the possible influence of incisor tooth movement on their

location. However, their widespread use justifies their inclusion here. The mean values of SNA and SNB (at ages 12 to 14) are 82 degrees and 80 degrees, respectively, and may be used to evaluate the anteroposterior position of the denture bases in relation to the cranial reference plane. The difference between the angles—the ANB angle—is perhaps of more clinical interest because it indicates the extent of discrepancy anteroposteriorly between the maxilla and mandible. The mean value of the ANB angle is 2 degrees. A high positive ANB angle indicates a forward-positioned maxilla, a retrognathic mandible, or a combination of these deviations. The tracing used in Fig. 19-8 shows an acceptable SNA angle of 81 degrees, a below average SNB angle of 75 degrees, and an ANB angle of 6 degrees. These figures indicate an anteroposterior skeletal dysplasia, with the problem involving a retrognathic mandible. It should be pointed out, however, that Fig. 19-7 (same patient) shows a facial angle of 87 degrees, which indicates normal anteroposterior chin position. Two variables are

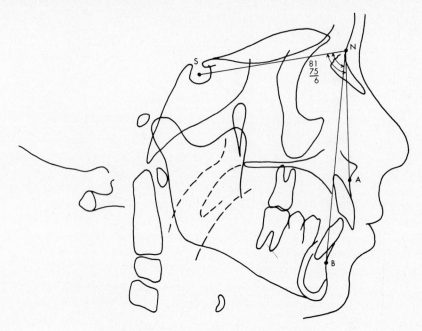

Fig. 19-8. SNA, SNB, and ANB angles.

involved here and should be evaluated. In patients with prominent "chin buttons," the facial plane that touches pogonion is not relating to the same part of the mandible as SNB. There also is considerable variability in the cant of the SN line in relation to the FHP. It appears that in the patient in these illustrations the SN line is canted upward anteriorly in relation to the FHP. These are normal variables but do demonstrate that the clinician must observe and understand the morphologic variation of the parts being evaluated. A negative ANB value indicates a prognathic mandible, a retropositioned maxilla, or a combination of these deviations.

Facial convexity may be measured by the horizontal relationship of point A to the facial plane (Fig. 19-9), measured horizontally in millimeters. The mean value for a 9-year-old is 2 mm, with a clinical variation of ±2 mm. Deviations greater than 3 mm behind the facial plane or 4 mm in front of it are indicative of an orthopedic problem in anteroposterior skeletal relations. In Fig. 19-9 the

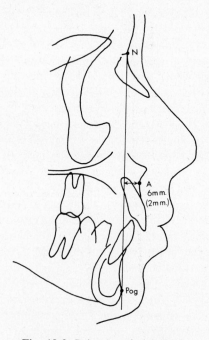

Fig. 19-9. Point A to facial plane.

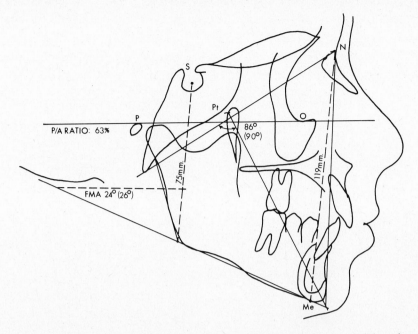

Fig. 19-10. Mandibular plane angle facial axis; posterior/anterior face height ratio.

measurement is 6 mm, which indicates skeletal profile convexity.

The measurements previously described are descriptive of anteroposterior profile relationships. Lower face morphology and to some extent vertical relationships may be evaluated with the mandibular plane angle. The angle is measured in relation to the FHP and is called the Frankfort mandibular angle (FMA). The mean value is 26 degrees with a clinical variation of ±6 degrees for the 9-year-old (Fig. 19-10). High mandibular plane angles may result from a short ramus, obtuse gonial angle, high position of the glenoid fossa, long anterior face height, or any combination of these. High mandibular plane angles are associated with vertical growth patterns and skeletal open bite. On the other hand, the low or flat mandibular plane angle is associated with deep bite and horizontal or sagittal mandibular growth. Low FMA angles are the result of a long ramus, acute gonial angle, short anterior face height, or any combination of these.

The facial axis, which extends from the Pt point through gnathion (Fig. 19-10), may be used to support findings from FMA evaluation. The Pt point is located on the posterosuperior aspect of the outline of the pterygomaxillary fissure at the lip of the foramen rotundum and represents a point of relative stability in relation to growth changes in the face. The facial axis is related to the BN line, with a mean value of 90 degrees and a clinical variation of ±3 degrees. There is no change with age from this 9-year-old norm. Values less than 90 degrees indicate lower face growth and tend to be more vertical, whereas higher than average values suggest a greater proportion of forward growth of the mandible.

The posterior/anterior face height ratio may also be used in vertical assessment (Fig. 19-10). Anterior face height is measured from nasion to menton and posterior face height from sella to constructed gonion. The normal ratio of posterior to anterior face height, expressed as a percentage, is 62%. A higher ratio indicates that posterior face height

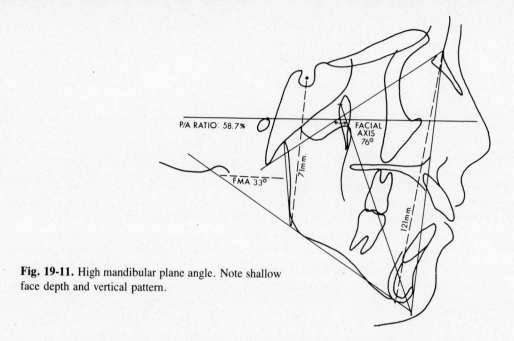

Fig. 19-11. High mandibular plane angle. Note shallow face depth and vertical pattern.

Fig. 19-12. Low mandibular plane angle. Note increased face depth and horizontal pattern.

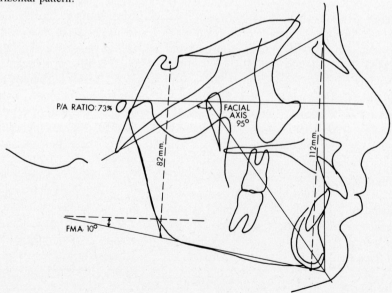

growth is increasing faster than anterior face height and is associated with deep bite. A lower than average ratio indicates a more rapid increase in anterior face height and would be associated with open bite.

Figs. 19-11 and 19-12 illustrate tracings showing high and low FMA angles, respectively, and the typical facial patterns associated with them. It is interesting to note that the high FMA angle is associated with a below average facial axis and a below average posterior/anterior face height ratio. Conversely, the low FMA angle (Fig. 19-12) is associated with a high facial axis and a high posterior/anterior face height ratio. The open bite and deep bite patterns are obvious visually, but the cephalometric data show the degree of severity and may confirm directional patterns of future growth change.

Dental assessment

In the dental assessment the upper and lower central incisors are related to their respective bony support and to the skeletal profile. The measurements are both angular and linear. The maxillary first permanent molars may be related linearly to the posterior outline of the maxilla.

In an anteroposterior linear assessment the incisal tips of the upper and lower central incisors are related to a line from point A to pogonion, which will be referred to as the A-Pog line or simply as A-Pog (Fig. 19-13). Mean values for the 9-year-old place the lower incisor tip 1 mm in front of the A-Pog line, with a clinical variation of ±2 mm, and the upper incisor tip 3 mm in front of the A-Pog line with the same clinical variation. There is no change in the mean with growth. Values larger than the mean are associated with dental protrusion, whereas smaller values indicate dental retrusion. In the example shown in Fig. 19-13, the lower incisor at 2 mm to A-Pog is in the acceptable range, whereas the upper incisor at 7 mm is protrusive.

The angular measurements used for incisor evaluation are the interincisal angle, the long axis of the lower incisor to the A-Pog line, and the long axis of the upper incisor to the FHP (Fig. 19-14). Various

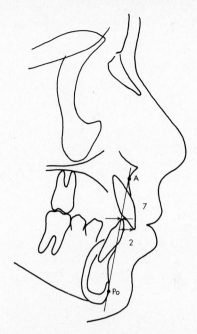

Fig. 19-13. Upper and lower incisor to APo line. Mean values are 3 mm for upper and 1 mm for lower.

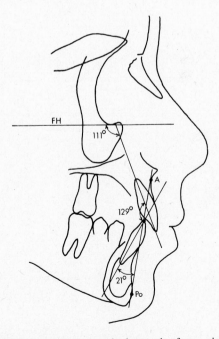

Fig. 19-14. Interincisal angle; long axis of upper incisor to FH; long axis of lower incisor to APo.

authors place the mean interincisal angle between 125 and 135 degrees. A larger interincisal angle results from very upright incisors and is associated with deep bite. Smaller than average interincisal angles are usually associated with dental protrusion. The lower incisor to A-Pog line angle (Fig. 19-14) provides a postural evaluation of the lower incisor with respect to its bony base and to the face. The mean value is 22 degrees with a clinical variation of ±4 degrees and no growth change. Larger values indicate procumbency of the incisor with associated instability and poor resistance to functional forces. Smaller values indicate an extremely upright lower incisor.

The long axis of the upper incisor related to the FHP (Fig. 19-14) shows a mean value of 110 degrees. Clinical variation is not noted. Larger than average angles indicate maxillary incisor protrusion. Smaller than average angles indicate very upright maxillary incisors.

The maxillary first permanent molar is related linearly to a perpendicular from FHP at the Pt point (Fig. 19-15). This vertical reference line is called pterygoid-vertical or simply PTV. The mean value for the distance from PTV to the distal outine of the maxillary first molar is 3 mm plus the age of the patient. The growth change is therefore 1 mm per year but only through the years of active growth. The measurement is useful in evaluating anteroposterior location of the maxillary dentition and in treatment planning considerations involving distal movement of maxillary molars.

Soft tissue assessment

A commonly used evaluation of soft tissue profile is the esthetic plane, or "E plane" (Ricketts), as shown in Fig. 19-16. The esthetic line extends from the tip of the nose to the tip of the chin. In an ideal profile the lower lip should be from 2 mm behind the line to just touching it. The upper lip should be slightly behind the lower lip in relation to the line.

Although this soft tissue evaluation may appear to be primarily an esthetic consideration, it is based

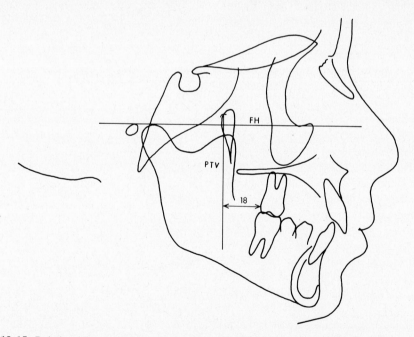

Fig. 19-15. Relationship of maxillary first molar to PTV. Mean value is age plus 3 mm. In this 12-year-old patient, the molar is forward and distal movement is practical if desired.

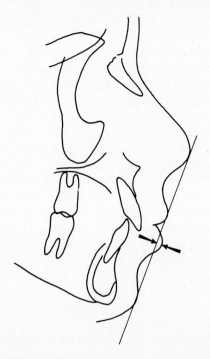

Fig. 19-16. Relationship of lower lip to esthetic plane.

on the fact that lip posture is influenced directly by the anteroposterior position of the teeth behind the lips. This is especially true in cases of maxillary incisor overjet and deep bite in which the protrusion and "roll" on the lower lip are the result of the maxillary incisor position. In Fig. 19-16 the lower lip extends beyond the esthetic plane, yet the lower incisor is normally related by all criteria. Reduction of maxillary incisor overjet and the deep bite would produce normal lip posture.

Analysis

The analysis used to evaluate tracings in the next few pages is actually a composite of measurements from several of the many analyses that have been developed. In my judgment they provide reasonable data on which the clinician can base diagnostic and treatment planning decisions. This is not to suggest that the measurements illustrated are the most accurate or significant, but they do represent a contemporary approach to cephalometric evaluation and have been found to be clinically useful.

Fig. 19-17 illustrates all the previously described

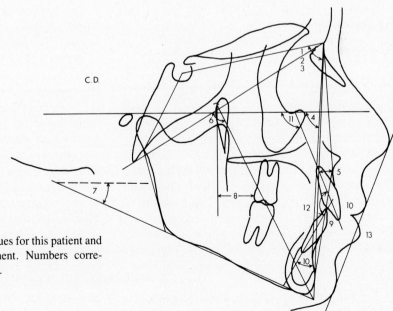

Fig. 19-17. See Table 19-1 for values for this patient and mean values for each measurement. Numbers correspond to numbered items in table.

Table 19-1. Comparison of means and clinical values for patient C.D.

	Mean	Growth change from age 9	C.D.
1. SNA	82°		81°
2. SNB	80°		75°
3. ANB	2°		6°
4. Facial angle	86° ± 3°	+1° per 3 yr	87°
5. Convexity	2 ± 2 mm	−1 mm per 3 yr	6 mm
6. Facial axis	90° ± 3°	No change	87°
7. FMA	26° ± 6°	−1° per 3 yr	24°
8. Upper molar to PTV	Age +3 ± 2 mm	1 mm per yr	18 mm
9. 1* to A-Pog	+1 ± 2 mm	None	2 mm
10. 1* to A-Pog	22° ± 4°	None	21°
11. 1† to FH	110°	None	111°
12. 1 to 1‡	125° to 135°	None	129°
13. Lower lip to E plane	−2 mm ± 2 mm	Decrease	+2 mm

*$\overline{1}$ designates lower central incisor.

†$\underline{1}$ designates upper central incisor.

‡$\underline{1}$ to $\overline{1}$ designates the angle formed by the intersection of their long axes.

measurements on patient "C.D." Table 19-1 lists each measurement numbered to correspond with the numbers on the tracing located at the site of each measurement. The table shows the means for a 9-year-old, the anticipated growth change, and the measurements of patient C.D. Because each measurement has been discussed, only a summary statement will be made. This patient, a 12-year-old boy, is essentially normal according to these cephalometric means except for midface skeletal convexity, maxillary dental protrusion, and deep bite.

To further develop the concepts of cephalometric analysis, two additional tracings will be evaluated. The first (Fig. 19-18) is of a girl, age 10 years, 9 months, with a history of chronic upper respiratory tract infection, enlarged tonsillar tissues, allergy, persistent mouth breathing, and an active tongue thrust. Skeletal profile analysis shows a retrognathic mandible, mild skeletal convexity, and marked dental protrusion. Facial depth is shallow, the mandibular plane is steep, and the posterior/anterior face height ratio is low. The low facial axis reading confirms the vertical pattern of the face and suggests that future growth will show no improvement. Because this vertical pattern is not a familial characteristic, it must be assumed that the oropharyngeal and nasopharyngeal health problems have contributed to its development. Posterior vertical growth has not kept pace with the increase in anterior face height, which probably was influenced by the abnormal respiratory and swallowing functions.

Treatment of Class II malocclusions in this pattern by attempts to move the maxillary teeth distally usually worsens the pattern by further increasing the divergence. This patient had teeth removed as a part of orthodontic treatment.

Fig. 19-19 illustrates a skeletal Class III pattern. The 90-degree facial angle is high for this 10-year-old girl. The negative ANB angle and the location of point A behind the facial plane document the concave profile associated with Class III patterns. The maxilla is normally positioned anteroposteriorly, whereas the mandible is forward. The body of the mandible is longer than the anterior cranial base, which together with the normal maxilla identifies the problem as excessive mandibular growth. The facial axis at 95 degrees is high and suggests continued strong forward growth in the lower face. With a familial occurrence of mandibular prognathism, the future treatment for this patient should include the possibility of surgical reduction.

These observations emphasize the importance of cephalometric techniques in evaluating and possibly forecasting future patterns of growth change in individual patients.

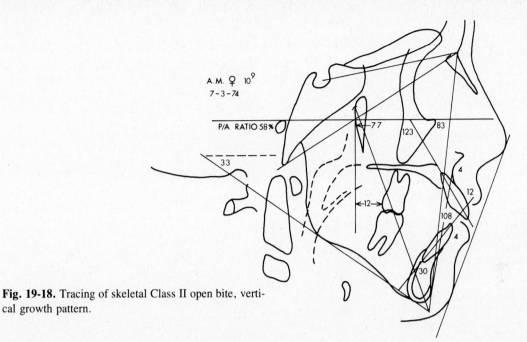

Fig. 19-18. Tracing of skeletal Class II open bite, vertical growth pattern.

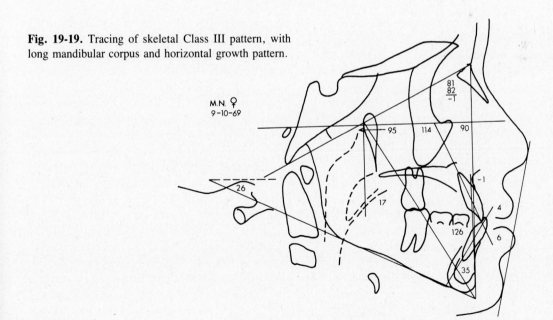

Fig. 19-19. Tracing of skeletal Class III pattern, with long mandibular corpus and horizontal growth pattern.

Growth evaluation

The growth of the human face has long been the subject of intensive study and research. Efforts to predict growth changes have recently begun to realize some success. It is not within the scope or purpose of this chapter to present an in-depth review of this function. However, certain basic principles of growth study and growth forecasting are described as they relate to the practice of dentistry. The interested reader is encouraged to review the works of Bjork, Enlow, and Ricketts for a more complete understanding of current knowledge in growth research.

The researcher begins with the cranial base and works out from there. To the clinician, however, the mandible generally is the determiner of facial pattern. Therefore the clinician asks, "Where is this mandible going to go, how far will it go, and when will this growth occur?" The primary variables are direction, increment, and time. This section deals briefly with the direction, or pattern, of growth change.

Four variables may be evaluated to obtain a general impression of predicted pattern of growth change in the lower face. The first is a measurement of the degree of divergence as represented by the "sum of posterior angles"—cranial base flexure, articular, and gonial angles. The second is the posterior/anterior face height ratio, which has already been discussed. The third is the morphology of the gonial angle. The fourth is the ratio of mandibular body length to the length of the anterior cranial base. The data used in evaluating these variables come from research by Bjork (1969), modified by Jarabak and Fizzell.

Fig. 19-20 illustrates a tracing with the measurements just described. The figures on the tracing are the norms or normal ranges for each variable. The mean value for the sum of the posterior angle is 396 degrees. Values of 400 degrees or higher indicate an opening or clockwise direction of change in mandibular growth. Values below the mean suggest a closing or counterclockwise pattern of change and would be associated with deep bite.

The posterior/anterior face height ratio has al-

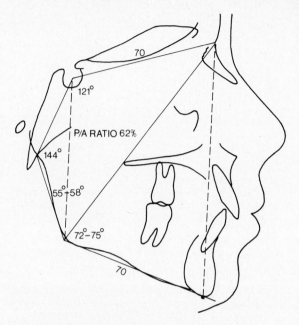

Fig. 19-20. Posterior angles, gonial angle, and posterior/anterior face height ratio.

ready been discussed, but it should be added that below average P/A ratios tend to accompany above average sum of posterior angle measurements.

The gonial angle is divided into an upper half and a lower half by a line from constructed gonion to nasion (Fig. 19-20). Constructed gonion is the intersection of the mandibular plane with a line tangent to the posterior border of the ramus. The average range is 55 to 58 degrees for the upper half and 72 to 75 degrees for the lower half. The upper half is a horizontal indicator, with high values suggesting increased horizontal growth. The lower half is a vertical indicator, with high values indicating a vertical growth pattern.

In ideal growth patterns the corpus length of the mandible (constructed gonion to menton) should equal the length of the anterior cranial base (sella to nasion) by maturity. Generally speaking, if the corpus length is within 4 mm of the anterior cranial base length by age 11, there is a good chance of achieving this ideal—especially in males. A corpus length greater than anterior cranial base length

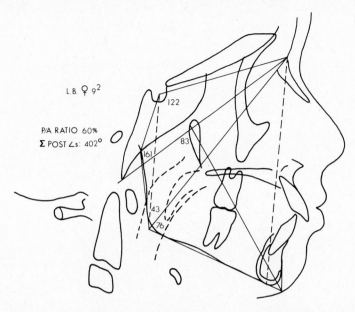

L.B. ♀ 9²

P/A RATIO 60%
Σ POST ∠s: 402°

122

83

161

143

76

Fig. 19-21. Tracing of pattern forecasting clockwise mandibular growth.

(Fig. 19-19) indicates excessive mandibular growth and probably a skeletal Class III pattern.

Another variable that should be added in this discussion is the facial axis (Ricketts and associates), as shown in Fig. 19-10. Below average measurements indicate a downward or vertical pattern, whereas above average values suggest an increased forward vector.

Fig. 19-21 is the tracing of a 9-year-old girl. Evaluation for pattern forecast shows a sum of posterior angles of 402 degrees, a P/A ratio of 60%, and a low upper half of gonial angle of 44 degrees. The corpus length is slightly less than the anterior cranial base length. Quite significant is the 83-degree facial axis. All of these measurements indicate a downward or clockwise pattern of growth change.

Approximately 20 months later another tracing of the same patient was made and superimposed over the earlier one. In this instance, the SN lines were superimposed and registered at sella. Fig. 19-22 shows the superimposed tracings and illustrates

the predicted downward and backward growth change in mandibular position.

Another method of superimposing to observe general growth change is shown in Fig. 19-23. The BN lines are superimposed and registered at the point where the facial axes intersect with the BN lines. The same result is observed with the pattern worsening by clockwise mandibular growth change.

Fig. 19-24 is the tracing of a 12-year-old boy. The pattern here is the opposite of the previous examples. The sum of posterior angles of 388 degrees and the high P/A ratio of 66% indicate a closing or counterclockwise pattern. The patient obviously has the deep bite associated with this pattern. The high value for upper half of gonial angle at 59 degrees indicates a strong possibility of a reasonable amount of forward growth at the chin. Fig. 19-25 shows almost 3 years of growth change, with the tracings superimposed on SN and registered at sella. The patient had treatment during this period, which hinged open the mandible slightly.

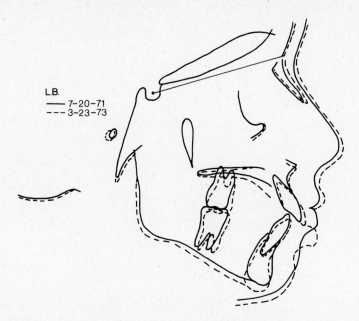

Fig. 19-22. Superimposed tracings showing clockwise mandibular growth change during 20 months of growth. Tracings are superimposed on SN and registered at sella.

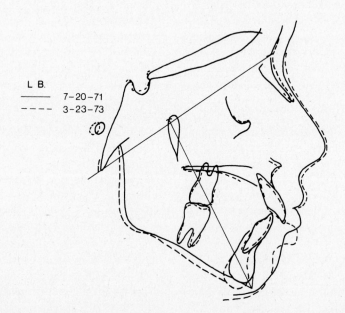

Fig. 19-23. Tracings superimposed on basion-nasion, registered at intersection of facial axes.

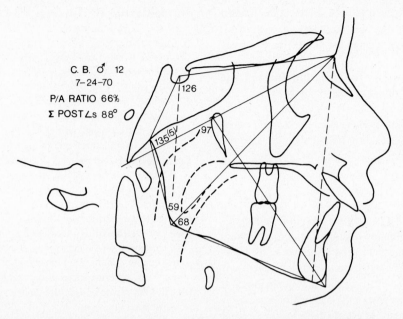

C. B. ♂ 12
7–24–70
P/A RATIO 66%
Σ POST∠s 88°

Fig. 19-24. Tracing of pattern forecasting counterclockwise mandibular growth change, with good prognosis for forward growth of the chin.

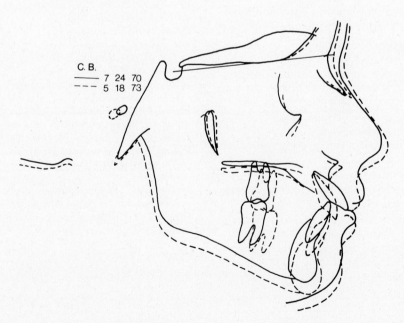

C. B.
——— 7 24 70
– – – 5 18 73

Fig. 19-25. Superimposed tracings showing counterclockwise pattern with forward growth. Tracings are superimposed on SN, registered at sella.

However, the forward growth vector in the mandible was strong enough to show a significant amount of anterior change in spite of that counteracting influence.

Clinical use of growth forecasting principles is important in establishing treatment objectives and outlining treatment plans. Treatment objectives and procedures that do not take into account existing growth patterns are unrealistic, to say the least.

Summary

This chapter has presented an overview of the basic principles of cephalometrics and their application in the evaluation of craniofacial morphology and growth assessment. The diagnostic and treatment planning advantages to the clinician are obvious. It should be stressed again that cephalometric evaluation is but a part of the diagnostic procedure. The clinician must use all available resources and apply sound judgment. Those who do not have access to a cephalometer should still become students of the human face. Many of the principles discussed here can be applied by careful observation, which will improve dental services and make dental practice more fascinating.

Glossary

A (subspinale) the deepest midline point on the premaxilla between the anterior nasal spine and prosthion.

ANS (anterior nasal spine) the tip of the anterior nasal spine as seen on the lateral film.

AR (articulare) the point of intersection of the contour of the external cranial base and the posterior contour of the condylar process.

B (supramentale) the most posterior point on the outer contour of the mandibular alveolar process.

Gn (gnathion) the midpoint between the most anterior and inferior points on the outline of the bony chin.

Go(gonion) *(constructed gonion)* the intersection of lines tangent to the mandibular base and to the posterior margin of the ascending ramus.

Me (menton) the most inferior point on the outline of the symphysis as seen on the lateral film.

N (nasion) the most anterior point of the nasofrontal suture as viewed from norma lateralis.

O (orbitale) the lowermost point on the inferior margin of the orbit.

P (porion) the "anatomic porion" is the outer upper margin of the external auditory canal.

PNS (posterior nasal spine) the tip of the posterior spine of the palatine bone in the hard palate.

Pog (pogonion) the most anterior point of the bony chin as seen on the lateral film.

Pt point the intersection of the inferior border of the foramen rotundum with the posterior wall of the pterygomaxillary fossa.

Ptm (pterygomaxillary fissure) the projected contour of the fissure on the lateral film; the anterior wall represents the maxillary tuberosity outline, and the posterior, the anterior curve of the pterygoid process.

S (sella) the center of the sella turcica as determined by inspection.

REFERENCES

Bjork, A.: Facial growth in man, studied with the aid of metallic implants, Acta Odontol. Scand. **13:**9-34, 1955.

Bjork, A.: Prediction of mandibular growth rotation, Am. J. Orthod. **55:**585-599, 1969.

Downs, W.B.: Variations in facial relations: their significance in treatment and prognosis, Am. J. Orthod. **34:**812, 1948.

Downs, W.B.: Analysis of the dento-facial profile, Angle Orthod. **26:**191, 1956.

Enlow, D.H.: Handbook of facial growth, Philadelphia, 1975, W.B. Saunders Co.

Jarabak, J.R., and Fizzell, J.A.: Technique and treatment with light-wire edgewise appliances, St. Louis, 1972, The C.V. Mosby Co.

Ricketts, R.M.: New perspectives on orientation and their benefits to clinical orthodontics. II., Angle Orthod. **46:**26-36, 1976.

Ricketts, R.M., and others: An overview of computerized cephalometrics, Am. J. Orthod. **61:**1-28, 1972.

Steiner, C.C.: Cephalometrics in clinical practice, Angle Orthod. **29:**8, 1959.

20 Management of space maintenance problems

RALPH E. McDONALD
DAVID R. AVERY

The damaging effects of the untimely loss of one or more of the primary teeth differ greatly in patients of the same age and stage of dentition. These effects present a problem that has not been accorded a thorough investigation. Conclusions drawn from observing small groups of children for a short period of time have resulted in diverse and contradictory opinions concerning the indications for space maintenance after the loss of a primary tooth. Despite this loss, a normal or at least a functional occlusion may have developed. However, if most patients with a premature loss of a primary tooth are observed in a critical manner, particularly children with some type of existing malocclusion, abnormal changes will be seen to take place that can be traced throughout the patient's life.

A study by Miyamoto, Chung, and Yee refers to the effect of the premature loss of deciduous canines and first and second molars on malocclusion of the permanent dentition. They studied 255 schoolchildren 11 years of age or older at the final examination of the permanent dentition. Malocclusion was evaluated by scoring malalignment (major and minor) and measuring crowding in the anterior teeth. Children who had a premature loss of one or more canines or molars more commonly received orthodontic treatment for the permanent dentition. The likelihood of need of treatment increased with the number of prematurely lost teeth. Children who had lost one or more deciduous teeth through age 9 had a greater than threefold increase in the fre-

quency of orthodontic treatment relative to the control group. Of those who did not receive orthodontic treatment, there was no detectable relationship of the premature loss of canines with the malalignment of permanent teeth. However, the premature extraction of molars had a significant effect on alignment and was especially associated with major malalignment of permanent teeth. No differences were noted in effects between the loss of the first and second deciduous molars. Crowding of the anterior teeth was directly affected by the premature loss of deciduous canines.

The dentist who treats children must become proficient in dentition analysis to make scientifically based predictions regarding the need to maintain space. Then, if necessary, the dentist can provide the service through the construction of an appliance.

A tooth is maintained in its correct relationship in the dental arch as a result of the action of a series of forces (Fig. 20-1). If one of these forces is altered or removed, changes in the relationship of adjacent teeth will occur and will result in drifting of teeth and the development of a space problem. Subsequent to these changes, inflammatory and degenerative changes will occur in the supporting tissues. The following is an example of forces that maintain the mandibular second primary molar in its correct relationship during the mixed dentition period. The first permanent molar exerts a mesial force on the second primary molar; the first pri-

529

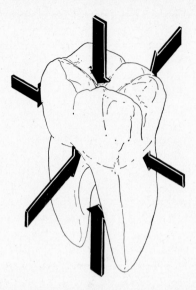

Fig. 20-1. Forces that act on a tooth to maintain its relationship in the arch. If one of these forces were removed, as would be the case if a tooth mesial to the tooth shown were extracted, forward tipping and mesial drifting would occur.

mary molar exerts an equal and opposite distal force; the tongue on the lingual aspect and the cheek musculature on the buccal aspect also exert equal and opposite forces; the alveolar process and the periodontal tissues produce an upward force; and the teeth in the opposing arch exert a compensating downward force. An alteration in one of the forces, as would occur if the first primary molar were extracted, would allow the second primary molar to drift forward under the influence of the first permanent molar. This force would be particularly strong if the first permanent molar were in an active state of eruption.

As a general rule, when a primary molar is extracted or prematurely lost, the teeth both mesial and distal to it tend to drift or be forced into the resulting space. Our observations indicate that the greatest amount of space closure may occur during the first 6 months after the untimely loss of a primary tooth. In many patients, however, a decrease in the space is evident within a matter of days. Therefore it is unwise to subscribe to the theory of

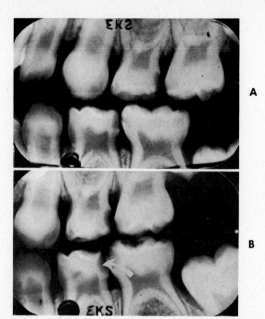

Fig. 20-2. A, Note the large carious lesions on the distal surface of the mandibular first primary molar. **B,** The second primary molar has drifted mesially into the space created by the carious lesion *(arrow)*. Several millimeters of space needed for the permanent teeth can be lost in this manner.

watchful waiting to determine whether the closure will occur because changes, particularly during certain stages of the development of the occlusion, take place within a matter of days or weeks.

The development of a carious lesion on the proximal surface of a primary molar can result in drifting of teeth and loss of space needed for the eruption of permanent teeth (Fig. 20-2).

Although there is lack of agreement regarding the frequency with which space closure will occur or a malocclusion will develop after the untimely loss of a primary or a permanent tooth, the following general factors will influence the development of a malocclusion:

1. *Abnormalcy of the oral musculature.* An abnormally high tongue position coupled with a strong mentalis muscle may be damaging to the occlusion after the loss of a mandibular

primary molar. A collapse of the lower dental arch and distal drifting of the anterior segment will be the result.

2. *Presence of oral habits.* Thumb or finger habits that provide abnormal forces on the dental arch have been shown to be responsible for initiating a collapse after the untimely loss of teeth.

3. *Existence of a malocclusion.* Arch length inadequacies and other forms of malocclusion, particularly the Class II, Division 1 variety, normally become progressively severe after the untimely loss of mandibular primary teeth.

4. *Stage of developing dentition.* In general more space loss is likely to occur if teeth are actively erupting adjacent to the space left by the premature loss of a primary tooth.

Planning for space maintenance

The following considerations are important to the dentist when space maintenance is considered after the untimely loss of primary teeth.

1. *Time elapsed since loss.* The time that has elapsed since the loss of a tooth should receive careful consideration. If space closure is to occur, it will usually take place during the first 6-month period after the extraction. In instances in which the dentist removes a primary tooth, if all factors indicate a need for space maintenance, it is best to provide an appliance as soon as possible after the extraction. In some cases it is possible to fabricate an appliance before the extraction and to deliver it at the extraction appointment. This is often the most desirable approach. Watchful waiting for space closure before planning space maintenance is not indicated.

The dentist often sees children who have had teeth removed months or even years before their first appointment with the dentist. Unfortunate changes in the occlusion may have already taken place. Even though space closure has occurred, it may occasionally be desirable to construct a space maintainer for no other reason than to aid in the reestablishment of normal occlusal function in the area. It may also be desirable to construct a space-maintaining appliance that will be active in regaining the lost space before holding it for the eruption of the permanent tooth.

2. *Dental age of the patient.* The chronologic age of the patient is not as important as the developmental age. The average eruption dates must not influence decisions regarding the construction of a space maintainer; there is too much variation in the eruption time of teeth. It is not unusual to observe premolars that have erupted by the age of 8 years. However, the extreme of the situation is a child 15 years old who still retains primary molars with the succeeding teeth in the final stages of development and eruption. Grøn studied the emergence of permanent teeth based on the amount of root development, as viewed on radiographs, at the time of emergence. She found that the majority of teeth erupt when three fourths of the root is developed, regardless of the child's chronologic age. A method based on these findings is a more reliable way of predicting the emergence of the succedaneous teeth than one based on average eruption ages. However, the age at which the primary tooth was lost can influence the emergence time of the succedaneous tooth. A number of studies have indicated that the loss of a primary molar before 7 years of age (chronologic) will lead to delayed emergence of the succedaneous tooth, whereas the loss after 7 years of age leads to an early emergence. The magnitude of this effect decreases with age. In other words, if a primary molar is lost at 4 years of age, the emergence of the premolar could be delayed by as much as 1 year; emergence will occur at the stage of root completion. If the same primary molar is lost at age 6, a delay of about 6 months is more likely; emergence will occur at a time when root development approaches completion.

3. *Amount of bone covering the unerupted tooth.* Predictions of tooth emergence based on root development and the influence of the time of the primary tooth loss are not reliable if the bone covering the developing permanent tooth has been destroyed by infection. In such a situation the emergence of the permanent tooth is usually accel-

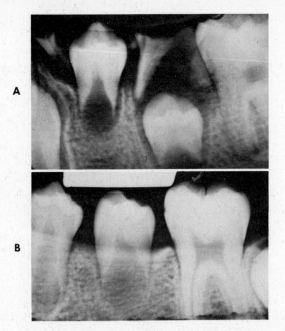

Fig. 20-3. A, Alveolar abscess associated with the second primary molar. **B,** The second premolar has erupted ahead of schedule and without the desirable amount of root formation.

erated. In some instances the tooth may even emerge with a minimum of root development (Fig. 20-3). However, when bone loss has occurred before three fourths of the root of the permanent tooth has developed, it is best not to rely on the emergence being greatly accelerated. Instead, the dentist should provide space maintenance and explain to the parent that the appliance might be needed for only a short time.

If there is bone covering the crowns, it can be readily predicted that eruption will not occur for many months; a space-maintaining appliance is indicated. A guide for predicting emergence is that erupting premolars usually require 4 to 5 months to move through 1 mm of bone as measured on a bitewing radiograph. This method of prediction is less reliable than that based on root development.

4. *Sequence of the eruption of teeth.* The dentist should observe the relationship of developing and erupting teeth to the teeth adjacent to the space created by the untimely loss of a tooth. For example, if a second primary molar has been lost prematurely and the second permanent molar is ahead of the second premolar in its eruption, there is a possibility that the permanent molar will exert a strong force on the first permanent molar, causing it to drift mesially and to occupy some of the space required by the second premolar (Fig. 20-4). A similar situation exists if the first primary molar has been lost prematurely and the permanent lateral incisor is in an active state of eruption. The eruption of the permanent lateral incisor will often result in a distal movement of the primary canine and an encroachment on the space needed by the first premolar (Fig. 20-5). This condition is frequently accompanied by a shift in the midline toward the area of the loss. In the mandibular arch a "falling in" of the anterior segment may occur and an increased overbite may result.

5. *Delayed eruption of the permanent tooth.* Individual permanent teeth are often observed to be delayed in their development and consequently in their eruption. It is not uncommon to observe partially impacted permanent teeth or a deviation in the eruption path that will result in abnormally delayed eruption. In cases of this type it is generally necessary to extract the primary tooth, construct a space maintainer, and allow the permanent tooth to erupt and assume its normal position (Fig. 20-6). If the permanent teeth in the same area of the opposing dentition have erupted, it is advisable to incorporate an occlusal "stop" in the appliance to prevent supraeruption in the opposing arch during the space maintenance period.

6. *Congenital absence of the permanent tooth.* In congenital absence of succeeding permanent teeth the dentist must decide whether it is wise to attempt to hold the space for many years until a fixed replacement can be provided or whether it is better to allow the space to close. It is important to request orthodontic consultation for patients of this type, particularly if a malocclusion exists at the time of the examination. If the decision is reached that the space should be allowed to close, there will

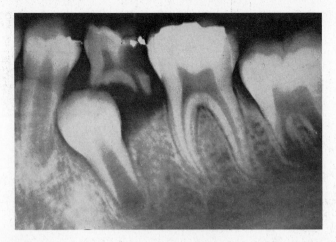

Fig. 20-4. The second permanent molar is exerting an active force on the first permanent molar, causing it to move mesially into the carious lesion on the second primary molar.

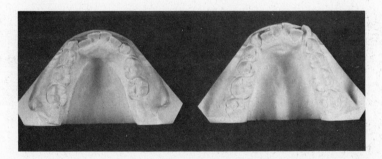

Fig. 20-5. The lower right first primary molar was lost before the eruption of the first permanent molar and the permanent lateral incisor. This loss resulted in a distal movement of the primary canine, a shift in the midline, and mesial drifting of the second primary molar. The lower right permanent canine was later blocked from its position in the arch as a result of space loss in that quadrant.

rarely if ever be bodily movement of the teeth adjacent to the space. Therefore the orthodontist should be called on to construct an appliance to guide the teeth into a desirable position.

7. *Presentation of problems to parents.* An important aspect of the problem of space maintenance is the presentation of existing problems to the parents. Dentists should take sufficient time to explain existing conditions and discuss the possibility of the development of a future malocclusion if steps are not taken to maintain the space or to guide the development of the occlusion. Parents should be informed of existing malocclusion and should be told how the loss of a primary or a permanent tooth will contribute to this condition. Dentists should likewise make it clearly understood that the space-maintaining appliance will not correct an existing malocclusion but will only prevent an undesirable condition from becoming worse or more complicated.

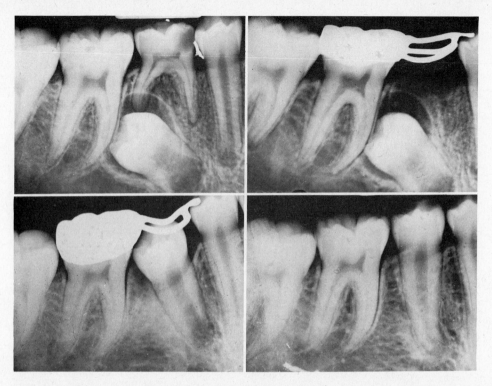

Fig. 20-6. Extraction of the second primary molar and space maintenance were indicated because of prolonged retention of the primary tooth and partial impaction of the second premolar. The second premolar eventually erupted into its normal position.

Tooth migration and arch changes during the development of the occlusion

The supervision of the developing dentition and the institution of preventive procedures, including space maintenance, require an understanding of the biogenetic course of the primary and permanent dentition. A review of the clinical studies by Baume will provide essential knowledge for the dentist who treats children.

Plaster study models of the primary dentitions of 30 children were taken at various developmental stages and were examined for changes in morphology. Two consistent morphologic arch forms of the primary dentition were found: either spaces between the teeth were present at all stages or the teeth were in proximal contact at all stages.

Spacing in the primary dentition was apparently congenital rather than developmental. The spaced arches frequently exhibited two distinct diastemata: one between the mandibular canine and the first primary molar and the other between the maxillary lateral incisor and the primary canine (Fig. 20-7). Baume referred to these spaces as "primate spaces."

Baume observed that from about the age of 4 years until the eruption of the permanent molars the sagittal dimensions of the dental arches remained essentially unchanged. A slight decrease in this dimension can occur either as the result of mesial migration of the primary second molar just after eruption or after the development of dental caries on the proximal surfaces of the molar teeth. Only minor changes in the transverse dimension of the maxillary and mandibular primary arches occurred during the period from 3½ to 6 years of age (Fig. 20-8).

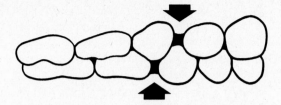

Fig. 20-7. Primate spaces between the maxillary primary lateral incisor and primary canine and between the mandibular primary canine and mandibular first molar. (Modified from Baume, L.J.: J. Dent. Res. **29**:129, 1950.)

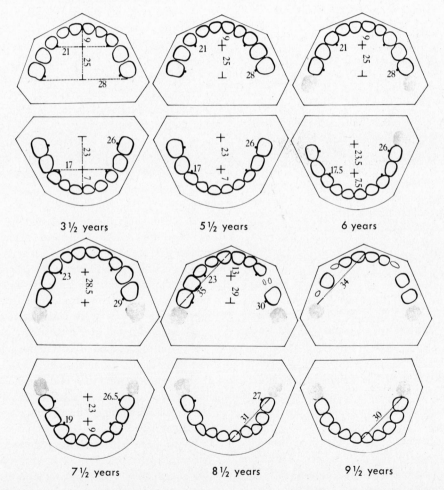

Fig. 20-8. Development of the primary dentition. No change occurred in the dimension of the arches between 3½ and 5½ years of age. Between 5½ and 7½ years of age there was a 2-mm increase in the intercanine width of both arches. There was approximately 4-mm forward extension of the upper arch and 2-mm extension of the lower arch. (Modified from Baume, L.J.: J. Dent. Res. **29**:341, 1950.)

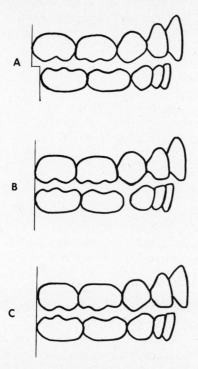

Fig. 20-9. A, Occurrence of terminal plane forming a mesial step that allows the first permanent molar to erupt into proper occlusion. **B,** Straight terminal plane with primate space; an early shift of mandibular molars into the primate space allows proper first permanent molar occlusion (early shift). **C,** Straight terminal plane without primate space; proper first permanent molar occlusion is not attained until the mandibular second primary molar exfoliates, which then allows the desirable mesial shift of the mandibular first permanent molar (late shift).

A comparative study of models of 60 children before and after the eruption of the permanent molars revealed three distinct kinds of normal molar adjustment:

1. The occurrence of a terminal plane forming a mesial step (Fig. 20-9, *A*), which allowed the first permanent molar to erupt directly into proper occlusion without altering the position of the neighboring teeth
2. The presence of a mandibular primate space and a straight terminal plane (Fig. 20-9, *B*),

which was conducive to proper molar occlusion by means of an early shift of the mandibular molars into this primate space on eruption of the first permanent molar
3. Closed primary arches and a straight terminal plane, which resulted in a transitory end-to-end relationship of the first permanent molars (Fig. 20-9, *C*) (Proper occlusion was effected through a late mesial shift of the mandibular molars subsequent to the shedding of the primary second molars.)

Moyers believes that the pattern of transition involving the straight terminal plane is normal but that the occlusion forming a mesial step is more ideal.

Fig. 20-10 illustrates the occurrence of a straight terminal plane. Proper permanent molar occlusion was achieved by a late mesial shift of the mandibular permanent molars.

A distal step, such as where the distal surface of the lower second primary molar is distal to the same surface of the maxillary molar, is abnormal and is indicative of a developing Class II malocclusion.

In a later study Baume evaluated the serial casts of 60 children. Observations were made at the time of eruption of the permanent incisors. A transverse widening of the mandibular arches occurred, representing a physiologic process to provide space for the erupting permanent incisors and their greater mesiodistal widths. This widening was brought about by lateral and frontal alveolar growth during the time of the eruption of the permanent incisors. The mean increase in intercanine width was greater in the maxillary arch than in the mandibular arch. The increase was also greater in previously closed upper or lower primary arches than in previously spaced arches.

In the mandibular arch the greatest tendency to lateral growth was noted during the eruption of the lateral incisors, whereas in the maxillary arch it occurred during the eruption of the central incisors. A "secondary" spacing of the maxillary primary incisors occasionally occurred when the still undeveloped maxillary arch was widened somewhat

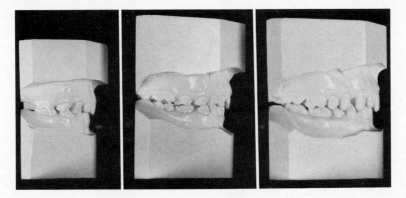

Fig. 20-10. Straight terminal plane in the primary dentition. An end-to-end relationship of the first permanent molars occurred after their eruption. A late mesial shift of the mandibular first permanent molars following loss of the primary molars allowed the development of a proper first permanent molar occlusion. (Courtesy Dr. Paul E. Starkey.)

on eruption of the mandibular permanent central incisors.

Spaced primary arches generally produced favorable alignment of the permanent incisors, whereas about 40% of the arches without spacing produced crowded anterior segments.

Determination of arch length adequacy before space maintenance procedures

The dentist faced with the problem of maintaining the space after the loss of an individual primary tooth or the multiple loss of primary teeth should look beyond the immediate state of the dentition and think in terms of the development of the dental arches and the establishment of a functional occlusion. This is particularly important during the primary and mixed dentition periods. The size of the permanent teeth that are yet to erupt, specifically the teeth in the dental arch anterior to the first permanent molars, should be determined. The amount of space that is needed for the proper alignment of the anterior permanent teeth should also be determined. Furthermore, the amount of mesial movement of the first permanent molars that will occur after the loss of the primary molars and the eruption of the second premolars should be taken into consideration.

It is a well-accepted fact that the available arch circumference (arch length), which is generally considered the distance from the mesial surface of the first permanent molar on one side of the arch to the mesial surface of the first permanent molar on the opposite side of the arch, is continually decreasing. Even in the course of orthodontic treatment, there is little that can be done to increase it. It should be recognized that the circumference decreases through the proximal wear and the mesial movement of the first permanent molars at the time of the exchange of teeth. Moorrees reported that the average arch length of an individual is smaller at 18 years of age than at 3 years of age. This is the result of a decrease in maxillary and mandibular dental arch length occurring between 10 and 14 years of age, caused by the exchange of primary molars for the first and second premolars. Mills completed measurements of dental arch breadth and length in 1253 children 6.6 through 19.5 years of age, all of whom had neutroclusion of molars. The maximum dental arch breadth appeared to be established before the eruption of the second premolars and canines. Dental arch length tended to decrease with age. Maxillary arch length in both sexes initially increased on the average by 1.05 mm. However, by about 11.5 years of age it began to decrease. In girls the maxillary arch length was 0.45 mm less at 19.5 years than at 6.6 years of age. In boys the maxillary arch length at age 19.5 years was about the same as at age 6.6 years.

The mandibular arch length for boys increased slightly, then decreased significantly with age. During the 12.9-year period of observation, mandibular arch length decreased 2.12 mm for girls and 5.06 mm for boys.

The arch breadth reached a peak between about the eleventh and thirteenth years of age and increased, on the average, 1.2 mm. By 19 years of age the breadth measurements had almost returned to their beginning measurements.

Barber believes that the goal should be the prevention of arch length loss in any degree, no matter how small. He points out that the combined mesiodistal widths of the primary teeth essentially equal the combined mesiodistal widths of their permanent successors in the same arch. Thus the leeway described by Nance between the combined mesiodistal widths of the primary canine, first and second molars, and their successors may be needed to allow the already erupted permanent incisors to unwind and alleviate anterior crowding in many individuals.

Arch length analysis*

Nance's analysis. Nance concluded, as a result of comprehensive studies, that the length of the dental arch from the mesial surface of one mandibular first permanent molar to the mesial surface of the corresponding tooth on the opposite side is always shortened during the transition from the mixed to the permanent dentition. The only time the arch length can be increased even during orthodontic treatment is when the incisors show an abnormal lingual inclination or when the first permanent molars have drifted mesially after the untimely loss of second primary molars. Nance further observed that in the average patient a leeway of 1.7 mm exists between the combined mesiodis-

---

*An alternative approach to arch length analysis is presented in Chapter 18.

tal widths of the primary mandibular canine and first and second primary molars and the mesiodistal widths of the corresponding permanent teeth, the primary teeth being the larger. This difference between the total mesiodistal width of the corresponding three primary teeth in the maxillary arch as compared with the three permanent teeth that succeed them is only 0.9 mm. Moorrees, however, showed that the loss of space in the mandible is 3.9 mm for boys and 4.8 mm for girls during the exchange of primary and permanent teeth.

For a mixed dentition arch length analysis similar to that advocated by Nance, the following materials are needed: sharp dividers, a set of periapical radiographs that have been taken with a meticulous technique, a millimeter rule, a piece of 0.026-inch brass ligature wire, a ruled 3×5 inch card for recording measurements, and a set of study models (Fig. 20-11). The width of the erupted four mandibular permanent incisors is first measured. The actual width should be determined rather than the space the incisors occupy in the arch. The individual measurements are recorded. The width of the unerupted mandibular canines and first and second premolars on the radiographs should be measured next. The estimated measurements are then recorded. If one of the premolars is rotated, the measurement of the corresponding tooth on the opposite side of the mouth may be used. This will give an indication of the space needed to accommodate all the permanent teeth anterior to the first permanent molars. The next step is to determine the amount of space available for the permanent teeth. This may be accomplished in the following manner. A piece of 0.026-inch brass ligature wire, contoured to arch form, is placed on the lower cast extending from the mesial surface of the first permanent molar on one side of the arch to the mesial surface of the first permanent molar on the opposite side. The wire should pass over the buccal cusps of the posterior teeth and the incisal edge of the anterior teeth (Fig. 20-12). From this measurement must be subtracted 3.4 mm, the amount by which the arch length may be expected to decrease as a result of the mesial drift-

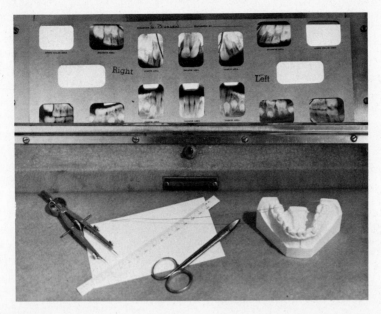

Fig. 20-11. Materials needed to complete the Nance mixed dentition analysis.

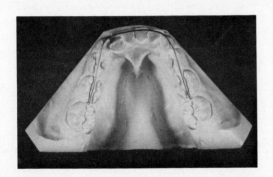

Fig. 20-12. Lower cast with a piece of brass ligature wire extending from the mesial surface of the first permanent molar through the contact areas of the teeth to the mesial surface of the opposite first permanent molar. This measurement will give an indication of the available arch length before the mesial movement of the first permanent molars.

ing of the first permanent molars. Thus by comparing the two measurements the dentist can predict with a fair degree of accuracy the adequacy or inadequacy of the arch circumference.

Some prefer to use a flexible millimeter rule to determine the available arch length. The ruler is contoured to the arch form in the same manner as the brass ligature wire, and the arch length is read in millimeters.

Moyers' mixed dentition analysis. The analysis advocated by Moyers has a number of advan-

tages. It can be completed in the mouth as well as on casts, and it may be used for both arches. The analysis is based on the fact that there is precise correlation of tooth size and that one may measure a tooth or a group of teeth and predict accurately the size of the other teeth in the same mouth. The mandibular incisors, since they erupt early in the mixed dentition and may be measured accurately, have been chosen for measuring to predict the size of the upper as well as the lower posterior teeth.

The following procedure has been suggested by

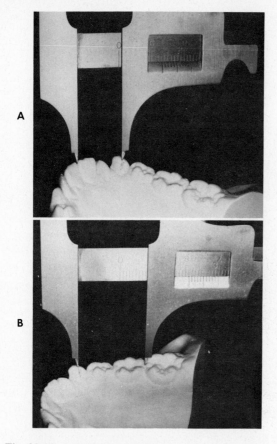

Fig. 20-13. A, Boley gauge has been set to a value equal to the sum of the widths of the permanent central and lateral incisors. A mark has been made on the cast where the distal tip of the Boley gauge has touched. **B,** A measurement from the point mark on the canine to the mesial surface of the first permanent molar indicates the amount of space available for the permanent canine and premolars after incisor alignment.

Moyers to determine the space available for teeth in the mandibular arch:

1. Measure the greatest mesiodistal width of each of the four mandibular incisors with the aid of a Boley gauge and record the value.
2. Determine the amount of space needed for the alignment of the incisors. This may be accomplished as follows: Set the Boley gauge to a value equal to the sum of the widths of the right central incisor and the right lateral incisor. Place one point of the gauge at the midline between the central incisors and let the other point lie along the line of the dental arch on the right side (Fig. 20-13, *A*). Mark on the tooth or the cast the precise point where the distal tip of the Boley gauge has touched. This represents the point where the distal surface of the lateral incisor will be when it has been aligned properly. Repeat the procedure for the opposite side of the arch.
3. Determine the amount of space available for the permanent canine and premolars after incisor alignment. This may be accomplished by measuring the distance from the point mark in the line of arch to the mesial surface of the first permanent molar (Fig. 20-13, *B*). This distance is the space available for the permanent canine and premolars as well as for first permanent molar adjustment.
4. Predict the combined width of the mandibular canines and premolars with the aid of the probability chart (Fig. 20-14). Locate at the top of the mandibular chart the value over a column of figures that most nearly corresponds to the sum of the widths of the *four* mandibular incisors. Immediately beneath the figure just located is recorded the range of values for all canine and premolar sizes that will be formed for incisors of the indicated size. Generally the figure at the 75% level is used, since this has been found to be most practical from a clinical standpoint.
5. Compute the amount of space remaining in the arch for first permanent molar adjustment. The estimated canine and premolar size value is subtracted from the measured space. From this value is subtracted the amount by which the first permanent molar is expected to shift mesially. It must be assumed that the first permanent molar will move mesially at least 1.7 mm.

After all the values have been recorded, a complete assessment of the space situation in both

Probability chart for predicting the sum of the widths of maxillary canines and premolars from mandibular permanent incisors

Mandibular incisors =	19.5	20.0	20.5	21.0	21.5	22.0	22.5	23.0	23.5	24.0	24.5	25.0
95%	21.6	21.8	22.1	22.4	22.7	22.9	23.2	23.5	23.8	24.0	24.3	24.6
85%	21.0	21.3	21.5	21.8	22.1	22.4	22.6	22.9	23.2	23.5	23.7	24.0
75%	20.6	20.9	21.2	21.5	21.8	22.0	22.3	22.6	22.9	23.1	23.4	23.7
65%	20.4	20.6	20.9	21.2	21.5	21.8	22.0	22.3	22.6	22.8	23.1	23.4
50%	20.0	20.3	20.6	20.8	21.1	21.4	21.7	21.9	22.2	22.5	22.8	23.0
35%	19.6	19.9	20.2	20.5	20.8	21.0	21.3	21.6	21.9	22.1	22.4	22.7
25%	19.4	19.7	19.9	20.2	20.5	20.8	21.0	21.3	21.6	21.9	22.1	22.4
15%	19.0	19.3	19.6	19.9	20.2	20.4	20.7	21.0	21.3	21.5	21.8	22.1
5%	18.5	18.8	19.0	19.3	19.6	19.9	20.1	20.4	20.7	21.0	21.2	21.5

Probability charts for computing the size of unerupted canines and premolars. The above chart is the maxillary arch. Measure and obtain the sum of the widths of the permanent mandibular incisors and find that value in the top horizontal column. Reading downward in that column, obtain the value for the expected widths of the canine and premolars corresponding to the level of probability you wish to use. Ordinarily, the 75% level of probability is used. The mandibular incisors are used for the prediction of both the mandibular and maxillary canines and premolar widths.

Probability chart for predicting the sum of the widths of mandibular canine and premolars from mandibular incisors

Mandibular incisors =	19.5	20.0	20.5	21.0	21.5	22.0	22.5	23.0	23.5	24.0	24.5	25.0
95%	21.1	21.4	21.7	22.0	22.3	22.6	22.9	23.2	23.5	23.8	24.1	24.4
85%	20.5	20.8	21.1	21.4	21.7	22.0	22.3	22.6	22.9	23.2	23.5	23.8
75%	20.1	20.4	20.7	21.0	21.3	21.6	21.9	22.2	22.5	22.8	23.1	23.4
65%	19.8	20.1	20.4	20.7	21.0	21.3	21.6	21.9	22.2	22.5	22.8	23.1
50%	19.4	19.7	20.0	20.3	20.6	20.9	21.2	21.5	21.8	22.1	22.4	22.7
35%	19.0	19.3	19.6	19.9	20.2	20.5	20.8	21.1	21.4	21.7	22.0	22.3
25%	18.7	19.0	19.3	19.6	19.9	20.2	20.5	20.8	21.1	21.4	21.7	22.0
15%	18.4	18.7	19.0	19.3	19.6	19.8	20.1	20.4	20.7	21.0	21.3	21.6
5%	17.7	18.0	18.3	18.6	18.9	19.2	19.5	19.8	20.1	20.4	20.7	21.0

Fig. 20-14. Moyers probability chart.

arches is possible. The chart illustrated in Fig. 20-15 is useful in recording the data.

Space maintenance for the first primary molar area

The effect of the untimely loss of the first primary molar on the occlusion depends to a degree on the stage of development of the occlusion at the time the loss occurs. If the first primary molar is lost during the time of active eruption of the first permanent molar, a strong forward force will be exerted on the second primary molar, causing it to tip into the space required for the eruption of the first premolar. Likewise, distal drifting of the primary canine is likely to occur if the loss occurs during the active stage of eruption of the permanent lateral incisor (see Fig. 20-5). Thus changes in the occlusion may extend as far as the midline after the

MIXED DENTITION ANALYSIS

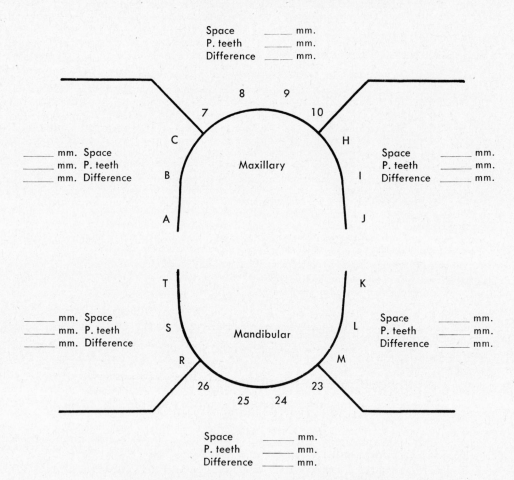

Fig. 20-15. Useful chart for recording arch length data.

loss of the first primary molar, with a shifting of the midline toward the space created by the untimely loss, a falling-in of the anterior segment on the affected side, and an increased overbite.

Band and loop maintainer. The advantages of the band and loop maintainer include ease of construction, requirement of a minimum of chair time, low cost of materials, and ease of adjustment of the loop to accommodate the changing dentition. Although the advantages outweigh the disadvantages, the dentist must realize that the band and loop

maintainer will not restore masticatory function in the area and that it will not prevent the continued eruption of the opposing teeth, which may or may not be considered an important factor. Any appliance involving a band should be removed each year, the tooth should be polished and inspected, topical fluoride should be applied, and the band should be recemented to prevent the possibility of a break in the seal and subsequent carious involvement of the tooth.

The preformed stainless steel band is used in the

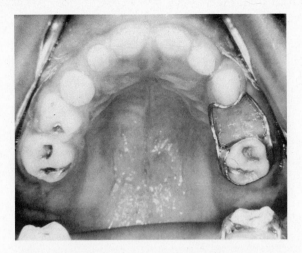

Fig. 20-16. Trial seating of a properly fitted and designed band and loop appliance. The appliance is ready to be cemented into place.

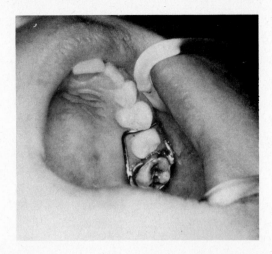

Fig. 20-17. Band and loop maintainer. The loop is sufficiently large to allow the eruption of the permanent tooth.

construction of the band and loop maintainer. If teeth have erupted anterior or posterior to the tooth that is to receive a band, it may be necessary to obtain separation with an elastic separator.

A band should be selected that will fit the tooth snugly on the occlusal one third to one half when applied with finger pressure. The band may be rocked into place with a band setter. On a maxillary tooth the band is rocked from the buccal surface over the lingual surface. On a mandibular tooth the band is rocked from the lingual surface over the buccal surface. A band biter and a band pusher are used for complete seating and adaptation of the band into the grooved areas on the buccal and lingual areas of the tooth.

A compound impression should be made of the abutment tooth, including the area of premature loss, and the tooth anterior to it. The band should be removed from the tooth with the band-removing pliers and placed securely in the compound impression area. The band is secured with a small amount of sticky wax on the mesial and distal surfaces. Stone is then poured into the impression to produce a working model.

A loop of 0.036-inch stainless steel wire is con-

toured to rest close to the tissue, touching the distal surface of the tooth anterior to the space at the gingival area. The loop should be sufficiently wide to allow for the eruption of the premolar. The loop is soldered to the band on the stone model, after which the maintainer is removed, polished, and prepared for seating in the mouth (Figs. 20-16 and 20-17).

Chrome steel crown and loop maintainer. The chrome steel crown and loop maintainer may be used if the posterior abutment tooth has extensive caries and requires a crown restoration or if the abutment tooth has had vital pulp therapy, in which case it is desirable to protect the crown with full coverage (Fig. 20-18). The loop may be cut off and the crown may be allowed to continue to serve as a restoration for the abutment tooth when there is no longer a need for the space maintainer.

The steel crown should be prepared as described in Chapter 12. However, before cementation, a compound impression is taken, the crown is removed from the tooth and seated in the impression, and the stone working model is prepared. A piece of 0.030-inch or 0.036-inch steel wire is used to prepare the loop, which is soldered to the crown

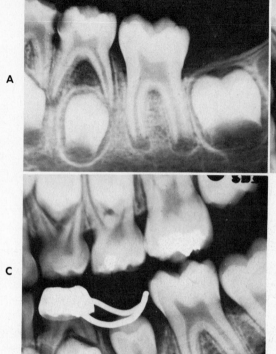

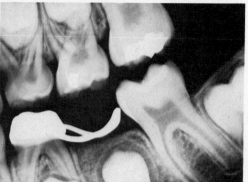

Fig. 20-18. A, Second primary molar that is indicated for extraction. Incomplete root formation and bone covering the crown of the premolar make space maintenance imperative. **B,** A crown and loop maintainer. **C,** The second premolar has emerged through the tissue. The loop may now be removed to allow for eruption of the tooth.

with silver solder and a borax type of flux. The advantages of the crown and loop type of maintainer are similar to those of the band and loop type. The ease of construction is apparent, and the cost of materials is incidental. The restoration does not, however, restore function, and it does not prevent the overeruption of teeth opposing the space. Furthermore, it is difficult to remove the crown and make adjustments in the loop. Some dentists prefer to adapt a band over a cemented crown restoration and construct a conventional band and loop appliance for easier removal and adjustment of the appliance.

Modified fixed bridge maintainer. When long-term space maintenance is anticipated, a modified fixed bridge casting may be used to maintain the relationship of teeth in the arch after the untimely loss of the first primary molar (Fig. 20-19). The

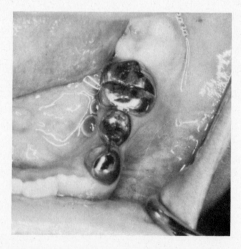

Fig. 20-19. A modified fixed bridge space maintainer has been constructed after the untimely loss of the first primary molar.

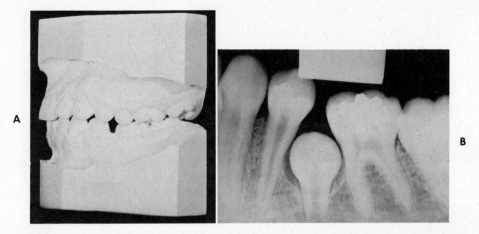

Fig. 20-20. A, Casts showing the result of the early loss of a mandibular second primary molar. **B,** Radiograph of an impacted second premolar. Space needed for the eruption of this tooth has been almost completely lost.

primary canine and second molar are prepared for full cast crowns; the maintainer may be cast in one piece. It should be recognized that the permanent canine may erupt before the first premolar. It may be necessary to cut the pontic away from the second primary molar crown and construct a band and loop maintainer before the eruption of the first premolar. Because of the greater difficulty of tooth preparation and the increased cost of materials, cast space maintainers are rarely used.

Space maintenance for the second primary molar area

The loss of the second primary molar will usually have less effect on the teeth in the anterior segment than the loss of a first primary molar. However, an irregularity will develop in the permanent molar relationship. The result of untimely loss of the second primary molar is invariably the mesial drifting of the first permanent molar and possible impaction of the second premolar (Fig. 20-20).

The space-maintaining appliances that are generally advocated when the second primary molar is lost are the band and loop and the passive lingual arch. The passive lingual arch is discussed later in

the chapter. The band and loop maintainer is more frequently recommended, with the band placed on the first permanent molar (Fig. 20-21). The first permanent molar is selected as the abutment tooth because it usually erupts before the second premolar. If the first primary molar is used as the abutment tooth, there is a possibility of its loss before the time when the space-maintaining appliance can be discarded. Occasionally, however, if the first and second premolars are developing at a comparable rate, the first primary molar may be used as the abutment tooth (see Fig. 20-18).

A passive soldered lingual arch is often the appliance of choice in the mandibular arch, especially if the permanent mandibular incisors exhibit crowding.

Loss of the second primary molar before the eruption of the first permanent molar

Mesial movement and migration of the first permanent molar will often occur before eruption in instances of premature loss of the second primary molar (Fig. 20-22). This is one of the most difficult problems that confront the dentist who provides services for children. A space maintainer that will guide the first permanent molar into its normal

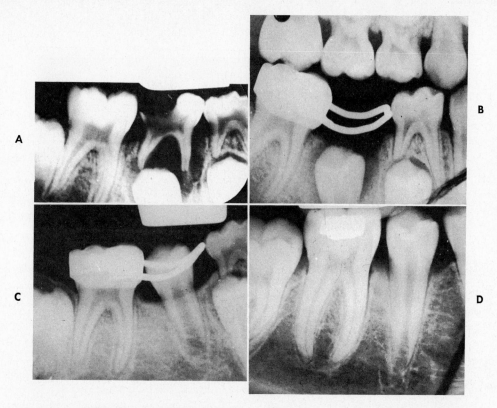

Fig. 20-21. A, Pulpless second primary molar is indicated for extraction. Although there was considerable loss of bone covering the crown of the second premolar, there was concern about space loss before eruption of the tooth. **B,** A band and loop maintainer has been constructed immediately after the removal of the pulpless primary tooth. **C,** The second premolar has erupted through the loop. The maintainer may now be removed. **D,** Adequate space has been maintained in the arch for the second premolar.

position is indicated. Drinkard and Oldenburg have offered a comprehensive discussion of this condition and its management. A variety of appliances have been recommended for this purpose, but all of them are somewhat complicated in their construction and need frequent maintenance to accomplish the desirable result.

Cast gold (Willett) distal shoe maintainer. The cast distal shoe maintainer was advocated for many years. The primary canine and first primary molars are used as the abutment teeth, which are prepared for the Willett overlay type of casting.

The abutment teeth may require preparation,

however, to reduce undercut areas, and there must be proximal cuts to break contact with adjacent teeth. The occlusal tooth surfaces should remain untouched, since the cusps of the teeth are exposed through the restoration. This allows the maintainer to be removed for inspection of the abutment tooth or modification of the appliance (Fig. 20-23). This appliance is rarely used today for the same reasons cited previously regarding the modified fixed bridge maintainer.

Crown and band maintainer with distal shoe extension. The crown and band maintainer with distal shoe extension advocated by Roche has

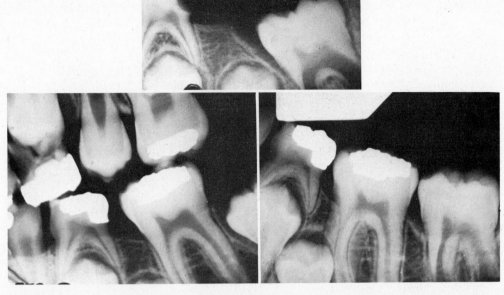

Fig. 20-22. A sequence of three radiographs showing the untimely loss of the second primary molar and mesial movement of the first permanent molar before its eruption. Eventually there was complete closure of the space needed for the second premolar.

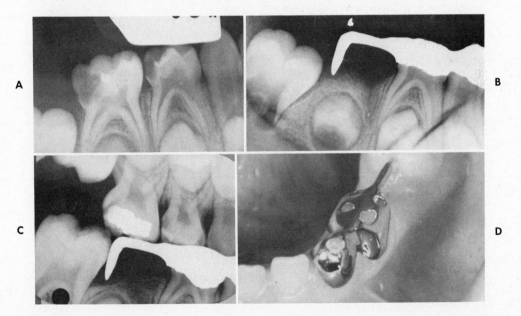

Fig. 20-23. A, Patient in whom a second primary molar must be removed before the eruption of the first permanent molar. **B,** An overlay–distal shoe type of maintainer was constructed and seated at the time of the second primary molar extraction. **C,** The maintainer has successfully guided the first permanent molar into a desirable position. **D,** After the eruption of the first permanent molar, the gold extension into the tissue may be removed and the maintainer recemented and allowed to remain in position until the eruption of the second premolar or as long as the abutment teeth are serviceable.

many advantages over the cast gold distal shoe appliance (Fig. 20-24). The first primary molar is used as the abutment tooth. The tooth is first prepared for a chrome steel crown. The crown should be adequately contoured and cemented to the first primary molar. The chrome steel crown provides a desirable retentive contour for the placement of a stainless steel band. Gold band and wire materials were recommended originally for the fabrication of this appliance. Gold provides an excellent appliance, but stainless steel materials have also been found satisfactory. The band is prepared as previously described and placed over the steel crown on the abutment tooth. A compound impression should then be taken, the band should be removed and placed in the impression, and a stone model should be prepared. If the second primary molar is scheduled for extraction but has not yet been

removed, it should be cut off the prepared model. A hole that simulates the position of the distal root of the tooth is made with a bur in the model. If the second primary molar has previously been removed, the positioning of the tissue extension may be determined with dividers and a bite-wing radiograph. The tissue-bearing wire loop is next contoured with 0.040-inch wire extending distally and into the prepared opening on the model. The free ends of the loop are soldered to the band. Next, the band and loop appliance should be removed from the model and the V of the tissue extension should be filled in and soldered with a piece of 0.040-inch wire. A knife edge should be formed at the apex of the V. If the second primary molar has previously been extracted, the maintainer may still be used. The sharpened distal shoe may be forced through a sterilized prepared area of the ridge.

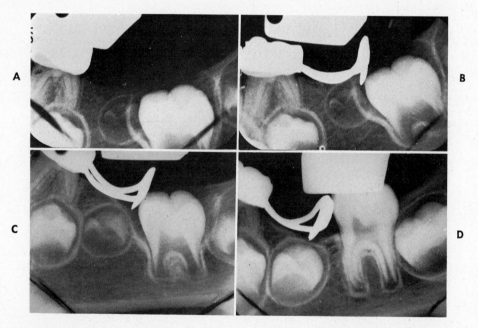

Fig. 20-24. A, The second primary molar has been extracted. The first permanent molar has migrated mesially several millimeters after the extraction. **B,** Crown and band appliance with a distal shoe to guide an unerupted first permanent molar into its normal position. Note the contour of the distal shoe to direct the first permanent molar distally and regain the lost space. **C,** Progress can be seen in the eruption of the permanent molar. **D,** The first permanent molar has erupted. The distal shoe tissue extension may now be removed.

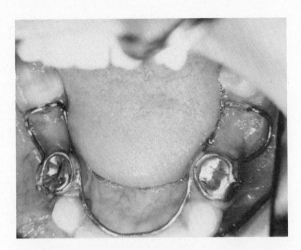

Fig. 20-25. A modified Roche distal shoe appliance to provide bilateral space maintenance and eruption guidance for the first permanent molars. The permanent molars are erupting properly, and the intragingival extensions may be removed.

Before final placement of the maintainer in the mouth, a radiograph of the appliance should be taken to determine whether the tissue extension is in proper relationship with the unerupted first permanent molar. Final adjustments in length and contour of the shoe may be made at that time. It has been observed that the soft tissue tolerates the extension of this type of appliance well, although a small metallic "tattoo" may result in the gingiva. A minimum of adjustment is required (Fig. 20-25).

Space maintenance for the primary canine area

Loss of the primary canine is infrequently caused by dental caries but may occur at the time of the eruption of the permanent lateral incisor. This problem and alternative types of treatment are discussed in detail in Chapter 21.

When the loss of the primary canine occurs prematurely and there has been no shift in the midline or space closure, a cast overlay, a band and loop, or a lingual arch with a spur can be used. The first primary molar is used as the abutment tooth (Fig. 20-26).

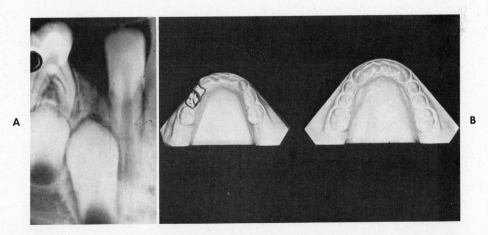

Fig. 20-26. A, Premature loss of a primary canine. **B,** A cast gold overlay was constructed as a space maintainer. Today the steel band and loop would be used to achieve the same results. The cast at the right shows that space has been maintained for the eruption of the permanent canine. An alternative treatment could have been the extraction of the right primary canine and the placement of a passive lingual arch, or the right canine could remain and a spur could be placed on the lingual arch distal to the left incisor.

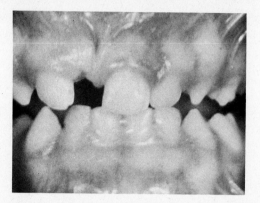

Fig. 20-27. Space closure within 6 weeks after the loss of a primary central incisor. The canines are in an active stage of eruption.

Space maintenance for the primary incisor area

Some dentists take the problem of the loss of primary incisors lightly, believing that space closure rarely occurs in the anterior part of the mouth. The dentist must critically evaluate each case from the standpoint of the rules previously mentioned. It is also important to consider the occlusion and the degree of spacing, if any, between the anterior teeth. If spacing is present, there is little possibility that drifting of the adjacent teeth will occur with resultant loss of space needed for eruption of the permanent tooth. However, if the anterior primary teeth were in contact before the loss or if there is evidence of an arch length inadequacy in the anterior region, a collapse in the arch after the loss of one of the primary incisors is almost certain (Fig. 20-27). In some patients even the primary canines drift mesially out of their normal relationship (Fig. 20-28).

The type of anterior space maintainer that is selected should depend on the age of the child, the degree of cooperation, the cleanliness of the mouth, and the wishes of the child and parents.

Removable partial dentures. Even when spacing is present, it may be desirable to construct a partial denture or a fixed appliance to reproduce the

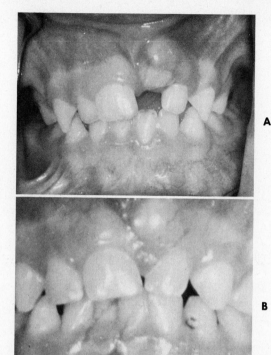

Fig. 20-28. A, Child with arch length inadequacy and some loss of space in the primary incisor area, which was noted at the time of the first examination. The tooth had been lost 10 months previously. **B,** Space closure continued and was accompanied by drifting of teeth through out the anterior area, including the canines.

desirable esthetic appearance, to reestablish function, or to prevent abnormal speech and tongue habits. Acrylic partial dentures have been successful in the replacement of maxillary anterior primary teeth (Fig. 20-29). Appliances of this type can be constructed for young children if there is a degree of cooperation and interest. It is unwise, however, to place a removable partial denture if there is an uncontrolled dental caries problem or if the child's mouth will not be kept clean enough to reduce the possibility of dental caries activity.

Fixed bridgework. Although it is not done often, a fixed bridge can also be constructed to

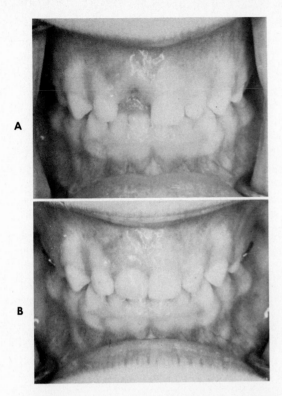

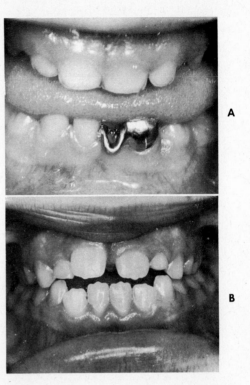

Fig. 20-29. A, This 3½-year-old child has lost a primary canine incisor as the result of a traumatic injury. A space maintainer should be constructed to prevent space closure and to restore normal appearance. **B,** An acrylic palatal retainer has been constructed. The placement of 0.028-inch steel clasps around the second primary molars aids in retention of the appliance.

Fig. 20-30. A, Cast gold overlay and loop maintainer is satisfactory for a young child. The abutment tooth requires little or no preparation. The canines are in an active stage of eruption. **B,** The lower permanent incisors have erupted in good relationship and alignment.

serve as a space maintainer after the loss of a maxillary primary incisor. Modified three-quarter crown preparations are made on the abutment teeth. A gold bar soldered to the castings is used to support an acrylic pontic. The pontic can be produced in wax and then reproduced in acrylic, or it can be built with quick-curing resin.

Gold overlay and loop. In the mandibular arch a gold overlay and loop type of maintainer can be used (Fig. 20-30). A passive lingual arch with spurs to prevent the drifting of teeth adjacent to the space may also be considered if there are adequate abutment teeth bilaterally.

Space maintenance for the permanent incisor area

The loss of anterior permanent teeth requires immediate treatment by the dentist if intra-arch changes are to be intercepted. Within a few days after the loss of a tooth as a result of trauma or the extraction of a severely traumatized tooth, the teeth adjacent to the space will begin to drift, and often within a few weeks several millimeters of space will be lost. Rather than allow the extraction area to heal and regain normal contour, the dentist should take an impression at the time of the initial appointment or within a few days. The temporary appliance can then be constructed and inserted within a matter of hours after the loss, preventing space closure.

If any degree of space closure has occurred after the loss of an anterior tooth, the space should be regained before the construction of a space maintainer. If the child has no other irregularities in the occlusion that require the attention of an orthodontist, the treatment can be completed by the pedodontist or the family dentist. A partial denture activating appliance can be used successfully in this procedure if there is no necessity for bodily movement of teeth (Fig. 20-31).

A thorough prophylaxis should precede the algi-

nate impression to produce an accurate stone model with good detail. Contoured steel cervical clasps constructed of 0.030-inch or 0.036-inch steel wire can be adapted to the first permanent molars to aid in retention of the appliance. Adams clasps of 0.028-inch or 0.030-inch wire are often used to gain a greater retentive quality (Fig. 20-32). Finger springs of 0.020-inch to 0.025-inch steel wire should be contoured for the teeth to be repositioned. The wire should be placed as far cervically as possible. The finger springs should be adjusted no more than 0.5 mm each 2 to 3 weeks. This procedure prevents an undesirable tissue reaction resulting from excessive pressure and produces slow,

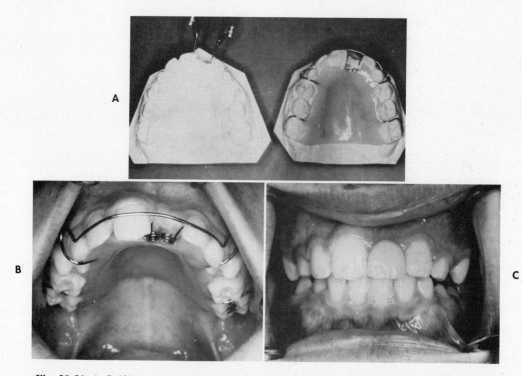

Fig. 20-31. A, Drifting and tipping of the maxillary anterior teeth have taken place within 3 months after the loss of the central incisor. The space must be regained before eruption of the permanent canines. **B,** A palatal retainer with a Hawley labial wire to aid in retention and finger springs to reposition the drifted teeth. Activation of the wires 1.5 mm every 2 or 3 weeks will result in desirable movement of the teeth. Repositioning of the teeth has been accomplished. A tooth can now be added to the appliance or a new appliance can be constructed and used until a fixed bridge can be inserted. **C,** A temporary replacement for the lost tooth.

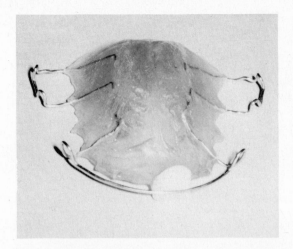

Fig. 20-32. Removable space-maintaining partial denture with Adams clasps that grasp the first permanent molars.

orderly movement of the teeth. A temporary tooth replacement may be made to improve the child's appearance. After the space has been regained, a new palatal retainer can be constructed to serve until the time a fixed replacement can be considered.

The loss of an anterior tooth occasionally occurs before the eruption of an adjacent tooth. For example, if a maxillary permanent central incisor is lost before the eruption of the lateral incisor, the lateral incisor will drift mesially during its eruption. The addition of an acrylic extension into the alveolus will normally be successful in guiding the unerupted tooth into position (Fig. 20-33).

The acid etch technique has made it possible to consider a very conservative approach for esthetic temporary fixed bridgework and space mainte-

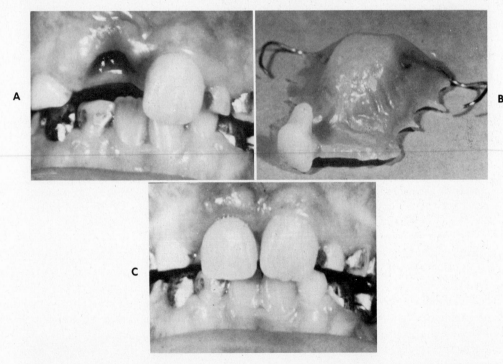

Fig. 20-33. A, Traumatic injury resulted in the loss of a permanent central incisor before the eruption of the lateral incisor. **B,** A palatal retainer was constructed within hours after the injury. An acrylic extension was added to the tooth to guide the eruption of the adjacent lateral incisor. **C,** The space maintainer in the mouth 24 hours after the injury.

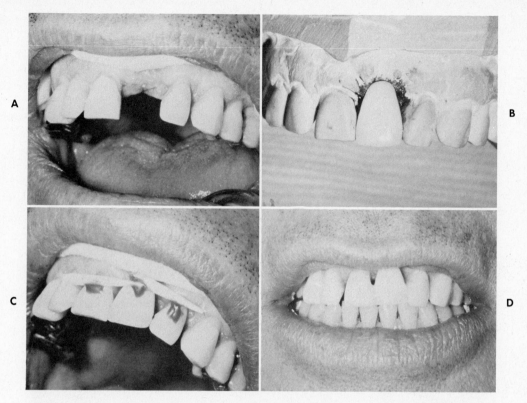

Fig. 20-34. A, Preoperative photograph of patient needing an esthetic temporary bridge to replace a missing maxillary left central incisor. **B,** Acrylic denture tooth of appropriate size and shade is ground to fit space on working model, and a horizontal slot is prepared on the lingual surface. **C,** The teeth are carefully isolated, and the abutment teeth are etched, rinsed, and dried. The pontic is stabilized in the proper position with wooden wedges and sticky wax from labial but cervical to proximal contact areas. Unfilled or composite resin is placed in the lingual slot of the pontic and completely around the embrasure areas. **D,** Finished temporary bridge. (Courtesy Dr. Norris Richmond.)

nance in some situations. An example of this approach is illustrated in Fig. 20-34. Although the example shown is of an adult who needed a long-term (over 6 months) temporary bridge, the technique is also applicable in older children and adolescents with a similar problem. The details of the acid etch technique are discussed in Chapter 17.

Temporary fixed bridgework is sometimes considered preferable to a removable appliance and can often be made for even the preteenage child. An acid etch fixed prosthesis used to replace miss-

ing permanent anterior teeth was described by Yanover, Croft, and Pulvey and by Denehy. It offers an alternative to conventional fixed bridgework and has many applications, especially in the younger age groups. The acid etch fixed prosthesis uses a lingual cast metal framework that supports fused procelain pontics. The perforated lingual cast framework is bonded to the abutment teeth by the acid etch resin technique. The design of the framework requires excessive contour on the lingual areas of the abutment teeth, but the bridge does not require tooth reduction. The technique does not require local anesthesia. The appliance is entirely supragingival, and the procedure is reversible. Yanover and associates and Denehy caution that the appliance may have limitations in situations where occlusal stresses are greater than usual, unless adequate occlusal clearance can be incorporated in the design of the bridge. If the prosthesis becomes dislodged or needs to be removed, it can usually be reattached without difficulty. The patient should be encouraged to practice good plaque control because the framework design is not one of "extension for prevention." Such a prosthesis is now considered a transitional appliance, but it should prove useful for young people. Chapman and Hamilton recently described the use of a similar prosthesis that preserved the natural diastemata between the pontic (replacing a maxillary lateral incisor) and the two abutment teeth.

Space maintenance for areas of multiple loss of teeth

The multiple loss of primary molars in the preschool or mixed dentition stage will invariably lead to severe mutilation of the developing dentition unless an appliance is constructed to maintain the relationship of the remaining teeth and to guide the eruption of the developing teeth. Cross-bite in the first permanent molar area and subsequent anterior drifting of the permanent molars have been observed to occur after the loss of the maxillary primary molars. Reduced masticatory function is undesirable from the nutritional standpoint. Also, the collection of plaque material and food debris after the loss of normal cleansing function will often result in increased dental caries activity and gingival inflammation.

Acrylic partial denture. The acrylic partial denture has been successful after the multiple loss of teeth in the mandible or the maxillary arch. This appliance, which is indicated when there has been bilateral loss of more than a single tooth, can be readily adjusted to allow for the eruption of teeth. If artificial teeth are included on the denture, an essentially normal degree of function will be re-

stored. However, the acrylic partial denture space maintainer is not without disadvantages. Breakage of the appliance is a potential factor, since the child patient may not exercise the necessary care. If the appliance is removed from the mouth for even a few days and is allowed to dry, changes in the denture base may occur, and the drifting of teeth may make it impossible for the child to replace the appliance unless extensive adjustments are made by the dentist.

The proper cleansing of the denture and the teeth is essential to reduce the possibility of the development of new carious lesions. Removable space-maintaining appliances of any type should not be constructed for child patients until the dental caries problem has been solved and until the dentist is reasonably certain that the patient will practice an acceptable degree of oral hygiene.

A partial denture space maintainer of the contoured clasp type is acceptable from the standpoint of simplicity of construction, functional requirements, and cost to the patient. The retention problem must be considered important, at least during the initial period of insertion. Stainless steel wire clasps are contoured for the primary canines, and 0.036-inch steel wire rests are contoured for the molars. If the permanent incisors are in an active state of eruption, it is desirable to remove the clasps after the child has become accustomed to wearing the appliance to allow the distal drifting and lateral movement of the primary canines and alignment of the permanent incisors. It is unlikely that there will be additional intercanine expansion in the older child. Therefore no adverse effect on the dental arch can follow the fixation of the primary canines before the eruption of the permanent successors (Figs. 20-35 and 20-36).

If the loss of one or both of the second primary molars occurs a short time before the eruption of the first permanent molars, the acrylic removable appliance may be considered in preference to one of the distal shoe maintainers described previously.

An "immediate" acrylic partial denture with an *acrylic distal shoe* extension has been advocated by

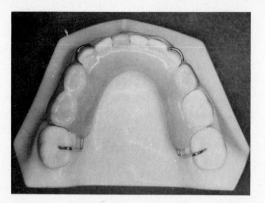

Fig. 20-35. Acrylic partial denture space maintainer to compensate for the untimely loss of three primary molars. The acrylic denture base material can be cut away to allow for the early eruption of one of the premolars before the maintainer is discarded. The acrylic may also be extended along the lingual tissues of the first permanent molars to incorporate retentive clasps for the molars if necessary.

Starkey and has been used successfully to guide first permanent molars into position (Figs. 20-37 and 20-38). The tooth to be extracted is cut away from the stone cast and a depression is cut into the stone model to allow the fabrication of the acrylic extension. The acrylic will extend into the alveolus after the removal of the primary tooth. The extension may be removed after the eruption of the permanent tooth.

The partial denture with a *cast framework* has an advantage of superior strength over the completely acrylic appliance (Fig. 20-39). A clearance of 1.5 to 2 mm should be provided between the bar and soft tissue to allow for expansion of tissue in the area as the permanent incisors move occlusally before their eruption. The cast partial denture may also be modified when permanent teeth begin to erupt.

Passive lingual arch. The soldered lingual arch is often the space maintainer of choice after the multiple loss of primary teeth in the maxillary or in the mandibular arch (Figs. 20-40 and 20-41). Although it does not satisfy the requirements of

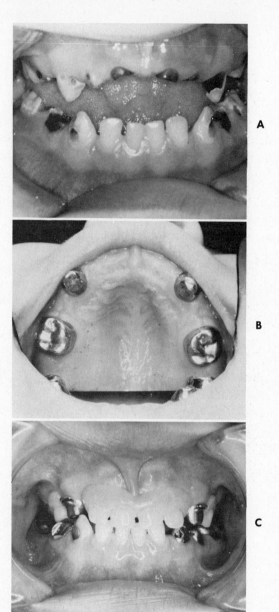

Fig. 20-36. A, This child requires removal of the maxillary primary incisors and the first primary molars. **B,** Chrome steel crowns have been placed on the primary canines and second molars. **C,** A maxillary partial denture restores function, improves appearance, and reduces the possibility of a tongue-thrusting habit.

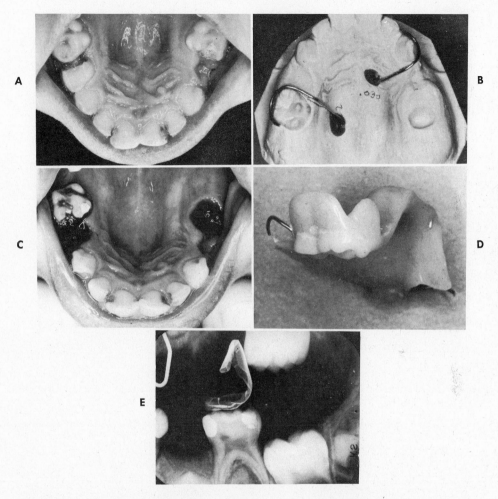

Fig. 20-37. A, Clinical and radiographic examination revealed the need to extract the maxillary left first and second primary molars. The photograph is a mirror image. **B,** The teeth indicated for extraction are cut away from the stone model. A depression is made on the second molar area for the acrylic distal shoe type of extension. **C,** The primary teeth have been extracted in preparation for the placement of the partial denture. **D,** Acrylic distal shoe extension. **E,** Lead foil has been placed over the tissue extension for the purpose of determining, with the aid of a radiograph, if the acrylic is positioned properly to guide the eruption of the first permanent molar. (Courtesy Dr. Paul E. Starkey.)

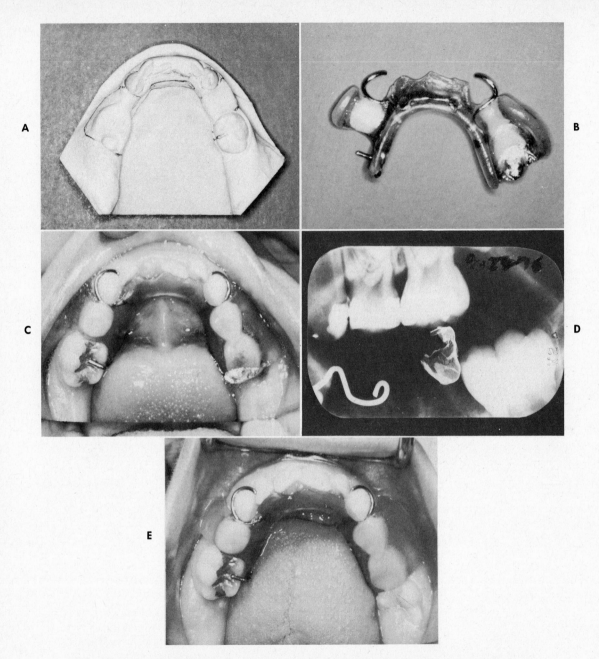

Fig. 20-38. A, Model prepared for fabrication of a mandibular acrylic distal shoe appliance. **B,** Tissue-bearing surface of appliance with lead foil adapted over the tissue extension. **C,** Mirror view of appliance during the trial insertion immediately after removal of the left second primary molar. **D,** Radiograph confirms the proper position of the tissue extension. **E,** Mirror view of the appliance and lower arch 6 months postoperatively. Favorable eruption of the left first permanent molar has occurred. When permanent molars are sufficiently erupted, the acrylic appliance may be replaced with a passive lingual arch to allow the anterior segment to "unwind." (Courtesy Dr. Hala Z. Henderson.)

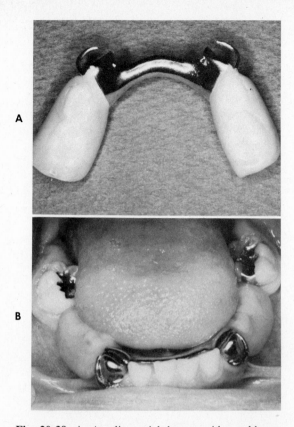

Fig. 20-39. A, Acrylic partial denture with a gold cast framework has been constructed after the removal of pulpless first and second primary molars. **B,** Chrome steel crowns have been placed on carious canines. A piece of 0.028-inch steel wire has been soldered to the cervical third of the crown to provide an undercut for the clasps.

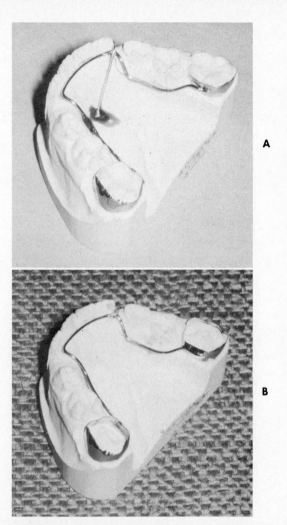

Fig. 20-40. A, Mandibular passive lingual arch wire and a spur to the distal surface of the right lateral incisor have been properly contoured and fixed to the working model with sticky wax in preparation for soldering. **B,** Soldered and polished appliance ready for trial insertion in the mouth.

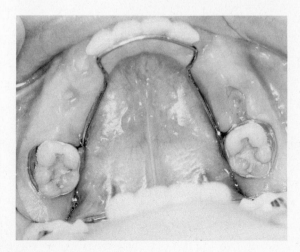

Fig. 20-41. Mirror view of a passive mandibular soldered lingual arch immediately after cementation. (Courtesy Dr. Theodore R. Lynch.)

restoring function, the appliance has many advantages that seem to outweigh this fact. The use of the lingual arch as a space-maintaining appliance essentially eliminates the problem of patient cooperation. There should be no breakage problem and no concern about whether the child is wearing the appliance. The problem of an increase in dental caries activity is considerably lessened. The lingual arch may be constructed from gold or steel. From the standpoint of durability, gold offers the advantage, but steel materials are considerably more economical.

The compound impression of the entire arch should be taken, the bands should be removed from the teeth and placed in the impression, and a stone model should be prepared. A 0.036-inch or 0.040-inch steel wire or a 0.040-inch or 0.045-inch gold wire should be contoured to the arch, extending forward and making contact with the cingulum portion of the incisor. In contouring the arch wires, thought should be given to the path of eruption of the premolar and anterior teeth in order that the arch wire will not interfere and necessitate time-consuming alteration of the appliance. The arch wire should be extended posteriorly along the middle third of the lingual surface of the molar band and soldered firmly in this position in an inactive state. A similarly designed lingual arch or one of the W-shaped variety can be used in the maxillary arch, as described in Chapter 21.

Two important considerations related to the use of the lingual arch require emphasis: the appliance, when used as a space maintainer, should be made entirely inactive to prevent undesirable movement

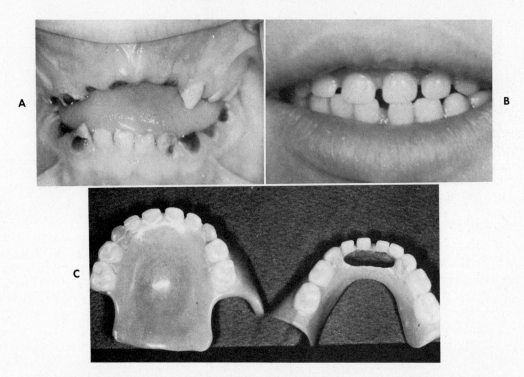

Fig. 20-42. A, Primary teeth have gross caries and pulpal involvement. **B,** Complete dentures were constructed after the extraction of all primary teeth. **C,** The dentures were modified after the eruption of the maxillary first permanent molars and the mandibular permanent incisors.

of the abutment teeth, and care must be exercised during the cementation procedure. Abutment teeth must be polished free of plaque material, dried, and maintained in this state during the cementation procedure. The manufacturer's directions must be followed during the mixing and the cementation to ensure a strong bond to the tooth structure.

Full dentures for children. It is occasionally necessary to recommend the extraction of all the primary teeth of a preschool-age child. Although this procedure was more common in the prefluoridation era, some children even today must have all of their teeth removed because of widespread oral infection and because the teeth are unrestorable. Preschool-age children can wear complete dentures successfully before the eruption of permanent teeth (Fig. 20-42).

The construction of dentures will result in an improved appearance and restored function and may be effective to some degree in guiding the first permanent molars into their correct position. The technique, although similar to that of complete denture construction for adults, is somewhat less complicated. A nonpressure alginate impression technique with No. 1 or No. 2 trays is satisfactory. Stone casts can be mounted after centric relationship has been obtained. Primary maxillary anterior teeth are manufactured for partial or complete dentures. Lower anterior denture teeth may be prepared from a set of small acrylic permanent teeth. The posterior border of the denture should be carried to an area approximating the mesial surface of the unerupted first permanent molar. The denture will have to be adjusted, a portion of it cut away as the permanent incisors erupt, and the posterior border contoured to guide the first permanent molars into position. When the permanent incisors and first permanent molars have erupted, a partial denture space maintainer or a lingual arch can be constructed to serve until the remaining permanent teeth erupt.

Appliances to regain space

The dentist frequently sees children whose first permanent molars have drifted mesially. Whether this problem can be managed by means of an uncomplicated procedure or demands the services of an orthodontist depends on a number of factors. It is generally agreed that the distal movement of first permanent molars other than minimal tipping can most satisfactorily be corrected with a headgear appliance that uses extraoral anchorage. The headgear technique is relatively uncomplicated and can be used successfully by any dentist with proper education and experience.

A number of removable appliances have been recommended for regaining space (tipping), particularly when the first permanent molars have drifted mesially. This usually occurs because the child does not receive regular dental care and space maintenance was not achieved at the proper time. It should be recognized, however, that when these appliances are used to reposition a molar, there will be a reciprocal force exerted to the teeth and supporting tissues anterior to the space, and the result may be an undesirable flaring of the anterior teeth. This is particularly true during the mixed dentition period when the permanent incisors are incompletely erupted and may be adversely influenced by even so-called minimal forces. Furthermore, the forward movement of the first permanent molars may be accompanied by movement of the unerupted second permanent molar, and any attempt to tip or reposition the first permanent molar may produce an impaction of the second molar.

The space-regaining procedure that involves tipping only the first permanent molar can be accomplished more easily in the maxillary arch than in the mandibular arch. The procedure should be limited to those situations in which the occlusion is of the Class I type, there is adequate anchorage, the second permanent molar is unerupted, and there is a favorable relationship of the second permanent molar with the first permanent molar. If the dentist concludes that conditions are favorable, an appliance similar to the type shown in Fig. 20-43 may be considered. Activation of the 0.025-inch steel wire should be approximately 0.5 mm each 3 or 4 weeks to encourage slow movement of the tooth that is to be repositioned.

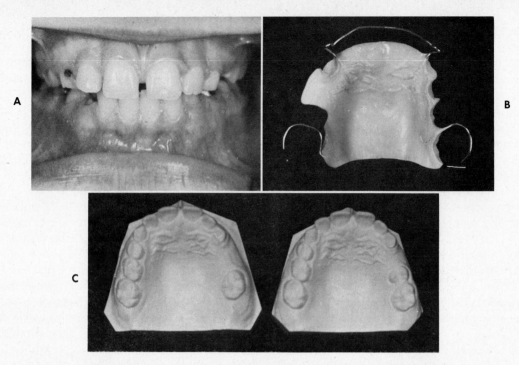

Fig. 20-43. A, Child with an essentially normal occlusion. However, a maxillary first permanent molar drifted forward after the untimely loss of primary molars. **B,** The appliance used to reposition the first permanent molar. **C,** Before and after models illustrate the regaining of space and the eruption of the second premolar into a desirable position.

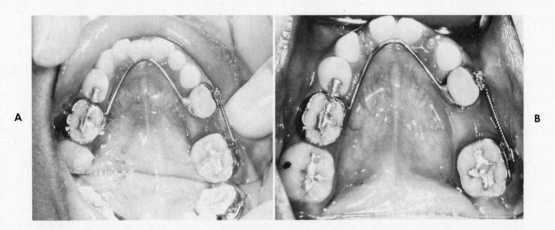

Fig. 20-44. A, Coil spring space-regaining appliance in place on the day it was inserted initially. **B,** Desired amount of space regaining accomplished in about 2 months. Although the entire amount of space loss was not regained, the first permanent molars on the affected side are in a Class I relationship. During this period of treatment the mandibular primary lateral incisors exfoliated normally and the position of the lingual arch wire encouraged some flaring of the erupting permanent central incisors.

Space regaining that requires distal tipping of a mandibular first permanent molar is a definite challenge. However, if favorable conditions exist, an attempt to regain space is certainly indicated. A fixed intraoral appliance with coil spring activation has been used successfully for this procedure (Fig. 20-44). Bilateral stability and anchorage may be provided with a soldered lingual arch. A 0.022-inch edgewise narrow twin bracket is aligned and welded to the buccal surface of the abutment band adjacent to the space before the lingual arch portion of the appliance is cemented into place. A band is also fitted to the first permanent molar to be tipped distally, and a 0.036-inch (or slightly smaller) buccal tube is properly aligned and welded to the band before it is cemented into place. A 0.022-inch round or a 0.016×0.022 inch rectangular wire is selected so it will slide freely in the buccal tube but can also be securely fixed to the bracket with ligature wire. The wire is cut to the desired length and adjusted to the alignment of the teeth by making smooth, gentle bends if necessary. A section of coil spring material (0.009×0.036 inch) approximately 2 mm longer than the space between the bracket and the tube is placed around the wire, and the entire assembly is fixed in position as illustrated. As the space opens, the wire and spring are replaced with longer sections at approximately 2-week intervals until the desired position is attained. The same appliance will often serve as a space maintainer by using a wire and a passive coil spring or by fixing a wire (tied in or soldered) to the two bands adjacent to the space.

Loss of the first permanent molar

The first permanent molar is unquestionably the most important unit of mastication and is essential in the development of functionally desirable occlusion. From the examination of the first permanent molar in a group of schoolchildren, much can be learned about the dental health level of the community and the effectiveness of the local dentist in providing adequate dental care and a preventive program for the children. Grainger and Reid report that in individual children caries susceptibility of the whole mouth can be correlated with the amount of decay in the first permanent molars.

Knutson, Klein, and Palmer believe that the first permanent molars are the most susceptible of all the permanent teeth to caries attack. As a result of unusually deep occlusal fissures, the bases of which are often incompletely coalesced, and the collection of plaque material, the first permanent molars often need restorations even before the tooth completes its eruption process and the entire occlusal surface becomes exposed to the oral cavity. If the dentist can engage the defects on the occlusal surface with a sharp explorer point, a pit and fissure sealant should be placed before the development of a definite carious lesion.

A carious lesion develops rapidly in the first permanent molar and occasionally progresses from an incipient lesion to a pulp exposure in a 6-month period. The loss of a first permanent molar in a child can lead to changes in the dental arches that can be traced throughout the life of the individual. These changes may be placed under three general headings: diminished local function, drifting of teeth, and continued eruption of opposing teeth.

Diminished local function. The loss of a mandibular first permanent molar can result in a reduction in chewing efficiency as great as 50%. Klapper and Wilkie demonstrated in a group of experimental animals that when the opposing molars were removed, the caries scores were more than twice as large as those in a control group. They concluded that normal interdigitation of opposing molars is important in retarding the initiation of dental caries or in reducing the rate of dental decay during the early stages. Children who lose a first permanent molar are aware of the loss of normal function. This loss is often followed by a shifting of the load of mastication to the unaffected side of the mouth. Such a shift will result in an unhygienic condition of the unused side of the mouth and perhaps in gingival inflammation and a breakdown of the supporting tissues. Uneven occlusal wear is often associated with the acquired habit of chewing on one side of the mouth, the side where there is greater efficiency (Fig. 20-45).

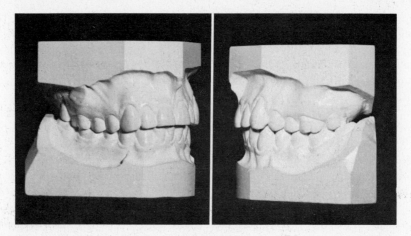

Fig. 20-45. Models of a patient who lost a mandibular permanent molar before the eruption of the second molar. A unilateral chewing habit developed. The teeth on the right side of the dental arch have shorter crowns as a result of increased occlusal wear.

Drifting of teeth. The second molars, regardless of whether they have erupted, start to drift mesially after the loss of the first permanent molar. A greater degree of movement will occur in children in the 8- to 10-year age group; in older children, if the loss occurs after the eruption of the second permanent molar, only tipping of this tooth can be expected. Although the premolars will undergo the greatest amount of distal drifting, all of the teeth anterior to the space, including the central and lateral incisors on the side where the loss occurred, may show evidence of movement. Contacts will open and the premolars, in particular, will rotate as they fall distally (Fig. 20-46). There is a tendency for the maxillary premolars to move distally in unison, whereas those in the lower arch may move separately. Traumatic occlusion will develop as a result of the drifting and rotation of these and other teeth in the area.

Continued eruption of opposing teeth. The mandibular first permanent molars apparently are more susceptible to decay and are more frequently lost than the maxillary first permanent molars.

When the maxillary first permanent molar loses its opponent, it will erupt at a faster rate than the adjacent teeth. As the first molar continues to

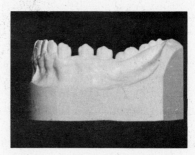

Fig. 20-46. Lower cast showing distal drifting of the premolars and mesial tipping of the second and third molars after the extraction of the first permanent molar.

erupt, it will be "squeezed" buccally. In later life the overerupted maxillary first permanent molar will show evidence of gingival recession, since it will receive the brunt of the toothbrushing procedure. Exposed sensitive dentin may also present a problem.

• • •

The treatment of patients involving the loss of first permanent molars must be regarded as an individual problem. A superimposed existing maloc-

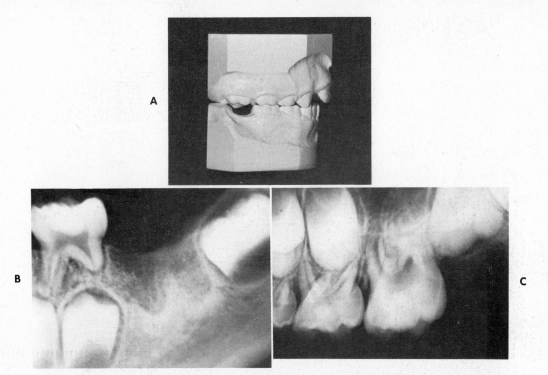

Fig. 20-47. A, Models of the dentition of an 8-year-old child who had a mandibular first permanent molar extracted. It would be virtually impossible to guide the second permanent molar into its normal position and at the same time prevent overeruption of the opposing first permanent molar. Therefore extraction of the opposing molar is often indicated. **B** and **C,** Position of the second permanent molars. If first permanent molars are removed at this age, reasonably good positioning of the second molars can be expected.

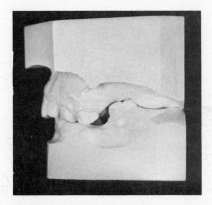

Fig. 20-48. Continued eruption of a mandibular first permanent molar after loss of its maxillary opponent.

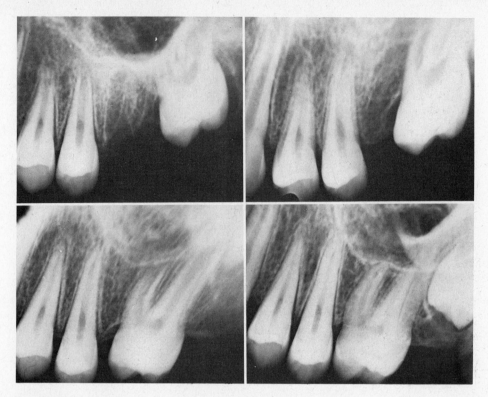

Fig. 20-49. Radiographs taken at 6-month intervals after a maxillary first permanent molar was lost before the eruption of the second permanent molar.

clusion, abnormal musculature, or the presence of oral habits can affect the result as in the case of the premature loss of primary molars.

Loss of the first permanent molar before the eruption of the second permanent molar. Although it is possible to prevent overeruption of a maxillary first permanent molar by placing a lower partial denture, there is no completely effective way to influence the path of eruption of the developing second permanent molar other than the use of an acrylic distal shoe extension from a partial denture as described previously. The second molar will drift mesially before eruption when the first permanent molar has been extracted. Repositioning this tooth orthodontically is possible after its eruption. However, the child must then be considered for prolonged space maintenance until the time when a fixed bridged can be constructed.

The removal of the opposing first permanent molar, even though the tooth appears to be sound and caries free, is often recommended in preference to allowing it to extrude or to subjecting the child to prolonged space maintenance and eventual fixed replacement (Figs. 20-47 and 20-48).

If the first permanent molars are removed several years before the eruption of the second permanent molars, there is an excellent chance that the second molars will erupt in an acceptable position (Fig. 20-49). However, the axial inclination of the second molars, particularly in the lower arch, may be slightly greater than normal (Fig. 20-50).

The decision to allow the second molar to drift mesially or to be guided forward in an upright position may be influenced by the presence of a third molar of normal size. If there is a question regarding the favorable development of a third molar on

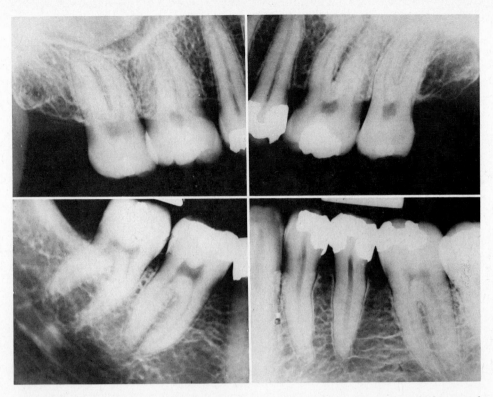

Fig. 20-50. Adult who had all four first permanent molars removed at approximately 9 years of age.

the affected side, repositioning the drifted second molar and holding it for fixed bridgework is the treatment of choice.

Loss of the first permanent molar after the eruption of the second permanent molar. When the first permanent molar is lost after the eruption of the second permanent molar, orthodontic evaluation is indicated, and the following points should be considered. Is the child in need of corrective treatment other than in the first permanent molar area? Should the space be maintained for fixed bridgework, or should the second molar be moved forward into the area formerly occupied by the first molar? The latter choice is often the more satisfactory, even though there will be a difference in the number of molars in the opposing arch. A third molar can often be removed to compensate for the difference. It is important to realize that without

treatment the second molar will fall forward within a matter of weeks (Fig. 20-51).

If it is decided that the space should be maintained, there are several ways in which the process may be accomplished:

1. *Cast overlay.* This type of space maintainer is essentially the same as the Willett overlay, except an occlusal bar and rest are added to maintain the relationship of the opposing teeth (Fig. 20-52). It is advisable to place a distoclusal restoration in the tooth that is to receive the rest to prevent the development of a carious lesion beneath the rest.

2. *Modified band and loop maintainer.* A well-adapted, heavy gold band strengthened by an additional quantity of solder with an attached loop, occlusal bar, and rest is often the maintainer of choice. However, retention may be

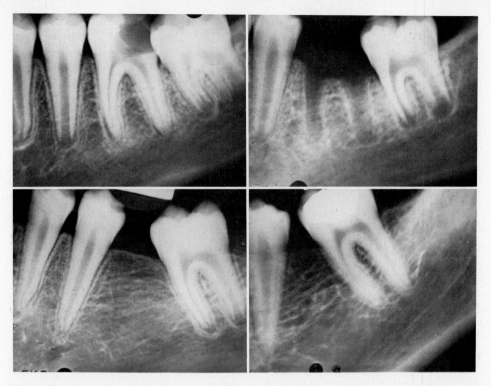

Fig. 20-51. Radiographs taken at 6-month intervals after the loss of a mandibular first permanent molar. Note the degree of tipping of the second molar and distal drifting of the premolars.

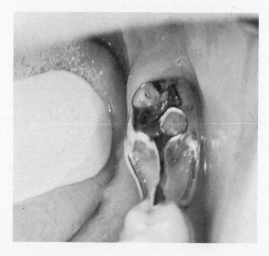

Fig. 20-52. Cast overlay type of space maintainer that can be used to maintain the relationship of adjacent teeth before the construction of a fixed bridge.

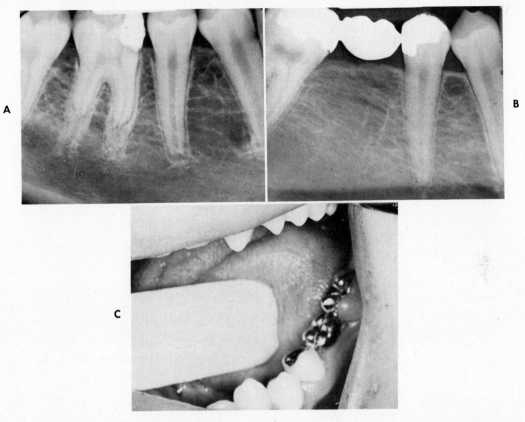

Fig. 20-53. A, First permanent molar recommended for extraction because it was not considered suitable for root canal therapy. Although the patient was only 14 years of age, the pulp chambers were relatively small and it was possible to prepare the teeth for bridge attachments. **B,** Radiograph of a fixed bridge. **C,** Photograph of the fixed bridge.

a problem with this maintainer and with the overlay type.

3. *Conventional fixed bridgework.* The belief that fixed bridgework cannot be considered before a definite age has been dispelled. Mink found that patients in the early teenage period can often be considered candidates for fixed bridgework. The size of the pulp in the abutment teeth is essentially the determining factor. Whenever the pulp has receded to the degree that inlay or full crown preparations can be completed, a fixed bridge can be constructed (Fig. 20-53). Although gingival re-cession will continue and margins of the restoration may become exposed, the modified fixed bridge will function satisfactorily into early adulthood.

4. *Etched casting resin bonded posterior bridge (modified fixed bridgework).* Recent reports of posterior bridgework bonded to abutment teeth with composite resin materials have been encouraging. The posterior resin bonded bridge, introduced by Livaditis and improved by Thompson and Livaditis, has opened a completely new approach to fixed posterior retainers. The basic prosthesis and

its application are similar to those described previously in the discussion of anterior bridgework. However, the posterior technique requires slight tooth enamel preparation to establish a correct path of insertion and occlusal rests for the cast metal retainer. Retention of the bridge is derived from the proximal parallelism of the preparation, etched enamel, and resin bonding. Preferably the case framework is electrolytically etched (instead of being perforated) to enhance the resin bonding to the metal.

Thompson and Livaditis reported on 15 successful 3-unit posterior bridges using this new approach. The bridges had been functioning in normal occlusion for 2 to 4 years. No debonding of the bridges had occurred, although wear of exposed resin was observed at the perforations of nonelectrolytically etched retainers. This technique seems especially suited for adolescents and young adults when a first permanent molar has been lost after the eruption of the second premolar and second molar.

REFERENCES

Ballard, M.L., and Wylie, W.L.: Mixed dentition case analysis: estimating size of unerupted permanent teeth, Am. J. Orthod. **33:**754-759, 1947.

Barber, T.K.: The crowded arch, J. South. Calif. Dent. Assoc. **35:**232-240, 1967.

Baume, L.J.: Physiological tooth migration and its significance for the development of occlusion. I. The biogenetic course of the deciduous dentition, J. Dent. Res. **29:**123-132, 331-337, 440-447, 1950.

Chapman, K.W., and Hamilton, M.L.: Maintenance of diastemas by a cast lingual loop connector and acid-etch technique, J.A.D.A. **104:**49-50, 1982.

Denehy, G.E.: Cast anterior bridges utilizing composite resin, Pediatr. Dent. **4:**44-47, 1982.

Drinkard, C., and Oldenburg, T.R.: Appliances for guiding first permanent molar eruption. In McDonald, R.E., and others: Current therapy in dentistry, vol. 7, St. Louis, 1980, The C.V. Mosby Co.

Grainger, R.M., and Reid, D.B.W.: Distribution of dental caries in children, J. Dent. Res. **33:**613-623, 1954.

Grøn, A.M.: Prediction of tooth emergence, J. Dent. Res. **41:**573-585, 1962.

Klapper, C.E., and Wilkie, E.: Influence on experimental dental caries after extraction of opposing molars, J. Dent. Res. (abs.) **37:**53, 1958.

Knutson, J.W., Klein, H., and Palmer, C.E.: Studies on dental caries. VIII. Relative incidence of caries in the different permanent teeth, J.A.D.A. **25:**1923-1934, 1938.

Livaditis, G.J.: Cast metal resin-bonded retainers for posterior teeth, J.A.D.A. **101:**926-929, 1980.

Mills, L.F.: Changes in dimension of the dental arches with age, J. Dent. Res. **45:**890-894, 1966.

Mink, J.R.: Personal communication, 1965.

Miyamoto, W., Chung, C.S. and Yee, P.K.: Effect of premature loss of deciduous canines and molars on malocclusion of the permanent dentition, J. Dent. Res. **55:**584-590, 1976.

Moorrees, C.F.A.: Growth changes of the dental arches: a longitudinal study, J. Can. Dent. Assoc. **24:**449-457, 1958.

Moyers, R.E.: Handbook of orthodontics for the student and general practitioner, ed. 2, Chicago, 1963, Year Book Medical Publishers, Inc.

Nance, H.N.: The limitations of orthodontic treatment. I. Mixed dentition diagnosis and treatment, Am. J. Orthod. **33:**177-223, 1947.

Roche, J.R.: Unpublished data, 1968.

Starkey, P.E.: Personal communication, 1967.

Thompson, V.P., and Livaditis, G.J.: Etched casting acid etch composite bonded posterior bridges, Pediatr. Dent. **4:**39-43, 1982.

Yanover, L., Croft, W., and Pulver, F.: The acid-etched fixed prosthesis, J.A.D.A. **104:**325-328, 1982.

21 Diagnosis and correction of minor irregularities in the developing dentition

RALPH E. McDONALD
DAVID R. AVERY

In the initial examination of a patient's mouth there is often a temptation to look first for obvious carious lesions. This is important because carious lesions progress rapidly in the child patient and the pulp may become involved within a few months after the lesion has started. It is more important, however, to begin the examination with an inspection of the soft tissues and to record deviations from normal. Next in order of importance is a consideration of the occlusion to determine whether the dentition has developed normally. If the condition of the soft tissues and the state of the occlusion are not observed early in the examination, the dentist may become so engrossed in charting carious lesions and in planning for their restoration that other important anomalies in the mouth are overlooked.

Irregularities in the occlusion are frequently observed in preschool-age children, in children with mixed dentition, and in teenagers. The irregularities may involve an actual skeletal anomaly that can be corrected only by major orthodontic treatment, or the defect may be of a so-called minor nature. Ideally, some irregularities should be treated in their incipient form; if this is done, a major malocclusion can often be averted.

How much orthodontics should be undertaken by practitioners other than orthodontists? This question has received much attention in recent years and has been the subject of considerable debate. The logical answer must be that dentists can do as much as they are qualified to do as a result of their education and experience.

In this chapter consideration is given to developmental irregularities that should be recognized by the dentist who provides dental care for children. Relatively uncomplicated treatment procedures are outlined that are based on the assumption that a correct diagnosis has been made, the cause of the problem is completely understood, and the dentist has an adequate knowledge of growth and development. A review of the material in Chapters 18 and 19, which deal with growth of the dental arches and the development of the occlusion, will be helpful in the diagnosis and treatment of the conditions described in this chapter.

Supernumerary teeth and accompanying malocclusion

Supernumerary teeth, which result from the continued budding of the enamel organ of the preceding tooth or from excessive proliferation of cells, can be responsible for a variety of irregularities in the primary and transitional dentition. The stage of differentiation determines whether a cyst, an odontoma, or a supernumerary tooth will result. In separate studies, Stafne and Schulze concluded that supernumerary teeth occur in approximately one in 110 children. The ratio of the prevalence in the maxilla and mandible is 8:1. The most common site for supernumerary teeth is in the maxillary incisor area. Supernumerary primary teeth (Fig.

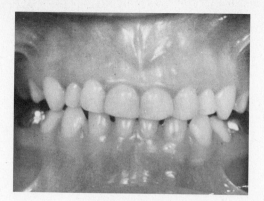

Fig. 21-1. Supernumerary maxillary primary incisors. There may be corresponding supernumerary permanent teeth. The teeth should be counted at the time of the clinical examination so that erupted supernumerary teeth will not be overlooked.

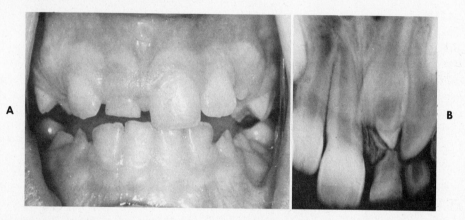

A
B

Fig. 21-2. A, Patient with an unerupted maxillary permanent incisor. Space closure is the result of delayed eruption. **B,** The radiograph shows a supernumerary tooth (mesiodens), which has delayed the eruption of the permanent incisor.

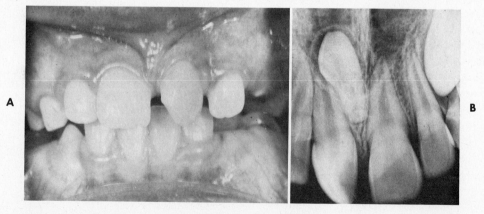

A
B

Fig. 21-3. A, Rotation and labioversion of a maxillary anterior tooth are often caused by the presence of a supernumerary tooth. The position of this tooth increases its susceptibility to fracture. **B,** Radiograph of a well-developed midline supernumerary tooth. Surgical removal of the tooth is indicated.

21-1) are apparently much less common than supernumerary permanent teeth. The occurrence of supernumerary teeth in several members of the same family is not uncommon. Therefore some investigators have suggested that this anomaly follows a familial pattern.

Supernumerary teeth, particularly in the maxillary anterior region, may prevent the eruption of adjacent permanent teeth (Fig. 21-2) or cause their ectopic eruption (Fig. 21-3). Both conditions frequently result in an irregularity of the developing occlusion that requires treatment. Stafne and also Montelius and Wahlquist reported cysts developing from unerupted supernumerary teeth.

Diagnostic techniques. The frequency with which supernumerary teeth are observed in children makes a full-mouth radiographic survey for preschool children imperative (before expected eruption of any permanent teeth). If a supernumerary tooth is observed, a special radiographic technique, as described in Chapter 6, can be used to localize the tooth. The decision can then be made whether to intervene surgically or to keep the tooth under observation.

Surgical removal of supernumerary teeth. The surgical removal of an unerupted supernumerary tooth is the eventual course of treatment. However, if the supernumerary tooth is not interfering with the symmetric development and eruption of adjacent teeth and if there is no evidence of the formation of a cyst, the correct decision may be to observe the tooth until the child is old enough to tolerate the procedure better. Many surgeons prefer to delay the surgery until permanent teeth erupt and until root closure is complete, provided there is no evidence of a developing irregularity in the occlusion.

The delayed eruption of one of the maxillary incisors as a result of a midline supernumerary tooth is relatively common. In this case the immediate surgical removal of the supernumerary tooth is recommended. At the time of the surgical procedure the bone and soft tissue should be removed from the incisal third of the tooth or teeth that are delayed in their eruption. An open pathway should be maintained, if possible, to hasten the eruption of the delayed tooth. A thin covering of dense scar tissue can delay eruption of a tooth indefinitely. The surgical procedure is described in detail in Chapter 29.

Because teeth move more rapidly during the time of cellular activity at the developing root end and because adjacent teeth may bypass the delayed tooth in the eruption pattern, early diagnosis and treatment are imperative in the majority of cases.

When permanent teeth have been delayed by supernumerary teeth, several years may elapse before the permanent tooth erupts into a desirable position. The permanent tooth in its eruption may deviate from its normal path or may rotate even if an open pathway is maintained. Thus orthodontic procedures may be necessary to treat the condition completely.

Correction of minor irregularities resulting from supernumerary teeth. Delayed eruption of maxillary anterior permanent teeth, resulting from the presence of a supernumerary tooth, will frequently result in an arch length inadequacy. Study models should be prepared and the occlusion should be carefully studied to determine whether the malocclusion is limited to the area of the supernumerary involvement. If there is a superimposed malocclusion, a comprehensive orthodontic evaluation is indicated.

If there is sufficient room within the arch to accommodate teeth delayed in their eruption, plans should be made to remove the supernumerary tooth, expose a portion of the crown of the unerupted permanent tooth, and regain space in the area (Fig. 21-4). Space may be regained with a removable palatal working retainer if treatment is undertaken before the development of the occlusion is complete. After the eruption of the permanent canines, it is usually not possible to regain sufficient space for the eruption of the incisors.

A midline diastema may result from a supernumerary tooth. If the axial inclination of the adjacent teeth is satisfactory, the diastema may be closed with a Hawley type of palatal appliance. If this

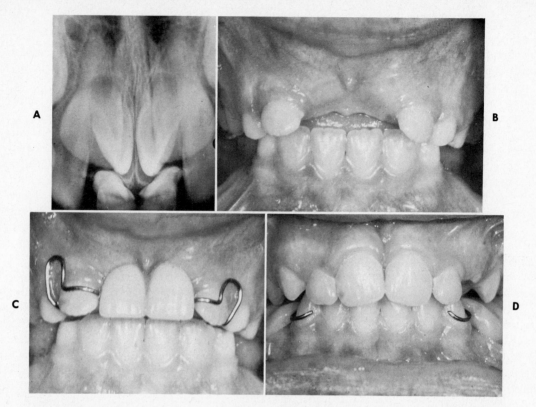

Fig. 21-4. A, Supernumerary teeth and retained primary central incisors are responsible for the delayed eruption of the permanent central incisors. The eruption of the permanent lateral incisors before the central incisors has resulted in space loss. **B,** Radiographs before this time would have revealed the reason for the delayed eruption of the central incisors. **C,** The supernumerary teeth have been removed, and a space-maintaining appliance has been placed to maintain the relationship of teeth in the arch during the period of eruption of the central incisors. **D,** The permanent teeth have erupted. Eruption often occurs slowly, and the area must be observed for many months.

treatment is undertaken, the practitioner should be aware of the limitations of the appliance and the possibility that the teeth may tip to some degree.

The labial displacement or rotation of an anterior tooth is often caused by a supernumerary tooth. This displacement may occur with or without the loss of arch length in the area. After a supernumerary tooth has been removed, the malaligned teeth should be brought into proper alignment. This, too, can usually be done with a palatal working retainer.

Anterior cross-bite in the primary and permanent dentition

Anterior cross-bite in the primary dentition is usually indicative of a skeletal growth problem and a developing Class III malocclusion. Anterior cross-bite (inlocking) of one or more of the permanent incisors, however, may be evidence of a localized discrepancy and a condition that almost without exception should be treated in the mixed dentition state or as soon as it is discovered. Delayed treatment can lead to serious complica-

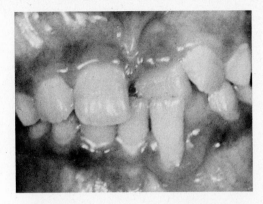

Fig. 21-5. Untreated inlocked central incisor has resulted in stripping of the tissue, pocket formation, and a loss in arch length.

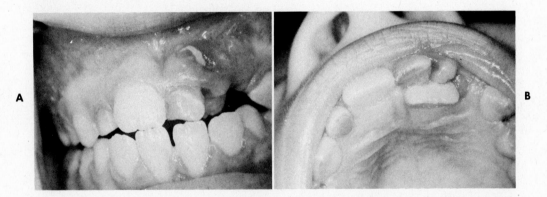

Fig. 21-6. A, Prolonged retention of a pulpless primary incisor has resulted in lingual eruption and inlocking of permanent tooth. Note exposed and unresorbed apex of necrotic primary incisor that has perforated the gingival tissues. **B,** Incisal view.

tions, such as loss of arch length, when adjacent teeth drift into the area. Traumatic occlusion with resultant stripping of the gingival tissue and pocket formation on the labial aspect of the lower opposing tooth is a common result (Fig. 21-5). Unsightly wear facets may also develop on the incisal and labial surfaces of the involved maxillary incisors. Anterior cross-bite is the result of a variety of conditions, including the following:

1. A labially situated supernumerary tooth may cause torsiversion and lingual deflection of an incisor, which may erupt in a rotated or a cross-bite relationship.
2. A traumatic injury to an anterior primary tooth may cause displacement of the developing permanent successor and eruption in cross-bite. If a primary incisor is delayed in its exfoliation because of a necrotic pulp resulting from trauma or caries, the tooth may act as a foreign body and cause deflection of permanent teeth in the area (Fig. 21-6). Pulpless primary teeth often do not undergo normal root resorption and can cause serious complications in the developing occlusion.
3. An arch length deficiency can cause the lingual deflection of permanent anterior teeth in their eruptive process. This is most often observed in the maxillary lateral incisor area. The premature eruption of permanent canines

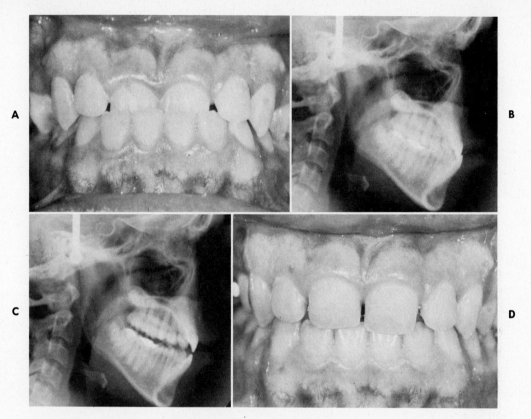

Fig. 21-7. A, Anterior cross-bite involving the maxillary central incisors. The canine and molar relationship is essentially normal. **B** and **C,** Lateral headplate films will aid in determining whether the defect is limited to the dental arch or includes structures beyond the alveolar process. Tracing and evaluation of the lateral films indicated that the facial pattern was within normal limits. At rest position, the incisors assume an end-to-end relationship. **D,** After treatment of the malocclusion with a bite plane.

in instances of arch length deficiency can cause a lateral incisor to be "squeezed" to the lingual side and to erupt in an inlocking relationship.

Properly articulated study models, full-mouth radiographs, and in some cases lateral headplate films should be used to complete the diagnosis (Fig. 21-7). With the information available from these records and as a result of a careful clinical examination, the dentist must decide whether the occlusion problem is a complex one requiring consultation with an orthodontist (Fig. 21-8). If the

dentist concludes, after a careful review of the records, that the following conditions are present, the problem may be considered as one in which uncomplicated (minor) treatment may be undertaken:

1. There must be sufficient room mesiodistally to move the inlocked tooth forward into its correct position. Furthermore, there should be sufficient overbite to hold the tooth in its new position in the arch; otherwise, a retainer will have to be worn indefinitely and the result of treatment will be unsatisfactory.

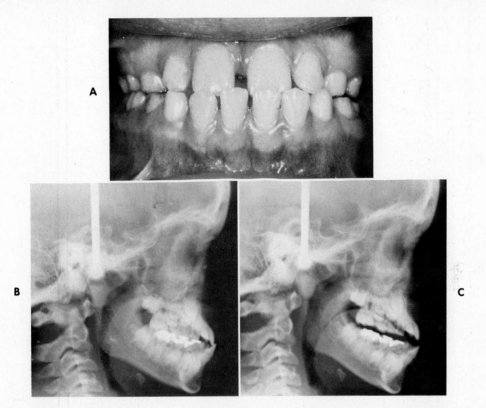

Fig. 21-8. A, Inlocked central incisors. The lateral incisors are in an end-to-end relationship in occlusion. **B** and **C,** Lateral headplate films, with the teeth in occlusion and at rest, show a marked deviation from the normal axial inclination of the upper central incisors to the lower central incisors, an excessively large mandible, and underdevelopment of the upper face. A case of this type requires major orthodontic treatment.

2. The apical portion of the inlocked tooth should be in relatively the same position as it would be if the tooth were in normal occlusion.
3. The patient should have normal occlusion in the molar and canine areas.

One of several treatment methods may be selected after an evaluation of such factors as patient cooperation, the degree of overbite that can be expected after the correction of the inlocking, the state of the development of the occlusion, and the sequence of eruption. After careful case analysis and a consideration of these points, the correct treatment method can be selected.

Tongue blade therapy. Children who are cooperative and have proper encouragement and guidance at home can correct an inlocked tooth with a narrow wooden tongue blade (Fig. 21-9). Teeth in their initial stage of eruption with a minimal degree of inlocking can often be repositioned within a 24-hour period with this technique.

The child is instructed to place the tongue blade behind the inlocked tooth and, using the chin as a fulcrum, to exert pressure on the tooth toward the labial side. This procedure should be practiced at least 10 minutes out of each hour as often as possible during the day. The incisal edge of the lower anterior teeth may be used as a fulcrum if these

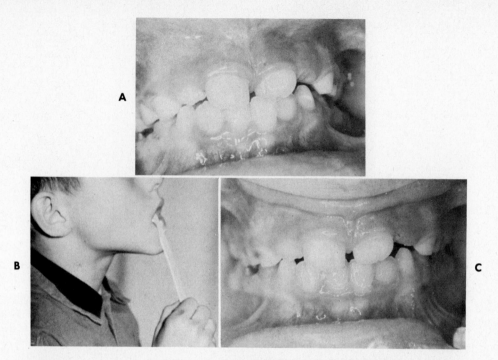

Fig. 21-9. A, Partially erupted central incisor with a minimum degree of inlocking. A tongue blade can often be used to correct the condition successfully. **B,** Tongue blade used to exert pressure on the inlocked tooth. **C,** Correction of the inlocked condition accomplished with the aid of the tongue blade.

teeth have erupted sufficiently to become stabilized in the arch. The results of this type of therapy are often disappointing because of poor cooperation between the child and the parents, despite the fact that they realize that a dental fee could be saved if they cooperated.

Lower cemented bite plane. An acrylic inclined plane cemented to the lower anterior teeth is an efficient way to reposition one or more inlocked anterior teeth. This may be the method of choice in treating inlocked central incisors when there is no anticipated need for a retainer. If there is a possibility that a maxillary retainer will be needed, one of the other appliances may be the best.

An acrylic bite plane can be constructed on a stone model produced from an accurate alginate impression (Fig. 21-10). Self-curing resin is applied to the model and covers the lower incisors and possibly the canines, depending on the degree of retention and stability that will be required. An inclined plane approximately ¼ inch in length is then added, extending lingually at a 45-degree angle to the long axis of the lower incisors.

Final adjustment of the plane is made before cementation in the mouth. Only the inlocked tooth is in contact with the plane, and there is no contact with the palatal tissue.

When the bite plane has been cemented, only the inlocked tooth contacts the inclined plane and the posterior teeth lack being in occlusion by 2 to 3 mm. This limits the time the appliance can be worn. Within 10 days considerable eruption of the posterior teeth will have occurred and a tendency toward an open bite in the anterior region will have been produced. Such a condition is normally undesirable.

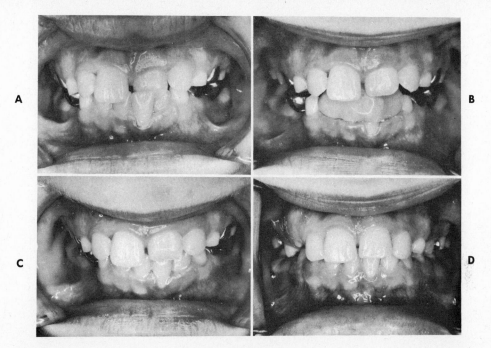

Fig. 21-10. A, Occlusion was essentially normal with the exception of the central incisor cross-bite. **B,** A lower cemented acrylic bite plane was used to reposition the inlocked tooth. **C,** The inlocked tooth has been moved into correct position, and there is sufficient overbite to maintain the new relationship. **D,** Four years after the treatment of the cross-bite. Note the improvement in the appearance of the tissue on the labial surface of the lower left central incisor.

An appointment should be made 24 hours after the delivery of the bite plane to adjust the height and contour of the plane so that other teeth will not come in contact with it.

The child should be instructed to attempt to follow a normal diet during the time the bite plane is worn. This will result in pressure being exerted on the inlocked tooth as an attempt is made to bring the posterior teeth into occlusion.

The activities of children who are wearing bite planes should be restricted to reduce the possibility of an accident that could result in a traumatic injury of the maxillary teeth. Teeth that occlude on an inclined plane are especially vulnerable to avulsion from a blow to the chin.

The inclined plane may be removed when the inlocked tooth has passed over the incisal edge of the lower incisors. At this point it must be decided

whether there is sufficient overbite to retain the tooth. The tooth has a strong tendency to return to its former position, particularly when the jaws assume rest position.

Removable palatal appliance. The use of the removable palatal appliance is indicated when one or two teeth, particularly lateral incisors, are inlocked or when there is an anticipated need for a retainer after treatment (Fig. 21-11). Occasionally the palatal appliance can be used at the same time for a space maintainer or for the correction of other minor irregularities in the arch. Since retention of this type of appliance may be a problem, adequate clasps must be added. It is rarely necessary to open the bite to correct the inlocked condition.

Soldered lingual arch (W appliance). The soldered lingual arch is used for the treatment of a cross-bite when other irregularities in the arch may

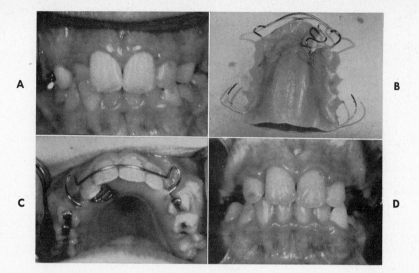

Fig. 21-11. **A,** Inlocked permanent lateral incisor. There was sufficient space to bring the tooth forward but a minimum amount of overbite; therefore the removable working retainer was selected. **B,** The appliance designed to correct the inlocked condition. **C,** Activation of the S-shaped wire at weekly intervals resulted in the labial movement of the inlocked tooth. **D,** The corrected occlusion at the time the appliance was discarded.

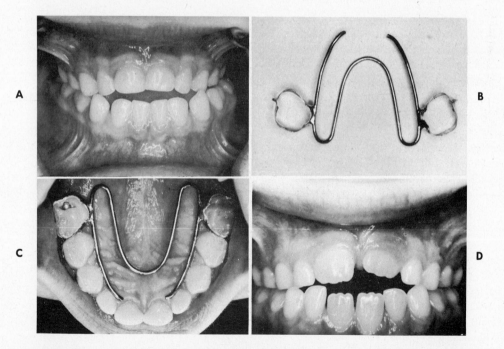

Fig. 21-12. **A,** Anterior open bite related to a thumb-sucking habit. There is a left buccal cross-bite involving the maxillary left primary canine and the first and second molars. **B,** The appliance. **C,** A mirror image of the cemented soldered lingual arch (W appliance). **D,** The cross-bite has been corrected and the lingual arch is worn as a retainer for 3 to 6 months. The buccal occlusion is good. There has been some improvement in the anterior open bite as a result of a less vigorous sucking habit.

simultaneously be corrected or when space maintenance in the primary molar area is indicated. If the cross-bite involves one or more of the anterior teeth and extends distally into the molar area, the lingual arch is the appliance of choice (Fig. 21-12). The lingual arch is frequently used to correct the cross-bite of a permanent lateral incisor. There is usually minimum overbite when the tooth has been repositioned; the lingual arch will serve effectively as a retainer until the tooth has erupted sufficiently to ensure its stability in the new relationship with the mandibular teeth.

Bands should be adapted to the first permanent molars. A compound impression of the maxillary arch and the completion of a stone cast are followed by the contouring of the W-shaped arch wire. Before the cementation of the arch wire, the free end should be activated approximately 1 mm and should be in contact with only the anterior inlocked tooth. If it is necessary to make additional adjustments, the appliance is removed from the mouth and adjustments are made at intervals of 2 to 3 weeks.

Johnson twinwire appliance. Graber (1972) reports that the twinwire attachment was introduced by Johnson in the 1930s. The philosophy behind its use was that two light wires placed in the same bracket would produce more physiologic tooth movement than one heavy wire. Although this appliance permits rapid reduction of rotations, it has limited use by orthodontists today because of problems of anchorage and control and also because the technique favors the nonextraction philosophy of reducing malocclusions. It is understandable that the limitations of the twinwire appliance would discourage its use by orthodontists who need maximum versatility in appliances for comprehensive care.

However, the twinwire appliance is very effective in reducing minor dental malalignments, such as anterior rotations or cross-bites in the absence of major malocclusions (Fig. 21-13). Sheppard describes the appliance and its application in Salzmann's textbook. The labial arch is composed of two 0.010-inch paralleled stainless steel wires drawn into end section tubes with a 0.035-inch outside diameter and a 0.022-inch inside diameter. The end sections then fit properly in 0.36-inch buccal tubes attached to the abutment molar bands. Establishing the correct angulation of the buccal tubes is critical to regulate the intrusive or extrusive forces applied to the anterior teeth by the twinwire appliance. Correction of minor anterior irregularities can usually be accomplished rapidly with this appliance.

Posterior cross-bite in the primary and mixed dentition

Cross-bite in the primary dentition, involving the second molar or even all of the teeth anterior to it, is not uncommon. In a study involving 515 children 3 to 9 years of age, Kutin and Hawes observed the prevalence of posterior cross-bite in the primary and mixed dentition to be 1:13, or 7.7%.

Schoenwetter believes that the use of instruments and manipulation during childbirth may cause both anterior and buccal cross-bites. In 27 cases of cross-bites observed by him, 25 of the children had been born with the use of obstetric instruments. Most of them had symmetric bilateral narrowing of the maxilla associated with a lateral deviation of the mandible as it moved from rest to occlusion.

Although it is often obscure, the cause can be different in the three general types of cross-bite—skeletal, dental, and functional. The irregularity in the occlusion of the young child may not be clear cut but may occur as a combination of all three of the classifications of buccal cross-bite. A careful clinical examination, supplemented by at least occlusion models and an observation of the mandible at rest, will be required for an accurate diagnosis.

Posterior cross-bite in the primary dentition is one of the types of malocclusion that usually is not corrected with continued development of the denture. In fact, occlusal interference and resultant shift into a cross-bite relationship can develop into a true skeletal defect if untreated. Likewise, if a cross-bite in the second primary molar area is untreated before the eruption of the first permanent molar, the first and even the second permanent

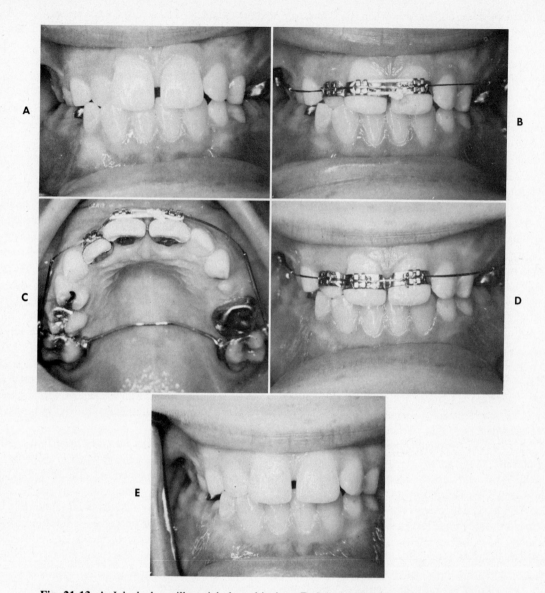

Fig. 21-13. A, Inlocked maxillary right lateral incisor. **B,** Johnson twinwire assembly in position, tightly ligated to lateral incisor but loosely ligated to central incisors. The elastic ligature was needed to close the midline diastema to provide adequate space for the crown of the lateral incisor to be tipped labially through proximal contact areas. **C,** Incisal view of appliance, showing how twinwire is activated by ligating tightly to inlocked lateral incisor and also showing soldered transpalatal arch wire attached to abutment molar bands for added stability. **D,** Correction occurred in 3 weeks. **E,** Corrected position of lateral incisor and recurrence of midline diastema 3 months postoperatively. The diastema will close naturally when the permanent canines erupt.

molars may erupt in this undesirable relationship. It became evident in the study by Kutin and Hawes that posterior cross-bite is not self-correcting and that untreated primary dentition cross-bite is followed by mixed dentition cross-bite. The treatment of primary dentition cross-bite favors development of normal occlusion in the mixed dentition.

A *skeletal* cross-bite results from a discrepancy in the structure of the bone of the mandible or maxilla. A basic discrepancy in the width of the arches may be noted. A narrow maxillary arch or a wide mandibular arch is often associated with a buccal cross-bite. The axial inclination of the molars in a favorable occlusion, as viewed from the distal aspect, will result in a flat occlusal plane relationship. In a skeletal cross-bite, however, there may be a lingual inclination of the maxillary teeth. Expansion of the maxillary arch in this situation would only result in a further lingual inclination of the roots and a buccal tipping of the crowns of the maxillary teeth.

A *dental* cross-bite results from a faulty eruption pattern; one or more of the posterior teeth erupt into a cross-bite relationship. There may be no irregularity in the basal bone. Once the teeth erupt, the occlusion locks them in position and drives them even further into a cross-bite relationship.

A low tongue position can result in unequal forces being applied to the maxillary posterior teeth and can allow them to assume a cross-bite relationship with the mandibular teeth. In patients who breathe through their mouths the tongue can assume a position in the floor of the mouth that results in a muscle imbalance and subsequent development of a buccal cross-bite.

There is some evidence as reported by Stewart, Hershey, and Warren that widening the hard palate of children with cross-bite to improve occlusion may improve breathing. The beneficial effects of this procedure on occlusion and appearance are obvious, but the secondary effects on the function of breathing are not until it is noted that nasal resistance to the passage of air is reduced and the flow of air increases.

It is also recognized that pressures such as those

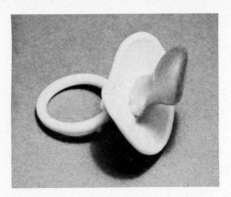

Fig. 21-14. NUK orthodontic exerciser.

exerted by aberrant sucking habits can easily be of sufficient intensity and duration to modify the conformation of the arch and be directly related to the development of a cross-bite. Rutrick believes that the use of the traditional slender-type pacifier can cause a cross-bite. He has observed that the NUK orthodontic exerciser* (Fig. 21-14), which is a broad-based pacifier, can be used as an activator appliance to cause an expansion of a narrow arch. When tongue pressure and sucking forces are applied to the pacifier by the young child, the maxillary arch over a period of months can be widened by several millimeters.

A *functional* cross-bite results from the mandible shifting into an abnormal but often more comfortable position. The presence of a functional cross-bite can be determined by observing the relationship of the arches in rest position. If there is no evidence of a discrepancy in the upper and lower midline when the mandible is at rest but there is a deviation of the mandible toward the side of the cross-bite when the teeth are brought into occlusion, the malocclusion should be considered functional. Also, when models of the upper and lower arches are examined separately, they should appear essentially symmetric. However, if there is a midline discrepancy that remains constant both at rest position and when the teeth are in occlusion, the condition is more serious and is indicative of a

*Reliance Products Corp., Woonsocket, R.I. 02895.

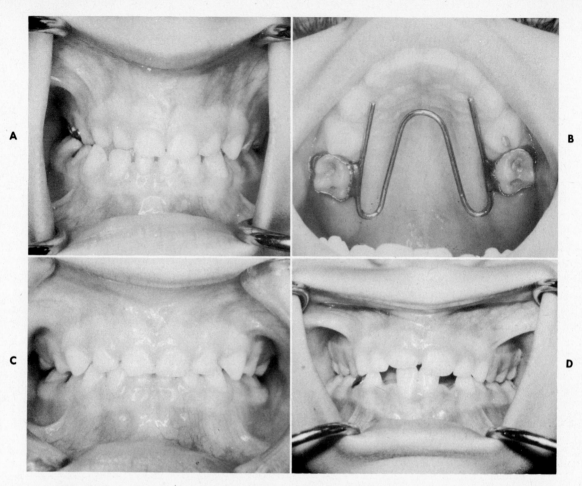

Fig. 21-15. A, Buccal cross-bite in the primary dentition involving the lateral incisor and all teeth posterior to it. In the rest position the dental midlines are normal, but in maximum interdigitation, as shown here, there is a 1.5-mm mandibular midline shift to the affected side. **B,** Soldered W lingual arch ready for cementation after activation and trial seating. **C,** The cross-bite was corrected in 6 weeks and the appliance was removed after 3 months of retention. Note that the dental midlines are properly aligned. **D,** After 3 years the first permanent molars are in proper relationship and the dental midlines remain properly aligned. There is no mandibular shift during closure.

skeletal deformity that will require major orthodontic treatment.

Some functional cross-bites can be corrected by reducing cuspal interference, particularly if the interference is responsible for the shift into the cross-bite relationship in the canine area. Occasionally equilibration involving a reduction of the inclined planes of the primary teeth, particularly the canine, may be all that is necessary to correct the condi-

tion. More frequently, however, the cross-bite can be corrected more quickly and easily with an appliance. If a critical examination of the occlusion reveals the presence of developing Class II or Class III malocclusion, the cross-bite may be corrected during the course of more comprehensive orthodontic treatment.

Soldered W lingual arch. The soldered W lingual arch is an efficient appliance for the correction of a cross-bite involving one or two teeth in the buccal segment or an entire buccal segment, or a bilateral cross-bite involving the posterior teeth (Figs. 21-12 and 21-15). Preformed stainless steel bands are adapted to the most distal teeth involved in the cross-bite, and a 0.036-inch or 0.040-inch steel wire is contoured to the arch. The wire should be free of the tissue by 1 to 2 mm, particularly in the molar loop areas, so that no impingement on the tissue will occur during activation of the wire.

If the cross-bite involves an entire quadrant, including the first permanent molar, the cross-bite of the first permanent molar is generally corrected first. The appliance should be activated by making a slight opening of the palatal loop with a corresponding adjustment in the molar loop area. The anterior extension of the wire should be free of the teeth anterior to the one to be moved buccally. Activation should be to the degree that the arch must be compressed by 1 to 2 mm to replace it on the banded teeth. By activating an appliance to move one or two teeth initially, the teeth on the opposite side of the arch are used for stabilization. Activation of the arch wire should be performed approximately every 3 weeks until the cross-bite has been corrected. In treating a bilateral cross-bite, symmetric activation and adjustment of the appliance should be made. The appliance is cemented in place during the active phase of treatment and retention and is removed only for activation and adjustment. It is allowed to remain as a retaining device for 3 to 6 months after completion of treatment.

Although the soldered W arch is a very stable appliance, its primary value is for situations that require only buccal or labial tipping of teeth. The "fixed-removable" W arch appliance and the quad-helix appliance provide greater versatility, and they are becoming more widely used for posterior cross-bite conditions.

Cross elastic technique. If a single posterior tooth is involved in a cross-bite—the first permanent molar or second primary molar, for example—the condition can often be corrected by use of cross elastics (Fig. 21-16). Preformed steel bands

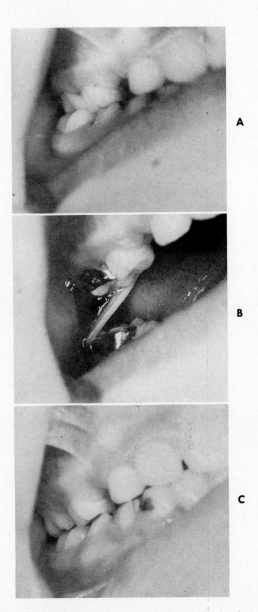

Fig. 21-16. A, Buccal cross-bite is limited to the first permanent molars on the right side. Correction of the cross-bite at this time will favorably influence the eruption of the second permanent molars. **B,** Molar bands with hooks and cross elastics are being used to correct the cross-bite. **C,** The molar cross-bite has been corrected in a 4-week period.

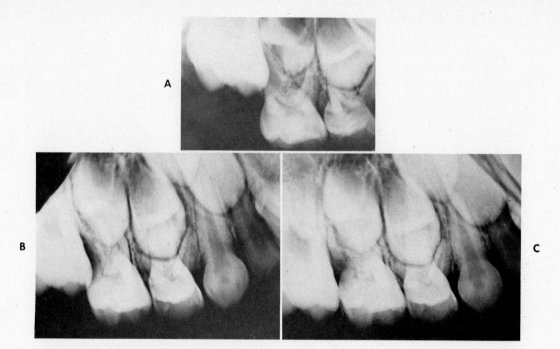

Fig. 21-17. A, Ectopic eruption of a maxillary first permanent molar. There is evidence of resorption of the distal buccal root of the second primary molar. **B** and **C,** Subsequent radiographs show continued resorption of the primary molar but normal positioning of the first permanent molar.

are adapted to the opposing molars that are in cross-bite. A wire loop is welded to the lingual surface of the upper band and the buccal surface of the lower band. The bands are cemented into place, and the child is shown how to place the elastics on the hooks. The elastics should be changed by the child or parent each day until the cross-bite has been corrected. Normally, a cross-bite involving two teeth can be corrected with cross elastics in 3 to 4 weeks. The corrected cuspal interdigitation will usually hold the teeth in their new relationship and there will be no need for a retentive appliance.

Problems related to the eruption of teeth

A variety of eruption problems arise during the transitional dentition period. Early diagnosis and treatment may prevent the development of a malocclusion of a more complicated nature. The dentist must be alert to the possibility of this and complicating sequelae.

Ectopic eruption of the first permanent molar. Critical examination of periapical and bitewing radiographs is important before the time of eruption of first permanent molars to detect evidence of ectopic eruption of these teeth. Frequently a first permanent molar, in instances of otherwise ideal occlusion, may be positioned too far mesially in its eruption with resultant resorption of the distal root of the second primary molar. The permanent molar may become hopelessly locked and may cause the premature exfoliation of the second primary molar or make it necessary to extract the affected tooth. The ectopically erupting first permanent molar may eventually right itself and erupt into its normal position after causing only minor destruction of the primary molar (Fig. 21-17).

Cheyne and Wessels reported that ectopic eruption occurs in approximately one in 50 children. Young observed that ectopic eruption of the first permanent molar occurred 52 times in 1619 boys and girls (3% of the time). The ectopic eruption occasionally occurred in more than one quadrant in the same mouth but was most often observed in the maxilla. In fact, only two ectopically erupting mandibular first permanent molars were noted. The anomaly was observed more frequently in boys (33 times) than in girls (19 times). Young further observed that 66% of the ectopically erupting molars finally erupted into their essentially normal position without the need for corrective treatment.

Carr observed a much more frequent occurrence of ectopic first permanent molar eruption in children with cleft lip and cleft palate. In children who underwent lip surgery at 6 to 8 weeks and palate closure at 24 months, 29% of the girls and 22.9% of the boys had ectopic eruption. Self-correction occurred in 22% of the children.

The cause of ectopic eruption of first permanent molars is not clearly understood, although one or more of the following conditions, as described by Pulver, may accompany this condition or may be related to it. Pulver's study of the problems revealed the following combination of factors:

1. Larger than normal mean sizes of all maxillary primary and permanent teeth
2. Larger affected first permanent molars and second primary molars
3. Smaller maxillae
4. Posterior position of the maxillae in relation to the cranial base
5. Abnormal angulation of eruption of the maxillary first permanent molar
6. Delayed calcification of some affected first permanent molars

Although ectopic eruption is most often discovered in the routine radiographic survey, the child may occasionally complain of neuralgic pain in the area of the impaction. The pain may be the result of resorption of the distal portion of the second primary molar, a break in the epithelial attachment that has allowed the ingress of oral fluids, and resultant pulpal inflammation. If this occurs, the primary tooth must be removed (Fig. 21-18).

When the impacted first permanent molar is unerupted or only partially erupted, the treatment of

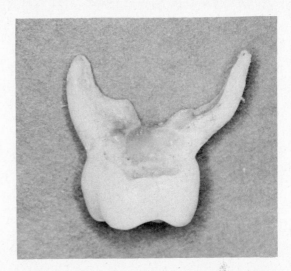

Fig. 21-18. Distal view of a maxillary second primary molar immediately after removal. An ectopic first permanent molar caused complete resorption of the distal-buccal root, portions of the palatal root, and the root trunk. Acute symptoms developed in the tooth.

choice is watchful waiting, since more than half of the teeth will eventually erupt into normal position.

After the occlusal surface of the first permanent molar becomes exposed in the oral cavity, the eruption path of the impacted tooth can often be favorably influenced by inserting a 0.026-inch brass ligature wire at the site of contact between the permanent and primary molars (Fig. 21-19). The brass ligature is completely looped through the contact area and is tightened with a No. 110 pliers. The free end of the wire is cut to 2 or 3 mm in length and is placed in the gingival crevice to reduce irritation to the buccal tissue. The wire should be tightened or a new one should be placed at 3-day intervals to cause distoclusal movement of the first permanent molar. If the contact opens during treatment to the degree that the wire can no longer be retained, a larger wire should be used or the patient should be seen in 3 or 4 days, at which time tight contact will have been reestablished and the ligature treatment can be resumed.

Humphrey has described another technique for correcting ectopically erupting first permanent mo-

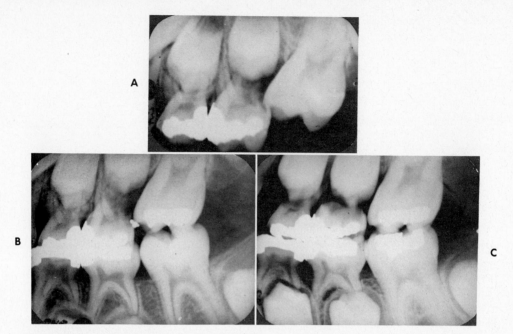

Fig. 21-19. A, Ectopic eruption of a maxillary first permanent molar. Note the resorption of the distal buccal root of the primary molar and the mesial drifting of the first permanent molar. **B,** A brass separating wire is being used to direct the first permanent molar into its normal position in the arch. **C,** The first permanent molar has been repositioned. The primary second molar has been retained to its normal exfoliation time.

lars. A preformed steel band is adapted to the second primary molar on the affected side. A soft wire (Elgiloy*) is adapted and soldered to the band; flux and silver bar solder are used, with the carbon point on the spot welder. An S-shaped loop is placed in the wire with a No. 139 pliers. The loop is opened slightly and is heat treated with a match flame (950° F) before cementation of the loop into place (Fig. 21-20). The distal extension of the wire is placed in an opening in the occlusal surface of the ectopically erupting molar. It may be necessary to remove the appliance for a second activation of the loop in a week or 10 days. An occlusal amalgam restoration is later placed in the first molar. Acid etch resin techniques have been developed since Humphrey's original report, and now the activating

*Rocky Mountain Metal Products, Denver, Colo. 80201.

wire may be stabilized in the central fossa of the first permanent molar and resin on etched enamel without opening the fossa.

Occasionally the affected second primary molar will be mobile as a result of its root resorption and the forces exerted by the ectopically erupting first permanent molar. The basic idea of the Humphrey technique may be incorporated into a bilateral lingual arch if additional appliance stability is desired. When adequate access to the mesial surface of the ectopic molar exists, the spring may also be designed to direct its distal force against the mesial surface of the tooth (Fig. 21-21).

Davis recommends the use of a helical spring for the correction of ectopically erupting permanent molars. A helical spring designed primarily for the separation of teeth before orthodontic banding can be adapted to correct most ectopic eruption patterns

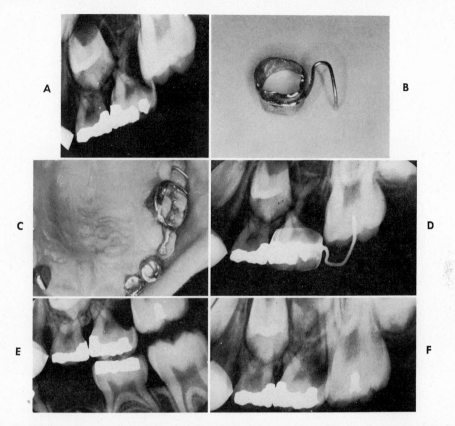

Fig. 21-20. A, Ectopic eruption of the maxillary first permanent molar. The first permanent molar is positioned too far mesially to unlock it with a brass separating wire. **B** and **C,** A band and S-shaped wire have been fabricated to reposition the first permanent molar. **D** and **E,** Radiographs demonstrating the distal repositioning of the first permanent molar. **F,** The first permanent molar has erupted into a favorable position.

of the maxillary and mandibular first permanent molars, provided there is sufficient dental development for its insertion. The advantages of this technique include prefabrication of the appliance, ease of insertion of the device, and patient comfort. The spring design gives an optimum force and rate for orthodontic movement and requires fewer patient visits and decreased chair time. A new spring rarely has to be inserted during treatment, only activated and stress relieved. The only disadvantage of the appliance is the time required to learn the technique and theory of design and to master the mechanics of its insertion.

The spring is constructed from 0.022-inch round stainless steel wire (orthodontic grade) and bent around a nontapered 0.040-inch cylinder beak of the pliers. The bending and activation scheme is illustrated in Fig. 21-22. Care should be taken not to scar the wire during bending. The length of the wire is determined by the buccolingual width of the tooth.

Insertion of the spring is most easily achieved by grasping the active arm of the spring adjacent to the helix with a modified bird beak pliers No. 800-418. The head of the spring is placed on the marginal ridge or near the middle of the contact area

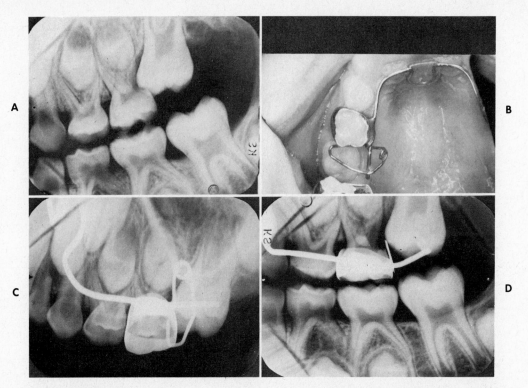

Fig. 21-21. A, Another example of ectopic eruption of the maxillary first permanent molar. **B,** Mirror view of lingual arch appliance with spring wire designed to properly redirect eruption of inlocked molar. The spring is shown in its passive position before engaging the working end against the mesial-buccal surface of tooth. **C,** Radiograph showing spring after it has been engaged in its active position. **D,** One month later the tooth was repositioned sufficiently to allow modification of the appliance. The spring was removed, and a distal extension guide plane was made by welding a piece of band material to the distal surface of the band.

and held firmly with a cervical force while the active arm is directed below the contact point of the ectopically positioned tooth. The dentist may insert the spring from either the buccal or the lingual side, whichever provides the greatest access. The buccal approach to insertion of the wire is usually more desirable. The patient is instructed to keep the helix of the spring at the gingival margin and is at liberty to adjust the helix occlusally should it impinge on the soft tissue.

Activation of the spring after it has been fitted consists of bending the free arm to touch or slightly

cross the occlusal arm, as illustrated in Fig. 21-22. Before final insertion, the bending stress should be relieved by heating the spring in an 800° F (377° C) oven for 4 minutes. This procedure allows a molecular realignment and should be followed at each activation period.

The spring should be left in place until the tooth has freed its contact with the adjacent tooth and is erupting in a normal manner. The patient should be seen every 5 to 6 weeks for an evaluation of the eruption progress and reactivation of the spring. Occasionally the teeth will separate sufficiently for

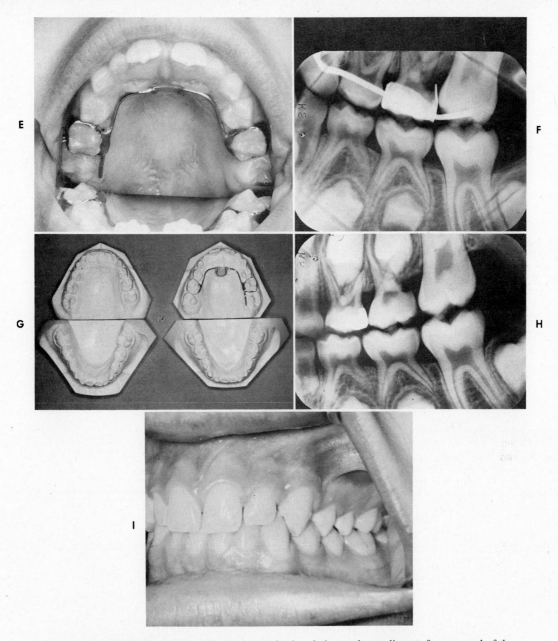

Fig. 21-21, cont'd. E, Position of erupting molar in relation to the appliance after removal of the spring. **F,** Radiograph demonstrating favorable eruption 4 months later. **G,** Preoperative and post-operative models showing corresponding positions of tooth before and after correction. **H,** Two years after treatment the first permanent molar is in a good position and the second primary molar has been retained. **I,** Good first permanent molar relationship in the permanent dentition 5½ years postoperatively.

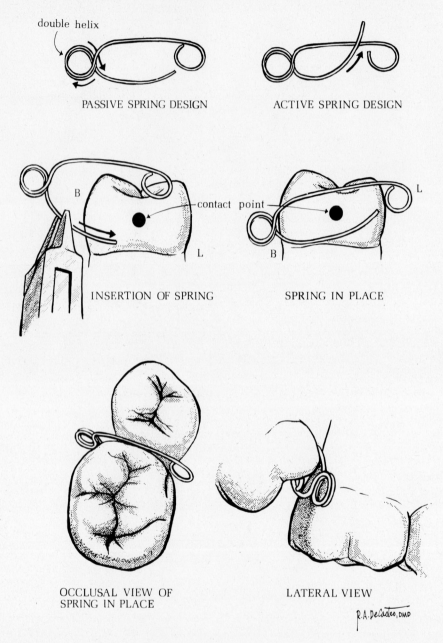

double helix

PASSIVE SPRING DESIGN

ACTIVE SPRING DESIGN

B

contact point

L

B

L

INSERTION OF SPRING

SPRING IN PLACE

OCCLUSAL VIEW OF
SPRING IN PLACE

LATERAL VIEW

R.A.DeCastro, DMD

Fig. 21-22. Helical spring of 0.022-inch stainless steel wire designed for the correction of ectopically erupting permanent molars.

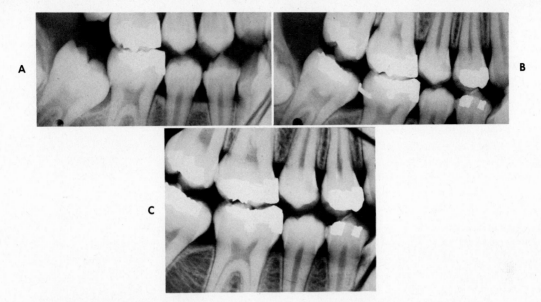

Fig. 21-23. A, Impacted second molar. The second molar should not be extracted; instead, an attempt should be made to upright the tooth. **B** and **C,** A brass separating wire has been used to successfully reposition the second permanent molar. Treatment was extended over a 12-month period.

the spring to become dislodged. The parent should be instructed to call for an appointment to determine if the ectopic condition has been corrected or if further treatment is recommended.

Removal of the spring is achieved by reversing the path of insertion or by the use of two Jacquette scalers. One is placed in the helix, and the other lifts the head of the spring from the contact point and then simultaneously lifts and pulls to remove.

The second primary molar may eventually have to be sacrificed because of extensive resorption and the development of pulpitis. However, it is to the child's advantage if the tooth can be retained until the first permanent molar erupts, since the first permanent molar will be in its correct relationship for space maintenance. An *immediate* band and loop maintainer is usually the appliance of choice if the second primary molar is extracted.

Impacted second permanent molars. Although no surveys have been made to indicate the frequency of impacted second permanent molars,

they apparently occur with considerably less frequency than impacted first permanent molars. When the condition occurs, it is generally in the mandibular arch. Insufficient arch length or excessive tooth mass is probably responsible.

Treatment involving the use of a brass ligature wire similar to that recommended for the correction of an ectopically erupting first permanent molar should be considered (Fig. 21-23). However, treatment will invariably follow a prolonged course. The removal of an impacted second permanent molar to allow the third molar to move forward and take its place is impractical, since the third molar will usually move into a similarly impacted position.

A removable appliance, or the Humphrey appliance, in combination with a ligature wire can be successfully used to upright an impacted mandibular second permanent molar. The appliance with an S-shaped wire extending distally into one of the occlusal pits of the molar is constructed when the crown of a tooth becomes exposed in the oral cavity. Adjustment of the wire at 3-week intervals will guide the molar distally during its eruption.

Ectopic eruption of the permanent lateral incisor. The primary canine is frequently lost prematurely at the time of the eruption of the permanent lateral incisor. The condition generally referred to as ''ectopic eruption'' is a problem that often has not been given adequate attention. In most children the lateral incisor erupts essentially in a normal manner, but because of excessive tooth mass or inadequate arch length, resorption begins on the mesial aspect of the root of the primary canine (Fig. 21-24). The process continues until the canine is prematurely lost (Fig. 21-25). Parents often fail to recognize the untimely loss, thinking it is just another front tooth that should be lost at approximately 7 years of age. In reviewing the pedodontic radiographic survey, the dentist should be alerted to the condition and should be prepared to manage the problem if an early loss of primary canines occurs. In a survey of 400 children in the transitional dentition period, Croxton found that 32 of them had 48 ectopically erupting permanent lateral incisors. Seventeen ectopically erupting teeth were noted in the maxilla and 31 in the mandible. In contrast to the ectopic eruption of the first permanent molar, this condition is probably seen only in children with some degree of arch length inadequacy.

If the child is seen at the time of the unilateral loss of the primary canine and if no shift in the midline has occurred, a space maintainer is indicated. A band and loop maintainer or a lingual arch with a spur can be used to prevent distal drifting of the lateral incisor (see Fig. 20-26). If the unilateral loss is accompanied by a severe crowding of the incisors and if a shift in the midline toward the area of the loss is evident, the corresponding canine on the opposite side of the arch should be extracted and a passive lingual arch should be used (see Fig. 20-40). Maintaining symmetry and preventing a shift in the midline and a ''falling-in'' of the anterior segment are important. Before deciding on a definite course of treatment, a careful analysis of the occlusion should be made and an orthodontist

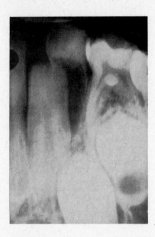

Fig. 21-24. Premature primary canine root resorption resulting from arch length inadequacy and ectopic eruption of the permanent lateral incisor.

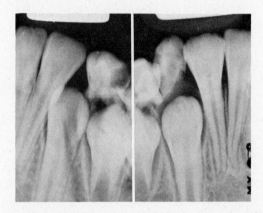

Fig. 21-25. Primary canine has been lost prematurely on the left side of the arch. The permanent incisor has driften distally into contact with the first primary molar. Extraction of the corresponding primary canine would have aided in maintaining symmetry in the arch.

should be consulted in regard to the need for future treatment.

If the problem of crowding in the lower anterior segment is identified before the premature loss of canines, the condition may be alleviated by a time sequence of ''slicing'' procedures on the remaining primary teeth as advocated by both Kramer and

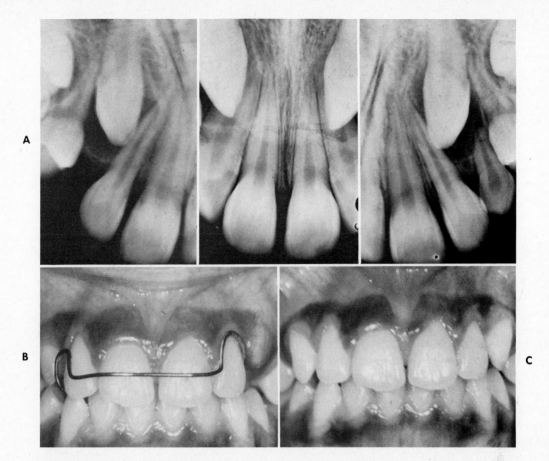

Fig. 21-26. A, Delayed eruption of maxillary permanent canines. The remaining primary canine was recommended for extraction. **B,** A Hawley type of retainer was constructed to maintain the relationship of other teeth in the arch during the eruption period of the canines. **C,** Satisfactory eruption of the permanent canines.

Wyatt. Additional space is created for favorable positioning of the lateral incisors by removing or slicing a portion of the primary canines on the mesial surface. The slicing procedure is repeated as indicated on additional primary teeth as the permanent teeth continue their eruption process in sequence. Slices are made at the appropriate time on the second primary molars to accommodate the eruption of the first premolars and canines. If the initial crowding in the lower arch is approximately equal to the leeway space of the arch, adequate space for all permanent teeth will be preserved

without appliances or extraction of permanent teeth. Wyatt recommends the slicing procedure even when the amount of tooth structure removed may require a pulpotomy on the primary tooth.

Impaction and delayed eruption of permanent canines. Mandibular third molars are the most frequently impacted teeth. Next in frequency are the maxillary permanent canines. Cohen believes that the impaction of the maxillary canine is related to the facts that this tooth has the longest period of development, follows the most dubious course in its eruption, and occupies several developmental positions in succession. Also, it can be easily deflected from its normal course of eruption. The prolonged retention of the primary canine is often thought to be responsible for causing the impacted condition.

In the radiographic and oral examination the dentist should look for evidence of asymmetric eruption of the maxillary canines. There is a tremendous advantage to early diagnosis of an abnormal sequence of eruption. A delay in the eruption of the canine can allow adjacent teeth to encroach on the space needed for the canine. This encroachment will contribute to the impacted condition.

If the canine is thought to be impacted, it should be localized in respect to adjacent teeth. If the canine is merely delayed in eruption or is out of normal sequence of eruption, a passive Hawley retainer is indicated to maintain the relationship of the adjacent teeth until the canine erupts (Fig. 21-26).

If the maxillary permanent canine is definitely impacted, surgical intervention is indicated. However, localization of the tooth by special radiographic technique is essential. The procedure described in Chapter 6 will be helpful in localizing the impacted tooth.

The available arch space for the canine should be compared with the size of the crown. The measurement of the opposite canine can be used or the measurement of the impacted canine can be made directly from the radiograph. If space for the tooth is adequate and if occlusion is essentially normal, the space should be maintained. Surgical exposure of the impacted canine and the maintenance of a pathway are normally the treatment of choice. If the deciduous canine is still present, it should be extracted. Sufficient soft tissue and bone should then be removed from the crown of the impaction to maintain an opening that will stimulate the eruption of the impacted tooth. The opening may initially be packed with surgical cement. A resin crown form filled with zinc oxide–eugenol on the canine crown has also been used successfully to stimulate eruption. A deep palatal impaction may move into an inlocked position or may require orth-

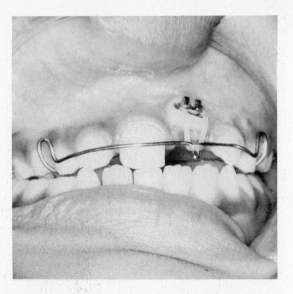

Fig. 21-27. Modified Hawley appliance used for anchorage as the previously impacted and surgically exposed central incisor is encouraged to erupt with light elastic. (Courtesy Dr. Paul Yim.)

odontic movement to bring it into a desirable relationship.

Guided eruption of anterior teeth. In the practice of dentistry for children, appliances to guide or to aid in the eruption of anterior teeth are frequently constructed. A traumatic injury to the primary anterior teeth can often cause delayed eruption of an anterior permanent tooth. The condition is often accompanied by drifting of adjacent teeth that must be repositioned and maintained in their new relationship until the eruption of delayed teeth can occur.

Labioversion and sometimes impaction of permanent maxillary incisors caused by prolonged retention or trauma of primary incisors, the presence of a supernumerary tooth, or an oral habit can be corrected and the permanent tooth can be guided into position with a removable appliance, a Hawley arch wire, or an appliance with anterior hooks and light rubber elastics (Figs. 21-27 and 21-28). The rubber elastics should exert approximately 10 g of pressure on the malpositioned tooth and should be

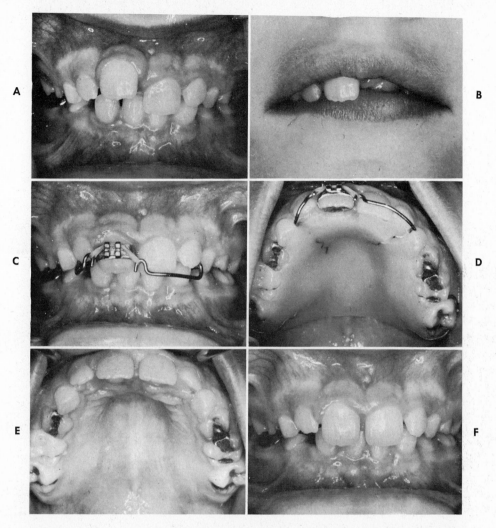

Fig. 21-28. A and **B,** Permanent central incisor is positioned labially as the result of a retained primary incisor. A lip habit has also influenced the abnormal position of the tooth. **C** and **D,** A palatal retainer with a labial wire, hooks, and light rubber elastics is used to reposition the incisor. **E** and **F,** The central incisor is in good relationship with the adjacent and opposing teeth.

replaced daily by the patient during the course of treatment. A band and bracket on the tooth will hold the elastics in their proper relationship.

The congenital absence of one or both of the maxillary permanent lateral incisors is a problem that requires careful analysis of the available arch length and the occlusion. It must be decided

whether there is sufficient arch length to maintain space for the lateral incisor replacement or whether the permanent canine should be allowed to drift mesially into the lateral incisor position and eventually be reshaped to resemble this tooth.

If the decision is made to maintain the space for an eventual fixed bridge replacement, the perma-

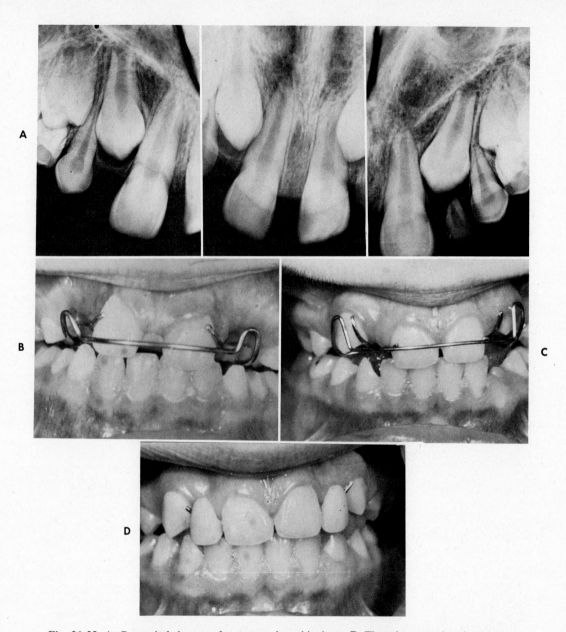

Fig. 21-29. A, Congenital absence of permanent lateral incisors. **B,** The primary canines have been extracted, and a working appliance has been constructed to close the diastema between the central incisors. **C,** Auxiliary wires have been added to the appliance to guide the permanent canines into a more favorable position. **D,** Space has been regained for an eventual fixed bridge in place of the lateral incisors. The removable retainer will be worn until the teeth are ready to receive fixed bridgework.

nent canine must be encouraged to erupt as close to its normal position as possible. The early removal of the primary canine will favorably influence the eruption of the permanent canine; however, it still may follow a mesial course. A palatal appliance with a wire to engage the canine as soon as it erupts and to redirect it will result in a desirable solution to the problem (Fig. 21-29).

Oral habits—their cause and correction

Bruxism. Bruxism, which is usually considered an oral habit of children, is a nonfunctional grinding or gnashing of the teeth. Reding, Rubright, and Zimmerman have reported that 15% of the children and young adults in their study group practiced bruxism to some degree. The habit is practiced most often at night and, if continued over a prolonged period of time, can result in abrasion of both the primary and the permanent teeth. When the practice is continued into adulthood, periodontal disease and even temporomandibular joint disturbances can result (Fig. 21-30).

Nervous children may develop bruxism, which may be continued consciously or unconsciously over an indefinite period of time. The dentist should approach the problem by seeking the cause. Ramfjord believes that occlusal interference may act as a trigger for bruxism, particularly if combined with nervous tension. Therefore occlusal adjustment should be the first approach to the prob-

lem if interferences are present. Sheppard recommends the construction of a palatal bite plate, which allows the continued eruption of the posterior teeth. This eruption is desirable if the teeth have been abraded by the habit. A vinyl plastic bite guard that covers the occlusal surfaces of all teeth, plus 2 mm of the buccal and lingual surfaces, can be worn at night to prevent continuing abrasion of the teeth. The occlusal surface of the bite guard should be flat to avoid occlusal interference. A guard of the type described in Chapter 26 may also be helpful in overcoming the habit.

In patients with no apparent severe psychogenic disturbance but with some degree of nervousness and restlessness, tranquilizing drugs have been helpful in overcoming bruxism. A dose of 25 mg of hydroxyzine (Atarax) 1 hour before bedtime has resulted in eventual discontinuation of the habit. Dramatic changes cannot be expected in only a few nights of medication with tranquilizing drugs, but over a period of several months remarkable progress has been observed.

Thumb-sucking. Various and conflicting theories have been presented to explain the cause of thumb-sucking in children, and there are equally conflicting recommendations in the literature for the correction of the habit. Thumb-sucking in an infant is a problem of concern to the pediatrician and the parents, since a feeding problem may occasionally be responsible for the initiation of the

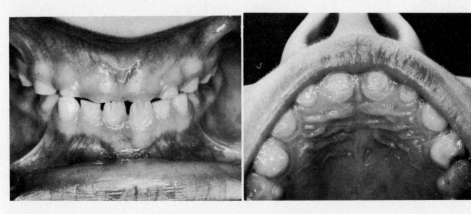

Fig. 21-30. Bruxism has resulted in severe abrasion of the maxillary primary anterior teeth.

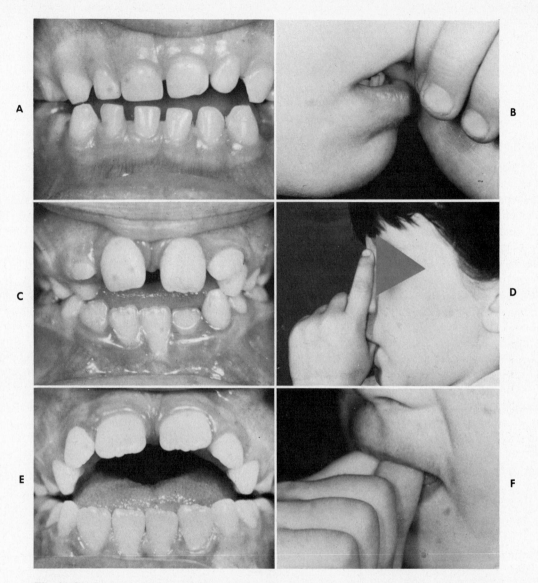

Fig. 21-31. Occlusion of three children with thumb-sucking and finger-sucking habits. **A,** An open bite in the primary dentition caused by the child placing the thumb between the anterior teeth. **B,** A photograph showing how the thumb was held between the teeth. The child apparently did not suck the thumb. **C,** An open bite and flared maxillary incisors caused by a thumb-sucking habit. **D,** During sucking the index finger was placed alongside the nose. Sucking was practiced for long periods of time. **E,** An open bite extending into the second primary molar, a result of the child sucking the thumb and index finger. **F,** An illustration of how the fingers were placed in the mouth.

habit. Thumb-sucking in infants has been related to rapid feeding or the presence of tension during the feeding period.

Although it has been frequently stated that thumb-sucking during the first 2 years is normal, many children never have this habit. Although it is true that many normal children suck their thumbs for short periods of time during infancy or early childhood, dentists are ill advised to tell parents not to worry, that the child will eventually quit, and that there will be no ill effects (Fig. 21-31). It is true that many children discontinue the habit during the preschool years, but some continue the habit into the school years and occasionally even into adulthood, as reported by Brody. Even if there is no ill effect on the occlusion, thumb-sucking is not a socially acceptable habit; therefore it should be tactfully discouraged as soon as there is evidence of the habit developing, regardless of the age of the child.

Salzmann (1974) believes that the effect of the sucking habit on the maxillary and mandibular bones and on the dental arches, including the occlusion of the teeth, depends on a number of factors, such as the frequency with which the habit is practiced, the duration of the time the habit lasts, the osteogenic development, the genetic endowment of the child, and the state of health of the child.

Traisman and Traisman observed 2650 infants and children from birth through 16 years of age. Of this number, 45.6% sucked their thumbs at some time during the observation period. However, 75% began during the first 3 months of life and approximately 25% began during the remainder of the first year. The average age at which the sucking stopped was 3.8 years. However, some stopped as late as 12 to 15 years of age.

Popovich and Thompson observed 1258 children at the Burlington Growth Centre; the group represented approximately 90% of the child population of Burlington, Ontario. Many of the children were seen annually from the ages of 3 to 12 years, and their oral habit and occlusion status were recorded at ages 3, 6, 9, and 12 years. There was a significant association between the prevalence of Class II malocclusion and persisting digit-sucking in the different age groups. Class II malocclusion increased from 21.5% at ages 3 and 4 to 41.9% at age 12. As the duration of the habit increased, the probability of a child developing a Class II malocclusion increased. If the habit was stopped early (before 6 years), the effects on occlusion were often transitory. In the serial sample none of the children who stopped a habit after the age of 6 years had a normal occlusion at age 12. Another interesting observation was that children who had used a pacifier had a significantly lower rate of thumb- and finger-sucking.

Cumley believes that prolonged thumb-sucking after the age of 4 years is usually a symptom that the child suffers from emotional starvation and uses the thumb for comfort and compensation. In some instances the child may use the habit as a means of revenge against the parent. Cumley believes that the best corrective measures are indirect adjustments, such as providing adequate rest and play outlets for the child. Most children will stop sucking the thumb by the age of 5 years. If the habit persists, parents should remember that children are capable of self-discipline and can be helped only by helping themselves.

Oral habits are not peculiar to any group of children, although Calisti, Cohen, and Falls reported that there were significantly more oral habits in the higher socioeconomic group than in the middle and low groups.

Although the dentist is frequently the first one and sometimes the only one consulted regarding the habit, thumb-sucking is often not a dental problem. It is the dentist's obligation, however, to look for evidence of the habit, attempt to determine the cause, describe the possible consequences should the habit be continued, and, in selected cases, attempt to aid the child in overcoming the habit.

If the infant has a thumb-sucking habit, correction may be possible when the child passes from the sucking to the chewing phase. A redirection from the sucking activity toward chewing activities may be achieved. It is often helpful to remove the

Patient _____ Age _____ Sex _____

Type of habit _____

Feeding during infancy

    (a) Breast _____ How long? _____

        When weaned to bottle? _____

    (b) Bottle _____ When weaned to cup? _____

Sleeping habits:

    (a) Daytime naps, regularity, duration, etc. _____

    (b) At night, number of hours, frequency of interruption, soundness, etc. _____

_____

Unusual fears _____

Toilet habits and training _____

Eating habits _____

_____

Home conditions:

    (a) Siblings—number and age _____

    (b) Mother's temperament _____

    (c) Father's temperament _____

    (d) Other persons in household _____

    (e) Occupation of mother _____

    (f) Occupation of father _____

School adjustments:

    (a) Social difficulties _____

    (b) Play habits _____

    (c) Scholastic difficulties _____

Fig. 21-32

General health of child:

   (a) Major childhood diseases _____

   (b) Number of colds and minor ailments annually _____

   (c) When does child get sick—winter, summer, throughout year? _____

   _____

Response under stress _____

At what age did habit start? _____

Has it been continuous since then? _____

   (a) Day, night, or both? _____

   (b) During television? _____

   (c) Frequency, persistence, intensity? _____

What methods have been used to stop habits? _____

Has child been nagged about habit by family or outsiders? _____

Similar habits or history of habits of others in family _____

_____

Attitude toward therapy?

   (a) Does child want to discontinue the habit? _____

   (b) Do the parents want an appliance constructed? _____

   (c) Does child know purpose of visit? _____

Additional comments:

                              Date completed _____

Fig. 21-32, cont'd

thumb from the mouth and replace it with a substitute, such as something chewable. In older children the use of visual aids may be helpful to show them how the thumb-sucking habit may spoil their mouths if it is continued.

One of the many recommended corrective approaches to thumb-sucking should not be considered until a careful history has been completed in an attempt to learn the cause. By talking to the child and the parents the dentist can usually determine whether the habit is related to an early feeding problem that is now carried on as an empty habit, is acquired in imitation of someone else, or is the result of a complex emotional problem. The modification of a questionnaire (Fig. 21-32) recommended by Graber (1972) has been valuable in developing a pattern of events leading to the development of the habit.

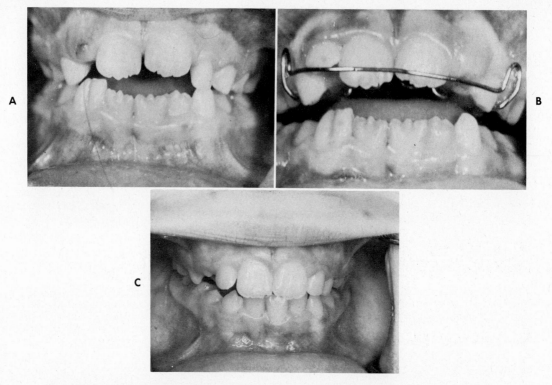

Fig. 21-33. A, Anterior open bite caused by a severe thumb-sucking habit. **B,** A passive type of reminder appliance was constructed after other problems in the patient's life were recognized and treated. **C,** The occlusion 18 months after the child had overcome the habit.

Thumb-sucking is frequently only one manifestation of the child's insecurity or maladjustment. The child may have a fear of the dark, fear of separation from the parents, or fear of animals or insects. The history will often reveal difficulty in toilet training; some children continue to wet the bed several years after starting school. Such things as an unwillingness to enter group activities at school may be brought out in the history. Conflicts in the home may also be related to the habit and to other problems of normal adjustment. The problem of thumb-sucking therefore may not be a single, isolated symptom but instead may be one of several symptoms related to conflicts and emotional instability resulting from a series of past events.

Corrective appliances for oral habits are indi-

cated only when it can be determined that the child wants to discontinue the habit and needs only a reminder to accomplish the task. If an appliance is used, it should be one that will not be painful or interfere with occlusion; instead, it should merely act as a reminder. A removable partial retainer with a series of smooth loops placed lingual to the incisors has often proved successful in helping the child overcome the habit (Fig. 21-33). The indiscriminate use of habit-breaking appliances, when the habit is the result of a deep-seated emotional problem, can result in a series of undesirable reactions. Korner and Reider reported that the insertion of a "hay rake" type of appliance in three children not only failed to stop the sucking habit but focused the child's attention on thumb-sucking. In addition, drastic new symptoms such as night terrors, day wetting, speech disorders, refusal to eat solids, belligerency, and irritability were observed.

An entirely different approach has been practiced by some dentists when it is evident that a child wants to discontinue the habit (Fig. 21-34). This approach involves cooperation by the parents and their consent to disregard the habit and make no mention of it to the child. In private conversation with the child, the dentist discusses the problem and its effect. The child is asked to keep a daily record on a card of each episode of thumb-sucking and to call the dentist each week and report on progress in stopping the habit. Over a period of a week a decrease in number of times that the habit is practiced is evidence that progress is being made and is indicative that the child will eventually discontinue the habit.

The parents' role in the correction of an oral habit is most important. Parents are often overanxious about the habit and its possible effects. This anxiety may result in nagging or punishment that often creates a greater tension and intensification of the habit. Changes in the home environment and routine are often necessary before the child can overcome the habit.

The problem of correction of thumb-sucking is therefore a complex one. The role of the dentist is often secondary in the correction of thumb-sucking, although he or she may be the first one approached. It is the dentist's duty to advise the parents of the possible dental effects and of the possible methods of correcting the habit. The dentist is also obligated to refer the family to proper medical or psychologic authorities for the treatment of more advanced cases.

Self-mutilation. Although there has been infrequent reference to self-mutilation in the dental literature, occasionally children purposely traumatize their oral structures. Plessett reported observing a 9-year-old girl of apparently normal intelligence who worked her maxillary primary canine and mandibular permanent incisors loose from their supporting tissues and removed them.

Self-mutilation probably occurs more frequently

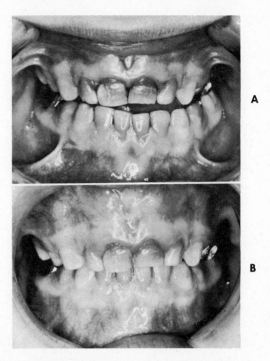

Fig. 21-34. A, Open bite is evident in the primary dentition resulting from a thumb-sucking habit. **B,** The child was encouraged by the dentist to discontinue the habit. There was self-correction of the open bite when the habit was discontinued.

than is realized because relatively few children will admit the act unless they are observed practicing it. Therefore the self-inflicted lesions may be incorrectly diagnosed. Dentists should be aware of the incidence of this condition and should approach the problem in the same manner as they do thumb-sucking. An attempt should be made to determine the cause. If it is found to be the result of local dental factors, it can be corrected. However, in the majority of children an emotional problem will be involved and the family must be directed to competent consulting services (Fig. 21-35).

Children as young as 4 years of age have been observed who have traumatized the free and attached gingival tissues with a fingernail, occasionally to the extent that the supporting alveolar bone has been destroyed (Fig. 21-36). A 14-year-old girl

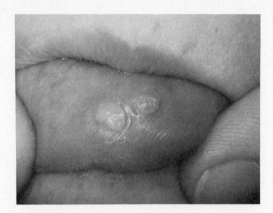

Fig. 21-35. A nervous habit of lip biting and sucking resulted in these chronic raised lesions on the mucous membrane of the lower lip. This is an example of mild self-mutilation that is reversible if the habit is controlled.

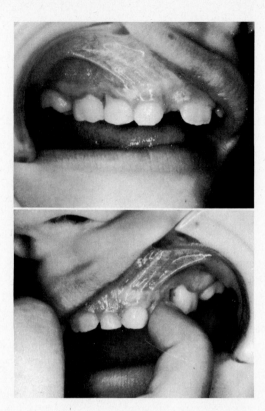

Fig. 21-36. The 6-year-old child has traumatized the gingiva between the maxillary primary molars with the index fingernail.

produced bilateral stripping of the buccal tissue in the maxillary premolar areas (Fig. 21-37) with her fingernail and a bobby pin. In addition, she bit the inner surface of her cheek and produced large necrotic areas. The parents were unaware of the habit and the cause of the ulcerated areas in her mouth, since the daughter did not reveal that they were self-inflicted. The history revealed an unhappy child, poorly adjusted to the home and school environment. Referral to a child guidance clinic was accepted by the child and the parents and resulted in a solution to the problem. The self-mutilation was apparently an escape from reality.

Tension and conflicts in the home can cause self-mutilation in young patients. Fisher reported that unhappiness and conflict in the home can be hidden more easily from a 15-year-old child than from a 15-week-old child.

Traumatic gingival recession in infants, the result of a dummy (pacifier) sucking habit, has been observed by Stewart and Kernohan. In the unconventional sucking habit a segment of the plastic shield is embraced by the infant's lower lip so that the inner surface of the shield bears against the labial aspect of the incisors and the gingival tissues (Fig. 21-38). If the shield is held in this position, the edge of the shield during sucking moves with an abrasive action, leading to gingival injury, recession, and loss of alveolar bone.

Role of myofunctional therapy in correction of tongue and swallowing habits. Abnormal tongue position and a deviation from the so-called normal movement of the tongue during swallowing have long been associated with anterior open bite and also with a protrusion of the maxillary incisors. Proffit has investigated the matter thoroughly and has published widely on the subject. According to him, three major problems are usually associated with the anterior tongue position, which is variously called tongue thrust, deviate swallow, visceral swallow, and infantile swallow. These problems are open bite, protusion of the incisors, particularly the maxillary incisors, and lisping.

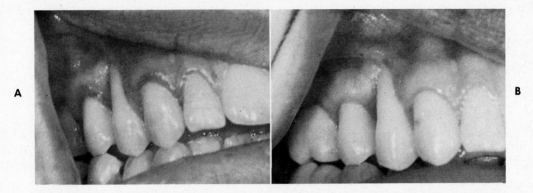

Fig. 21-37. A, Stripping of the free and attached tissue from the buccal side of the premolar and exposure of the root surface were accomplished with a fingernail and a hair pin. The patient had a psychologic problem and was referred to a child guidance clinic. **B,** After the treatment of the emotional problem the habit was discontinued. Although the soft tissue inflammation was reduced, there was no regeneration of tissue over the root surface.

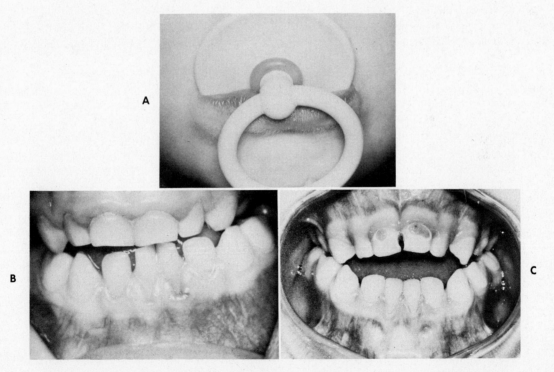

Fig. 21-38. A, An unconventional manner of pacifier sucking may lead to gingival trauma and recession. **B** and **C,** Two children with gingival recession in lower incisor region. Note anterior open bite in **C.** (From Stewart, D.J., and Kernohan, D.C.: Traumatic gingival recession in infants: the result of a dummy sucking habit, Br. Dent. J. **135:**157-158, 1973.)

According to data from the National Center for Health Statistics, the prevalence of anterior open bite in children between the ages of 6 and 11 is approximately 6%.

Proffit believes that since there is a relatively high prevalence of anterior tongue positioning in children, this condition is often improperly labeled as tongue thrust or deviate swallowing. He also believes that there are two major reasons: that relating to the physiology of the child (maturation) and that relating to anatomy (growth).

It has long been recognized that normal infants position the tongue anteriorly in the mouth, both at rest and during swallowing. The first physiologic priority at birth is that an airway be established so that respiration can begin. Accomplishment of this priority requires holding the tongue forward and down. The set of postural relationships of the oral and pharyngeal structures established in the first few minutes of life in response to respiratory requirements is maintained thereafter.

In an infant the normal swallow is characterized by strong lip activity to seize the nipple, placement of the tongue tip against the lower lip beneath the nipple, and relaxation of the elevator muscles of the mandible so that the mouth is wide open. As oral function matures, there is a gradual activation of the elevator muscles of the mandible so that the mandible is brought up toward what ultimately will be occlusal contact of the teeth. This act occurs while the tongue tip is still placed against the lower lip. Physiologic transition in swallowing begins during the first year of life and normally continues over the next several years. A mature swallow pattern is characterized by relaxation of the lips, placement of the tongue behind the maxillary incisors, and elevation of the mandible all the way to the point of posterior tooth contact; this is not usually observed before age 4 or 5 years. Proffit believes that children who are in the normal transitional stages of swallow maturation tend to be labeled as "tongue thrusters" or deviate swallowers." Children seen in this state of development are often considered for myofunctional therapy, but this procedure should be seriously questioned.

Some preschool children with a forward tongue position during swallow most likely have not yet learned to follow the adult pattern.

Proffit and Mason believe that several factors enter into the normal maturation in the swallow pattern. A child with a thumb-sucking habit may delay the transition toward adult swallowing and could thus be labeled a "tongue thruster" in the early mixed dentition years. A change to the adult swallow pattern will not occur until the sucking habit is corrected, but spontaneous transition toward the adult swallowing often occurs.

It is also recognized that anterior tongue positioning can result from airway problems both in the nose and in the pharynx. Lymphoid tissue grows quickly in children. Furthermore, enlarged tonsils in a young child are a fairly common finding. Often it is necessary for these children to carry the tongue forward and rotate the mandible open to provide mechanical clearance for breathing and swallowing. It should also be recognized that chronic allergic conditions and nasal infections and mechanical blockage by turbinates or a deviate nasal septum can lead to chronic mouth breathing. The resulting respiratory obstruction may produce tongue thrusting and perhaps a malocclusion.

Proffit believes that the only rationale for myofunctional therapy in the child with the tongue thrust who has neither speech problems nor a malocclusion would be that this therapy would prevent development of such problems in the future. He further suggests that the simplest guideline for dealing with the child who has a malocclusion and anterior tongue position is to treat the malocclusion, not just the tongue thrust. Myofunctional therapy in his view is one adjunctive method for treatment of the clinical problem. Proffit firmly believes that tongue thrust behavior does not usually cause malocclusion. For most patients with malocclusions, skeletal relationships and other factors are important components of the etiology. Therapy therefore must be directed at more than just the tongue. To the extent that myofunctional therapy is indicated, it should be aimed at alterations in resting posture of the tongue and not focused only on swallowing. Proffit believes that postponing tongue therapy until treatment of the malocclusion is begun has the following major advantages:

1. In the absence of obvious predisposing factors, correction of the malocclusion will usually result in a disappearance of tongue thrust without any particular therapy directed to it.
2. Postponing tongue therapy gives the child a maximum opportunity to complete the swallow pattern transition.
3. For children who are older and do not show spontaneous progress toward adult swallowing and for whom therapy is indicated to promote changes in resting tongue position, the therapy seems most effective if it is carried out along with orthodontic treatment.

Although appliances are often recommended for the treatment of tongue thrust, functional therapy should first be attempted. Andrews recommends that the patient be instructed to practice swallowing correctly 20 times before each meal. Holding a glass of water in one hand and facing a mirror, the child takes a sip of water, closes the teeth into occlusion, places the tip of the tongue against the incisive papilla, and swallows. This is repeated and each time is followed by the relaxation of the muscles until the swallowing progresses smoothly.

The use of a sugarless mint has also resulted in successful management of simple tongue thrusting. The child is instructed to use the tip of the tongue to hold the mint in the roof of the mouth until the mint melts. As the mint is held, saliva will flow and make it necessary for the child to swallow.

After the patient has trained the tongue and muscles to function properly during the swallowing process, a mandibular lingual arch with a crib or an acrylic palatal retainer with a "fence" may be constructed as a reminder to position the tongue properly during swallowing (Fig. 21-39).

It has often been suggested that a decreased lip capability and reduced circumoral muscular tonus could produce a malocclusion (open bite) similar to that sometimes associated with a tongue-thrusting habit. Barber and Bonus conducted a study in which 20 tongue-thrusting children exercised their lips twice daily by pulling on a string attached to a button placed in the labial vestibule. They observed no significant changes in the incisor tooth relationships after periods of circumoral myofunctional exercise. Evidence was obtained that the circumoral musculature can be strengthened through exercise and that the lip musculature nearly retains the tonus obtained by exercising for as much as 18 months after cessation of exercise. Barber and Bonus did not observe any significant change in the dental relationship in the children after prolonged myofunctional exercise of the circumoral musculature.

The occurrence of an anterior open bite is often related, initially at least, to a thumb- or finger-sucking habit. After the space has been created in the anterior region, it is retained by the tongue being thrust forward or the tongue merely occupying the space. Gellen has observed that if an open bite has its origin in the primary dentition and later closes spontaneously, the initial closure begins by 10 years of age in 90% of the children. Thus the dentist may be justified in waiting until the child's tenth birthday before taking active steps to correct the anterior open bite.

Serial extraction for the child patient

There has been considerable controversy and misunderstanding regarding the definition of "serial extraction" and indications for its practice. This has been true not only among general practitioners but also among pedodontists and orthodontists.

Dewel has suggested that the procedure referred to as "serial extraction" involve the orderly removal of selected primary and permanent teeth in a predetermined sequence. Its use is indicated only in dental arches that are structurally inadequate for the developing teeth and when there is little or no hope of ever attaining a normal size and proportion.

Serial extraction is indicated primarily in severe Class I malocclusion in the mixed dentition that has

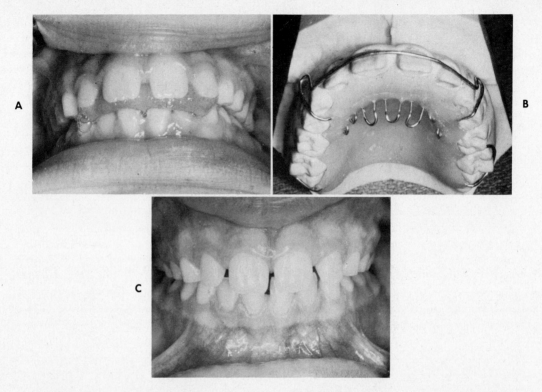

Fig. 21-39. A, Anterior open bite resulting from a tongue-thrust habit. **B,** A removable palatal retainer was constructed to prevent the tongue from being thrust forward during the swallowing process. **C,** The tongue-thrusting habit has been overcome. The occlusion is greatly improved.

insufficient arch length for the amount of tooth material. Salzmann (1966) believes that with our present knowledge it is not always possible to predict at an early age that there will be insufficient space to accommodate all of the permanent teeth in normal alignment. Dewel agrees that growth is often unpredictable; no one can be certain that it will be unfavorable to the development of the occlusion. Many children with an arch length inadequacy have spectacular growth when least expected. Such children have often been treated successfully by the orthodontist without sacrificing four permanent teeth.

Many dentists have unrealistically believed that serial extraction would solve all Class I occlusion problems. Too often they have been disillusioned to learn that serial extraction in itself rarely creates

an acceptable occlusal relationship and that certain adverse reactions will result if the procedure is not followed by adequate orthodontic treatment.

Ringenberg emphasizes that bimaxillary protrusion is not an indicator for serial extraction. Serial extraction primarily benefits children who demonstrate an arch length discrepancy. If the discrepancy is less than 7 mm throughout the arch, the dentition should be allowed to develop past the serial extraction stage and until all first premolars have erupted.

It is generally agreed that a malocclusion for which serial extraction treatment may be considered is characterized by severe crowding of the anterior teeth, premature loss of one or more of the primary canines, midline deviations, impacted or displaced lateral incisors, and gross deficiency in

Table 21-1. Developing malocclusion in the mixed dentition: diagnosis and treatment

Clinical condition	Significance	Radiographic findings	Treatment suggestions
Overretained primary teeth	May prevent normal eruption of permanent tooth; may produce cross-bite; space loss may occur in anterior area because of drifting of adjacent teeth	1. Supernumerary tooth preventing normal exfoliation of primary tooth and eruption of permanent tooth 2. Missing or unerupted permanent teeth 3. Abnormal or incomplete root resorption of primary tooth preventing normal exfoliation	1. Remove supernumerary tooth; space management (space regainer or maintainer) may be required 2. Maintain primary tooth or remove and manage the space 3. Remove primary tooth; space management may be required
Delayed eruption of permanent tooth after loss of primary tooth	Allows drifting of adjacent teeth and possible extrusion of opposing teeth	1. Missing or unerupted permanent tooth 2. Supernumerary tooth preventing eruption of permanent tooth 3. Impacted permanent tooth resulting from drifting of adjacent teeth or arch length inadequacy 4. Apparent fibrous barrier	1. Manage space (maintain, regain, or close space) as required; may eventually require fixed bridge 2. Remove supernumerary tooth; space management may be required 3. Regain space if possible; other space management techniques may be required, including extraction in preparation for orthodontics 4. Expose the crown; space management may be required
Premature loss of primary molars	Allows drifting of adjacent teeth with loss of arch length and possible extrusion of opposing teeth Eruption of premolars may be early or delayed depending on several conditions at time of loss	1. Unerupted premolars 2. Missing premolars	1. Manage space as required 2. Manage space; may ultimately require orthodontics and a fixed bridge
Premature loss of primary canine	A midline shift with loss of space for the permanent canines may occur; may indicate an arch length deficiency	Before premature exfoliation, root resorption may be noted on the mesial aspect of the primary canines; this resorption results from the erupting permanent lateral incisors	May extract primary canine on opposite side of arch; place lingual arch with spur to prevent further midline shift and incisor collapse

Modified from Myers, D.R.: J. Dent. Child. **41**:445-447, 1974.

Continued.

Table 21-1. Developing malocclusion in the mixed dentition: diagnosis and treatment—cont'd

Clinical condition	Significance	Radiographic findings	Treatment suggestions
Mandibular incisor crowding	May indicate arch length inadequacy; may produce a periodontal disturbance	Overlap of incisors, possible resorption of mesial surface of primary canine root	Analyze mixed dentition to determine arch length adequacy; consider early removal of primary canines and placement of lingual arch or sequential slicing of primary teeth to allow alignment of incisors
Ankylosed primary molar	If crown is below occlusal plane, it allows tipping of adjacent teeth and possible extrusion of opposing teeth; erupting premolar may be deflected or impacted	Tooth may be below occlusal plane; may observe an abnormal root resorption pattern and absence of periodontal ligament space; may also observe deflection of erupting premolar	
		1. Permanent successor present but no immediate threat of adjacent teeth tipping or of the premolar being deflected	1. Retain primary molar and observe it for normal root resorption and eruption of premolar; inform parents of need for periodic observation
		2. Permanent successor present and the possibility of adjacent tipping or premolar deflection an immediate concern	2. Extract ankylosed tooth; manage space as required
		3. Permanent successor absent	3. May retain primary molar as long as arch integrity or periodontium is not compromised; if tooth does not normally exfoliate, it will ultimately require extraction, space management, and probably a fixed bridge
Premature occlusal contacts	Is most common in primary canine area; may produce mandibular shift and functional cross-bite	None	Selective grinding; appliance therapy to correct cross-bite may be required
Anterior open bite	May be associated with thumb habit, abnormal swallowing pattern, or abnormal tongue position	May appear as curvature in maxillary anterior area, especially on panoramic film	Evaluate for thumb or finger habit or tongue thrust; incorporate habit correction therapy with or without orthodontic correction

Table 21-1. Developing malocclusion in the mixed dentition: diagnosis and treatment—cont'd

Clinical condition	Significance	Radiographic findings	Treatment suggestions
Ectopic eruption of first permanent molar	Interferes with normal eruption of first permanent molar; space loss and impaction of second premolar are possible	Resorption on distal surface of second primary molar roots; mesial surface of first permanent molar may appear locked below distal surface of second primary molar	Brass separating wire or helical spring; extraction of second primary molar and space regaining appliance may be required
Supernumerary teeth	Local malocclusion; interferes with normal eruption of permanent teeth	May initially be diagnosed on radiograph	Extraction or surgical removal; manage space as required
Abnormal tooth size or shape	Localized malocclusion or esthetic problem	May initially be diagnosed on radiograph	Recontour; full coverage or extraction and replacement; acid etch resin technique may be useful to build contour in some cases, such as peg-shaped lateral incisor
Interproximal caries	Eventual loss of primary tooth or loss of tooth structure and arch length loss	Early diagnosis depends on radiographs	Restorative dentistry and home care
Diastema between maxillary central incisors	Often represents normal stage of dental development before eruption of maxillary canines; may be related to tooth size discrepancy, abnormal labial frenum, or mesiodens	1. Tooth size discrepancy 2. Missing laterals 3. Heavy frenum 4. Mesiodens present	1. Orthodontic evaluation 2. Orthodontic evaluation 3. Frenectomy; may be postponed until after canine eruption; low frenum attachment with associated esthetic or periodontal problem may dictate early surgical procedure (see Chapter 1) 4. Extraction or surgical removal; consider closing space

arch length. Gingival recession and possibly alveolar destruction along one or both of the lower incisors may be present. A careful arch length analysis should be completed as described in the preceding chapter to determine the extent of the arch length inadequacy.

The primary canine is removed first in the serial extraction procedure, then the first primary molar, and finally the first premolar. The interval between extractions varies from 6 to 15 months. A passive lingual arch should be used to maintain the position of the mandibular first permanent molar and to prevent the incisors from tipping lingually. A Hawley type of maintainer is often the choice in the maxillary arch. After the removal of the primary canines, there is a degree of self-correction in the position and alignment of the permanent incisors.

Dewel advocates an alternative extraction sequence in the borderline malocclusion when there is still the possibility that extraction of the first premolar can be avoided, with the anticipation that growth may yet be sufficient to accommodate all the teeth. A first primary molar is extracted 6 to 12 months before the extraction of the primary canine, the purpose being to encourage the first premolar eruption and to retard canine eruption. If growth exceeds expectations, as it occasionally does, there will be no need to extract the first premolar.

The placement of an appliance in the mouth during the serial extraction sequence often implies to the parents that orthodontic treatment is being undertaken and that the entire malocclusion problem will be solved. It must be recognized that, without follow-up orthodontic treatment, serial extraction can be followed by persistent spacing at the extraction sites and the development of a closed bite. The lower incisors may tip lingually, the canine may tip distally, and the second premolar may tip mesially; all of these are undesirable.

Serial extraction has a place in dental practice; however, the procedure requires exceptional diagnostic skill and careful supervision of the developing occlusion. This subject is also discussed in Chapter 18.

Throughout the text there are references to the diagnosis and treatment of conditions that have the potential for creating an irregularity in the occlusion. The "minor treatment" procedures are discussed particularly in Chapters 20 and 21.

An excellent outline of clinical conditions seen in the developing dentition that may adversely influence the occlusion has been offered by Myers. A modification of his table is included in this chapter (Table 21-1). The amount of treatment undertaken by the dentist who has not had formal orthodontic training should be based on the dentist's background and experience in managing such cases. The table is intended to serve as a guide in the prevention, treatment, and referral of irregularities in the developing dentition.

REFERENCES

Andrews, R.G.: Tongue thrusting, J. South. Calif. Dent. Assoc. **28:**47-53, 1960.

Barber, T.K., and Bonus, H.W.: Dental relationships in tongue-thrusting children as affected by circumoral myofunctional exercise, J.A.D.A. **90:**979-988, 1975.

Bell, R.A., and LeCompte, E.J.: The effects of maxillary expansion using a quad-helix appliance during the deciduous and mixed dentitions, Am J. Orthod. **79:**152-161, 1981.

Brody, E.B.: Thumbsucking in an adult, J.A.M.A. **189:**971, 1964.

Calisti, L.J.P., Cohen, M.M., and Falls, M.: Correlation between malocclusion, oral habits, and socio-economic level of preschool children, J. Dent. Res. **39:**450-454, 1960.

Carr, G.E.: Ectopic eruption of the first permanent maxillary mollar in cleft lip and cleft palate children, J. Dent. Child. **32:**179-188, 1965.

Cheyne, V.D., and Wessels, K.E.: Impaction of permanent first molar with resorption and space loss in region of deciduous second molar, J.A.D.A. **35:**774-787, 1947.

Cohen, M.I.: Recognition of the developing malocclusion, Dent. Clin. North Am., pp. 299-311, July 1959.

Croxton, W.L.: Unpublished data, 1960.

Cumley, R.W.: Why do children suck their thumbs? Psychiatr. Bull. **5:**50-53, 1955.

Davis, W.B.: Personal communication, 1972.

Dewel, B.F.: Serial extraction: requirements and responsibilities, Dent. Abs. **12:**522-523, 1967.

Ewan, G.E.: Locating impacted cuspids using the shift technique, Am. J. Orthod. **41:**926-929, 1955.

Fisher, G.D.: Growth and development of the child, J. Dent. Child. **25:**69-83, 1958.

Gellen, M.E.: Anterior open bite: serial observations of 37 young children, J. Dent. Child. **33:**226-237, 1966.

Graber, T.M.: The finger sucking habit and associated problems, J. Dent. Child **25:**145-151, 1958.

Graber, T.M.: Orthodontics principles and practice, ed. 3, Philadelphia, 1972, W.B. Saunders Co.

Humphrey, W.P.: A simple technique for correcting an ectopically erupting first permanent molar, J. Dent. Child. **29:**176-178, 1962.

Korner, A.F., and Reider, N.: Psychologic aspects of disruption of thumbsucking by means of dental appliance, Angle Orthod. **25:**23-31, 1955.

Kramer, W.S.: Personal communication, 1982.

Kutin, G., and Hawes, R.R.: Posterior cross-bites in the deciduous and mixed dentitions, Am. J. Orthod. **56:**491-504, 1969.

Montelius, G.A., and Wahlquist, N.F.: Supernumerary tooth bud which developed into a cyst, Northwest Dent. **25:**151-165, 1946.

Myers, D.R.: A table of clinical and radiographic clues to developing malocclusions in the mixed dentition period, J. Dent. Child. **41:**445-447, 1974.

Plessett, D.N.: Auto-extraction, Oral Surg. **12**:302-303, 1959.

Popovich, F., and Thompson, G.W.: Thumb and finger sucking: its relation to malocclusion, Am J. Orthod. **63**:148-155, 1973.

Proffit, W.R.: Myofunctional therapy: what is its proper role? In Goldman, H.M., and others, editors: Current therapy in dentistry, vol. 6, St. Louis, 1977, The C.V. Mosby Co.

Proffit, W.R., and Mason, R.M.: Myofunctional therapy for tongue thrusting: background and recommendations, J.A.D.A. **90**:403-411, 1975.

Pulver, F.: The etiology and prevalence of ectopic eruption of the maxillary first permanent molar, J. Dent. Child. **35**:138-146, 1968.

Ramfjord, S.P.: Bruxism: a clinical and electromyographic study, J.A.D.A. **62**:21-44, 1961.

Reding, G.R., Rubright, W.C., and Zimmerman, S.O.: Incidence of bruxism, J. Dent. Res. **45**:1198-1204,1966.

Ringenberg, G.M.: Serial extraction: stop, look and be certain, Am. J. Orthod. **50**:327-336, 1964.

Rix, R.E.: Deglutition and the teeth, Dent. Rec. **66**:105-108, 1946.

Rutrick, R.E.: Crossbite correction with a therapeutic pacifier, J. Dent. Child. **41**:442-444, 1974.

Salzmann, J.A.: Serial extraction in general practice (editorial), Am. J. Orthod. **52**:145-146, 1966.

Salzmann, J.A.: Orthodontics in daily practice, Philadelphia, 1974, J.B. Lippincott Co.

Schoenwetter, R.F.: A possible relationship between certain malocclusions and difficult or instrument deliveries, Angle Orthod. **44**:336-340, 1974.

Schulze, C.: Incidence of supernumerary teeth, Dent. Abs. **6**:23, 1961.

Sheppard, I.M.: The treatment of bruxism, Dent. Clin. North Am., pp. 207-213, 1960.

Stafne, E.C.: Supernumerary upper central incisors, Dent. Cosmos **73**:976-980, 1931.

Stewart, B.L., Hershey, H.G. and Warren, D.W.: Changes in nasal airway resistance after rapid maxillary expansion, Int. Assoc. Dent. Res. p. 876, 1974.

Stewart, D.J. and Kernohan, D.C.: Traumatic gingival recession in infants: the result of a dummy sucking habit, Br. Dent. J. **135**:157-158, 1973.

Straub, W.J.: Malfunction of the tongue. The abnormal swallowing habit: the cause, effects and results in relation to orthodontic treatment and speech therapy, Am. J. Orthod. **46**:404-424, 1960.

Traisman, A.S., and Traisman, H.S.: Thumb and finger sucking: a study of 2650 infants and children, J. Pediatr. **52**:566-572, 1958.

West, E.E.: Pitfalls in serial extraction. In Cook, J.T., editor: Transactions of the Third International Orthodontic Congress, London, 1975, Crosby Lockwood Staples.

Wyatt, W.E.: A two-phase slicing technique for space allocation, Int. J. Orthod. **10**:125-130, 1972.

Young, D.H.: Ectopic eruption of the first permanent molar, J. Dent. Child. **24**:153-162, 1957.

22 Genetic aspects of dental anomalies

DAVID BIXLER

The study of molecular biology in our scientific world is often considered to be the ultimate biologic challenge, ideally providing answers to perplexing biologic problems. In our present state of knowledge, however, most of the diseases affecting the dentofacial complex cannot be relegated to the molecular level for their solution. Despite this inadequacy in our knowledge, this is the direction of research effort today in dentistry. For this reason the pertinent features of this molecular approach, which is encompassed by the broad term "biochemical genetics," are considered here.

One cannot help but be fascinated by the fact that the single, fertilized ovum contains within its cell wall the complete potential for development into the incredibly complicated human organism. This process comes about by growth, which involves cell division and differentiation. The term "differentiation" has been given many definitions, depending on the situation in which it is used. The definition that has greatest significance and meaning to the molecular biologist is a progressive specialization, and hence limitation, of cell function. The reader can immediately infer from this definition that the molecular biologist views the fertilized egg as having all the necessary equipment to produce muscle cells, nerve cells, liver cells, or any of the myriad other cells that make up the adult human organism. Two questions immediately present themselves: what is this equipment and how does it function? In the answers to these two questions lie the story of genetics and the domain of the molecular biologist.

The equipment of the fertilized egg that enables it to regulate differentiation of the cell into the total organism is its genetic material. It has been demonstrated that this material is deoxyribonucleic acid (DNA). The genetic material, then, may be visualized as a message that instructs the cell in how to become one cell type or another. Obviously, the genetic message is different for different species, since all species exhibit overt structural differences. Equally important is the fact that the message is stable—horses never give rise to humans or vice versa.

To answer the second question ("How does the inherited [genetic] equipment function?"), we must first state what it is that makes one cell type different from any other type. This fundamental difference is defined in terms of the kind of protein that each cell manufactures. Therefore protein synthesis, not that of fat or carbohydrate, is the critical element that determines cell function and cell type. Muscle cells produce actomyosin; connective tissue cells produce collagen; liver cells produce various enzymes; intestinal cells also produce enzymes but of a different kind.

Only in the past few years have we been able to state with certainty that the genetic material, DNA, controls the function—and hence differentiation—of a cell by specifying what proteins it will produce. Thus for each cell type, some genes are turned "on" and many, many others are turned "off." The cell consists of two main areas: the nucleus, which houses the DNA, and the cytoplasm, where the metabolic and synthetic activities of the cell take place. DNA in the nucleus conveys its message for protein synthesis to the cytoplasm, where this process takes place by a complicated and yet highly efficient system. It makes a copy of its message in the form of ribonucleic acid (RNA), which is passed into the cytoplasm from the nucleus. At the ribosome this message-containing RNA directs the synthesis of the proper proteins.

Several different types of RNA participate in this complicated process of protein synthesis, each with its own specific function; it is beyond the scope of this chapter to discuss these details. The reader may find them in any standard textbook of biochemistry. The key to the thinking of today's molecular biologist is summarized in the following statements:

1. The genetic message in the coded DNA is transmitted from cell generation to cell generation when the DNA molecules are replicated (or duplicated).
2. Cell function is determined by production of specific RNA molecules made from the DNA master, and these in turn direct protein synthesis.
3. Cell function is specified by the protein molecule it manufactures.

With the preceding material in mind, it now becomes evident that genetic disease can also be termed "molecular disease." An individual who is afflicted with an inherited disease is one who is carrying an alteration in DNA such that the altered cells will produce an abnormal protein, abnormal amounts of protein, or both. This process of abnormal protein production, by virtue of its alteration in cell function, results in a clinical disease that we recognize as a specific inherited disease.

Genes and chromosomes

The genetic material, DNA, that controls the production of a single protein (or polypeptide chain) is called a gene. There are thousands and thousands of human genes, each one regulating the production of a specific polypeptide. These genes are grouped in units called chromosomes. Such a packaging arrangement has great advantage to the cell when it divides, since it is much simpler for the cell to equally partition a few chromosomes into two daughter cells than it would be to similarly sort out thousands of genes.

Humans have 46 chromosomes. Each chromosome has a paired mate that is referred to as the homologue. Genes on homologues control the same genetic trait and, with the single exception of those genes on the sex chromosomes, there are at least two genes that control each inherited trait. Thus the human chromosome complement actually consists of 23 pairs of chromosomes. Twenty-two of these pairs are designated the autosomes; the remaining pair, the X and the Y chromosomes, are named the sex chromosomes.

One of the more rapidly developing areas of interest in the field of human genetics is cytogenetics, the study of human chromosomes. This interest has been stimulated by the development of techniques whereby cytogeneticists can culture cells of organisms in vitro and can examine chromosomes under the microscope for alterations in size, shape, and fine structure. It was just such a technique of chromosome analysis (karyotyping) that led LeJeune, Turpin, and Gautier in 1959 to demonstrate that the fundamental defect in Down syndrome is the presence of an extra chromosome in the affected individual's karyotype. Thus the typical child with Down syndrome has 47 chromosomes. Since 1959, several disease states have been specifically ascribed to alteration in chromosome number. However, this quickly proved to be only one aspect of chromosomal alteration in humans. Refined karyotyping techniques revealed that the *structure* of chromosomes, as well as their *number,* could be altered. These various structural alterations have been given the following descriptive designations:

1. Deletion—the absence of a piece of chromosome
2. Duplication—the insertion of an extra fragment into a chromosome from its now deficient homologue
3. Inversion—the breaking of a chromosome in two places and subsequent rejoining with the middle piece inverted
4. Translocation—the attachment of a broken

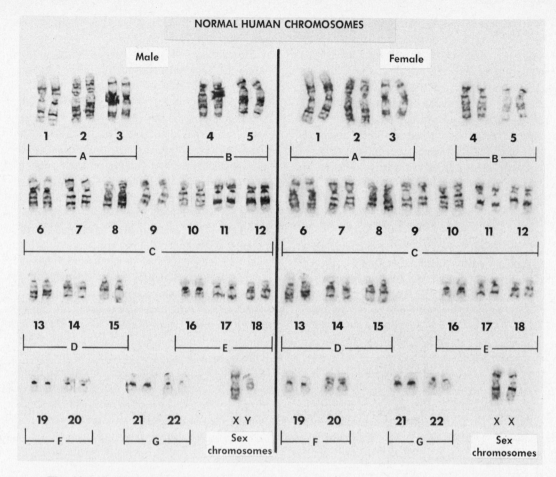

Fig. 22-1. Banded karyotypes of a normal human male *(left)* and female *(right)*, also indicating group designations according to Denver nomenclature.

piece from one chromosome to another, but nonhomologous, chromosome

With the identification of all these alterations in both chromosome number and structure, a nomenclature system for the various chromosomes based on their morphology became a necessity. The currently accepted system, called the Denver nomenclature, is based primarily on chromosome identification by overall size and individual anatomic characteristics.

A series of techniques for elucidating chromosome structure has been developed that employs enzymatic digestion followed by special staining procedures. The net result of these techniques, each of which appears to indicate chromosome morphology in a different way, is the production of a series of bands in the chromosome itself. (Fig. 22-1 shows the karyotypes of a normal human male and female.) Hence, the designation is made of "banded" chromosomes when they are prepared by these procedures. The essential point is that the bands of each chromosome are characteristic and reproducible, thereby permitting absolute identification of each chromosome and resolution and

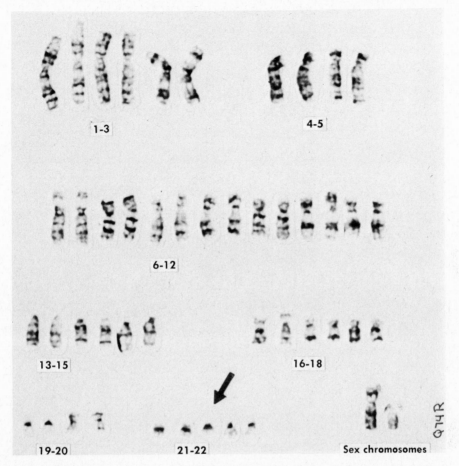

Fig. 22-2. Banded karyotype of a male with trisomy of chromosome 21, or Down syndrome.

description of internal structural defects not heretofore recognizable. As might be expected, the sensitivity of banding procedures to identify chromosome structure has expanded the number of chromosome defects known to be responsible for human malformations from a handful to more than 100, and the list grows almost daily.

Each chromosome consists of thousands of genes. It is easy to see how an extra piece—or a missing piece—of a chromosome could involve many cell functions and hence result in a clinically identifiable disease state. As might be expected, disease states resulting from gross chromosomal alterations have a complicated clinical picture involving multiple organ systems. This is readily apparent in Down syndrome.

When an extra chromosome is present, the condition is spoken of as *trisomy* of the chromosome in question, for example, Down syndrome (trisomy 21). Fig. 22-2 shows the karyotype of a male who has Down syndrome. The extra chromosome belonging to the G group is readily apparent. *Monosomy* of an autosome, or a missing autosomal chromosome, had not been thought to be compatible with life until one such affected individual was recently reported with an apparent G group monosomy. On the other hand, monosomy of the sex chromosomes does occur, is compatible with life,

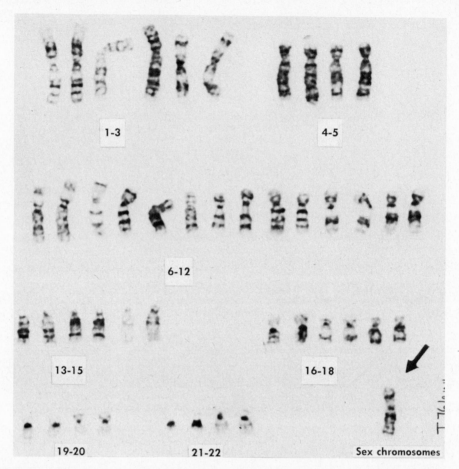

Fig. 22-3. Banded karyotype of a female with a missing X chromosome, or Turner syndrome.

and typically affects development of both internal and external sex organs of the individual. The best-known example of this is Turner syndrome, which occurs in about one of every 10,000 live births. These individuals are phenotypic females who are missing an X chromosome and are chromosomally designated as XO. They are typically short of stature, lack secondary sex characteristics, and are sterile. The Turner syndrome karyotype is shown in Fig. 22-3. Table 22-1 summarizes the better-known chromosome aberrations that produce clinical disease.

Chromosome abnormalities are an important cause of spontaneous abortion. About 15% of all recognized pregnancies end in spontaneous abortion. The incidence of chromosome abnormalities in the abortuses is greater than 50%. However, the reader should be cognizant of the fact that only 0.3% to 0.5% of all live-born infants have a chromosome abnormality. Clinicians agree that even though these aberrations are relatively rare, they remain a significant cause of mental and physical defects in humans.

Hereditary traits in families

When hereditary traits in families are considered, it is convenient to think of two broad classes of gene-controlled traits. *Monogenic* traits are pro-

Table 22-1. A summary of the more common chromosomal aberrations

Type	Specific alteration	Clinical result
Aneuploidy	Trisomy 21	Down syndrome
	Trisomy 18	Edwards syndrome
	Trisomy 13	Patau syndrome
	Extra X chromosomes	In females: XXX, XXXX, XXXXX syndromes
		In males: Klinefelter syndrome—XXY, XXXY, and XXXXY
	Monosomy, autosomal	Nonviable (?)
	Monosomy, X chromosome	In females: Turner syndrome, XO
		In males: nonviable, YO
Translocation	14/21, 21/21, or 21/22	Translocation carrier (normal phenotype) or mongoloid
Deletion	Ring chromosome	Variable
	Short arm chromosome No. 5	Cri du chat syndrome
	Philadelphia chromosome (No. 22)	Chronic granulocytic leukemia

duced and regulated by a single gene. These traits are usually easy to recognize in families, and the transmission of the trait from one family member to the next follows simple mendelian principles of dominant, recessive, autosomal, or sex-linked inheritance. Few such simply inherited traits appear in the population more frequently than once in a thousand individuals. *Polygenic* traits are controlled by many genes at different loci. Polygenic traits are common and are illustrated by examples such as intelligence, skin color, and height. Such traits do not show clear-cut differences between "normal" and "affected" persons as often as do monogenic traits; instead, they show a continuous or quantitative distribution of the trait in the population. Recently the term "multifactorial inheritance" has been employed to describe traits that do not fit simple mendelian inheritance patterns. A multifactorial inheritance disorder is one that is determined by a combination of genetic and environmental facts. The term "polygenic" is often used interchangeably with multifactorial, but this is incorrect. Polygenic is a term that should be restricted to conditions controlled by a large number of genes, each with a small effect and working additively. The definition of multifactorial inheritance and its relationship to human disease are considered on pp. 628 to 630.

Monogenic inheritance. The investigation of human genetics is primarily an observation of spe-cific traits in families and a study of family pedigrees. At this point is is necessary to introduce some terms that may be unfamiliar to the reader but that are essential to an understanding of the study of genes in families.

The first affected individual in a family who brings that family to attention is referred to as the proband or propositus. This individual is the index case. Brothers and sisters are referred to as siblings or sibs. Thus a sibship consists of all the brothers and sisters in a single family unit. The clinical appearance of a given trait for an individual, such as eye color or height, is that individual's *phenotype,* whereas the specific genetic makeup that controls that phenotype is the *genotype.*

In an earlier section the point was made that the human chromosome complement consists of 22 homologous pairs of autosomes and one pair of sex chromosomes. Because of homologue pairing, there are at least two genes, one located on each member of the homologous pair, that control each phenotypic trait. Genes at the same locus on a pair of homologous chromosomes are alleles. When both members of a pair of alleles are identical, the individual is *homozygous.* When the two alleles at a given locus are different, the individual is *heterozygous.*

A gene that expresses a particular phenotype in single dose is a *dominant* gene. If the gene must be present in double dose (homozygous) to express a

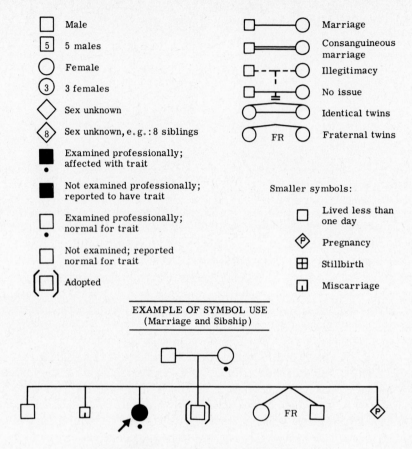

Fig. 22-4. Pedigree symbols used in family studies.

phenotype, it is a *recessive* gene. The reader should note that it is actually the phenotype that is dominant or recessive and not the gene itself. The terms "dominant gene" and "recessive gene," though, are commonly used by geneticists in describing inherited traits in families, and the common usage will be continued here.

Family data for the study of inherited traits are conveniently summarized by making a pedigree, which is a shorthand method of classifying the data. The symbols commonly used in constructing a pedigree are summarized in Fig. 22-4. The observable inheritance patterns followed by monogenic traits within families are determined by (1) whether the trait is dominant or recessive, (2) whether the gene is autosomal (on one of the autosomes) or sex linked (on a sex chromosome), and (3) the chance distribution in offspring of the genes passed down from parents by means of the gametes (sperm and ova). The simple patterns of monogenic inheritance seen in families are presented in the following discussion. A final portion is devoted to facts that may alter these simple patterns and make them more difficult to discern.

Autosomal dominant inheritance. An excellent example of autosomal dominant inheritance is dentinogenesis imperfecta. Although the specific molecular defect has not been elucidated, the clin-

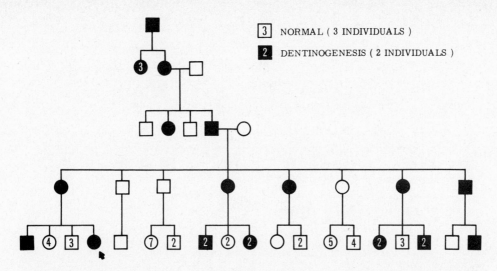

Fig. 22-5. Pedigree of a family with dentinogenesis imperfecta, an autosomal dominant trait.

ical manifestations of this single gene defect are well known and the trait appears as an autosomal dominant in all families that have been reported. Thus the gene producing the defective dentin may be represented by D,* and the normal dentin recessive allele by d. The homozygous dominant (DD) and heterozygous dominant (Dd) individuals both have defective dentin, and the homozygous recessive (dd) individual has normal dentin. Affected individuals are most likely to be heterozygous (Dd) rather than homozygous (DD) because of the rarity of the D gene. This situation is true for *all* rare dominant traits. For simplicity, all individuals with a rare dominant condition may be considered heterozygous.

A pedigree of what may be the largest family in the United States affected with dentinogenesis imperfecta is shown in Fig. 22-5. Matings of the two genotypes, Dd (affected) and dd (normal), can be expected to produce only two kinds of offspring, affected and unaffected in an equal ratio (Fig. 22-6). Since gamete combination is random, all possible gamete combinations produce affected and unaffected offspring in equal numbers.

---

*Capital letters typically designate dominant genes, and lower case letters designate recessive genes.

Parent (Dd)

Gametes	D	d
Parent (dd) d	Dd	dd
d	Dd	dd

Fig. 22-6. Mating types, gametes, and offspring genotypes for dentinogenesis imperfecta, an autosomal dominant trait.

From pedigrees such as that seen in Fig. 22-5, the following general criteria for making the diagnosis of autosomal dominant inheritance may be formulated:

1. The trait appears in each generation.
2. On the average, 50% of the offspring of affected parents will also be affected.
3. Unaffected parents do not have affected offspring. There are two important exceptions: a fresh gene mutation in one of the parental gametes and nonpenetrance (see p. 628).

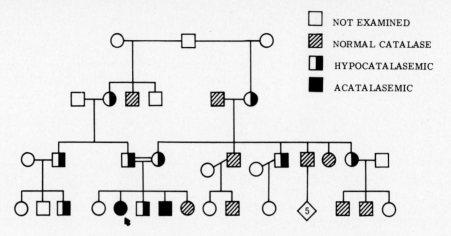

Fig. 22-7. Pedigree of a family with acatalasia, an autosomal recessive trait.

4. The occurrence and transmission of the trait are not affected by sex: males and females are equally likely to have or transmit the trait.

Autosomal recessive inheritance. An autosomal recessive trait is one that is expressed by the individual who has both altered recessive alleles present and is thereby homozygous. The most common pedigree for this type of inheritance shows two normal parents who have an affected child. The trait may also appear in siblings of the proband but rarely in relatives outside the sibship. There are many clinical examples of this kind of inheritance, but a well-described example of interest in dentistry is acatalasia.

In acatalasia there is a deficiency of the enzyme catalase, which is normally present in blood, skin, liver, muscle, bone marrow, and mucous membrane. The chemical reaction catalyzed by catalase is $2H_2O_2 \rightarrow 2H_2O + O_2$; thus individuals with abnormal enzyme do not metabolize these peroxides. Although systemic signs of the deficiency are absent, the oral cavities of affected (homozygous) individuals show a severe, gangrenous stomatitis. It has been reasoned that oral lesions are the result of accumulation of peroxides produced by bacteria and that these peroxides oxidize the blood coming to the oral tissues and deprive them of both oxygen and nutrition.

If the defective gene for catalase formation is designated by the letter c, then C may represent the normal allele that is dominant to c. Affected individuals have the genotype cc. Unaffected individuals may be either CC or Cc. Since it is commonly two phenotypically normal but heterozygous parents who have children affected with rare recessive diseases, considerable interest has been shown by molecular chemists and geneticists in identifying these "carriers." Individuals who are heterozygous for the defective catalase gene can be identified biochemically by assaying their catalase blood level. These heterozygous carriers are found to have blood catalase levels intermediate between the homozygous normal individuals and the affected individuals. In the heterozygotes the normal allele (C) can apparently produce enzyme in approximately normal amounts, whereas the mutant gene (c) can produce little or no active enzyme. The net effect is a blood level of enzyme in the heterozygote that is about half that of the normal homozygote. Fig. 22-7 shows a pedigree of a family with a catalase deficiency as reported by Nishimura and associates.

Acatalasia is a rare recessive disease whose frequency in the Japanese population, in which it was originally discovered, has been estimated to be approximately one in 10,000. Because of the rarity of this disease, affected individuals almost invariably come from two normal but carrier (heterozygous) parents. The pedigree in Fig. 22-7 also illustrates another important feature of rare recessive diseases. Parents of affected children are often found to be related by blood. The resultant marriage is described as consanguineous (note double line connecting parents in Fig. 22-7). Such blood-related parents are most likely to have obtained the same rare recessive gene from the ancestor they have in common. This explains the observed higher frequency of parental consanguinity in rare recessive disorders.

Fig. 22-8 illustrates the types of offspring that may be produced by two parents who are both heterozygous for the recessive acatalasic gene, c. It can be seen that three different genotypes can be produced from such matings: CC (homozygous normal), Cc (heterozygous normal but gene carrier), and cc (homozygous affected). Thus, on a random chance basis, two parents heterozygous for a single recessive gene will produce offspring in the phenotypic ratio of three normal children to one affected child. The following criteria characterize autosomal recessive inheritance:

1. The trait typically appears only in siblings, not in parents or other relatives.
2. On the average, one fourth of the siblings of an affected individual will be similarly affected.
3. The rarer the trait, the more likely that the parental mating is consanguineous.
4. Males and females are equally likely to be affected.

Sex-linked (or X-linked) recessive inheritance. Genes on the sex chromosomes can be considered unequally distributed to males and females. This inequality is the result of two facts: (1) males have one X and one Y chromosome, whereas females have two X chromosomes, and (2) the only genes known to be active on the Y chromosome are concerned with the preferential development of the male reproductive system. For these reasons, then, males are hemizygous for all X-linked genes, meaning that they have only half (or one each) of the X-linked genes. Since females have two X chromosomes, they may be either homozygous or

		Parent (Cc)	
Gametes		C	c
Parent (Cc)	C	CC	Cc
	c	Cc	cc

Fig. 22-8. Mating types, gametes, and offspring genotypes for acatalasia, an autosomal recessive trait.

heterozygous for X-linked genes, just as with autosomal genes.

Interesting genetic combinations are made possible by the male hemizygous condition. Since only one gene locus of each kind on the X chromosome is represented in the male, even recessive genes in single dose may express themselves phenotypically and thereby behave as though they were dominant genes. On the other hand, X-linked recessive genes must be present in double dose in females to express themselves. Consequently, rare X-linked recessive diseases are practically restricted to males and are infrequently seen in females.

Fig. 22-9 shows a pedigree of a family with anhidrotic ectodermal dysplasia, a genetic disorder that is inherited as an X-linked recessive trait. Affected males show hypotrichosis, absence of sweat glands, decreasing salivary flow, and multiple missing permanent teeth. Heterozygous females show minimum effects, if any.

It can be noticed from this pedigree (Fig. 22-9) that an affected father (I-1) does not pass the gene to his sons but must pass it to all his daughters, who are then carriers or heterozygotes. If a carrier daughter (II-5) marries a normal male (II-6), four genotypes are possible in the offspring and in equal proportions: affected male (III-5), normal male (III-8), normal female (III-7), and carrier female (III-6). This type of mating is the most common for X-linked recessive disorders producing affected male offspring. Because half the daughters of this

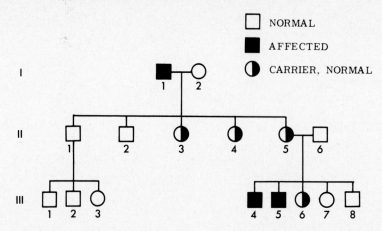

Fig. 22-9. Pedigree of a family with anhidrotic ectodermal dysplasia, a sex-linked recessive trait.

mating (carrier female by normal male) will also be heterozygous carriers, it is possible by chance for a sex-linked recessive gene to be passed along through a long series of carrier women before finally making its appearance in an affected male.

The criteria for diagnosing an X-linked recessive trait may be summarized as follows:

1. Since the gene cannot be passed from father to son, affected fathers almost never have affected sons. (The reader is left to figure out the rare situation when this could occur.)
2. All daughters of an affected male receive his X-linked genes. Therefore affected males transmit the trait to their grandsons through their daughters.
3. The incidence of the trait is much higher in males than in females. This is typified by the disease hemophilia, which is also caused by a sex-linked recessive gene.

It should be noted that genes on the X chromosome may behave differently in males and females. For example, heterozygous females may show significant clinical expression of a single recessive gene. The reason for this apparent contradiction is lyonization, a biologic process that is named after its discoverer, Mary Lyon, and that occurs only in females. All female cells have two X chromo-

somes, but it is now clear that genes on one of the two X chromosomes are inactivated at about the blastula stage of development. If the individual is heterozygous for an X-linked trait, two populations of cells result, some with genes on the X_1 that are active, the remainder with genes on the X_2 that are active. When by chance the X chromosome with the deleterious gene is left active in a significant proportion of the cells, its expression may be observed in the female. Chance dictates that this does not occur frequently, but since all females are, by definition of lyonization, *mosaic* with regard to X-linked traits, occasionally the phenotypic expression of such heterozygous recessive genes appears. In the case of anhidrotic ectodermal dysplasia, female carriers may show patchy areas of skin that do not sweat and also may have varying degrees of oligodontia, typically less severe than that seen in males.

Sex-linked dominant inheritance. Although there are several inherited types of amelogenesis imperfecta, one of the hypoplastic types is inherited as a sex-linked dominant trait. This dental disease involves an enamel defect that can be described as a failure of the ameloblasts to lay down sufficient organic enamel matrix. The result is that all teeth of both dentitions show a well-

mean (or average) for the trait; statistical concepts applied to any normal distribution curve may also be applied to the study of the trait (for example, 2 standard deviations from the mean will include 95% of the population).

This point of continuous variation is emphasized because the most common diseases with which the dentist must deal are probably multifactorial traits—dental caries, periodontal disease, and malocclusion. This means that only the extremes of variation will be readily apparent to the clinician, for example, the rampant-caries child or the caries-free adult. In this latter instance, if one did not understand the concept of multifactorial inheritance, it might be concluded that such individuals represent a single gene–controlled, discrete phenotype. This is frequently not the case.

A most important feature of traits produced by polygenes is that they are susceptible to environmental modification. A phenotype controlled by the concerted action of 100 genes is much more likely to be altered and modified by the existing environment than is one controlled by only one or even several genes. For example, dental caries is the interaction product of three essential factors: a cariogenic diet, a caries-producing bacterial flora, and a susceptible tooth. These three factors encompass a variety of biologically complicated entities such as saliva, plaque, tooth matrix formation, and crystallization. It should be easy to visualize that the development of these complex elements must involve a great number of genes. Environmental modification, such as properly timed systemic fluoride supplementation, produces a considerable alteration in the phenotype without changing the basic genetic constitution of the individual. The reader can probably think of numerous additional environmental modifications that can produce a markedly altered dental caries experience without changing an individual's genes. By contrast, a single gene trait, such as amelogenesis imperfecta, shows little environmental modification and routinely exhibits a characteristic phenotype in all individuals who carry the gene.

Two concepts are commonly used to help in the identification of polygenic inheritance: (1) the closer the blood relation, the higher the phenotypic resemblance, and (2) the mean value of a polygenic trait in the *offspring* tends to be about halfway between the mean value for the *parents* and the mean value for the *general population*. Offspring thereby tend to "return" to the mean value of the population, regardless of the phenotypic extremes of the parents.

Multifactorial inheritance in human diseases. In many common disorders (such as diabetes, schizophrenia, and hypertension) and the major common congenital malformations (such as spina bifida, anencephaly, and cleft lip and cleft palate) there is a definite familial tendency. This is shown by the fact that the proportion of affected relatives is greater than the general population incidence. However, this proportion is much less than would be expected for a monogenic trait, and the explanation most commonly offered is that these are multifactorial traits. As previously stated, the definition of a multifactorial trait is one that is partly the result of the combined effects of many genes (polygenes) and partly the result of an interaction of these polygenes with the environment—hence the term "multifactorial." Environment is defined as those nongenetic circumstances that render an individual more or less susceptible to a disease state. In contrast to monogenic traits, whose characteristics have been summarized in preceding paragraphs, polygenic diseases have the following characteristics:

1. Each person has a liability for a given polygenically controlled disease, and that liability is the sum of the polygenic and environmental liability.
2. For many polygenic diseases there is discontinuous distribution of phenotype (for example, cleft versus noncleft). It is assumed that the "dose" of liability (genetics plus environment) has to exceed a threshold amount before the affected phenotype appears. All persons past the threshold have the phenotype. A graphic representation of this idea is shown in Fig. 22-11.
3. Because dosage (of several genes) is involved, the incidence of the trait in near rel-

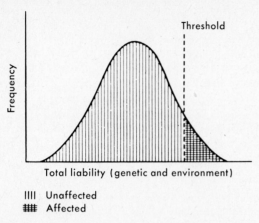

Fig. 22-11. Multifactorial model for inheritance of cleft lip and palate.

atives *decreases* much faster than expected for a *monogenic* trait. However, because relatives do have genes in common, the trait incidence in relatives is still higher than expected for the general population.

The consequence of these features of multifactorial diseases is that the disease risk to offspring of an affected parent is low. For example, the recurrence risk for monogenic dominantly inherited traits is 50% and for recessive traits is 25% but for a multifactorial (polygenic) trait is typically less than 10%. Thus it is essential for the geneticist to distinguish monogenic traits from multifactorial traits, since genetic counseling is quite different in the two situations; recurrence is high in the former instance and low in the latter.

Twin studies in genetic research

Toward the end of the nineteenth century, Galton recognized that twins could be most useful for evaluating the nature-nurture argument that was raging at that time. Today, the essentiality of considering both heredity and environment in any analysis of the individual is recognized. Nevertheless, interest in the twin method for study of the relative importance of heredity and environment in humans has been increasing over the past 25 years. One likely explanation for this renewed interest is

that many human traits are polygenic, are susceptible to environmental modification, and are thereby difficult to study with conventional methods. The twin method allows an approach to the study of such traits.

The twin study method is based on the principle that human twins are of two types: *monozygotic* (or identical) twins resulting from a single ovum fertilized by a single sperm and *dizygotic* (or fraternal) twins resulting from fertilization of two ova by two sperm. It is axiomatic that monozygotic twins have identical genotypes, whereas dizygotic twins are no more closely related to each other than are any two siblings. From this conclusion it follows that differences between monozygotic twins result from environmental differences, whereas those between dizygotic twins result from differences in both heredity and environment. Additional utility of dizygotic twins lies in their comparison with nontwin sibling pairs for a given trait. At least theoretically, the environmental contribution to dizygotic twin differences is more uniform for both members than it is for the nontwin sibling pairs, particularly if the twins are of the same sex.

To use the twin method, it is necessary (1) to distinguish between the two types of zygosity (usually done by blood typing) and (2) to obtain a sample of monozygous and dizygous twins with a definable level of comparability in their environment. If the twin pair is identical for the trait in question (regardless of their zygosity), they are described as *concordant*. If they are unlike for the trait, they are *discordant*. Such intrapair differences are usually expressed in percentage figures for a group of twins being evaluated. For example, monozygous twins show about a 40% concordance (alikeness) for cleft lip with or without cleft palate, whereas dizygous twins show only a 5% concordance.

Genetic aspects of dental caries

It is clear from many dietary studies, notably the Vipeholm study by Gustafsson and associates, that individual variation in susceptibility to dental caries exists even under identical, controlled conditions. This implies that because of genetic differences, certain environmental factors are potentially more cariogenic for some people than for others. This is not to say that dental caries is an inherited disease; rather, genetic influences may modify the overt expression of this disease in the individual.

Several investigators have studied the genetic aspects of dental caries in humans, using both the twin and the family pedigree approach for study material. Because dental caries is an age-dependent process, much of the reported data cannot be compared because of age differences in the various population groups studied. Nevertheless, the family observations by Klein and by Klein and Palmer are worth noting. Their findings indicated that children show a remarkable similarity in caries experience to their parents when the parents' susceptibility is the same (either high or low). However, when caries susceptibility of two parents is unlike, the children's susceptibility tends to be more like that of the mother than the father. This finding was particularly evident in daughters.

Since genetics is the study of variation, the more common a genetic trait is, the more difficult it is to demonstrate its genetic character. Böök and Grahnén attempted to maximize differences in caries experience within families by selecting caries-free, 20-year-old men and studying caries experience within their families. These results were compared with data from similarly selected families in which the propositus (index case) had an unknown and, ideally, random dental caries experience. Their results showed that parents and siblings of caries-free propositi had significantly lower DMF rates when compared with the "control" families. However, no significant correlations in caries experience were found between parents and children in families in either the low or average caries experience group. The authors concluded that the observed differences are hereditary and are probably of a polygenic nature.

Studies of twins by Dahlberg and Dahlberg; Mansbridge; Horowitz, Osborne, and De George; Goodman and associates; and Caldwell and Finn also indicate that genetic factors contribute significantly to individual differences in caries susceptibility. However, most authors agree that this genetic component of dental caries is a minor one in comparison with the overall effect of environment. Little has been done to relate caries susceptibility to specific biochemical differences in individuals, although Goodman and associates reported significant differences between monozygotic and dizygotic twins in salivary flow, pH, and amylase activity.

It is worth noting that Hunt, Hoppert, and Rosen have succeeded in establishing caries-resistant and caries-susceptible strains of rats by inbreeding techniques. The resistant strain was challenged by oral inoculation with cariogenic bacteria. This was accomplished by nursing resistant offspring with susceptible mothers. The resistant phenotype was maintained in spite of the environmental challenge, thus demonstrating its genetic nature. These results confirm the hypothesis of a definite genetic component in dental caries, at least in experimental animals.

The foregoing summary points to multifactorial causation in the susceptibility to human dental caries. Wide deviations of dental caries susceptibility may, however, be determined by single genes. For example, certain types of extreme susceptibility to dental caries (rampant caries) or high resistance to dental caries may eventually prove to be monogenic traits. Green (1959) suggested that certain individuals with high resistance to dental caries—designated by him as "immune"—have a specific immunoglobulin in their saliva that conveys immunity by lysing the cariogenic bacterial cells. It has been suggested by Warren that this immune phenotype is inherited; preliminary data on 74 individuals in five families indicate that high resistance to dental caries is transmitted as an autosomal dominant trait. Specific biochemical evidence in saliva will probably prove to be necessary, however, to clearly delineate this type of caries resistance from other types that are environmentally induced, such as dental fluorosis.

In summary, susceptibility to human dental caries is controlled to a significant but minor degree by heredity. This genetic control is undoubtedly multifactorial in nature, and such a polygenic background strongly implies considerable environmental modification. Specific types of dental caries susceptibility representing the extremes of variation of this trait may prove to be monogenic traits, but at present the evidence is insufficient for a clear statement of such inheritance.

Genetic aspects of periodontal disease

The clinical entity of periodontal disease is generally accepted as a local inflammatory disease with possible underlying systemic factors. This disease is so widespread in human populations and has such widely varying clinicohistopathologic features as to suggest that multiple diseases with multiple causes are being lumped together. Baer has suggested that there is evidence for several clinically variant types of periodontal disease generally subclassified by age of onset, severity of bone loss, oral hygiene, and presence or absence of local factors. One might well visualize the continuum of this disease as ranging from a localized gingivitis to a generalized periodontitis with severe bone and tooth loss. Periodontists agree that this disease has both inflammatory and degenerative pathologic features.

With this description in mind, it is easy to understand why genetic studies of this common problem have been neglected. As is true for dental caries, periodontal disease is common, occurs with a continuum of expressivity, and is greatly influenced by environmental conditions such as diet, occlusion, and oral habits. All of these features fit the description of a multifactorial type of disease or at least the susceptibility to it.

Family pedigree studies of periodontal disease are few and suffer from broad, uncritical diagnosis of the conditions studied. If one considers that all these studies are reporting on the same entity, however, tentative comparisons may be made. In a study of 47 families with periodontal disease, Dickmann reported that the condition appeared to be transmitted as a dominant trait. Rojahn differentiated between gingivitis and periodontitis but also

concluded that a dominant mode of inheritance was evident. If a child had the disease, in 87% of the instances a parent was similarly affected. On the other hand, it was reported by Gorlin and associates (1967) that there may be a significant positive relationship between the severity of gingivitis in Japanese children and consanguinity in the parents. As discussed previously, if consanguinity is proved important, recessive genes seem to be implicated.

Studies of periodontal disease in twins are conspicuous by their absence. Reiser and Vogel reported that dizygous twins were more frequently discordant for subgingival calculus deposition than were monozygous twins. This finding may be important, since it points to one of the proposed causes of periodontal disease (calculus formation) and thereby emphasizes a single causative aspect of the disease.

Racial differences can be used as indicators of a genetic basis for certain traits. Such differences in the prevalence of periodontal disease have been suggested; blacks seem to have a higher incidence than whites. This is confirmed in part by findings with a triracial isolated population (black-white-Indian) that has been reported to have a high prevalence of periodontal disease.

In contrast to dental caries, periodontal disease has not had a well-established animal model in which a genetic basis could be demonstrated. Such a model is important for demonstrating both a clear-cut mode of inheritance and disease pathogenesis. However, it seems probable that periodontal disease in its broadest sense will prove to be multifactorial in nature, perhaps with specific subtypes such as periodontosis proving to be simple mendelian traits. Better phenotypic definition through study of pathogenesis of the disease, application to the animal model, and, finally, pedigree studies in humans seems to be the most probable sequence of events leading to an understanding of the hereditary nature of this complex disease.

Papillon-Lefèvre syndrome and familial juvenile periodontitis. Two disorders involving destruction of the periodontium in childhood and

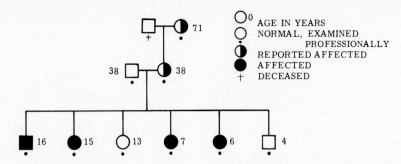

Fig. 22-12. Pedigree of family with juvenile periodontitis, a dominant trait.

early loss of permanent teeth are the heritable traits of Papillon-Lefèvre syndrome and familial juvenile periodontitis. Although uncommon, these disorders are important because they represent a phenotypically uniform type of disease that differs sharply from the common form of periodontal destruction seen in adults that is multifactorial in nature and whose hereditary component is almost certain to be multigenic. Such examples strengthen the idea that within the nonspecific category of periodontal disease are specific, well-defined, single gene–caused diseases.

The synonym of Papillon-Lefèvre syndrome, keratosis palmoplantaris with periodontopathia, is descriptive and highlights the diagnostic features. Early in life, usually between 2 and 4 years of age, affected individuals exhibit reddened, scaly, and rough palms and soles; inflamed gingivae; and horizontal alveolar bone destruction, usually beginning after eruption of the second primary molars. The first two features are directly related to the hyperkeratosis. Once the primary dentition has been shed as a result of the periodontal bone loss, the gingival tissues return to normal until the permanent dentition makes its appearance; the inflammatory and degenerative processes are repeated.

This rare syndrome is inherited as an autosomal recessive trait; typically the parents are unaffected and there is a negative family history for this condition other than the affected individual and possibly some siblings of the individual. Treatment is symptomatic and palliative. Full dentures are usu-

ally worn by the time the individual reaches puberty.

Familial juvenile periodontitis is the other childhood periodontal disease that may be manifested as an inherited trait. In this disease alveolar bone loss is vertical, is more selective than the bone loss of Papillon-Lefèvre syndrome, and occurs principally around the permanent first molars and the central and lateral incisors. Benjamin and Baer have developed diagnostic criteria for this disease. In one young individual of an affected family seen in the Indiana University Dental Genetics Clinic, bone loss was observed around the primary molars and incisors. Those affected with this condition lose their teeth early in life but usually not before young adulthood.

This disease has been frequently observed as a single, isolated instance in a family. Such observations make genetic hypotheses difficult. Fig. 22-12 shows a pedigree with several affected persons in which the mode of inheritance seems to be dominant. The mother gave a history of severe periodontal disease but reported few cavities. Some of her teeth "fell out," and the remaining teeth were removed when she was 27 years old. Similarly, the maternal grandmother was reported to have had periodontal destruction and loss of all teeth in her twenties. Melnick, Shields, and Bixler have performed a segregation analysis of published families and two new ones they have studied. Their results support an X-linked dominant mode of inheritance for the periodontitis phenotype.

In 1980, Saxén carried out a family study of juvenile periodontitis in 31 propositi and their first-degree relatives. Three different genetic analytic approaches were employed. The conclusion from this study is that the published data are compatible with the hypothesis that juvenile periodontitis is inherited in an autosomal recessive mode.

Obviously, these two inherited types of periodontal disease represent wide departures from the more common form in their age of onset, pattern of attack, and severity. It is hoped that detailed study of their pathogenesis will provide insight into the more chronic but treatable form of periodontal disease that is observed in well over half of the adult population.

Genetic aspects of malocclusion

The study of occlusion pertains to relationships between teeth in the same dental arch, as well as between the two dental arches when the teeth come together. Many factors are involved in the definition of normal occlusion, and it is not possible in this chapter to discuss all of them. Some of the most important orofacial parameters of occlusion are (1) the size of the maxilla, (2) the size of the mandible—both ramus and body, (3) the arch form, (4) the anatomy of teeth, including malformations, (5) congenitally missing teeth, and (6) the rotation of teeth.

All of these are important elements that must be included in the concept of occlusion. Most important for our purposes, all have been described as having a genetic background. Soft tissues have not been included in this list, but clearly they also play a significant role in developing the occlusal pattern.

Malocclusion is perhaps somewhat easier to define. One may simply say that malocclusion is a significant deviation from normal occlusion. However, this description is useful only if one considers the multiple factors or polygenic nature implicit in such a definition of malocclusion. In any case, it must be emphasized that the concepts of normal occlusion and malocclusion are dynamic and involve interrelationships of many factors, not a few of which have been shown to be heritable traits.

Dental anthropologists tell us that malocclusions are uncommon in pure racial stocks. In the Philippine Islands, for example, malocclusion is almost nonexistent. Population groups that are genetically homogeneous tend to have ''normal'' occlusion; however, in populations that are mixtures of different racial strains the incidence of jaw discrepancies and occlusal disharmonies is significantly greater. This latter point has been demonstrated in the experiments of Stockard and associates in which an animal model was used. They produced gross orofacial deformities in dogs by crossbreeding different inbred strains. It seems probable that racial crossbreeding in humans may resemble the conditions of these experiments and may result in an increase of orofacial malrelations.

In a previous section the use of twins for the study of inherited traits was discussed. Studies of occlusion in twins have also been made. Lundström made an intensive analysis of specific dentofacial attributes in twins and concluded that heredity played a significant role in determining the following characteristics: (1) tooth size, (2) width and length of the dental arch, (3) height of palate, (4) crowding and spacing of teeth, and (5) degree of overbite. To this list one might well add soft tissue position, conformation, and abnormalities.

Kraus, Wise, and Frei made a cephalometric study of triplets in an attempt to assign specific craniofacial morphologic features to heredity. The authors looked at the lateral profile of the head and cranial vault, the outline of the calvarium, the cranial base, and the facial complex, which included both the upper and lower face and the maxillomandibular relationship. In addition, they selected 17 individual measurements of single portions of a given bone (for example, posterior border of ramus) for comparison in these triplets. Their findings may be summarized by this statement: morphology of an individual bone is under strong genetic control, but the environment plays a major role in determining how various bony elements are combined to achieve a harmonious or disharmonious craniofacial skeleton.

This conclusion offers an explanation for the remarkable differences sometimes seen in the facial patterns of identical twins and emphasizes the important role of environment in their development.

These reports and others that have been reviewed by Kraus and associates indicate the following conclusions:

1. There is a relative conformity of dentofacial patterns within different races.
2. An even greater similarity exists among family members.
3. A high degree of structural similarity is noted in individuals of identical genetic composition (twins and triplets).

Litton and associates have reported Class III malocclusion to be a heritable trait that is probably polygenic in nature. Harris has shown that the craniofacial skeletal patterns of children with Class II malocclusions are heritable and that there is a high resemblance to the skeletal patterns in their siblings. He concluded that the genetic basis for this resemblance is probably polygenic. Interestingly, Harris used the family skeletal patterns as predictors for making a treatment prognosis in the child with a Class II malocclusion.

Thus it seems apparent that occlusion with all of its variable components is a polygenic trait. Thus it is subject to considerable environmental modification, as are all polygenic traits. In a few isolated instances we have specific information about genetic control of specific traits (for example, missing teeth, occlusal patterns, tooth morphology, and even mandibular prognathism), but these are exceptions and we do not obtain sufficient information to make accurate predictions about the development of occlusion simply by studying their appearance in parents. Admittedly, family patterns are frequently apparent, but predictions must be made cautiously because of the genetic and environmental variables, which are unknown and difficult to evaluate. Noyes has stated that even if he knew a particular malocclusion to be of genetic cause, he still would not alter his orthodontic treatment plan because orthodontic treatment does not change the fundamental architecture of the face. The long-range goal of orthodontic treatment, then, would appear to be to permit the face to grow

according to its fundamental pattern with minimum obstruction from environmental influences, habits, and functional pathologic factors, which may work against achievement of the individual's full genetic endowment.

Genetic aspects of cleft lip and palate

Less than one fourth of all cases of cleft lip and palate are multiple occurrences in near relatives of a single family. That is, they are familial cases. The remainder are isolated instances that do not show familial predisposition. Studies of the cleft lip and palate phenotype in twins indicate that monozygous twins have about 40% concordance, whereas dizygous twins show only a 5% concordance. These two pieces of information give strong evidence for a hereditary basis for the cleft lip and palate trait. Despite numerous extensive investigations, however, no simple mendelian pattern of inheritance is readily apparent. This has led to the proposal by different authors of a variety of genetic modes of inheritance including dominance, recessiveness, sex linkage, and various modifying conditions such as incomplete penetrance and variable expressivity. There are two important reasons for this confusing situation: (1) Some of the occurrences are, in fact, nongenetic and thus should not be included in a genetic analysis; unfortunately, these cases are seldom clearly recognized and are difficult to prove. (2) There is a failure to recognize individuals who carry genes for clefting but are not cleft themselves. Such is the present status of the hereditary aspects of cleft lip and palate.

In spite of these problems, however, recurrence risk figures have been assembled by several investigators and these are in close agreement. They provide the genetic counselor with the necessary information for enquiring parents. The following statements represent a summary of current thought concerning the hereditary basis for cleft lip and palate:

1. Cleft lip either with or without cleft palate (designated CL ± CP) is a different entity from isolated cleft palate (designated CP). The latter clefting entity has a different embryologic history and developmental timing, and it appears to be

more susceptible to induction by environmental teratogens.

2. At least three subgroups of clefts can be defined for both entities, CL ± CP and CP: syndromes with clefts, nonsyndromic sporadic cases, and nonsyndromic familial cases. Let us consider each briefly.

Syndromes with clefts. These are cases of children who have clefts plus other major and minor malformations that collectively comprise a syndrome. Well-known examples are the Pierre Robin and Treacher Collins syndromes. Inheritance patterns for syndromes vary from nonheritable forms (such as frontonasal dysplasia) to chromosome defects (trisomy 13) and to monogenic traits (van der Woude syndrome). All children with multiple malformations should be considered as having a possible syndrome, and its specific designation should be sought in syndrome texts to learn its heritability.

Nonsyndromic sporadic cases. These are isolated occurrences of clefts without other malformations. There is reason to believe that most of these cases are the result of gene-environment interaction and therefore will have little chance to recur in the family. Several intrauterine conditions and drugs are known to predispose to clefts; thus maternal history becomes important for these cases.

Nonsyndromic familial cases. These familial cases of clefts have a high heritability, and although they make up only 10% to 15% of all cleft types, they must be looked for to provide the correct genetic counseling. Inheritance appears to be dominant with incomplete penetrance.

3. To overcome the discrepancies in the CL ± CP genetic hypotheses, several workers have attempted to demonstrate that the proposed gene for this trait has variable expression, showing itself in one person as a cleft and in another as a soft or hard tissue discrepancy, but not a cleft, in the clefting area. Such discrepancies have been termed "microforms" or incomplete manifestations of gene action. Pits of the lip, raphe of lip, asymmetric nasal shape, missing or pegged maxillary lateral incisors, bifid uvula, and many others have been proposed to be microforms. Even ocular hypertelorism, which is frequently seen in cleft lip and palate patients, has been suggested as a microform of gene expression.

A fundamental approach to the study of any human hereditary problem is concerned with identifying individuals in a population who carry a gene for a given affliction but who do *not* clearly demonstrate the typical phenotype for that gene (designated nonpenetrance). This statement correctly implies the great importance of phenotypic definition in such genetic studies. The cleft lip and palate problem provides a perfect example. When incomplete manifestations of gene action such as those described are used as evidence for a clefting gene in families, autosomal dominance with decreased penetrance is a reasonable genetic hypothesis for CL ± CP.

4. Recurrence risks for cleft lip and palate have been reported in which microforms are not considered. These data are frequently used by genetic counselors and represent the population mixture of all three groups of clefts presented in No. 2 on this page. Thus they are *average* risk figures. They are summarized in Table 22-2.

These data show that the recurrence risk for either CL ± CP or CP is low when the parent has the condition (column 2) or when a sibling is already affected (column 1). Note that in the absence of any other affected individuals in the family, these cases might be classified sporadic (or nongenetic) and therefore have a recurrence risk equal to that of the general population, which is less than 2% for clefts. Column 3 must be classified as the familial cases, since there are at least two affected persons among the near relatives. In a recent review of the genetics of cleft lip and cleft palate, Bixler (1981) noted that three subgroups of CL ± CP and CP can be recognized. These are designated as (1) syndromic, (2) isolated, and (3) familial. Excluding the small proportion of syndromic cases of clefting, since they have multiple and varied causes, good evidence suggests that the sporadic (single) cases of CL ± CP and CP are etiologically different from the familial (multiple) ones. This indicates that geneticists should no longer pool population cleft data on recurrence

Table 22-2. Recurrence risks for cleft lip with or without cleft palate (CL ± CP) and isolated cleft palate (CP)

	Mating type		
	□—○ → ■ ?	■—○ → ?	□—● → ● ?
Fogh-Andersen			
CL ± CP	4%	2%	14%
CP*	12%	7%	17%
Curtis and Walker			
CL ± CP	4%	4%	19%
CP*	2%	6%	14%
Curtis, Fraser, and Warburton			
CL ± CP	4%	—	17%
CP*	7%	—	15%

*Isolated cleft palate data were obtained from families with cleft individuals, in addition to the immediate family unit.

risks to provide genetic counseling, as is illustrated in Table 22-2. If the parent is a sporadic case in the family, instead of providing an overall 4% to 5% recurrence risk for that parent's next child, the recurrence risk is about 0.1%. If other family members are also affected, this represents a familial case and the recurrence risk is as high as 16%. Resolution of this counseling problem will come only when genetic marker studies are done on biochemical traits under known genetic control that are either linked to or closely associated with clefting. At several institutions in the United States studies are already in progress that are looking for such a linkage relationship between the major histocompatibility complex (HLA) and CL ± CP and CP. If a linkage is found, such a biochemical marker would greatly reduce genetic counseling problems in this area.

These data make the point that both clefting traits have a strong hereditary component that does not appear to conform with simple mendelian modes of inheritance. The reason for this is unclear but is partly the result of failure of genetic investigators and counselors to identify the three subgroups of each cleft type (see No. 2 on p. 636), to analyze data based on that classification, and then to provide the counseling on that basis.

Genetic counseling

Information about heredity, all too often incorrect, has been provided for families with children showing unusual congenital defects since the development of communication. The advice of friends, enemies, and neighbors in many instances has been effective in altering reproductive behavior of the family in question. Although such ill-founded advice has a precedent in time, in our modern society we like to believe that enlightened attitudes and accurate information will avoid such mystical approaches to science. Since advice about heredity will inevitably be sought and given, it would seem that the professional geneticist is in a better position to give it than even one's best friend. This brings us to the consideration of the requirements for a counselor in hereditary problems.

First of all, this person must have a working knowledge of human genetics. Genetic modes of inheritance, gene interaction in families and human populations, and chromosomal abnormalities with all of their consequences are a few of the important subjects to be comprehended by the genetic counselor. With this armamentarium, facts and figures can be sorted out and presented intelligently to the people being counseled.

The second and perhaps equally important requirement for a genetic counselor is a deep respect for the attitudes, sensitivities, and reactions of the people being counseled. It is not enough to make a diagnosis and then lay out the bare facts of the problem. Admittedly, such facts are usually presented in some detail and are only rarely withheld, but the framework in which they are presented is very important. Only when the counselor knows that the facts are understood and are not being distorted by the patients—either consciously or unconsciously—can he or she assume that a service is being done. Feelings of guilt, fear, hostility, and resentment are frequently encountered at the counseling table. A mother of a newborn child with a cleft lip and palate may suddenly find herself rejected by her husband when he retrospectively discovers that her great-uncle Charlie was similarly afflicted. This husband may come to the counselor convinced that a ''bad gene'' present on his wife's side of the family has been concealed from him. Only after a careful discussion of the nongenetic causes of cleft lip and palate, the frequent failure of individuals who carry genetic traits to show them, and the prospective or empiric risks of two normal parents having children afflicted with any congenital abnormality can the genetic counselor finally communicate the nature of the problem to the clients. All this must be couched in tact and sensitivity, for perhaps in no other area of human existence do we feel so personally responsible as in the area of conception and childbearing.

Finally, the genetic counselor must have a sincere desire to teach the truth to the full extent that it is known. By careful attention to responses, the feedback necessary for evaluation of success in communication can be obtained, a technique used by all good teachers.

Genetic defects affecting the teeth frequently carry social stigmata. Instances are known in which tooth defects such as dentinogenesis imperfecta and amelogenesis imperfecta have caused young girls to avoid dating and marriage and even to deliberately suppress all smiles, with the consequence of greatly hampered personality development. Nothing illustrates the feelings of guilt for such an inherited defect as dramatically as the case of a mother whose daughter had suffered through high school with a severe disfiguring enamel defect. This defect was known in the family to be an inherited type. The daughter, after having her teeth removed, married and had a son whom she and her mother brought to the Indiana University Dental Genetics Clinic for examination and genetic counseling. At the onset the grandmother made it clear that her desire was to have her grandson sterilized if examination proved him to have teeth like his mother's. Her irrational comment was, ''I won't go through that again!'' Unfortunately, such emotional, illogical reactions are not rare. Dental treatment offers much for such individuals; at least emotional torment resulting from unacceptable appearance can be avoided. *Nevertheless,* the genetic counselor must be sure that individuals affected with the hereditary conditions completely understand their risks for having similarly affected children. The decision on whether to have children is a practical consideration for the parents and should be reached only after carefully weighing the information supplied by the counselor. This decision is *not* in the realm of the genetic counselor, and the counselor should refrain from giving either positive or negative influences.

The question can be asked, ''Is the dentist equipped to give genetic counsel?'' Under certain conditions the dentist may function adequately as a genetic counselor. The dentist must first be sure of the diagnosis. Incorrect diagnosis can only lead to incorrect and, at best, inadequate genetic counsel. Second, the dentist must have information as to the hereditary aspects of the condition in question. Table 22-3 has been constructed to give the dentist specific genetic information about the more common oral conditions seen in children.

Finally, the dentist must be able to communicate this information in its proper perspective to the patient. Undoubtedly, the general practitioner functions daily in this role but perhaps is not cognizant of it. Parents frequently comment that their child's susceptibility to tooth decay is not unexpected since their own teeth were similarly af-

Table 22-3. Some genetic traits associated with the dento-oro-facial complex and their modes of inheritance

Genetic trait	Frequency in population	Mode of inheritance*
Amelogenesis imperfecta, hypocalcification type	1:20,000	AD
Amelogenesis imperfecta, local hypocalcification type	1:40,000	AD
Amelogenesis imperfecta, hypoplastic type	1:40,000	SLD
Amelogenesis imperfecta, hypomaturation type	1:40,000	SLR
Ankyloglossia	1:300	Familial (AD?)
Bifid nose (median cleft face)	Rare	?
Bifid or cleft uvula	1:100 white	AD
	10:100 Indian, Japanese	
Cleft, median alveolar and diastema	Rare	?
Cleft lip with or without cleft palate	1:800 white	Familial (polygenic)
	1:500 Japanese	
	1:2500 black	
Cleft palate alone	1:2500 white	Familial (AD)
Darier disease (keratosis follicularis)	Rare	AD
Dentinogenesis imperfecta, Types I-III	1:8000	AD
Dentin dysplasia, Types I-III	1:50,000	AD
Ectodermal dysplasia (hypohidrotic)	Rare	SLR
Fibrous dysplasia of jaws (cherubism)	Rare	AD
Freckles (ephelis), susceptibility to	1:10	AD
Gingival fibromatosis, hereditary	Uncommon	AD
Glossitis, median rhomboid	1:500	?
Hereditary hemorrhagic telangiectasia	1:50,000	AD
Hereditary macrocheilia	Prevalent in blacks; uncommon in whites	AD
Hypertrichosis	Rare	AD
Hypodontia of primary dentition (usually mandibular incisor)	1:1000	Polygenic?
Hypodontia of permanent dentition	Common	Familial (polygenic)
Hypophosphatasia	Uncommon	AR, AD
Ichthyosis vulgaris	Rare	SLR
Lip, commissural pits of	1:50	AD
Lip, lower, pits and fistulas of	1:25,000	AD
Maxillary lateral incisors	1:20	D
Micrognathia	1:500	?(familial)
Missing premolars	1:10	D
Missing third molars	1:4	D
Mucosa, white folded dysplasia of	Rare	AD
Rickets, vitamin D–resistant	1:20,000	SLD
Taurodontism	Rare in whites; common in Eskimos, Indians, and South African natives	Familial
Teeth, fused (gemination)	1:500	AD
Tongue, fissured	1:10 (mild cases)	?
Tongue, geographic	1:50	Familial
Tongue, scrotal	As high as 1:5	AD
Torus mandibularis	1:20	AD
Torus palatinus	As high as 1:4	AD

*AD, autosomal dominant; AR, autosomal recessive; SLD, sex-linked dominant; SLR, sex-linked recessive; D, dominant.

fected. In this instance, the dentist must be careful to differentiate the *familial* problem, with all of its environmental ramifications, from the *hereditary* one. Only a sound knowledge of the cause of dental decay, as well as those heritable traits that may modify it, will prevent the dentist from perpetuating erroneous concepts.

Correction of erroneous ideas is not the only area in which the dentist may function as a genetic counselor. Not infrequently, parents are concerned about certain dentofacial variations or abnormalities and may request specific factual information from the dentist. If a child has a hereditary tooth defect and if the parent is so informed, the typical parent will be concerned about the possibility of having additional, similarly affected children and their oral health prognosis with and without treatment. The individual dentist who is familiar with the condition in question and knows the family well enough to communicate easily with them certainly should do so, since he or she bears the professional responsibility for the oral health of this family. On the other hand, if the slightest doubt exists concerning any of these qualifications, the dentist should refer the family to a genetics clinic, preferably one with a dentist on its staff. A great service can be performed and rapport can be established for future dental treatment when the patient and the patient's family know that extra effort is expended in the interest of their oral health.

REFERENCES

Baer, P.: Personal communciation, 1972.

Benjamin, S.D., and Baer, P.M.: Familial patterns of advanced alveolar bone loss in adolescence (periodontosis), J. Am. Soc. Psychosom. Dent. Med. **5:**82-88, 1967.

Bixler, D.: Genetic counseling in dentistry, J. Dent. Educ. **40:**645-649, 1976.

Bixler, D.: Genetics and clefting, Cleft Palate J. **18:**10-18, 1981.

Bixler, D., Conneally, P.M., and Christen, A.G.: Dentinogenesis imperfecta: genetic variations in a six generation family, J. Dent. Res. **48:**1196-1199, 1968.

Bixler, D., Fogh-Andersen, P., and Conneally, P.M.: Incidence of cleft lip and palate in the offspring of cleft parents, Clin. Genet. **2:**155-159, 1971.

Blumel, J., and Kniker, W.T.: Lawrence-Moon-Bardet-Biedl syndrome, Tex. Rep. Biol. Med. **17:**391-410, 1959.

Böök, J.A., and Grahnén, H.: Clinical and genetical studies of dental caries. II. Parents and sibs of adult highly resistant (caries-free) propositi, Odontol. Rev. **4:**1-53, 1953.

Caldwell, R.C., and Finn, S.B.: Comparisons of the caries experience between identical and fraternal twins and unrelated children, J. Dent. Res. **39:**693-694, 1960.

Coccia, C.T., McDonald, R.E., and Mitchell, D.F.: Papillon-LeFevre syndrome: precocious periodontosis with palmar-plantar hyperkeratosis, J. Periodontol. **37:**408-414, 1966.

Coccia, C.T., Bixler, D., and Conneally, P.M.: Cleft lip and cleft palate: a genetic study, Cleft Palate J. **6:**323-336, 1969.

Curtis, E.J., and Walker, N.F.: Etiological study of cleft lip and cleft palate, The Research Institute of the Hospital for Sick Children, University of Toronto, 1961.

Curtis, E.J., Fraser, F.C., and Warburton, D.: Congenital cleft lip and palate, Am. J. Dis. Child. **102:**853-857, 1961.

Dahlberg, G., and Dahlberg, B.: Über Karies und andere Zahnveränderungen bei Zwillingen, Uppsala Läkerf. Forh. **47:**395-416, 1942.

Dickmann, A.: Die Verebung der Paradentose (dissertation), München, 1935.

Fogh-Andersen, P.: Incidence of harelip and cleft palate, Copenhagen, 1942, Nyt Nordisk Forlag.

Galton, F.: The history of twins as a criterion of the relative powers of nature and nurture, Fraser's Magazine, 1875.

Goodman, H.O. and others: Heritability in dental caries, certain oral microflora and salivary components, Am. J. Hum. Genet. **11:**263-273, 1959.

Gorlin, R.J., Sedano, H., and Anderson, V.E.: The syndrome of palmer-plantar hyperkeratosis and premature periodontal destruction of the teeth—a clinical and genetic analysis of Papillon-LeFevre syndrome, J. Pediatr. **65:**895-908, 1964.

Gorlin, R.J., Stallard, R.E., and Shapiro, B.L.: Genetics and periodontal disease, J. Periodontol. **38:**5-10, 1967.

Grant, R., and Falls, H.F.: Anodontia; report of a case associated with ectodermal dysplasia of the anhidrotic type, Am. J. Orthod. **30:**661-672, 1944.

Green, G.E.: A bacteriolytic agent in salivary globulin of caries-immune human beings, J. Dent. Res. **38:**262-275, 1959.

Green, G.E., and others: A study of the genetics of immunity to human dental caries, Forty-First General Meeting of International Association for Dental Research, Pittsburgh, 1963.

Gustafsson, B.E., and others: Vipeholm dental caries study: the effect of different levels of carbohydrate intake on caries activity in 436 individuals observed for 5 years, Acta Odontol. Scand. **11:**232, 1954.

Harris, J.E.: Genetic factors in the growth of the head: inheritance of the craniofacial complex and malocclusion, Dent. Clin. North Am. **19**(1):151-160, 1975.

Horowitz, S.L., Osborne, R.H., and De George, F.V.: Caries experience in twins, Science **128:**300-301, 1958.

Hunt, H.R., and Hoppert, C.A.: Inheritance of susceptibility to caries in albino rats *(Mus norvegicus)*, J. Am. Coll. Dent. **11**:33-37, 1944.

Hunt, H.R., Hoppert, C.A., and Rosen, S.: Genetic factors in experimental rat caries. In Sognnaes, R.F., editor: Advances in experimental caries research, Washington, D.C., 1955, American Association for the Advancement of Science.

Kallman, F.J.: Twin data in the analysis of mechanisms of inheritance, Am. J. Hum. Genet. **6**:157-162, 1954.

Kerr, C.B., Wells, R.S., and Cooper, K.E.: Gene effect in carriers of anhidrotic ectodermal dysplasia, J. Med. Genet. **3**:169-176, 1966.

Klein, H.: The family and dental disease. IV. Dental disease (D.M.F.) experience in parents and offspring, J.A.D.A. **33**:735-743, 1946.

Klein, H., and Palmer, C.E.: Studies on dental caries. V. Familial resemblance in caries experience in siblings, Public Health Rep. **53**:1353-1364, 1938.

Kraus, B.S., Wise, W.J., and Frei, R.A.: Heredity and the craniofacial complex, Am. J. Orthod. **45**:172-217, 1959.

Lejeune, J., Turpin, R., and Gautier, J.: Le mongolisme: premier exemple d'abérration et autosomique humaine, Ann. Genet. **1**:41-49, 1959.

Litton, S.F. and others: A genetic study of Class III malocclusion, Am. J. Orthod. **58**:565-577, 1970.

Lundström, A.: Tooth size and occlusion in twins, Stockholm, 1948, A.B. Fahlcrantz Boktrycheri.

Mansbridge, J.N.: Hereditary and dental caries, J. Dent. Res. **38**:337-347, 1959.

McKusick, V.A.: Heritable disorders of connective tissue, ed. 4, St. Louis, 1972, The C.V. Mosby Co.

Melnick, M., Shields, E.D. and Bixler, D.: Periodontosis: a phenotypic and genetic analysis, Oral Surg. **42**:32-41, 1976.

Metrakos, J.D., Metrakos, K., and Baxter, H.: Clefts of the lip and palate in twins, including a discordant pair whose monozygosity was confirmed by skin transplants, Plast. Reconstr. Surg. **22**:109-122, 1958.

Moore, G.R.: Hereditary as a guide in dentofacial orthopedics, Am. J. Orthod. **30**:549-554, 1944.

Nishimura, E.T., and others: Carrier state in human acatalasemia, Science **130**:333-334, 1959.

Noyes, H.J.: A review of the genetic influence on malocclusion, Am. J. Orthod. **44**:81-98, 1958.

Osborne, R.H., and De George, F.V.: Genetic basis of morphological variation, Cambridge, Mass., 1959, Harvard University Press.

Rank, B.K., and Thompson, J.A.: Cleft lip and palate in Tasmania, Med. J. Aust. **47**:681-689, 1960.

Reiser, H.E., and Vogel, F.: Über die Erblichkeit der Zahnsteinbildung beim Menschen, Dtsch. Zahnaezrtl. **13**:1355-1358, 1958.

Rojahn, H.: Familienuntersuchungen bei Paradentose (dissertation), Heidelberg, 1952.

Rushton, M.A.: Hereditary enamel defects, Proc. R. Soc. Med. **57**:53-58, 1964.

Saxēn, L.: Heredity of juvenile periodontitis, J. Clin. Periodontol. **7**:276-288, 1980.

Schulze, C., and Lenz, F.: Über Zahnschmelzhypoplasie von unvollständig dominatem geschlectsgebunden Erbgang, Z. Menschl. Vererb. Konstitutionsl. **31**:14-114, 1952.

Singh, A., Jolly, S.S., and Kaur, S.: Hereditary ectodermal dysplasia, Br. J. Dermatol. **74**:34-37, 1962.

Smith, S.M., and Penrose, L.S.: Monozygotic dizygotic twin diagnosis, Ann. Hum. Genet. **19**:289-293, 1955.

Stockard, C.R. and others: The genetic and endocrine basis for differences in form and behavior, Am. Anat. Memoirs 19, 1941.

Takahara, S.: Progressive oral gangrene, probably due to lack of catalase in the blood (acatalasemia): report of nine cases, Lancet **2**:1101-1104, 1952.

Wallace, J.R.: Hereditary dentinogenesis imperfecta, J. Pediatr. **65**:128-130, 1964.

Warren, L.A.: A family study of exceptional resistance to dental caries (thesis), Indianapolis, Indiana University, 1968.

Weinstein, E.D., and Cohen, M.M.: Sex-linked cleft palate: report of a family and review of 77 kindreds, J. Med. Genet. **3**:17-22, 1966.

Weinstein, P.R., and Green, G.E.: Clinical and bacteriological studies of caries-immune human beings, J. Dent. Res. **36**:690-694, 1957.

Witkop, D.J.: Hereditary defects in enamel and dentin, Acta Genet. **7**:236-239, 1957.

23 Dental problems of the handicapped child

THEODORE R. LYNCH
JAMES E. JONES
JAMES A. WEDDELL

A handicapped child is one who has a mental, physical, or social condition that prevents the child from achieving full potential when compared to other children of the same age. Approximately 9 million children and adults in the United States are affected by some form of handicapping condition. Recently the term "disabled" has been used to describe these individuals; it includes all handicapping conditions that a health professional might encounter.

Many disabled children are best managed initially by a multidisciplinary team in which a dentist is available to evaluate intraoral status and to make recommendations for care. A child can then be referred to a dental practitioner whom the family chooses, if a preference is indicated. The initial management by the team can help to prepare the family practitioner to treat the child.

Disabled children present challenges that require special preparation before the dentist and the office staff can provide acceptable care. In addition, parental anxiety concerning the problems associated with a disabled child frequently delays dental care until significant oral disease has developed. Unfortunately, some dentists feel uncomfortable providing treatment for disabled children, which may also result in the loss of a greatly needed service.

The purpose of this chapter is to discuss some of the disabling conditions that a dentist is most likely to encounter in children in a private dental practice.

If a dentist becomes familiar with a child's special needs and with the parents' concerns, the dental management of the child's case can be quite gratifying.

Dental examination

The initial dental examination for a disabled child is not unlike the initial examination described in Chapter 1. Special attention should be given to obtaining a thorough medical and dental history. The names and addresses of medical or dental personnel who have previously treated the patient are necessary for consultation purposes.

The first dental appointment is usually the most important and can "set the stage" for subsequent appointments. As previously noted, parental anxiety about a child's dental treatment may be a significant factor. By scheduling the patient early in the day and by allowing sufficient time to talk with the parents and the patient before initiating any dental care, a practitioner can establish a good relationship with the parents and patient. This initial demonstration of sincere interest in the child often proves beneficial throughout the entire treatment process.

Radiographic examination

Adequate radiographic records are essential in planning dental treatment for a handicapped child. Through appropriate behavior management of the

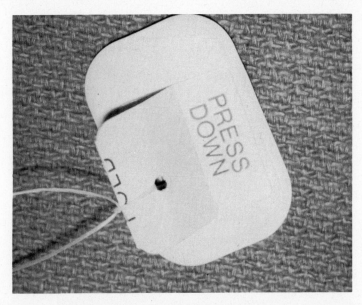

Fig. 23-1. Bite-wing radiograph secured with floss.

child, a dentist can usually perform a complete radiographic examination of the teeth. Occasionally, assistance from the parent or from dental auxiliaries may be necessary to obtain the films. Better cooperation may be elicited from some children by delaying radiographs until the second visit, when they will be more familiar with the dental office and will have found it to be a friendly place.

When possible, a panoramic film, bite-wing and anterior occlusal films, and any necessary periapical radiographs should be made for all new patients. On recall visits, radiographic examination should include bite-wing films at least every 12 months, or at the dentist's discretion, and selected periapical films should be made of any areas that appear suspicious. Intraoral films with bite-wing tabs are used for all bite-wing and periapical radiographs. An 18-inch length of floss is attached through a hole made in the tab, as shown in Fig. 23-1, to facilitate retrieval of the film if it falls toward the pharynx. If the patient cannot remain motionless for a panoramic film, a pedodontic radiographic survey may be made as an alternative.

Regardless of the types of radiographs to be made, the patient should wear a lead apron with a thyroid shield, and anyone who helps to hold the patient and the film steady should wear an apron and gloves lined with lead (Fig. 23-2).

Preventive dentistry

Prevention is the most important consideration in ensuring good dental health for any dental patient. However, an effective preventive dental program is particularly important for a disabled child because of predisposing social, economic, physical, and medical factors that make good dental care harder to obtain even though it is necessary. The dentist should perceive the patient's needs and assume the responsibility for formulating an individual program for the child and adequately communicating to the parents and the patient how such a program can be effected. Because a clear perception of the situation by everyone involved is essential for a successful preventive program, adequate communication is vital.

Home care. The parents (or the guardian) have

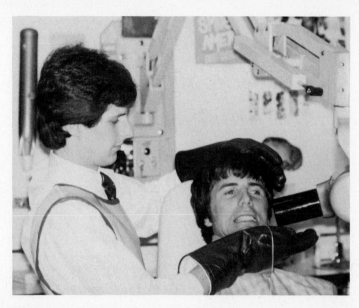

Fig. 23-2. Extra assistance in holding the patient's head steady to prevent movement while a radiograph is being taken.

the initial responsibility for establishing good oral hygiene in the home. Reinforcement of good home dental care is provided through mass media (newspapers, radio, television), communication with other people, and school activities (such as health classes, PTA meetings, and observation of National Dental Health Month). This supplementary support relieves the dentist of the sole responsibility for explaining the need for home dental care and increases the receptivity of the parent and child to such a program.

Home dental care should begin in infancy; the dentist should instruct the parents to gently cleanse the incisors daily with a soft cloth or an infant toothbrush. For older children who are unwilling or physically unable to cooperate, the dentist should teach the parent or guardian correct toothbrushing techniques and positions that safely restrain the child when necessary. Fig. 23-3 shows several positions for toothbrushing that permit firm control and support of the child, adequate visibility, and convenient positioning of the adult, with reason-

able comfort for both. Some of the positions most commonly used for children requiring oral care assistance are as follows:

1. The standing or sitting child is placed in front of the adult so that the adult can cradle the child's head with one hand while using the other hand to brush the teeth.
2. The child reclines on a sofa or bed, with the head angled backward on the parent's lap. Again, the child's head is stabilized with one hand while the teeth are brushed with the other hand.
3. The child's buttocks are placed on one parent's lap, with the child facing that parent, while the child's head and shoulders lie on the other parent's knees, thus allowing the first parent to brush the teeth.

These positions are particularly valuable for children with handicapping conditions. If a child cannot be adequately restrained by one person, then both parents, and perhaps siblings, may be required to complete the home dental care proce-

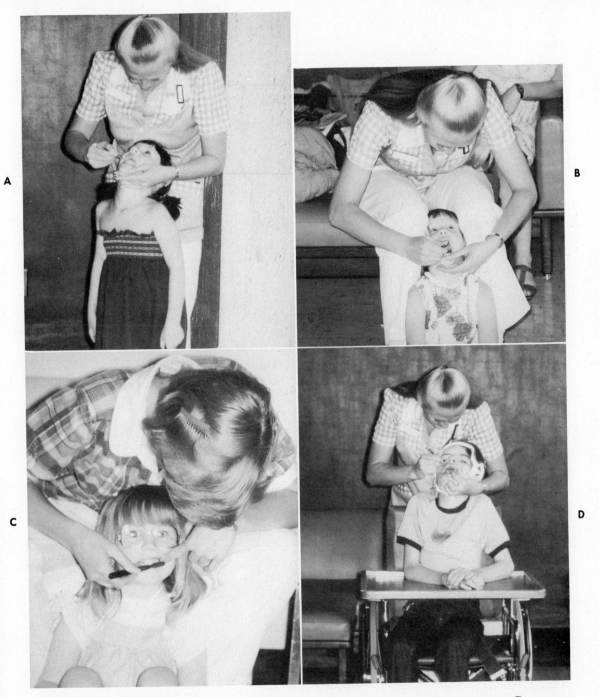

Fig. 23-3. Common positions for plaque removal. **A,** Standing. **B,** Sitting with knee support. **C,** Sitting. **D,** Upright wheelchair.

Continued.

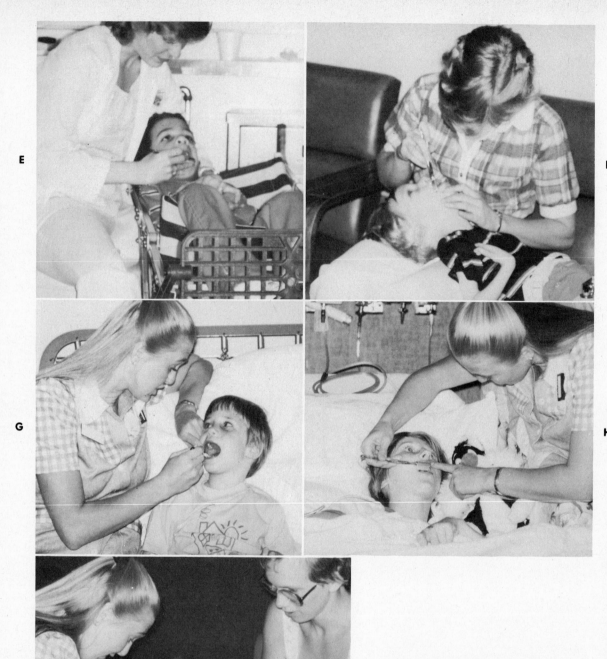

E

F

G

H

I

Fig. 23-3, cont'd. E, Reclining wheelchair. **F,** Reclining on couch. **G,** Raised bed position. **H,** Reclining in bed. **I,** Face-to-face lap position.

dures. If a child is institutionalized, the staff should be instructed in the proper dental care regimen for the child. Wrapped tongue blades may be of benefit in helping to keep a child's mouth open while plaque is being removed.

Some parents and health care centers have encouraged handicapped children to assume the responsibility for their own oral hygiene, but the results are usually poor. Parents should be cognizant of the fact that unsupervised oral hygiene procedures in handicapped or very young children can have serious dental consequences. The amount of supervision and assistance provided by the parents should depend on the child's willingness to cooperate and ability to maintain good oral hygiene.

The brushing technique for handicapped patients should be effective and yet simple for the individual performing the brushing. One technique often recommended is the horizontal scrub method because it is easy and can yield good results. This technique consists of gentle horizontal strokes on cheek, tongue, and biting surfaces of all teeth and gums. A soft, multitufted nylon brush should be used.

Fig. 23-4 illustrates various grips that may be added to a toothbrush to help persons with poor fine motor skills to grasp the brush more firmly. While many types of grips are available, using the patient's hand to custom-design a handle has often had good results (Fig. 23-5). Electric toothbrushes have also been used effectively by handicapped children, but their use does not necessarily result in better plaque removal than manual brushes.

The plaque control program developed by the dental services program at James Whitcomb Riley Hospital for Children, in Indianapolis, can be used at home by patients and parents. The Riley Plaque Score (RPS) provides a method for determining the level of success achieved by the patient in removing dental plaque (Fig. 23-6). The dentist can introduce the RPS to the parents and the patient by giving them a question-and-answer handout that explains dental terminology and the necessity for plaque removal. The parents are shown how to apply a pink disclosing solution to the child's teeth

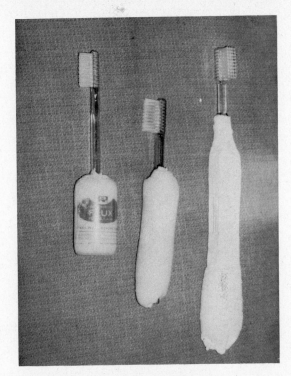

Fig. 23-4. Toothbrush handles.

and instructed in the use of a small, disposable mouth mirror and an ordinary flashlight to examine all areas of the mouth. The RPS is then determined according to the amount of pink stain on the teeth. If a tooth being scored is without plaque (white), the score is 0. If the cervical third of the tooth contains plaque (pink), the score is 1. If half or more of the tooth is pink, the score is 2. If the entire crown is covered with plaque, the score is 3. To complete the plaque score, six teeth that are likely to demonstrate plaque formation are selected from six different areas of the mouth—the upper and lower right and left posterior segments and the upper and lower anterior segments. The sum of the scores from the six teeth is the child's RPS. Clinical records at Riley Hospital indicate that children whose RPS is 3 or below have fewer carious lesions and soft tissue problems than those whose RPS is above 3. The RPS and similar evaluation

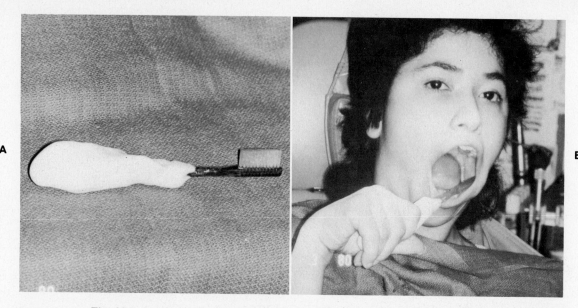

Fig. 23-5. A, Custom-designed acrylic handle. **B,** Patient using the custom handle.

tools are quite effective in helping handicapped children and their parents maintain adequate oral hygiene.

Diet and nutrition. Diet and nutrition influence dental caries by affecting the type and virulence of the microorganisms in dental plaque, the resistance of teeth and supporting structures, and the properties of saliva in the oral cavity. A proper diet, as outlined in Chapter 16, is essential to a good preventive program for a handicapped child. As discussed in Chapter 7, the diet should be assessed by reviewing a diet survey with the parent, realizing that allowances must be made for certain conditions that require dietary modifications. For example, conditions associated with difficulty in swallowing, such as severe cerebral palsy, may require the patient to be on a pureed diet. Patients with certain metabolic disturbances or syndromes, such as phenylketonuria (PKU), diabetes, or Prader-Willi syndrome, will have diets that restrict specific foods or total caloric consumption. Whatever the special circumstances, any dietary recommendations should be made on an individual basis after

proper consultation with the patient's primary physician or dietitian. Particular emphasis should be placed on discontinuation of the bottle by 12 months of age and cessation of at-will nursing after teeth begin to erupt, to decrease the likelihood of caries.

Fluoride therapy. The judicious use of fluoride supplements, which are effective agents in reducing the incidence of dental decay, is very important in the comprehensive management of any dental patient. Special emphasis should be placed on ensuring adequate systemic fluoride for a disabled patient. The dentist should first determine the concentration of fluoride in the patient's daily water supply. If the level of fluoride is between 0.7 and 1 ppm, no supplementation is normally required. A dentifrice containing a therapeutic fluoride compound should be used daily. Some clinicians who treat disabled patients having chronically poor oral hygiene and high decay rates suggest a daily rinsing regimen with 0.05% sodium fluoride (NaF) solution. In certain cases, chewing a 2.2-mg NaF tablet (1 mg fluoride) or a 1.1-mg NaF tablet is

RILEY PLAQUE SCORE

PATIENT'S NAME _____ DATE _____

PURPOSE (Why we do a RPS?)
1. To measure the amount of plaque present in your mouth
2. To determine and evaluate your oral hygiene status at any specific time

MATERIAL (What do we need to do a RPS?)
1. Trace (or a similar staining and disclosing aid)
2. A mirror (preferably a small mouth mirror)
3. A light source (flashlight or penlight)

INSTRUCTIONS (How do we do a RPS?)
1. Put 4-5 drops of Trace under or on your tongue.
2. Sip some water and swish the Trace all around.
3. Be sure to cover every tooth in your mouth with the red solution.
4. With a mirror and light source, check for red areas.
5. Remove the red areas (plaque) with your brush and floss as you were shown.
6. Restain with Trace and reexamine.
7. Brush and floss until all plaque is removed.

GRADING SCALE

0	1	2	3
No plaque	1/3	2/3	All covered

YOUR SCORE

Upper back tooth right side	Upper front tooth	Upper back tooth left side
Lower back tooth right side	Lower front tooth	Lower back tooth left side

TOTAL SCORE:

_____ 0-3—VERY GOOD!!
_____ 4-7—Good
_____ 8-11—Average; work harder
_____ 12-18—Not adequate to prevent
            cavities and gum infections

GRADE:

COMMENTS: _____

Thanks for your help.   RILEY HOSPITAL DENTAL CLINIC

See you next visit!   Dental Health Educator _____

Fig. 23-6

recommended daily to provide both topical and systemic effects, although a mild mottling of the teeth may occur in a young patient who also ingests fluoridated water. In most instances the benefits of a reduction in decay are far more significant than the mild fluoride mottling that may result.

If the dentist is not sure of the fluoride level of the patient's drinking water, an analysis to determine the level is indicated. Most state health departments have facilities available to determine the level of fluoride in water. Once the level has been documented, a determination of the need for fluoride supplementation can be made. The amount of systemic fluoride supplementation necessary, along with the various forms available (drops, tablets, rinses), is outlined in Chapter 7. Whether the patient lives in a fluoridated area or a non-fluoridated area, a topical fluoride should be applied after a semiannual professional prophylaxis.

Regular professional supervision. Close observation of susceptible patients and regular dental examinations are important in the treatment of disabled patients. Although most patients are seen semiannually for professional prophylaxis, examination, and topical fluoride application, certain patients can benefit from examinations every 3 to 4 months. This is particularly true of patients who are confined to institutions in which dental health programs are inadequate.

Management of a handicapped child during dental treatment

The previously mentioned principles of behavior management (Chapter 2) are even more important in treating a handicapped child. Since hospital visits or previous appointments with a physician frequently result in the development of apprehension in the patient, additional time with the parent and the child is needed to establish rapport and dispel the child's anxiety. If patient cooperation cannot be obtained, the dentist must consider alternatives such as physical restraints and premedication to perform necessary dental procedures.

Physical restraint. Although the benefits and importance of physical restraints have been documented, one should keep in mind that the use of premedication, as discussed in Chapter 10, can reduce the amount of physical restraint required. Physical restraint is only one means of behavior control to achieve an adequate level of dental treatment. Parents must, of course, be informed and give consent before the use of physical restraints. They should have a clear understanding of the type of restraints used and the reason for their use. In many cases, during the initial examination and conference with the parents, the use of restraints should be included in the explanation of the overall management approach for the child.

Physical restraint is a useful and effective way to facilitate the delivery of dental care for patients who need help controlling their extremities, such as infants and patients with certain neuromuscular disorders. Physical restraint is also useful for managing extremely resistant patients who need dental care but who are not candidates for general anesthesia. The dentist may choose to use a simple restraint or combined restraints to manage severely handicapped patients. Common mechanical aids for maintaining the mouth in an open position are shown in Fig. 23-7.

Padded and wrapped tongue blades are easy to use, disposable, and very inexpensive. Frequently, parents of a handicapped child are given such tongue blades to aid with home dental care. The Molt Mouth Prop* can be vital in the management of a difficult patient for a prolonged period. It is made in both adult and children's sizes, allows accessibility to the opposite side of the mouth, and operates on a reverse scissor action. Its disadvantages include its expense and the possibility of lip and palatal lacerations as well as luxation of teeth if it is not used correctly. Caution must be exercised to prevent injury to the patient, and the prop should not be allowed to rest on anterior teeth. The patient's mouth should not be forced open beyond its natural limits because of discomfort and a tendency of the patient to panic, which would result in

---

*H-U Friedy, Chicago, Ill. 60618.

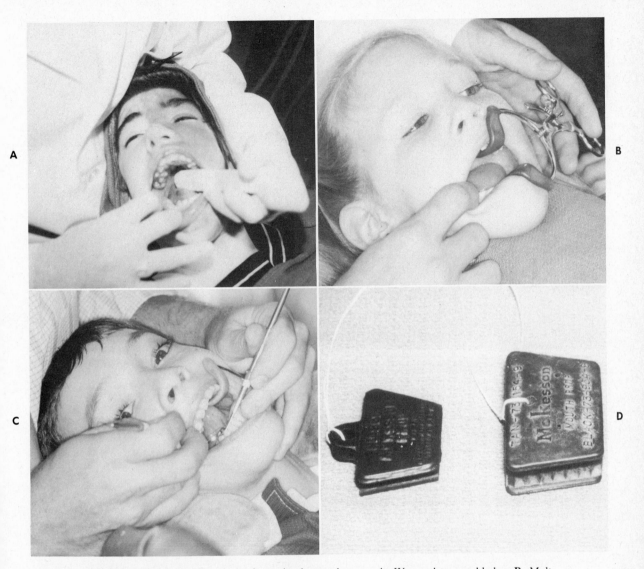

Fig. 23-7. Physical aids to keep the patient's mouth open. **A,** Wrapped tongue blades. **B,** Molt Mouth Prop being inserted. **C,** Molt Mouth Prop in proper position. **D,** McKesson bite blocks.

further patient resistance and might also compromise the patient's airway.

A finger splint, or interocclusal thimble, which also prevents mouth closure, is inexpensive and fits on the dentist's finger (see Fig. 1-13). Its main disadvantage is limited mobility of the dentist's hand once the splint is in place and functioning. Rubber bite blocks* can be purchased in various sizes to fit on the occlusal surfaces of the teeth and stabilize the mouth in an open position. The bite blocks should have floss or string attached for easy retrieval if they become dislodged in the mouth.

---

*McKesson Co., Moncks Corner, S.C. 29461.

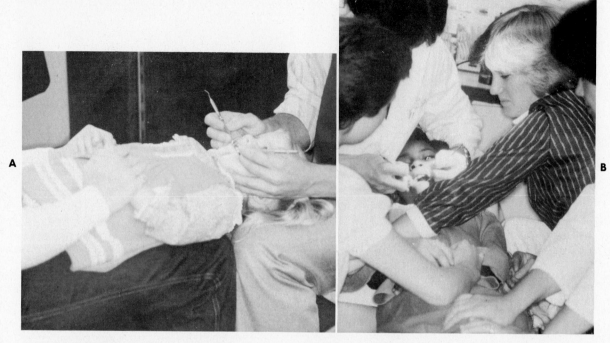

Fig. 23-8. Assistance for physical restraint. **A,** Parental aid during an examination. **B,** Additional assistance during the dental procedure.

Body control is gained through a variety of methods and techniques. For severely retarded or very young children, parents and dental assistants can assist in the control of movements during dental procedures, as shown in Fig. 23-8. Usually, however, for the severely retarded, better working conditions and a more predictable patient response are obtained through the use of body restraints.

The following are some commonly used physical restraints:

Body
Pedi-Wrap
Papoose Board
Triangular sheet
Safety belt
Extra assistant
Extremities
Straps
Towel and tape
Extra assistant

Head
Head positioner
Extra assistant
Forearm-body support

The Papoose Board* (Fig. 23-9) has several advantages. Simple to store and use, it is available in sizes to hold both large and small children. It has attached head stabilizers and is reusable. However, it does not fit the contours of a dental chair (a homemade pillow is needed). Since it covers the patient's diaphragm, a stethoscope is necessary to monitor respiration during premedication appointments. An extremely resistant patient may develop hyperthermia if restrained too long, and of course any restrained patient requires constant attendance and supervision.

Mink describes the bed sheet technique (triangular sheet) and its use in controlling an extremely

---

*Olympic Medical Corp., Seattle, Wash. 98108.

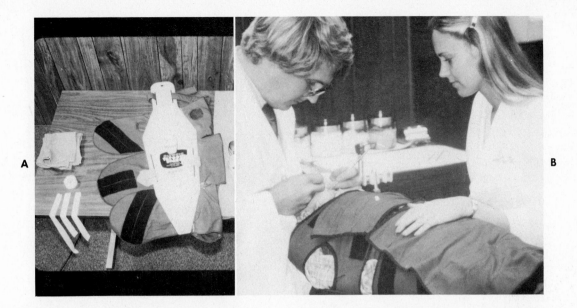

Fig. 23-9. A, The Olympic Papoose Board. **B,** Papoose Board in use.

resistant child. It is inexpensive and allows the patient to sit upright during radiographic examinations. Its disadvantages include the frequent need for straps to maintain the patient's position in the chair, the difficulty of its use on small patients, and the possibility of airway impingement should the patient slip downward unnoticed. Hyperthermia may be another problem during long periods of restraint. Again, the need for constant supervision is emphasized so that these problems may be avoided.

The Pedi-Wrap* (Fig. 23-10), which does not have head supports or a backboard, also comes in various sizes, allows some movement while still confining the patient, and, because of its mesh-net fabric, permits better ventilation, lessening the chances of the patient developing hyperthermia. Although it is expensive, it costs less than the Papoose Board. It, too, requires straps to maintain body position in the dental chair and constant supervision to prevent the patient from rolling out of the chair.

A patient's head position can usually be successfully maintained through the use of forearm-body pressure by the dentist (Fig. 23-11). Other options include an additional assistant to stabilize the child's head, head positioners (for example, the Papoose Board), or a plastic bowl (doggie bowl) to provide position guidance.

The child's arms and legs can be immobilized with help from the parent or the dental assistant, with Posey straps,* or with a towel combined with adhesive tape (Fig. 23-12). If movement of the extremities is the only problem, having a dental assistant restrain the child is very helpful. Posey straps are inexpensive, fasten to the arms of the dental chair, and allow limited movement of the patient's forearm and hand. This limited movement frequently prevents overreaction by resistant or retarded patients. A towel, wrapped around the patient's forearms and fastened with adhesive tape (without impeding circulation), is often helpful for an athetoid-spastic cerebral palsy patient, who tries desperately but without success to control body

---

*Clark Associates, Charlton City, Mass. 01508.

*Posey Co., Pasadena, Calif. 91107.

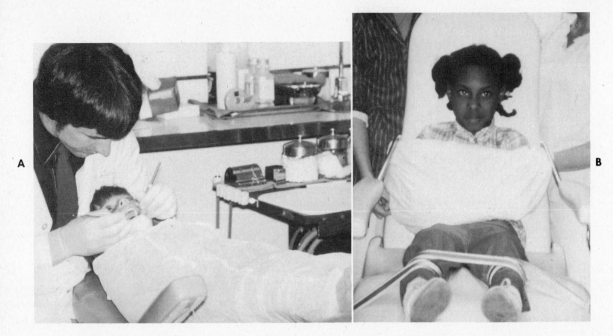

Fig. 23-10. Physical restraints for control of body and extremities. **A,** Patient in a Pedi-Wrap restraint. **B,** Patient confined in a triangular sheet with leg straps.

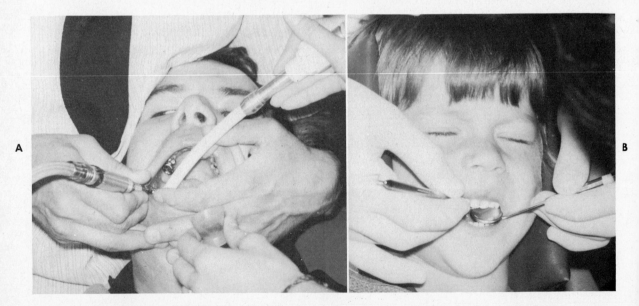

Fig. 23-11. Physical aids for head stabilization. **A,** Proper positioning of the dentist's hands, forearm, and body. **B,** Use of the Papoose Board head restraint.

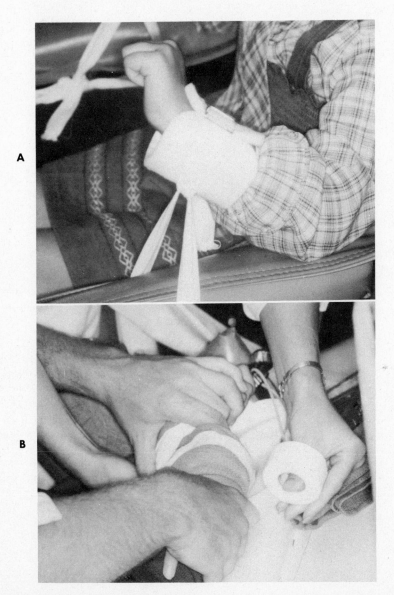

Fig. 23-12. Physical restraints for the extremities. **A,** Posey strap on wrist. **B,** Towel and tape on forearm.

movements. Such restraints actually encourage relaxation and prevent undesired reflexes by keeping the patient's arms in the midline of the body.

Physical restraints should never be used as punishment. An explanation of their benefits should be presented by the dentist before their use, if communication with the patient is possible. The mouth prop can be identified as a "tooth chair," the Pedi-Wrap as a "safety robe," or a restraining strap as a "safety belt," allowing the patient to feel secure rather than threatened. A careful explanation should be given to the parents about how physical restraints allow the needed dental work to be done while minimizing the possibility of accidental injury to the patient. If a child requires extensive dental treatment and cooperation cannot be achieved by routine psychologic, physical, or pharmaco-

logic measures, the use of general anesthesia in a controlled atmosphere, as discussed in Chapter 11, is recommended.

Mental retardation

Mental retardation is a general term applied to persons whose intellectual development is significantly lower than that of normal individuals and whose ability to adapt to their environment is consequently limited. The condition varies in severity and etiology. A classification of mental retardation is presented in Table 23-1. Mental retardation has been identified in approximately 3% of the U.S. population. For many years the potential abilities of the intellectually handicapped were poorly understood, and they were often treated as inferior individuals. They were described with the terms

Table 23-1. Classification of mentally retarded persons

| Degree of mental retardation | IQ | | School classification | Communication | Special requirements for dental care |
	SB*	WISC-R†			
Mild	67-52	69-55	Educable mentally retarded (EMR)	Should be able to speak well enough for most communication needs	Treat as normal child, mild sedation or nitrous oxide–oxygen analgesia may be beneficial
Moderate	51-36	54-40	Trainable mentally retarded (TMR)	Vocabulary and language skills such that the child can communicate at a basic level with others	Mild to moderate sedation may be beneficial; restraints and positive reinforcement; general anesthesia may be indicated in severe, generalized dental decay
Severe or profound	35 and below	39 and below	Nontrainable	Mute or communicates in grunts; little or no communication skills	Same as for moderately retarded

*Stanford-Binet General Intelligence Test
†Wechsler Intelligence Scale For Children—Revised

"idiot" (IQ below 25), "imbecile" (IQ of 25 to 50), and "moron" (IQ of 50 to 70). With the formation, in 1968, of the President's Committee on Mental Retardation, emphasis was placed on education of the mentally retarded to increase their social and civic responsibilities, motor skills, and independence within society. Attitudes toward the mentally retarded are now becoming more favorable.

Although a child who scores 2 standard deviations below the mean on the Stanford-Binet (SB) test or the Wechsler Intelligence Scale for Children—Revised (WISC-R) may have some degree of retardation, individuals are not usually classified as retarded on the basis of IQ alone. An individual who demonstrates both social incompetence and intellectual deficiency is considered mentally retarded.

A mildly retarded child is one who, because of low intelligence, cannot derive full benefit from regular education. In the academic environment these children are classified as educable mentally retarded (EMR). Educational programs for such children are generally simplified versions of regular school programs and usually lead to literacy and attainment of skills necessary for employment. Most children in this group, which accounts for approximately 80% of all mentally retarded individuals, will function acceptably as adults.

Children who are capable of some education and partial independence but who are not expected to experience full independence as adults are classified as moderately mentally retarded. Educational programs for such children, who are known as trainable mentally retarded (TMR), usually focus on basic skills. Classrooms are often designed and furnished like a home, and the curriculum includes dressing, grooming, cooking, table setting, feeding, and cleaning. It is hoped that these individuals will be able to take care of their own needs while usually living within a sheltered atmosphere with trained personnel who will help them with problems that they may not be able to cope with on their own.

A severely or profoundly retarded child often is not trainable and requires constant supervision by trained support personnel. These individuals are often confined to institutions because of their special needs. In recent years programs have been initiated in many institutions to facilitate language acquisition in children with IQ scores of 35 and under. Many individuals who were previously mute or communicated only in grunts are now acquiring first approximations of words. Their social behavior has also shown improvement.

Dental treatment of a mentally retarded person. Providing dental treatment for a mentally retarded individual requires adjusting to social, intellectual, and emotional immaturity. A short attention span, restlessness, hyperactivity, and erratic emotional behavior characterize mentally retarded patients undergoing dental care. The dentist should assess the degree of mental retardation by consulting the patient's physician or the staff of the institution if the patient does not live with the parents.

The following procedures have proved beneficial in establishing dentist-patient rapport and reducing the patient's anxiety about dental care:

1. Give a brief tour of the office before attempting treatment. Introduce the patient to the office staff. This will familiarize the patient with the personnel and office design and reduce the patient's fear of the "unknown."
2. Speak slowly and in simple terms. Make sure explanations are understood by asking the patient if there are any questions.
3. Give only one instruction at a time. Reward the patient with compliments after the successful completion of each procedure.
4. Listen carefully to the patient. Retarded individuals often have trouble in communication, and the dentist should be particularly sensitive to gestures and verbal requests.
5. Keep appointments short. Gradually progress to more difficult procedures (anesthesia and restorative dentistry) after the patient has become accustomed to the dental environment.

6. Schedule the patient early in the day, when the dentist, the staff, and the patient will be less fatigued.

With adequate preparation the dentist and the staff can provide a valuable service. By thoroughly understanding the patient's degree of mental retardation and abilities and by exercising patience and understanding, the dentist should have no significant problems in delivering dental care.

Down syndrome (trisomy 21 syndrome, mongolism)

Down syndrome is the best-known chromosomal syndrome. The overall incidence in the general population is estimated to be 1.5 in 1000 births. Because the risk of having a child with Down syndrome is greater among older women, some researchers have suggested an environmental cause. Factors potentially linked to the increased incidence of Down syndrome in older women include maternal exposure to diagnostic irradiation of the abdomen and "overripeness" of the ovum because decreased frequency of coitus leads to delayed fertilization. The majority of Down syndrome individuals (95%) have trisomy 21; translocations and mosaic presentations are also documented.

Approximately 12,000 children are born with Down syndrome in the United States each year. It is estimated that they account for about 10% of the mentally retarded individuals living in institutions. A dentist who routinely treats children or works in an institution should be familiar with the physical characteristics of Down syndrome (Table 23-2).

Medical conditions that increase the mortality of children and infants with Down syndrome include cardiac disease, increased incidence of abnormalities of the white blood cells, and increased incidence of acute and chronic infections of the upper respiratory tract. The incidence of cardiac disease associated with Down syndrome is about 40%. Septal defects, especially of the endocardial cushion, are particularly common. The incidence of leukemia in young individuals who have Down syndrome is 10 to 20 times greater than in the general population. The increased incidence of leukemia in Down syndrome infants is not maintained in later life. Congenital heart disease and respiratory tract infections are the most common causes of death in Down syndrome children during the first 5 years of life.

Individuals with Down syndrome are usually moderately to severely retarded. Most Down syndrome individuals are affectionate and cooperative and present the dentist with no unusual conditions in providing dental care. In the more apprehensive patients, mild sedation may be beneficial. General

Table 23-2. Physical characteristics of Down syndrome

Features	Comments
Body growth	Small stature; retardation in appositional and endochondral growth
Head	Brachycephalic with relatively flat occiput
Eyes	Upward, outward slant and epicanthal folds; speckling of the iris (Brushfield spots) frequently present
Osseous orbits	Smaller than normal
Nose	Flat, underdeveloped nasal bridge
Tongue	Macroglossia; scrotal tongue in approximately 50% of Down syndrome individuals
Neck	Broad, short neck
Hands and feet	Simian crease; short, broad hands; incurved fifth finger; first and second toes widely spaced
Skin	Occasionally dry; eczema and hyperkeratosis common
Muscle tone	Hypotonia in infancy, becoming less pronounced as the individual ages
Teeth	Microdontia and conical teeth; overretention of deciduous dentition; aberrant eruption patterns, with anodontia, oligodontia, or supernumerary teeth possible

anesthesia should be considered if severe resistance to dental treatment is encountered.

Learning disabilities

For years, students who consistently had difficulty achieving a level of academic performance concomitant with their intellectual capacity were unfortunately labeled "retarded." Today the term "learning disabled" is applied to children who exhibit a disorder in one or more of the basic psychologic processes involved in understanding or using spoken or written language. Learning disabilities affect between 3% and 15% of the population. They occur four times more frequently among boys than among girls.

In 1968 the National Advisory Committee on Handicapped Childen of the U.S. Department of Health, Education and Welfare stated that learning disabilities "may be manifested in disorders of listening, thinking, talking, reading, writing, spelling or arithmetic. They include conditions which have been referred to as perceptual handicaps, brain injury, minimal brain dysfunction, dyslexia and developmental aphasia." It should be emphasized that learning disabilities do not include learning problems caused mainly by hearing, visual, or motor handicaps, mental retardation, emotional disturbance, or environmental conditions.

The cause of learning disabilities remains unclear. Physiologic factors, such as minimal brain injury or damage to the central nervous system, have been implicated. Because learning disabilities appear more frequently in some families than in others, a genetic factor has also been suggested. Of special importance is the possibility that severe emotional disturbances can develop as a result of learning disabilities. It is this potential that has prompted early diagnosis and treatment of affected individuals.

Most children with learning disabilities accept dental care and cause no unusual management problems for the dentist. If a child is resistant, analgesia and sedation techniques can be used with success.

Autism

Autism is a severely incapacitating disturbance of mental and emotional development that causes problems in learning, communication, and relating to others. This lifelong developmental disability manifests itself during the first 3 years of life, is difficult to diagnose, and has no cure. Until recently autism was believed to be an emotional disability. In the 1980 *Diagnostic and Statistical Manual of Mental Disorders,* published by the American Psychiatric Association, autism is listed as a neurologic disorder. It is now believed to be caused by a physical disorder of the brain.

Autism occurs in approximately five of every 10,000 births and is four times more common in boys than girls. Autistic children look like normal children and have normal life spans. However, they have a limited capacity to communicate, socialize, and learn. Approximately 60% of diagnosed autistic individuals have IQ scores below 50, 20% between 50 and 70, and only 20% greater than 70. Special educational programs that employ behavior modification techniques designed for a specific individual have proved helpful in training autistic children. Counseling the family on effective management techniques in the home is essential in the overall training of autistic individuals.

Dental management of an autistic child depends on the degree of mental retardation and the child's language development. Such children often have little effective contact with other people and experience profound difficulties in relating to other individuals, objects, and events. Sedative drugs have been beneficial in treating autistic individuals.

It has been observed that the sound of a high-speed handpiece is particularly upsetting to an autistic individual. Precautions should therefore be taken to reduce the sound level to which the person might be exposed.

Cerebral palsy

Cerebral palsy is one of the primary crippling conditions of childhood. The incidence of cerebral palsy in the United States, for all ages, is 1.5 to 3 cases per 1000 individuals. One newborn in approximately 200 live births will be afflicted with this condition. Cerebral palsy is not a specific disease entity but rather a collection of disabling disorders caused by insult and permanent damage to the brain in the prenatal and perinatal periods, during which time the central nervous system is still maturing. A person with cerebral palsy characteristically has a motor disability that is manifested as a loss or impairment of voluntary muscle control. This disability might involve muscle weakness, stiffness, or paralysis; poor balance or irregular gait; and uncoordinated or involuntary movements.

Although many recognized conditions result in damage to the motor centers of the brain, in at least one third of cases of cerebral palsy there is no discernible cause. It has been well established that any factor contributing to decreased oxygenation of the developing brain can be responsible for brain damage. In addition, causal relationships have been established between cerebral palsy and complications of labor or delivery, infections of the brain such as meningitis and encephalitis, toxemias of pregnancy, congenital defects of the brain, kernicterus, poisoning with certain drugs and heavy metals, and accidents resulting in trauma to the head. There is an appreciably high correlation between premature births and cerebral palsy (approximately one third of all infants born prematurely have a demonstrable nervous system abnormality).

There are various types of cerebral palsy, which are distinguished according to the neuromuscular dysfunctions observed and the extent of anatomic involvement. Some individuals may have almost imperceptible symptoms. Others will be severely handicapped, with no appreciable use of the muscles of their limbs and other voluntary muscles. It is imperative to keep in mind that two patients with the same type of cerebral palsy may evidence very disparate symptoms. The following terms are commonly used to designate involved areas of the body:

1. Monoplegia—involvement of one limb only
2. Hemiplegia—involvement of one side of the body
3. Paraplegia—involvement of both legs only
4. Diplegia—involvement of both legs with minimum involvement of both arms
5. Quadriplegia—involvement of all four limbs

The following outline provides a classification of cerebral palsy according to the type of neuromuscular dysfunction, with a few of the basic characteristics of each type:

I. *Spastic* (approximately 70% of cases)
   A. Hyperirritability of involved muscles, resulting in exaggerated contraction when stimulated
   B. Characterized by tense, contracted muscles (For example, in spastic hemiplegia, which accounts for one third of all children with cerebral palsy, the hand and arm are flexed and held in against the trunk. The foot and leg may be flexed and rotated internally, resulting in a limping gait with circumduction of the affected leg.)
   C. Limited control of neck muscles, resulting in ''head roll''
   D. Lack of control of the muscles supporting the trunk, resulting in difficulty in maintaining upright posture
   E. Lack of coordination of intraoral, perioral, and masticatory musculature; possibility of impaired chewing and swallowing, excessive drooling, persistent spastic tongue thrust, and speech impairments

II. *Dyskinetic* (athetosis and choreoathetosis) (approximately 15% of cases)
   A. Constant and uncontrolled motion of involved muscles
   B. Characterized by a succession of slow, twisting, or writhing involuntary movements (athetosis) or quick, jerky movements (choreoathetosis)
   C. Neck musculature frequently involved, resulting in excessive movement of the head (Hypertonicity of these muscles may cause the head to be held back, with the mouth constantly open and the tongue positioned anteriorly or protruded.)

D. Possibility of frequent, uncontrolled jaw movements, causing abrupt closure of the jaws or severe bruxism

E. Perioral musculature frequently hypotonic, with mouth breathing, tongue protrusion, and excessive drooling

F. Facial grimacing

G. Chewing and swallowing difficulties

H. Speech problems

III. *Ataxic* (approximately 5% of cases)

A. Involved muscles unable to contract completely, so that voluntary movements can only be partially performed

B. Poor sense of balance and uncoordinated voluntary movements—for example, stumbling or staggering gait or difficulty in grasping objects

C. Possibility of tremors and an uncontrollable trembling or quivering on attempting voluntary tasks

IV. *Mixed* (approximately 10% of cases)

A. Combination of characteristics of more than one type of cerebral palsy—for example, mixed spastic-athetoid quadriplegia

Two additional forms of cerebral palsy have been described but occur very infrequently. In *hypotonia* the muscles are flaccid—that is, there is an inability to elicit muscle activity on volitional stimulation. In *rigidity* the muscles are in a constant state of contraction. The condition is characterized by prolonged periods in which the muscles of the extremities or trunk remain rigid, resisting any effort to move them.

In many patients with cerebral palsy, certain neonatal reflexes may persist long after the age at which they normally disappear. These "primitive reflexes" are usually modified or are progressively replaced as the subcortical dominance of the infant's behavior is suppressed by higher centers of the maturing central nervous system. Infantile reflexes are manifested as a sudden extension and/or flexions of the limbs, with assumption of characteristic postures. Three of the most common such reactions, which a dentist should recognize, are as follows:

1. *Asymmetric tonic neck reflex.* If the patient's head is suddenly turned to one side, the arm and leg on the side to which the face is turned will extend and stiffen. The limbs on the opposite side will flex.

2. *Tonic labryinthine reflex.* Should the patient's head, while the patient is supine, suddenly fall backward, the back may assume the position known as postural extension; the legs and arms will straighten out, and the neck and back will arch.

3. *Startle reflex.* This reflex, which is frequently observed in persons with cerebral palsy, consists of sudden, involuntary, often forceful bodily movements. As the term implies, this reaction is produced when the patient is surprised by such stimuli as sudden noises or unexpected movements by other people.

Since the motor involvement in cerebral palsy results from irreversible damage to the developing brain, there may also be other symptoms of organic brain damage. The fact that these other symptoms are frequently seen underscores the premise that the term "cerebral palsy" does not denote one specific disease entity. Rather, it is a complex of disabling conditions, the clinical manifestations of which depend on the extent and location of damage to the brain. The following are some common manifestations:

1. *Mental retardation.* Approximately 60% of persons with cerebral palsy demonstrate some degree of mental retardation.

2. *Seizure disorders.* Seizures are an accompanying condition in 30% to 50% of cases; they occur primarily during infancy and early childhood. Most seizures can be well controlled with anticonvulsant medications.

3. *Sensory deficits or dysfunctions.* Impairment of hearing is more common than in the normal population, and eye disorders affect approximately 35% of individuals with cerebral palsy. The most common visual defect is strabismus.

4. *Speech disorders.* More than half of patients with cerebral palsy have some speech problem—usually dysarthria, an inability to articulate well because of lack of control of the speech muscles.

5. *Joint contractures.* Individuals with spasticity and rigidity will demonstrate abnormal limb postures and contractures during growth and at maturity, primarily because of disuse of muscle groups.

No intraoral anomalies are unique to individuals with cerebral palsy. However, several conditions are more common or more severe than in the normal population:

1. *Periodontal disease.* Periodontal disease occurs with great frequency in individuals with cerebral palsy. There is an obvious correlation between the severity of the disease and the patient's oral hygiene. Oftentimes the patient will not be physically able to brush or floss adequately. When oral hygiene measures must be provided for the individual, they may be done infrequently and inadequately. The type of diet may also be significant; children who have difficulty chewing and swallowing tend to eat soft foods, which are easily swallowed and are high in carbohydrates. Cerebral palsy patients who take phenytoin to control seizure activity will generally have a degree of gingival hyperplasia. Again, the thoroughness of oral hygiene measures is proportional to the severity of the hyperplasia.

2. *Dental caries.* The data are conflicting relative to the incidence of dental caries in cerebral palsy patients compared with the general population. With the exception of institutionalized patients, the incidence of caries does not seem to be significantly greater among persons with cerebral palsy.

3. *Malocclusions.* The prevalence of malocclusions in patients with cerebral palsy is approximately twice that of the general population. Commonly observed conditions include marked protrusion of the maxillary anterior teeth, excessive overbite and overjet, open bites, and unilateral cross-bites. A primary cause may be a disharmonious relationship between intraoral and perioral muscles. Uncoordinated and uncontrolled movements of jaws, lips, and tongue are observed with great frequency in patients with cerebral palsy.

4. *Bruxism.* Bruxism is commonly observed in patients with athetoid cerebral palsy. Severe occlusal attrition of the primary and permanent dentition may be noted, with the resulting loss of vertical interarch dimension. Temporomandibular joint disorders may be sequelae of this condition in adult patients.

5. *Trauma.* Individuals with cerebral palsy are more susceptible to trauma, particularly to the maxillary anterior teeth. This situation is related to the increased tendency to fall, along with a diminished extensor reflex to cushion such falls, and the frequent increased flaring of the maxillary anterior teeth.

To an uninformed dentist, a person with cerebral palsy who has involuntary movements of the limbs and head might be perceived as an uncooperative and unmanageable patient. In addition, patients who have unintelligible speech, uncontrollable jaw movements, and spastic tongue are often erroneously assumed to be intellectually retarded. A clinician who is not knowledgeable about cerebral palsy and other physically and mentally handicapping conditions may feel uncomfortable about treating such patients and may, in fact, refuse to do so.

In providing treatment for children with cerebral palsy, it is imperative that a dentist evaluate each patient thoroughly in terms of personal characteristics, symptoms, and behavior and then proceed as conditions and needs dictate.

The dentist should never assume the degree of a child's physical or mental impairments without first acquiring the facts. A thorough medical and dental history is very important, and the parent or guardian should be interviewed before the initiation of any treatment. Only through such personal communication can valuable insight be obtained about the patient's particular physical and behavioral characteristics. It may also be beneficial to consult the patient's physician regarding the patient's medical status.

A patient with cerebral palsy who has involuntary head movements is cognizant of the need to minimize these movements while receiving dental care. Paradoxically, the patient's own endeavors to control these movements may only exacerbate the problem. Therefore it is imperative that all dental personnel be empathic about the fears and frustrations that such an individual experiences. The importance of maintaining a calm, friendly, and professional atmosphere cannot be overemphasized.

The following suggestions are offered to the clinician as being of practical significance in treating a patient with cerebral palsy:

1. Consider treating a patient confined to a wheelchair in the wheelchair. Many patients express such a preference, and it is frequently more practical for the dentist. For a young patient, the wheelchair may be tipped back into the dentist's lap.

2. If a patient is to be transferred to the dental chair, ask about a preference for the mode of transfer. If the patient has no preference, the two-person lift is recommended.

3. Make an effort to stabilize the patient's head throughout all phases of dental treatment.

4. Try to place, and maintain, the patient in the midline of the dental chair, with arms and legs as close to the body as feasible.

5. Keep the patient's back slightly elevated, to minimize difficulties in swallowing (it is advisable not to have the patient in a completely supine position).

6. On placing the patient in the dental chair, determine the patient's degree of comfort and assess the position of the extremities. Do not force the limbs into unnatural positions. Consider the use of pillows, towels, and other measures for trunk and limb support.

7. Use physical restraints judiciously for controlling flailing movements of the extremities.

8. For control of involuntary jaw movements, choose from a variety of mouth props and finger splints. Patient preference should weigh heavily, since a patient with cerebral palsy may be very apprehensive about the ability to control swallowing. Such appliances may also trigger the strong gag reflex that many of these patients possess.

9. To minimize startle reflex reactions, avoid such stimuli as abrupt movements, noises, and lights without forwarning the patient.

10. Introduce intraoral stimuli slowly to avoid eliciting a gag reflex or to make it less severe.

11. Consider the use of the rubber dam for restorative procedures, a highly recommended technique.

12. Work efficiently and minimize patient time in the chair to decrease fatigue of the involved muscles.

Deafness

Deafness is a handicap that is often overlooked because it is not obvious. Total deafness is not common, but a dentist is likely to treat hearing-impaired children who have varying degrees of deafness. Almost inevitably, speech is affected. If an impairment is severe enough that dentist and child cannot communicate verbally, the dentist must use sight, taste, and touch to communicate and to allow the child to learn about dental experiences. Table 23-3 shows how speech and psychologic problems relate to various degrees of hearing loss. Many times, mild hearing losses are not diagnosed, leading to management problems because of misunderstanding of instructions, while children with more severe hearing losses already possess psychologic and social disturbances that make dental behavior management more complex. No abnormal dental findings are associated with deafness.

The following are known causes of hearing loss:

Table 23-3. Implications of auditory relative to International Standards Organization (ISO) reference levels*

ISO (db)	Handicap	Speech comprehension	Psychologic problems in children
0	Insignificant	Little or no difficulty	None
>25	Slight	Difficulty with faint speech; language and speech development within normal limits	May show a slight verbal deficit
>40	Mild-moderate	Frequent difficulty with normal speech at 1 m; language skills are mildly affected	Psychologic problems can be recognized
>55	Marked	Frequent difficulty with loud speech at 1 m; difficulty understanding with hearing aid in school situation	Child is likely to be educationally retarded, with more pronounced emotional and social problems than in children with normal hearing
>70	Severe	Might understand only shouts or amplified speech at 1 foot from ear	The prelingually deaf show pronounced educational retardation and evident emotional and social problems
>90	Extreme	Usually no understanding of speech even when amplified; child does not rely on hearing for communication	The prelingually deaf usually show severe educational retardation and emotional underdevelopment

Modified from Goetzinger: The psychology of hearing impairment. In Katz, J., editor: Handbook of clinical audiology, ed. 2, Baltimore, 1978, The Williams & Wilkins Co.

*Reference levels are decibels of threshold in normal young patients.

Prenatal factors
    Viral infections, such as rubella and influenza
    Ototoxic drugs
    Congenital syphilis
    Heredity (for example, Waardenburg syndrome)
Perinatal factors
    Toxemia late in pregnancy
    Prematurity
    Birth injury
    Anoxia
    Erythroblastosis fetalis
Postnatal factors
    Viral infections, such as mumps, measles, chickenpox, influenza, poliomyelitis, meningitis
    Injuries
    Ototoxic drugs, such as aspirin, streptomycin, neomycin, kanamycin

The following should be considered when treating a hearing-impaired patient:

1. Prepare the patient and the parent before the first visit, via a "welcome" letter that states what is to be done.
2. Through the parent, determine during the initial appointment how the patient desires to communicate, which will go far in decreasing the child's fears.
3. Assess speech and language ability and degree of impairment by taking a complete medical history.
4. Face the patient and speak at a natural pace and directly to the patient without shouting. Exaggerated facial expressions and the use of slang make lipreading difficult. Even the best lip-readers comprehend only 30% to 40% of what is said.
5. Watch the patient's expression. Make sure the patient understands what the dental equipment is, what is going to happen, and how it will feel.

6. Reassure the patient with physical contact; hold the patient's hand initially, or place a hand reassuringly on the patient's shoulder.
7. Employ the tell-show-do approach. Allow the patient to see the instruments, and demonstrate how they work—for example, vibrations of the handpiece, scratching of the explorer, scooping of the excavator, and texture of the rubber dam.
8. Use smiles and reassuring gestures to build up confidence and reduce anxiety.
9. Avoid blocking the patient's visual field.
10. Adjust the hearing aid (if the patient has one) while the handpiece is in operation, since a hearing aid will amplify all sounds. Many times the patient will prefer to have it turned off.

Blindness

Blindness affects over 15 million people today and will affect an estimated 30 million people by the year 2000. The list that follows gives some of the known causes of blindness; however, in over 35% of those affected the cause is either unknown or unreported. Blindness is not an all-or-none phenomenon; a person is considered to be affected by blindness if the visual acuity does not exceed 20/200 in the better eye, with correcting lenses, or if the acuity is greater than 20/200 but accompanied by a visual field of no greater than 20 degrees.

Prenatal causes
Optic atrophy
Microphthalmus
Cataracts
Colobomata
Dermoid and other tumors
Toxoplasmosis
Cytomegalic inclusion disease
Syphilis
Rubella
Tuberculous meningitis
Developmental abnormalities of the orbit

Postnatal causes
Trauma
Retrolental fibroplasia
Hypertension
Premature birth
Polycythemia vera
Hemorrhagic disorders
Leukemia
Diabetes mellitus
Glaucoma

Blindness may be only one aspect of a child's disability. For example, a patient with congenital rubella may be afflicted with deafness, mental retardation, congenital heart disease, and dental defects, as well as blindness resulting from congenital cataracts. Blindness is one disorder that may result in frequent hospitalizations, separation from family, and slow social development. Since a blind child's capabilities are difficult to assess, many times such a child may be considered developmentally delayed.

Consideration must be given to every developmental aspect of a blind child. Many times, early in development the parents experience guilt and either overprotect or reject the child, resulting in a lack of development of self-help skills and delayed development in general, which is often misinterpreted as mental retardation. Assessment of parental attitudes is of primary importance in behavioral management. In addition, blind children may exhibit self-stimulating activities such as eye pressing, finger flicking, rocking, and head banging. Therefore assessment of the child's socialization is useful in managing dental behavior.

A distinction should be made between children who at one time had sight and those who have never seen and thus do not form visual concepts. More explanation is needed for children in the latter category to help them perceive the dental environment. Dentists should realize that congenitally blind children need a greater display of affection and love early in life and that they differ intellectually from children who are not congenitally blind. While explanation is accomplished through touching and hearing, reinforcement takes place through smelling and tasting. The modalities of listening, touching, tasting, and smelling are extremely important for blind children, in that they help these children to learn coping behavior. Once speech is developed, reports indicate that the other senses assume heightened importance and that other development can occur that is comparable to what takes place in children with sight.

Reports also reveal that motor activity affects the development of language and perception. Blind children tend to have more accidents than other children during the early years while they are acquiring motor skills.

Hypoplastic teeth and trauma to the anterior teeth have been reported with greater than average frequency in blind children. Such children are also more likely to have gingival inflammation because of their inability to see and remove plaque. Other dental abnormalities occur with the same frequency as in the normal population.

Before initiating dental treatment for a blind child, the dentist should keep the following points in mind:

1. Determine the degree of visual impairment. For example, can the patient tell light from dark?
2. If the patient is accompanied by a companion, find out if the companion is an interpreter. If he or she is not, address the patient.
3. Avoid expressions of pity or references to blindness as an affliction.
4. In maneuvering the patient to the operatory, ask if the patient desires assistance. Do not grab, move, or stop the patient without verbal warning.
5. Describe the office setting. Always give the patient adequate descriptions before performing treatment procedures.
6. When making physical contact, do so reassuringly.
7. Introduce other office personnel very informally.
8. Allow the patient to ask questions about the course of treatment and answer them, keeping in mind that the patient is highly individual, sensitive, and responsive.
9. Allow a patient who wears eyeglasses to keep them on for protection and security.
10. Avoid sight references.
11. Rather than using the tell-show-do approach, invite the patient to touch, taste, or smell, recognizing that these senses are acute.
12. Describe in detail instruments and objects to be placed in the patient's mouth.
13. Demonstrate a rubber cup on the patient's fingernail.
14. Holding the patient's hand often promotes relaxation.
15. Since strong tastes may be rejected, use smaller quantities of dental materials with such characteristics.
16. Explain the procedures of oral hygiene and then place the patient's hand over yours as you slowly but deliberately guide the toothbrush.
17. Use audiocassette tapes and braille dental pamphlets explaining specific dental procedures to supplement information and decrease chair time.
18. Announce exits from and entrances to the dental operatory cheerfully. Keep them minimal, and avoid unexpected loud noises.
19. Limit the patient's dental care to one dentist.
20. Maintain a relaxed atmosphere.

The provision of dental care to a blind child is facilitated by an in-depth understanding of the patient's background. A team approach by all health professionals involved in the care of the child is ideal. Disease prevention and continuity of care are of utmost importance.

Heart disease

Heart disease can be divided into two general types: congenital and acquired. Because individuals with heart disease require special precautions during dental treatment (such as antibiotic coverage for prevention of subacute bacterial endocarditis), a dentist should closely evaluate the medical histories of all patients to ascertain their cardiovascular status.

Congenital heart disease. The incidence of congenital heart disease is approximately nine in 1000 births. The following is the relative incidence of congenital heart defects (data from the Toronto Heart Registry):

Defect	Percent
Ventricular septal defect	22
Patent ductus arteriosus	17
Tetralogy of Fallot	11
Transposition of the great vessels	8
Atrial septal defect	7
Pulmonary stenosis	7
Coarctation of the aorta	6
Aortic stenosis	5
Tricuspid atresia	3
All others	14

The cause of a congenital heart defect is obscure. Generally it is a result of aberrant embryonic development of a normal structure or the failure of a structure to progress beyond an early stage of embryonic development. Only rarely can a causal factor be identified in congenital heart disease. Maternal rubella and chronic maternal alcohol abuse are known to interfere with normal cardiogenesis. If a parent or a sibling has a congenital heart defect, the chances that a child will be born with a heart defect are about 5 to 10 times greater than average. Congenital heart disease can be classified in two groups: acyanotic and cyanotic.

Acyanotic congenital heart disease. Acyanotic congenital heart disease is characterized by minimum cyanosis, or no cyanosis, and is commonly divided into two major groups. The first group consists of defects that cause left-to-right shunting of blood within the heart. This group includes ventricular septal defect and atrial septal defect. Clinical manifestations of these defects can include congestive heart failure, pulmonary congestion, heart murmur, labored breathing, and cardiomegaly. The second major group consists of defects that cause obstruction—for example, aortic stenosis and coarctation of the aorta. The clinical manifestations can include labored breathing and congestive heart failure.

Cyanotic congenital heart disease. Cyanotic congenital heart disease is characterized by right-to-left shunting of blood within the heart. Cyanosis is often observed even during minor exertion. Examples of such defects are tetralogy of Fallot, transposition of the great vessels, pulmonary stenosis, and tricuspid atresia. Clinical manifestations can include, in addition to cyanosis, hypoxic spells, poor physical development, heart murmurs, and clubbing of the terminal phalanges of the fingers (Fig. 23-13).

Acquired heart disease

Rheumatic fever. Rheumatic fever is a serious inflammatory disease that occurs as a delayed sequela to pharyngeal infection with group A streptococci. Rheumatic fever is a commonly diagnosed cause of acquired heart disease in patients under 40 years of age. The mechanism by which the group A *Streptococcus* initiates the disease is unknown. The infection can involve the heart, joints, skin, central nervous system, and subcutaneous tissue. In general the incidence of rheumatic fever is decreasing. However, the incidence following exudative pharyngitis in epidemics is approximately 3%. (The incidence is much lower when the streptococcal pharyngitis is less severe.)

Although rheumatic fever can occur at any age, it is rare in infancy. It appears most commonly between the ages of 6 and 15 years. Rheumatic fever is most prevalent in temperate zones and high altitudes and is more common and severe in children who live in substandard conditions. The clinical symptoms of rheumatic fever vary. In 1944, Jones proposed a set of diagnostic critera that is still used today (Table 23-4).

Cardiac involvement is the most significant pathologic sequela of rheumatic fever; carditis develops in approximately 50% of patients. Cardiac involvement can be fatal during the acute phase or can lead to chronic rheumatic heart disease as a result of scarring and deformity of heart valves.

Infective bacterial endocarditis. Infective bacte-

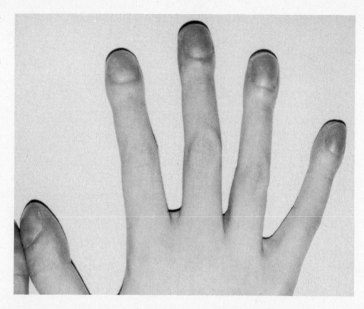

Fig. 23-13. Hand of a 9-year-old boy with tetralogy of Fallot. Clubbing of the terminal phalanges is apparent.

Table 23-4. Jones criteria in diagnosis of rheumatic fever (revised)

Major manifestations	Minor manifestations	Supporting evidence
Carditis	Fever	Evidence of preceding
Polyarthritis	Arthralgia	streptococcal infection
Chorea	Previous history of rheumatic fever or rheumatic heart	Positive throat culture
Erythema marginatum	disease	for group A *Streptococcus*
Subcutaneous nodules	Elevated erythrocyte sedimentation rate or positive C-reactive protein	
	Prolonged PR interval	

From American Heart Association: Circulation **32**:664, 1965. By permission of the American Heart Association, Inc.

rial endocarditis is one of the most serious infections of humans. It is characterized by microbial infection of the heart valves or endocardium in proximity to congenital or acquired cardiac defects. Infective bacterial endocarditis has been classically divided into *acute* and *subacute* forms. The acute form is a fulminating disease that usually occurs as a result of microorganisms of high pathogenicity attacking a normal heart, causing erosive destruction of the valves. Microorganisms associ-

ated with the acute form include *Staphylococcus aureus,* group A *Streptococcus,* and *Pneumonococcus.* In contrast, subacute bacterial endocarditis usually develops in persons with preexisting congenital cardiac disease or rheumatic valvular lesions. The subacute form is commonly caused by viridans streptococci. Surgical placement of prosthetic heart valves can also predispose a patient to subacute infective endocarditis; heart valve infections occur in 1% to 2% of such patients.

Embolization is a characteristic feature of infective endocarditis. Microorganisms introduced into the bloodstream may colonize on the endocardium at or near congenital valvular defects, valves damaged by rheumatic fever, or prosthetic heart valves. These vegetations, composed of microorganisms and fibrous exudate, may separate and, depending on whether the endocarditis involves the left or right side of the heart, be propelled into the systemic or pulmonary circulation.

The clinical symptoms of subacute bacterial endocarditis include low, irregular fever (afternoon or evening peaks) with sweating, malaise, anorexia, weight loss, and arthralgia. Inflammation of the endocardium increases cardiac destruction, with murmurs subsequently developing. Painful fingers and toes and skin lesions are also important symptoms. Laboratory findings can include leukocytosis with neutrophils and normocytic, normochromic anemia. The erthrocyte sedimentation rate is rapid.

Transient bacteremia is an important initiating factor in subacute bacterial endocarditis. Procedures known to precipitate transient bacteremias include the following:

1. Dental manipulation or extractions
2. Tonsillectomy
3. Rigid bronchoscopy
4. Urinary tract instrumentation
5. Use of intravenous catheters
6. Cardiac surgery and insertion of valvular prostheses

Any dental patient who has a history of congenital heart disease or rheumatic heart disease or who has a prosthetic heart valve should be considered susceptible to subacute bacterial endocarditis. The American Heart Association recommendations for prevention of bacterial endocarditis are presented in Fig. 23-14.

With adequate prophylactic antibiotic therapy, routine restorative and surgical dental procedures can be safely completed. Before initiating care, the dentist should obtain a thorough history, perform a physical examination, formulate a complete treatment plan, and discuss the treatment with the child's physician or cardiologist. Oral premedication and nitrous oxide–oxygen analgesia have proved beneficial in reducing anxiety in such patients. Cardiopulmonary resuscitation equipment should be readily available during the appointment. If a general anesthetic is indicated for the treatment of such a patient because of severe dental disease, the procedure should be completed in a hospital, where adequate supportive care is available if needed.

The following considerations are especially important in treating patients who are susceptible to subacute bacterial endocarditis:

1. Pulp therapy for primary teeth is not recommended because of the high incidence of associated chronic infection. Extraction of such teeth and appropriate fixed-space maintenance are preferred.
2. Endodontic therapy in the permanent dentition can usually be accomplished successfully if the teeth are carefully selected and the endodontic therapy is adequately performed. Teeth that have a poor or questionable endodontic prognosis should be removed.
3. In patients with cardiac pacemakers but without existing congenital or acquired heart disease, prophylactic antibiotic coverage to prevent subacute bacterial endocarditis is not indicated. If a cardiac defect is documented, appropriate antibiotic therapy is essential.
4. A dentist who feels uncomfortable in treating patients who are susceptible to infective endocarditis has a responsibility to refer them to someone who will provide the necessary care.

Hemophilia

The most common congenital blood coagulation disorders that are capable of producing serious bleeding episodes are factor VIII deficiency (hemophilia A) and factor IX deficiency (hemophilia B or Christmas disease). Deficiencies of other coagulation factors are seen infrequently and account for less than 5% of all such disorders.

Hemophilia A, or classical hemophilia, affects

Name: _____

needs protection from
BACTERIAL ENDOCARDITIS
because of an existing
HEART CONDITION

Diagnosis: _____

Prescribed by: _____

Date: _____

**For Dental Procedures and also for Tonsillectomy,
Adenoidectomy, and Bronchoscopy**

I. For most patients: PENICILLIN	**a) Intramuscular plus Oral** **Adults:** 600,000 units of procaine penicillin G mixed with 1,000,000 units of aqueous crystalline penicillin G intramuscularly 30-60 minutes prior to procedure, followed by 500 mg penicillin V orally every 6 hours for 8 doses. **Children:** 30,000 units aqueous penicillin G/kg mixed with 600,000 units of procaine penicillin intramuscularly (not to exceed adult dose). For children less than 60 lbs. the dose of penicillin V is 250 mg every 6 hours for 8 doses. **b) Oral only** **Adults:** 2.0 gm of penicillin V 30-60 minutes prior to procedure and then 500 mg every 6 hours for 8 doses. **Children less than 60 lbs.:** 1.0 gm of penicillin V orally 30 minutes to one hour prior to procedure and then 250 mg orally every 6 hours for 8 doses.
II. For those allergic to penicillin (may also be selected for those receiving oral penicillin as continuous rheumatic fever prophylaxis): ERYTHROMYCIN	**Adults:** 1.0 gm orally one and one-half to two hours prior to procedure and then 500 mg every 6 hours for 8 doses (or Regimen IV). **Children:** 20 mg/kg orally one and one-half to two hours prior to procedure and then 10 mg/kg (not to exceed adult dosage) every 6 hours for 8 doses (or Regimen IV).
III. For those patients at higher risk of infective endocarditis (especially those with prosthetic heart valves) who are not allergic to penicillin: PENICILLIN plus STREPTOMYCIN	**Adults:** IM penicillin as outlined above in I.a, plus streptomycin 1.0 gm IM, both given 30-60 minutes before procedure, then penicillin V 500 mg orally every 6 hours for 8 doses. **Children:** Timing of doses is same as for adults. Aqueous penicillin dose is 30,000 units/kg mixed with 600,000 units procaine penicillin. Streptomycin dose is 20 mg/kg (not to exceed adult dosage). For children less than 60 lbs., the dose of penicillin V is 250 mg every 6 hours for 8 doses.

| IV. For higher risk patients (especially those with prosthetic heart valves) who are allergic to penicillin:
VANCOMYCIN intravenously and ERYTHROMYCIN orally | **Adults:** Vancomycin 1 gm IV over 30-60 minutes, begun 30-60 minutes before procedure, then erythromycin 500 mg orally every 6 hours for 8 doses.
Children: Timing of doses is same as for adults. Dose of vancomycin is 20 mg/kg. Dose of erythromycin is 10 mg/kg every 6 hours for 8 doses (not to exceed adult dose). |

**For Gastrointestinal and Genitourinary Tract
Surgery and Instrumentation
And Also For Any Surgery of Infected Tissues**

| I. For most patients:
PENICILLIN or AMPICILLIN plus STREPTOMYCIN or GENTAMICIN | **Adults:** 2 million units of aqueous penicillin G IM or IV or 1.0 gm ampicillin IM or IV plus gentamicin 1.5 mg/kg (not to exceed 80 mg) IM or IV or streptomycin 1.0 gm IM. This should be given 30-60 minutes before procedure. Repeat every 8 hours for 2 additional doses if gentamicin is used, or every 12 hours for 2 additional doses if streptomycin is used.
Children: Same timing of medications as adult schedule. Dosages are aqueous penicillin G 30,000 units/kg or ampicillin 50 mg/kg; gentamicin 2.0 mg/kg (not to exceed adult dosage). |
| II. For patients allergic to penicillin:
VANCOMYCIN plus STREPTOMYCIN | **Adults:** 1.0 gm vancomycin IV given over 30-60 minutes plus 1.0 gm streptomycin IM, each given 30-60 minutes before procedure. Doses may be repeated in 12 hours.
Children: Timing as above. Doses are vancomycin 20 mg/kg and streptomycin 20 mg/kg (not to exceed adult dosage). |

NOTE: IN PATIENTS WITH SIGNIFICANTLY COMPROMISED RENAL FUNCTION, ANTIBIOTIC DOSAGES MAY NEED TO BE MODIFIED. INTRAMUSCULAR INJECTIONS MAY BE CONTRAINDICATED IN PATIENTS RECEIVING ANTICOAGULANTS.

Adapted from: The Report of the Committee on Rheumatic Fever and Bacterial Endocarditis. American Heart Association, 1977.

Please refer to the original report for more complete information as to which patients and which procedures require prophylaxis. These joint American Heart Association-American Dental Association recommendations are published in the following sources: "Prevention of Bacterial Endocarditis", a brochure printed by the American Heart Association; *Circulation* 56:139A, 1977. *J Am Dent Assoc* 95:600, 1977.

American Heart Association
7320 Greenville Ave • Dallas, Texas 75231

78-004-C
79-150M
10-80-150M

The Council on Dental Therapeutics of the American Dental Association has approved this statement as it relates to dentistry.

Accepted
COUNCIL on DENTAL THERAPEUTICS
AMERICAN DENTAL ASSOCIATION

Fig. 23-14. Patient education card supplied to all patients with congenital and rheumatic heart disease at James Whitcomb Riley Hospital for Children.

about 20 in 100,000 males in the United States. It is inherited as an X-linked recessive trait. Therefore all males who possess the defective X chromosome have clinical manifestations of the disease, whereas females are carriers and generally do not have bleeding problems (Fig. 23-15). In approximately 30% of cases of classical hemophilia a familial history of hemophilia cannot be documented.

Another bleeding disorder, frequently confused with classical hemophilia, is von Willebrand dis-

ease. The classical inheritance pattern of this disorder is via an autosomal dominant gene, affecting females as well as males. Individuals with von Willebrand disease have both decreased factor VIII activity and an abnormality of platelet function. Platelets do not adhere to damaged vessel walls in a normal manner.

Patients with von Willebrand disease who have normal or only mildly deficient levels of factor VIII activity may be asymptomatic all of their lives. Their medical history may be unremarkable

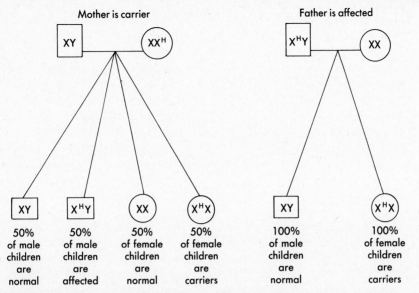

Fig. 23-15. Patterns of inheritance of hemophilia A. With each pregnancy there is a 50% chance that a son will have hemophilia A or that a daughter will be a carrier.

except for an increased frequency of nosebleeds or excessive bleeding from minor cuts. The disease may even go undetected in some individuals until they undergo a surgical procedure such as tooth extraction or tonsillectomy. However, patients with severe von Willebrand disease may show the same clinical manifestations seen in classical hemophilia.

The hallmark of hemophilia is hemorrhaging into joints and muscles, although the severity and subsequent clinical manifestations of the disease will vary according to the amount of functionally available factor (Table 23-5).

The mainstay of therapy for hemophilia is a purified concentrate of the missing factor, extracted from blood plasma. Ten years ago whole blood or plasma had to be used to replace the deficient factor. The newer concentrates are particularly advantageous because they are generally accessible, are easier to handle and store, and have more consistent potencies. The dosage, frequency of administration, and total duration of therapy depend on the location and severity of the bleeding episode. Multiple administrations may be necessary because the

Table 23-5. Classification of hemophilia

Degree of severity	Percent of factor VIII or IX available	Characteristics
Severe	<1	May be frequent spontaneous bleeding into joints and muscles
Moderate	1-5	Occasional spontaneous joint bleeding; minor trauma may initiate hemorrhage
Mild	5-35	Significant hemorrhage only after major insult, such as dental extraction

half-life of the factor concentrate is short (approximately 12 hours for factor VIII and 18 to 20 hours for factor IX).

The use of ϵ-aminocaproic acid (EACA, Amicar*) as an adjunct to factor replacement therapy has proved to be of great value in the management

*Lederle Laboratories, Pearl River, N.Y. 10965.

of patients with hemophilia, particularly those requiring dental extractions. In a hemophilic patient there is a normal fibrinolytic mechanism but the generation of thrombin necessary for clot formation is retarded and inadequate. Therefore loose, friable clots are formed, which may be readily dislodged and quickly dissolved. The fibrinolytic mechanism is effectively inhibited by EACA, allowing more stable clots to organize and mature.

One of the most serious complications encountered by a hemophiliac is the formation of inhibitor, antibodies formed against the host clotting factor. Inhibitor develops in approximately 10% of patients; its presence is manifested as a decreased ability of a patient to respond to replacement therapy. The management of a patient who has developed inhibitor is variable. With low titers, the effects may be overcome by large doses of concentrate. For very high titers, exchange transfusions may be indicated. The effects of inhibitor may also be "bypassed" through the use of prothrombin complex concentrates (PCC). However, the effectiveness of PCC may be extremely variable, with no correlation to the dosage or frequency of administration.

The dental treatment of a patient with hemophilia, or any other coagulation deficiency, necessitates a thorough understanding of the patient's disorder. The dentist must be fully cognizant of those procedures than can be performed with ensured safety and those in which complications might arise. It is very important that the nature of the child's disorder be determined through personal interviews with the parent or guardian and the child's physician. For a patient with severe hemophilia, it is imperative that the dentist confer with the patient's hematologist or primary care physician to formulate an appropriate treatment plan. Before any dental procedure the dentist should know the answers to the following questions:

1. What specific type of hemostatic disorder does the patient have?
2. What is the severity of the disorder?
3. How frequent are the bleeding episodes?
4. How are they controlled, and how well are they controlled?

5. Is the patient enrolled in a program whereby replacement therapy may be administered at home?
6. Does the patient have inhibitor?
7. Does the patient have a history of hepatitis?
8. Has the patient had recent screening tests for hepatitis?

The actual procedures employed in treating a patient with hemophilia should not differ significantly from those performed for a normal individual. It is especially important to avoid tissue laceration or other intraoral trauma. The following points may also be of value:

1. The relief of anxiety has been shown to be beneficial in maintaining hemostasis, since there appears to be a direct relationship between emotional factors and an increase in fibrinolysis. If patient apprehension is significant, premedication or nitrous oxide–oxygen inhalation analgesia may be considered. Hypnosis has also proved beneficial for some individuals. NOTE: Intramuscular administration of hypnotic, tranquilizing, or analgesic agents is contraindicated because of the possibility of hematoma formation.

2. In the absence of factor replacement, intraligamental injections may be used. The anesthetic is administered along all four axial surfaces of the tooth by placement of the needle into the gingival sulcus and the periodontal ligament space. Local infiltration anesthesia may be safely administered after a single infusion of factor replacement, as long as a hemostatic level greater than 25% to 30% is achieved. Block anesthesia is not recommended, even with factor replacement.

3. The teeth can usually be polished with a rubber cup without replacement therapy. Minor hemorrhaging can be readily controlled with local measures such as direct pressure with a moistened gauze square. For minor hemorrhaging that persists several minutes, the topical application of bovine thrombin may be of value. Depending on the hemorrhaging anticipated and the severity of factor deficiency, replacement therapy should be considered before subgingival scaling.

4. Most restorative procedures and pulp ther-

apy on deciduous teeth can be successfully completed without discomfort to the child through the use of acetaminophen with codeine in conjunction with nitrous oxide–oxygen inhalation analgesia.

5. To prevent trauma to the oral mucosa, particularly the highly vascular sublingual tissues, particular care must accompany the placement of intraoral radiographic films and the use of high-speed suction or saliva ejectors.

6. The use of the rubber dam will greatly assist in the management and protection of soft tissues. The selection and placement of clamps are important. Those with subgingival extensions, such as the 8A or the 14A, should be avoided.

7. Conventional pulp therapy is preferable to tooth extraction. Intrapulpal injections may be safely used to control pain. Hemorrhaging does not present significant problems and is readily controlled with pressure from cotton pledgets.

8. In the absence of replacement therapy, electrosurgical procedures are generally not recommended for a hemophilic patient because of the possiblity of spontaneous hemorrhaging for several days after such a procedure.

9. Primary teeth commonly exfoliate without significant hemorrhaging. However, the sharp margins of incompletely resorbed roots may lacerate the enveloping gingiva, thereby inducing hemorrhaging. This bleeding can usually be controlled by local measures subsequent to the atraumatic extraction of the remaining tooth. The bleeding can often be stopped by direct finger and gauze pressure that is maintained for several minutes. The direct topical application of hemostatic agents, such as bovine thrombin or Avitene,* may be advantageous in initiating hemostasis. An intraoral bandage of Stomadhesive† may be placed directly over the wound for further protection from the oral environment. For routine extraction of primary teeth, factor replacement may be necessary. The patient's physician should be consulted.

10. Total joint replacement, usually of the hip or knee, may be performed in hemophilic patients to restore function and alleviate the pain associated with arthritis that has developed secondarily to multiple, severe hemarthroses. A major concern in total joint arthroplasty is the increased susceptibility of the joint to acute infections resulting from bacteremias. Therefore patients with joint implants should be given antibiotics prophylactically before all dental procedures in which bacteria could be introduced into the bloodstream.

11. In the absence of quantitative hepatitis screening tests, a patient with hemophilia in whom factor replacement has been necessary should be assumed to be a carrier of hepatitis B surface antigen, and appropriate precautions should be taken.

Should the child with hemophilia sustain oral trauma, or if oral surgical procedures are anticipated in which there may be excessive bleeding, the following modalities of therapy are suggested:

1. Hemorrhaging associated with laceration of oral mucous membranes will usually respond to a single dose of factor concentrate that raises the level of factor to 50% of normal. The administration of EACA at the time of infusion and continued administration until epithelialization is complete will usually eliminate the need for subsequent infusion of factor concentrates.

2. Lacerations that require suturing may necessitate repeated dosages of factor replacement in which a level of at least 25% of normal is maintained. EACA should be administered at the time of initial factor infusion and continued until the wound is well healed.

3. When the extraction of primary or permanent teeth is planned, factor VIII is generally infused to a level of 100% of normal and a loading dose of EACA is administered. A maintenance dosage of EACA is maintained postsurgically for 7 to 10 days. The extraction of the teeth may begin within 1 hour after infusion and should be completed as atraumatically as possible. Adjunctive local measures to control hemorrhaging should be considered. Apart from direct pressure, packing the apical third of the socket with an oxidized cellulose

---

*Microfibrillar collagen hemostat (Avitene), distributed by American Critical Care, McGraw Park, Ill. 60085; manufactured by Avicon, Inc., Humacao, P.R. 00661.
† E.R. Squibb & Sons, Inc., Princeton, N.J. 08540.

material impregnated with bovine thrombin may be helpful. In general, the use of sutures should be avoided if possible.

The patient must be given very specific and thorough instructions for postoperative home care. This should include a strict diet for the first 2 weeks—for example, during the first 72 hours a clear, liquid diet is necessary. Dairy products should be discouraged, since they can leave a film residue. For the next week, a soft, pureed diet is recommended. After 10 days, the patient may begin to consume a more normal diet.

Leukemia

Malignancy is second only to accidents as the leading cause of death in children. Leukemia is a malignancy of the hematopoietic tissues in which there is a disseminated proliferation of abnormal leukocytes in the bone marrow. These immature-appearing, undifferentiated "blast" cells replace normal cells in bone marrow and accumulate in other tissues and organs of the body.

Leukemia is classified according to the morphology of the predominant abnormal white blood cells in the bone marrow (Table 23-6). These types are

Table 23-6. Childhood leukemias

Type	Age at onset	Prognosis	Treatment drugs
Acute lymphocytic (ALL)		94% remission induction	Vincristine, L-asparaginase, prednisone, 6-mercaptopurine, methotrexate, and others
	3-5 yr	Good risk (87% NED* at 60 mo)	
	6-10 yr	Average risk (67% NED at 60 mo)	
	<1 or >12 yr	Poor risk (44% NED at 60 mo)	
Acute nonlymphocytic† Myelocytic (AML) (myelomonocytic, monocytic)	Older children and adolescents	80% remission induction; 25% NED at 25 mo	Prednisone, daunomycin, ara-C, vincristine, 5-azacytidine
Di Guglielmo (erythroleukemia)		Generally very poor	
Chronic myelocytic			Busulfan, hydroxyurea
Juvenile	Infants and toddlers	Median survival less than 9 mo	
Adult	Older children and adolescents	Chronic phase about 2½ to 3½ yr; then death in blast crisis, usually of AML, which is very resistant to therapy	
Chronic lymphocytic	Not seen in children		

Courtesy Thomas D. Coates, M.D., Pediatric Hematology/Oncology Division, James Whitcomb Riley Hospital for Children, Indianapolis.

*NED, no evidence of disease.

† Bone marrow transplantation is the treatment of choice. Each sibling has one chance in four of being a perfect match. The patient is put into remission with standard chemotherapy before the transplantation. Of AML patients receiving transplants in their first remission, 60% show no evidence of disease after 2 years.

further classified as acute or chronic, depending on the progression of the clinical course and the degree of differentiation, or maturation, of the predominant abnormal cells.

Acute leukemia accounts for about half of all childhood malignancies; of these, approximately 80% are lymphocytic (ALL). Chronic leukemia in children is rare, accounting for less than 2% of all cases.

Leukemia afflicts about five in 100,000 children in the United States. The peak incidence is between 2 and 5 years of age. Certain groups of children have demonstrated an increased risk for leukemia: those born with certain chromosomal abnormalities (for example, Down syndrome and Bloom syndrome), the identical twins of children with leukemia, and children with known immunologic deficiencies. There is no known cause of leukemia, although ionizing radiation, certain chemical agents, and genetic factors have been implicated.

The clinical manifestations of acute leukemia are extremely variable. They either represent complications of the disease itself, such as anemia, thrombocytopenia, and granulocytopenia, or are the result of a leukemic cell infiltration of tissues and organs. The onset of the disease may be insidious, being characterized by history of increased irritability, lethargy, persistent fever, vague bone pain, and easy bruising. Some of the more common findings on initial physical examination are pallor, fever, tachycardia, adenopathy, hepatosplenomegaly, petechiae, cutaneous bruises, gingival bleeding, and evidence of infection.

In approximately 90% of the cases of acute leukemia a peripheral blood smear reveals anemia and thrombocytopenia. In about 65% of cases the white blood cell count is low or normal, but it may be greater than 50,000 cells/mm^3.

The following terms are used with some frequency in the ensuing discussion of the treatment and prognosis of childhood leukemia:

1. *Complete remission*. The bone marrow morphology is normal (less than 5% blast cells), the peripheral blood values and morphology are normal, and the physical examination findings are normal.

2. *Incomplete remission*. There is a persistent abnormality in bone marrow morphology (increased numbers of blast cells) and/or in the results of a physical examination (adenopathy, hepatosplenomegaly, petechiae).

3. *Relapse*. The clinical picture is the same as that of an incomplete remission, except that the abnormalities are noted after the patient has obtained a complete remission.

The basic principles and objectives of treatment, as well as the modalities used in attaining them, are at present fairly uniform. However, these so-called treatment regimens vary considerably in the type and number of drugs used, the sequence and specific times that the drugs or radiation is administered, and the duration of treatment.

When a new case of leukemia is diagnosed, the patient is hospitalized and therapy is directed toward stabilizing the patient physiologically, controlling hemorrhaging, identifying and eliminating infection, evaluating renal and hepatic functions, and preparing the patient for chemotherapy.

The goal of chemotherapy is to induce, and subsequently maintain, a complete remission. The initial phase of therapy, referred to as "induction," incorporates the use of a combination of antileukemic drugs at staggered intervals during a regimen (Fig. 23-16 and Table 23-7). The drugs should rapidly destroy the leukemic cells and yet maintain the regenerative potential of the nonmalignant hematopoietic cells within the bone marrow. Combination chemotherapy will induce a complete remission in approximately 90% of patients with ALL, usually within 4 weeks (a bone marrow aspiration is performed on day 28 of drug therapy).

When the patient has attained a first remission, the cranial vault and testes are irradiated prophylactically to prevent central nervous system and testicular relapse and thus prolong the complete remission. This stage is referred to as "central nervous system intensification."

The third stage, referred to as "maintenance," is accomplished by intense combination chemotherapy. Various drugs are used at specific intervals for a period of 2 to 2½ years. Bone marrow

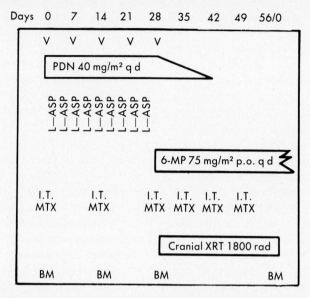

Fig. 23-16. Induction and central nervous system intensification phases of a regimen for the treatment of acute lymphocytic leukemia. Methotrexate is administered intrathecally to help destroy leukemic cells within the central nervous system. This is necessary because antileukemic drugs do not readily cross the blood-brain barrier. (Courtesy Thomas D. Coates, M.D.)

aspiration is performed approximately every 3 months to monitor the efficacy of treatment, since any relapse is usually manifested in the bone marrow. However, as previously mentioned, the central nervous system and the testicles are also primary sites of relapse.

The prognosis for a child with acute leukemia has improved dramatically within the last 15 to 20 years. Twenty-five years ago, there would have been no need to discuss dental treatment for a child with leukemia at any length because such cases were invariably fatal, most within 6 months of diagnosis. With the development of new and better antileukemia drugs, the use of intensive combination drug therapy, the incorporation of radiation therapy, and improvements in diagnostic techniques and general supportive care, complete cures are apparently being achieved.

Several variables are considered to be of prognostic importance at the time a child is diagnosed as having leukemia. For example, a low initial white blood cell count, minimal adenopathy, and normal liver and spleen size in a white child between 3 and 5 years of age would be favorable prognostic signs. A black child less than 2 years of age or older than 10 years of age, with a high initial white blood cell count and hepatosplenomegaly, would have a much poorer prognosis. The overall 5-year survival of children with ALL is 65% to 70%. At least half of these individuals remain in prolonged remission and are, it is hoped, cured.

The prognosis for patients with nonlymphocytic leukemia is still poor. Although successful induction into a first remission takes place in approximately 70%, the duration of remission is usually 12 to 18 months at best.

Oral manifestations of leukemia. Pathologic changes in the oral cavity as a result of leukemia occur frequently. Oral signs and/or symptoms suggestive of leukemia have been reported in as many

Table 23-7. Major chemotherapeutic agents and their side effects

Agent	Nausea	Bone marrow suppression	Hair loss	Stomatitis/ulcers	Renal	Neurologic
Cyclophosphamide (Cytoxan)	Moderate	Moderate 7 days after dose; spares platelets somewhat	Yes	No	Hemorrhagic cystitis	
Methotrexate	Moderate at high dose	Yes	Yes (depends on the dose)	Yes (may involve whole GI tract)	Yes	Leukoencephalopathy with radiation
6-Mercaptopurine	Not at usual dose	Yes	Usually not	Rare	No	No
Cytosine arabinoside (ara-C)	Yes	Yes	Yes	Yes		
Vincristine	No	Rare	Yes	Rare; jaw pain		Peripheral neuropathy
Actinomycin D*	Yes	Yes, 7 days after dose	Yes	Yes		
Doxorubicin*†	Severe	Marked 10 to 14 days after dose	Yes	Yes		
L-Asparaginase‡	Yes	No	No	No	Rare	Seizures
Dimethyltriazenoimadazolecarboxamide (DTIC)	Yes	Yes (may be delayed)	Yes	No		
Cis-diaminodichloroplatinum (CPDD, cis-platinum)	Severe	No	No	No	Progressive renal failure	Peripheral neuropathy
Prednisone	No	No	No	No	No	Pseudotumor psychoses

Courtesy Thomas D. Coates, M.D.
*These cause severe skin burns if they leak from the vein.
† Major cardiac toxin.
‡ L-Asparaginase may cause pancreatitis and diabetes.

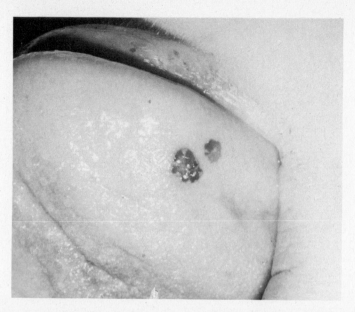

Fig. 23-17. Two small ecchymoses on the lateral border of the tongue in a 10-year-old white girl with acute lymphocytic leukemia. The platelet count was 22,000 cells/mm³. (Courtesy Dr. Bruce W. Vash.)

as 75% of adults and 29% of children with leukemia. The lower incidence of oral manifestations in children can be attributed in part to the early age at diagnosis and the high percentage of ALL in the pediatric age group. The incidence of ALL peaks at 3 years of age, when preexisting inflammatory and degenerative changes are comparatively less frequent.

Abnormalities in or around the oral cavity have been reported in all defined types of leukemia, and no age group is spared. Oral pathoses are, however, more commonly observed in acute leukemias than in chronic forms of the disease. Oral findings suggestive of leukemia are also more common in nonlymphocytic leukemias.

The most frequently reported oral abnormalities attributed to the leukemic process include regional lymphadenopathy, mucous membrane petechiae and ecchymoses, gingival bleeding, gingival hypertrophy, pallor, and nonspecific ulcerations. Manifestations seen occasionally are cranial nerve palsies, chin and lip paresthesias, odontalgia, jaw pain, loose teeth, extruded teeth, and gangrenous stomatitis. Each of these findings has been reported in all types of leukemia. Regional lymphadenopathy is the most frequently reported finding. Gingival abnormalities, including hypertrophy and bleeding, are more common in patients with nonlymphocytic leukemia, whereas petechiae and ecchymoses are more common in ALL.

Like the systemic manifestations of leukemia, oral changes can be attributed to anemia, granulocytopenia, and thrombocytopenia, all of which result from the replacement of normal bone marrow elements by undifferentiated blast cells, or to direct invasion of tissue by these leukemic cells. Proliferation of leukemic cells in the bone marrow and their appearance in the peripheral blood in increased numbers can lead to stasis in small vascular channels. The subsequent tissue anoxia results in areas of necrosis and ulceration, which, in a granulocytopenic individual, can readily become in-

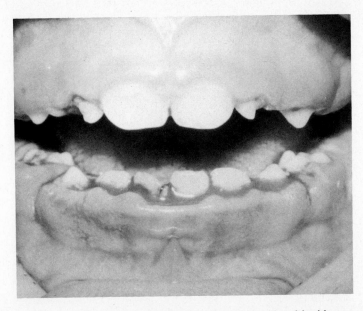

Fig. 23-18. Spontaneous gingival hemorrhaging in a 2-year-old white girl with acute myelocytic leukemia. The platelet count was less than 10,000 cells/mm^3. (Courtesy Dr. Bruce W. Vash.)

fected by opportunistic oral microorganisms. A thrombocytopenic person, having lost the capacity to maintain vascular integrity, is likely to bleed spontaneously. Such bleeding results in petechiae or ecchymoses of the oral mucosa or frank bleeding from the gingival sulcus (Figs. 23-17 and 23-18). The propensity for gingival bleeding is markedly increased in persons with deficient oral hygiene, since accumulated plaque and debris are significant local irritants.

Direct invasion of tissue by an infiltrate of leukemic cells can produce striking gingival hypertrophy (Fig. 23-19). Such gingival changes can occur despite excellent oral hygiene. Infiltration of leukemic cells along vascular channels can result in strangulation of pulpal tissue and spontaneous abscess formation as a result of infection or focal areas of liquefaction necrosis in the dental pulp of clinically and radiographically sound teeth. In a similar fashion, the teeth may rapidly loosen as a result of necrosis of the periodontal ligament.

Skeletal lesions caused by leukemic infiltration of bone are common in childhood leukemia. The most common finding is a generalized osteoporosis caused by enlargement of the haversian canals and Volkmann's canals. Osteolytic lesions resulting from focal areas of hemorrhage and necrosis and leading to loss of trabecular bone are also common.

Evidence of skeletal lesions is visible on dental radiographs in up to 63% of children with acute leukemia. Manifestations in the jaws include generalized loss of trabeculation, destruction of the crypts of developing teeth, loss of lamina dura, widening of the periodontal ligament space, and displacement of teeth and tooth buds (Fig. 23-20).

None of the oral changes that have just been discussed are pathognomonic signs of leukemia; all are also associated with numerous local or systemic disease processes. A diagnosis of leukemia therefore cannot be based on oral findings alone. Such

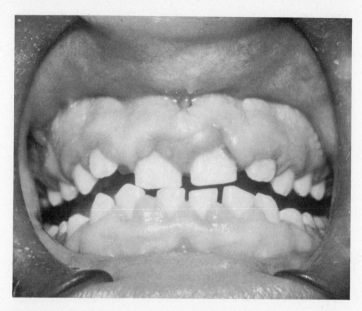

Fig. 23-19. Massive gingival hypertrophy, which biopsy showed to be leukemic infiltrate in a 16-year-old white male with acute monocytic leukemia. (Courtesy Dr. Bruce W. Vash.)

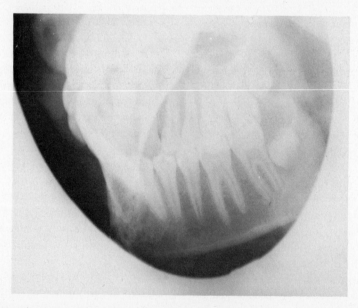

Fig. 23-20. Right lateral jaw radiograph of a 14-year-old white boy with acute myelocytic leukemia. Note generalized loss of trabeculation in the mandible, thinning and loss of lamina dura about the mandibular molar and premolar teeth, and destruction of the cortical lining of the mandibular and maxillary third molar tooth crypts. (Courtesy Dr. Bruce W. Vash.)

changes should, however, alert the clinician to the possibility of malignancy as the underlying cause.

Dental management of patients with leukemia. Before any dental treatment for a child with leukemia, the child's hematologist and oncologist or primary care physician should be consulted. The following information should be ascertained:

1. Primary medical diagnosis
2. Anticipated clinical course and prognosis
3. Present and future therapeutic modalities
4. Present general state of health
5. Present hematologic status

It is also very important to establish, via consultation with the patient's physician, when dental treatment may be most propitious, and to schedule the patient accordingly. The proposed procedures should be discussed to determine if they are appropriate.

For a child whose first remission has not yet been obtained, or one who is in relapse, all elective dental procedures should be deferred. It is, however, essential that potential sources of systemic infection within the oral cavity be controlled or eradicated whenever they are recognized (for example, immediate extraction of carious primary teeth with pulpal involvement).

Routine preventive, restorative, and surgical procedures can usually be provided for a patient who is in a complete remission yet undergoing a chemotherapeutic regimen. The time when such procedures may be completed without complications will depend on the specific agents administered and the time of administration. Before the appointment—preferably the same day—a blood cell profile (complete blood count) and platelet count should be taken to confirm that the patient is not unexpectedly at undue risk of hemorrhage or infection. A patient who has been in complete remission for at least 2 years and no longer requires chemotherapy may be treated in an essentially normal manner. A preappointment blood workup is not necessary.

Pulp therapy on primary teeth is contraindicated in any patient with a history of leukemia. Endodon-

Table 23-8. Clinical importance of platelet counts*

Count (cells/mm^3)	Significance
200,000-400,000	Normal
50,000-100,000	Bleeding time is prolonged, but patient would tolerate most routine procedures
20,000-50,000	At moderate risk for bleeding; defer elective surgical procedures
>20,000	At significant risk for bleeding; defer elective dental procedures

Courtesy Thomas D. Coates, M.D.

* The indication for platelet transfusion is *bleeding*. Do not use platelet transfusion prophylactically unless the patient is septic or a surgical procedure is planned. If the count is less than 20,000 to 30,000 cells/mm^3, the patient should probably be given prophylactic platelets before dental procedures. Indiscriminant use of platelets may lead to the development of antiplatelet antibodies.

tic treatment for permanent teeth is not recommended for any patient with leukemia who may have a chronic, intermittent suppression of granulocytes. Even with the most exacting technique, an area of chronic inflammatory tissue may remain in the periapical region of endodontically treated teeth. An area of low-grade, chronic inflammation in a normal patient is generally well tolerated, but in an immunosuppressed, neutropenic patient the same area can act as an anachoretic focus, with devastating sequelae. The decision to perform an endodontic procedure on a patient who has been in prolonged complete remission and who is not undergoing chemotherapy must be borne by the dentist.

A platelet level of 100,000/mm^3 is adequate for most dental procedures (Table 23-8). Routine preventive and restorative treatment, including non-block injections, may be considered when there are at least 50,000 platelets/mm^3. With inadequate oral hygiene, unhealthy periodontal tissues, and the presence of local irritants, hemorrhage from the gingival sulcus may be observed when platelet counts are between 20,000 and 50,000/mm^3. Such

Table 23-9. Clinical importance of white blood cell counts

AGC*	Significance
>1500	Normal
500-1000	Patient at some risk for infection; defer elective procedures that could induce significant transient bacteremia
200-500	Patient must be admitted to hospital if febrile and given broad-spectrum antibiotics; at moderate risk for sepsis; defer all elective dental procedures
<200	At significant risk for sepsis

Courtesy Thomas D. Coates, M.D.

*All numbers refer to absolute granulocyte count:

$$AGC = \frac{(\% \text{ PMN} + \% \text{ Bands}) \times \text{Total white count}}{100}$$

hemorrhaging is usually noted only after manipulation of the tissues, such as during toothbrushing. If there are fewer than 20,000 platelets/mm^3, all the intraoral mucosal tissues may show clinical evidence of spontaneous hemorrhaging (for example, petechiae, ecchymoses, or frank hemorrhage). No dental treatment should be performed at such a time without a preceding prophylactic platelet transfusion. Good oral hygiene must be maintained while the platelet count is at this level, but it may be necessary to discontinue the use of a toothbrush and to substitute moist gauze wipes, supplemented by frequent saline rinses.

The absolute granulocyte count (AGC) is an indicator of the host's ability to suppress or eliminate infection. It is calculated with the following formula: AGC = (% of neutrophils + % of bands) × Total white count ÷ 100. The clinical significance of the AGC is presented in Table 23-9. If the AGC is less than 1000/mm^3, elective dental treatment should be deferred. A leukemic patient with a low AGC may require prophylactic broad-spectrum antibiotics before certain dental procedures. The patient's physician should be consulted as to the appropriate drugs and dosages.

Infection is the primary cause of death in approximately 80% of children with leukemia.

Bleeding is the second most common cause. Therefore the primary objective of dental treatment in a child with leukemia should be the prevention, control, and eradication of oral inflammation, hemorrhage, and infection.

Not infrequently, initial oral manifestations of bleeding or infection are observed in association with an unhealthy periodontium. In patients with leukemia who are granulocytopenic or are being treated with corticosteroids, the true degree of periodontal inflammation or infection may be masked, since the cardinal signs of inflammation may not be apparent. There is a much greater propensity for gingival bleeding when the periodontium is unhealthy. When oral hygiene is neglected and local irritants are present, spontaneous hemorrhaging from the gingival sulcus may be observed if the patient is thrombocytopenic.

Needless to say, it is imperative that a patient who is diagnosed as having leukemia be enrolled in a good preventive dental care program, wherein special emphasis is placed on the initiation and maintenance of a comprehensive oral hygiene regimen. The use of a soft nylon toothbrush for the removal of plaque is recommended, even if the patient is thrombocytopenic. As long as the gingiva remains in a healthy state and its manipulation by brushing does not induce significant hemorrhage, it is not appropriate to discontinue the use of a toothbrush because of the platelet level alone. The practicality of flossing must be assessed on an individual basis.

It is important that significant local irritants be removed. Scaling and subgingival curettage should not necessarily be perceived as elective dental treatment in all patients. This is especially true if the anticipated clinical course may place the patient at high risk of hemorrhage and infection. Patients with classical leukemic gingivitis experience varying degrees of discomfort. The use of warm saline rinses several times each day may assist in the relief of symptoms.

Erosive or ulcerative lesions are common in children with leukemia. These lesions are often associated with the use of certain chemotherapeutic

Table 23-10. Topical obtundents for oral pain (frequently used at James Whitcomb Riley Hospital for Children)

Combination	Administration	Indications
1 part Kaopectate and 1 part Benadryl elixir	Swish 5-10 ml for 1 min, then expectorate	Generalized stomatitis, mild discomfort
1 part Benadryl elixir, 1 part Maalox, 1 part viscous Xylocaine 2%, plus cherry or vanilla flavoring*	Swish 5-10 ml for 1 min, then expectorate	Generalized stomatitis, moderate pain
Orabase with benzocaine, or viscous Xylocaine 2%,* or Dyclone 0.5%	Apply locally to lesions with cotton swab	Discrete, painful lesions

*Use should be supervised to prevent Xylocaine toxicity.

agents (see Table 23-7), especially methotrexate. The lesions may be an early indicator of drug toxicity. With a reduction in dosage or after discontinuation of administration, these lesions usually disappear within a few days. Treatment is directed toward the relief of discomfort (Table 23-10).

In a patient who is granulocytopenic, trauma may result in ulcerative lesions occurring especially along the lateral border of the tongue and buccal mucosa. The clinical course of these ulcerations is generally benign, although the time necessary for healing may be prolonged. Topical obtundents for pain may be the only treatment indicated.

Infrequently, deep lesions will bleed spontaneously or as a result of trauma. Local measures, such as the topical application of bovine thrombin or Avitene, and the placement of an oral adhesive for protection, may be beneficial.

For a patient who is physically debilitated or who is in relapse, septic, and severely granulocytopenic, ulcerative lesions necessitate close observation. Such lesions may serve as a nidus for the proliferation of microorganisms, leading to potentially fatal viral, fungal, or bacterial infection. Therefore these ulcerative lesions should be cultured, with subsequent sensitivity testing, and antibiotic therapy should be initiated or modified accordingly.

Candidiasis is common in children with leukemia, who are especially susceptible to this fungal infection because of (1) general physical debilitation, (2) immunosuppression, (3) prolonged antibiotic therapy, (4) chemotherapy, and (5) poor oral hygiene. The topical use of nystatin in either of the following forms can be particularly beneficial:

1. Nystatin oral suspension, 100,000 units/ml. Swish 5 ml for 5 minutes and then swallow. Repeat every 6 hours. Continue for 48 hours after lesions disappear.
2. Nystatin popsicle, 500,000 units each. Slowly consume one popsicle every 6 hours.

The nystatin popsicle was formulated to increase the acceptance of this oral antifungal antibiotic by pediatric patients (Fig. 23-1). Children enjoy the novel form in which the medicine is administered. The taste is greatly improved, and the bitter aftertaste that occurs with the oral solution is eliminated. Since at least 5 minutes is required for the popsicle to be consumed, maximum topical benefit is ensured. For patients with intraoral lesions the coldness may provide temporary relief of discomfort.

For patients who are thrombocytopenic or at risk of intermittent episodes of thrombocytopenia because of chemotherapy or active disease, the dentist should avoid prescribing drugs that may alter platelet function, such as salicylates (aspirin).

A patient with leukemia who has received transfusions of blood products should be assumed to be a carrier of hepatitis B surface antigen unless

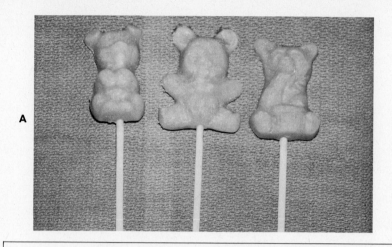

A

B

```
           NYSTATIN POPSICLES: THERAPY MADE DELICIOUS


INDICATIONS:  For patients exhibiting symptoms of oral infection with
   Candida albicans

ADVANTAGES:
          •Sustained release dosage—average 5-10 minutes to consume
          •Novelty, more acceptable, not typical "medicine"
          •Coldness—soothing, anesthetic effect on sore, ulcerated oral tissues
          •Decreased after-taste because of freezing

Nilstat Solution formulation:

     260 cc Nilstat Solution (Lederle Laboratories)
     780 cc sterile, deionized water
     15 drops red food color
         Yields sixty-nine 15-cc popsicles

Nystatin Powder formulation:

     30 million units Nystatin Powder (American Cyanamid Company)
     75 cc black cherry concentrate (Nu-Life)
     900 cc sterile, deionized water
     128.6 cc sorbitol 70% solution
     540 mg saccharin, sodium
         Yields seventy-three 15-cc popsicles

MATERIALS:
          •15-cc chocolate lollipop molds (cake supply store)
          •Paper lollipop sticks (cake supply store)—wooden or plastic sticks
               may lacerate already denuded tissues
          •Rope wax to stabilize sticks in molds
          •Plastic sealable bags

     After thorough mixing of either formulation, solution is poured into
        molds with lollipop sticks stabilized in wax

     Freezing of nystatin does not alter efficacy

RECOMMENDED DOSAGE:  For children and adults:  One popsicle (500,000
        units) q.i.d.
```

Fig. 23-21. A and **B,** The nystatin popsicle is a novel way of administering an otherwise unpleasant-tasting medicine. (Courtesy Dr. Keith L. Ray.)

appropriate tests prove otherwise. Measures to prevent the possible transmission of hepatitis to dental personnel and other patients should be instituted.

Solid tumors

Solid tumors account for approximately half of the cases of childhood malignancy. These include Wilms tumor, osteosarcoma, rhabdomyosarcoma, and neuroblastoma. Many of the same medical complications noted in acute leukemia are manifested by children with solid tumors, hemorrhage and infection being the most notable.

Most of the concepts and treatment modalities that have been previously discussed are used in the medical management of patients with solid tumors. Chemotherapy and radiation therapy are employed with considerable frequency. Some of these tumors may also be surgically excised.

In general, the dental management of patients with solid tumors is similar to that of patients with acute leukemia.

REFERENCES

Abildgaard, C.E.: Current concepts in the management of hemophilia, Semin. Hematol. **12:**223-232, 1975.

American Heart Association: Jones criteria (revised) for guidance in the diagnosis of rheumatic fever, Circulation **32:**664, 1965.

Benda, C.: Down syndrome: beginning of end, Roche Rep. **7:**1-5, 1970.

Benz, G., Bradeis, W.E., and Willich, E.: Radiological aspects of leukemia in childhood, Pediatr. Radiol. **4:**201-213, 1976.

Brown, J.P.: The efficacy and economy of comprehensive dental care for handicapped children, Int. Dent. J. **30:**14-27, 1980.

Brownstein, M.P.: Dental care for the deaf child, Dent. Clin. North Am. **18:**643-650, 1974.

Burket, L.W.: A histopathologic explanation for the oral lesions in the acute leukemias, Am. J. Orthod. Oral Surg. **30:**516-523, 1944.

Canion, S.: Dental care of the handicapped child. In Forrester, D.J., Wagner, M.L. and Fleming, J., editors: Pediatric dental medicine, Philadelphia, 1981, Lea & Febiger.

Curtis, A.B.: Childhood leukemias: initial oral manifestations, J.A.D.A. **83:**159-164, 1971.

Curtis, A.B.: Childhood leukemias: osseous changes in jaws on panoramic dental radiographs, J.A.D.A. **83:**844-847, 1971.

Danforth, H.A., Snow, M., and Stiefel, D.J.: Dental management of the cerebral palsied patient, Project DECOD, Seattle, 1978, University of Washington.

Engar, R.C., and Stiefel, D.J.: Dental treatment of the sensory impaired patient, Seattle, 1977, Disability Dental Instruction.

Feasby, W., and Wright, G.: The special child patient. In Wright, G.Z., editor: Behavior management in dentistry for children, Philadelphia, 1975, W.B. Saunders Co.

Fey, M.R., and Turley, P.K.: The handicapped child. In Davis, J.M., Law, D.B., and Lewis, T.M., editors: An atlas of pedodontics, ed. 2, Philadelphia, 1981, W.B. Saunders Co.

Goepferd, S.J.: Leukemia and its dental implications, J. Dent. Handicap. **4:**44-49, 1979.

Hobsen, P.: The treatment of medically handicapped children, Int. Dent. J. **30:**6-13, 1980.

Hughes, J.G.: Synopsis of pediatrics, ed. 5, St. Louis, 1979, The C.V. Mosby Co.

Johnston, R.B., and Magrab, P.R.: Developmental disorders: assessment, treatment, education, Baltimore, 1976, University Park Press.

Kanner, L.: Childhood psychosis: initial studies and new insights, Washington, D.C., 1973, V.H. Winston & Sons.

Kanner, L., and Lesser, L.: Early infantile autism, Pediatr. Clin. North Am. **5:**711, 1958.

Kaplan, E., and others: Prevention of bacterial endocarditis, AHA Committee Report, Circulation **56:**139, 1977.

Kisby, L.: Understanding the blind child, J. Pedod. **2:**67-72, 1977.

Lambert, B.G., and others: Adolescence: transition from childhood to maturity, ed. 2, Monterey, Calif., 1978, Brooks/Cole Publishing Co.

Lambert, E.C., and Hahn, A.R.: The pediatrician and congenital heart disease, J. Pediatr. **70:**833-847, 1967.

Lebowitz, E.J.: An introduction to dentistry for the blind, Dent. Clin. North Am. **18:**651-669, 1974.

Liebert, R.M., Odom, R.D., and Poulos, R.W.: Language development in the mentally retarded. Final Report, R.D.-2952-5, Social and Rehabilitation Service, Washington, D.C., 1971, U.S. Department of Health, Education and Welfare.

Ligh, R.Q.: The visually handicapped patient in dental practice, J. Dent. Handicap. **4:**38-40, 1979.

Lynch, M.A., and Ship, I.I.: Initial oral manifestations of leukemia, J.A.D.A. **75:**932-940, 1967.

McCandless, B.R., and Trotter, R.J.: Children: behavior and development, ed. 3, New York, 1977, Holt, Rinehart & Winston.

Mercer, J.R.: The eligible and the labeled, Berkeley, 1973, University of California Press.

Michaud, M., and others: Oral manifestations of acute leukemia in children, J.A.D.A. **95:**1145-1150, 1977.

Miller, O.R., and others: Smith's blood diseases of infancy and childhood, ed. 4, St. Louis, 1978, The C.V. Mosby Co.

Mink, J.R.: Dental care for the handicapped child. In Goldman, H.M., and others, editors: Current therapy in dentistry, vol. 2, St. Louis, 1966, The C.V. Mosby Co.

Morsey, S.L.: Communicating with and treating the blind child, Dent. Hyg. **65:**288-290, 1980.

National Advisory Committee on Handicapped Children: Special education for handicapped children, First Annual Report, Washington, D.C., 1968, U.S. Department of Health, Education and Welfare.

Nelson, W.E., and others, editors: Nelson's textbook of pediatrics, ed. 11, Philadelphia, 1979, W.B. Saunders Co.

Nowak, A.J.: Dentistry for the handicapped patient, St. Louis, 1976, The C.V. Mosby Co.

Pear, B.L.: Skeletal manifestation of the lymphomas and leukemias, Semin. Roentgenol. **9:**229-240, 1974.

Phillips, S., Liebert, R.M., and Poulos, R.W.: Employing para-professional teachers in a group language training program for severely and profoundly retarded children, unpublished manuscript, State University of New York at Stony Brook, 1972.

Pinkham, J.R.: The handicapped patient. In Braham, R.L., and Morris, M.E., editors: Textbook of pediatric dentistry, Baltimore, 1980, The Williams & Wilkins Co.

President's Committee on Mental Retardation: The problem of mental retardation, DHEW Pub. No. (OHD) 75-22003, Washington, D.C., 1975, U.S. Government Printing Office.

Recent advances in dental care for the hemophiliac. In Powell, D., editor: Proceedings of a workshop conference, Orthopaedic Hospital, Los Angeles, 1979.

Rituo, E.R., and Freeman, B.J.: National society of autistic children definition of the syndrome of autism, J. Pediatr. Psychol. **2:**146, 1977.

Robbins, S.L.: Pathologic basis of disease, Philadelphia, 1974, W.B. Saunders Co.

Rosenstein, S.N.: Dentistry in cerebral palsy and related handicapping conditions, Springfield, Ill., 1978, Charles C Thomas, Publisher.

Segelman, A.E., and Doku, H.C.: Treatment of the oral complications of leukemia, J. Oral Surg. **35:**469-477, 1977.

Silver, L.: Familial patterns in children with neurologically based learning disabilities, J. Learn. Disab. **4:**349-358, 1971.

Stafford, R., and others: Oral pathoses as diagnostic indicators in leukemia, Oral Surg. **50:**134-139, 1980.

Stewart, R.E., and others: Pediatric dentistry, St. Louis, 1982, The C.V. Mosby Co.

Strauss, A.A., and Kephart, N.C.: Psychopathology and education of the brain injured child: progress in theory and clinic, vol. 2, New York, 1955, Grune & Stratton, Inc.

Swallow, J.N., and Swallow, B.G.: Dentistry for physically handicapped children in the International Year of the Child, Int. Dent. J. **30:**1-5, 1980.

Tarnopol, L.: Delinquency and minimal brain dysfunction, J. Learn. Disab. **3:**200-207, 1970.

Thomas, L.B., and others: The skeletal lesions of acute leukemia, Cancer **14:**608-621, 1961.

The treatment of hemophilia. Series published by The National Hemophilia Foundation, Medical and Scientific Advisory Council, New York, 1975-1982.

Tunis, W., and Dixter, C.: Dentistry and the hearing impaired child, J. Pedod. **3:**321-334, 1979.

Weetman, R.M.: Acute leukemia in childhood. In Introduction to pediatrics. Educational manual, Department of Pediatrics, Indiana University School of Medicine, Indianapolis, 1974.

Wender, P.H.: Minimal brain dysfunction in children, New York, 1971, John Wiley & Sons, Inc.

Wessels, K.: Oral conditions in cerebral palsy, Dent. Clin. North Am., pp. 455-468, 1960.

White, G.E.: Oral manifestations of leukemia in children, Oral Surg. **29:**420-427, 1970.

Williams, B.J.: Practical oral hygiene for handicapped children, J. Dent. Child. **46:**408-409, 1979.

Wilson, J.A.R.: Diagnosis of learning difficulties, New York, 1971, McGraw-Hill Book Co.

Wing, L.: Early childhood autism: clinical, educational and social aspects, Oxford, 1976, Pergamon Press, Inc.

Wintrobe, M.W., editor: Harrison's principles of internal medicine, ed. 8, New York, 1977, McGraw-Hill Book Co.

24 The team approach to cleft lip and palate management

LaFORREST D. GARNER

W. BAILEY DAVIS

The number of cleft lip and palate babies being born in the United States is increasing. According to Grace, the ratio was one in 800 live births in 1942, but Ivy reports that the ratio since then has increased to one in 762. Although some of these anomalies appear to be genetically determined, most are of unknown cause or are due to teratogenic influences. The dental care of the cleft lip or cleft palate child is professionally stimulating and is a rewarding experience when the patient is satisfactorily habilitated.

The cleft palate team

The value of the team approach to the treatment of cleft lip or cleft palate has been pointed out by Halfond, Spriestersbach, Vincent, Kobes, and Pruzansky. The team requires the integrated skills of a pediatrician, a plastic surgeon, a pedodontist, an orthodontist, a social worker, a prosthodontist, and an otolaryngologist. Others included in the team are a psychologist, a medical geneticist, a periodontist, and an oral surgeon. Each participant plays an important role in the treatment of the child. The integrated program of surgery, speech training, dental habilitation, and social adjustment for each individual child requires careful planning and periodic reevaluation of the patient's developmental changes and response to treatment. The organization of the cleft lip and palate team is presented in Fig. 24-1.

No attempt will be made to discuss in detail the role of each member of the team. The roles of some of the team members, including pediatrician, social worker, plastic surgeon, periodontist, oral surgeon, and prosthodontist, are obvious. The contributions of the speech therapist and the geneticist in the management of children with cleft palate and children with other anomalies are discussed in Chapters 22 and 25. The two members of the team who contribute the most to the dental care and habilitation of the cleft palate patient are the pedodontist, or perhaps the family dentist, and the orthodontist.

The child's habilitation should proceed without difficulty if each member of the team carefully considers each phase of the treatment and places it in proper perspective. Improper coordination of treatment is usually reflected by unsatisfactory results.

Classification of cleft lip and palate

The condition described by the expression "clefting of the lip and palate" is subject to many variations. Discussion of a particular case of the congenital anomaly requires either a detailed picture or a description of the involved structures. The principal differences occur not only in regard to the degree of clefting but also in regard to the quantitative and qualitative adequacy of the tissues of the clefted parts. Veau has proposed what is probably the simplest and most commonly used classification of the variations of cleft lip and cleft palate

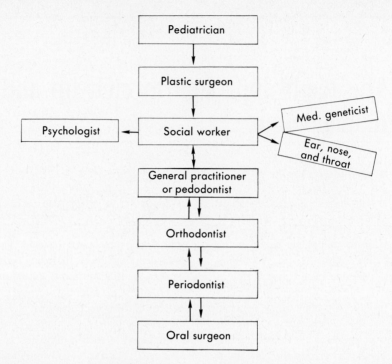

Fig. 24-1. Schematic outline of the patient's route through a cleft palate rehabilitation clinic.

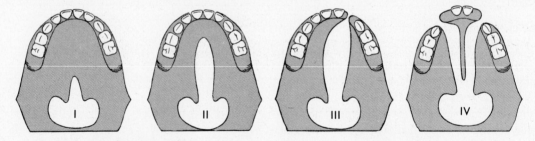

Fig. 24-2. Veau's classification: *I,* clefts of the velum; *II,* clefts of hard and soft palates; *III,* unilateral complete clefts of alveolus and secondary palate; *IV,* bilateral complete clefts of alveolus and secondary palate.

(Fig. 24-2). He describes four classes of cleft palate: Class I involves only the soft palate; Class II involves the soft and hard palates but not the alveolar process; Class III involves both the soft and hard palates, and the alveolar process on one side of the premaxillary area; Class IV involves the soft and hard palates and continues through the alveolus on both sides of the premaxilla, leaving it free and often mobile. Class III and Class IV are usually associated with clefting of the lip. Veau classifies clefts of the lip as follows: Class I, a unilateral notching of the vermilion border but not extending into the lip; Class II, a unilateral notching of the vermilion border with the cleft extending into the

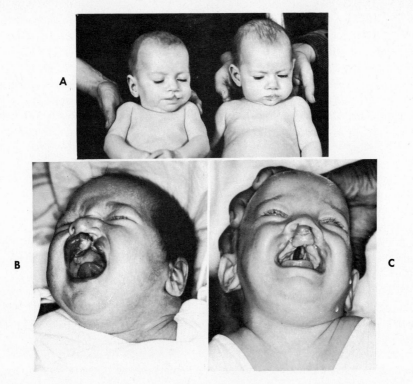

Fig. 24-3. A, Baby on the right has a Type I cleft lip. Baby on the left has a Type II cleft lip. **B,** Type III cleft lip and palate. A unilateral complete cleft lip and palate. **C,** Type IV bilateral complete cleft lip and palate.

lip, but not including the floor of the nose; Class III, a unilateral clefting of the vermilion border of the lip, extending into the floor of the nose; Class IV, any bilateral clefting of the lip, whether this be incomplete notching or complete clefting (Fig. 24-3).

The submucous cleft of the palate should be mentioned, since it does not appear in Veau's classification; this is a variation of the isolated cleft of the palate. It is significant because it is frequently overlooked as a cause of feeding difficulty or nasal regurgitation during infancy and of unintelligible speech in childhood. The condition may be expected if there is a bifid uvula. However, the diagnosis can be easily made if there is a palpable V-shaped notch at the midline posterior border of the hard palate. In addition to the notching, a thin translucent membrane may replace the median portion of

the soft palate. The soft palate also frequently appears short in the anteroposterior dimension.

It should be mentioned that clefts of the lip and palate are frequently elements in the multiple-congenital-anomaly syndromes affecting the head and neck as described by Gorlin and Pindborg. The examiner should always rule out possible associated anomalies when a child has a cleft of the lip or palate.

Pedodontic treatment

The routine dental treatment of the cleft palate patient is not really different from the dental treatment of other children of comparable age. The preventive and restorative needs of the child can be managed by a dentist who understands the developmental problems associated with the cleft defects and who is aware of the long-range treatment objectives. If there is a difference in dental care for the cleft palate patient, it is related to the greater urgency for a comprehensive preventive program, as described in Chapter 7. Restorative procedures are usually considered routine except for the management of hypoplastic and morphologic defects, as described in Chapter 4. Unfortunately, the dental health of many children with cleft palate or cleft lip has been neglected. These children often have not been seen in the dental office as early as other children, and during their first examinations there is often evidence of dental neglect and irreparable damage to the teeth. The parents may have been preoccupied with the child's previous surgical procedures and may have overlooked routine dental care. On occasion, a dentist has hesitated to perform even routine dental care because of the fear of interfering with surgical procedures. A mobile malformed premaxilla can be of great concern to a dentist who has not had experience in treating a cleft palate or cleft lip child. The importance of an early dental examination and a thorough restorative and preventive program cannot be overemphasized as a part of such a child's total habilitation.

Orthodontic treatment

Orthodontic treatment for cleft lip and palate patients can be divided into four phases, which correspond to stages in the child's dental development.

Maxillary orthopedic treatment (Stage I—birth to 18 months). The maxillary orthopedic phase of treatment is concerned with the alignment of the maxillary segments into a near normal relation, before cheiloplasty. The realignment of severely expanded segments greatly facilitates primary lip closure. Normal alignment of the affected segments has encouraged some surgeons to place otogenous bone into the cleft to produce a bony union of the segments. Maxillary orthopedics has its greatest success when it is carried out in the first few weeks of life, before surgery.

The maxillary orthopedic technique has been described by Rosenstein and Jacobson, Hotz, and McNeil. The technique can be carried out by a generalist, a pedodontist, an orthodontist, a maxillofacial prosthodontist, or a surgeon.

The technique involves producing a study cast of the infant's maxilla from an alginate impression. The usual methods of impression taking should be followed; however, the infant should be held by an assistant in an upright position. A word of caution: if the patient turns blue (becomes cyanotic), the airway is probably blocked with the alginate impression material. Care should be taken to prevent this blockage from occurring by having the infant supported in an upright position by an assistant. Having suction available is a necessity to remove impression material from the nasal passageway and pharynx. On the fabricated cast an obturator is constructed as an active or passive appliance. The technique and subsequent arch changes are illustrated by the following case,* which involved a unilateral complete cleft lip and palate in a female patient, 1 month of age.

The series of photographs (Fig. 24-4, *A* to *G*) depicts the treatment of this patient. Fig. 24-4, *A,* shows the study cast, with a 13-mm bony defect and ridge outlines. The appliance seen in Fig. 24-4, *B,* has soft-cushion rebase cold-cure acrylic† placed in all undercuts into the palatal defects and regular cold-cure acrylic covering the ridge and palatal areas. This appliance serves passively in the patient to allow segment molding following lip closure, which has been done, and doubles as a feeding appliance. The appliance acts as an obturator, feeding adjunct, and orthopedic retainer following surgical lip closure.

C and *D* of Fig. 24-4 show the study cast and the clinical view of the patient with the appliance in place and the butt joint established. An autogenous bone graft was done 2 months after the stage of treatment shown in Fig. 24-4, *D.* The occlusal radiograph of this patient 2 years after the graft can be seen in Fig. 24-4, *E.* This radiograph shows an

*This case report was made available by Dr. S.W. Rosenstein.

†Dura Base, Reliance Dental Manufacturing Co., Chicago, Ill. 60643.

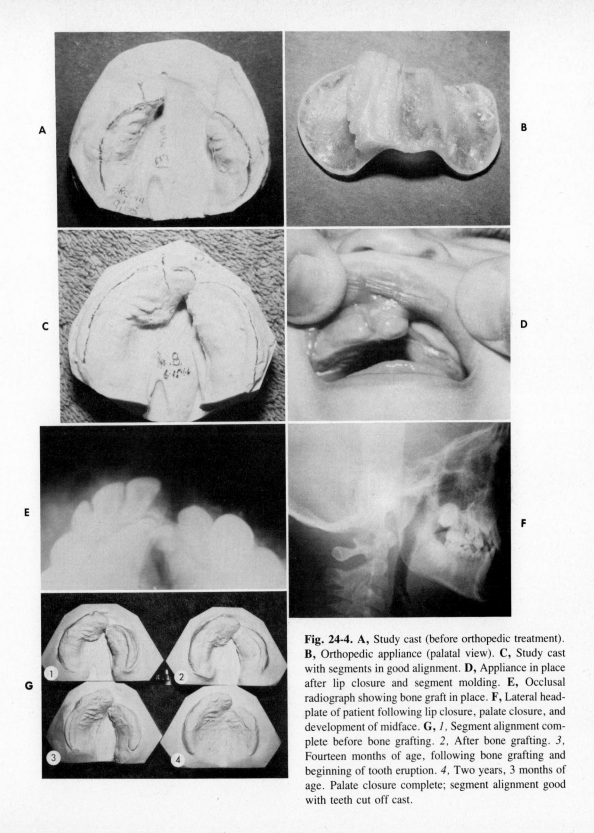

Fig. 24-4. A, Study cast (before orthopedic treatment). **B,** Orthopedic appliance (palatal view). **C,** Study cast with segments in good alignment. **D,** Appliance in place after lip closure and segment molding. **E,** Occlusal radiograph showing bone graft in place. **F,** Lateral headplate of patient following lip closure, palate closure, and development of midface. **G,** *1,* Segment alignment complete before bone grafting. *2,* After bone grafting. *3,* Fourteen months of age, following bone grafting and beginning of tooth eruption. *4,* Two years, 3 months of age. Palate closure complete; segment alignment good with teeth cut off cast.

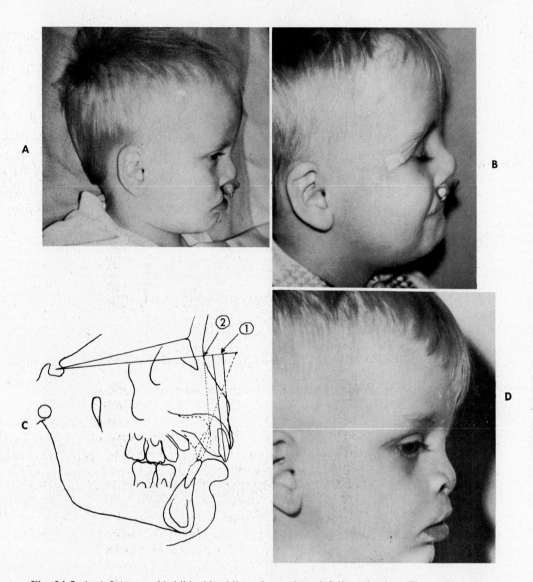

Fig. 24-5. A, A 2½-year-old child with a bilateral complete cleft lip and palate. The profile before orthodontic repositioning of the premaxillary segment. **B,** The profile after orthodontic repositioning of the premaxillary segment. **C,** Cephalometric evaluation of the distal movement of the premaxilla. **D,** Postsurgery profile view of the child. **E,** Appliances used in treating this patient include an acrylic cup, elastic bands, and high-pull headgear. **F,** Headgear appliance in place.

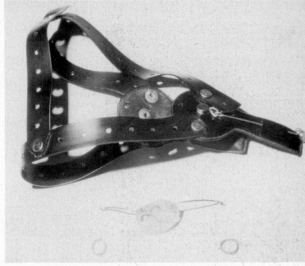

E

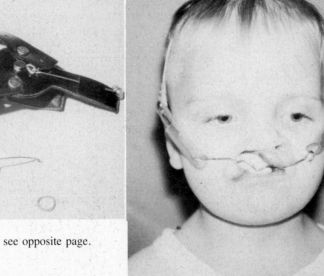

F

Fig. 24-5, cont'd. For legend see opposite page.

incisor developing in the area of the graft site. Fig. 24-4, *F,* a lateral cephalometric radiograph, shows the development of an acceptable facial profile. The final photographs of the study cast (Fig. 24-4, *G*) illustrate the ridge alignment; the top left was taken before the bone grafting, but after lip closure, at 6 months of age; the top right was taken after the bone grafting, at 1 year of age; the bottom left shows eruption of the incisors (the cast has been cut off so that the ridge contour can be viewed) at 14 months of age; and the bottom right shows palate closure, canine incisors, and erupted molars at 2 years, 3 months of age.

A recent study of infants who were born with complete clefts of the palate, with or without lip clefts, and who were seen in the James Whitcomb Riley Hospital for Children at the Indiana University Medical Center by Garner, Swartz, and Severns, points out the fact that, at least in this population, early obturation before lip or palate closure improves by 90% the ability to nurse and thrive, as compared with other feeding techniques commonly

used. For this reason these authors strongly recommend that maxillo-orthopedic techniques be carried out in infants with complete palate clefting.

Primary dentition treatment (Stage II—2 to 5 years of age). Orthodontic treatment during this stage consists of repositioning maxillary segments or correcting dental cross-bites in an attempt to allow the dentition to develop in a normal relationship. Unilateral complete and bilateral clefts of the lip and palate most frequently require orthodontic treatment during the period of the primary dentition. Children with these defects have lateral facial asymmetries as well as exaggerated convexities of the profile. Orthodontic repositioning of the premaxilla posteriorly, through retraction of the teeth, is best accomplished by means of extraoral appliances. To illustrate this treatment rationale, a 2½-year-old boy with bilateral complete cleft lip and palate (prepalate and palate) is shown before and after treatment (Fig. 24-5). The headplate tracing illustrating the radiographic change can be noted. It should be emphasized that early orthodontic treat-

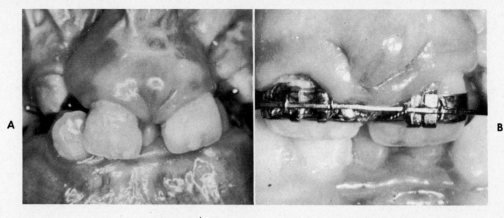

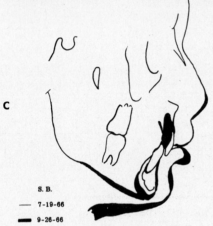

Fig. 24-6. A, Pretreatment position of the maxillary central incisors illustrating 100% overbite of the mandibular incisors. **B,** An orthodontic appliance was used in accomplishing the depression of the premaxilla and the incisors. **C,** A lateral headplate tracing superimposed on the cranial base illustrates changes in lip contour and overbite.

ment often requires lengthy retention of appliances and may aggravate problems with dental caries, in addition to taxing patient cooperation. At the time of definitive treatment, it is difficult for an orthodontist to be confronted with poor patient cooperation resulting from an appliance program that has been in effect since early childhood. Careful selection of patients for early treatment is mandatory to prevent these problems.

Mixed dentition treatment (Stage III—6 to 10 or 11 years of age). Ectopic eruption, protruding premaxilla, rotated permanent central incisors, and deep overbite and overjet are commonly observed during the mixed dentition stage in children with cleft lip and palate (Fig. 24-6). The third phase of orthodontic treatment consists of segment align-

ment and correction of traumatic occlusion. Patients with severe unilateral cleft lip and palate or with bilateral complete cleft lip and palate frequently have a cross-bite of the posterior and anterior maxillary segments. This problem can be corrected in the mixed dentition by palatal expansion and by an appliance to flare the maxillary anterior teeth (Fig. 24-7). Retention of corrected segments and teeth also presents a serious problem and must be considered in the long-range treatment. Patient fatigue must be prevented and should be an important consideration in extensive therapy. Growth analysis must be carefully predicted to avoid the need for retreatment of a problem in the permanent dentition that was hastily treated in the mixed dentition. If there is no evidence of traumatic occlu-

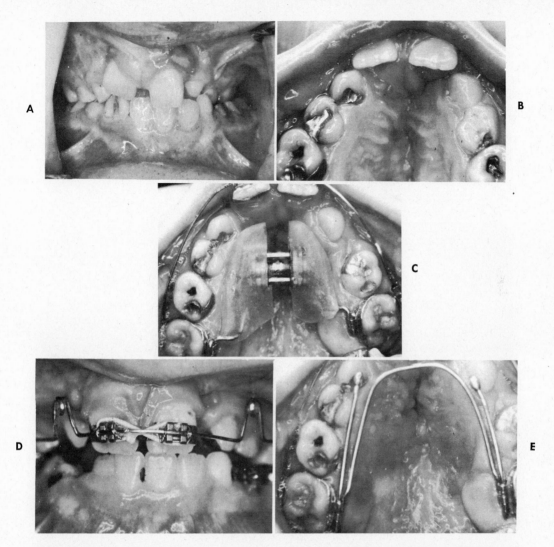

Fig. 24-7. A, Occlusion before treatment. There is a diastema between the central incisors and a left buccal cross-bite. **B,** An occlusal view of the maxillary arch. **C,** The jack screw appliance used for sutural expansion. The labial arch wire was designed for advancing the arch length and flaring the central incisors. **D,** The labial spring used for flaring the incisors. **E,** A removable lingual arch wire was used to retain posterior widths.

sion, in many cases treatment is best postponed until the permanent dentition phase or deferred until the growth pattern can be determined.

Permanent dentition treatment (Stage IV—12 to 18 years of age). Orthodontic treatment for the teenage cleft palate–cleft lip patient (permanent dentition) requires the same consideration as that for other children, with the exception of alignment and spacing in the cleft area. Each child must have a careful orthodontic evaluation before treatment. The prosthodontist should always be consulted so that definitive restorative care and retention can be

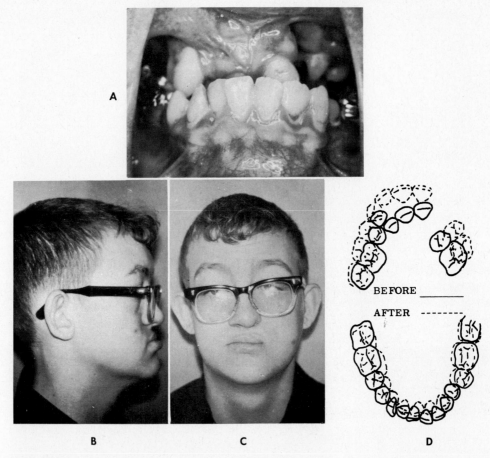

Fig. 24-8. A, Anterior and bilateral cross-bite. **B** and **C,** The pretreatment facial profile was concave and asymmetric to the right side. **D,** An occlusogram of the occlusion before and after orthodontic alignment of the teeth and arches.

planned in advance. Fig. 24-8 illustrates the comprehensive tooth movement and facial esthetic changes that resulted from treatment of a unilateral complete cleft of the lip and palate (prepalate and palate) (Type III) in a boy 14 years of age.

The patient had an anterior and bilateral posterior cross-bite. The facial profile was concave and asymmetric to the right side. On clinical examination a 2-mm mesial shift of the mandible was recorded, and the vertical dimension was found to be 6 mm overclosed. An occlusogram of the maxillary and mandibular arches was made and the

inadequacies in arch length were recorded, as well as rotations of the mandible in the projected treatment position. The cephalometric analysis indicated a concave skeletal profile and an Angle Class III malocclusion. There was a maxillomandibular discrepancy to occlusal plane of 6 mm.

Treatment consisted of rotating the mandible downward and backward 2 degrees; the position of the most prominent lower central incisor was to be retracted 5 mm and the maxillary incisor flared 8 mm to correct the 13-mm anterior cross-bite. To accomplish this correction, the two mandibular

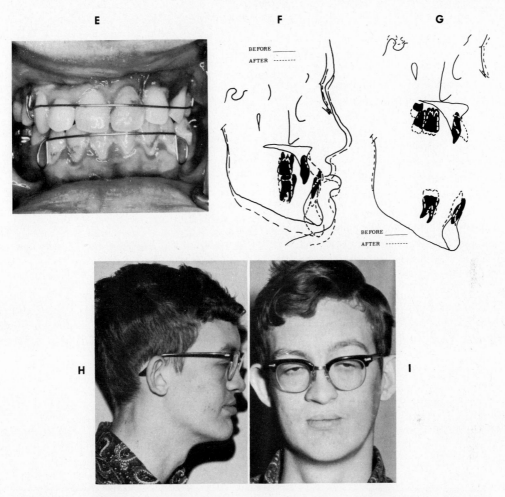

Fig. 24-8, cont'd. E, The occlusion after the correction of the anterior and posterior cross-bite. The retainers are in place. **F,** Composite cephalometric tracings registered on cranial base and illustrating changes in profile and tooth positon. **G,** Maxillary and mandibular superpositions illustrating changes in the positions of individual teeth. **H and I,** The posttreatment profile and frontal photographs.

first premolars were removed surgically, and bands were placed on the remaining teeth in both arches. Kloehn extraoral headgear (cervical-type) appliances were placed on the lower first molars to aid the eruption of the posterior teeth and to prevent their mesial movement during the retraction of the six anterior teeth en masse. The maxillary teeth were banded, the buccal segments expanded, and the anterior teeth advanced with an open-coil spring to make space for the lingually locked lateral incisor.

The results of the orthodontic treatment can be seen on the occlusogram. The original positions of the teeth are recorded in solid lines, and posttreatment positions are recorded in dotted lines.

The clinical frontal view of the occlusion after treatment shows the anterior and posterior cross-bite corrected, with a maxillary Hawley retainer in position, replacing the missing lateral incisor and canine. The hinging action of the mandible can be seen by using a cephalometric tracing with the cranial base superpositioned. The mandible was rotated downward and backward 2 degrees, and the skeletal profile was improved from −18 to −12 degrees. Maxillary and mandibular superpositional tracings are also included to illustrate changes in the positions of individual teeth. The positions of the maxillary and mandibular incisors and molars before treatment are represented by solid lines; dotted lines represent posttreatment positions.

In Fig. 24-8, *E*, gross plaque and poor oral hygiene are evident. Poor oral hygiene is one of the problems occasionally observed in cleft lip and/or palate patients. Often they are conscientious about keeping appointments for regular dental visits and orthodontic adjustments, until it becomes time for a finished prosthesis, when they lose interest in their dental health. Such was the case with this patient.

REFERENCES

Conway, H., and Wayner, K.S.: Incidence of clefts in New York City, Cleft Palate J. **3:**284-290, 1966.

Garner, L.D., Swartz, B., and Severns, P.: Maxillo-orthopedics—adjunct feeding appliance, J. Ind. Dent. Assoc. **61:**7-10, 1982.

Gorlin, R.J., and Pindborg, J.J.: Syndromes of the head and neck, New York, 1964, McGraw-Hill Book Co.

Grace, L.: Frequency of occurrence of cleft palates and harelips, J. Dent. Res. **22:**495-497, 1943.

Halfond, M.M.: The team approach: cum grano salis, Cleft Palate Bull. **11:**62-63, 1961.

Harkins, C.S., and others: A classification of cleft lip and palate, Plast. Reconstr. Surg. **29:**31-39, 1962.

Hotz, R., editor: Early treatment of cleft lip and palate, Berne, 1964, Hans Huber, Medical Publisher.

Ivy, R.H.: Modern concept of cleft lip and palate management, Plast. Reconstr. Surg. **9:**121-129, 1952.

Kobes, H.R., and Pruzansky, S.: The cleft palate team: a historical review, Dent. Abs. **5:**501-502, 1960.

McNeil, C.K.: Orthodontic procedures in the treatment of congenital cleft palate, Dent. Rec. **70:**126, 1950.

Moorrees, C.F.A.: Normal variation in dental development determined with reference to tooth eruption status, J. Dent. Res. **44**(suppl.):161-173, 1965.

Pruzansky, S.: Factors determining arch form in clefts of the lip and palate, Am. J. Orthod. **41:**827-851, 941 (correction), 1955.

Pruzansky, S.: The multidiscipline approach of the treatment of cleft palate in children, Cleft Palate Bull. **10:**99, 1960.

Rosenstein, S.W., and Jacobson, B.N.: Early maxillary orthopedics: a sequence of events, Cleft Palate J. **4:**197-204, 1967.

Spriestersbach, D.C.: Professional survival groups, Cleft Palate Bull. **12:**63-66, 1962.

Veau, V.: Treatment of the unilateral harelip, Int. Dent. Cong. Eighth Trans., pp. 126-131, 1931.

Vincent, C.J.: The pedodontist in cleft palate rehabilitation, Cleft Palate Bull. **10:**68-69, 1960.

25 Pedodontics and speech pathology: speech and language performance in children

BERND WEINBERG

A dentist may be the first professional person consulted for professional advice concerning children with speech and language problems. It is therefore desirable for dentists to be knowledgeable about and have access to information concerning (1) the normal sequence of development of speech and language in young children, (2) the process by which speech is produced, (3) the major types of speech and language disorders, and (4) the professional diagnostic and therapeutic services available to children with communication disorders. This chapter is designed to provide dentists with basic information about these aspects of communication behavior during childhood. Appropriate references are also provided for those interested in further study.

The speech process

Speech may be defined as the ordered utterance of a language. The speech mechanism involves the various systems, structures, and cavities seen in Fig. 25-1. Several basic processes—respiration, phonation, resonance, and articulation—are coordinated to produce the dynamic acoustic modulations of speech.

The initial requirement for speaking is an energy source, which is provided by the respiratory system. Normal speech demands a readily available, adequate, well-controlled, and systematically directed airstream. Air is rapidly inhaled, and speech is typically produced during a more lengthy period of expiration.

Phonation, a sound-generating process, results from vibratory activity of the vocal folds. During the production of voiced sounds the vocal folds vibrate as exhaled air is forced between them. The exhaled airstream is interrupted by the vibratory pattern of the vocal folds, and the emanating air puffs create sound. The sound generated by the larynx is not what is heard as speech. Rather, this sound, referred to as a ''source excitation,'' serves

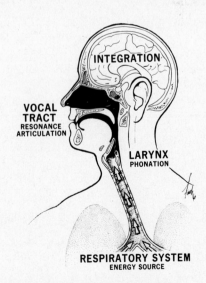

Fig. 25-1. The speech mechanism.

699

as acoustic material from which some speech sounds are later developed.

The processes concerned with shaping or modifying source sounds into identifiable speech sounds are resonance and articulation. Since the cavities of the vocal tract can be resonated, source sounds are modified through selective alteration of the size and shape (configuration) of the vocal tract.* Thus resonance is a cavity function that contributes significantly to the production of speech. Depending on the configuration of the vocal tract, certain frequencies of the source are selectively amplified or attenuated.

The term "articulation" refers to the placement and movement of the lips, teeth, tongue, mandible, palate, and associated structures during speech. Articulatory behavior alters the configuration of the vocal tract, thereby determining some of its resonant properties. These actions also form the well-defined and systematically varied oral and pharyngeal constrictions necessary for consonant production.

The term "integration" refers to activity within the nervous system and to the operation of important auditory mechanisms and "servomechanisms" that coordinate the processes involved in the production of speech and regulate the dynamic features of speech.

Speech can be studied in terms of its acoustic properties, its perception, and its anatomic and physiologic aspects. Speech can be thought of as an acoustic signal that results from various anatomic and physiologic factors. Speech sounds have special physical properties. However, the properties of each sound are influenced by the speech sounds that precede and succeed it. The articulation of speech is a dynamic process involving the generation of acoustic signals that vary in frequency, duration, and intensity. Some of these variations assist the listener in differentiating between sounds; other variations make it difficult for

listeners to discriminate between sounds. Speech perception, however, depends on factors other than the acoustic signals. For example, the adequacy of the listener's auditory system, the nature of the perceptual environment, and the linguistic orientations of the speaker and the listener influence the perception of speech. The introduction of perception into the description of the speech process is a reminder that communication is a reciprocal activity; it involves both the reception and the expression of acoustically transmitted information.

Language and speech development in childhood

The acquisition of language and speech during childhood represents a unique facet of human growth and development. Information about normal aspects of language acquisition is essential for understanding humans in general, for describing the intellectual and cognitive development of children in particular, and for providing standards that distinguish normal from deviant or disordered language function.

It is important for dentists and other professionals who see children to appreciate the special significance of language development. For example, language and cognition are clearly related. Since language function may predict future intellectual or cognitive endowment, an appraisal of language function should be an essential feature of the evaluation of infants and young children. A dentist, particularly a pedodontist, is in a position to see children with potential developmental disabilities or problems, and deviant or delayed language development accompanies many childhood disorders.

The initial utterance of a human infant is the birth cry. The cries of newborns have been used to evaluate their well-being and their neurologic status. As the infant develops, cry sounds become varied, assuming certain acoustic and temporal patterns, and soon the infant's mother can distinguish a pain cry from a hunger cry. Thus, early cry vocalizations are used by the infant to meet the fundamental demands of communication.

---

*The vocal tract consists of the cavities and structures above the glottis or the opening between the vocal folds.

In the early months of life, infants exhibit alerting responses—responses that verify that a child recognizes sound. These include Moro responses, blinking, movements of the body or body parts, and alterations in the respiratory or heart rate in response to sound. During the first months of life, cooing (the sustained production of long vowels) becomes superimposed upon or interspersed with differentiated cries. At around 4 to 5 months of age, children display orienting responses—for example, turning the head toward the mother's voice or toward a stimulus (such as a bell ring) located either above or to the side of the head.

Between 4 and 6 months of age, most children begin producing sounds that resemble speech. The magnitude of these sounds, known as babbling, increases during the first year of life. Babbling often sounds like speech, seems to occur in sentence-like sequences, and seems to be associ-ated with appropriate variations in emphasis, intonation, and pitch. Babbling sounds are often not interpretable or understood. Typically, children begin producing their first words between 10 and 15 months of age. The frequency of babbling declines as understood words emerge. Gesture language, exemplified by waving "bye-bye" or playing "pat-a-cake," often is present late (9 to 11 months) in the first year of life.

Most children begin speaking with single words. Typically they begin to put words together during the second year of life, and the length and linguistic complexity of this process increase as they grow older. Children exhibit extensive variation in the rate at which they master new words, the intelligibility of their speech, the rate and nature of spontaneous imitation, and the diversity of linguistic structures produced in this process.

It is now evident that sometime during the sec-

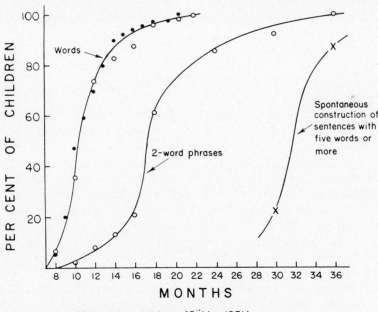

Fig. 25-2. Emergence of various developmental milestones in the acquisition of language. (From Lenneberg, E.H.: The natural history of language. In Smith, F., and Miller, G.A., editors: The genesis of language, Cambridge, Mass., 1966, The M.I.T. Press.)

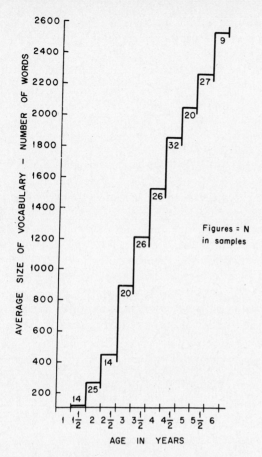

Fig. 25-3. Average vocabulary size of 10 samples of children at various ages. (From Lenneberg, E.H.: The natural history of language. In Smith, F., and Miller, G.A., editors: The genesis of language, Cambridge, Mass., 1966, The M.I.T. Press.)

vocabulary, particularly around the third birthday, is illustrated in Fig. 25-3.

Language milestone	Months of age
Alerting	1
Social smile	1½
Cooing	3
Orient to voice	4
Orient to bell (looks to side)	5
Babbling	6
Orient to bell (looks to side, then up)	7
Gesture	9
Orient to bell (turns directly toward bell)	10
"Da da," "ma ma" (appropriately)	10
One word	11
One-step command (with gestures)	12
Two words	12
Three words	14
One-step command (without gestures)	15
Four to six words	15
Immature jargoning	15
Seven to 20 words	18
Mature jargoning	18
One body part	18
Three body parts	21
Two-word combinations	21
Five body parts	23
Fifty words	24
Two-word sentences (noun/pronoun inappropriately and verb)	24
Pronouns (I, me, you, and so forth inappropriately)	24

One purpose of this chapter is to give dentists who deal with children a better understanding of language development, deviance, and disorder. Milestone or normative data have been presented to provide the dentist with a basis for determining whether a child has problems that are likely to preclude or delay language acquisition and lead to a communication disorder. Individual differences are important, and the ages at which children reach milestones vary extensively. Young children follow various paths to attain the common goal of speaking a language. Hence, it is important to note that milestone data highlight commonalities of development and not individual differences.

At the same time, it is clear that auditory and language milestones do exist. Reliable information

ond year of life, normal children produce words relatively often and provide evidence of thought; that is, they pretend and recall. Certain important language development milestones are reached in a sequential fashion and at relatively constant ages in normally developing youngsters. Some characteristic stages of language development in children are presented in Fig. 25-2 and in the following list.* The rapid increase in the size of a child's

*Modified from Capute, A.J., and Accardo, P.J.: Clin. Pediatr. **7:**847, 1978.

QUESTIONS FOR OBTAINING ACCURATE
PARENTAL REPORTING OF LANGUAGE AND
AUDITORY MILESTONES

1. When did your infant first recognize the presence of sound by blinking, startling, moving any part of the body, and so on?
2. When did your infant smile at you when you talked to him or stroked his face?
3. When did your infant produce long vowel sounds in a musical fashion?
4. When did your infant turn to you when you spoke to him? (Rule out any visual clues.)
5. When did your infant first babble? (Demonstrate.)
6. When did your infant first wave bye-bye or play pat-a-cake?
7. When did your infant first begin to use "da da" or "ma ma" appropriately?
8. When did your infant say his first word other than "da da" and "ma ma"?
9. When did your infant begin to follow simple commands such as "Give me _____" or "Bring me _____" accompanied by a gesture?
10. (12 months) How large is your child's vocabulary?
11. (14 months) How large is your child's vocabulary?
12. When was your infant able to follow simple commands without any accompanying gesture?
13. (15 months) How large is your child's vocabulary?
14. When did your infant begin to jargon—to run unintelligible "words" together in an attempt to make a "sentence" or speak as if in a foreign language?
15. (18 months) How large is your child's vocabulary?
16. When did your child's jargoning begin to include several intelligible words?
17. How many body parts can your child point to when named? Which ones?
18. (21 months) How many body parts can your child point to when named? Which ones?
19. When did your child start to put two words together? (Demonstrate.)
20. (23 months) How many body parts can your child point to when named? Which ones?
21. (24 months) How large is your child's vocabulary?
22. When did your child start to combine a noun or pronoun with a verb?
23. When did your child use three pronouns but inappropriately?

Modified from Capute, A.J., and Accardo, P.J.: Clin. Pediatr. **7:**847, 1978.

---

about these milestones often can readily be obtained from parents, specifically mothers. Questions dentists can ask mothers concerning milestone data are summarized in the box above. Significant (9 to 12 month) delay in the attainment of milestones is an important indicator of potential abnormality. For example, significant language delay can be said to exist for any child who is not saying single words by 24 months, who is not using simple words that are intelligible by 36 to 42 months, or who is solely babbling or imitating speech at 24 to 30 months. Referral for evaluation is justified in such cases.

As is the case in regard to physical growth and temperament, children exhibit great variation in their language development. Differences in the rate at which the biologic maturing process proceeds and in the experiences children have bring about differences in the age at which they begin to talk, in the rate at which linguistic development proceeds, and in the approaches children implement to acquire linguistic behavior. Unfortunately, there are instances when a delay in language acquisition or the nature and frequency of differences characterize a child's language development as deviant or disordered.

Language development may be deviant or delayed in several ways. For example, it may be delayed, yet follow normal patterns. As shown previously, deviance depends on linguistic maturity in relation to a child's age. Deviance also depends on the number of aspects of language production and comprehension that differ from normal. For example, the speech of a child with an articulation problem may not appear as disordered as it would if this difficulty were combined with deviant grammar.

Many preschool- and school-age children show delayed or deviant language development. Some exhibit problems only in producing the sounds of speech (articulation problems). Others display a more fundamental type of deviance or delay—one that is not restricted merely to production of the sounds of speech. Such a problem may be related to comprehension or to the production of grammar. For example, deficits in hearing may exert a profound effect on language acquisition. Deaf children are typically handicapped in the development of several language skills. Two other examples of conditions marked by substantial language deviance or delay are mental retardation and infantile autism. Finally, there are children with language deviance or delay who do not have any of these major developmental disorders.

The sounds of the English language

The efficient transmission and reception of information are the fundamental purposes of human communication. A useful method of attempting to understand the code involved in communication is to describe the sounds of oral language.

There is a considerable body of evidence to support the view that individual speech sounds probably do not constitute the basic units of speech production or perception. In other words, speech is probably not produced or perceived by serially ordering individual sounds to form words, phrases, and sentences in a fashion akin to stringing beads to form a necklace. Thus, although we generally think of spoken words as if they were made up of separate speech sounds, the acoustic patterns of these words are continuous and cannot readily be segmented into component units corresponding to the individual sounds. However, for explanatory purposes speech can be artificially divided into isolated sound units. Basic understanding of how individual speech sounds are produced and of their developmental pattern of emergence will enhance the dentist's understanding of the speech process. Such understanding will facilitate the dentist's attempts to evaluate and refer patients who are having difficulty in producing speech sounds.

The two major categories of speech sounds in the English language are vowels and consonants. The production of vowels and diphthongs (vowel combinations) necessitates the formation of fairly consistent vocal tract configurations. During vowel production the larynx generates a source sound that is resonated by the cavities of the vocal tract. The distinctive shape of the vocal tract modifies the laryngeal sound source in characteristic ways to produce a specified vowel. Vowels are produced with minimum constriction of the vocal tract—that is, they are produced in a relatively "open" vocal tract—and they result from air cavity resonance.

On the other hand, consonants are generally produced by constricting or obstructing the vocal tract in specific ways at particular locations. Consonant sound production requires constricting, obstructing, or modulating the outgoing breath stream or laryngeal sound, or both, in a "closed" vocal tract. The voiceless consonants have as their sole sound source the modulation of the respiratory airstream resulting from a constriction or an obstruction. During voiced consonant production the laryngeal sound source is added to these breath stream modulations.

The consonant sounds are extremely important because they represent the information-bearing elements of speech and because they contribute significantly to speech intelligibility. As might be expected, consonant misarticulations are more frequent than vowel misarticulations. Consonant misarticulations are of major concern to both dentists and speech pathologists, since consonants carry such a high information-bearing load.

The consonant sounds may be classified according to place of production, manner of production, and voicing component (Table 25-1). The place of production is the location of the constriction or occlusion within the vocal tract—that is, the place where the breath stream is impeded or stopped momentarily as it is directed through the vocal

Table 25-1. Speech sound classification

Speech sound	Voicing	Primary resonating cavity and/or air flow receptor	Principal place and manner of articulation	Sample word
p	Voiceless	Oral	Bilabial contact—plosive	*p*ie
b	Voiced	Oral	Bilabial contact—plosive	*b*oy
m	Voiced	Oral and nasal	Bilabial contact—nasal	*m*an
t	Voiceless	Oral	Lingual-alveolar contact—plosive	*t*ie
d	Voiced	Oral	Lingual-alveolar contact—plosive	*d*og
n	Voiced	Oral and nasal	Lingual-alveolar contact—nasal	*n*o
l	Voiced	Oral	Lingual-alveolar contact—glide	*l*ady
f	Voiceless	Oral	Labial-dental contact—fricative	*f*our
v	Voiced	Oral	Labial-dental contact—fricative	*v*ery
th (θ)	Voiceless	Oral	Lingual-interdental contact—fricative	*th*in
th (ð)	Voiced	Oral	Lingual-interdental contact—fricative	*th*is
k	Voiceless	Oral	Lingual-velar contact—plosive	*k*ey
g	Voiced	Oral	Lingual-velar contact—plosive	*g*o
ng (ŋ)	Voiced	Oral and nasal	Lingual-alveolar to lingual-velar contact—nasal	ri*ng*
h	Voiceless	Oral	Glottal constriction—glottal	*h*ow
w	Voiced	Oral	Widening labial aperture—glide	*W*ales
hw (ʍ)	Voiceless	Oral	Widening labial aperture—glide	*wh*ale
s	Voiceless	Oral	Tongue tip or tongue blade production; narrow, central, lingual-alveolar orifice; lateral lingual-dental/alveolar seal—fricative	*s*ee
z	Voiced	Oral	Tongue tip or tongue blade production; narrow, central, lingual-alveolar orifice; lateral lingual-dental/alveolar seal—fricative	*z*oo
sh (ʃ)	Voiceless	Oral	Central lingual-alveolar/palatal orifice; lateral lingual-dental/alveolar seal—fricative	*sh*oe
r	Voiced	Oral	Widening lingual-palatal aperture—glide	*r*ing
j	Voiced	Oral	Widening lingual-palatal aperture—glide	*y*es
ch (tʃ)	Voiceless	Oral	Lingual-alveolar contact to central lingual-alveolar orifice—affricative	*ch*air
ʒ	Voiced	Oral	Central lingual-palatal/alveolar orifice; lateral lingual-dental/alveolar seal—fricative	a*z*ure
dʒ	Voiced	Oral	Lingual-alveolar contact to central lingual-palatal/alveolar orifice; lateral lingual-dental/alveolar seal—affricative	*J*ack
Vowels				
i	Voiced	Oral		h*ea*t
ɪ	Voiced	Oral		h*i*t
ɛ	Voiced	Oral		h*ea*d
æ	Voiced	Oral		h*a*d
ʌ	Voiced	Oral		h*u*d
ɑ	Voiced	Oral		f*a*ther
ɔ	Voiced	Oral		*a*ll
ʊ	Voiced	Oral		p*u*t
u	Voiced	Oral		c*oo*l
o	Voiced	Oral		t*o*ne
e	Voiced	Oral		t*a*ke

tract. The major places of consonant production are the lips (bilabial consonants), the lips and anterior teeth (labial-dental consonants), the tongue and teeth (lingual-interdental consonants), the tongue and palate (lingual-palatal or lingual-velar consonants), and the glottis (glottal consonants).

The following is a classification of consonants on the basis of manner of production:

1. *Plosive or stop-plosives* (/p/,/b/,/t/,/d/,/k/, and /g/). Plosive consonants are produced by occluding the vocal tract at a certain location, building up air pressure behind this site, and subsequently opening the site to release a pressure pulse.

2. *Fricatives* (/f/,/v/,/th/,/s/,/z/,/ʒ/, and /sh/). Fricative consonants are produced by directing the airstream through a well-defined constriction within the vocal tract. Fricative sounds result from turbulence or "friction" produced within the constriction. Unlike plosive consonant production, fricative consonant formation does not require complete occlusion of the vocal tract.

3. *Affricatives* (/ch/ and /dʒ/). Affricate consonants are produced by combining the plosive and fricative manners of production. The acoustic event, however, is perceived as a single speech sound.

4. *Glides* (/l/,/w/,/r/, and /j/). Glides are produced in a relatively open vocal tract and result primarily from air cavity resonance. During the production of glides the speech articulators are in motion. Glides are characterized by continuous changes in acoustic properties during the course of their production. They are in many respects similar to vowels.

5. *Nasals* (/n/,/m/, and /ng/). Nasal sounds are produced by directing air and sound through the nose and creating resonance within both the oral and nasal cavities. The nasal sounds differ from all other speech sounds in that the nasal cavities are added to the oral and pharyngeal portions of the vocal tract during their production.

Discussions of consonant production frequently present sounds in pairs called cognates. Approximately half of the consonants are produced by supplementing articulatory activity with vocal fold vibration (voiced consonants); the other half are produced in the absence of vocal fold vibration (voiceless consonants). Each pair of cognates consists of a voiced consonant and its corresponding voiceless consonant—that is, the consonant produced when the vocal fold vibration is removed.

Speech articulation development

The gradual emergence of sound units and the acquisition of speech articulation skills represent a maturational process. The sequential development of the articulatory process is shown in Fig. 25-4. Such normative data can be used by the dentist to evaluate a patient's speech articulation skills. Vowels are the first speech sounds to be fully mastered. Most children are able to correctly articulate vowels by 3 to 3½ years of age. The consonant sounds require more time to master. Cross-sectional, normative studies have shown that for some children consonant sound maturation is not complete until 8 years of age.

Thus, speech sound errors in children 8 years of age and older are highly significant, while such errors in 5-year-old children may or may not indicate an articulatory disorder, since proficiency in the production of all speech sounds is not expected.

Speech disorders: a broad classification

Human speech may be categorized and studied in terms of three primary factors: (1) the phonetic units of speech, (2) the rhythmic features of speech, and (3) the pitch, loudness, and voice-quality characteristics of speakers. Speech pathologists frequently classify speech disorders according to these principal divisions; they describe speech as defective or disordered when one or more of these features differs significantly from what is normal for the age, sex, and psychosocial environment of the speaker. When a disorder involves a primary disturbance in the articulation of speech sounds, the defect is a speech articulation

Age level

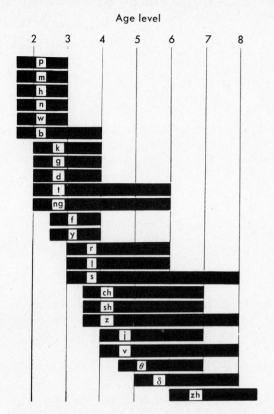

Fig. 25-4. Estimates of average age and upper age limits of consonant production. The solid bar corresponding to each sound starts at the median age of customary articulation; it stops at an age level at which 90% of all children are customarily producing the sound. (From Sander, E.K.: J. Speech Hear. Disord. **37**:55-63, 1972.)

problem. When significant differences from normal are heard in pitch, loudness, or voice quality, the defect is a voice disorder. When a disorder involves a disturbance in the rhythmic features of speech, the problem is stuttering.

Disorders of speech articulation. Speech articulation disorders are the most common type of speech problem. Speech sound errors may result from a number of factors: hearing loss, poor auditory discrimination, oral malformations, sensory-motor impairment, intellectual retardation, emo-

tional disorders, and faulty learning. In general, speech sound errors are sound substitutions ("wabbit" for rabbit), sound omissions ("ca" for cat), or sound distortions (lisping).

The common belief that articulation disorders in children are related to dental deviations often causes parents to seek the professional advice of dentists. Dentists, physicians, parents, and speech therapists may inadvertently attach etiologic significance to dental deviations observed in children exhibiting speech sound misarticulations without first determining that there are logical relationships between the dental deviations and the sound errors. As a general rule, children compensate for minor dental deviations.

That the teeth have a normal function during the production of speech cannot be contested. Certain differences in oral structure may preclude or hinder the formation of appropriate vocal tract constrictions required for speech. It has generally been assumed that the teeth play a role in the production of the labial-dental consonants /f/ and /v/, the lingual-interdental consonants /θ/ and /ð/, and the lingual-alveolar consonants /s/, /z/, /ʒ/, /sh/, /ch/ and /ʤ/.

Developmental studies have shown that missing teeth are common among children during the period of speech articulation development. The period from 5 to 12 years of age is characterized by deciduous tooth resorption and shedding and by eruption of the permanent dentition. It has been shown that many of the fricative sounds are being developed and stabilized during the period from age 5 to age 8 (Fig. 25-4). Disruptions in the dentition may contribute to articulation errors in sounds that are developing, as well as in sounds that have already been established.

No significant relationship has been found between the adequacy with which the /sh/, /z/, /f/, /v/, and /th/ sounds are produced and the absence or presence of incisors in 6- to 8-year-old children. The majority of children with missing incisors are able to produce these sounds correctly; that is, they are able to manipulate the tongue and associated structures in ways that enable them to produce these consonants in a normal manner. Moreover, many first-grade children are unable to articulate some of these sounds correctly even with their incisors present. This latter finding emphasizes the developmental nature of the acquisition of speech articulation and indicates that some sounds are late-developing units not dependent on dental elements for their maturation.

Absence of incisor teeth is, however, significantly related to problems with /s/ sound production in some children. It must be remembered that the loss of incisors represents only one possible etiologic factor related to defective /s/ sound production.

There has been only a limited amount of substantive research on the relationship between malocclusion and speech articulation. Clinical experience suggests that severe malocclusion may be associated with defective /s/ articulation skills. However, minor malocclusion is frequently not associated with speech articulation errors. For example, patients with Class II, Division 1 malocclusion may produce the bilabial consonants (/p/,/b/, and /m/) in a labial-dental manner because of difficulties in achieving lip closure. Although no difference may be heard during the production of these sounds, careful observation of such patients may reveal compensatory speech mechanisms. Further research is needed for early identification of children whose dentition may contribute to articulatory problems.

Dental deviations must always be functionally related to specific speech sound misarticulations. The absence of dentition should generally not be causally related to problems in bilabial (/p/,/m/, /b/), lingual-velar (/k/,/g/,/ŋ/), lingual-palatal (/r/, /j/,/k/,/g/, and /ng/), glottal (/h/), or vowel production. Speakers usually compensate for the loss of dental elements during the production of the labial-dental consonants (/f/ and /v/) and the lingual-interdental consonants (/th/), to the point that no differences can be heard. In some children the absence of incisors may influence the production of /s/ and other sibilant speech sounds. When speech sound errors are heard during sibilant sound artic-

ulation, the dentist should consider the dental condition of the patient as one of a number of possible contributing factors. However, when children have difficulty producing other consonant sounds, the dentist should look for factors other than the dentition. It is doubtful that dental therapy alone will correct a speech defect in children who cannot compensate adequately for dental abnormalities. In such cases dental therapy may allow a patient to profit more from speech therapy.

On rare occasions, a dentist or a physician examines a child with a short lingual frenum. It may be tempting to relate this difference in oral structure to the child's speech. In some cases, a short lingual frenum may prevent the normal interdentalization of the tongue during /th/ production or may preclude the normal tongue tip elevation for production of /t/,/d/,/n/,/l/,/ch/, and /dʒ/. However, children usually adapt readily to this problem and produce these sounds in an acceptable fashion. Restrictions of the lingual frenum rarely affect the speech patterns of children. Surgical release of such a restriction may enable a child to produce certain consonants in the normal place of articulation. However, factors other than speech typically determine the need for the surgical release of a short lingual frenum.

Minor differences in lip form and function also do not represent major factors in speech articulation errors. A listener can rarely detect differences in the production of bilabial and labial-dental consonants when minor deviations of the lips are present. This view is consistent with the finding that individuals with repaired clefts of the lip have essentially normal speech. Clinical experience suggests that persons with short or taut upper lips or with unusually great facial height compensate with greater lower lip movement to effect normal speech.

Complete diagnostic evaluations of children with speech articulation disorders are essential. Conclusions must be based on thorough studies of the factors responsible for speech sound errors, an awareness of the maturational features of speech articulation in children, an appreciation of the acoustic, anatomic, and physiologic mechanisms that underlie speech, and an ability to delineate the type and consistency of speech sound errors exhibited.

Speech problems associated with velopharyngeal impairment. Studies of the form and function of the palate and pharynx have done much to provide an area of common interest between speech pathologists and dentists. In particular, multidisciplinary research and ''team'' management of children with cleft lip and palate have brought the two disciplines toward the significant realization that each is concerned with oral and pharyngeal form and function. Dentists play an important role in the management of cases involving children who have speech problems associated with velopharyngeal impairment. Thus, basic information concerning the function of the palate and pharynx during speech and a description of the most frequent speech problems associated with abnormalities of velopharyngeal form and function are presented here.

During tidal respiration the soft palate is typically in contact with the dorsum of the tongue, a basic motor mechanism that serves to protect the pharyngeal airway. During tidal breathing the velopharyngeal isthmus (which is situated between the soft palate and the posterior pharyngeal wall) is open (Fig. 25-5).

The relationships between the palate and pharynx during deglutition and speech differ markedly from the relationships between these structures during respiration. For example, during speech the velopharyngeal mechanism functions as a valve to control the degree of coupling between the oral-pharyngeal and nasal cavities. When the soft palate (or velum) is elevated, it approximates the pharyngeal walls, thereby closing the velopharyngeal port. Closing of the velopharyngeal port is accomplished primarily by elevation of the velum, together with medial movement of the lateral pharyngeal walls.

During the production of normal speech, the velopharyngeal valve mechanism either precludes coupling or allows for various degrees of coupling between the nasal and oral-pharyngeal cavities of the vocal tract. During the production of nasal consonant sounds in English, the velum is lowered, permitting coupling between the nasal and oral-pharyngeal cavities. During the production of the

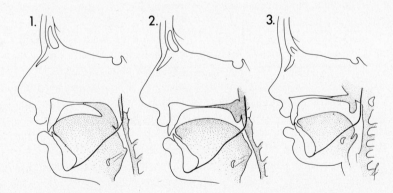

Fig. 25-5. Lateral cephalometric drawings demonstrating velopharyngeal relationships during speech and tidal respiration in normal persons. *1*, Adult subject during tidal respiration. Note patency of velopharyngeal isthmus and pharyngeal airway and contact between soft palate and tongue. *2*, Adult subject sustaining voiceless fricative consonant. Note prominent levator eminence, absence of uvular participation in isthmus closure, and length of velopharyngeal contact. *3*, Eight-year-old child sustaining voiceless fricative consonant. Note superior locus of closure and influence of adenoidal mass.

other speech sounds, the velum is normally elevated to preclude coupling entirely (for example, during the production of fully oral stops and fricatives) or to permit minimal degrees of nasal coupling (for example, during the production of vowels).

Thus during speech the mechanism of closing the velopharyngeal port is of utmost importance (Fig. 25-5). The achievement of isthmus closure effectively eliminates the nasal cavities as resonators, allows airflow to be directed primarily through the oral portion of the vocal tract, and permits, unless there are inappropriate system leaks, the necessary production of intraoral pressure. During nasal consonant production the velopharyngeal isthmus is open, and the nose is appropriately coupled to the vocal tract. Under these conditions the nasal cavities contribute their resonant characteristics to the total acoustic output of the tract.

Velopharyngeal port closure should be expected during the production of fully oral stops and fricatives. The following are characteristics of port closure:

1. Isthmus closure takes place at approximately the level of palatal plane.
2. During closure, contact is generally made between the middle third of the soft palate and the posterior pharyngeal wall.
3. The area of contact between the soft palate and the pharynx is several millimeters long. During velopharyngeal closure the palate does not merely touch the pharyngeal wall, but instead comes into contact with the pharynx over a considerable length.
4. During closure, a prominent levator eminence can frequently be seen. In younger children, isthmus closure may be assisted by the adenoidal mass. In such cases the necessity for generous palatal elevation is not present and the levator eminence may not be visualized. In young children the location of closure may be superior (contact between the superior portions of the soft palate and adenoidal mass) rather than posterior (contact between the palate and posterior pharyngeal wall).

5. During speech, velopharyngeal closure is achieved without appreciable assistance from the aerodynamic components of speech or from tongue elevation.
6. Maximum velar activity is elicited during the production of high vowels, voiceless plosives, and voiceless fricatives. The pattern of isthmus closure and narrowing is influenced by the effects of preceding and succeeding speech sounds and by the rate at which speech is delivered.
7. Normal velopharyngeal function requires adequate movement of the soft palate and pharynx, normal spatial and dimensional relationships between the structures that affect closure, and an anatomically intact palate.

Various abnormalities and conditions may produce velopharyngeal incompetence. Velopharyngeal incompetence results in specific differences from normal speech, while incompetence during deglutition may lead to nasal spill. In general, the inability to achieve velopharyngeal closure can be attributed to one or more of three factors: (1) clefts of the palate; (2) abnormalities in the dimensions of, and/or the spatial relationship between, the structures that influence closure; or (3) impairment of palatal or pharyngeal motion (Fig. 25-6).

In patients with congenital or acquired palatal clefts, isthmus closure cannot be accomplished because the palate is not intact. Impairment of velopharyngeal motion has been demonstrated in individuals having poliomyelitis, muscular dystrophy, myasthenia gravis, cerebral palsy, or other neuromuscular problems. Insufficient palatal elevation may sometimes be observed after cleft palate surgery. Abnormalities in dimension and spatial relationship between structures that accomplish closure have been demonstrated in persons having insufficient soft palate length, large nasopharynges, or ventral displacement of palatal structures. In such persons, structures may be intact and may demonstrate adequate motion, but the palate may be hypoplastic or the pharynx may be too large for isthmus closure to be accomplished.

The three factors that cause velopharyngeal in-

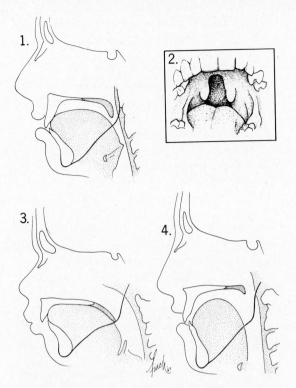

Fig. 25-6. Cephalometric and photographic illustrations demonstrating three general factors responsible for velopharyngeal incompetence. *1,* Adult subject during speech demonstrating impairment of palate motion. *2,* Unoperated cleft palate in a 7-year-old child. *3* and *4,* Subjects exhibiting abnormalities in dimension, spatial relationship, or both, between structures that affect isthmus closure. Note increased distance between posterior nasal spine and tubercle of atlas (increased skeletal nasopharyngeal depth) and abnormal position of the tubercle of the atlas in *3.* Observe deficient soft palate length in *4.*

competence may be present in isolation or in conjunction with one another. For example, an infant born with a cleft palate initially lacks structural integrity of the palate. However, after palatal surgery the same youngster may have an impairment of palate motion or insufficient palate length, or both.

There is a large body of data to support the view that impairment of velopharyngeal function is associated with two major types of speech disturbance:

(1) defective consonant articulation, including nasal emission of air, and (2) excessive nasalization, or hypernasality. Hypernasality continues to be related to an undesirable and inappropriate magnitude of nasal coupling during vowel production. Although speech pathologists, dentists, surgeons, and others continue to attempt to identify the presence or absence of excessive nasality and the severity of nasalization, there is a substantial body of data to indicate that such judgments are of questionable validity and reliability. There simply is no evidence to support the view that individual raters of nasalization can provide reliable or valid judgments about its severity. This situation suggests that management decisions for children with potential velopharyngeal inadequacy should not be made on the basis of nasality judgments.

In addition to nasality, speech articulation problems are common among speakers who cannot adequately close the nasopharynx. Individuals with cleft palate are generally retarded in articulation skills. In speakers with velopharyngeal incompetence, certain types of speech sounds are more likely to be defective. For example, vowels are seldom found defective when judgments are made of their phonetic acceptability; however, as already stated, those vowel productions are frequently hypernasal. Speakers with velopharyngeal insufficiency have more difficulty with fricative and stopplosive consonants than they do with glides and nasals. In general, such speakers produce consonants correctly more frequently when they occur in isolation than when they occur as component elements of blends. Voiceless consonants are more frequently misarticulated than their voiced cognates, and sound omissions occur more frequently than sound substitutions or distortions.

Speakers with velopharyngeal incompetence may also develop unusual or atypical speech articulation mechanisms. For example, speakers having cleft palate may substitute sounds formed at the glottis for plosive sounds normally produced in the mouth. Other unusual articulation methods involve the production of consonants within the pharynx. For example, during sibilant sound production speakers with velopharyngeal insufficiency may retract the dorsum of the tongue or the epiglottis to form a constriction with the adjacent pharyngeal wall.

During the production of these unusual speech articulation movements, the speaker forms a constriction inferior to the velopharyngeal isthmus. These movements represent atypical constriction formations within the vocal tract, which produce acoustic signals different from those of the intended speech sound. In general, these movements are used for sounds that require velopharyngeal closure and maintenance of intraoral pressure.

Most articulation errors in speakers with cleft palate are related to inadequate velopharyngeal function and to the associated inability to produce sufficient intraoral breath pressure during speech. Children with velopharyngeal insufficiency also exhibit articulation errors that are related not to their velopharyngeal incompetence, but rather to maturational factors.

Articulation testing continues to provide a reliable, noninvasive way to assess velopharyngeal adequacy for speech. Other useful forms of appraisal include case histories, oral-facial examinations, radiologic studies, and aerodynamic evaluations. These forms of evaluation are generally available in medical centers or universities that have staff members who are interested in investigating speech disorders or who are responsible for the clinical management of disabilities associated with cleft lip and/or palate.

Abnormalities of the lips, teeth, and dental arches do not account for the majority of articulation errors made by children with velopharyngeal insufficiency. Children with cleft palate have a higher incidence of hearing loss than normal children. In isolated cases, hearing loss or dental abnormalities may contribute to articulation problems, but neither should be regarded as a factor responsible for a large proportion of the speech articulation errors in this population of speech-impaired children.

Voice disorders. Significant voice disorders can occur in school-age children. To understand such disorders, the dentist must understand the laryngeal and respiratory mechanisms related to vocal fre-

quency, intensity, and quality. The frequency of sound is related to an important perceptual attribute of sound, called pitch. The perceived pitch of a voice is closely related to the lowest, or fundamental, frequency of vibration of the vocal folds. The frequency of vocal fold vibration is determined in part by the effective vibrating mass of the vocal folds, their stiffness or elasticity, and their effective vibrating length. For example, the more massive the vocal folds, other factors being constant, the more slowly they will vibrate, and the lower the perceived pitch of the voice will be. Theoretically, in two sets of vocal cords having the same effective vibrating mass and the same measures of elasticity or stiffness but having different vibrating lengths, the more lengthy folds will vibrate more slowly. In reality, however, lengthening the vocal folds causes a decrease in the cross-sectional area (and thus in the mass) of the vibrating cords, as well as an increase in tension, thereby increasing the pitch of the voice.

The intensity of sound is closely related to another important attribute of the way we hear sound, called loudness. Sound of a given frequency can vary in loudness or intensity. The perceived loudness of a voice is related in part to subglottic pressure. The degree of loudness is partially determined by the amount of pressure generated below the vocal folds during phonation. If the subglottic pressure is high during sustained phonation, other factors being constant, the perceived loudness of the voice is increased; if the subglottic pressure is low, the voice is perceived as soft.

The perceived quality of a voice is related in a complex manner to the vibratory pattern of the vocal cords and to the resonant characteristics of the vocal tract. If the breath stream is not completely interrupted during a portion of each vibratory cycle of the folds, breathiness may result.

Voice disorders result from a large variety of physical, psychologic, and behavioral factors. Voice disorders are heard as significant alterations in pitch, loudness, or quality.

Speech pathologists usually refer to the pitch of the voice in terms of the frequency of the voice with respect to the musical scale. The dentist should identify and refer for evaluation children who regularly use pitch levels that are unusual or inappropriate in terms of age, sex, and psychosocial environment. There are several primary types of pitch disorders. First are those defects in which a child speaks in pitch ranges that are consistently higher than normal for persons of the same age, sex, and psychosocial environment—for example, a 16- or 17-year-old male who still talks in the high-pitched range appropriate to a young, preadolescent boy. Second are those voice disorders associated with the use of pitch levels that are significantly lower than expected for a child's age, sex, and environment. A young girl whose extremely low-pitched voice simulates that of an older boy represents this type of pitch disorder. A third type is illustrated by a child who exhibits little or no variation in pitch (monotone), who uses pitch levels inappropriate to the meaning of an utterance, or whose pitch variations are excessive. Pitch disorders may be related to organic factors (hormonal disorders or structural anomalies of the larynx) or to functional factors (emotional conflict or psychiatric disturbance).

Disorders involving loudness may be classified in a similar manner: speech that is produced with inadequate or excessive loudness with respect to the speaking environment; speech produced with loudness variations that are inappropriate to the meaning, context, or environment; and disorders of loudness precipitated by various organic problems (for example, hearing loss) or functional conditions.

The voice quality disorders may be represented by a continuous scale extending from aphonia (no phonation—whispered speech) to abnormalities characterized chiefly by breathiness or hoarseness. Although the terms used to describe abnormalities of voice quality remain poorly defined, a dentist should recognize hoarseness and breathiness as principal indications of laryngeal dysfunction. Chronic hoarseness may be the first symptom of a pathologic condition in the larynx.

A significant feature of vocal behavior that is of particular interest to the pedodontist is the voice changes associated with pubertal growth. The change of voice during puberty results primarily from the accelerated growth of the larynx, the vocal folds, and the vocal tract. Dramatic changes begin with the onset of puberty. The growth of the larynx, which takes place gradually during childhood, is greatly accelerated by hormonal influences. During puberty the male vocal folds grow approximately 1 cm, while an increase of approximately 3 to 4 mm occurs in the female. The cartilaginous structures of the larynx increase in size simultaneously.

As a consequence of the developmental enlargement of the larynx, voice change occurs. In boys the lower pitch range drops approximately one octave, while in girls only a two- or three-tone decrease may occur. Male adolescent voice changes typically occur between 14 and 16 years of age. Girls undergo a voice change approximately 2 years earlier than boys.

Factors related to voice change are extremely important in understanding some of the voice disorders of adulthood. Conspicuous abnormalities related to precocious or delayed pubertal voice change identify important voice disorders deserving referral by the patient's dentist.

A number of pathologic conditions may influence laryngeal function and voice during childhood. A dentist should regard abnormal vocal characteristics as possible indications that something is fundamentally wrong with the larynx or with the manner in which the child uses the vocal apparatus. Abnormal voice may be the first symptom of a pathologic condition of the larynx. A child who has an obvious voice disorder should be referred to a competent otolaryngologist for medical evaluation. Under no circumstances should voice therapy for such a child be undertaken by a speech pathologist until the child has been evaluated by a physician. Some pathologic conditions or functional disorders are not reversible by voice therapy and may in fact be aggravated by such therapy. Other conditions are partially or totally reversible through voice therapy rehabilitation.

Stuttering. Slightly less than 1% of the school-age population in the United States stutters. Stuttering typically begins in childhood; the majority of children who stutter exhibit symptoms between 2½ and 4 years of age. A general characteristic of this disorder is a remarkable fluctuation in speech fluency. A stuttering child may speak fluently at times, but on other occasions may exhibit a severe lack of fluency. Stuttering occurs more frequently among males than females, tends to run in families, and is unexpectedly common among children who are identical twins.

Stuttering is characterized by breakdowns (repetitions, prolongations, and hesitations) in the rhythm or fluency of speech. It is important to emphasize that normal speakers experience some fluency breaks during speech. Thus stuttering involves more than the fluency breakdowns themselves. Children who stutter develop fears, reactions, and anxieties about speech. They become aware that their manner of speaking is unusual, and they begin to exhibit symptoms of struggle behavior.

Stuttering has been described in terms of what a speaker does in attempting not to stutter. The disorder apparently develops in essentially normal children and is in part precipitated by factors that induce struggle behavior during speech. Various organic, hereditary, personality, and psychosocial factors may play roles in precipitating, maintaining, ameliorating, or aggravating the problem. The mechanism of development of struggle behavior and the mechanism by which certain factors precipitate fluency breakdown in the speech of young children are not yet known.

Children regarded as stutterers have not been found to be neurotic or severely maladjusted. There has been no substantial support for the hypothesis that consistent differences exist between stuttering and nonstuttering children with respect to physical abnormalities or personality. No distinctive nonspeech characteristics distinguish stutterers from normal speakers.

The pedodontist should be concerned about a child who begins to experience an obvious breakdown in speech fluency, who begins to avoid verbal communication, becomes withdrawn, or refuses to speak in environments that previously were not threatening, or who exhibits struggle behavior during speech. Not all types of speech breakdown merit careful observation; for example, everyone experiences simple pauses or moments of indecision in speech. The pedodontist should also be particularly sensitive to the reactions of parents of children who have problems with fluency. For example, if the parents of such a child express concern about the child's speech, professional consultation is desirable.

Tongue thrust. Dentists and speech pathologists share an interest in the management of children with an allegedly deviant pattern of deglutition called tongue thrust swallowing.

In response to a growing concern about the creation of clinical programs involving myofunctional therapy and the involvement of speech pathologists in these programs, the American Speech-Language-Hearing Association sought an assessment of the status of management procedures related to tongue thrust. After a comprehensive study of relevant literature and a thorough evaluation of clinical methods, a Position Statement on Tongue Thrust was adopted. This statement, originally published in the journal *ASHA* in May 1975, is reprinted below.

Review of data from studies published to date has convinced the Committee that neither the validity of the diagnostic label tongue thrust nor the contention that myofunctional therapy produces significant consistent changes in oral form or function has been documented adequately. There is insufficient scientific evidence to permit differentiation between normal and abnormal or deviant patterns of deglutition, particularly as such patterns might relate to occlusion and speech. There is unsatisfactory evidence to support the belief that any patterns of movements defined as tongue thrust by any criteria suggested to date should be considered abnormal, detrimental, or representative of a syndrome. The few suitably controlled studies that have incorporated valid and reliable diagnostic criteria and appropriate quantitative assessments of therapy have demonstrated no effects on patterns of deglutition or oral structure. Thus, research is needed to establish the validity of tongue thrust as a clinical entity.

In view of the above considerations and despite our recognition that some dentists call upon speech pathologists to provide myofunctional therapy, at this time, there is no acceptable evidence to support claims of significant, stable, long-term changes in the functional patterns of deglutition and significant, consistent alterations in oral form. Consequently, the Committee urges increased research efforts, but cannot recommend that speech pathologists engage in clinical management procedures with the intent of altering functional patterns of deglutition.

Unfortunately, the issues surrounding this topic remain essentially unchanged today.

The dentist and the speech pathologist: general considerations

The maturation of speech and language ability is one of the most important features of child development. Since speech is a form of learned behavior, it is influenced by numerous factors. Although most children attain normal speech ability without difficulty, 5% to 10% do not. Abnormalities of speech often are symptoms of physical or psychosocial disturbances that may affect a child's general growth, development, and learning. Since speech is an important measure of human adaptation, a speech defect may handicap a child personally, socially, and educationally, even when other developmental factors appear normal.

This chapter is intended not to transform dentists into practicing speech pathologists but rather to provide dentists with basic information concerning speech and language behavior during childhood, since they are frequently asked to make clinical decisions about this important aspect of child development. Comprehensive programs of prevention and identification of speech disorders in childhood, followed by rehabilitation, can then be instituted. Participation in such a program clearly includes dentists, even though primary responsibility rests with specialists in communication disorders and other child health disciplines.

There are many speech pathologists in hospitals, universities, rehabilitation centers, public schools, and private practice. At present, speech pathologists can be certified for clinical competence by the American Speech-Language-Hearing Association and can be licensed to practice in most states. Information concerning the availability of speech pathologists can be obtained from the American Speech-Language-Hearing Association, 10801 Rockville Pike, Rockville, Maryland 20852.

REFERENCES

Aronson, A.: Clinical voice disorders, New York, 1980, Thieme-Stratton, Inc.

Bloom, L., and Lahey, M.: Language development and language disorders, New York, 1978, John Wiley & Sons, Inc.

Borden, G.T., and Harris, K.S.: Speech science primer, Baltimore, 1980, The Williams & Wilkins Co.

Brown, R.: A first language: the early stages, Cambridge, Mass., 1973, Harvard University Press.

Bzoch, K.R.: Communicative disorders related to cleft lip and palate, Boston, 1971, Little, Brown & Co.

Denes, P., and Pinson, E.: The speech chain, New York, 1973, Doubleday & Co., Inc.

Hixon, T.J., Shriberg, L.D., and Saxman, D.H.: Introduction to communication disorders, Englewood Cliffs, N.J., 1980, Prentice-Hall, Inc.

Van Riper, C.: The nature of stuttering, Englewood Cliffs, N.J., 1971, Prentice-Hall, Inc.

26 Special restorative problems in adolescent patients

ROLAND W. DYKEMA
CHARLES J. GOODACRE
DONALD M. CUNNINGHAM

Many of the dental problems of adolescents result from fractured, lost, or missing permanent teeth. The etiologic factors may be trauma, caries, periodontal disease, or congenital abnormalities (Fig. 26-1). The treatment in many instances requires crowns, fixed bridges, or removable partial dentures.

Many adolescents are handicapped psychologically by the unsightliness of missing or broken teeth or by the presence of conspicuous clasps on poorly designed removable partial dentures.

Chronologic age is of minor importance in determining and executing a plan of treatment for an adolescent patient. If the teeth involved are fully erupted, have achieved complete root formation, and may be prepared adequately without causing irreversible damage to the pulp, successful restorations or replacements can usually be made (Fig. 26-2). Extensive repair of individual teeth and successful replacement of missing teeth may be accomplished for patients as young as 12 to 14 years of age. However, a patient must be able to cooperate fully during and after treatment. This requires the ability to tolerate long appointments, hold still for several minutes while impression materials are setting, exercise adequate care for temporary restorations, and maintain good hygiene around restorations and prostheses as well as in the rest of the mouth. All of these conditions make it highly desirable that complex treatment for adolescent patients be performed as expeditiously as possible.

Finally, it must be understood that an adolescent is more likely to sustain trauma to the oral structures than an adult is; thus there is greater risk of damage to restorations and prostheses than there is for an adult patient.

Treatment of fractured teeth

Resin restoration. The incisor is the tooth most often fractured as the result of trauma. If only the mesial or distal incisal angle is missing, a resin restoration may suffice. The techniques for placing resin restorations are described in detail in Chapter 17. When the incisal third or half of the crown has been fractured, the jacket or metal-ceramic crown is generally the restoration of choice.

Jacket crown supported by cast post and core. When a fracture involves the pulp and root development is complete, a routine pulpectomy and filling of the root canal with gutta-percha are indicated (Fig. 26-3). This procedure will permit the construction of a cast core retained by a post in the root canal before crown construction (Fig. 26-4). Most pulpless permanent incisors should be prepared to receive a post and core in order to reduce the incidence of fracture resulting from the unusually heavy stress load that is associated with the functioning of the incisors (Figs. 26-5 and 26-6). However, in the case of an athletically

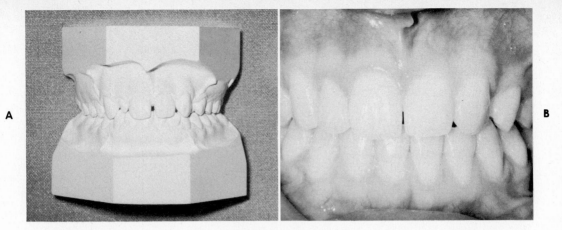

Fig. 26-1. A, Diagnostic casts before orthodontic treatment and restoration of malformed right lateral incisor. **B,** Orthodontic treatment completed. The maxillary right lateral incisor has been restored with a collarless metal-ceramic crown.

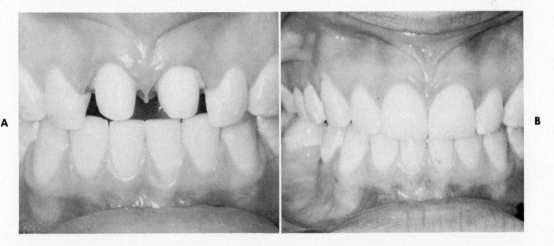

Fig. 26-2. A, Young patient with traumatically injured, vital central incisors prepared for metal-ceramic restoration. **B,** Maxillary central incisors restored with collarless metal-ceramic crown.

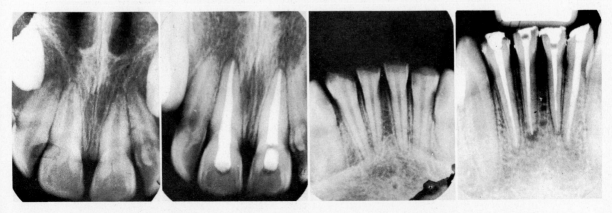

Fig. 26-3. Radiographs of traumatically injured maxillary and mandibular incisors at time of injury, left, and after endodontic therapy, right.

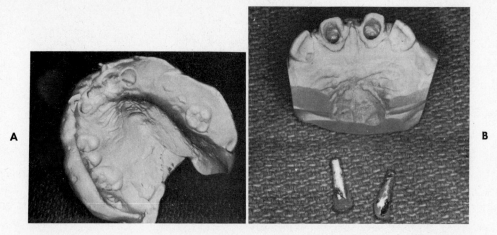

Fig. 26-4. A, Silicone impression of enlarged root canals of the maxillary central incisors. **B,** Working cast and gold cast posts and cores.

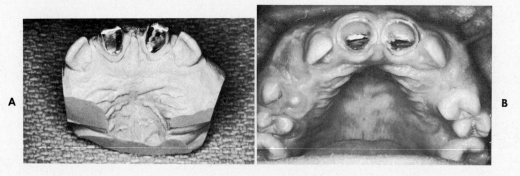

Fig. 26-5. A, Cast posts and cores on working cast. **B,** Cast posts and cores cemented.

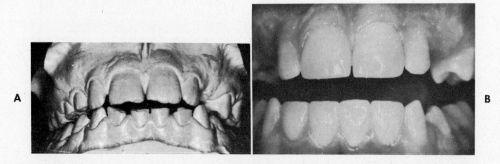

Fig. 26-6. A, Diagnostic casts before treatment. **B,** Photograph after cementation of posts and cores and porcelain jacket crowns.

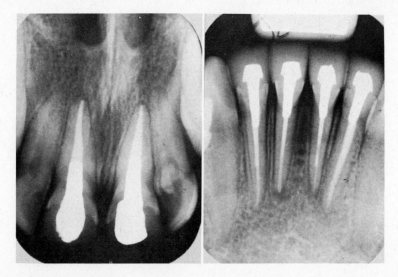

Fig. 26-7. Posttreatment radiographs. Cast posts and cores have been constructed to support jacket crown restorations.

inclined patient, rebuilding a pulpless tooth without the use of a post in the prepared pulp canal might be considered to avoid irreparable damage in the form of root fracture should the restored tooth be subjected to trauma.

In cases of pulpal involvement when the root is not yet completely formed, a pulpotomy followed by placement of a temporary crown is indicated. Subsequently, when root formation is complete, a pulpectomy is performed, followed by construction of the post and core and the jacket or veneered gold crown (Fig. 26-7). The jacket crown is the preferred restoration, with two major exceptions— when adverse occlusal relationships exist and when retention is a problem. If occlusion occurs on the cingulum or cervically to it, the metal-ceramic gold crown is indicated because such an occlusal relationship often results in fracture of a porcelain jacket crown or deformation, accompanied by loss of fit, of an acrylic resin jacket crown. When a prepared tooth is short or has a tapering form, the metal-ceramic crown will achieve the greater retention that is afforded by a cast restoration.

When the post and core are constructed, the post should extend into the root canal so that its length

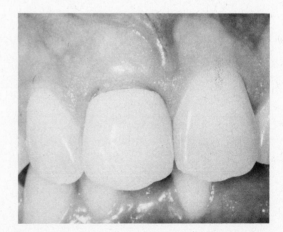

Fig. 26-8. Gingival contour at age 25 resulting from subgingival crown placement at age 8. The gingival crest is not positioned as far apically as on the unrestored central incisor, and its form is rounded and thick rather than having the normal knife-edge configuration.

equals or exceeds the length of the proposed jacket or metal-ceramic crown. This will provide adequate retention and the greatest resistance to fracture. Any coronal tooth structure remaining after normal preparatory procedures should be preserved, and the core should be constructed to complete the normal form. This will materially increase the resistance of the post and core to rotational dislodging forces (Fig. 26-7).

Whenever possible, cervical margins should not be extended into the gingival sulcus. If oral hygiene is inadequate, subgingival margins may produce accelerated gingival recession or interfere with the normal cervical relocation of the gingival tissues as the patient matures. Either occurrence produces an esthetic liability (Fig. 26-8).

Construction of fixed bridges

The loss of a permanent first molar is a dental problem frequently seen in adolescents. The loss of this tooth is generally due to caries but may also be the result of the severe vertical bone destruction seen in juvenile periodontitis. In cases in which the second molar and the second premolar are in ideal positions and occlusion, an inlay fixed bridge may be used. To prevent tipping of the teeth adjacent to the edentulous area, space maintenance must be provided immediately after extraction and must be continued until the bridge has been cemented into place.

If tipping or tilting has occurred, the abutment teeth must be repositioned orthodontically or alignment must be achieved through the use of full crowns or partial veneer crowns. However, pulp size may not permit the amount of tooth reduction necessary to align preparations made on tipped teeth. In such cases, realignment of the abutments by orthodontic procedures is mandatory.

Inlay retainers. If inlays are used as retainers, the preparations should be as deep axially and pulpally as pulp size and position permit. The occlusal and proximal steps should be wider than those normally prepared for a single restoration. A post hole about 1.5 mm deep is used in the pulpal floor near the marginal ridge opposite the proximal

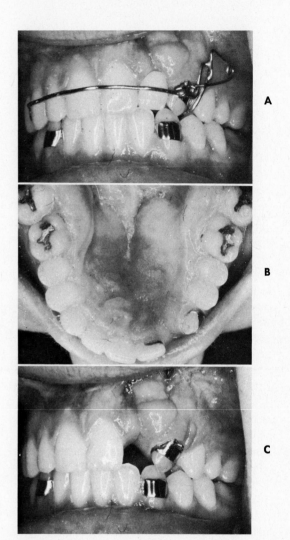

Fig. 26-9. A, Orthodontic retainer, maxillary left lateral incisor replaced, and mechanism for retaining canine position. **B,** Palatal view (mirror). Inflammatory gingival hyperplasia is present. **C,** Anterior view of edentulous area.

step. These modifications are made to increase retention, to provide adequate bulk of metal for strength, and to allow solder joints of proper form, position, and dimension.

Full crown retainers. When a full crown is indicated on a second molar, a gingivoplasty may be necessary to adequately expose the distal surface for preparation. When a partial veneer crown is to be used on a mandibular second premolar, an auxiliary groove is made to include the distal third of the buccal surface. This affords additional retention and resists lingual displacement of the retainer better than do proximal grooves or boxes alone, which necessarily must be rather short on most mandibular premolars.

Bridge pontics. Bridge pontics usually can be of conventional design, but meticulous attention must be paid to the amount of ridge coverage, with the area of contact being minimized, and the embrasures should be as large as possible while meeting the demands of esthetics.

Because pin facings are not as available as they were in the past and because many technicians do not offer pontics using pin facings as part of their services, the metal-ceramic pontic has come into common use. A highly versatile replacement, it combines the esthetic benefits of porcelain with the strength of metal, and it is often adaptable to spaces that are difficult to manage with manufactured facings. However, one must be prepared to use post-ceramic soldering procedures, since adolescent abutment teeth often do not permit the additional tooth reduction required for the metal-ceramic retainer (see Fig. 26-11, *B* and *C*).

The sanitary pontic, with a porcelain ridge-contacting surface, or a pontic that is constructed entirely of gold (used when vertical space is limited), is usually indicated as the replacement for a mandibular molar or second premolar, because its convex tissue surface is easily cleansed.

Occasionally an incisor is congenitally missing or is lost prematurely, resulting in an edentulous area that is an esthetic liability as well as a space maintenance problem (Fig. 26-9). In most cases a fixed bridge not only serves for space maintenance

but also provides an acceptable solution to the esthetic problem.

Pin-ledge and partial veneer crown retainers. If the proposed anterior abutments are sound and are in the correct positions, pin-ledge retainers or partial veneer crowns are generally indicated as the retainers (Fig. 26-10). Adequate preparations can usually be executed, although it may be necessary to use shorter pins and shallower grooves than would be used when restoring adult teeth (Fig. 26-11). When caries or existing restorations have weakened the proposed abutments or when enamel hypoplasia is present, a full crown restoration is often required for strength, esthetics, or both.

Acrylic resin bridge. When full-coverage retainers are indicated but pulp size will allow only minimal reduction, an acrylic resin bridge may be the restoration of choice. The all-acrylic resin bridge offers the maximum in esthetics and requires the least removal of tooth structure, but because of its inferior physical properties it must be considered a temporary restoration (3 to 5 years). The acrylic veneered cast restoration offers greater longevity but is still considered an interim restoration (Fig. 26-12). By the time replacement is needed, however, enough pulpal recession has usually occurred that sufficient tooth reduction can be accomplished to permit the use of a metal-ceramic crown as the retainer (Fig. 26-13).

Metal-ceramic bridge. In partially edentulous mouths, when crown length and tooth form demand and pulp size permits, metal-ceramic restorations are often useful. Fig. 26-14 illustrates a case of ectodermal dysplasia in which crown form dictated full coverage and metal-ceramic restorations were used. Fig. 26-15 illustrates a case of dentinogenesis imperfecta that demanded full coverage for both functional and esthetic reasons. (See Chapter 4 for a description of dentinogenesis imperfecta.)

Construction of removable partial dentures

In a partially edentulous mouth in which a fixed bridge cannot be used, a removable partial denture becomes a restoration of necessity. Indications for

Text continued on p. 727.

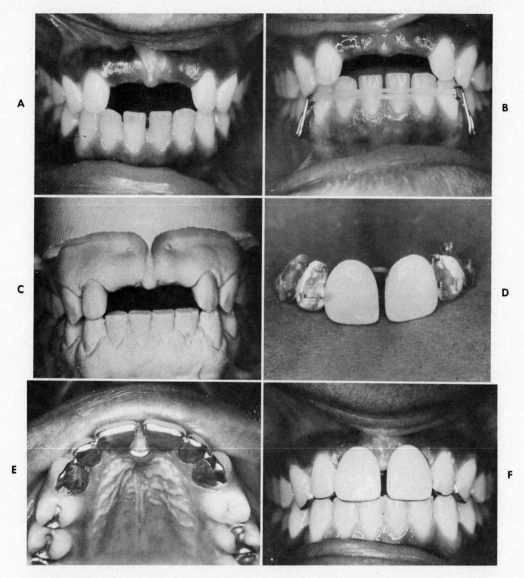

Fig. 26-10. A, Patient 15 years of age with large maxillary anterior bridge space and spacing of mandibular anterior incisors. **B,** Orthodontic appliance with rubber ligature to reposition maxillary incisors lingually to establish proximal contacts. **C,** Casts showing repositioned incisors after they have been shortened to offset the additional length obtained by uprighting that occurred during orthodontic movement. **D,** Completed bridge using four pin-ledge retainers. A 17-gauge wire loop was used as a connector between the central incisor pontics, since the space was too large to avoid a diastema. **E,** Palatal view of completed bridge. **F,** Labial view of completed bridge. (From Johnston, J.F., Phillips, R.W., and Dykema, R.W.: Modern practice in crown and bridge prosthodontics, ed. 3, Philadelphia, 1971, W.B. Saunders Co.)

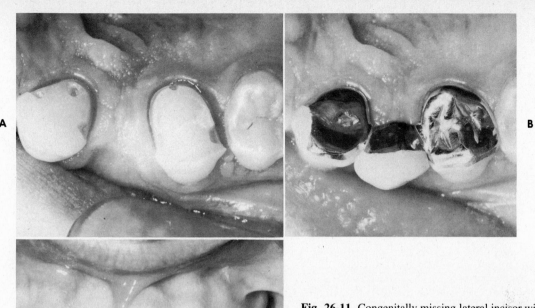

Fig. 26-11. Congenitally missing lateral incisor with the canine in the lateral incisor position. A fixed partial denture was constructed using partial coverage retainers and a metal-ceramic pontic. **A,** Mirror view of preparations using conservative grooves, boxes, and pinholes. **B,** Mirror view of cemented prosthesis. **C,** Anterior view of cemented prosthesis.

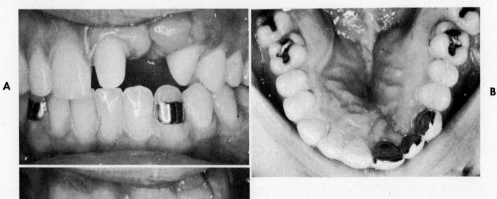

Fig. 26-12. **A,** Abutments prepared for full crown restorations. **B,** Mirror view of temporary resin veneered bridge replacing the left maxillary lateral incisor. **C,** Anterior view of temporary fixed bridge.

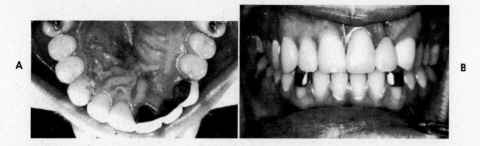

Fig. 26-13. A, Mirror view of permanent metal-ceramic bridge replacing the left maxillary lateral incisor. **B,** Anterior view of permanent fixed bridge replacing the left maxillary lateral incisor.

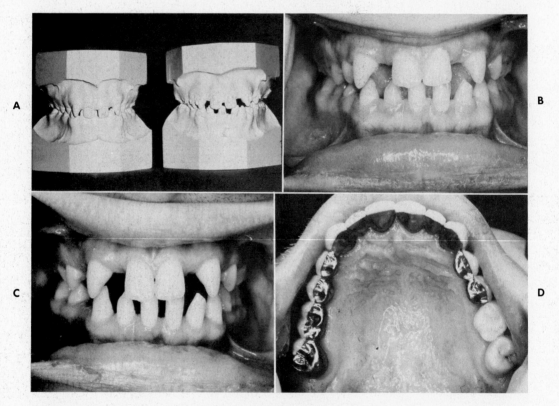

Fig. 26-14. A, Casts of patient exhibiting incomplete dental manifestation of hereditary ectodermal dysplasia. Left: casts before orthodontic treatment. Right: progress casts near completion of orthodontic treatment. **B,** The patient shown in **A** after orthodontic treatment. Note vertical overbite correction and space adjustment to facilitate prosthetic treatment. Additional illustration of the treatment may be seen in **C** through **H. C,** After periodontal treatment. Gingivoplasty was done to gain crown length and improve tissue contours. **D,** Mirror view of maxillary arch after prosthetic treatment.

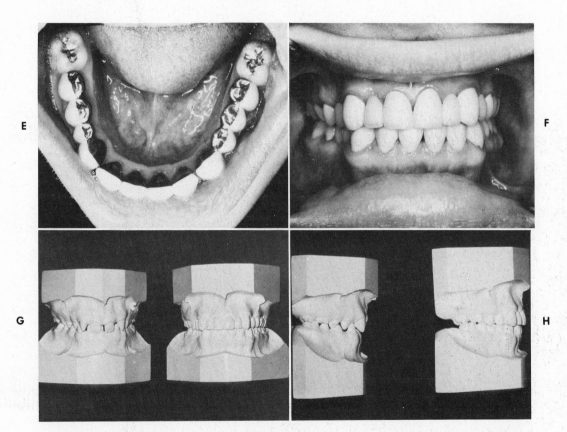

Fig. 26-14, cont'd. E, Mirror view of mandibular arch after prosthetic treatment. **F,** Anterior view in occlusion after prosthetic treatment. Metal-ceramic and fixed partial dentures were employed to correct abnormal tooth form, replace congenitally missing teeth, and restore occlusion. **G** and **H,** Anterior and right lateral views of casts before and after treatment.

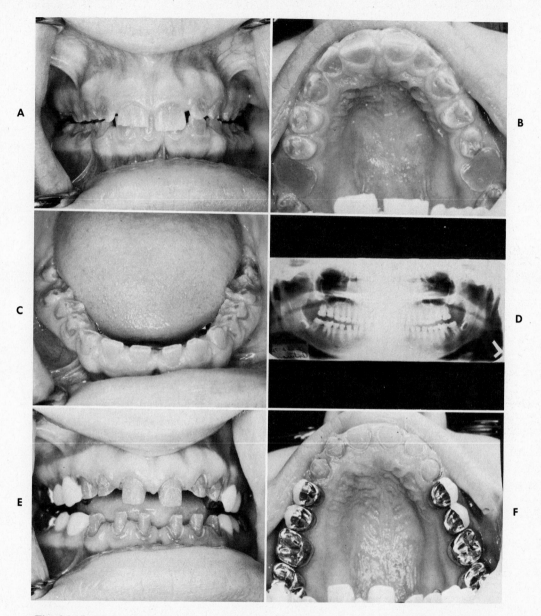

Fig. 26-15. Dentinogenesis imperfecta. **A,** Frontal view before treatment. **B,** Mirror view of maxillary arch; extreme wear of first permanent molar and enamel fracture on several teeth. **C,** Mandibular arch showing enamel fracture and wear of permanent teeth. **D,** Panoramic radiography before treatment. **E and F,** Frontal and occlusal mirror views of preparation on incisors and canines.

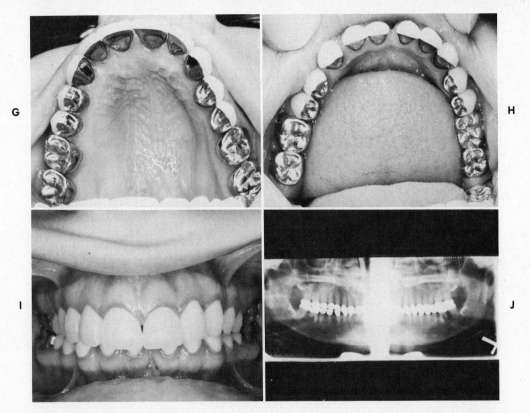

Fig. 26-15, cont'd. G and **H,** Mirror views of maxillary and mandibular arches showing permanent metal-ceramic full crown restoration. **I,** Frontal view of completed restorations in occlusion. **J,** Panoramic radiograph after treatment.

a partial denture generally result from congenital malformations in which only a few, widely spaced permanent teeth develop or from severe traumatic injuries that have caused teeth to be lost (Figs. 26-16 to 26-28).

When treatment is planned for an adolescent patient who needs a removable partial denture, there are at least three major objectives: (1) the restoration of the functions of mastication and speech, (2) the restoration of dental and facial esthetics, and (3) the preservation of the remaining teeth and their supportive tissues.

The function of *mastication* can be restored by providing correct, harmonious, and nondestructive occlusal relationships between the supplied teeth and the opposing remaining natural dentition. The presence of the equipment for proper speech can be ensured if the parts of the partial denture are given correct form, dimension, and position in their relationships to the tongue, cheek, and lips.

The restoration of *esthetics* is often the most important personal consideration for adolescent patients. Artificial teeth of compatible shade, size, and form, naturally arranged and positioned, enhance dental esthetics. In addition, the correct form and size of the base of a partial denture are necessary to ensure the restoration of normal facial contours (Fig. 26-28).

The *preservation of the remaining teeth* and their supportive tissues is the most important objective

Text continued on p. 732.

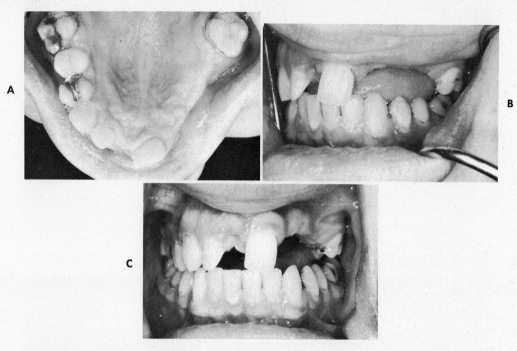

Fig. 26-16. A, Mirror view of maxillary arch. Multiple teeth have been lost in this young adult as a result of a gunshot accident. **B,** Left lateral view in centric occlusion. **C,** Anterior view in centric occlusion.

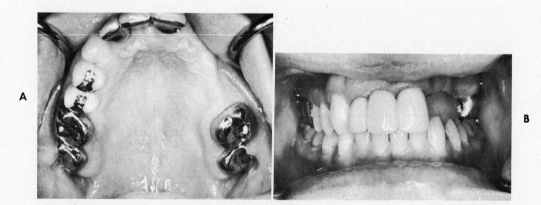

Fig. 26-17. A, Palatal view of maxillary arch of patient seen in Fig. 26-16 after mouth preparation that consisted of periodontal therapy (gingivoplasty) and construction of crowns, fixed bridge, and inlays. **B,** Anterior view in occlusion. Missing right central incisor replaced with fixed bridge, thereby splinting the lone-standing left central incisor and eliminating a troublesome anterior modification space.

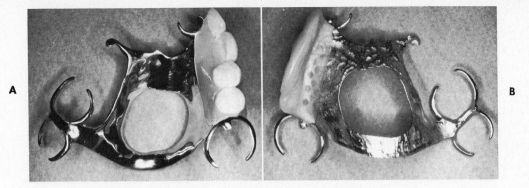

Fig. 26-18. A, Removable partial denture replacing the missing left maxillary lateral incisor, canine, and first and second premolars. **B,** Tissue surface view of removable partial denture. Note amount of base material needed to replace lost alveolar bone.

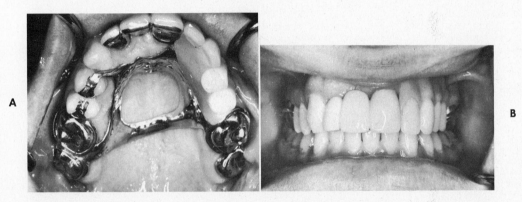

Fig. 26-19. A, Palatal view of maxillary arch with removable partial denture in position. Minor connector and auxiliary occlusal rest have been employed to ensure rigidity of major connector. **B,** Anterior view in occlusion with removable partial denture in positon.

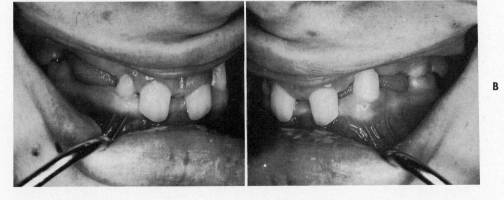

Fig. 26-20. Oligodontia as a result of hereditary ectodermal dysplasia. **A** and **B,** Right and left lateral views in occlusion (note overclosure).

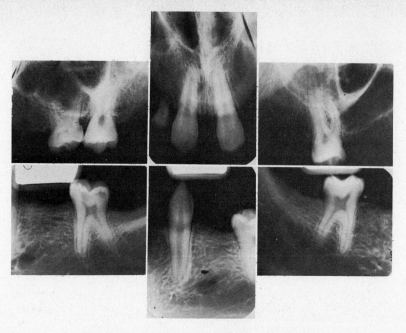

Fig. 26-21. Radiographs of patient in Fig. 26-20.

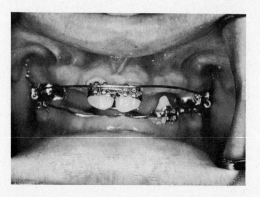

Fig. 26-22. The patient in Fig. 26-20 after 18 months of orthodontic therapy to erupt molars and depress left mandibular canine and to eliminate the diastema between the maxillary central incisors. Additional illustrations of the treatment may be seen in Figs. 26-23 thru 26-28.

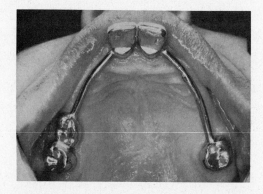

Fig. 26-23. Mirror view of maxillary arch after mouth preparation. Cross-arch splinting was achieved with full crown restorations joined with an 11-gauge round bar.

Fig. 26-24. Mandibular arch after mouth preparation. Cross-arch splinting using thimble crowns joined with an 11-gauge round bar.

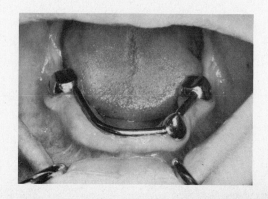

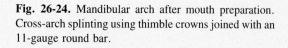

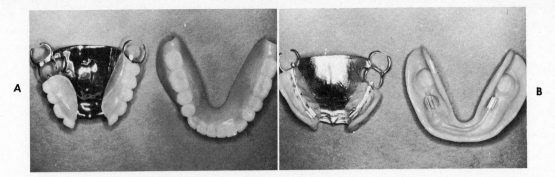

Fig. 26-25. A, Maxillary removable partial denture and mandibular superimposed complete denture. B, Tissue surface view of prostheses. (The snap-on attachments create retention by grasping the 11-gauge bar.)

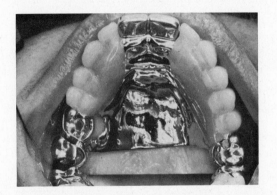

Fig. 26-26. Mirror view of maxillary removable partial denture in position.

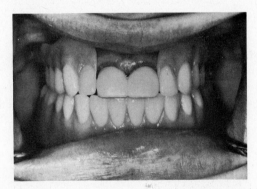

Fig. 26-27. Anterior view in occlusion of maxillary partial denture and mandibular superimposed complete denture.

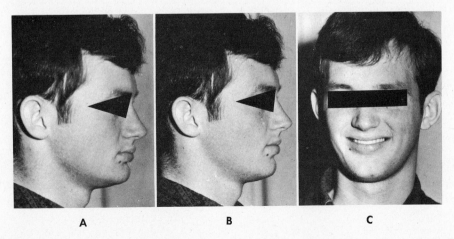

Fig. 26-28. A, Lateral profile view without prosthesis. B, Lateral profile view with prosthesis. C, Anterior full-face view with prosthesis.

of all but is unfortunately the one least often achieved. If this objective is to be realized, there must be adequate mouth preparation, correct partial denture design, accurate fabrication of that design, periodic professional follow-up care, and continued proper home care by the patient.

Mouth preparation. Mouth preparation consists of operations or procedures necessary to create an oral environment that will furnish proper support and retention for the removable partial denture and that will prevent the development of forces or processes that are harmful to the remaining teeth and their supportive tissues. These preparatory procedures may involve all phases or branches of dentistry.

Surgical preparation. Surgery may be necessary in the eradication of soft tissue or osseous pathoses and can range from uncomplicated extraction of teeth to complex procedures.

Periodontal preparation. Adolescents often require periodontic procedures, particularly to increase crown length and to improve tissue contours in order to achieve ideal results in restorative and prosthetic treatment (Figs. 26-16 and 26-17).

Endodontic preparation. Endodontic therapy makes possible the preservation of teeth that have been damaged by caries or trauma, and that are strategic to the support and retention of a proposed partial denture.

Orthodontic preparation. Orthodontic procedures can be used to reposition severely malpositioned teeth, which would otherwise require extraction. Orthodontic procedures are particularly indicated for teeth that are vital to an adequate plan of treatment (Fig. 26-22).

Restorative dentistry. Finally, restorative dentistry is most often indicated for long-term restoration of extensively carious teeth and for producing a crown form that is ideal for support and retention. Lone-standing or periodontally weakened teeth may be splinted by means of fixed bridges or crowns soldered together to better distribute forces to the supportive alveolar bone and thereby prevent future periodontal failure.

Construction of crowns and bridges. The con-struction of crowns and bridges in the preparation of a mouth for removable partial dentures requires exactness in form and contour and must be coordinated with the indicated design. To satisfy these requirements, an indirect technique of fabrication, together with the intelligent use of a surveying instrument (parallelometer), is a necessity (Figs. 26-17, 26-23, and 26-24). These procedures can be done by using either reversible hydrocolloid or rubber impression materials. Full-arch impressions should be made, and the resultant casts should be mounted on an instrument capable of simulating jaw movements. The wax patterns for the crowns are built to ideal form and proper occlusal and contact relationships. The casts are then removed from the articulator and are taken to a dental surveyor for alteration of the areas that will provide proper support, adequate retention, and positive reciprocation of the partial dental framework.

Partial denture design. The design of the removable partial denture must be so conceived and implemented that stress loads transmitted to the remaining teeth and the periodontium are within physiologic limits. The directing of forces axially on the abutments by means of occlusal rests will aid in the achievement of this objective. The use of the minimum retention necessary to resist reasonable dislodging forces and the reciprocation of the retentive clasp arms during insertion and removal of the partial denture further contribute to preservation of the periodontal structures. Proper form and dimensions of connectors to achieve rigidity and the tapering of retentive clasps for flexibility will ensure the most favorable distribution of stress loads across the arch and will reduce the degree of tilting and the severity of rotational forces exerted against the abutments (Figs. 26-18, 26-19, and 26-25 to 26-28).

When free-end bases are necessary, the design should be such that the maximum denture-bearing area is used so that the force per unit area on the residual ridge is minimal. The artificial teeth must have a harmonious occlusal relationship with the opposing dentition and must be made of a material that is nondestructive. When the opposing denti-

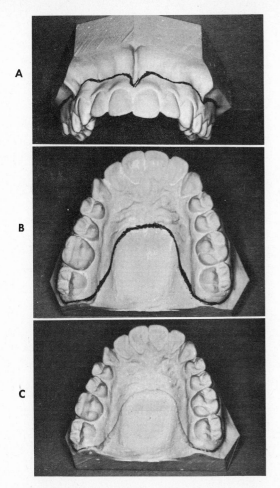

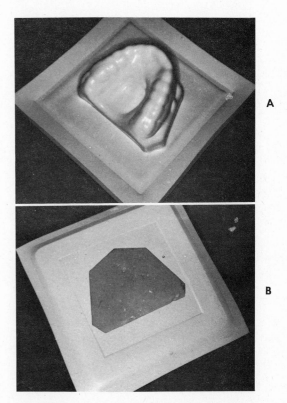

Fig. 26-29. A and **B,** Frontal and palatal views of maxillary cast with outline of proposed mouth guard. **C,** Palatal view with proposed peripheral area beaded on cast.

Fig. 26-30. A, Occlusal and, **B,** bottom views of maxillary cast after the mouth guard material has been adapted to the cast.

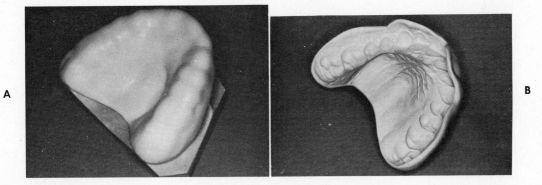

Fig. 26-31. A, Occlusal view and, **B,** tissue surface view of trimmed and polished mouth guard with full palatal coverage.

tion consists of natural teeth or gold restorations, the artificial teeth should be plastic, gold, or a combination of these materials. Porcelain artificial teeth should be reserved for situations in which the opposing dentition consists of other porcelain teeth or porcelain restorations.

Recall program

The treatment for an adolescent does not end with the insertion of the indicated restorations. Periodic recall appointments for inspection, maintenance, repair, or replacement are a necessity if longevity of service is to be expected. For patients who have removable partial dentures, relining or rebasing should be performed when indicated. When jacket crowns or metal-ceramic restorations are used in an adolescent, replacement will be needed periodically as gingival recession occurs. Patients with fixed bridges should be inspected periodically for soft tissue reaction to pontics, evidence of occlusal wear, and response of the supportive tissues to the added stress loads.

Every adolescent patient not only should be taught proper oral hygiene and home care of prosthetic restorations but also must be motivated until adequate performance is routinely achieved. In the absence of periodic maintenance and adequate home care, restoration failure is inevitable.

When indicated, a patient should be taught the use of aids such as the floss threader and the interproximal brush to enhance oral hygiene efforts.

Protective mouth guards

Although this chapter is concerned with restorative problems in adolescents, emphasis should always be placed on the prevention of oral disease and injury. The number and severity of traumatic injuries to the teeth and jaws can be significantly reduced by the faithful use of protective mouth guards by athletes who are engaged in contact sports. Several effective, easily constructed, and inexpensive mouth guards are available.

A mouth guard may be custom made by vacuum molding over a stone cast of the maxillary arch (Figs. 26-29 and 26-30). The mouth guard sheet material (0.15 inch thick) is placed in a molding machine, which softens the material by heat and closely adapts it to the dry stone cast in 3 to 5 minutes by vacuum. After the adapted material has cooled, the cast is removed and the excess material is trimmed off with heavy shears. The borders are finished and polished with fine-grit carborundum arbor bands and with wet pumice on a rag wheel (Fig. 26-31).

Maximum retention is obtained by covering the entire hard palate; if there is interference with speech, however, a portion of the palatal area of the guard can be removed.

The use of mouth guards by many high school athletes has convinced us that they can be worn with comfort and can serve as effective safeguards against injuries to the teeth and jaws.

REFERENCES

Dykema, R.W., Cunningham, D.M., and Johnston, J.F.: Modern practice in removable partial prosthodontics, Philadelphia, 1969, W.B. Saunders Co.

Johnston, J.F., Phillips, R.W., and Dykema, R.W.: Modern practice in crown and bridge prosthodontics, ed. 3, Philadelphia, 1971, W.B. Saunders Co.

Mink, J.R.: Crown and bridge for the young adolescent, Dent. Clin. North Am., pp. 149-160, March 1966.

Scures, C.C.: Porcelain baked to gold in pedodontics, J. Dent. Child. **30:**9, 1963.

27 Oral infections and skin diseases

WILLIAM G. SHAFER

A variety of specific and nonspecific infections manifest themselves by lesions of the oral cavity, and many have accompanying skin lesions. Some of these oral lesions are prodromal and forecast a more widespread involvement, whereas others only reflect a widespread involvement already present. Still other infections are confined to the oral cavity. For obvious reasons, these oral lesions must be recognized promptly and diagnosed correctly so that treatment, if indicated, can be instituted without delay.

Specific infections

Scarlet fever. Scarlet fever, or scarlatina, is predominately a disease of children caused by a β-hemolytic *Streptococcus* that elaborates an erythrogenic toxin. The portal of entry is usually the pharynx; after an incubation period of 3 to 5 days, pharyngitis, tonsillitis, headache, fever, chills, nausea and vomiting, and an associated cervical lymphadenopathy develop. Within 2 or 3 days the typical bright red exanthem or skin rash appears.

The oral manifestations, called "stomatitis scarlatina," consist of an intense congestion of the oral mucosa, palate, and throat. The tonsils are usually swollen and may be ulcerated. The "strawberry tongue" develops early in the course of the disease and appears as a white-coated tongue with numerous small red projecting knobs representing edematous, hyperemic fungiform papillae. This white coating is soon lost, and the entire tongue appears bright red, still with the swollen papillae. This condition has been termed a "raspberry tongue." The

disease terminates within a week to 10 days, the skin desquamates, and the oral tissues resume their normal appearance.

Diphtheria. Diphtheria, a disease predominately of children, is caused by *Corynebacterium diphtheriae,* the Klebs-Loeffler bacillus. It is transmitted chiefly by droplet infection or direct contact. After an incubation period of a few days, fever, headache, malaise, nausea and vomiting, and subsequently a sore throat develop.

The oral manifestations consist of a typical patchy "diphtheritic membrane" over the tonsils, pharynx, and larynx and occasionally on the palate, gingivae, and other oral mucous membranes. This diphtheritic membrane is a fibrinous exudate forming over ulcerated surfaces; if it is stripped off, it leaves a raw, bleeding surface. In addition, the soft palate sometimes becomes temporarily paralyzed, with a consequent nasal regurgitation of liquids when the patient is drinking. The disease terminates within a few weeks.

Pyogenic granuloma. The pyogenic granuloma is a distinct entity that appears to result when minor trauma provides a pathway for invasion of nonspecific microorganisms to which there is a characteristic tissue response as a result of the low virulence of the organisms.

There is no predilection for occurrence in any particular age group. Lesions occur at any time from infancy to old age. The pyogenic granuloma can develop at any site in the oral cavity, although the vast majority of lesions occur on the gingiva (Fig. 27-1). The lesion usually appears as an elevated superficial mass, with a sessile or peduncu-

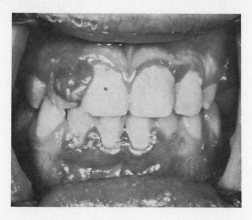

Fig. 27-1. Pyogenic granuloma. The lesion in this child is essentially a mass of hyperplastic vascular granulation tissue that developed rapidly and bled readily.

lated base, that begins suddenly, grows rapidly, reaches full size in a short period of time, and then remains stationary for an indefinite period. Such lesions vary in color from dark red or purple to pale red, depending on the age and vascularity of the lesion. The early lesions are painless, soft, smooth or lobulated, and frequently ulcerated, and they have a tendency to hemorrhage. Older lesions more closely resemble a fibroma.

The pyogenic granuloma is treated by conservative surgical excision and, if the lesion is situated on the gingiva, careful scaling and polishing to remove any source of irritation. If it is adequately excised and if irritation is removed, the lesion seldom recurs.

Herpangina. Herpangina or aphthous pharyngitis, a disease caused by a group A coxsackievirus, occurs in epidemic fashion, usually in the summer, and affects chiefly young children. After an incubation period of 3 to 5 days, a sore throat, headache, fever, nausea, vomiting, and abdominal pain develop.

The oral manifestations are the chief feature of the disease; these consist of the development of small ulcers on the pharynx, the faucial pillars, the palate, and sometimes the tongue. These ulcers are not extremely painful, although dysphagia may be present, and they heal within a few days.

The disease is self-limited, has no complications, and needs no treatment. A permanent immunity usually develops after the disease subsides.

Acute lymphonodular pharyngitis. Acute lymphonodular pharyngitis is another mild coxsackievirus type A viral infection that commonly occurs in children and young adults. It is similar to herpangina in that its onset is characterized by malaise, fever, chills, and sore throat. Within a few days multiple small inflamed nodular lesions develop, particularly on the soft palate and fauces. These nodules consist of small hyperplastic lymphoid aggregates. The disease is self-limited, has no complications, needs no treatment, and usually produces immunity against further attacks.

Hand-foot-and-mouth disease. Hand-foot-and-mouth disease is also a coxsackievirus type A viral infection that commonly occurs in children. The disease has no relationship to hoof-and-mouth disease, despite the similarity in names.

Clinically, the disease is characterized by a maculopapular or vesicular erythematous eruption of the hands, feet, and "diaper area." Oral lesions are also present; they consist of multiple scattered superficial ulcers, commonly on the tongue, palate, and buccal mucosa. At least on some occasions, the oral lesions have appeared a few days before the skin eruptions.

Although the disease is generally mild and of short duration, infection by this virus has led on occasion to serious complications, sometimes even death.

Measles. Measles, or rubeola, is an acute, contagious viral disease affecting chiefly children and often occurring in epidemic pattern. The portal of entry is the respiratory tract after transmission by direct contact or droplet infection. After an incubation period of 8 to 10 days, malaise, fever, cough, conjunctivitis, and photophobia develop, and finally maculopapular lesions of the skin appear on the face and spread to the trunk and extremities.

The oral lesions, called "Koplik's spots," are a prodromal manifestation of the disease and characteristically occur 2 to 3 days before the development of the skin lesions. Koplik's spots reportedly occur in more than 95% of persons with measles.

Koplik's spots characteristically develop on the buccal mucosa and appear as small, bluish white macules surrounded by a bright red margin; the spots increase in number and coalesce in small patches. A generalized inflammation, sometimes with ulceration, may also develop in the oral mucosa. Koplik's spots generally disappear by the time the skin lesions appear. The only treatment for the disease is rest and supportive care.

Rubella. Rubella, or German measles, presents no significant oral manifestations except for occasional red macules of the palate and tonsillar enlargement.

Chickenpox. Chickenpox, or varicella, is a viral disease that is most common in winter and spring and predominately affects children. The same virus in adults causes herpes zoster, or "shingles." The portal of entry is probably the respiratory tract. After an incubation period of about 2 weeks, headache, fever, nasopharyngitis, and anorexia develop, followed by maculopapular or vesicular lesions of the skin beginning on the trunk and spreading to involve the face and extremities. The skin eruptions develop in crops; as some are healing, others are developing. Occasionally the lesions become infected and actual pustules form.

The oral manifestations consist of papular or vesicular lesions developing chiefly on the palate, buccal mucosa, and pharynx. These commonly rupture to leave small eroded ulcers. The skin lesions heal within 7 to 10 days by crusting and desquamation. The oral lesions disappear in about the same period of time. No treatment is necessary, and complications are rare.

Cat-scratch disease. The cause of cat-scratch disease is unknown, although considerable evidence points toward a viral origin. The disease occurs predominately in children and young adults, following a bite or scratch on the skin by a household cat. Apparently the cat is only the carrier of the disease, since the animal itself is not sick. However, not all patients give a history of exposure to a cat. Within a few days after a scratch, a papule or vesicle develops at the site of the injury; 1 to 3 weeks later a severe regional lymphadenitis occurs. The lymph nodes are painful, and the over-lying skin may be inflamed. At this time the patient also usually has a headache, fever, chills, nausea, and abdominal pain. The lymphadenopathy may persist as long as 6 months, the nodes gradually becoming necrotic and suppurative. However, the disease is self-limited and the prognosis is good.

The disease has significance in dentistry because cervical lymphadenopathy that has been present after a cat-scratch on the face has been mistakenly diagnosed as being caused by dental infection. The possibility of cat-scratch disease must always be considered in a case of unexplained regional lymphadenopathy.

Mumps. Mumps, or epidemic parotitis, is an acute contagious viral infection that affects both children and adults; it is characterized by a unilateral or bilateral swelling of the salivary glands. Transmission is by droplet infection. After an incubation period of 2 to 3 weeks, headache, fever, chills, nausea, vomiting, and pain in the region of the salivary glands develop. The glands then become swollen, and they have a firm elastic consistency. The disease regresses within about a week. A variety of serious complications may arise from mumps, particularly in adults.

Nonspecific "mumps." Enlargement of the major salivary glands occurs in a variety of conditions not related to the viral infection of epidemic parotitis; these conditions sometimes produce considerable difficulty in diagnosis and differentiation from epidemic parotitis because of their clinical similarity. Such salivary gland enlargement is seen in (1) chronic nonspecific sialadenitis, most frequently a result of salivary duct calculus with a subsequent bacterial infection; (2) acute postoperative parotitis, usually a result of dehydration and xerostomia after a surgical operation with a subsequent ascending bacterial infection through the duct into the gland; (3) nutritional "mumps," a poorly understood condition commonly found in patients with multiple signs of nutritional deficiency, particularly of protein and the vitamin B complex group; (4) chemical "mumps," an idiosyncratic reaction to organic or inorganic iodide compounds used in the treatment of a variety of diseases, including myxedema; (5) Mikulicz disease and Sjögren syndrome, probably as a result of a salivary gland autoimmune reaction; and (6) fibrocystic disease (mucoviscidosis) of the pancreas, in which salivary gland enlargement is a consistent and almost universal finding.

Dermatologic diseases

Many primary dermatologic diseases also produce lesions in the oral cavity, sometimes as a prodromal manifestation but more frequently as an accompaniment of the disease. However, dermatologic diseases are relatively uncommon in children, and only the more common ones are discussed here.

Erythema multiforme. The cause of erythema multiforme is unknown, although an eruption of the disease is often associated with the administration of one of a variety of common drugs, with a bacterial infection, or even with some viral infections, including herpes simplex. Erythema multiforme is chiefly a disease of adolescents and young adults.

The skin lesions are characteristically asymptomatic erythematous macules or papules, sometimes vesicles or bullae, which develop in a symmetric pattern over the extremities, trunk, and face. These lesions, which are usually only a few centimeters or less in diameter, develop rapidly, persist for a few days to a few weeks, and then gradually disappear.

The oral lesions usually develop about the same time as the skin lesions and also consist of macules, papules, and vesicles that often become eroded or ulcerated and covered by a fibrinous exudate. The lesions are usually painful and may involve a large portion of the oral cavity. The oral lesions regress at the same time as the skin lesions. Corticosteroids and antibiotics are frequently used in treatment. Significantly, recurrences over a period of years are common.

Stevens-Johnson syndrome. Stevens-Johnson syndrome is now considered to be only a severe form of erythema multiforme. This syndrome includes, in addition to the cutaneous and oral lesions, lesions of the eyes and genitalia. The cutaneous and oral lesions are identical to those of erythema multiforme. The eye lesions generally consist of conjunctivitis, which may lead to corneal ulceration. The genital lesions are usually a nonspecific urethritis or vaginitis. Because of the multiple organ involvement, this disease has sometimes been referred to as a mucocutaneous-ocular syndrome.

Epidermolysis bullosa. Epidermolysis bullosa, an uncommon dermatologic disease, is characterized by the appearance of vesicles or bullae on the skin or mucous membranes, which develop spontaneously or following mild trauma. There are several different types of epidermolysis bullosa, but most of them exhibit a definite hereditary pattern.

Clinically, the disease is usually manifested at birth or shortly thereafter. In children with this disease, vesicles and bullae develop at sites of pressure or irritation. The bullae rupture and usually heal by scarring.

The oral cavity is similarly involved by the formation of vesicles or bullae after even the mildest irritation or trauma. Large areas of mucous membrane may be denuded with relative ease. These oral ulcerations are generally painful. The condition makes routine restorative procedures and rubber dam application difficult.

There is no known treatment for epidermolysis bullosa; it cannot be controlled. Many of those affected die early in life, although some survive into adulthood.

Mucocutaneous lymph node syndrome, or Kawasaki disease. Mucocutaneous lymph node syndrome was first described in Japan in 1967; it was recognized in the United States in 1974. The cause is unknown, but it has been suggested that it is viral in origin, a collagen-vascular disease, or possibly immunologic, although heredity is recognized as playing some role.

The majority of patients are children, in whom fever, conjunctivitis, lymphadenopathy, and an exanthematous rash develop with erythema of the hands and feet and subsequent desquamation of the fingers and toes. The most serious sequelae are cardiac complications, such as coronary thrombosis or coronary artery aneurysm.

The oral manifestations of the disease consist of a diffuse erythema of the oral and pharyngeal mucosa, with the development of a "strawberry" tongue and dryness, redness, and fissuring of the lips. Occasionally there is gingival ulceration. This disease must be carefully distinguished from erythema multiforme and related conditions.

There is no specific treatment for the disease, and it is generally self-limited. However, deaths do occur occasionally.

REFERENCES

Allen, A.C.: The skin, ed. 2, New York, 1967, Grune & Stratton, Inc.

Burnett, G.W., and Schuster, G.S.: Oral microbiology and infectious disease, Student ed., Baltimore, 1978, The Williams & Wilkins Co.

Krugman, S., and Katz, S.L.: Infectious diseases of children, ed. 7, St. Louis, 1981, The C.V. Mosby Co.

Lever, W.F., and Schaumburg-Lever, G.: Histopathology of the skin, ed. 5, Philadelphia, 1975, J.B. Lippincott Co.

Perlman, H.H.: Pediatric dermatology, Chicago, 1960, Year Book Medical Publishers, Inc.

Shafer, W.G., Hine, M.K., and Levy, B.M.: A textbook of oral pathology, ed. 3, Philadelphia, 1974, W.B. Saunders Co.

28 Oral tumors

WILLIAM G. SHAFER

Benign and malignant tumors occur with unfortunate frequency in the oral cavities of both children and adults. Because the majority of the patients with whom pedodontists deal have purely dental problems, pedodontists are often forgetful of the need to be constantly aware of the possible presence of neoplasms, and they often minimize the probability with which such lesions may be encountered. Certain neoplasms obviously occur with far greater frequency than others. Nevertheless, it must always be remembered that *any* tumor can occur in children. For example, although intraoral epidermoid carcinoma is predominantly a disease of elderly adults, it can and does occur in children. Cases have even been recorded of oral epidermoid carcinoma present in newborn infants. Thus a high index of suspicion must always be maintained when carrying out an oral examination of a young patient.

Only tumors that occur in children with considerable frequency are discussed here. That a tumor is not included in this chapter by no means implies that it may not be encountered at any time in a pedodontic patient.

Benign tumors

Papilloma. The papilloma is the oral counterpart of the common skin wart, or verruca vulgaris; however, it is not known to be caused by a virus as are some skin warts. The papilloma occurs in even young children and may develop at any site in the oral cavity. In children it is most common on the soft palate near the uvula, on the gingiva, and on the tongue (Fig. 28-1). The typical papilloma measures a few millimeters to a centimeter in diameter and is a pedunculated growth with a roughened surface made up of numerous fingerlike projections.

The papilloma should be surgically excised, including the mucosa from which the base of the pedicle projects. It seldom recurs.

Intraoral viral warts. Intraoral warts are also seen occasionally. These appear to have been autoinoculated from other lesions—usually from lesions on the hands. They should be treated in the same fashion as the papilloma.

Fibroma. The fibroma is probably the most common benign soft tissue tumor of the oral cavity. However, it is likely that the majority of lesions designated as fibromas actually represent a reactive fibrous connective tissue hyperplasia that occurs in response to some irritation, rather than a true neoplasm. Undoubtedly, some fibromas represent healed or sclerosed pyogenic granulomas.

The oral fibroma occurs at any age and at any site. It is usually a firm, elevated lesion with a smooth surface and a sessile base. The color is that of the normal mucosa, or sometimes a fibroma is slightly reddened as a result of superimposed inflammation. The lesion seldom recurs after surgical excision.

Peripheral giant cell granuloma. The peripheral giant cell granuloma is not a true neoplasm but rather a reaction of the tissues to injury, possibly trauma. The lesion occurs only on the gingiva or alveolar ridge and is usually a sessile (or sometimes a pedunculated) growth that often appears to be originating from deeper underlying structures, either the periodontal ligament or the mucoperios-

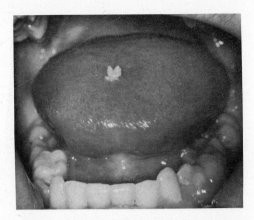

Fig. 28-1. Papilloma. This papilloma of the tongue shows the typical fingerlike projections comprising the lesion.

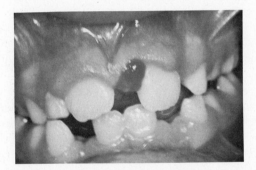

Fig. 28-2. Peripheral giant cell granuloma. The lesion in this 6-year-old child developed immediately after the loss of the primary incisor.

teum. It is usually dark red or purplish (indicative of its vascular nature), and it may show ulceration of the surface (Fig. 28-2).

The lesion can occur at any age but is commonly seen in children, about 25% occurring in persons younger than 20 years of age. Although there does not seem to be any predilection for occurrence between maxilla and mandible, the lesion is usually limited to the gingiva anterior to the molar area. In most reported series of cases, females are affected more frequently than males, usually in a ratio of at least 2:1; the reason for this is unknown.

The histologic picture of the peripheral giant cell granuloma is striking. The mass is composed of a loose fibrous connective tissue interspersed with large numbers of young fibroblasts, small capillaries, and varying numbers of multinucleated giant cells, sometimes within the lumen of the blood vessels. An inflammatory cell infiltrate is also usually present, as well as considerable hemosiderin pigment, particularly on the margins of the lesions (indicative of old hemorrhage). Trabeculae of bone are frequently found at the base of the lesion, indicating superficial involvement of alveolar bone, although this is not usually evident in a radiograph of a dentulous patient.

This lesion should be treated by surgical excision. Care must be taken to remove the entire base of the lesion. If the excision is too superficial, recurrence may be expected. However, extraction of adjacent teeth is seldom if ever warranted, although this was strongly advocated at one time to prevent recurrence.

Central giant cell granuloma. The central giant cell granuloma bears a remarkable histologic similarity to the peripheral giant cell granuloma, yet there is little evidence available to suggest that the two lesions are related. Most authorities do agree that the central lesion also is probably not a true neoplasm but rather a reaction to some type of injury, possibly trauma. It has been suggested that the lesion may represent an exuberant attempt at repair of a hematoma of bone. Whether this represents the true pathogenesis must await further study.

The central giant cell granuloma occurs centrally within bone; the mandible is affected about twice as frequently as the maxilla. This is predominantly a disease of children; about 60% of the cases occur before the age of 20 years. As with peripheral giant cell granuloma, females are affected more frequently than males in a ratio of about 2:1. Here also, this sex predilection lacks an explanation. It would be most unlikely that females would be subjected to traumatic injury to the jaws more frequently than males. Pain is not generally a feature of the lesion, and many of the small lesions are

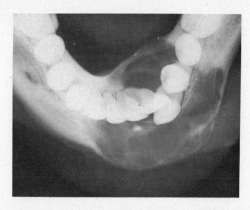

Fig. 28-3. Central giant cell granuloma. This 14-year-old girl had swelling of the mandible, which showed an expansile, multilocular lesion on the radiograph.

discovered accidentally during routine radiographic examination or following a complaint of mild discomfort. The larger lesions produce bulging of the cortical plates, and the swelling is the usual complaint.

The radiograph typically reveals a poorly circumscribed, expansile radiolucency with thinning but seldom perforation of the cortical plates of bone. The larger lesions usually present a multilocular appearance, thus resembling the ameloblastoma as well as many other lesions of the jaws (Fig. 28-3).

The microscopic appearance of the central giant cell granuloma is identical to that of the peripheral counterpart, and the two cannot be distinguished except by the clinical description of the location of the lesions.

One additional important fact should be pointed out concerning the microscopic appearance of the central giant cell granuloma. The lesion is histologically indistinguishable from the bone lesion of hyperparathyroidism or von Recklinghausen disease of bone (osteitis fibrosa). Therefore every patient with a diagnosis of central giant cell granuloma should have a serum calcium analysis to rule out the possibility of the jaw lesion representing bony involvement of hyperparathyroidism. This is particularly true in adults, since the parathyroid

adenoma, the most common cause of hyperparathyroidism, is more common in adults than in children. Nevertheless, such adenomas do occur in young persons, as does secondary hyperparathyroidism.

The treatment for this lesion is surgical excision. Healing is almost invariably prompt, and recurrence is rare.

Hemangioma. The hemangioma is considered by most authorities to represent, at least in the majority of cases, a congenital developmental abnormality or hamartoma rather than a true neoplasm. Most hemangiomas are present at birth, although some are not clinically manifested until later in life.

The oral hemangioma may occur in any location, although the tongue is by far the most common site, followed by the lips, gingiva, and buccal mucosa. When the tongue is involved, the lesion may be focal or more commonly may diffusely infiltrate the superficial and deep musculature of much of the tongue.

A central hemangioma of the maxilla or the mandible is rare. Unfortunately, there is nothing radiographically suggestive of the true nature of the radiolucency, and surgical exploration of such lesions may result in severe loss of blood or even death because of inability to stop the profuse hemorrhage.

The two chief histologic forms of hemangioma are the capillary and the cavernous. The former is composed of tiny capillaries, usually with marked endothelial cell proliferation, and the latter of large cavernous blood-filled spaces.

Many congenital hemangiomas need no treatment, since they may undergo spontaneous involution within the first few years of life. Lesions that do not regress may be treated in a variety of ways, including the injection of a sclerosing solution, surgical excision, electrocautery, or x-radiation, although this last form of treatment is not advisable for the oral hemangioma. If a hemangioma is small, no treatment is necessary.

Encephalotrigeminal angiomatosis. Encephalotrigeminal angiomatosis, also called Sturge-We-ber syndrome, is an unusual and unfortunate congenital form of hemangioma. It is characterized by a diffuse hemangioma of the skin area supplied by the trigeminal nerve and by hemangiomas of the leptomeninges over the cerebral cortex with intracranial convolutional calcifications. The cranial involvement often leads to neurologic manifestations of epileptic-like seizures and mental retardation. Oral involvement is also common in the form of hemangiomas of the buccal mucosa, gingiva, and sometimes the underlying bone. Treatment of the soft tissue hemangiomas is the same as for other hemangiomas, and the cerebral lesions are a neurosurgical problem.

Lymphangioma. The lymphangioma is the lymphatic vessel counterpart of the hemangioma, and it is also congenital in the majority of cases. It is far less common than the hemangioma. The oral lymphangioma may also occur at any site but most commonly involves the tongue, buccal mucosa, or lips (Fig. 28-4). The lesion may appear as a diffuse smooth or nodular enlargement, particularly in tongue and lip involvement, or as multiple elevated papillary nodules of the same color as the surrounding mucosa, particularly in involvement of the buccal mucosa. Unilateral tongue involvement is relatively common. Some lesions are deep red because of an admixture of hemangioma with the lymphangioma element. Lymphangiomas of the alveolar ridges in neonates have also been reported. These are described as blue-domed, fluid-filled lesions that, at least on occasion, undergo spontaneous regression (Fig. 28-5). The microscopic appearance of the lymphangioma is similar to that of the hemangioma, except that the vessels are lymphatics filled with lymph fluid rather than blood vessels filled with blood.

Treatment is not necessary unless the lesion is large or disfiguring, in which case sclerosing agents or surgical excision is used.

Congenital epulis of the newborn. The congenital epulis of the newborn is an unusual tumor of unknown histogenesis. As the name indicates, the lesion is present at birth and appears as a pedunculated mass on the anterior maxillary or, less

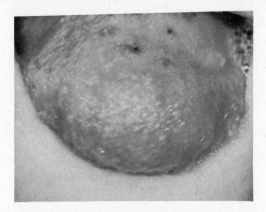

Fig. 28-4. Lymphangioma. In this child the macroglossia was of such an extent that the tongue could not be completely retruded into the mouth. The entire tongue was involved by the lymphangioma.

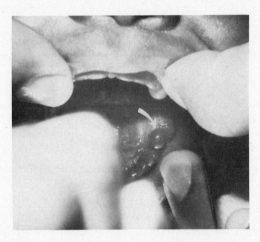

Fig. 28-5. Lymphangioma of the neonate. The lesion is present on the alveolar ridge. (From Levin, L.S.: Pediatrics **58**:881, 1976.)

commonly, mandibular ridge. Most reported series of cases indicate that at least 90% of lesions occur in infant girls.

The congenital epulis is histologically nearly identical to the granular cell myoblastoma, being composed of large cells with a granular eosinophilic cytoplasm. However, pseudoepitheliomatous hyperplasia of the overlying epithelium is not present as in the myoblastoma.

The lesions are treated by surgical excision and seldom recur.

Melanotic neuroectodermal tumor of infancy. The melanotic neuroectodermal tumor of infancy, once thought to be odontogenic in origin, is now recognized as a neuroectodermal lesion on the basis of histochemical evidence and the urinary excretion of a catecholamine similar to that occurring with other known neuroectodermal tumors.

The lesion is interesting in that nearly all reported cases have occurred in infants under the age of 6 months. The majority of the oral tumors have occurred in the maxilla rather than the mandible. Histologically identical tumors have been reported in other parts of the body, including the skull, shoulder, epididymis, and uterus. Clinically, these tumors appear as a rapidly growing nonulcerated pigmented mass that shows radiographic evidence of invasion of bone and resembles malignant neoplasm in this regard. Despite the apparently serious clinical and radiographic features of this lesion, it seldom recurs after even a relatively conservative surgical excision. However, a very rare malignant form has been reported that has resulted in metastases and death.

Malignant tumors

Malignant lymphoma group. The malignant lymphoma group of diseases consists of a series of neoplasms, all derived from certain cells of the reticuloendothelial system. Numerous classifications of these diseases have been proposed in recent years, none of which has found universal acceptance. At present, the lymphomas, excluding lymphocytic and monocytic leukemias, are simply placed in the main categories of non-Hodgkin and Hodgkin types. The non-Hodgkin type comprises those diseases formerly called lymphocytic lymphoma or lymphosarcoma and histiocytic lymphoma or reticulum cell sarcoma. The Hodgkin type of lymphoma remains in its classical form. The diagnosis of the specific type of malignant lymphoma present can be determined only through microscopic study of the lesional tissue, combined with a complete hematologic examination and bone

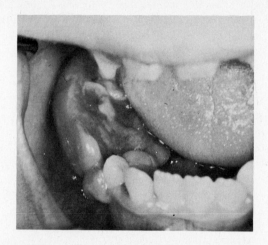

Fig. 28-6. Lymphocytic lymphoma. In this 8-year-old girl a soft tissue tumor developed at the site of a recently extracted primary molar. She died within a month. (From Shafer, W.G., Hine, M.K., and Levy, B.M.: A textbook of oral pathology, ed. 3, Philadelphia, 1974, W.B. Saunders Co.)

marrow analysis. Of the malignant lymphoma group, children are involved more frequently by the lymphocytic types, Hodgkin disease, and the leukemias than by any of the others. However, intraoral involvement in Hodgkin disease is uncommon.

The typical lymphoma begins with a painless lymphadenopathy, often of the cervical nodes. The tonsils, nasopharynx, and other focal areas in the oral cavity, such as the gingiva, are also common sites of involvement (Fig. 28-6). Such an oral lesion usually appears as a rapidly growing mass that frequently causes loosening and premature exfoliation of the teeth if it involves the jaws.

Burkitt (African jaw) lymphoma, a specific form of lymphoma, was first discovered in Africa but is now known to occur in the United States. The great majority of cases involve children. Significantly, Burkitt lymphoma is now recognized as being caused by the Epstein-Barr virus, the same virus that causes infectious mononucleosis and possibly nasopharyngeal carcinoma in adults.

The clinical manifestations of the leukemias do not differ significantly from those of the other lymphomas. The oral lesions, however, consist of spontaneous gingival bleeding, diffuse gingival hyperplasia, or both, more frequently than in the other lymphomas. In addition, petechiae and multiple ulcerations of the oral cavity are relatively common. Loosening of the teeth and premature exfoliation sometimes occur as a result of involvement of the periodontal ligament and the alveolar bone.

There is no uniformly successful treatment for any of the diseases in the malignant lymphoma group, although x-radiation and chemotherapy are resulting in long-term remissions and apparent cures in some cases.

Ewing sarcoma. Ewing sarcoma is a malignant neoplasm that develops centrally in bone. The cell of origin has never been determined. This is a disease of the young, occurring almost exclusively between the ages of 5 and 25 years.

Ewing sarcoma is first manifested by pain and swelling of the involved bone, often followed by pathologic fracture. Either the maxilla or the mandible is involved in up to 15% of cases.

Radiographically, the lesion appears as an irregular diffuse radiolucency, which commonly produces a subperiosteal reactive new bone formation with an onion-ring pattern.

The disease is usually treated by x-radiation, sometimes coupled with surgical excision. The prognosis is grave, and most patients die within a short time.

Osteosarcoma. Osteosarcoma is a primary malignant tumor of bone derived from osteoblasts. It may affect any bone in the skeleton. About 7% of cases arise in the jaws. Many of these cases develop in individuals under the age of 20 years. The lesions are approximately twice as common in the mandible as in the maxilla, and in most series males are affected more frequently than females.

Pain and swelling are early clinical manifestations of the neoplasm. It is interesting that a high percentage of cases of osteosarcoma involve a definite history of trauma preceding the development of the tumor. The lesions generally grow rapidly and may or may not produce ulceration of the mucosa. Loosening of the teeth is also an early manifestation of the disease.

The radiographic appearance of osteosarcoma depends on the histologic nature of the tumor. Some are sclerotic, some are lytic, and others are mixed. Some cases of osteosarcoma are characterized by the classic "sun-ray" appearance on the radiograph; this is seen in only about 25%. Regardless of whether the lesion is sclerotic or lytic, it is invariably poorly defined and generally expansile. One of the earliest significant radiographic changes occurring in osteosarcoma is a symmetric widening of the periodontal ligament space around one or more teeth, visible on a periapical dental radiograph.

The tumor is treated in a variety of ways, but radical surgery produces the best survival rate. Even at best, however, the 5-year survival rate is less than 40%. About 50% of all osteosarcomas of the jaws ultimately metastasize.

Rhabdomyosarcoma. The rhabdomyosarcoma is the malignant tumor of striated muscle cells. One form of this tumor, the embryonal rhabdomyosarcoma, occurs far more frequently in young children than in adults and is more common in the head and neck region than in any other site. The oral lesions generally begin as a rapidly growing, nonulcerated mass of the mucosa, commonly the soft palate, which soon ulcerates and may rapidly fill the oral cavity. This tumor is treated by radical surgical excision, sometimes accompanied by x-radiation. The survival rate is generally less than 10%.

Odontogenic cysts

The odontogenic cysts are lined with epithelium derived from the epithelium of the odontogenic apparatus in varying stages of its development. These are true cysts, inasmuch as they are all pathologic epithelium-lined cavities that usually contain fluid or semisolid material. Because of the close microscopic similarity between the various odontogenic cysts, the correct diagnosis of type can be made only by studying the histologic, clinical, and radiographic findings, along with all pertinent facts of the lesion's history.

Primordial cyst. The primordial cyst develops in place of a tooth, apparently through cystic degeneration of the stellate reticulum before any enamel or dentin has formed. Thus the epithelial lining is derived essentially from the inner and outer enamel epithelium. It is the least common of the odontogenic cysts.

The primordial cyst may develop in place of any tooth. However, it is most common in the site of the third molar, followed by the maxillary and mandibular premolars and the maxillary canine. Without an adequate history one cannot make a definitive diagnosis of a primordial cyst, since a cyst that appears to be primordial could be a residual dentigerous cyst or even a residual radicular cyst *if* a tooth had once been present in the area. The majority of primordial cysts are discovered accidentally during routine radiographic examination, although they may become large enough to produce expansion and swelling of the jaw.

Radiographically, the lesion appears as a well-circumscribed radiolucency in the area of a missing tooth. Histologically, the epithelial lining is of the stratified squamous type, usually thin and commonly keratinizing. In the latter situation the lesion is classified as an odontogenic keratocyst.

A primordial cyst should be surgically removed when discovered. Although too few cases have been reported in the literature to be certain of the potential of this cyst, there is no reason to believe that it would not behave similarly to the dentigerous cyst.

Dentigerous (follicular) cyst. The dentigerous cyst develops around the formed crown of an impacted tooth, presumably through accumulation of fluid between the crown of the tooth and the reduced enamel epithelium. In many cases it is impossible to determine just when the normal follicular space ceases and the pathologic dentigerous cyst begins. A dentigerous cyst is exceedingly rare in association with primary teeth. It is most commonly found in association with permanent mandibular third molars and maxillary canines, since these are the most frequently impacted teeth.

Clinically, the majority of dentigerous cysts are

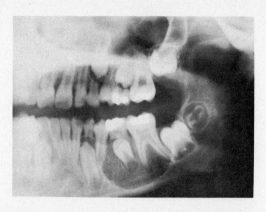

Fig. 28-7. Dentigerous cyst. This 10-year-old child was found during routine radiographic examination to have a large dentigerous cyst associated with the crown of an unerupted mandibular second premolar.

discovered accidentally during routine radiographic examination. However, a significant number of these cysts, particularly those associated with the third molar, become large enough to cause expansion of cortical plates of bone and facial swelling. It is not rare for these cysts to involve even the entire ramus of the mandible as well, and displacement of the impacted crown against the inferior border of the mandible is relatively common. Such cysts also frequently displace adjacent teeth and may even cause resorption of roots of adjacent teeth on which the cyst impinges.

The radiographic appearance of a dentigerous cyst will vary depending on the size of the lesion. In general, it appears as a well-circumscribed radiolucency associated with an impacted tooth that may or may not be displaced (Fig. 28-7).

Histologically, the dentigerous cyst is similar to the primordial cyst in that it is lined by a thin stratified squamous epithelium that occasionally shows keratinization, in which case it, too, should be called an odontogenic keratocyst. It has been proved beyond question that this epithelium has the potential to undergo transformation into an ameloblastoma; numerous such cases have been reported. When a transformation occurs, it usually cannot be determined by gross examination of the tissue. Such a transformation has been seen in dentigerous cysts in young children. For this reason it is imperative that every dentigerous cyst that is surgically removed be submitted to an oral pathologist for microscopic examination. It is also recognized that the epithelium of dentigerous cysts has the potential for undergoing transformation into epidermoid carcinoma and mucoepidermoid carcinoma; such cases have been reported in children. Therefore it is strongly recommended that all dentigerous cysts be surgically removed and examined when discovered.

Odontogenic cyst–basal cell nevus–bifid rib syndrome. The odontogenic cyst–basal cell nevus–bifid rib syndrome, which has been described as a hereditary syndrome, consists of multiple odontogenic keratocysts of the jaws, multiple basal cell nevi of the skin, and a bifid rib, as well as any of a large number of other skeletal anomalies. Whenever a patient with multiple keratinizing jaw cysts is found, the possible presence of the other components of the syndrome should be investigated, although some patients have only solitary cysts. This syndrome may be discovered in children as well as in adults. It is important to recognize that a significant percentage of affected persons develop a particular type of brain tumor, a medulloblastoma. Furthermore, it is reported that persons who have the syndrome do not respond to the administration of parathyroid hormone.

The odontogenic keratocyst, irrespective of whether it is associated with the syndrome, has an unusually high recurrence rate after surgical enucleation.

Odontogenic tumors

Tumors derived from various components of the odontogenic apparatus during different stages of odontogenesis are relatively common lesions. It is interesting that certain of these specific lesions have a remarkable predilection for occurrence in children, while others are uncommon during this period of life. At the present time there is no reasonable explanation for this peculiarity in occurrence; it does not appear to be related to differentiation of the tissues involved. Thus tumors that are composed of well-differentiated dental tissues as well as of poorly differentiated or embryonic dental tissues are common in children.

No completely acceptable classification of odontogenic tumors is currently available. However, a workable classification divides this group of neoplasms into three main groups—ectodermal origin, mesodermal origin, and mixed-tissue origin—with respect to the odontogenic apparatus.

Ectodermal tumors. Ectodermal tumors include the tumors originating from the ameloblasts, stratum intermedium, stellate reticulum, or any of their histogenetic derivatives.

Ameloblastoma. The ameloblastoma is one of the most common odontogenic tumors. Although about half of these tumors occur between the ages of 20 and 40 years, they arise in persons of any age, including even young children. Regardless of the age at occurrence, approximately 80% of the tumors occur in the mandible and the majority of these are in the molar-ramus area. Radiographically, the tumor appears as an expanding radiolucency that may present a multilocular pattern if it becomes sufficiently large. However, since many other central lesions of the jaws present an identical radiographic picture, this should not be considered pathognomonic.

The ameloblastoma has been described as a slowly destructive, locally invasive, and persistent tumor of bone. For this reason the lesion is difficult to eradicate by a completely conservative surgical procedure. To prevent recurrence of the tumor, complete surgical removal is necessary. Because of the invasive nature of the tumor, removal is sometimes difficult to accomplish without sacrificing a considerable portion of the jaw.

Adenomatoid odontogenic tumor. The adenomatoid odontogenic tumor, previously called the adenoameloblastoma, is an unusual odontogenic tumor that bears little if any similarity to the ameloblastoma. The majority of these tumors occur before the age of 21 years. In fact, the lesion is relatively common even in children under 10 years of age. The lesion develops with equal frequency

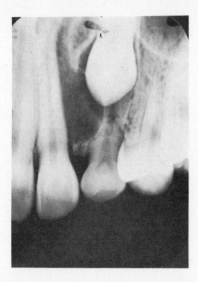

Fig. 28-8. Adenomatoid odontogenic tumor. This tumor resembled a dentigerous cyst associated with an unerupted tooth and was diagnosed only by microscopic examination of the tissue after its surgical removal.

in the maxilla and the mandible. In further contrast to the ameloblastoma, the adenomatoid odontogenic tumor occurs in the anterior segment of the jaws in the vast majority of cases. The tumor is commonly associated with the crown of an impacted or unerupted tooth, although many cases appear to originate within a cyst of unexplained origin (Fig. 28-8).

Radiographically, this tumor is a well-circumscribed radiolucency that is seldom larger than 2 to 3 cm in diameter. Inasmuch as calcification occasionally occurs within this tumor, a speckled radiopaque appearance may be seen on the radiograph.

The tumor derives its name from its unusual histologic picture of ductlike or adenomatoid structures composed of cuboidal or columnar epithelial cells scattered throughout the tumor mass of polyhedral epithelial cells that often have a whorled pattern. The elaboration of an enameloid matrix material is relatively common within the tumor mass. In contrast to most other odontogenic tumors, this lesion is almost invariably encapsulated.

For this reason the tumor is easily removed by surgical enucleation, and seldom if ever is there a recurrence.

Mesodermal tumors. Mesodermal tumors include the tumors originating from the dental papilla, the dental follicle, or the periodontal ligament or any of its derivatives.

Peripheral odontogenic (ossifying) fibroma. The peripheral odontogenic fibroma is a lesion that develops only on the gingiva or alveolar ridge; it occurs most frequently in children and young adolescents. It appears clinically as a focal overgrowth of the gingiva and thus resembles a fibroma, peripheral giant cell granuloma, or pyogenic granuloma of this location (Fig. 28-9). It derives its name from the fact that, when viewed microscopically, the lesion is highly cellular, being composed of fibrous connective tissue interspersed with large numbers of young proliferating fibroblasts and scattered or focal trabeculae of osteoid, bone, cementum, or even dystrophic calcification. This bone is not continuous with the underlying alveolar bone but rather represents a metaplastic change in the connective tissue of the lesion itself.

The lesion is treated by surgical excision. However, recurrence of this tumor after excision is fairly common.

Central odontogenic fibroma. The central odontogenic fibroma is a relatively uncommon odontogenic tumor of which little is known because of the paucity of reported cases in the literature. It apparently occurs in young persons, most frequently children. The portion of the odontogenic apparatus from which the tumor originates is not known.

A radiograph shows a central odontogenic fibroma to be a destructive, expansile, central lesion; it may occur in any segment of the maxilla or mandible (Fig. 28-10). It is apparently a relatively slow-growing tumor. The few cases reported seem to indicate that it is best treated by conservative surgical excision and that there is little tendency toward recurrence.

Odontogenic myxoma. The odontogenic myxoma is a mesodermal tumor of the jaws that is almost certainly of odontogenic origin, since many

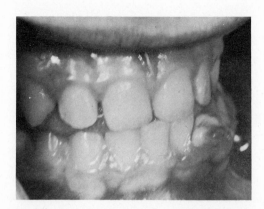

Fig. 28-9. Peripheral odontogenic (ossifying) fibroma. This lesion of the gingiva clinically resembles a fibroma, a peripheral giant cell granuloma, and the pyogenic granuloma.

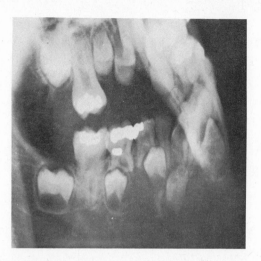

Fig. 28-10. Central odontogenic fibroma. This tumor was discovered during routine radiographic examination and was causing displacement of the developing premolars.

cases are known to have occurred in the jaws and a histologically similar lesion is practically unknown in other bones of the skeleton. The tumor, which appears to be most common between the ages of 10 and 30 years, has no predilection for maxilla or mandible or any site within the jaw. Interestingly, many of these tumors are associated with missing or impacted teeth, although this is not invariably true.

The odontogenic myxoma is clinically and radiographically similar to the central odontogenic fibroma in that it is a relatively slow-growing, destructive, expansile lesion central in bone that may present a multilocular appearance if sufficiently large. Histologically the lesion is deceptive, appearing as a relatively acellular, loose lesion composed of delicate collagen fibrils embedded in a large bulk of amorphous, mucoid material.

In many instances surgical excision of the tumor is difficult because of its slimy mucoid nature. This loose nature of the tumor and ensuing difficulty in complete removal and the fact that it does infiltrate between bony trabeculae account for the moderate recurrence rate of the lesion.

Caution must be exercised in accepting a diag-

nosis of odontogenic myxoma by pathologists who are not completely familiar with this tumor. It has been found that many pathologists make such a diagnosis when the tissue examined represents only the normal dental papilla of a developing tooth in which the calcified crown has been removed, and the uncapped papilla excised separately. This normal papilla does bear some resemblance to the odontogenic myxoma, but this mistake is not made by an experienced oral pathologist. In addition, the dental follicle around some impacted teeth is relatively thick and may be composed of a loose, fibrous, myxomatoid tissue resembling the myxoma, and this has also caused mistakes in diagnosis.

Central cementifying fibroma. The central cementifying fibroma is a lesion that is now accepted by most authorities as an odontogenic neoplasm. Although it may occur at any age, it is most common in young adults but may be found even in young children. It appears to develop more frequently in the mandible than in the maxilla. Clinically, the lesion is generally asymptomatic until a firm swelling of the jaw is noted, frequently accompanied by displacement of teeth. In most cases the lesion grows slowly.

The radiographic appearance of the tumor is variable and depends on the degree of calcification within the mass. Some lesions appear as a well-circumscribed, expansile radiolucency with little or no evidence of calcification, whereas others are well-circumscribed, expansile, dense radiopacities.

Histologic examination of this tumor shows it to be composed of a highly cellular fibrous mass interspersed with varying amounts of droplet calcification that resembles cementicles or "cementum drops." In some tumors these droplets are sparse; these are the radiolucent lesions. In others the droplets form the bulk of the tumor; these tumors are radiopaque on a radiograph.

This tumor is usually well circumscribed and rather easily excised surgically, and it seldom recurs. Occasional lesions seem less well circumscribed, present more difficulty in complete excision, and thus may recur.

Mixed-tissue tumors. Mixed-tissue tumors are those that contain odontogenic ectodermal and mesodermal components, both of which appear to be participating in the neoplastic process.

Ameloblastic fibroma. The ameloblastic fibroma is characterized by the simultaneous proliferation of odontogenic epithelium and connective tissue without the formation of either enamel or dentin. Although the simple ameloblastoma is also composed of epithelium and connective tissue, there are certain microscopic differences between the two lesions that clearly distinguish them. This differentiation is distinctly supported by the clinical differences between the two tumors.

The ameloblastic fibroma generally occurs at a far earlier age (average age about 14 years) than the ameloblastoma. The majority of cases occur in the molar area of the mandible. The tumor grows slowly by expansion and seldom shows evidence of local invasion. The first clinical manifestation may be a swelling of the jaw, although in many cases the tumor remains small and is discovered accidentally during routine radiographic examination. The radiographic appearance is usually a well-circumscribed radiolucency, but there are no radiographic features that characterize this tumor. The tumor is treated by simple surgical excision and, since it usually is well circumscribed, seldom recurs.

Odontoma. Although the term "odontoma" actually means any odontogenic tumor, it has come to refer to a specific lesion composed of enamel, dentin, and pulp tissue. This is often referred to as a "compound composite odontoma" when the calcified mass has some superficial anatomic similarity to normal teeth and as a "complex composite odontoma" when the mass has no anatomic similarity to teeth but consists only of a jumbled mass of calcified dental tissue.

The odontoma, as differentiated and restricted a lesion as it is, more closely resembles a developmental anomaly such as a hamartoma rather than a true neoplasm. Either type of odontoma may be discovered at any age and at any tooth-bearing site in the maxilla or the mandible. Most odontomas remain small and asymptomatic and are discovered accidentally on routine radiographic examination. An odontoma may occasionally reach sufficient size to produce expansion of bone and noticeable swelling. This is particularly true if an odontoma should develop a dentigerous cyst similar to a dentigerous cyst developing around the crown of an impacted tooth.

There is seldom any difficulty in the radiographic diagnosis of the compound composite odontoma, because of the resemblance of the components to miniature teeth. However, the complex composite odontoma may be radiographically indistinguishable from the ameloblastic fibro-odontoma, a highly calcified adenoameloblastoma, or even an osteoma. Both types of odontoma often occur in association with an impacted or unerupted tooth. On occasion, particularly in children, a developing odontoma may be found on a radiograph. This may cause difficulty in diagnosis, since the lesion may be predominantly a radiolucency with linear calcifications representing beginning calcification of the enamel and dentin matrix.

All odontomas should be surgically removed when discovered and submitted for microscopic examination to confirm the diagnosis. The lesion does not recur.

Ameloblastic fibro-odontoma. The ameloblastic fibro-odontoma, formerly referred to as an "ameloblastic odontoma," is basically a tumor composed of an ameloblastic fibroma associated with an odontoma.

This tumor has all the clinical features of the ameloblastic fibroma and occurs in the molar area of the mandible, chiefly in children. However, such a tumor may become extensive and produce considerable swelling and facial asymmetry. Radiographically, the lesion resembles an odontoma, although there is usually an associated radiolucency of variable size representing the soft tissue component of the tumor.

The ameloblastic fibro-odontoma is benign and seldom recurs after even rather conservative surgical excision. However, a rare variant of this lesion, an ameloblastic odontoma, which is a simple ameloblastoma developing in association with an odontoma, behaves as aggressively as the simple ameloblastoma and does have potential for recurrence.

Salivary gland tumors

Tumors of the major salivary glands are generally outside the province of the dentist with regard to diagnosis and certainly with regard to treatment. However, tumors of the intraoral accessory salivary glands are distinctly the responsibility of the dentist; the frequency with which these occur, even in children, is often not appreciated.

It should be remembered that accessory salivary gland tissue normally occurs in nearly every anatomic site in the oral cavity: upper and lower lip, hard and soft palate, buccal mucosa, retromolar area, floor of mouth, and tongue. Tumors can develop from these glands in any of these locations. It has been found that intraoral salivary gland tumors are about evenly divided between benign and malignant lesions.

The diagnosis of the exact type of salivary gland tumor depends entirely on microscopic examination. Clinically, however, the benign tumors are usually slow-growing, nonulcerated, painless lesions, whereas the malignant lesions generally are more rapidly growing, ulcerated, and often pain-

ful. Therefore any soft tissue tumor mass occurring in a location where salivary gland tissue is found must always be suspected of being such a tumor. The occurrence of such tumors, including the malignant tumors, in young children unfortunately is not rare. On many occasions these have been mistaken for dental infection and have been treated as such until the tumor has become advanced.

Mucus retention phenomenon. The mucus retention phenomenon, or mucocele, is not a neoplasm but may appear as a tumorlike swelling. It develops as a result of traumatic severance of an accessory salivary duct, such as that produced by biting the lip or pinching the lip accidentally with extraction forceps. After disruption of the duct, saliva continues to flow from the connecting acini, pools in the loose connective tissue, and forms the typical retention "cyst." However, this is not a true cyst, since it does not have an epithelial lining. Contrary to a widely accepted idea, this lesion is not caused by obstruction of a duct.

The mucus retention phenomenon may occur in any location where accessory salivary gland tissue is found. Actually, over half of all the occurrences are on the lower lip, with the buccal mucosa and the floor of the mouth being the next most common sites (Fig. 28-11). Involvement of the upper lip is

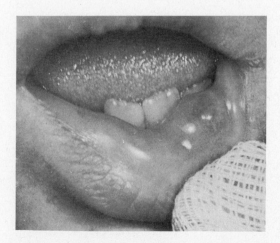

Fig. 28-11. Mucus retention phenomenon. This mucocele occurred as a fluctuant swelling of the lip.

exceedingly rare. The condition occurs at any age but is particularly prevalent in children and has even been recorded at birth.

A mucocele may form deep in the tissue and appear as a firm or fluctuant nodule or more commonly may develop superficially just beneath the epithelium, where it appears as a bluish, fluid-filled blister or vesicle. The lesions vary in size from a few millimeters to a centimeter or more in diameter. A mucocele may persist for a considerable period of time if untreated. If the lesion is incised, the fluid will drain out, but the lesion will refill as soon as the point of incision heals.

Histologically, the lesion consists simply of a mucus-filled cavity surrounded by a granulation tissue wall with no epithelial lining.

The mucus retention phenomenon is treated by surgical excision of the entire lesion or by surgically unroofing the lesion. Recurrence is relatively uncommon.

Ranula. A ranula is a form of retention cyst that occurs in the floor of the mouth in association with the ducts of the submaxillary or sublingual gland.

Although it may arise in the same fashion as a mucus retention cyst, partial obstruction may also play a role, since the majority of ranulas are lined by epithelium.

The clinical appearance of a ranula is that of a slowly enlarging, painless or slightly discomforting, fluctuant mass on one side of the floor of the mouth. Because of its size, the lesion is best treated by unroofing rather than by total excision. Recurrence is occasionally seen.

REFERENCES

Dargeon, H.W.: Tumors of childhood, New York, 1960, Harper & Row, Publishers, Inc.

Gorlin, R.J., and Goldman, H.M., editors: Thoma's oral pathology, ed. 6, St. Louis, 1970, The C.V. Mosby Co.

Gorlin, R.J., Chaudhry, A.P., and Pindborg, J.J.: Odontogenetic tumors: classification, histopathology, and clinical behavior in man and domesticated animals, Cancer **14**:73-101, 1961.

Shafer, W.G., Hine, M.K., and Levy, B.M.: A textbook of oral pathology, ed. 3, Philadelphia, 1974, W.B. Saunders Co.

Willis, R.A.: The pathology of tumors of children, Springfield, Ill., 1962, Charles C Thomas, Publisher.

29 Oral surgery for the child patient

CHARLES E. HUTTON

No greater joy or feeling of accomplishment can come to a dentist than that which results from the successful treatment of a child. The gaining of a child's confidence, the diagnosis of the child's ills, the elimination of the source or potential source of disease and pain, and the winning of the child's admiration are the first steps toward developing a healthy dental patient who is appreciative of good dentistry and who will be an apostle for dentists.

Possibly the greatest problem that exists in the surgical treatment of children is behavior management. Unfortunately, if a behavior problem exists, it is usually not the fault of the patient. The dentist may be as fearful of the child as the child is of the dentist. Many parents are not capable of properly preparing the child for the dental experience. Many children rely on untimely tales heard from unthinking relatives and playmates.

The art of working with children is inborn in some but must be acquired by others. Every dentist who has the desire, however, can become a friend of young patients. Complete honesty, kindly patience, a show of understanding, and firm control are essential. A well-adjusted child, properly prepared by the parents and managed with these attributes, will experience no emotional or physical stress.

A tense or maladjusted child, poorly prepared or having experienced pain or deceit in the past, may require a great deal of conditioning before even the simplest operation can be performed.

It must be remembered that all surgical procedures require adequate anesthesia; if a patient is properly premedicated and comfortable and if the tissues are handled gently, extensive operations can be performed with local anesthesia. When the fears of the patient are insurmountable, when an understanding of the situation is impossible, or when the procedure is complicated, general anesthesia is indicated.

It should also be emphasized that no surgical procedure should be done without the permission of the parent or guardian, who should have a basic understanding of what is to be done, why it is being done, and what complications can occur.

Extraction of teeth

Indications for extractions for children are much the same as for adult patients: unrestorable caries, apical disease, fractures of crowns or roots, prolonged retention of primary teeth because of improper root resorption or ankylosis, and supernumerary teeth.

Radiographic surveys of teeth to be extracted are of prime importance. The dentist should observe the size and contour of the primary roots, the amount and type of resorption, the relation of roots to succedaneous teeth, and the extent of disease.

The armamentarium for exodontic procedures is much the same as for adults, even though all anatomic structures are smaller. Special forceps for primary teeth offer some convenience; however, they are not necessary to perform any of the extractions Large adult forceps, such as the 99C, 53 R & L, and "cowhorns," and large foot and pick elevators are contraindicated in a child patient. Fig. 29-1 shows some of the forceps used for removal of primary teeth.

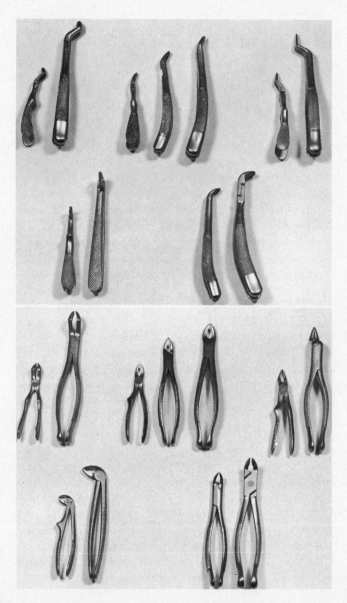

Fig. 29-1. Comparison of the size and shape of standard forceps and those smaller in size designed for the removal of primary teeth.

When permanent teeth are being removed from a child's mouth, the same basic techniques as those applied to adults are used. The young, elastic bone structures and incomplete root development will usually facilitate an extraction that would be difficult after maturity.

Fracture of slender roots is common, especially when the premolar teeth have projected well into the bifurcation of the molars and have caused uneven resorption (Fig. 29-2). Fractured roots should be removed, provided damage to the permanent bud can be avoided. Fig. 29-3 shows slender, delicate apexolevers that can be used judiciously in removing these roots. The mosquito hemostat may also be useful for grasping small fragments.

Anterior teeth should be luxated to the labial during the extraction procedure—because of the lingual position of the permanent teeth—and then rotated slightly and delivered to the labial.

Posterior teeth should be luxated with buccal and lingual pressures, and then delivered to the lingual. Occasionally, because of the great curvatures of roots, a mesial or distal path may be found.

Surgical removal of teeth

Ankylosed teeth. Ankylosed primary teeth, which occur frequently in children, need special mention because of their surgical potential. From a practical clinical point of view, there are two types of ankylosed teeth.

First are those that present clinical signs of ankylosis, such as "submerging" or failing to keep pace with the eruption of the other teeth in their quadrant. These teeth may be slightly out of occlusion (Fig. 29-4), or they may be completely within the alveolar process yet show evidence of having once been in the mouth (Fig. 29-5).

Second are those teeth that have all or nearly all of the root resorbed but that show no sign of mobility when pressure or leverage is applied and exhibit a solid sound on percussion. These teeth may be virtually welded to the surrounding bone, and there may be considerable difference in the degree of ankylosis as pertains to removal. These teeth will eventually become "submerged," but not all submerged teeth will clinically show these more complicating signs of ankylosis.

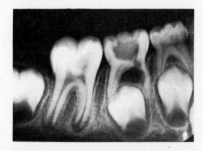

Fig. 29-2. Internal resorption and irregular root resorption may result in root fracture during extraction.

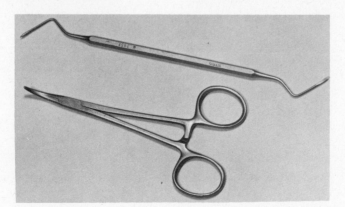

Fig. 29-3. Fine double-end apexolever and mosquito hemostat.

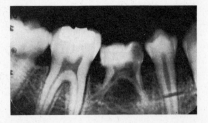

Fig. 29-4. Ankylosed second primary molar. Bone is continuous with areas of root resorption. A second premolar is absent.

One cannot entirely predict from radiographic and clinical examination what difficulties may be encountered in the removal of ankylosed teeth. A forceps extraction, when practical, should first be attempted; a dentist will frequently be pleasantly surprised to discover that only a millimeter or two of bone is maintaining a tooth. If luxation is not accomplished with reasonable forceps pressure, the dentist may then be faced with a formidable surgical procedure.

The crown is first removed by making a horizontal, round bur cut just below the cervical margin of the crown and inserting a straight elevator to fracture the crown. The remaining portions of the tooth are then encircled with the aid of a No. 8 bur, with bone being taken away until removal of the tooth is possible. Frequently the difference between tooth structure and bone cannot be determined clinically, and a block dissection must be carried out. In these instances undue destruction of bone and trauma to the underlying tooth and adjacent teeth must be avoided. It may be necessary to check the surgical progress by radiographic examinations.

Impacted teeth. Removal of impacted or unerupted primary teeth in young patients is sometimes necessary. Teeth that have received trauma (Fig. 29-6) may, as a result, be unerupted and may be obstructing the progress of the permanent teeth. Occasionally, unerupted premolars are removed in the course of orthodontic treatment.

Impacted permanent canines (Fig. 29-7) pose a special problem in developing dentitions. For such an impaction, surgical exposure of the crown is

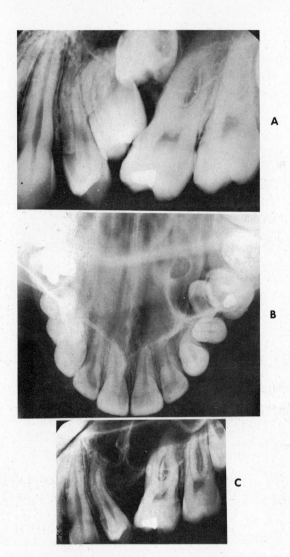

Fig. 29-5. A, Ankylosed second primary molar. Failure to observe this condition and to correct it at the proper time has resulted in mesial movement of the permanent molars and impaction of the second premolar. Surgical removal of the ankylosed tooth is indicated. **B,** An occlusal radiograph showing the position of the ankylosed molar. **C,** A postoperative radiograph.

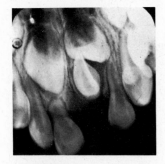

Fig. 29-6. Primary central incisor has been depressed as a result of a traumatic injury. The tooth has not re-erupted. There is evidence of injury to the permanent incisor.

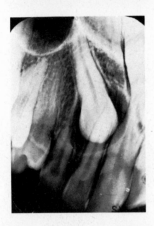

Fig. 29-7. Impacted permanent canine had an enlarged follicle. There was evidence of resorption of the root of the lateral incisor. Surgically uncovering the crown of the canine and guiding it into proper position is desirable.

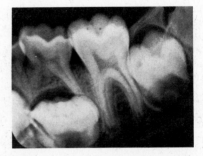

Fig. 29-8. Malformed second premolar in a 9-year-old boy required early surgical removal to avoid possible damage to adjacent teeth.

indicated and orthodontic guidance of the tooth may also be necessary. Every effort should be made to save impacted canines in young patients, because properly positioned canines contribute significantly to the long-term stability of the entire dental arch. Sometimes, however, an impacted canine may be so poorly positioned in the jaw, or it may be discovered so late, that surgical removal becomes the best form of treatment.

Malformed teeth (Fig. 29-8) and occasionally third molars should be removed at an early age.

The surgical approach to these problems should include the creation of an adequate mucoperiosteal flap to avoid damage to the blood supply of the tooth, followed by conservative bone removal.

Once a tooth is uncovered so the crown can be seen, multiple sectioning of the crown with a No. 8 carbide bur will facilitate removal through conservative windows in the bone, thus minimizing the chance of injury to adjacent structures. Complete debridement of all follicular tissues and incompletely calcified apical tissues is important. The edges of the remaining bone are smoothed with files, and closures are made with silk or absorbable sutures.

Supernumerary teeth. Supernumerary teeth are frequently observed during the examination of children. Such teeth may be observed singly or they may be multiple (Fig. 29-9). They are most commonly found in the anterior maxillae; how-

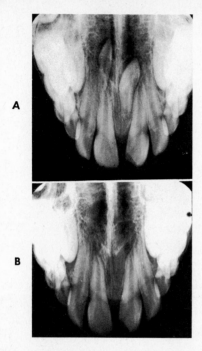

Fig. 29-9. A, Two supernumerary teeth were discovered in a 9-year-old patient when radiographs were taken of the fractured incisor. **B,** The 5-month postoperative radiograph demonstrates good healing in the area.

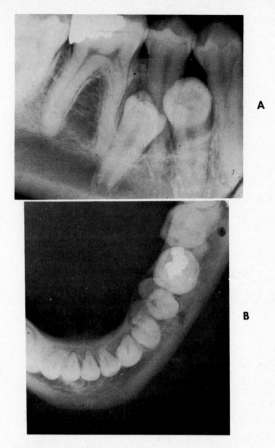

Fig. 29-10. A, Supernumerary premolars. **B,** An occlusal radiograph is useful in localizing the supernumerary teeth.

ever, they are occasionally seen elsewhere, such as in the lower premolar regions (Fig. 29-10) or even in the molar regions.

Anterior maxillary supernumerary teeth in a young patient are of great concern to a dentist because of the problems they can create. These teeth, which may be evident radiographically at any age from the newborn period to adulthood, rarely erupt into the mouth and are usually located palatally to the primary roots and in a position to prevent the proper eruption of the permanent central or lateral incisors. Unless the child is having regular dental examinations with periodic radiographs, the most common evidence of their presence is the retention of one or more maxillary primary anterior teeth or failure of eruption of one or more permanent teeth.

Each case involving a supernumerary tooth must

be diagnosed and evaluated according to its own peculiarities, but in general the earlier such teeth are removed the better. Occasionally, surgical access to the area is difficult, and undue hazards to the permanent teeth are present. In these instances the dentist can observe the progress of the dentition with the aid of radiographs and can hope that growth and development will provide better surgical conditions.

Before attempting surgical removal, the dentist must accurately locate the positions of the unwanted teeth in relation to the root ends of the primary teeth and erupted permanent teeth, the unerupted permanent teeth, the floor of the nose, the maxillary sinus, and other structures. It must also be noted that supernumerary teeth are not always small and malformed; indeed, it may be difficult to determine which teeth should be sacrificed and which should be saved. The interpretation of periapical, occlusal, cross-sectional, panoramic, and cephalometric radiographs can usually provide the answer, but occasionally the dentist must surgically expose the crowns and then decide which tooth or teeth to sacrifice. Radiographic techniques that are useful in locating teeth before surgical removal are described in detail in Chapter 6.

Palatally positioned supernumerary teeth are commonly approached by way of an anterior palatal flap. The incision is made at the lingual necks of the anterior teeth and is carried posteriorly far enough to gain adequate exposure of the palate. Judicious bone removal is done with well-cooled round carbide burs. Anatomic perspective must be kept in mind at all times. When the crowns are uncovered, the dentist should positively identify each tooth by position and form before removal. Small supernumeraries can usually be elevated intact, whereas large teeth require sectioning to minimize bone destruction. Gentle but complete curettage is necessary to remove all follicular and noncalcified tissues. Closures are made by suturing around the teeth.

Management of unerupted teeth by means other than extraction

Not all teeth that are delayed in eruption into occlusion need to be removed. Procedures may be taken to encourage or force their eruption into the arch. This is especially true of impacted maxillary canines, although the same principles can be applied to any teeth whose eruption is thought to be seriously delayed.

The important factors in the surgical encouragement of the eruption of teeth are (1) early diagnosis and treatment, (2) provision of adequate space for passage through the bone and soft tissue, (3) maintenance of adequate space for the tooth's proper placement in the arch, and (4) watchful patience.

In general, as soon as it is discovered that a tooth is delayed in its eruption, the crown should be surgically exposed, and an eruption path through bone and soft tissue should be created and maintained until eruptive activity is observed.

The treatment of a maxillary canine, which is one of the most common teeth to be delayed in its eruption, involves removal of the retained primary canine and the establishment of a pathway to the crown area. For a labially impacted canine, little difficulty is encountered in opening a window overlying the crown and in maintaining exposure during the eruptive process. Usually, however, unerupted canines lie high in the palate and frequently have moved anteriorly so that the lateral incisors provide a hazard during surgical exposure.

The surgical approach is much the same as that made in preparation for removal of a tooth. An incision is made around the lingual margins of the anterior teeth in each direction for a sufficient distance to gain adequate exposure. A well-cooled round carbide bur is used to remove the bone overlying the crown, with care being taken to avoid damage to the enamel. When possible, the entire periphery of the crown should be exposed and 1 mm of bone surrounding it removed. When the crown lies close to the roots of the incisor teeth, this amount of exposure may not be possible. When the angulation of the tooth is such that a path of eruption can be established in the alveolar bone, this should be accomplished with the aid of a rongeur and burs. A window is then created in the mucoperiosteal flap overlying the exposed crown, and the flap is returned to its proper position and retained there by sutures around the anterior teeth.

Some means of preventing closure of the intended eruptive path is then established. The area may be packed with surgical cement, iodoform gauze, cotton plugs coated with zinc oxide–eugenol, or similar materials. The important factor is the placement of a hygienic, nonirritating material that can be removed without difficulty. If a deep surgical defect is present, the pack will maintain itself; if a shallow cavity is present, the packing may require temporary suturing. When the crown lies just under the mucous membrane, no packing is necessary.

Such a pathway in the tissue should then be maintained for as long as is practical. Close observation will reveal how well the packing is maintaining itself and whether a fresh, clean replacement is needed.

Although it is desirable to direct the tooth toward the proper position in the arch, from a surgical viewpoint the important factor is to gain enough exposure and eruption in any direction so that an orthodontic appliance can be used to assist in guiding the tooth into its proper place.

Teeth that are delayed in their eruption or that are impacted show a wide variety of responses to the uncovering. Some teeth respond almost immediately and erupt into the mouth in a few weeks; others may take several months and may even require a second surgical exposure if they become covered again with tissue or appear to stop in their eruptive course. Occasionally teeth do not respond to the surgical procedure. If no progress is noted after a reasonable period of observation, such as 6 months, an appliance may be attached to the tooth and slight traction may be applied. When enough access to the crown is available, a small-gauge wire loop may be placed around the crown, twisted snugly, and brought into the mouth for attachment to a traction device. This procedure is not always possible; in such an event a small bur hole can be made in the crown and the wire can be placed in the hole and held with amalgam or cement. (Other techniques, making use of devices cemented to the surface of the crown or small jeweler's chains placed around the crown, have been advocated, but these are less successful.)

These procedures for bringing unerupted teeth into the mouth are usually highly successful; however, timing is of the utmost importance. One must not become impatient and induce too rapid eruption, or the tooth may become pulpless. As long as progress is being noted, it is best to practice watchful waiting.

Infections

The occurrence of infections in and about the oral tissues is well known to all dentists. A child is susceptible to the same organisms as an adult, the inflammatory responses are the same, and the same general principles of infection control and treatment apply.

Acutely infected tissues are usually swollen and tender or painful, and oral infections may be accompanied by trismus and general malaise. The oral examination therefore must be carried out with gentle finesse lest the child become fearful of the inevitable subsequent examinations.

In the diagnosis of inflammatory lesions of the mouth, especially in children, the dentist must keep in mind that the oral tissues may reflect a systemic pathologic condition that has not yet been manifested otherwise. It behooves a diagnostician, then, not to jump to the conclusion that a lesion is of dental origin until complete oral and radiographic examinations have been performed.

Acute dental infections. An acute apical infection resulting from a nonvital or degenerative pulp may be confined to the alveolar process, may break through the cortical barrier and involve the periosteum, or may invade the surrounding soft tissue and result in cellulitis. One of three results will become evident—resolution, localization, or overwhelming infection.

An immediate decision often must be made as to whether the offending tooth is to be extracted or treated endodontically. If the tooth must be sacrificed, appropriate antibiotic therapy is instituted. Penicillin is the drug of choice, but erythromycin or tetracycline may be administered, with the child dosage adjusted according to age, size, and severity of infection, and in accordance with the manufacturer's recommendation. Older children can take oral tablets or liquid preparations; young children may require intramuscular administration. A child with acute cellulitis may need a sedative in addition to antibiotics and pain medication. Fever, malaise, and oral pain may result in low fluid intake and a generalized acute illness; thus close observation is indicated (Fig. 29-11).

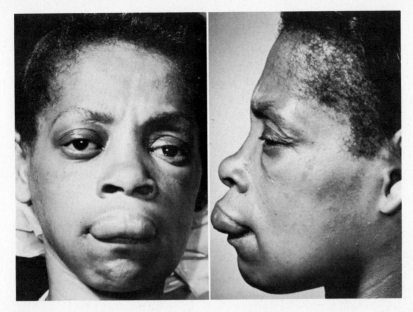

Fig. 29-11. Acute cellulitis of the upper lip resulting from a maxillary anterior dental infection.

One need not wait until the acute exacerbation has completely subsided before extraction can be done, as was formerly taught. However, a traumatic extraction or one performed at the time when the infection is most virulent may have severe local and systemic consequences. The timing of an extraction during an acute inflammatory process is based on exacting clinical judgment; when there is doubt, the surgery should be delayed until the process is known to be under control.

If pus seems to be localizing, heat should then be applied intraorally, extraorally, or in both ways to hasten localization so that incision and drainage may be performed (Fig. 29-12). After surgery, the administration of antibiotics should be continued until the signs and symptoms of infection disappear.

Chronic dental infections. Chronic infections are usually manifested by apical pathology (as shown by radiographic examination) or by a sinus tract that is draining through the alveolar process into the mouth. Antibiotic therapy is not usually necessary in the treatment of this phase, since heal-

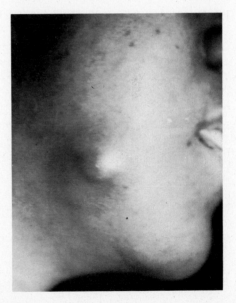

Fig. 29-12. Localized pointed infection ready for incision and drainage.

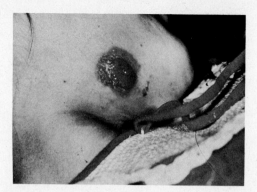

Fig. 29-13. Facial pyogenic granuloma resulting from chronic extraoral drainage owing to multiple incision and drainage procedures without removal of the offending first permanent molar.

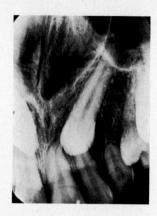

Fig. 29-14. Early evidence of a dentigerous cyst involving the maxillary canine.

ing is rapid after the removal of the source of infection. Gentle curettage should be accomplished after extraction, but in the case of a primary tooth, injury to the underlying tooth bud must be avoided.

Occasionally, the path of drainage of a chronic infection will find its way to the cutaneous surface of the face, especially the anterior portion of the mandible. When such a draining area results from an infected tooth, antibiotic therapy and extraoral surgical closures will fail completely until the source of the infection has been removed. It is not uncommon for such a drainage tract to undergo multiple surgical closures, with the area breaking down again within a few days or weeks of each procedure (Fig. 29-13).

Cysts of the jaws

Dentigerous cyst. Any of the odontogenic cysts may occur in children, but the dentigerous cyst is the most common. Such cysts may be associated either with unerupted permanent teeth or with supernumerary teeth (Fig. 29-14). Fissural cysts are rarely found in children, but traumatic or hemorrhagic cysts are common, especially in active young boys (Fig. 29-15). Although a traumatic cyst is usually unilateral and solitary, a lesion can become bilateral. Fig. 29-16 illustrates such a sit-

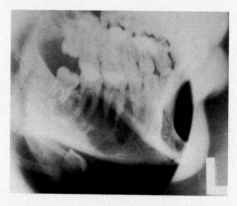

Fig. 29-15. Traumatic cyst of the mandible of a 15-year-old boy with a history of trauma 5 years previously. The cavity contained neither fluid nor tissue.

uation. Initially, two small lesions had developed in the regions of the right and left mandibular lateral incisors. Even though the patient was receiving regular dental care and orthodontic treatment, for 3 years these radiolucent areas were merely "watched." During this time the two lesions coalesced to form a single large lesion, which became a potential hazard to all six mandibular anterior teeth.

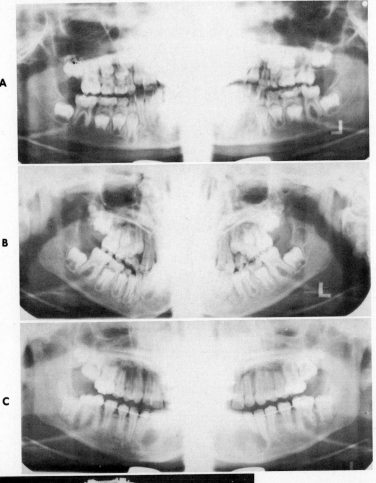

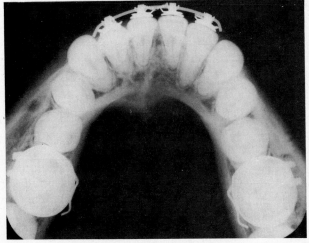

Fig. 29-16. A, Panoramic radiograph of a patient 8 years of age reveals the suggestion of developing bilateral lesions in the mandibular lateral incisor regions. **B,** A subsequent radiograph shows progression to definite lesions bilaterally. **C,** Panoramic radiograph made just before surgical intervention, when the patient was 11 years old, shows coalition of the lesions with displacement of the four incisor teeth and possible involvement of the left canine. **D,** Radiograph taken 13 months postoperatively shows healing of the lesion, intact cortical bone, and successful realignment of the incisors.

Radiolucent areas of the jaws should be given further diagnostic studies. The lesion should be aspirated to determine whether the area is filled with clear cystic fluid or is infected. Occasionally, bloody fluid is aspirated or no fluid is found, which may indicate a traumatic cyst. If tissue is present, a biopsy may be advisable before the extent of surgery required is determined.

The primary objective in the treatment of jaw cysts in children is the same as in adults: complete enucleation of the cyst wall. For dentigerous cysts, excision of the unerupted tooth as well ensures removal of all the potentially harmful epithelium. However, in developing dentitions a special effort should be made to save any involved permanent teeth that are needed to help preserve the integrity of the dental arch. In the case of a dentigerous cyst such as the one shown in Fig. 29-14, surgical enucleation of the cyst wall and exposure of the crown should be coordinated with orthodontic treatment to properly align the involved permanent canine in the arch. It is known that dentigerous cysts are lined with squamous epithelium, which has the potential to undergo neoplastic transformation. Therefore postoperative observation should continue until the tooth is fully erupted and complete healing can be demonstrated. In some cases the cystic lesion may already be so expansive at the time of discovery, especially around unerupted third molars, that the surgeon has no choice but to sacrifice the tooth. When large cyst cavities involve the roots of adjacent teeth, enucleation may be possible without devitalizing these teeth; otherwise, root canal therapy can maintain the teeth.

Because of the belief that a large percentage of ameloblastomas begin within odontogenic cyst walls (Fig. 29-17), I do not recommend a Partsch procedure for large cysts, although many authorities recommend this course of treatment.

When a suspected cyst cavity is surgically explored and no lining or soft tissue contents are found, the diagnosis of traumatic cyst is certain and the operation should be discontinued lest sound teeth be unnecessarily devitalized.

Eruption hematoma or eruption cyst. A cyst-like lesion peculiar to the eruption trauma of either

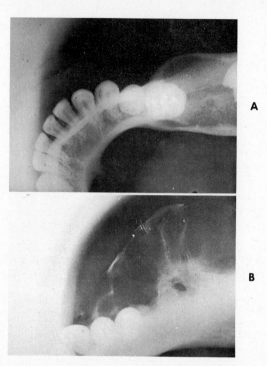

Fig. 29-17. A, Dentigerous cyst of the mandible of a 13-year-old girl. **B,** Ameloblastoma developed in the area 5 years later.

primary or permanent teeth may develop on the alveolar ridge and may be of considerable concern to a parent. Such a lesion occurs as the result of hemorrhage into the follicle of an erupted tooth that has projected through the alveolar bone but has not yet perforated the mucous membrane.

These lesions are frequently seen in erupting molar areas of young children; they resolve spontaneously when the involved teeth finally penetrate the gingival tissues. Occasionally a patient with an eruption cyst may benefit from treatment to reduce significant tissue enlargement that hampers function and causes prolonged soreness. When a lesion develops in the anterior segment, it may also be unsightly and especially disconcerting to the patient or the parents (Fig. 29-18). When indicated, treatment is simply surgical excision of the overlying mucous membrane to drain the fluid and expose the crown.

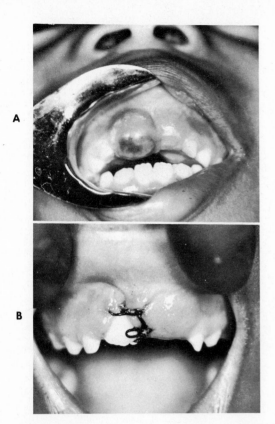

Fig. 29-18. A, "Eruption cyst" over the maxillary incisor area. **B,** Postoperative photograph showing the relationship of the tooth to the lesion.

Neoplasms

Oral pathology is discussed in Chapter 28, where one is made aware that children are susceptible to a wide variety of lesions—inflammatory and neoplastic, odontogenic and nonodontogenic, benign and malignant. A dentist must be aware of the differences between the various oral lesions and must be prepared to take the necessary steps to arrive at a diagnosis.

Peripheral lesions usually afford good access for biopsy. Although there are occasional indications for cytologic smears, most lesions require an adequate biopsy to establish a diagnosis.

Biopsy procedure. Small lesions (a few millimeters in diameter) require *excisional biopsies*. Elliptic incisions are made around the lesion, af-

fording a safe margin of normal tissue. The depth of the incision is determined by the clinical appearance and the feel of the lesion, but the incision should at least enter the subcutaneous layer. Using curved mosquito hemostats, the examiner should perform blunt dissection under the base of the lesion. This affords less chance of cutting through the base and minimizes deep hemorrhaging.

Large lesions require *incisional biopsies* from the area or areas that are most representative of the tumor. The incision should be deep enough to include the basal layer if possible, and if practical it should include the transition cells between normal and abnormal tissues. A pathologist needs not only representative tissue but enough tissue so that the tissue block can be properly processed and examined.

Central lesions that are radiolucent may be aspirated for diagnostic purposes. A needle of at least 18 gauge on at least a 5-ml aspirating syringe is inserted in the lesion from the site of best access. If a heavy cortical layer of bone overlies the lesion, a mucoperiosteal flap is reflected and access for the needle is made with a small round carbide bur. If the fluid does not establish the diagnosis, or if no fluid is found, a window is made overlying the lesion, and tissue is enucleated for biopsy purposes.

Abnormal frenum

The maxillary labial frenum may be a troublesome piece of anatomy, and there is diversity of thought concerning which types need excision and at what age it should be done. The diagnosis and surgical treatment of an abnormal frenum are discussed in Chapter 4.

Wounds and injuries

Active children are susceptible to a variety of injuries, and the soft and hard tissues of the mouth are frequent recipients of trauma. Displaced teeth require a careful diagnosis to determine if a lesion is present or if the displacement is due to trauma or to other factors (Fig. 29-19).

Although the management of injuries of the teeth and supporting tissues is discussed in Chapter 17, it

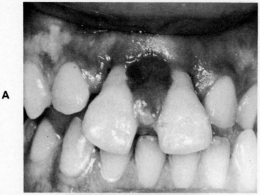

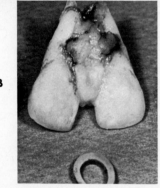

Fig. 29-19. A, Inflammatory lesion and displaced central incisors. There was no evidence of alveolar bone support. **B,** When the teeth were removed from the soft tissue attachment, a rubber band was found around the root apices that had been used in an attempt to correct a diastema between the central incisors.

is important to emphasize the need for long-term follow-up examinations of any tooth-bearing site that has received trauma. Developing tooth buds may react in many unfavorable ways following their disturbance. Fig. 29-6 illustrates malformation of a permanent incisor as a result of traumatic displacement of the overlying primary incisor.

It is not within the scope of this chapter to relate details of the treatment of oral lacerations and fractured jaws; however, discussion of some basic principles follows.

Fractures of the mandible and maxilla. Fractures of the maxilla are rare in children; when they do occur, they are usually the result of severe trauma, and the surgeon is faced with a complex of bony injuries and soft tissue damage.

Fractures of the mandible occur with enough frequency that a pedodontist or a general practitioner is likely to be called on for diagnosis or treatment.

A complete radiographic survey is indicated in all suspected fractures; this should include at least right and left lateral oblique radiographs and posterior-anterior views (Fig. 29-20). The use of panoramic radiographs, which has become popular in many dental offices in the past few years, may be a good substitute for the right and left lateral oblique projections. It is still necessary, however, to view fractures in a sagittal plane with a second radiograph. Bilateral fractures occur with such frequency that all fractures should be considered bilateral until proved otherwise. A fractured condylar neck may accompany a body or ramus fracture, and bilateral condylar neck fractures often result from a blow at the symphysis region. These injuries may go undiagnosed without proper radiographic views.

Early treatment is important, since tissues of children heal rapidly and a malunion can begin in a week's time.

Primary teeth do not lend themselves to a wiring procedure in stabilization as well as do permanent teeth. A mixed dentition may present only a few teeth for attachment of fixation wires. Permanent teeth in children may easily be moved or even extracted as a result of intermaxillary traction if an appliance is not properly designed and placed. Thus the treatment of mandibular fractures may present problems of immobilization. Occasionally splints must be constructed.

Open reductions on displaced angle fractures or occasionally on body fractures may be indicated. In these cases extreme caution must be exercised to avoid damage to tooth buds.

Any fracture that involves a developing tooth bud requires long-term follow-up care, since cystic degeneration, malformation of the tooth, or failure of the tooth to erupt can occur.

Soft tissue injury. Lacerations of the lips, the

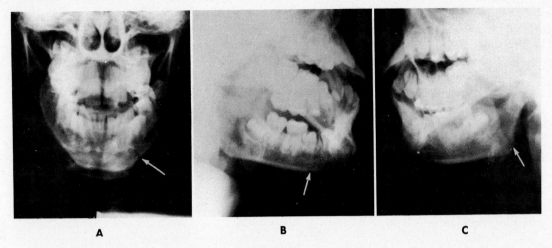

A   **B**   **C**

Fig. 29-20. Radiographs demonstrating mandibular fractures. These three views are essential for diagnosis and treatment of the fractures. **A,** A posterior-anterior radiograph showing bilateral fractures of the mandible. **B** and **C,** Right and left oblique radiographs of the mandible showing the fractures.

buccal mucosa, tongue, or the floor of the mouth require close examination. The view that intraoral lacerations should not be closed because of the danger of infection has long been abandoned. As a general rule, if a laceration is deep enough that healing must be by second intention, closure of the wound is indicated.

Areas of laceration should be debrided and cleansed of foreign material, the edges freshened if needed, and closures made using small (3-0 or 4-0) silk sutures. Other nonabsorbable suture materials (for example, nylon) are difficult to keep tied in the mouth, and their cut ends are more irritating to oral tissues; therefore they are less desirable than silk. In young or uncooperative children absorbable sutures should be employed to simplify the postoperative visit. Many new types of material are available, and choosing one is primarily a matter of personal preference, the handling properties desired, and cost. However, the twisted-strand collagen materials (such as gut and chromic gut) are also difficult to keep tied in mobile oral tissues or other areas where children can reach the sutures with their fingers. Therefore the surgeon is advised to use synthetic absorbable materials, such as poly-

glycolic acid. This suture material is braided to resist coming untied, and its strength permits a smaller diameter to be used.

Systemic conditions: influence on surgical procedures

A complete medical history should be obtained from the parent or guardian before surgical procedures are performed. There are a few medical conditions that present special problems, but these are not necessarily contraindications to minor surgery. Children are exposed to a myriad of infectious diseases that, although usually not serious, do produce periods of high fever, malaise, dehydration, and discomfort. These infections include measles, mumps, chickenpox, influenza, and whooping cough. If a child is known to have been exposed to one of these diseases, or if at the time of a dental appointment any of the early signs or symptoms of such a condition are present, dental treatment should be delayed unless a true emergency exists. Then it is wise to consult the child's pediatrician or family physician.

Rheumatic fever and congenital heart deformities. A patient who has any type of congenital heart deformity or a history of rheumatic fever requires special attention before and after surgical or endodontic treatment.

When a threat of bacterial endocarditis exists, the recommendations of the American Heart Association as to the protective needs of the patient should be followed. Penicillin remains the drug of choice for most patients. For those suspected to be allergic to penicillin, erythromycin is the drug of choice. However, since the philosophy of prophylaxis for bacterial endocarditis is constantly changing and new antibiotics continue to be developed, specific recommendations may be revised frequently. Current information is available from either the American Heart Association, 7320 Greenville Avenue, Dallas, Texas 75231, or the Council on Dental Therapeutics, American Dental Association, 211 East Chicago Avenue, Chicago, Illinois 60611. The recommendations in effect at the time of this writing are included in Chapter 23.

Glomerulonephritis. Elimination of oral infection is important for children with acute or chronic glomerulonephritis. If extraction or endodontic therapy is necessary, it should be performed during a period of kidney disease quiescence with antibiotic prophylaxis and with the consultation of the attending physician.

Hemophilia. Surgical procedures, when necessary for a young hemophiliac patient, may present a grave situation. Such procedures should always be performed in a hospital, under the direction of well-qualified oral surgeons and hematologists.

Much progress has been made in the diagnosis and treatment of the various types and degrees of hemophilia, but a child patient who is faced with a dental extraction remains in a serious situation. Proper dental care to prevent the need for an extraction is the best treatment.

Leukemias. The oral manifestations of leukemia in children may often be the first indication of the disease as well as the chief complaint of the patient. The role of the dentist in maintaining oral hygiene and preventing oral infection may be of primary importance in maintaining the patient's comfort and proper nutritional needs. Proper use of mouthwash, customized toothbrushing technique, oral prophylaxis, and effective caries control will do much to promote the child's comfort and to prevent infection.

Hospital procedures

Most dental procedures are best performed in a dental office with the aid of a local anesthetic. There are occasions, however, when hospitalization is necessary. Major surgical procedures, systemic complications, and operations requiring lengthy general anesthesia are examples of indications for hospitalization.

Because dentists are generally not hospital oriented, they should not attempt to admit, treat, and discharge patients without special training. Hospital rules and regulations, operating room decorum, and record keeping are essential, and they are best learned during a hospital rotating internship or a hospital pedodontic or oral and maxillofacial surgery training program.

The Joint Commission on Hospital Accreditation requires that a physical examination and a medical history be completed for any patient who is admitted to a hospital. The examination must be performed by a physician, except in those instances in which an oral and maxillofacial surgeon is deemed qualified to perform it for his or her own patient. Thus the attending dentist must work in close cooperation with the family physician, internist, or other medical specialist. However, if the primary purpose of hospital admission is dental care, the dentist must be knowledgeable enough in patient care and hospital conduct and procedure to assume the full responsibility for the patient. This includes the coordination and scheduling of admission and operating times, laboratory requests and evaluations, medications and other orders, appropriate consultation requests, complete physical examination, examination of the oral cavity and adjacent structures, history, daily progress notes, operative dictations, and discharge procedures.

Each hospital has its own code of conduct. Although the codes of different hospitals are similar, they vary to some extent; the dentist must be familiar with the code in each hospital where work is to be done.

With the exception of extraoral surgery, most dental procedures cannot be performed under aseptic conditions. However, since proper rules of sterility must be maintained in the operating room under all conditions, the dentist must be familiar with and able to practice the most strict operating room techniques.

The dentist must be aware of fire and explosion hazards in the operating room, especially with the use of some dental equipment. All equipment and personnel should be properly grounded. When electrical equipment is to be used that has not been specifically designed for operating room use, its hazards should be discussed with the anesthetist as well as with the chief operating room nurse, so that the proper precautions can be taken.

Further discussion of the preparation of pedodontic patients for treatment under general anesthesia and operating room protocol appears in Chapter 11.

REFERENCES

American Heart Association: Committee report on prevention of bacterial endocarditis, Circulation **65A:**139, 1977.

Hooley, J.R.: Hospital dentistry, Philadelphia, 1970, Lea & Febiger.

Kruger, G.O., editor: Textbook of oral and maxillofacial surgery, ed. 5, St. Louis, 1979, The C.V. Mosby Co.

Report of Councils and Bureaus: Prevention of bacterial endocarditis: a committee report of the American Heart Association, J.A.D.A. **95:**600-603, 1977.

Shafer, W.G., Hine, M.K., and Levy, B.M.: A textbook of oral pathology, ed. 3, Philadelphia, 1974, W.B. Saunders Co., pp. 236-284.

30 Practice management and health education

JAMES R. ROCHE

Philosophy of providing dental care for children

Each decision by a dentist that has a bearing on office environment, policy, or procedure or the assignment of staff responsibility should be directed toward the goal of rendering effective and pleasant service for children. All aspects of office routine should be continuously reevaluated to ensure that they contribute to that goal. If they do not, they should be modified or eliminated. Also, since the effective delivery of pedodontic services requires substantial overhead expense, an appropriate level of financial return must be maintained if proper standards of care are to be observed.

A critical responsibility of a practitioner of child dental care is to guard against delivery of treatment that is of an unacceptable quality or that is unnecessary. Proper standards of restorative care must be maintained, such as preventing overhang of restorative material, providing proper proximal contours, and ensuring that no exposed cavosurface margins of a preparation exist. Other responsibilities include maintaining a workable preventive dentistry program that is tailored to the needs of individual parents and children, keeping adequate clinical and radiographic records, and when indicated, forming diagnostic models of acceptable quality. Since interceptive orthodontic procedures are an integral part of child dental care, maintaining adequate records is vitally important. Likewise, formulating clearly defined treatment plans and performing treatment with appropriate justifi-

cation are necessary in guarding against the provision of unnecessary care. A practitioner's analyses of the results of treatment can also contribute significantly to the consistent rendering by the office staff of treatment that is necessary and of an acceptable quality.

A thorough oral examination, an accurate diagnosis, and effective treatment supported by preventive measures are essential in the treatment of a child patient. Emotional guidance is provided as needed, and dental services are conducted in the most efficient and pleasant manner commensurate with the child's behavior and the parents' attitudes. The dentist should periodically assess procedures used by the office staff in behavioral guidance for child dental care and identify wasted time and motion.

The dentist must keep abreast of new methods for refining diagnoses, new information about the biologic responses of tissues, and improvements in the mechanical techniques of treatment. Continuing education and study of the literature will result in frequent alteration of treatment procedures and office management techniques. So that the dentist can concentrate on providing care for children, practice management principles must be established clearly and followed by the office staff; otherwise, the dentist's diagnostic and treatment capabilities will be diminished by interrupting problems. The pedodontic service must guide both the child and the parents through the dental procedures and office routine. Parents will have questions pertaining to their child's dental needs, financial arrangements, and scheduling of the next visit. The child will require guidance to accept needed dental treatment and be motivated to perform proper home preventive measures.

Since the largest office expense in child dental care results from providing auxiliary personnel, the administrative principle of continuously evaluating the efficiency of the assisting staff's performance is indispensable to a successful practice. The dentist's philosophy concerning practice management, the value of good dental health for children, and the parents' important role in health education must be clearly understood by the entire staff.

Compliance as a key to practice management and health education

In order for a dentist's philosophy of care for children to be adequately implemented, each staff member must follow office policies and procedures as set forth in the office manual. First, staff members must be thoroughly familiar with all policies or procedures pertinent to their own responsibilities, in addition to policies or procedures of general application throughout the office. Second, they must be able to apply their skill and judgment to conform to the guidelines established in the manual. To encourage compliance, the dentist should teach the staff members their individual responsibilities are important. When direct or indirect supervision of a staff member's performance identifies deviations from the established guidelines, the dentist may be able to regain the compliance of the staff member by clarifying specific duties, explaining the reason for the policy or procedure, and showing a sincere interest in the staff member's contribution to the practice. Improved performance is the likely result of the practitioner's expression of genuine interest in an individual's special talent and potential.

Likewise, a dentist is desirous that the parent accept the treatment proposed for the child, see that the child keeps the appointment, and pay the fee. In addition, it is reasonable for the practitioner to expect that the parent will guide the child's oral hygiene practices, ensure that the child receives proper nutrition (particularly as it relates to dental health), and return the child for periodic recall procedures. This kind of cooperation by parents can be enhanced by the following measures:

1. Identifying the desired action by the parent
2. Helping parents to understand that they are responsible for complying with the recommendations of the office staff
3. Explaining the consequences of noncompliance for their child
4. Communicating sincere interest in the parent and the child

The compliance of a young child or a teenager with preventive oral health procedures may be successfully promoted if members of the family show support for recommendations by the dentist and staff members concerning personal oral hygiene and nutrition.

Initial communication with parents

At the time the parent makes the initial contact by telephone, the receptionist should project the dental office staff's true interest in the child patient. One way to accomplish this is by offering correct information in a friendly manner in response to inquiries. The receptionist should be aware of the value of this initial conversation with the parent, since the receptionist represents the dentist and the other staff members.

A friendly telephone voice conveys a cordial feeling toward the parent. The receptionist should speak clearly, using a natural and well-modulated tone, and should converse in an efficient but unhurried manner. Indecision, abruptness, giddiness, or confused answers may send the parent elsewhere. A receptionist who is scheduling an appointment or recording a payment when a parent telephones should answer the telephone promptly but request the caller to hold the call. On returning to the telephone, the receptionist should thank the caller courteously for waiting.

The telephone conversation between the receptionist and the parent may provide important information regarding the level of dental health understanding of the parents. The parents' chief concerns, and possibly their anxieties about dental care, often become evident during the initial conversation. The name and telephone numbers of the new patient, in addition to the patient's address and age and the name of the person recommending the dentist, can be recorded in a small alphabetical loose-leaf notebook. In addition to the basic information, significant parental requests or comments should be recorded. This convenient file provides a handy reference for recording information on the chart at the time of a child's first visit to the office.

Management of time

Appointment procedures. To guide parents in choosing the most desirable hour for their child's appointment, the receptionist must be prepared with information to justify the scheduling. The receptionist's duty of controlling the appointment schedule is essential in efficient practice management for child patients. Offering an alternative appointment shows consideration for the parents' other commitments and guides them into accepting an appointment favorable to the scheduling policy.

Since it is the parent who authorizes treatment and supervises the child's home care, two persons are to be considered at each appointment: the parent and the child.

Office policies and educational communications for parents should be described in detail in a procedure manual and should be delegated to the appropriate auxiliary staff member. The delegation of responsibilities will require a significant investment of the dentist's time in a detailed office training program. This initial investment, however, will result in the rewarding benefit of additional health service for the patient and the parent. Policies relating to scheduling, parent guidance, payment arrangements, health educational methods and materials, insurance claim applications, and printed office forms should be evaluated semiannually.

Scheduling only one appointment at a time for each child increases the control over the appoint-

ment book. Single appointments for children provide the flexibility of altering treatment plan sequences if any of the following situations occur: tardiness, illness or accident, erratic behavior by a child, unscheduled parental consultation, or an immediate need to change treatment procedures and assign additional appointment periods. Scheduling appointments on a one-at-a-time basis also reduces the tendency of parents to cancel for trivial reasons if they have the security of multiple appointments. In addition, such a scheduling plan more evenly distributes patients during popular appointment hours.

Today it is not uncommon for both parents of a child patient to be employed. This situation presents a special problem because it is desirable that at least one parent accompany a child to the office. The regular office hours may need to be altered to retain in the practice child patients whose parents are both employed. To accommodate working parents, patients may have to be scheduled for appointments during very early morning hours on certain days and late afternoon hours on others.

Another consideration in scheduling appointments is the day or afternoon during the workweek that the practitioner designates for activities other than patient care. It has been theorized that the first several hours of the first working day of the week are characterized by much less efficient performance by all office staff members than are later hours of the day. It is therefore recommended that the day or half-day designated to be free of patient care occur at the beginning or end of the workweek, instead of breaking the week into two portions of patient care. It is desirable that patient appointments be concentrated in successive days, instead of diminishing work efficiency with a day off.

Failed or canceled appointments. Missed or canceled appointments that cannot be reassigned to other patients result in significant reductions in patient service and office income. Maintaining a full appointment schedule and a currently accurate call list is a vital responsibility of the receptionist.

Reminding the parent by telephone the day before a child's scheduled appointment and maintaining a call list to fill in canceled appointments are essential for the economic use of time. Phone calls between 7:30 AM and 9:00 AM will usually reach parents before they leave for work or become involved in other activities. In addition, obtaining business phone numbers from employed parents can be helpful in confirming a child's appointment. This early morning call by the receptionist ensures that the child will be in the office the next day at the appropriate hour and reinforces the expected prompt participation by the parent.

In addition to the loss in treatment productivity, failed or canceled appointments lead to other serious problems, such as the child suffering pain, loss of arch length, or the need for more extensive treatment. Parents who do not schedule another appointment for their child present an important concern to the dentist and the business office. This "lost patient" phenomenon may occur in the following ways. Common situations in which parents, through neglect or deliberate choice, do not schedule additional appointments for their children include the following: (1) during the current appointment in which the child is receiving treatment, (2) during the conversation in which they cancel their child's appointment, and (3) during the period following a failed appointment. Although the parent has the responsibility and the freedom of choice to schedule the next appointment for a child, the dentist must share in this responsibility to ensure that the child will continue to receive treatment appropriate to need.

What approach should be taken in dealing with this problem of the "lost patient," whose chart may be filed away for weeks or months, resulting in the delay of needed treatment and the possibility that payments due on the open account will be overlooked?

If a parent does not schedule another appointment for a child during the current appointment, the receptionist should immediately attach a metal tab of a designated color to the top edge of the patient's ledger card. The same colored tab, indi-cating "patient without appointment," should be applied to the ledger cards of other patients whose parents have canceled or failed to keep appointments and who have not scheduled other visits. The next step in dealing with failed appointments or appointments that are canceled on the day of the appointment is for the receptionist to immediately notify the chairside assistant. The assistant promptly notifies the dentist, and this may make additional treatment time available for the child currently receiving care. The assistant also records failed appointments and late cancellations on the child's chart. This important information may identify a habit profile of certain parents, which may lead the dentist to analyze the case and perhaps refer a child to a colleague in the hope that different office personalities or a dental office at a more convenient location for the parent might improve the parent's cooperation in regard to the child's dental appointments.

Patients without appointments provide a means of filling canceled appointments and therefore permit the treatment of some children to be continued at an earlier time. If a parent does not accept an appointment offered on this basis or is unwilling to schedule another appointment, the receptionist should ask the parent directly whether he or she plans to have the child continue as a patient in the office. If the response is negative, the case should be audited by the dentist, the account adjusted, the parent immediately notified of any balance due, and the chart placed in the inactive file.

The dentist must realize that even the most conscientious receptionist may occasionally fail to attach the appropriate metal tab to a ledger card. Consequently, the receptionist's month-end duties should include evaluating the last entry on each patient's ledger card to determine if a date for the next appointment has been recorded or if the date of appointment has passed (see Fig. 30-7). Any untabbed ledger cards without future appointments should then be tabbed, and they will be included in the telephone calls to parents who are without appointments for their children.

Metal tabs of a designated color, placed on the

top edges of patients' ledger cards, are also used to identify parents who have a receptive attitude toward bringing their children to the office to make use of canceled appointments. Tabs of different colors denote patients on the call list who are in urgent need of care, parents who can bring their children to the office on a 24-hour notice, or parents who can use canceled appointment time only on particular days of the week. A card on the front of the file holder provides an index to the various colored tabs. The ledger contains telephone numbers and is always kept at the receptionist's desk. The colored tabs are easily evaluated and altered with respect to future appointments and parents' availability.

Lost charts. Locating misfiled charts can require a significant expenditure of time and cause staff frustration. In spite of careful attention, charts are occasionally misfiled. Time can be saved and frustration reduced by a system of filing charts by number rather than by patient name and using a different color or combination of colors on the outer edges of chart folders for every 500 charts. For example, charts numbered 1 through 499 could have a wide, easily visible red mark on the edge of the folder. Therefore a chart filed in the wrong section could easily be identified, or at least the area of hunting for a lost chart would be limited to a group of 500 charts.

Filing by number requires the formation of a master list of sequential numbers with assigned patient names and the additonal step of referring to the master list to locate an individual file. On the other hand, refiling charts should be quicker when it is done by number rather than by the patients' names, and there should be less chance of error.

Daily treatment schedule. The daily treatment schedule of patients should be prepared and duplicated by the receptionist at least 1 week in advance and grouped with the appropriate patient charts. This procedure ensures that the daily treatment schedule and charts are in readiness in the event that the receptionist becomes ill or the receptionist's routine duties are altered unexpectedly by child or parent management problems, emergency

situations, or an unusually large number of incoming telephone calls. It then takes only a few minutes to check a previously prepared treatment schedule and add or delete an appointment. Notation of each canceled appointment on the patient's chart will give the receptionist an indication of which parents habitually cancel. Records demonstrate that parents who have established periodic cancellation patterns are also the ones who complain about extended intervals between appointments.

The daily treatment schedule may be attached with small magnets to the fronts of the metal paper towel containers, at eye level. This practice enables the dentist and the auxiliary personnel to review efficiently, during the hand-washing procedure, the expected sequence of patients and each preindicated treatment.

Maintaining a supply inventory. Significant loss of time and serious interference in the performance of the business office and treatment rooms occur because of depleted supplies. Detailed inventory lists with maintenance levels of all clerical and treatment supplies must be reviewed on a routine schedule by the staff member who has been delegated this responsibility. Each item is placed on an individual inventory card. All information necessary for ordering supplies should appear at the top of this card, including complete name of the item, strength of a medicament if applicable, maintenance level, amount to order, and name, address, and telephone number of the supplier. The front of the card should be divided into three columns so that date of ordering, quantity requested, and price can be clearly recorded. On the reverse side of the card the dated periodic inventory is acknowledged by the assistant's initials. When the supply decreases to the maintenance level, the card is removed from the loose-leaf binder or card file and given to the receptionist for ordering.

The reception area

A dental office serving pedodontic patients should consider the age range of the persons using the facilities. The reception area is designed to be

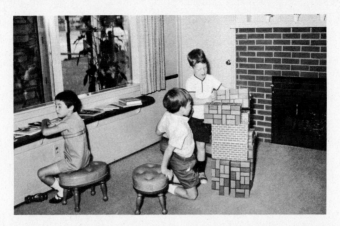

Fig. 30-1. A reception area with objects of interest to children provides a familiar environment.

patient and parent oriented, not dentist centered. An attractive and comfortable environment should be designed for both children and parents. The interests of patients of preschool age through the late teenage period need to be considered, as well as the interests of adults. The decor of the reception area deserves careful planning with these various age groups in mind. Before the dentist turns the decoration of the reception area over completely to an interior decorator, thought should be given to the excessively stimulating, excitable atmosphere that may be unwisely created by the use of many bright colors and designs. Neutral colors, such as beige or light shades of green or blue, for wall decor promote a tranquil feeling and permit the use of attractive color accessories, such as pictures, wallpaper murals, chair cushions, and magazine holders. Various decorating themes can be used. A travel theme could be created by means of maps and pictures of foreign countries. Other interesting themes might be education, history, transportation, science, animals pictured in their natural habitat, seasons, or holidays.

The reception area should be well lighted, preferably with ceiling or wall-attached fixtures. There should be comfortable seating for parents, and the room should be easy to clean.

Objects of interest for all ages of children will provide an inviting atmosphere. Children are attracted to picture or reading books and magazines; publications should be selected for various age levels and should include a wide range of topics. Toys and publications can promote a child's interest, provide a homelike atmosphere, and indirectly convey to the child that the staff is interested in him or her. Selected toys, preferably of large size, including building blocks, have proved to be the main attraction for children of all ages (Fig. 30-1). These articles should be inspected periodically by the receptionist for sharp or displaced parts, thereby eliminating the hazards of a reception room accident.

A child's first visit

Proper management of a child's first visit can cultivate good rapport between the parents and the office staff and can provide support for the consultation period. The relationship between the dentist and the parent is based on confidence, which can best be nurtured initially by a receptionist who has been informed of the potential behavior patterns and concerns of parents and children (Fig. 30-2). The motivation of the parent to proceed with scheduling another appointment with a particular dentist can be compared to a principle in sales promotion. Sales executives stress the importance of

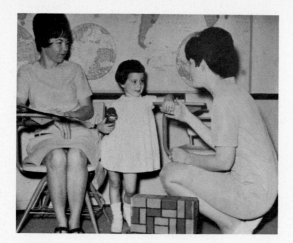

Fig. 30-2. Greeting the child at eye level in a leisurely manner improves communication between the young patient and the receptionist.

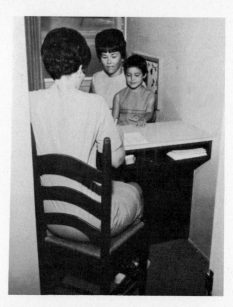

Fig. 30-3. Obtaining information for the dental records provides the receptionist with an opportunity to make friends with the child and to evaluate the patient's initial response to the dental office.

the initial contact between a business representative and a prospective customer; they emphasize that a consumer's first impressions are the most memorable.

Obtaining basic information and a health history. While the parents and the receptionist are seated comfortably in a private area of the business office, the receptionist should complete the basic information and health history forms efficiently and courteously. All staff members should understand that accurately recording a child's medical and dental histories is essential to an analysis of health conditions that relate to oral care. At this time the parent should read and sign the form granting consent for treatment. The receptionist's sincere interest in the child and the parent projects a similar feeling on the part of the entire office staff. Certain potential problems of child management related to fear or defiance can be alleviated greatly by the receptionist's initial dialogue with and effective management of the parent (Fig. 30-3). Identifying the degree of parental fear of dentistry may assist in preparing the dentist and the staff for the child's reactions to dental procedures.

Getting acquainted. When the dentist is available, the parent and the child are escorted into a

private area with a nonclinical atmosphere to meet the dentist and the hygienist. Usually the dentist's consultation room is used for this get-acquainted meeting. After the dentist and the hygienist have greeted the child and the parent, the dentist reviews the health history and probes into any known or suspected disorders or inappropriate health practices. Also, the dentist inquires into the parent's main dental concern or complaint and briefly explains to the parent the usual procedures involved in the examination procedures, such as prophylaxis, examination, and radiographs.

Proper behavior guidance of the child and the parent is the key to examining the oral tissues of a child patient. Adequate management of the child patient at this early point in the office visit promotes the acceptance of dental procedures and helps to prevent or minimize the development of behavior problems.

Occasionally parents do not understand the reasons for their child's need for a thorough and carefully performed examination of the oral tissues. Each staff member should be prepared to explain to parents that the examination procedures are the basis for forming a diagnosis and are important in helping to establish rapport with the child.

Both the dentist and the hygienist, as well as other staff members, should be aware of the signs of contagious skin diseases, such as impetigo and ringworm, that children and adolescents sometimes contract. In addition, as the face, the back of the head, and the neck are inspected for these conditions, the patient's hair should be checked for head lice. Each office staff member should be able to identify signs of potentially transferable conditions in pedodontic patients. (If a patient with such a condition is scheduled for a visit, appropriate safeguards should be used by all personnel treating the child, such as draping the patient and wearing sterile gloves. In general, such a situation occurs only in an emergency. If pedodontic care can be postponed, the patient should be rescheduled for an appointment after receiving treatment from a physician.)

Next, the hygienist accompanies the child to the treatment room. Although this is generally an uneventful transfer, misunderstandings on the part of the child can occur at this point. The child's confidence can be strengthened if the hygienist maintains a positive attitude toward the child's dental needs and the value of good dental health and establishes an atmosphere of naturalness, friendliness, and truthfulness.

The question of separating the child and the parent at this point is frequently raised. On occasion, auxiliary personnel may not clearly understand the reasons for separating the parent and the child. Making this separation has the following advantages:

1. It helps the dentist and staff members devote their entire attention to the child in the treatment room.
2. It permits the dentist to uncover anxieties that the parent may have about dentistry in general or that day's visit in particular.
3. It helps the child devote undivided attention

to the dentist or staff member rendering care.
4. It communicates to the child an environment of normalcy, as a result of the parent's permitting the child alone to accompany the hygienist to the treatment room.

Some dentists may desire to have parents in the treatment room with their children. Under these circumstances it is important that the auxiliary personnel understand the influence a parent may have on a child's cooperative behavior and on the staff member who is rendering the care. Furthermore, each member of the staff should know the office procedure to follow in the event of parental intervention in the guidance of a young patient's behavior during dental care.

While the transfer to the treatment room is taking place, the dentist continues to answer the parent's questions and to alleviate any parental anxieties. Informing the parent of the dental needs of the child is essential to providing any service, and this conversation strengthens the relationship between the dentist, the auxiliaries, and the parent.

As the child is walking from the consultation area to the treatment room, the dentist and the hygienist should observe and record the patient's gait to identify physical abnormalities that might have relevance to the child's general health, as well as to oral health.

Special procedures for children under 2 years of age. Examination of a child's oral structures shortly after 12 months of age and again before the age of 2 years gives the dentist an opportunity to diagnose early dental caries, record normal eruption, and emphasize an effective preventive oral health plan. As with older children, the child's health history is obtained through an interview with the receptionist, and the parent signs a form granting consent for treatment. Shortly thereafter, the dentist greets the child and the parent in the consultation area and investigates aspects of the health history that might be relevant to oral conditions or treatment. Then the parent and the child are transferred to a treatment room. The assistant places the parent in a comfortable reclining position in the

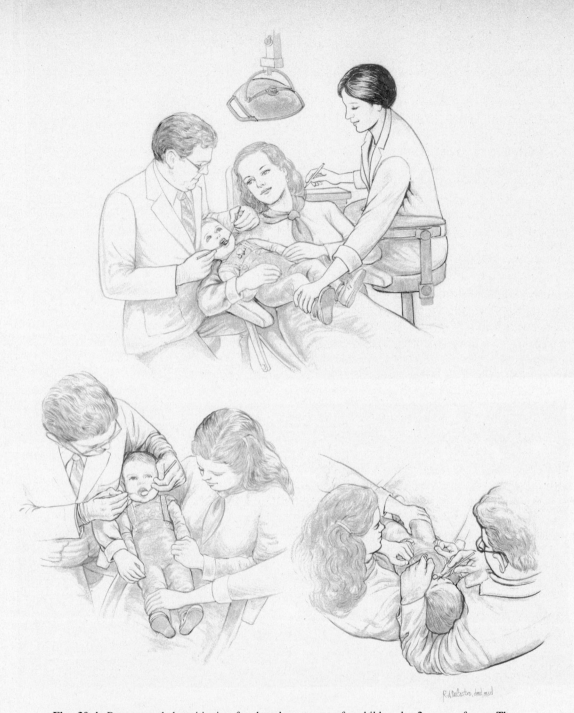

Fig. 30-4. Recommended positioning for dental treatment of a child under 2 years of age. The patient is seated on the mother's lap with the head resting against the mother's shoulder and upper arm. The mother is in a positon to restrain the child by wrapping her arms around the young patient's arms and chest. The chairside assistant is seated higher than the dentist and thus is in position to efficiently and safely hand the required instruments to him. She is also in position to grasp the child's feet or arms if they become free of the parent's restraint. The dentist cradles the child's head in his arm (holding the head firmly between his lower arm and chest) to prevent sudden head movements.

dental chair. The child is seated on the parent's lap, with the child's head resting against the parent's shoulder and upper arm (Fig. 30-4). The parent should be in a position to restrain the child by placing his or her arms around the child's arms and chest. The assistant should be seated higher than the dentist to hand the dentist the required instruments safely and effectively. The assistant should also be ready to grasp the child's feet or possibly arms if the parent loses his or her hold. The child's head should be cradled in the dentist's arm to prevent excessive head movements.

The examination begins with a slow digital inspection of the child's soft tissues, which may result in an amazingly good response. It is recommended that the dentist wear sterile rubber gloves for this procedure. This precaution eliminates the possibility of the dentist's fingernails traumatizing the soft tissue of the very young child. A sharp explorer, an unmarred front-surface mirror, and adequate light are aids for detecting incipient carious lesions. Breaks in the continuity of the enamel surface that feel soft under firm pressure with the explorer may be considered to be carious lesions. The assistant may pass a dry cotton roll to the dentist for use in drying the occlusal fissures of the primary molars or the labial surfaces of the incisors. Usually only light, "on guard" restraint of the patient's feet is required with the assistant's left hand, which permits the assistant to efficiently record the dentist's dictation during the examination of the soft tissues and the dentition.

Usually parents of children under 2 years of age readily accept a dentist's recommendations in regard to preventive home measures.

The role of the hygienist

The hygienist can make an outstanding contribution to the dental care of a child. The hygienist has the potential to acclimate the child to the dental instruments and the initial procedures.

To help the child develop confidence and to assist the dentist in the treatment of the child, the hygienist needs a general knowledge of how children might react to the initial dental experience.

The hygienist can save valuable time for the dentist by being able to convey an atmosphere of naturalness and confidence and to demonstrate the primary instruments. Accomplishing a dental prophylaxis may be an important step in introducing or reconditioning the child to oral health procedures. While the dentist is performing restorative care or conducting a consultation with the parents of another child, the hygienist can effectively provide a dental prophylaxis. Removal of all debris from the teeth is an important requisite for conducting an efficient examination of the dentition. Cleaning the teeth should be considered one of the more pleasant experiences of oral health care. It also provides an opportunity to compliment the patient on being a good helper. In addition, after the prophylaxis the hygienist can be in an excellent position to facilitate the young patient's cooperation with procedures that may cause anxiety, such as securing radiographs, applying topical fluoride, and taking impressions for diagnostic models.

Dentist's examination

After the prophylaxis, the dentist's examination of the child's mouth begins. It should follow a systematic approach. The staff member recording the dentist's dictation of findings should be aware of the sequence in which tissues are to be evaluated. As mentioned before, the evaluation includes the child's hair, back of head, face, neck, and gait. Also, the child's hands are observed for signs of related dental conditions, such as digital sucking. A dentist will probably tend to examine the oral structures in this order: buccal tissues, gingiva, tongue, floor of mouth, palate, occlusion, and finally the teeth. Next the dentist will determine the need for radiographs on the basis of signs and symptoms revealed during the examination.

Radiographic examination

Radiographs for children who present behavior problems are completed with no little effort and usually with a considerable expenditure of time. A young patient's lack of understanding, fear of discomfort, gagging, or other barriers to completing adequate radiographs may be diminished by presenting the procedure with confidence and performing one or more "fake-take" exercises. A hygienist or an assistant can motivate the child into the necessary quiescence for the completion of the diagnostic radiographs. Also, a hygienist or an assistant can be trained in the technique of taking a complete mouth radiograph with panoramic radiographic equipment.

Behavior evaluation

The hygienist or the assistant enters on the chart a concise evaluation of the child's actions and responses to instruction and procedures. These notations will be of value to the dentist in planning the chair time required to complete the indicated treatment plan.

For the dentist and the office staff to evaluate behavior adequately, it is important that they be aware of the objectives of child management and the criteria for evaluating behavior guidance during child dental care. Objectives of child management include (1) making the child comfortable, (2) providing freedom from pain, (3) performing the procedures safely, (4) carrying them out efficiently, and (5) having the child and the parent accept the procedures.

The dentist and the staff members may use the following guide to judge their own competence in managing child patients:

1. *Good voice technique.* This is demonstrated by good control and modulated tone.
2. *Effective acclimation procedures.* "Show and tell" is well used, and the child feels comfortable.
3. *Appropriate application of firmness.* The dentist uses firmness at the proper time and to the proper degree.
4. *Awareness of child's concerns.* Attention is given to the child's concerns, and the staff shows appropriate friendliness.
5. *Communication.* Rapport is achieved through the staff members' skills in obtaining appropriate verbal, visual, or physical responses from the child.
6. *Reinforcement.* Appropriate behavior is rewarded.
7. *Positive approach.* The dentist and the staff members show confidence and decisiveness.
8. *Logical statements and questions.* The entire office staff seems always to say just the right thing.
9. *Truthfulness.* Comments are honest, forthright, and well phrased.
10. *Ample time.* Good planning is evident, and ample time is provided for procedures.
11. *Efficiency of treatment.* An excellent amount of treatment is accomplished, considering the child's behavior.
12. *Medication.* Medication is used knowledgeably and with discretion.
13. *Positive reaction.* On the completion of dental procedures, the reaction of the child is positive, and the patient is not unduly fearful of dentistry.

In evaluating the management of parents in the office, the dentist and the staff will want to ensure that rapport is achieved with parents and that the office staff demonstrates attentiveness to parents and instills confidence. Such rapport is necessary for satisfactory dental treatment of young children.

A child's behavior should be evaluated and recorded on the chart at every visit. This important regular record of the child's responses to dental care will provide baseline data for (1) diagnosing the beginning, subtle signs of inappropriate behavior and (2) charting descriptions of the child's actions that show improvements or remain unchanged. It is also important for the receptionist and other staff members to record the parent's reactions to the child's dental care.

Business office transactions

As a child's treatment is nearing completion, the next appointment can be scheduled by the receptionist with the parent. This procedure allows the receptionist to allay parents' concern about dentistry and to receive and screen questions regarding

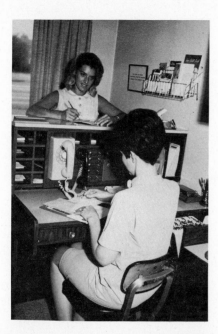

Fig. 30-5. The business office should be designed for orderly management of records. A counter constructed to check-writing height is convenient for the parent and provides partitioned areas for the intercommunication equipment and stationery. A holder attached to the wall near the parent's viewing level contains complimentary educational pamphlets. A recessed file to the right of the receptionist contains the patient ledger cards.

treatments. Also, the parent can present the payment and be ready to leave on completion of the child's treatment (Fig. 30-5).

The accounting system. An efficient and accurate accounting system should be used in the dental office. At each visit the receptionist should give the parents a current statement of their account. A statement-receipt form should contain date of service, charge, amount of payment, current balance, previous balance, and child's name (Fig. 30-6). By using carbon tape attached to the back of the statement-receipt form, the receptionist can transfer these entries automatically to the individual patient ledger, and by means of a pegboard and carbon paper the figures can be transferred to the office day sheet. The statement-receipt form may also

contain (in the description box of the accounting portion of the slip) the date and time of the child's next visit. This information can also be transferred automatically onto the individual ledger card along with the other entries (Fig. 30-7). Subsequently, by quickly referring to the patient's ledger card a staff member can determine the date of the next visit expeditiously, without a fatiguing search of the appointment book.

A quick daily proof of the business office's financial transactions may be obtained by comparing the totals of the financial day sheet. The total of the charge and previous balance columns should equal the total of the credit and balance columns.

Computers or computer services can provide an alternative to conventional systems for managing financial and other information about a child patient's dental care. Careful analysis needs to be conducted to determine whether this alternative would be cost effective in a particular practice for handling financial records, including dental insurance claims and patient statements, as well as for appointment scheduling, recall data, and diagnostic and treatment records.

Treatment planning and fee determination

The treatment plan should be formulated and the consultation planned during a reserved period when patients are not scheduled and when the dentist is free from distractions.

The child's medical history and past dental health experiences are reviewed; an orderly analysis is made of oral findings. Either the receptionist or the chairside assistant can expedite the preparation of the treatment plan by reading from the child's chart the findings of the comprehensive visual and tactile dental examination. Simultaneously, the dentist evaluates the radiographs and dictates the integration of the findings for each dental condition. The assisting staff member records the indicated treatment on the treatment plan outline. The completed form includes a summary of the findings and the proposed treatment, with the priority of procedures and the proposed grouping of treatments specified. This form also lists esti-

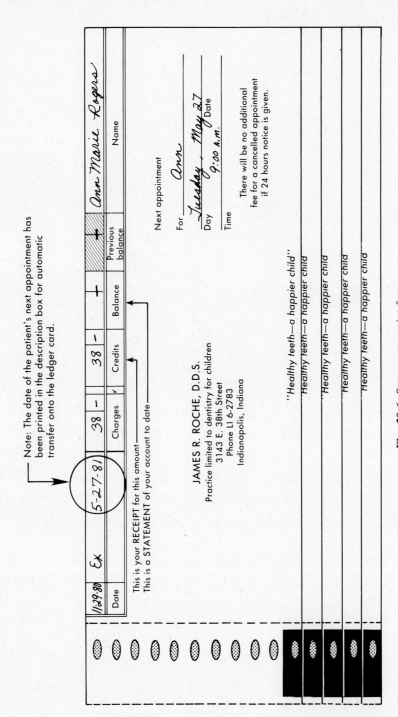

Fig. 30-6. Statement-receipt form.

Name:	Rogers, Ann Marie			Birth: 9-18-74			
Address:	5209 East 47th Avenue			Tel: 546-2783 Res.			
City:	Indianapolis, Indiana			264-7868 Bus.			
	Father Ronald W.						

Date	Description		Charges	✓	Credits	Balance	Previous balance
11-21-78	Ex	12-6-78	44 —		44 —	—	—
12-6-78	CC	1-19-78	224 —		46 —	178 —	—
1-19-79		2-10-79			46 —	132 —	178 —
2-10-79		2-28-79			46 —	86 —	132 —
2-28-79		3-28-79			46 —	40 —	86 —
3-21-79		5-8-79			40 —	—	40 —
5-8-79	Ex	11-27-79	24 —		24 —	—	—
11-27-79	Ex	6-6-79	38 —		38 —	—	—
6-6-80	Ex	6-24-80	24 —		24 —	—	—
6-24-80	CC	11-29-80	32 —		32 —	—	—
11-29-80	Ex	(5-27-8)	38 —		38 —	—	—

Note: The date of the patient's next appointment has been transferred to the description column for quick reference.

Fig. 30-7. Patient ledger card.

mated total expense, anticipated number of visits, and suggested payment for each visit. This prepared treatment plan outline provides the receptionist with the information for conducting the preliminary case consultation with the parent at the time of the child's next appointment.

If study models and diagnostic tests have been completed, they can help substantiate a diagnosis. Determining the diagnosis, evaluating the child's behavior, outlining a sequence of treatment, and considering the prognosis associated with the various conditions with and without treatment form the basis for the later consultation with the parent. The planning conference with the staff member should include a review of the parents' anxiety about dental care and a determination of the amount of dental health education that they will need.

In addition to the amount of time required for a child's treatment and the office overhead expense, the judgment and physical effort involved in managing a child, as a result of the child's behavior, contribute to the formula for establishing a fee.

A child's second visit

When the parents return the child to the office for a second visit, it can be assumed that they generally approved of the staff's management of the initial procedures.

Treatment consultation. The pedodontic case consultation is a meeting, first between the office personnel and the parents and then between the dentist and the parents, to present the findings, including diagnosis, treatment plan, and recommendations. This conference time provides an opportunity for the office staff and parents to discuss the child's current dental health and future dental needs and to inform the parents of their financial responsibilities in regard to the dental treatment.

The consultation should be held in an attractive private room, and the parents should be seated at eye level with the staff member. The dialogue should be unhurried and the atmosphere relaxed. The parents' undivided attention is important; they can easily be distracted by the patient or other children in the family or they may be "clock watch-

ing" because of concern for their previously scheduled activities. A wall-attached magnetic board on which creative designs can be produced may assist in entertaining the children and reducing interruption during the case consultation (Fig. 30-8).

Receptionist's preliminary presentation. During the consultation period at the second visit, the receptionist can effectively direct the parents' thinking toward their child's dental needs. By using the summarized notes from the treatment plan outline, the receptionist can explain in easily understood terms the dentist's findings and recommendations. This prelude to the dentist's presentation can include the following, when applicable: a definition of indicated pulp therapy, the meaning of plaque control, an explanation of space management appliances, the purpose of fluorides, reasons for restoring primary teeth, the number and severity of carious lesions, the expense involved, and the number of visits required. Barriers to communication may be reduced if the receptionist is alert to parental misconceptions regarding the purpose and method of treatment.

An educational series of slides with tape narrations may be selected by the receptionist to correspond to the major points of the diagnosis and treatment for each child. Such a programmed presentation can amplify the receptionist's verbal outline and help the parents visualize the details of their child's treatment. The 3M Sound-Slide system* is an example of audiovisual equipment that may be used to quickly tailor instruction about an individual child's needs to the parents' level of dental information. This system consists of a projector-recorder that is capable of handling 35-mm transparency slides. A magnetic sound track mounted on each slide holder can record and play back up to 35 seconds of narration. Thirty-six slide holders can fit into a slide cartridge, which can automatically advance to the next slide and accompanying sound track. Slides can be reprogrammed without disrupting audio synchronization.

---

*3M Brand Model 525 Projector-Recorder, 3M Co., Visual Products Division, St. Paul, Minn. 55144.

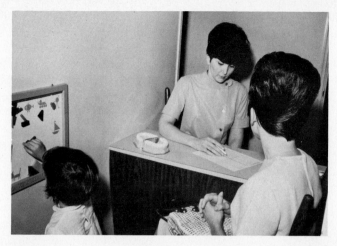

Fig. 30-8. When something of interest, such as the magnetic wall board, is provided for the child, the parent's attention can be more easily focused on the receptionist's preliminary consultation.

The receptionist's preliminary presentation can be helpful in guiding the parents' thinking and in helping them to formulate questions while they are still in the office. Another advantage of the receptionist's presentation is that it facilitates participation by the parent. Parents will convey thoughts and questions to the staff that they would not readily express to the dentist. The receptionist's interpretation of the parents' questions and remarks can alert the dentist to their degree of understanding and also to the level of anxiety that the parents have about their child's dental needs. Subsequently, the dentist's explanation of the treatment plan and comments about the child's radiographs can be concise and more meaningful and better understood by the parents. After this preliminary consultation, the receptionist assists the parent in selecting and establishing financial arrangements from the various methods that the dentist has established.

Adequate management of the initial consultation with the parents requires a training program for the receptionist, who needs instruction in the objectives of pedodontics and the various treatment procedures. The receptionist should be tested during practice sessions for the ability to inform parents about their child's oral health and for effectiveness in answering common questions regarding the dentist's proposed treatment.

The chairside assistant and the hygienist should also be trained in case presentation so that they can conduct the preliminary consultation if the receptionist is ill.

Unlike many sales situations, in which the prospect may be indifferent at first to the explanation of a product or service, during the dental consultation the parents usually show favorable interest in their child's dental health. This initial favorable acceptance of the office by the parents results from their confidence in the referring dentist, physician, or acquaintance.

Dentist's consultation. During the consultation with the parents the dentist may review the major diagnosis or may elaborate on specific details, such as type of infection, severity of dental caries, reasons for pain, nature of oral defects, and child's behavior during the dental procedures. The type of presentation depends on the parents' questions and their overt response to the receptionist's preliminary presentation. The dentist may illustrate the location of oral findings with the use of a large model of the dentition. Color photographs may be used to communicate the principles involved in, for example, ectopic eruption of teeth or the placement of space management appliances. The consultation by the dentist should include accurate information, which should be presented to the parents in a manner understandable to them. The dentist should control the consultation period efficiently, since the charge for this procedure usually includes the fee for the examination, diagnosis, treatment planning, and the interpretation of radiographs.

If the consultation period is to be conducted efficiently, control of the parents' conversation is important; this is accomplished by anticipating questions and reactions. What the dental staff will do for the child is of interest to parents, and a statement of this, with specific descriptions of services and their value, is an appropriate motivator to the reception of the needed care. The dentist needs to project his or her interest in the child and to convey this positive attitude to the parents. However, as with other health services, overpromising results can lead to parental dissatisfaction. The amount of education that will be necessary for parents to understand their child's dental condition depends on the parents' dental information level. Their understanding of the dentist's recommendations may be enhanced or clouded by their own past dental experiences and their concern for the child's dental needs. Identifying the true meaning of the parents' questions may be difficult. Disagreement with the treatment plan may indicate a misunderstanding regarding the meaning of the findings and the value of the proposed care. The parents' dissatisfaction with the proposed treatment may originate from a concern for the expense or for the plans available for payment.

The consultation is tailored to the specific dental findings, the child's behavior, and the attitude of the parents. The parents' emotional shock after a traumatic dental injury to their child may impede communication. The parents will be upset regarding the child's disfigurement, and they will not be in a responsive frame of mind to receive an entire treatment outline and the possible alternatives. The parents' anxiety while their child is suffering from a toothache is also a barrier to good communication, and the presentation of a comprehensive treatment plan and expected results should be postponed.

If the parents are argumentative or demanding or have a low level of dental information, the dentist will require additional time and patience to communicate the findings and the proper treatment program. Since the child's dental health is the main goal, unfavorable parental behavior needs understanding instead of disregard. A parent who is extremely talkative may be a poor listener. A slightly ill or temporarily upset parent may necessitate postponement of the consultation procedure. An unresponsive parent may be shy, dentally uneducated, or defiant. Questions regarding the personal dental experiences of a parent of this type may help the dentist to classify the parent's behavior and may assist in communication. A parent with a fearful attitude toward dentistry will usually express these fears during the consultation, and such a parent should be encouraged to do so if the child patient or the child's siblings are not present in the room. This ventilation of parental anxieties may reduce the barrier to effective communication concerning the child's present condition and needed care.

Education in home health measures

Following the dentist's consultation with the parent, both the child and the parent are escorted by the receptionist into the dental health education area.

Teaching proper oral hygiene procedures. Home preventive measures need enthusiastic presentation. Motivating the child to brush and floss the teeth adequately and the parents to supervise the child's efforts intelligently should be a continuous teaching process. Effective teaching will minimize the time spent with the child and the parent and maximize the level of oral hygiene.

The instruction should include easily understood objectives and might begin with the following steps:

1. Use visual aids to show parents the role bac-

terial plaque plays in the dental caries process.

2. Define plaque.
3. Explain to parents that the objective will be to remove all plaque from the child's teeth and control future deposits.

Then it might be appropriate to say something like, "Let's start with brushing. In order to efficiently remove large deposits of plaque, good brushing technique is important."

Teaching methods should be flexible enough to take into account the dexterity of the parent and the child, their attitudes toward dental health, and the age of the child. The teaching approach should be modified for parents of mentally or physically handicapped children, perhaps with special instruction given in how to stabilize the child's head and position the brush satisfactorily.

If the parent of a preschool child indicates that he or she feels familiar with toothbrushing technique or otherwise gives the impression of resisting instruction, the parent can be given a new toothbrush and asked to brush the child's teeth. The hygienist can observe the procedure and then disclose the remaining plaque deposits with a tablet or solution containing erythrosine (F.D.C. Red No. 3) after the parent has finished. Learning by discovery may provide the best means of motivating parents.

In cases of fair to poor brushing performance, remedial instruction will be necessary. For such parents and for all parents who indicate that they are unfamiliar with proper brushing technique, the following teaching method should be useful.

The hygienist presents a new junior-type brush to the child and tells the parent why the dentist recommends that particular style.

Using a brush and a model of the dentition, the hygienist acquaints the parent with the correct positioning of the brush and the proper stroke for a section of two or three teeth. The parent is then instructed to position the child and the brush for the same section of teeth, in the manner that has just been demonstrated by the hygienist. As the parent moves from one section of teeth to the next, the hygienist offers corrections and continues to guide

the parent by initially positioning the child's head, placing the brush, and briefly demonstrating the wielding of the brush before the parent brushes. For each section of teeth throughout the dentition, the hygienist observes the parent's skill, reinforcing proper technique or correcting inadequate performance.

The hygienist demonstrates a method of applying disclosing solution to the child's teeth, points out remaining plaque deposits, and shows the parent how to remove some of the disclosed plaque by more careful control of the brush. The parent then attempts to remove some of the easily seen debris. Guiding the parent through the more difficult areas as identified by the disclosing solution should help the parent to develop brushing skill. To avoid interfering with the instruction on flossing that is to follow, the hygienist at this point answers any questions the parent may have about proper brushing technique and reemphasizes its importance.

Since some areas in the child's dentition will show remaining deposits of plaque, the hygienist can explain the value of using dental floss. "Have you ever flossed your own teeth?" may be an appropriate question to ask the parent. If the response is yes, the parent is given a strip of floss and asked to demonstrate the technique on the child, with the instructor offering compliments or corrections. A parent who is unfamiliar with flossing is given a suitable length of floss; the hygienist demonstrates the wrapping of floss on the fingers, and then supervises the technique of the parent. The hygienist flosses a section of the model, then applies floss to the same area in the child's mouth. The parent repeats the flossing for the same area on the model to become acquainted with the feel of the floss passing through the interproximal contacts and to learn how to prevent gingival irritation. The parent then moves to the next section in the child's mouth and systematically proceeds with each section under the hygienist's guidance.

Disclosing solution is then reapplied to the child's teeth, this time by the parent, and the hygienist assists in evaluating remaining debris.

A similar educational method is followed in the

case of an older child, except that the parent only supervises the oral hygiene techniques and reinforces the correct procedures.

Evaluation sessions. Frequent evaluative sessions with the hygienist or assistant who manages the plaque control program may help increase parent and patient compliance. Soon after the oral hygiene instruction, a visit should be scheduled to evaluate the progress of the home cleaning procedures. During this appointment, the parent stains the child's teeth with disclosing solution and performs the brushing procedure. The hygienist notes the areas that need to be gone over again and provides the necessary reinforcement or reinstruction in brushing technique. The parent then proceeds to the flossing technique, reapplies the disclosing solution, and evaluates the results. Compliments may increase the meticulousness of the parent's efforts, and constructive criticism will emphasize the need for careful technique.

The frequency of appointments for evaluating the level of oral hygiene can be determined on the basis of demonstrated performance and the record of oral cleanliness. If the child's plaque score remains unsatisfactory, the staff member will need to determine if the problem is due to lack of skill on the part of the child or parent in the use of toothbrush or floss or to failure to include oral hygiene measures in the daily activities at home. If a child has consistently poor oral hygiene, the parent should keep a diary showing the specific times toothbrushing and flossing were performed by or for the child during a period of 1 or 2 weeks. Also, it is helpful if the office staff member determines what events take place immediately before and after the oral hygiene practices that could influence the effectiveness of plaque control.

The motivation of the parent and the child cannot be expected to last. The office staff must seek constantly to sustain interest in the continued practice of plaque control. For example, providing instruction concerning the parent's own oral hygiene, including evaluative sessions, may help to promote proper oral hygiene habits for the child.

Toothbrushing and flossing techniques are described in greater detail in Chapter 15.

Diet considerations. If a survey of the child's diet is not to be completed at this time, in a private environment the hygienist may explain the relationship between diet and dental caries and present to the parents the American Dental Association booklet *Diet and Dental Health*. The hygienist can provide a diet consultation with parents who have completed a diet record of their child's 7-day food intake. Appraisal of the frequency of eating refined carbohydrates from the child's diet record can provide a substantial basis for the consultation. Better cooperation will be obtained from the parents in completing an accurate diet survey if the objective of the survey is explained to them beforehand. The parents should understand that the dentist is concerned with the child's eating habits and the types of food the child eats as they relate to the decay process. If the parents believe that their ability to manage their child's diet is being questioned, they may be reluctant to provide a reliable survey and may resist subsequent dietary recommendations. In each case the dentist must be convinced of the value of using the diet record as an educational measure before the parents are asked to take time to complete the forms.

The importance of selecting foods from the four basic food groups should be stressed. Advising parents to completely eliminate the child's between-meal snacks may not be practical. Educating parents as to special snacks that do not contain refined carbohydrates, such as open-faced meat sandwiches, cheese and meat cubes, and fresh fruit, is recommended.

Another educational method involves the hygienist performing caries activity tests for the child. These tests may help the parents to better understand the variables in the caries process and may motivate them to attentively guide their child's diet.

The hygienist maintains control of the printed material used in acquainting the parents with the important effects of diet on oral health and marks the specific topics of interest. This helps to hold the parents' attention and encourages them to refer to the selected information when they return home.

During a child's "teething" period, the parents

generally appear eagerly interested in dental health education, and they can be receptive to learning how diet may affect oral health. For instance, the parents of an 18-month-old child will probably pay close attention when the hygienist tells them about the hidden sugars in such dietary favorites as raisins, soft drinks, and ice cream.

Additional instructions. Parents of children who are already receiving care in the dental office usually welcome information about the age at which their younger child should first visit the office. Since diagnosis is the key to preventive services for children, advising parents that their child should have a first dental examination shortly after 12 months of age may be one of the most effective means of reducing the progression of dental caries and establishing orderly home preventive measures. Furthermore, during the consultation period for a child under 2 years of age, the receptionist can present programmed instruction in first-aid measures for any future dental traumatic injuries, such as controlling bleeding from soft tissues around teeth. The instruction should also stress the value

of consulting a dentist and establishing baseline radiographic records of the injury.

Receptionist's make-ready procedures

Each time a child visits the office, the receptionist will transfer the child and the parent from the reception room to the dental health education area. The oral hygiene skills will be evaluated as described on p. 788. On completion of the oral hygiene procedures, if further treatment has been scheduled, the receptionist will accompany the child directly to the treatment room, seat the patient, properly adjust the chair, place on the child a protective plastic apron with a paper napkin collar, and provide articles that will occupy the child's interest while the other staff members are completing the previous child's care (Fig. 30-9). Chairside interest materials may include items such as a creative magnetic board, comic, picture, or cartoon books, or talking toys, depending on the child's age and interests. This will complete the receptionist's duties in regard to receiving and making the child ready for the dentist or the hygienist. The

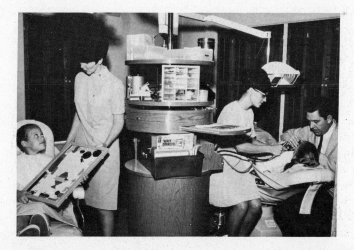

Fig. 30-9. Performance of the assistant at chairside is more important than make-ready or clean-up responsibilities. If possible, the chairside assistant should be seated at a higher level than the dentist with a convenient view of the treatment. Grouping all instruments and materials according to use on revolving shelves permits the assistant to remain at chairside during the treatment procedures. While the treatment is being completed, the receptionist positions the next child and provides articles of interest.

receptionist will then return to the dental health education area and escort the parent to the reception room.

Duties of the chairside assistant

Delegation of specific duties to the chairside assistant can contribute to the efficiency and pleasantness of pedodontic treatment. It is imperative that the assistant be aware of children's limited experience, short attention span, and inability to communicate feelings. Evaluation of the effectiveness of a dental assistant for child patients is based ultimately on chairside performance. Obviously, preparation of instruments in advance and the efficient manipulation of materials permit the assistant to concentrate on the dentist and the child (Fig. 30-9).

Make-ready procedures. As the dentist examines a patient in the hygienist's operatory, an assistant who is free of child supervision responsibilities will give top priority to make-ready procedures for the treatment of the next patient. From the proposed treatment indicated on the daily worksheet, the assistant places the appropriate instruments in readiness. The procedure manual provided for the assistant should list the articles generally required for various treatments. Before the dentist comes into position at chairside, the assistant will adjust the dental light properly and reposition the child if necessary.

Chairside procedures. Attendance at chairside and assisting the dentist with procedures that directly involve the young patient are the first priorities of the assistant. One of the most valuable aids that a chairside assistant can render during pedodontic care is the discreet handing of the local anesthetic syringe. The precise timing with which the assistant passes the syringe to the dentist can enhance the psychologic presentation of the injection. By practicing alertness, the dental assistant can be ready with moderate restraint to help protect the young patient from self-harm if the child suddenly decides to rebel. Close supervision of a handicapped child by the assistant can be helpful in preventing interference as a result of reflex move-ments or erratic responses during an injection or an operative procedure.

Chairside education. The chairside assistant can help develop a climate of naturalness and friendliness toward the child in the treatment room. The assistant can further condition the young patient and save the dentist time by explaining the use of the rubber dam and the expected sensation after a local anesthetic has been administered. Where state dental laws are not restrictive, a trained dental assistant can save a significant amount of time for the dentist by placing the rubber dam on the child while the dentist is examining the hygienist's patient or consulting with a parent.

The chairside assistant should refrain from conversation with the child during the dentist's instructions to the patient; however, the experienced team of dentist and assistant can develop a "psychologic script" of well-chosen words to lead the child through the indicated procedures.

Economy of motion. Treatment procedures are performed more efficiently when the assistant is continuously stationed at chairside. When the assistant leaves the chairside position and the procedure is therefore interrupted, additional time will be required for the assistant to become reoriented to the particular step in the procedure. In such a situation the dentist's efficiency is also decreased because the dentist must look away from the operating site to the instrument tray in order to maintain continuity in the procedure. Motion economy can be increased by grouping and storing instruments and materials according to their use, in reach of the chairside assistant when seated (Fig. 30-9). The organized readiness of instruments and the rendering of treatment are supported by cleaning and sterilizing complete instrument setups at specific intervals during the treatment schedule and by keeping different setups separate from each other. The staff should periodically monitor the sterilization of instruments to ensure that the sterility of instruments is not being compromised as the result of an effort to be efficient. Defective or misused sterilizers can be detected by a sterilization monitoring service, such as that provided by the Department of Oral

Microbiology at Indiana University School of Dentistry.

The placement of amalgam restorations for children may be expedited by having the chairside assistant deliver portions of the amalgam directly to the cavity preparation.

Delegating to an assistant all duties supportive of the restorative procedure will result in greatly increased efficiency, especially when a child's behavior deviates from the ideal.

Near the completion of each child's appointment, the dentist can dictate to the chairside assistant the details of the performed treatment, as applicable: amount of anesthetic used, location of treatment, size of pulpal exposure, condition of the tissue, specific materials used, name of each procedure performed, details of child behavior, and intended treatment for the next visit. The assistant records these details directly on the chart. This information helps the receptionist to answer questions immediately after the treatment and to schedule the next visit. Before the child's next visit, the receptionist transfers the planned treatment from the chart to the daily treatment schedule (see p. 774).

Proper chairside assisting in pedodontic care could be considered confining, since a patient should not be left in a room unattended. The assistant has the responsibility of watching the child to prevent misadventures such as falling from the dental chair or investigating, out of curiosity, potentially hazardous dental equipment, instruments, or medicaments. The assistant should also be present to detect symptoms of syncope or other unfavorable reactions to dental treatment, which do not occur frequently. In the absence of the dentist from the treatment room, the continued presence and friendly conversation of the assistant may prevent anxiety and, in the case of an older child, provide an opportunity to strengthen friendship.

Additional duties delegated to auxiliaries

Where state dental laws have been amended to permit trained auxiliary personnel to perform reversible procedures, the productivity of patient care can be increased. These expanded duties for auxiliary personnel may include making study model impressions or performing restorative procedures, including positioning and removal of matrix bands, placement and carving of restorations, and removal of rubber dam material. Delegating these technical procedures to auxiliaries gives the dentist additional time to perform diagnostic and irreversible procedures.

Traumatized young permanent teeth require repeated electrical vitality tests to determine the reliability of the child's response. The hygienist can perform the vitality tests and present the data to the dentist for analysis. The important procedure of polishing restorations also can be assigned to the hygienist. The maintenance of a dry field around bands, crowns, or fixed space management appliances after cementation, and the subsequent removal of cement, can be delegated to the hygienist. After a removable appliance has been seated initially and properly adjusted by the dentist, the hygienist or the assistant can instruct the child about the management of the appliance and the maintenance of good oral hygiene. The staff member can use a large hand mirror to aid in the instruction and supervise the child's efforts. This guidance can help the patient to develop dexterity in positioning the retaining wires of the removable appliance and thus gain a feeling of security.

Routine instructions for care following an extraction can be given to the parent by an assisting staff member. The receptionist will need to encourage the parent to observe the young child for several hours after the office visit to prevent the anesthetized oral tissues from becoming lacerated as a result of inadvertent biting. In addition, after restorative procedures a half-section of 6-inch No. 2 cotton roll can be inserted between the child's teeth on the anesthetized side. With a portion of the long cotton roll extending out of the child's mouth, the child can be encouraged to continuously bite down on the cotton roll rather than biting the lip or oral tissues. Furthermore, the cotton roll can remind the parent to continue to observe the child postoperatively.

Delegation of as many routine technical procedures as possible will free the dentist for diagnostic, consultative, and supervisory functions.

Final rinsing of the mouth, washing of the face, and mellowing of a problem child's lingering expression of unhappiness can be supervised by the assistant or the hygienist. The time of dismissal of the child from the treatment area will ultimately depend on the receptionist's schedule of activities. It is important that the receptionist's business with the parent be completed before the child is dismissed from the treatment area. Therefore the assistant or the hygienist should notify the receptionist when the child is ready to be dismissed. If the receptionist is arranging an appointment, providing a preliminary case presentation, receiving a payment, or performing another high-priority service, a child who is ready for dismissal should be escorted to an area within the treatment room and invited to enjoy this waiting period with toys or books. This "holding area" of the treatment room need not be large, but it should be located to provide easy surveillance by the assistants or hygienists until the receptionist can conveniently dismiss the patient.

Dialogue of the assisting staff

The auxiliary personnel should use language that is understandable to young patients. Instructions and comments by the staff should be consistent with a child's limited vocabulary and experiences. An assistant should refrain from the type of dialogue that could embarrass a child by making fun of the young patient's transitory speech imperfections or laughing at the child's limited ability in self-expression. To develop a true dialogue, staff members should listen to a patient because it is through a child's expressions that we learn the best avenue of communication. When giving instructions to a child, the chairside assistant should be alert to the child's reactions and should quickly modify any verbal, facial, or physical communication that may have provoked an unfavorable response.

Auxiliary personnel sometimes develop a habit of discussing personal matters in the presence of a child. However, the discussion of such matters should be confined to the lunch period or a lounge area. Conversation by the staff related to other children, parents, and office policies and problems should be handled in a discreet manner to avoid the possibility of a parent or a child misinterpreting the conversation as pertaining to them. Policies regarding conversation should be emphasized in each staff member's procedure manual.

Open communication must be present between the dentist and the staff at all times. Staff members must feel free to tell the dentist about any displeasure that they may feel, or a parent may express, about the operation of the office.

Misunderstandings by the staff can many times be prevented if the dentist will give reasons for certain assigned duties. However, it is sometimes necessary for staff members to follow the dentist's concise instructions during patient care without detailed reasons being given immediately. Fulfillment of these duties would be based on the loyalty and confidence that the auxiliary personnel feel toward the dentist.

Selecting and training auxiliary personnel

Staff members who assist in the management of child patients should have particular capabilities in addition to the usual desirable traits of personality and character. They will need to communicate with children of various ages by using appropriate vocabulary and referring to topics of appropriate interest. Not all persons are desirous of developing such a relationship, especially with preschool patients. The staff members must be capable of maintaining objective understanding and calm guidance in the face of the various behavior patterns exhibited by children. Each person in an office where children are treated should possess a mature emotional attitude that respects children and that classifies a child's occasional insulting remarks as expressions of the situation rather than as something personal.

The auxiliary personnel must also be able to take a tolerant and objective attitude toward disturbing parental behavior.

After preliminary screening, applicants who appear to have the qualifications for the position may be invited to observe office procedures for a day. This policy not only permits a potential employee to project himself or herself into the office operation but also enables the dentist and the staff to evaluate the applicant under a stressful situation. A trial employment period usually provides an opportunity to determine whether the person has the interest and emotional maturity necessary for assisting with the dental care of child patients.

Training and maintaining an office staff that is capable of instructing parents and measuring up to the dentist's standards for consultation procedures are constant problems. Efficient pedodontic care must be supported by at least two assisting staff members. Significant time may be required to train assistants for the special psychologic rapport needed in conducting a young patient, with limited experience, through the procedures pleasantly. They will need instruction in the various reactions of children to dental care. They must learn to recognize the reasons for the occasional unfavorable reaction to the dental experience. Short terms of employment can be expensive to the office and represent a poor investment in time and energy.

The procedure manual: an approach to a problem. Finding time to develop an effective manual of office procedures is often difficult. Yet this administrative project is essential because it (1) provides an orderly and disciplined approach to oral health care of children by the office team, (2) establishes a clear reference point during individual or group conferences with staff members, (3) communicates to the office staff the dentist's philosophy of practice, and (4) instructs new personnel in specific office procedures and responsibilities.

Office procedure manuals tailored to the needs of a particular office are much more effective than commercially prepared models, which will not coincide with an individual dentist's philosophy of practice. A separate procedure manual should be prepared for each staff position. Each manual will contain information pertinent to the specific position of receptionist, hygienist, or assistant, as well as information relevant to all staff positions. The principal divisions of the manuals would be as fol-

lows: major activities; specific duties; working conditions; general office policies; and reference section, including sample forms and lists of materials, guidelines on communication in the dental office, and a list of abbreviations and symbols.

Although the mechanism for developing the manuals may vary from office to office, the following outline provides a workable approach:

1. The dentist lists the major activities of each staff position, using scratch paper and double spacing for easy alteration.

   Example: Major activities of the receptionist: represents the entire office to the public; conducts financial transactions; schedules appointments; monitors the telephones; controls communications between the dentist, other office personnel, parents, and patients

2. The dentist lists specific duties for each auxiliary staff member. These duties will vary for each staff member, but they may be placed under one of the following categories: opening duties, daily responsibilities, closing duties, weekly duties, and monthly duties.

   Examples:

   a. Opening duties for the receptionist: opens business office and reception room: (1) turns on lights, intercom, and music; (2) verifies cash drawer; (3) distributes daily treatment schedule and charts

   b. Daily responsibilities for the receptionist: in preparation for a preliminary case presentation, selects an educational series of slides with tape narrations to correspond with the major points of the diagnosis and treatment of a child

   c. Closing duties for the hygienist: runs all contra-angles and prophylaxis angles in cleaner and lubricant (refer to reference section of manual, p. 15, for instructions)

   d. Weekly duties for the assistant: inventories weekly supplies (refer to reference section of manual, p. 12, for procedure)

e. Monthly duties for the receptionist: reviews patient ledger cards to identify patients without appointments

3. The dentist specifies working conditions.

Example: Sick leave: 1 day a month with pay, with paid sick days not accumulating to more than 5 days per year

4. The dentist carefully delineates general office policies. A copy of these policies will be placed in each staff member's manual.

Examples:

a. All personnel are to be present, in uniform, and ready to begin work at the time stated in the individual staff member's section on working conditions.

b. Any change in office procedure or treatment technique must be approved by the dentist.

5. The dentist gives the preliminary outline of each manual to the appropriate staff member for suggestions and for comments about clarity. Obtaining this important input from the auxiliary staff will help the dentist to understand the needs and expectations of the staff members.

6. While the auxiliary personnel are evaluating the preliminary outlines for the procedure manual, the dentist compiles a list of reference items appropriate to each position.

Examples:

a. For the receptionist: chart, health history form, parental consent for treatment form, patient ledger card, statement-receipt form, sample letters regarding delinquent accounts

b. For the hygienist: sample forms for instructing parents on the completion of diet records, handout on nutrition counseling

c. For the assistant: itemized instructions regarding procedures for sterilization, cleaning and lubricating of hand-

pieces, and tray setups (including photographs of completed tray arrangements of instruments)

In addition to these reference items, the dentist lists his wishes concerning verbal communication in the dental office.

Examples:

a. Each staff member should speak clearly and in a modulated voice.

b. Words or phrases that promote anxiety in a patient, such as *hurt, needle, drill, pull,* and *leave mother,* should be avoided. Instead, language should be used that will help guide a child through the procedures in a tranquil manner.

A list of abbreviations and symbols used by the particular dentist will complete the content of the reference section.

Examples: c̄ = with; s̄ = without; L = local anesthetic; CC = case consultation; Rec = recall; △ = amalgam

7. As the staff members complete their evaluations of the preliminary outlines, the lists of reference items are given to the appropriate staff members. Each staff member then assembles the sample forms and materials appropriate to his or her position and completes each form as a hypothetical case. These items are then added to the reference section.

8. Following the staff members' study of the manuals, the dentist makes revisions to improve clarity, as needed, and to incorporate reasonable suggestions. The procedure manuals are then typed in duplicate, with one copy of the appropriate manual being provided for each staff member and one for the dentist. Each manual is contained in a loose-leaf workbook, which allows for a convenient exchange of pages.

9. Each staff member is asked to review his or her typed manual and to formulate any questions.

10. The dentist confers with the staff members individually and discusses the sections on

major activities, specific duties, and working conditions for each position.

11. At the completion of the individual conferences, a staff meeting is conducted, and the rest of the manual is reviewed.
12. The procedure manual is then complete.
13. Each year the dentist and the staff members individually review the manuals before a staff conference, and suggestions for revision are solicited. During the staff conference each item of general application is reviewed, and additions, deletions, or substitutions are made. The conference should be completed within 30 to 45 minutes. Pages containing changes are retyped and inserted in the respective manuals.

A period of several weeks will be required for the dentist and the staff to complete the development of an office procedure manual for child care. However, the time it takes for the dentist and the staff to complete the 12 steps involved in establishing the initial manual represents a good investment, since it will lead to increased productivity, cooperation, and enjoyment.

Although the staff members are responsible for performing specific duties proficiently, they are required to maintain a working understanding of each other's assignments. In the event of illness, there should be a prearranged agreement on alternative duties for each staff member. In addition, instructing each staff member in another's specific responsibilities will assist the dentist in training new personnel when replacements are required.

Record keeping: a critical requirement

Since the complete value of child dental care may not become clear until several years after treatment, accurate, complete, and legible records are essential (Fig. 30-10). Uniform and understandable records are necessary if summaries of findings and treatments are to be written in the future.

Processing the results of treatment is a major responsibility of dentists who care for child patients. Thorough record keeping by the entire office staff is a critical requirement for fulfilling the practitioner's obligation to analyze accurately the success or failure of individual and overall treatment procedures. In guiding the office staff in proper record keeping, the dentist should explain how the records identify the oral findings and the diagnosis. The term "diagnosis" needs to be clearly understood by the staff so that when the dentist specifies, during dictation, a disease, traumatic injury, or abnormality, indicating the location and citing the cause, the staff member will realize that this important prerequisite to treatment has been established. Careful handling and effective filing by the office staff of properly trimmed pretreatment, interim, and posttreatment study models, as well as study models produced after the immediate posttreatment period, are essential. Particularly when space management or tooth movement is involved, the immediate availability at the dental chair of the patient's series of study models enables the dentist to compare relationships of teeth and to assess subtle changes. In addition, during the consultation of the receptionist or the dentist with the parent, an organized library of study models can be used to help the parents understand oral conditions similar to those of their own child.

Staff members must realize the value of the proper processing and careful filing of radiographs because these records serve as important reference points in the dentist's periodic evaluation of treatment efforts such as restorative care and pulp therapy.

Routine record keeping requires updating a child's health history at each appointment. The parental response to the receptionist's question "Has there been any change in your child's health since his last visit?" should be recorded on the patient's chart each visit. The patient's health history form should be revised at each recall visit, through the receptionist's interview of the parent.

Office policies concerning auxiliary personnel

Determining office policies and selecting procedures for the child patient are the responsibility of the dentist. However, the dentist should promote an attitude of reciprocal trust with his office staff.

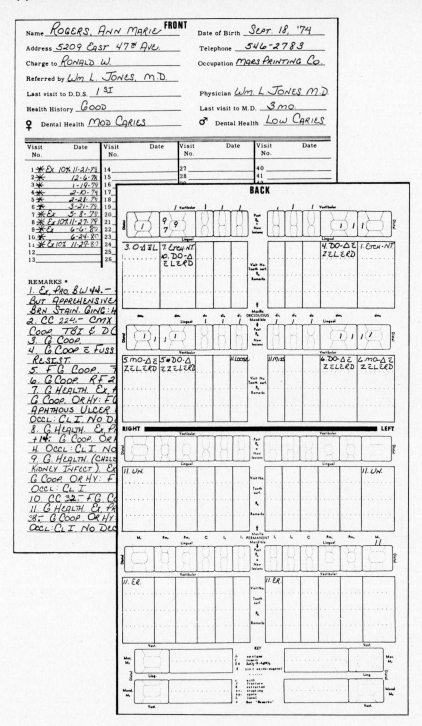

Fig. 30-10. For legend see opposite page.

A tranquil association between the dentist and the office personnel requires a mutual and definite understanding of assigned duties and expected performance. Each staff member's loose-leaf procedure manual should contain the office policies in regard to illnesses of personnel and expected personal appearance and office conduct, a calendar of the forthcoming year's expected working days and hours and vacation periods, and an outline of duties to be performed when patients are not in the office.

The performance of office responsibilities by the staff periodically warrants the dentist's expression of confidence and, when indicated, constructive criticism. Postponing intended correction of inadequate auxiliary performance will only allow problems to accumulate.

One method of maintaining an adequate office operation is to hold staff conferences. The personnel should be aware of the dentist's policy of scheduling periodic conferences, and they should be encouraged to compile items of concern and given the freedom to offer recommendations for improvement.

In a group practice, before office policies and procedures can be determined the dentists will need to have an understanding as to whether auxiliary personnel will be shared. If a group of dentists decides to share auxiliary personnel, the dentists could function as a board of directors in formulating office policies and agreeing on uniform procedures. In that event the chief responsibility for office management could rotate semiannually among the members of the group.

Office policy in regard to emergency care

Occasionally a child requires immediate attention, causing an interruption in the day's preassigned schedule. If treatment of an acute condition can be postponed until the regular emergency period for that day, treatment of the previously scheduled children will not have to be jeopardized by alterations in length of their treatment times. The dentist will need to be sensitive to the parent's concept of emergency care. If the child does not require attention in the office right away, it is important that the parents understand clearly the reasons for postponing the treatment. Even though a specific period is reserved each day for emergency services, the staff may need to extend their working hours occasionally to care for patients with traumatic dental injuries or toothaches.

Recall appointments

Recall visits for child patients can be the key to preventive dental care. A reliable receptionist can assure the dentist of fulfilling his or her obligation to parent and child by scheduling an appropriate recall visit at the time the child's current treatment plan is completed. Contacting parents by telephone or mail is also helpful in managing a productive recall system.

At a recall appointment, the hygienist presents a junior-type brush to the parent—or to the patient in the case of an older child—and assesses the oral hygiene skills of the parent or the child to encourage proper toothbrushing and flossing habits. After the recall examination, the dentist would certainly want to consult personally with the parent and

---

Fig. 30-10. A child patient's chart. This 8½ x 14 inch printed page of heavy paper stock allows the recording of oral findings and treatment for 52 patient visits. The front contains the basic information. Each examination series is color coded. (For example, visits 1 to 6 are recorded in green, visit 7 in red, visit 8 in blue, visits 9 and 10 in black, and visit 11 in green.) The back of the chart provides a diagrammatic representation of the primary and permanent dentitions. Carious lesions are indicated by placing the visit number that corresponds to the examination date in the appropriate diagrammatic area. The visit number and the treatment provided are recorded below in the corresponding area of the diagram. Superimposing recall findings on the original chart (using the appropriate color coding) permits an efficient and orderly review of the previous findings and treatment, confining the progressive record to a single page.

explain briefly the current findings. Examining recall patients and new patients and counseling parents are continuous activities in a progressive practice. By using appropriate auxiliary personnel and properly spacing the treatment of patients, the dentist can provide his or her services to the patients who need them. The dentist can give attention to recall or new patients while the chairside assistant is involved with dismissal or make-ready procedures for another patient or the dentist is delaying treatment of a child until there are signs of profound local anesthesia.

After a series of recall appointments that have shown a child's oral health to involve no complications and his or her dentition to be developing properly, the patient should be considered for referral back to the family dentist, or, if there is no family dentist, a general practitioner who is interested in child care should be chosen. This referral procedure enables the child to receive routine periodic recall care by the family dentist or another practitioner and gives the pedodontist greater freedom to treat complicated pedodontic cases. This referral procedure emphasizes the importance of pedodontics as a specialty.

The value of practice management and health education

The quality and effectiveness of a dentist's service to children can be improved through the study of practice administration and health education methods. A dentist who establishes definite policies and procedures and delegates duties in an appropriate manner to a well-trained staff will be able to devote most of his or her attention and effort to the children.

REFERENCES

American Dental Association, Council on Dental Practice: Computers in dental practice, Chicago, 1981, The Association.

Cooper, T.M., and DiBiaggio, J.A.: Applied practice management: a strategy for stress control, St. Louis, 1979, The C.V. Mosby Co.

Domer, L.R., Snyder, T.L., and Heid, D.W.: Dental practice management: concepts and application, St. Louis, 1980, The C.V. Mosby Co.

Katz, S., McDonald, J.L., Jr., and Stookey, G.K.: Preventive dentistry in action, ed. 3, Upper Montclair, N.J., 1979, D.C.P. Publishing.

Roche, J.R.: Preventive pedodontics. In Bernier, J.L., and Muhler, J.C., editors: Improving dental practice through preventive measures, ed. 3, St. Louis, 1975, The C.V. Mosby Co.

Sackett, D.L., and Haynes, R.B.: Compliance with therapeutic regimens, Baltimore, 1976, The Johns Hopkins University Press.

Weinstein, P., and Getz, T.: Changing human behavior: strategies for preventive dentistry, Chicago, 1978, Science Research Associates, Inc.

31 Community dental health

CHARLES W. GISH

What does a dentist say when the principal of the local school, the president of the city council, or a welfare director calls and says, "The most urgent health problem we have is the condition of our children's teeth. What can we do about it?" or "What more can we do than we are currently doing?" The dentist's answer depends on several factors, but certainly knowledge and understanding of community dental health are paramount in providing the professional guidance the community should receive from its dentists. This chapter is meant to assist the dentist in providing proper leadership to the community in establishing better dental health for its citizens.

Dental health has been caught behind an iron curtain of public apathy for too many years. This situation is rapidly changing, however, and people are accepting dental care as one of the health essentials of life. People are more aware of their dental needs and are turning their potential demand for dental service into an effective desire for dental care. Not only are individuals more aware and appreciative of good dental health, but communities are becoming vitally concerned as well. This can be witnessed by the increasing number of dental insurance plans, fluoridation programs, dental care programs for indigent persons, and many other activities. As dentistry gains this desired attention and respect, it must fulfill its total responsibility to people. Dental health may be an individual responsibility, but dental health education is the responsibility of the dental and teaching professions, which must teach the public how to keep dental disease at a minimum. In times of economic

problems it is even more important to keep dental health education before the public to help maintain an acceptable level of dental health.

In organizing and implementing a dental health program within a community, the dentist must step back from the details and specifics for individuals and look at the entire community. The dentist must be concerned with dental health measures that will provide the maximum amount of good for the maximum number of people. He or she must concentrate on establishing clear priorities and guidelines for action, just as diagnosis and treatment priorities must be established for a patient in private practice.

Although the diagnosis and treatment of dental disease are entirely the dentist's responsibility, dental health is much more than a dentist's problem. It is a problem of vital concern to the entire community and should be approached in this manner. The dental profession exists because of the services rendered to people through dentists; these certainly must include services that can be rendered on a community basis. Dentists must take advantage of community opportunities to improve dental health, if the public is to look upon oral disease as having greater significance than a "bad tooth" that can be treated mechanically.

Community interest in dental health is an important expression of concern by the community for a disease whose prevention and proper treatment require expert professional guidance. Although dentistry has developed noteworthy scientific knowledge and skills in patient treatment, perhaps the emphasis has been so directed to the development of these skills and knowledge that there has been some failure to improve the distribution of dental services. In general, dentistry provides only for those persons who go to a dental office for treatment on a regular basis. In the past, this has included less than 50% of the population. In industry the distribution or sale of a product is as important as the product itself. The dental profession can improve the distribution of its services only through the actions of dentists in their respective communities. Organized dentistry may be commended for actively engaging in an access program and institutional advertising. However, local commitment is essential in creating an effective demand for dental services.

Approaching the community

How does the dental society (or the local dentist) respond and function in community dental health? What are the opportunities for the individual dentist in developing dental health programs for the community? Certainly the dental society should see that dentists are appointed to the state and local boards of health; these dentists should make dental health a significant part of the total community health activity. Another activity for the dental society is to see that a dentist serves on any council or committee in the community concerning itself with health; for example, dentists should serve on current health care programs for indigent persons and welfare agencies. Another important community function is for the dental society to assign a dentist or dental committee as a consultant to each school system. This dentist or committee should make known to the school administration those services that are available. If there is a university or college that prepares teachers in the community, a local dentist should be appointed as a consultant to the administration and appropriate faculty members. Consultation should also be provided to nursing homes and the geriatric population. The dental society should have a speaker's bureau to provide speakers on dental health to community groups, and the existence of this bureau should be properly publicized. The dental society and each dentist

have a further responsibility—to handle requests from individuals and groups for dental health education materials and aids. The American Dental Association catalogue contains many educational materials, and it should be available for ready reference (Fig. 31-1). State and local health departments have films, materials, and services available for both lay and professional groups. A list of these should be available in each dental office. All dentists in a community are needed for an active dental health program through their dental society, especially during National Children's Dental Health Month in February of each year. They must be alert to current and future dental manpower needs of the community. "Dental manpower" means all members of the dental health team and their proper utilization. Methods of payment for services that are available to the community should be discussed at dental society meetings. These matters all provide opportunities to function in community dental health.

In this chapter community dental health is discussed in terms of activities for the school, the home, the dental office, and the community. First, however, a discussion of community dental health problems and needs is important.

Community dental health evaluation and determination of needs

Documenting dental disease. Dental disease is usually divided into four basic categories:
1. Dental caries—disease of the teeth themselves
2. Periodontal disease—disease of the supporting tissues of teeth
3. Oral neoplasms—proliferative diseases of oral soft tissues
4. Malocclusion—not a true disease, but rather a malpositioning of the teeth in relation to one another or of one jaw to the other

There are specific indices for documenting dental caries that should be familiar to the dentist. The DMF index is used for documenting decayed, missing, or filled permanent teeth; the def index provides the most generally accepted method for

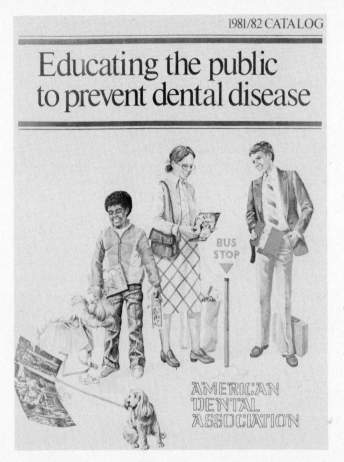

Fig. 31-1. The American Dental Association catalogue describes the wide variety of material available; it is distributed by the association as part of its program of service to the public and to the dental profession. (Copyright by the American Dental Association. Reprinted by permission.)

recording decayed, extracted because of caries, and filled primary teeth.

Several indices have been suggested for measuring inflammation and results of inflammation on the supporting tissues of teeth. One of the most usable indices is the periodontal index (PI). This has been discussed by Russell and is described in Chapter 14 of this book.

An oral hygiene index (OHI) has been developed by Greene and Vermillion; it provides an assessment of tooth debris and calculus. This index is specifically useful in studying the relationship between periodontal disease and oral cleanliness.

Oral cancer incidence is reported by either of two simple indices, the number of new cases per 100,000 persons per year or the number of deaths per 100,000 persons per year. Abnormalities other than the four dental disease categories, such as cleft lip and cleft palate, are reported on the basis of the number of children affected out of the total number of live births per year.

Indices for documenting malocclusion are not as well established as indices for other dental problems, nor have they been widely used in establishing the true extent of malpositioning of the teeth and jaw. Two malocclusion indices are the Oral

Facial Index by Poulton and Aaronson and the Malalignment Index of VanKirk and Pennell.

A few communities with high natural fluoride levels may be concerned about fluorosis. For evaluating the water supplies of these communities, refer to the community fluorosis index originated by Dean and Elvove. New fluorosis indices may be developed. The hazard posed by fluorosis resulting from high natural fluoride levels must be evaluated in terms of the degree of risk, defluoridation costs, and so on. Low fluoride levels certainly appear to present a much greater hazard than mild fluorosis.

The problem of dental disease. The problem of dental disease is multifold. Dental caries affects almost 100% of the population; it affects approximately 80% of children by 10 years of age. As stated in previous chapters, caries can begin in the infant. After the age of 2, new carious lesions occur at the rate of approximately one newly involved tooth or two surfaces per child per year. By age 14 there are 100 missing permanent teeth per 100 children. Less than 40% of the affected teeth are restored. (The above data are for nonfluoridated areas; children in fluoridated communities have approximately half the level of caries.)

Gingival involvement leading to disease of supporting bone and tissue is experienced by a much greater number of children than is usually thought. I have examined many third-, fourth-, and fifth-grade children and have found 50% and more with significant gingival inflammation. Malocclusion has been estimated to involve approximately 50% of the child population. Oral cancer (including lip) develops in about 25,000 persons in the United States each year. The current survival rate is about one third to one half in a 5-year period. This can be greatly improved through early diagnosis. One child is born with cleft lip or cleft palate out of every 800 births.

These data give general information that can be used in discussing dental disease problems. For specific community dental caries information, a baseline dental survey is recommended.

Conducting a dental survey. In establishing priorities of approach, a baseline survey can be of significant value. A dental survey is the most effective way of determining the dental health condition and overall needs of children (or other groups) in a community. It can provide a basis for developing a sound dental health program and for evaluating achievements in dental health in the future. A dental survey should be planned, executed, and interpreted so that it will be an educational experience for the entire community. Many groups can participate; through the pooling of community resources, the greatest benefit can be derived. Proper planning and execution of a survey can greatly increase awareness of the extent and importance of dental disease in the community.

A survey, like any other dental health activity, should be discussed and agreed on by the local dental society and the dentists concerned. Then, clearances and plans should always be made with the superintendent of schools and discussed with principals, teachers, and school nurses. It is also advisable to make the physicians in the community aware of the survey.

A community is never too large and is seldom too small to conduct a survey. In smaller communities all children may be included; in larger communities a sample of the population may be surveyed. For reliable data on dental caries, it is desirable to have at least 100 persons in every age group surveyed. It is always desirable to have a statistician assist, if possible, with sampling techniques, to ensure adequate representation of the total population.

Specific instructions should be written for all persons participating in the survey. The dentists making the survey should ensure consistency by defining all procedures and data to be recorded. It is often helpful to call on the dental health division of the state or local health department for assistance in planning.

Since dental caries is the most prevalent and most often evaluated dental problem, some of the details of a caries survey are outlined here. Many aspects of a dental caries survey, however, are applicable to any dental survey. In recording the number of DMF teeth, remember that a tooth can be counted only once. A tooth cannot be counted as both filled and decayed. If a tooth has been restored and caries is also detected, count it as decayed (do not also count it in the filled column). In recording decayed teeth, caries must be defined. For example, be sure the explorer goes into carious tooth substance and not just into a deep groove or pit. It is important to be consistent. Missing permanent teeth should include those that have been extracted because of caries, plus those so badly broken down that they are indicated for extraction (these are not counted in the decayed column). Filled permanent teeth are those that have been restored with no caries now evident. Only data for permanent teeth should be recorded unless plans have been made to record data for primary teeth in a special column. Data for caries in permanent teeth and primary teeth should not be combined. It is important to define what is meant by ''this child needs dental care'' or ''this child needs referral,'' so that consistency exists among all examiners.

For a sample dental inspection form, see Fig. 31-2. If dental referrals are to accompany the survey, see Fig. 31-3 for a sample referral card.

The inspections will move more rapidly if lists are prepared in advance and pupils are presented in the order listed. The following additional points assist in the survey:

1. Clerical aid should be available from students, PTA members, or community groups.
2. It is advisable to use a mirror and an explorer instead of a tongue blade, for example, to obtain accurate data.
3. Sterilization facilities must be available for the mirrors and explorers.
4. Towels are needed to dry instruments and hands.
5. A washbasin containing a hand sterilization solution or a foam hand sterilizer should be used after each patient.
6. Parental consent is usually not necessary for the inspection, but local policy should be investigated.

7. Assistance in planning and in summarizing data is usually available from the staffs of state or local boards of health.

Such a survey will provide data that can be meaningfully summarized for the community. These data will include percentage of children needing dental care, average number of teeth affected by caries at different ages (average DMF), percentage of teeth affected that have been restored, tooth mortality rates (missing permanent teeth per 100 children), and percentage of children who are caries free.

In the total evaluation of children's dental health in a community, much more is involved than simply the determination of the prevalence of dental disease. Additional considerations might include (1) determination of the adequacy of dental manpower, (2) level of use of dental services, (3) provisions for financial assistance for children of indigent families, (4) dental facilities and their adequacy for the care of children, (5) availability of private office facilities to all persons, (6) preventive programs that are in operation and feasibility of others, (7) groups or agencies in the community that concern themselves with dental health, (8) additional agencies or groups that are in a position to be concerned with improving dental health, and (9) fluoridation of the water supply.

These are topics that should be carefully evaluated when a community dental health program is implemented.

Promotion of dental health through the schools

School dental health policies. It has already been mentioned that each school system should have a dentist appointed as a consultant. One of the first activities of the consultant should be the establishment of school dental health policies. Most schools have school health policies, but few spell out specific *dental* health policies. The dental policies set forth in most school health policies are necessarily condensed and brief and do not take into consideration many important aspects of a school dental health program. The purpose of this

DENTAL INSPECTIONS

Sheet no. _____ Use separate sheet for <u>each age group</u> (Permanent teeth only).

City _____ Grade _____ Date _____

County _____ Age _____ School _____
(Years—last birthday)

Name	Sex	D	M	F	DMF	Care needed Yes / No		Comments
Total								

Fig. 31-2. Dental inspection sheet for use in conducting dental surveys.

SCHOOL DENTAL PROGRAM

To parents or guardians:

_____ has received a dental inspection as part of the school dental program.

_____ Immediate dental care is needed.

_____ No immediate dental care is observed. However, this examination is not as complete as one performed by a dentist in his office. We would urge 6 month visits to the family dentist.

Your child's happiness and success depend upon early recognition and treatment of dental disease. Good health, good teeth, and good appearance go together. As a part of this health program, we strongly urge you to take an active part in the care of your child's dental health:

1. See your dentist regularly.

2. Restrict the use of sweets.

3. Brush and floss properly each day.

4. Use fluorides to prevent decay.

Fig. 31-3. Dental referral card that can be used in conjunction with dental surveys.

section is to list in detail suggested policies to incorporate into a school dental health program. Although dental health policies in a community should be finalized by the local dental society, the following are examples of items to be considered.

Dental health services

1. A program of preschool examinations should be established. This can be best accomplished by the family dentist. Such a program helps ensure the early initiation of periodic dental care.

2. A dental health status report should be kept with the cumulative health record of each child. Pertinent information regarding the child (medical history, name of family dentist) should be included in this health record.

3. Periodic dental examinations should be encouraged by the schools through a program of education for the parents and the child. The program should be based on prevention and long-term oral hygiene practices rather

than on actual dental treatment in the school. The school curriculum should be planned to give dental health instruction the time proportionate to its importance.

4. Policies dealing with dental emergencies arising in school or during extracurricular activities should be worked out by the dental society and the school administration.

5. A representative of the local dental society should be appointed as consultant to the school dental program.

6. Consideration should be given to allowing students time during the school day to keep dental appointments, especially if no other time is available.

7. Schools should be strongly encouraged to eliminate sales of candy and sweetened beverage in the school. The dental society should be instrumental in helping to establish a school food and beverage program that contributes to the nutritional needs of the child.

8. Teachers should not attempt to provide

emergency treatment in school. A child should be referred directly to the family dentist.

9. Dental societies should work with schools in providing a mouth protector program for athletes.

10. Dental societies and school authorities should work with other community agencies in such activities as supporting a fluoridation program, encouraging the topical application of fluoride in rural areas where water systems cannot readily be fluoridated, and developing a policy on dental care for underprivileged and handicapped children.

11. In rural areas where water systems cannot be fluoridated easily, school water supplies can be fluoridated. The optimum level is four to five times that for community fluoridation in the area. Results show 35% to 40% fewer DMF teeth.

12. Specific operational policies should be established by the local dental society. These might include toothbrushing programs and dental inspection and referral programs. These are valuable in providing an estimate of group needs and problems, in facilitating community planning in meeting these demands, and in providing the baseline data needed in the evaluation of a dental health program. Also included should be a topical fluoride treatment program within the schools. This could be a self-application program that is conducted on a group basis. Such a program could involve the use of a fluoride rinse, a preventive paste, or a fluoride dentifrice.

Health instruction

1. Teacher institutes (in-service education) on dental health should be conducted periodically. These should include discussion of dental problems, programs, progress, and educational materials and their use.

   a. The state or local board of health is often happy to carry out this training or to provide guidance for such a program.

   b. The state or local board of health is also able, in most cases, to provide or recommend approved dental health educational materials.

2. A policy should be developed to follow up the dental institutes with further classroom instruction for teachers, in an effort to improve the teaching of dental health practices.

3. Proper instruction should be given for the systematic daily removal of bacterial plaque that forms on the teeth.

Dental health education. A school dental health program should also include a suggested formal approach to teaching dental health in the classroom. The teacher should maintain the principal student contact; however, the dentist or dental hygienist should serve as an active supporting resource person. It has been shown that the dentist can be a valuable asset in motivating children to improve their dental health practices, through periodic planned lectures or talks to school groups. The dentist serves as the expert resource person to strengthen the teacher's classroom instruction program. In schools without dental personnel such as a dental hygienist, the school or health department nurse serves an important role as an intermediary resource person. The nurse should have models, filmstrips, posters, pamphlets, demonstration kits, science fair projects, and flip charts readily available for teachers to use. The materials could be used on a rotating basis by different teachers and even different schools. The visual aids and demonstration materials should be attractive, effective, durable, and simple to use.

It is important for the dentist to be interested in dental health teaching and to sincerely *show* this interest by assisting teachers in the improvement of their skills. The most appropriate way for teachers to receive the basic concepts of dental health is through their college training; however, this often does not occur, and the dentist must in some way be responsible for giving the teacher the opportunity to become specifically familiar with dental health concepts. The extent of a teacher's potential problem in understanding some specifics about dental health should not be underestimated. The dentist should give each teacher sincere attention. This is important in developing proper attitudes and personal dental health practices by the teacher. Skill in plaque control can lead to improvement in the teacher's own oral health and can be passed on to the classroom. The dentist should see that a favorable and even an enthusiastic climate exists among the school administrators and faculty members for improving background skills in the teaching of dental health. Such enthusiasm will usually extend throughout the school system and result in more effective teaching. The teachers should set a good example by maintaining good dental health themselves, for the successful teaching of dental health involves more than the giving of knowledge. Phases of education beyond the giving of knowledge are essential; that is, the development of good attitudes about this knowledge should result in favorable action. A behavioral response must be achieved.

A teacher should have some basic concepts in dental health, and these should come from some formal background in dental health education. This suggests activities and training in colleges and universities that prepare teachers, for it has been my experience that many teachers have little if any formal preparation or background in teaching dental health. (For additional information on dental health education for schools, consult state or local health agencies or write to the American Dental Association.)

The dentist, either as an individual or as a representative of the dental society, should approach the colleges and universities preparing teachers and see that basic dental health concepts for teachers are made available. This should be a planned and formal approach and should involve the administration and appropriate department heads and faculty members of the school. The dentist should be well prepared with a concise, well-planned program for inclusion in the college or university curriculum. It need not be a course in itself but could successfully be part of several existing courses. A dental representative of the state or local health department may be of assistance in preparing the dentist's presentation.

Dental health kit for teachers. A dental health kit for teacher education is shown in Fig. 31-4. This kit was planned and prepared by a state dental association and the division of dental health of a state board of health. The kit was presented to every teacher education college and university in the state. Its use and value were demonstrated at formal meetings in each college and university, and a local dentist was appointed in each community as a consultant to the school. A follow-up evaluation has shown the kit to be an effective method of bringing basic dental health concepts to prospective teachers. Other colleges and universities could benefit from such a kit.

In-service program for teachers. It is important for the dentist and auxiliary personnel to introduce educational materials to teachers. This is true regardless of whether the materials are supplied by the schools themselves, by the dental society, or by a commercial source such as a dentifrice manufacturer. An effective way for dentists to introduce a dental health education program and appropriate materials is through an in-service teacher-training program on dental health. Such a program would be presented with the following purposes:

1. To increase awareness on the part of school personnel of dental disease problems and the important role schools and teachers can play in dental health education
2. To review available dental health teaching aids that can be used for explaining technical information in the classroom
3. To inform teachers of resources available and the methods used in other schools and communities for effectively teaching dental health

The program is conveniently divided into three areas: the problems of dental disease in schoolchildren and suggested ways in which teachers may help improve dental health; diet and dental health, with a snack demonstration; and materials available to aid teachers in preparing, presenting, and teaching dental health.

A dental in-service program is best presented by a team consisting of a dentist, a nutrition consultant, and a health education consultant. However,

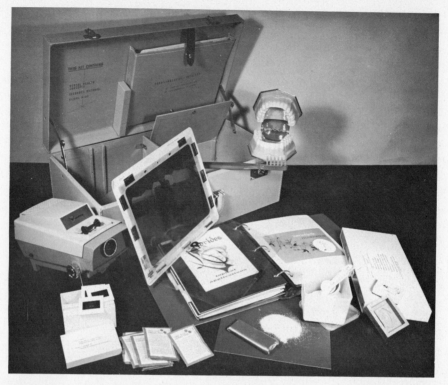

Fig. 31-4. Self-contained dental health kit for teacher education and presentation of basic dental health concepts.

the nutrition and health education components may be combined and presented by a dental hygienist or another dentist. The length of the total program should be held to 1 to 1½ hours. The program is usually held after school; however, it is highly desirable for the principal or superintendent of schools to dismiss school early on the day of the in-service program so that part of the teachers' time is regular school time or time set aside for such teachers' meetings. A low-carbohydrate demonstration snack prepared and served by the home economics class or the PTA just before the program starts accomplishes two important purposes: it is relaxing and creates a receptive atmosphere for the teachers and it demonstrates many low-carbohydrate foods for snacks that everyone can enjoy. The dental society may wish to pay the

small expense involved in the cost of the food. The snacks should be low in sugar and high in protein (for example, cheese and meat cubes, celery stuffed with peanut butter, small open-faced sandwiches, peanuts, diced vegetables, unsweetened fruit juice). They should be served buffet-style.

Preschool dental examinations. The school should require that each child have a dental examination by the family dentist before entering school. This lends emphasis to establishing early and regular visits to a family dentist. Beyond the examination, it is the responsibility of the family and the dentist to arrange for continuing treatment.

Restriction of sweets. No candy or sweetened beverages should be sold in the school. The dental society should be instrumental in establishing a school food and beverage program that contributes to the nutritional and dental needs of schoolchildren. Often candy or sweetened beverage vending machines or sales are in schools for economic reasons. These must be weighed against the time children lose from school because of dental diseases produced by the sweets. There are now many attractive substitutes for sweets that are high in food appeal and essential food value. Fresh fruit, milk, nut, and other vending machines are now available, and the profits from these are just as great as, if not greater than, the profits resulting from the sale of sweets. High-protein, low-carbohydrate snacks should be used for all classroom parties or activities where food is served. When such a snack program is actually put into effect, the comments from teachers and children are much more favorable than when sweet snacks are served.

School caries preventive program. The school should also have an active caries prevention program for its students. The search for a caries preventive procedure available to all children continues to be a major challenge to the dental profession.

Mercer and Gish point out that despite tremendous advances in caries prevention through fluoridation of community water supplies and the use of topical fluoride procedures by dentists, dental hygienists, and school programs, dental caries in children is still a significant problem. It has been recognized for many years that a major breakthrough in further prevention of caries would be possible if there were available to all school-age children a simple, effective caries preventive procedure that could be used on a broad basis in school. Such a program is now available through the administration of an effective fluoride compound by the children themselves. This group procedure could have tremendous importance in the prevention of dental caries. The essential criteria for such a program would include the following: that the therapeutic procedure be effective and safe; that the program be capable of reaching large numbers of children; that the procedure be economical and relatively simple to execute; that it require minimum use of professional manpower; that the program result in as little interference as possible in the school curriculum and community routine; that it complement the recall, home care, and office preventive program of a child's family dentist; that the procedure provide a benefit without any further action on the part of the patient; and that it be accepted satisfactorily by the child.

Such a program might operate in any of several ways. For example, all schools could set aside 15 to 20 minutes each semester, on a day that could be called "School Dental Health Day." Children in every classroom in a school, a community, or even a state would brush their teeth for 5 to 6 minutes, under supervision, with a prophylaxis paste. Dentists and dental hygienists would provide the overall instructions, and each classroom teacher, with a parent helper, would supervise the brushing. This would be not only an active group dental caries prevention program but also an effective dental health education program. The child would keep the toothbrush for home care (Figs. 31-5 and 31-6).

Since the use of a toothbrush is important to the prevention of periodontal disease, applying a caries-preventing fluoride with a toothbrush seems desirable. However, a current, widely known practice for administering topical fluorides is the use of fluoride rinses applied weekly in the classroom. The solution is mixed in the school and distributed to the children by the classroom teacher. Another method of applying topical fluoride in school is through daily brushing with an effective fluoride dentifrice. A multiple topical fluoride program is discussed in Chapter 7.

Regardless of the type of self-applied fluoride program, the program should be administered by the dental division of a state health department, by a dental school, or by similar dental authority, which should outline specific methods of use, storage, and so on.

Dental plaque control should also be taught to teachers and children. This should be done on the basis of students' skills and their specific capabilities for behavioral response. Both teachers and

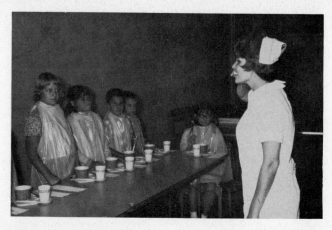

Fig. 31-5. Children receiving instruction for self-application of a preventive paste.

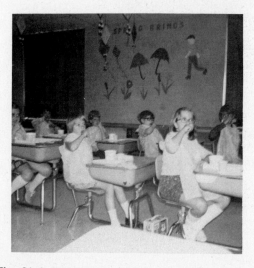

Fig. 31-6. Self-application programs using preventive paste or rinse can be supervised in the classroom.

children should learn to identify plaque and effectively remove it. Plaque control can be carried out on a daily basis in the classroom.

"Blanket" referral. A program that has proved to be effective in many schools is "blanket" referral of children to their family dentists. In this program, all children are given referral cards (Fig. 31-7) to take home and subsequently to the dentists, who sign the cards upon completion of examination, treatment, or both. The signed cards are then returned to the school nurse, school hygienist, or classroom teacher, who plays an important role in following up the referrals with the child and parents. It is advisable to spread the referrals throughout the year as much as possible to prevent too great an influx of children into dental offices at one time. An effective follow-up procedure in the school through the nurse, hygienist, or teacher is important for good results. A teachers' in-service program can often be used to good advantage in introducing a blanket referral program.

Mouth protectors. Since the National Alliance Football Rules Committee in 1962 made the wearing of an internal mouth protector mandatory for all high school athletes engaged in interscholastic football, there is no question that the number of injuries to athletes' teeth and supporting soft tissues has been greatly reduced. Many types of protectors have been used, but the important element is that dentists and schools provide athletes with mouth protectors that afford good protection and comfort with minimum inconvenience. Dentists have made a great contribution to athletes by helping to preserve their natural dentitions. The following facts should be kept in mind when a mouth protector program is being organized and carried out:

DENTAL HEALTH REFERRAL CARD

A program to promote
better dental health of school children

FOR STUDENTS — Section I

Pupil's name _____ Grade _____ Age _____

School _____ Town _____ County _____

To parent or guardian:

Your child's health, comfort, happiness, progress in school, and personal appearance may be seriously affected by neglecting his teeth. Three kinds of care are necessary to protect your child's dental health—adequate nutrition, mouth cleanliness, and regular supervision by the dentist. Part of our school health program is to promote better dental health. The school and your family dentist can assist you in this responsibility if you will take your child and this card to your family dentist for an examination and explanation of your child's dental needs. THIS CARD SHOULD BE SIGNED BY THE DENTIST AND RETURNED TO THE TEACHER BY YOUR CHILD.

Date _____

Teacher or
School Nurse _____

FOR DENTIST — Section II

A. I have examined the teeth of the above student and find no restorations, extractions, or cleaning needed. _____

B. I have completed the necessary dental work for the student. _____

Date _____ _____ D.D.S.

DOCTOR: Please do not sign card unless necessary work is actually completed.

Fig. 31-7. "Blanket" dental referral card may be used for referring all schoolchildren to their family dentists.

1. If possible, the fitting of mouth protectors should be done by local dentists. If this is impossible, a dental professional should at least supervise their fitting.
2. Except in a few situations, a mouth protector should be fitted over the upper teeth.
3. An athlete's teeth should be checked and found to be in sound condition before a mouth protector is fitted.
4. A mouth protector should be worn at all times, in practice sessions as well as during games.
5. A coach who believes in the value of mouth protectors, and emphasizes their importance, will find that athletes accept them more graciously.
6. A mouth disinfectant should be made readily available to athletes.

One method of constructing a mouth protector is described in Chapter 26.

Science fair. Many schools now hold science fair exhibitions, the winners of which compete in regional, state, and national fairs. A science fair is an excellent opportunity for dentistry to contribute substantially to the building of a growing reservoir of students who may someday choose a career in dentistry. Local and state dental associations should have committees to organize dental society support for local and regional fairs. Literature should be provided for students, outlining possible dental projects and offering the assistance of local dentists to help students develop projects. Local dental societies can provide judges for regional fairs and recognize winners who have chosen dental topics. The students with the best dental projects in regional science fairs are invited to represent their regions and local dental societies at the state science fair and/or the state dental association meeting.

Science fairs are important in developing potential dentists. Thus an active approach should be made to the schools, and encouragement and assistance should be given students with dental science projects.

Home care opportunities for dental health

A desirable objective of a community dental health program is to influence people to visit their family dentists on a regular basis and to assume responsibility for good oral hygiene habits and practices. This also should be a prime objective of a dental office; the dentist and the dental staff must be key persons in developing this attitude in children and their parents.

A school dental health program should also influence children to maintain good oral hygiene through proper home care. For elementary children, it is desirable that a specific message be sent home requesting support for the teaching lesson given at school. A good home care program includes proper toothbrushing and flossing daily for cleansing the mouth of plaque, restriction of the intake of refined sugars, safety precautions to prevent injuries to teeth, and strict adherence to routine recall appointments with dentists.

A suggestion for parents in good home nutrition would be to place the foods children should have for snacks in the places they look for snacks. These foods should include more than just celery and carrot strips. Something more attractive and appealing should be available: cheese and meat cubes, diced fresh fruits and vegetables, open-faced sandwiches, melon, peanuts, fruit punch, shishkabobs, and many other attractive, palatable low-carbohydrate items.

Every known preventive measure should be used in caries control; certainly one measure should be

the use of a professionally acceptable dentifrice. An American Dental Association–approved fluoride dentifrice that constitutes a daily topical preventive should be used. Such a dentifrice contributes to the total caries prevention program for children. This type of dentifrice is recommended in communities with fluoridated water as well as in those without fluoridated water.

Dental office aspects of community dental health

It has already been stated that the dental office should provide sound dental health education for the child and the parent. For children in the elementary grades, the mother is usually the main motivating factor toward good oral hygiene practices. Special emphasis should be given to developing her dental health awareness. Nutritional counseling and patient education should be used routinely.

All dental offices caring for children should also practice a full preventive program. A good office preventive program includes an effective recall procedure, for good surveillance of a child's dental health, and the use of multiple topical procedures and plaque control techniques. The currently recommended multiple procedure for both fluoride and nonfluoride areas involves the use of a prophylaxis paste, a topical fluoride treatment, and a fluoride dentifrice. The office use of multiple fluoride techniques is described in detail in Chapter 7.

Several dental offices that routinely use the recommended multiple fluoride topical procedure every 6 months report that of every 10 patients seen during recall only one or two need appointments for operative dentistry. Dentists using such a procedure also report significant increases in the numbers of patients in their practices and much better use of auxiliary personnel. These dentists further point out that they had to gear their offices to the greater patient volume and the more extensive recall systems.

Patients should also be taught to use a disclosing solution or tablet to identify dental plaque. They should be able to remove plaque through proper flossing between the teeth and brushing systematically and thoroughly. A dental hygienist or a disease control therapist can provide this instruction.

Diet surveys that include proper evaluation and discussion with parents should be available through the dental office. Seven-day surveys can be made and evaluated on the basis of the four food groups, the total number of exposures to sugar, the frequency of the exposures, and the form of sugar consumed. The results of a survey are discussed with the parent from the standpoint of specific diet recommendations. The procedure for conducting a diet survey has been outlined in Chapter 7.

Dental office experiences should make patients feel that if they want to know something about dental health or dentistry, they can come to the dental profession for the answers.

Community action

Good dental health cannot be bestowed on people by schools, the PTA, government, or any other group, but the community and dentists working together can certainly provide the opportunity for good dental health. If this is true, what are the most significant things that can be done on a community basis to improve dental health?

Fluoridation. There is no question that fluoridation of the community water supply should be the item of first importance. Fluoridation comes close to being the ideal public health measure for the prevention of dental disease, since it is highly effective and feasible and requires no specific motivation on the part of the individual. Much has been said about the organization and implementation of such a program, but I wish to state my own opinions on this subject, which are based on personal experience.

Fluoridation of the community water supply is the responsibility of the governing body of the community. In order for fluoridation to be achieved, this body must be sufficiently influenced to proceed with the measure. Personal experience has shown that perhaps the most effective way to influence a city council is to have people of stature in the community go before the council and request fluoridation. These people must follow through at subsequent council meetings to ensure final approval and implementation. One must develop a situation whereby a council member, looking out over a strong community representation at a council meeting, cannot politically or honestly vote against fluoridation or voice objection to the measure. Fluoridation *is* that convincing a caries-preventive measure, and the governmental body must be made to realize this fact.

In communities where support for fluoridation cannot be readily obtained, the following activities are suggested for achieving fluoridation:

1. Contact every local dentist and physician, so that they are aware of the current approach being made, and ask their support.
2. Distribute fluoridation material and information through personal contact as often as possible. Do not overlook, however, mass distribution by dentists, physicians, nurses, and health departments.
3. Prepare articles for local news media.
4. Have the community health officer and his or her staff actively encourage fluoridation.
5. Have the dental society send the mayor, city council, or town board a letter outlining the benefits of fluoridation and why the community should have it. Also, refer to other communities that have fluoridation and to groups that support the measure.
6. Have other organizations in the community send supporting letters to the governing body.
7. Provide specific assistance, materials, and know-how on fluoridation to key community leaders and groups.
8. See that these key persons and groups follow through by contacting the governing body.
9. Obtain sound engineering counsel on costs, procedures, and so on.
10. Encourage equipment companies and consulting engineers to automatically include

fluoridation in their plans for communities.

11. Know the opposition, and plan a program to counter their arguments in a positive manner.

12. Have all groups and key persons in the community follow up with actual appearances at council meetings and express their wishes for fluoridation.

13. Work!

I have purposely listed thirteen points so that no one will forget number 13. There is no substitute for WORK!

Dental health emphasis for specific groups. It has already been stated that dentists should take an active part in community activities, especially those involving the health of the community. A dentist, through his or her knowledge of areas related to health and well-being, can be a valuable asset to boards and committees whose functions are related to community health activities. A dentist should serve as a resource person for all groups or institutions in the community that are concerned with oral health—for example, schools (including universities and colleges), welfare agencies, health departments, special institutions, and hospitals. This overall community approach can ensure that dental health education receives appropriate emphasis. Dental expertise should certainly be available to all state health planning agencies. Where dental health education programs already exist, their concepts, utilization, and results should be evaluated. Where programs do not exist, dental health problems should be assessed and programs initiated as indicated. Keep in mind that *a dental health education program is intended not merely to disseminate information but to develop attitudes about dental health that will produce favorable action.*

After the implementation of a community preventive and education program, a good school program, and an effective office preventive practice that benefits all children, attention should be given to increasing the availability of dental care to specific segments of the population.

Indigent persons. Local dental societies and dentists should develop methods of rendering dental services to welfare and indigent groups on a regular and comprehensive basis. All dentists in the community should be aware of the guidelines and principles for care for these patients, which have been prepared by the American Dental Association and state and local dental societies in cooperation with sponsoring agencies. Besides the usual welfare and indigent programs, there are often voluntary programs that provide some type of dental service. However, there is often a lack of any real coordination among the various programs. There may be local, federal, and state low-income family programs as well as local voluntary services and interests that include dental care. Overall local coordination is essential to understanding and operating an effective comprehensive program. One way to coordinate some of these plans might be to utilize all funds through the local health department on a contract basis. In this way the health department could more effectively meet the needs of the community. A working arrangement with all welfare-related agencies could be established so that all parties involved would have the same understanding of eligibility criteria, extent of services, and many other operational aspects. Financial agreements or contracts could be made between the local health department (or agency providing services) and the various sources of the funds, rather than having the funds go directly and independently to groups or individuals in the community. Other methods of contracting for care could include prepayment mechanisms such as those provided by the Dental Service Corporation, Blue Shield, or private insurance companies.

The local dental facilities, which usually consist of the dentists' offices, should be utilized fully in providing dental services. The dentists of the community, if they want to keep all dental treatment in their offices, must make arrangements to treat patients regardless of ethnic, economic, or educational background. The funding agency for the recipients, on the other hand, should make payment on a fee-for-service basis. This, for all practical purposes, means that a fee must be the same as the dentist would charge any other patient. The dental society should provide a review committee to review all problems of a financial nature, and the society would provide a counseling committee to consider any grievances in regard to the quality of work. Through such a program, the dentists would be responsible for professional aspects of dental care. Problems with equipment, supplies, and personnel would thus be eliminated from the welfare, indigent, or other agencies. Funds from welfare or other financial sources would not be spent until services had been rendered. If this approach did not accomplish the desired result, the establishment of dental facilities or other methods for providing care to indigent persons would have to be pursued. This could present problems. In any event, it is important to have effective liaison between the local dental society and the welfare department or other groups concerned with the welfare of indigent persons. This again necessitates the dental society's having representation on appropriate boards and participating in comprehensive dental health planning.

Any program that provides dental services to indigent or low-income persons should strive to produce the greatest return, in terms of improved community health, for tax money spent. Since public welfare funds are seldom sufficient to provide complete dental care for all clients, some priority for treatment must be established. Relief of pain and control of acute infection, regardless of age of the patient, must claim top priority; however, the primary interest of the dental profession should be dental care for children. Through early and regular care of primary teeth and regular care during the first several years of the permanent dentition, dentistry can make a great contribution to an individual's oral and general health. The cost of providing essential dental services for children is small compared to later costs resulting from neglect. A generation of children who have had good dental care should appreciate good dental health and have an interest in maintaining that health. Their dental care as adults thus will not be a burden to themselves or to the community.

The ideal plan should provide eligible recipients complete freedom in choosing ethical practicing dentists to provide treatment. The plan should also provide a system of review by which the dental profession can guarantee the funding agency and its clients the high degree of professional service they deserve. Through this review committee, the dental society would be given control over the area of the contract about which it is most qualified to render judgment—professional services. It has been the experience of many communities that freedom of choice of dentist, participation of the most qualified professionals, and quality treatment can best be ensured if a standard of remuneration compatible with the community can be maintained. This is a controversial subject, and it must be dealt with on a basis of mutual understanding. It is important that the funding agency understand the value of the treatment being rendered and the pitfalls of cut-rate professional services and that the dental society understand the source of monies with which the agency operates and the budgetary requirements it must meet.

Although indigent patients represent a small segment of the average dental practice, the proper treatment of this population nevertheless represents a real responsibility of the profession. Sincere interest and enlightened activity in regard to this matter will constitute a valuable service to the community and to dentistry. The priorities and the extensiveness of dental services should be determined in accordance with the needs of the community and the funds available.

Handicapped persons. Another aspect of a community dental health program is the provision of services for handicapped persons. Each state or region should have a health center for complete and competent care of handicapped persons (perhaps within a distance of 50 to 150 miles). Ideally, however, not all patients should be treated in these highly sophisticated centers. Such a center is not always practical, since the costs involved in transporting a child to one are often much greater than the cost of treatment itself.

A training program for care of the handicapped should be established by a health center, dental school, health department, or other appropriate agency, and each community, through its dental society, should carefully select a dentist or dentists to attend. The dentist (or dentists) would return to the community so that referrals might be made locally for care of handicapped people. In a complex case, arrangements could be made for the patient to visit the specialized treatment center for complete diagnosis and treatment planning. Most of the subsequent treatment could then be carried out in the community by the local dentist who has been trained in the care of the handicapped.

Persons in institutions. Many communities have state hospitals and institutions that maintain a dental facility for patients. These are usually mental, correctional, or special institutions. The persons in these institutions deserve dental services that are in keeping with the high standards of the dental profession. The state dental association should appoint a committee on dental care programs in the state institutions to work with appropriate state agencies (especially the dental health division of the state health department) and local dentists. A working arrangement must be established for realistic surveys, evaluations, and recommendations for each dental facility. Equipment, supplies, personnel, salaries, policies, records, forms, priorities, program development, and all other aspects of the dental facility and service must be considered. For more details about such an operation, refer to the article by Mercer and Gish in the *Journal of Public Health Dentistry*.

Methods of payment. A dentist who is concerned with community dental health must consider the various methods of payment that are available for dental services. Payment programs have become an important aspect of extending dental care to greater numbers of people. Various types of payment plans are available to the public and the dental profession, and their advantages and disadvantages should be discussed. For further information consult the Health Insurance Council (which represents some 700 insurance companies), the American Dental Association's Council on Dental Care Programs, and the National Association of Dental Service Plans.

Professional activities

Dentists should continuously assess the availability of dental manpower in their communities. They should give assistance to school careers programs, science fair programs, and other community activities designed for recruitment and education of dentists, dental hygienists, dental assistants, and dental laboratory technicians. As dentistry serves the young people in the community, so someday will dentistry be served.

The dental society should hold regular meetings and provide programs to keep the practices of their members current. Each dentist should make a special point to attend dental society meetings, to take postgraduate courses, and to participate in special programs in a continual effort to improve services to patients.

Summary

What are a dentist's obligations to society, to patients, and to the profession? What defines a professional person? The answers to these questions could well summarize community dental health.

Community dental health must be a part of every dental practice. Dentistry is a profession, and it exists as a profession because it has been granted this privilege by people who trust and respect the services they receive from dentists and their staffs. Certainly these services must include those rendered on a community basis. Dentists must provide full programs of prevention and dental health education, as well as opportunities for treatment in the office, in the home, in the school, and throughout the community.

REFERENCES

Bernier, J.I., and Muhler, J.C.: Improving dental practice through preventive measures, ed. 2. St. Louis, 1970, The C.V. Mosby Co.

Dean, H.T., and Elvove, E.: Some epidemiological aspects of chronic endemic dental fluorosis, Am. J. Public Health **26:**567-575, 1936.

Greene, J.C., and Vermillion, J.R.: The simplified oral hygiene index, J.A.D.A. **68:**25-31, 1964.

Kasey, E.H.: Curriculum planning in dental health: problems, processes, and prospects. Proceedings of a New England

Conference on Dental Health Education, Woodstock, Vt., 1966.

Mercer, V.H.: Incorporation of preventive dentistry into office practice. In Bernier, J.L., and Muhler, J.C.: Improving dental practice through preventive measures, ed. 2, St. Louis, 1970, The C.V. Mosby Co.

Mercer, V.H., and Gish, C.W.: Continuing role of the Indiana State Dental Association in the improvement of dental programs in state institutions, J. Public Health Dent. **28:**2-4, 1968.

Mercer, V.H., and others: Self-application of fluoride as a community preventive measure: rationale, procedures, and three year results, J.A.D.A. **90:**388-397, 1975.

Mollenkopf, J.P.: A report on mouth protectors for high school football players in Indiana, personal communication, 1967.

Poulton, D.R., and Aaronson, S.A.: The relationship between occlusion and periodontal status, Am. J. Orthod. **47:**690-699, 1961.

Russell, A.L.: A system of classification and scoring for prevalence surveys of periodontal disease, J. Dent. Res. **35:**350-359, 1956.

VanKirk, L.E., and Pennell, E.A.: Assessment of malocclusion in population groups, Am. J. Public Health **49:**1157-1163, 1959.

Williford, J.: Oral hygiene improvement through dental health education, thesis, Indianapolis, 1966, Indiana School of Dentistry.

Yacovone, J.: Education for dental health basic concepts for a health education program in the schools, R.I. Med. J. **49:**469-472, 546-548, 1966.

Young, W.O., and Striffler, D.F.: The dentist, his practice, and his community, Philadelphia, 1964, W.B. Saunders Co.

Index